Pharmaceutical **Chemistry**

Commissioning Editor: *Pauline Graham*
Senior Development Editor: *Ailsa Laing*
Project Manager: *Frances Affleck*
Designer: *Charles Gray*
Illustration Manager: *Bruce Hogarth*

Pharmaceutical Chemistry

Edited by

David G Watson BSc PhD PGCE

Reader in Pharmaceutical Sciences, Strathclyde Institute of Pharmacy and Biomedical Sciences, School of Pharmacy, University of Strathclyde, Glasgow, UK

CHURCHILL LIVINGSTONE

ELSEVIER

Edinburgh London New York Oxford Philadelphia St Louis Sydney Toronto 2011

CHURCHILL
LIVINGSTONE
ELSEVIER

ISBN 978-0-443-07232-1
International ISBN 978-0-443-07233-8

British Library Cataloguing in Publication Data
A catalogue record for this book is available from the British Library

Library of Congress Cataloging in Publication Data
A catalog record for this book is available from the Library of Congress

Notices

Knowledge and best practice in this field are constantly changing. As new research and experience broaden our understanding, changes in research methods, professional practices, or medical treatment may become necessary.

Practitioners and researchers must always rely on their own experience and knowledge in evaluating and using any information, methods, compounds, or experiments described herein. In using such information or methods they should be mindful of their own safety and the safety of others, including parties for whom they have a professional responsibility.

With respect to any drug or pharmaceutical products identified, readers are advised to check the most current information provided (i) on procedures featured or (ii) by the manufacturer of each product to be administered, to verify the recommended dose or formula, the method and duration of administration, and contraindications. It is the responsibility of practitioners, relying on their own experience and knowledge of their patients, to make diagnoses, to determine dosages and the best treatment for each individual patient, and to take all appropriate safety precautions.

To the fullest extent of the law, neither the Publisher nor the authors, contributors, or editors, assume any liability for any injury and/or damage to persons or property as a matter of products liability, negligence or otherwise, or from any use or operation of any methods, products, instructions, or ideas contained in the material herein.

Printed in China

Contents

Preface

Western medicine advanced very slowly until the late 19th century, borrowing many of its ideas from the ancient Greeks. The idea that diseases could be cured by balancing the four humours persisted well into the 19th century and thus standard medical practice consisted of the use of bleeding and purges. Many of the life-threatening diseases of earlier centuries were due to microbial infection and since the germ theory only developed in the mid 19th century doctors had no real concept of the underlying causes of the diseases they were treating. This did not mean that physicians could not by careful observation come up with effective treatments however, for example, Jenner discovered vaccination without knowing anything about immunology or viruses.

So the history of modern drug discovery is surprisingly short. In 1930 a doctor would have only had about ten drugs which could be regarded as therapeutically efficacious in modern terms: morphine, codeine, ephedrine, aspirin, procaine, quinine, digoxin, some vitamins and the recently isolated hormones insulin and thyroxine. In addition, in the age before antibiotics there were various toxic complexes of heavy elements such as arsenic, mercury and antimony, which were useful for treating bacterial and parasitic infections. They would not be regarded as acceptable medicines nowadays unless there was no alternative. Between 1930 and 1975 drug discovery occurred at an enormous rate – this was before many of the very strict regulations for pharmaceutical products came into force. In the last 25 years the pace of drug discovery has been much slower, apart from in the niche area of biotechnologically produced drugs.

A major emphasis of the book is on the way that drugs interact with bio-molecules within the body. Although the understanding of this has grown rapidly in the past 25 years this has not been reflected in drug discovery, and it is hard to predict what the next phase of drug discovery will be. There are still significant challenges in areas such as cancer, neurological diseases and the management of mental illness. In the developing world there is a need for better drugs to treat parasitic diseases. A current buzzword is personalised medicine, where treatments are tailored to the individual, but such approaches demand a high level of resourcing. There is no doubt that medical technology will advance through the use of stem cells and the increasing sophistication of both cultured and engineered replacement body parts. Perhaps the focus in drug development will shift further towards targeting, delivery and incorporation into devices.

I would like to thank my colleagues for their contributions to this book. In addition I owe a great debt to two previous authors, both from the School of Pharmacy at Strathclyde – Professor John Stenlake, whose two textbooks on molecular pharmacology contain a huge amount of fundamental information, and Dr Walter Sneader, whose books *Drug Prototypes and Their Exploitation* and *Drug Discovery* provide the ultimate authority of the history of drug discovery from ancient times into the modern era.

Dave Watson
Glasgow

Contributors

Muhammed Hashem Alzweiri BSc PhD
Pharmaceutical analysis, Faculty of Pharmacy, The University of Jordan, Amman, Jordan

Simon D Brandt PhD PGCert LTHE FHEA MRSC MFSSoc
Senior Lecturer in Analytical Chemistry, School of Pharmacy and Biomedical Sciences, Liverpool; John Moores University, Liverpool, UK

John Connolly BSc PhD
Senior Lecturer, Strathclyde Institute of Pharmacy and Biomedical Sciences, University of Strathclyde, Glasgow, UK

Geoffrey Coxon BSc(Hons) MSc PhD
Lecturer in Medicinal Chemistry, Strathclyde Institute of Pharmacy and Biomedical Sciences, University of Strathclyde, Glasgow, UK

Christine Dufès PharmD PhD
Lecturer in Drug Delivery, Strathclyde Institute of Pharmacy and Biomedical Sciences, University of Strathclyde, Glasgow, UK

RuAngelie Edrada-Ebel BSc MSc DrRerNat AMRSC
Lecturer, Strathclyde Institute of Pharmacy and Biomedical Sciences, University of Strathclyde, Glasgow, UK

Muhammad Anas Kamleh BSc PhD
Doctor of Pharmacy, Damascus University, Syria

Simon P Mackay BPharm(Hons) PhD MRPharmS CChem MRSC
Professor of Medicinal Chemistry, Strathclyde Institute of Pharmacy and Biomedical Sciences, University of Strathclyde, Glasgow, UK

Jeffrey Stuart Millership BSC PhD FRSC CChem
Senior Lecturer in Pharmaceutical Chemistry, School of Pharmacy, Queen's University Belfast, UK

Alexander Balfour Mullen BSc(Hons) PhD MRPharmS
Professor, Strathclyde Institute of Pharmacy and Biomedical Sciences, University of Strathclyde, Glasgow, UK

Ahmed Saadi Ahmed BSc PhD
PhD Student in Pharmaceutical Analysis at Strathclyde University, Glasgow, UK

Justice Nii Addy Tettey BPharm(Hons) MSc PhD PgCert MPSGh FHEA FRSC
Chief, Laboratory and Scientific Section, Division of Policy Analysis and Public Affairs, United Nations Office on Drugs and Crime, Vienna, Austria

Clive G Wilson BSc PhD
JP Todd Professor of Pharmaceutics, Strathclyde Institute of Pharmacy and Biomedical Sciences, University of Strathclyde, Glasgow, UK; President, European Federation of Pharmaceutical Sciences

Chapter | 1 |

Bond type and bond strength

David G Watson

CHAPTER CONTENTS

INTRODUCTION AND SYNOPSIS

Of the 110 or so elements there are only about 22 which occur naturally in biological systems. The use of therapeutic agents introduces about another half dozen. In earlier centuries before the advent of selective antimicrobial agents the use of the toxic elements mercury and antimony was very popular to treat the then, more or less, incurable diseases of syphilis and malaria. If a cure was effective it was often a pretty close run thing with its opposite.

The structure of living systems is largely based on four elements: carbon, hydrogen, oxygen and nitrogen, the greatest part of any organism being hydrogen and oxygen in the form of water (*ca.* 70% of the human body). The predominant type of chemical bond which holds the structure of an organism together is the covalent bond which is formed when two atoms share their electrons. Covalent bonds vary in strength and properties according to the elements involved in the bond. One method of classifying the elements, which join together to form bonds, is according to their electronegativity. The electronegativity value for an element provides a measure of its affinity for electrons and hence its ability to attract a negative charge or conversely to give up some electron density and hold a positive charge. The electronegativity of some of the more common elements in biology is shown in Table 1.1; the derivation of electronegativity values is discussed later in the chapter.

Covalent bonds are usually formed between non-metals, with the more electronegative element in the bond attracting negative charge and creating a dipole (see Box 1.1).

Bonds formed between metals and non-metals are ionic because of their large differences in electronegativity. In an ionic bond the electrons are not shared, the less electronegative element gives the more electronegative element its electron(s) and then they are held together in the bond by the attraction of the resultant opposite charges. A third type of bond is due to weak van der Waals forces which are strongest between bulky chemical groups. Figure 1.1 shows some examples of bond types using an example which approximates to the binding of adrenaline to a β_2-adrenergic receptor where it interacts with several amino acid side chains on the G-protein.

Collectively, the making and breaking of various bond types drives the machinery of living organisms. Thus, for instance, the binding of calcium ions to certain proteins causes a change in their shape which results in muscle contraction. Similarly, the binding of a biologically active molecule such as acetylcholine to its receptor protein on muscle cell changes the shape of the pores in the muscle cell membrane, allowing sodium ions to enter the cell.

Table 1.1 Electronegativities of the biological elements

Metals	Non-metals
Na 0.9	H 2.1
Mg 1.2	C 2.5
Si 1.8	N 3.0
K 0.8	O 3.5
Ca 1.0	F 4.0
Mn 1.5	P 2.1
Fe 1.8	S 2.5
Co 1.9	Cl 3.0
Cu 1.9	Se 2.4
Zn 1.6	I 2.5

Box 1.1 **Dipoles**

$\overset{\delta-}{C}$—$\overset{\delta+}{H}$ 0.4 Debye

$\overset{\delta+}{C}$—$\overset{\delta-}{O}$ 0.7 Debye

A bond between two different atoms always has a dipole moment in which the negative end of the dipole is centred on the electronegative atom. When two dipoles are in different molecules they can interact to form a weak reversible bond and these types of bonds are very important in drug action. A dipole moment is conveniently expressed in Debye (units in charge/metre). The dipole moments for C–H and C–O are shown above; the dipole–dipole interactions between positively charged atoms and oxygen in drug molecules are of more significance than those with carbon.

This initiates a chain of events which results in entry of calcium ions into the cell and hence muscle contraction. Drug molecules act by altering the natural functioning of the machinery of the cells within the body (or pathogen), ideally, in order to repair an imbalance that is causing disease. Pharmaceutical chemistry concerns itself with which components within the structure of a molecule cause it to affect cells in a particular way. This brief introduction mentions several concepts relating to bond type which we will now discuss in more detail.

Q Self Test 1.1

Examine the structure of adrenaline and the precision with which it binds to the receptor. Which of the following drugs might mimic the actions of adrenaline and which could block its action? Where do you think the blocking drugs might bind most strongly to the receptor?

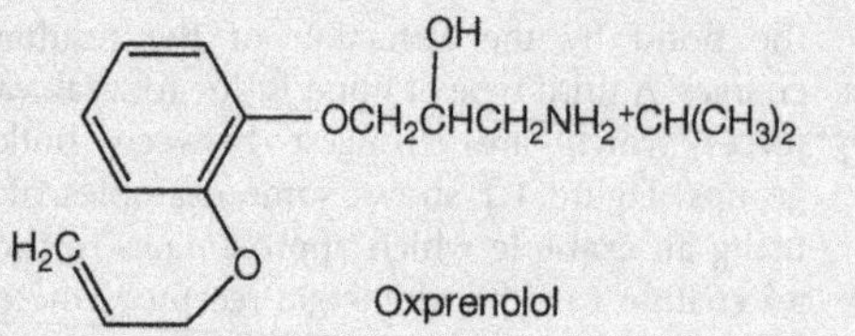

Oxprenolol

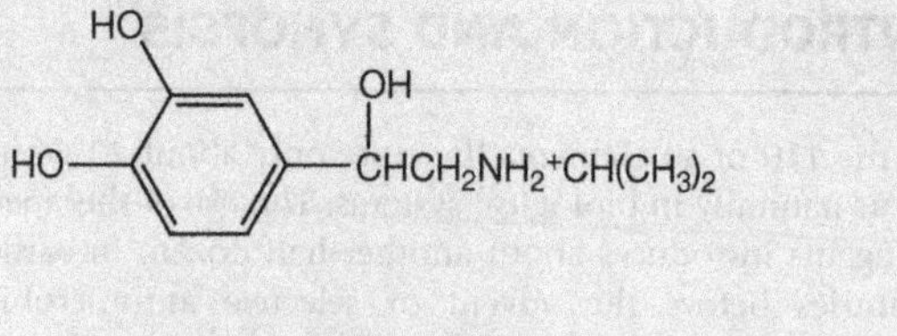

Isoprenaline

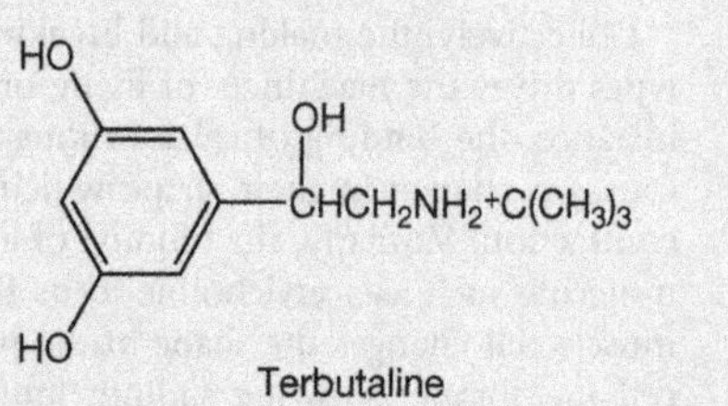

Terbutaline

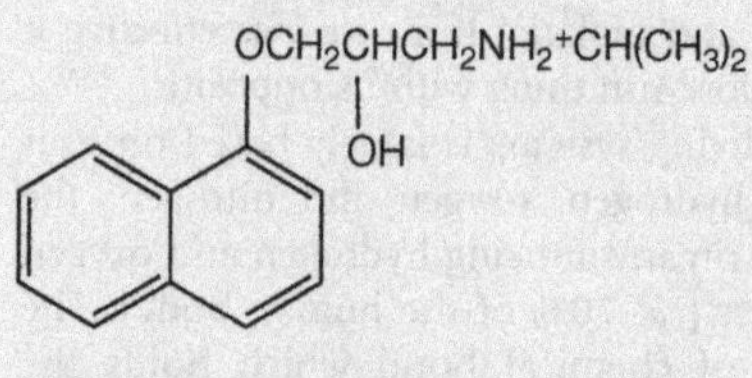

Propranolol

Figure 1.1 Interaction of adrenaline with amino acids within its receptor protein.

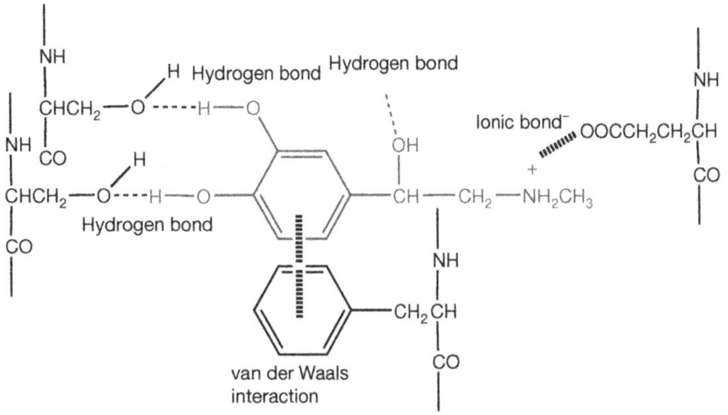

COVALENT BONDS

Covalent bonds are the strongest type of bond and are not usually involved directly in drug action. In fact, in most circumstances the formation of such bonds with a drug would give cause for concern because of the potential for alteration DNA and which could be potentially carcinogenic. However, there are circumstances in which the formation of a covalent bond is the therapeutic target for a drug. This is most notably the case for the alkylating agents used in cancer chemotherapy which are designed to form covalent bonds with the DNA of the cancerous cells and prevent them growing. As one might imagine, this process is also damaging to healthy cells within the body.

What is a covalent bond?

The theory of chemical bonding can be very complex and is worthy of several volumes in itself, but a basic knowledge will be sufficient for our purposes (see Box 1.2). The modern understanding of chemical bonding derives from quantum mechanics. A bond is formed when an atom shares its electrons with another atom. According to quantum mechanics, the electron behaves like a light wave and when electrons are shared they can either reinforce each other or cancel each other out in the way that light waves do when they destructively interfere. The waveform of an electron is known as a molecular orbital. The simplest atom is the hydrogen atom and when two hydrogen atoms join together they provide the simplest situation in which two molecular orbitals combine. Figure 1.2 shows the overlap between in-phase and out-of-phase hydrogen orbitals to form a bond.

The in-phase orbitals produce a viable σ–bond which holds the atoms together and the out-of-phase orbitals produce an σ* anti-bonding orbital in which there is no overlap between the atomic orbitals. Since the bonding between the two hydrogen atoms, or indeed any pair of atoms, is due to an electronic wave phenomenon one way of examining bonds is by observing their interaction with electromagnetic radiation.

A pair of hydrogen atoms requires high energy/short wavelength radiation at about 150 nm (8.3 eV) to break the bond between them. Formation of the anti-bonding orbital can be represented as shown in Figure 1.3 where the two electrons

> **Box 1.2 The electron volt**
>
> An electron volt is a measure of force, albeit a very tiny amount of force.
>
> 1 eV = $1.602176487(40)\times10^{-19}$ Joules. One Joule is approximately the energy required to lift a small apple quickly up 1 metre, or is the amount of energy required to heat 800 mL of dry, cool air through 1 degree Celsius.

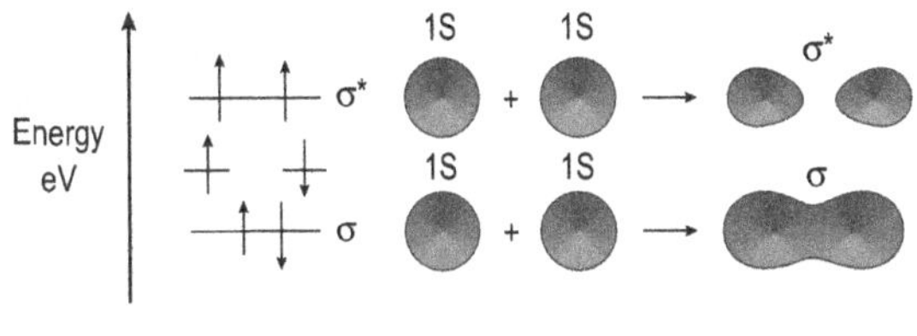

Figure 1.2 Bond formation between hydrogen atoms.

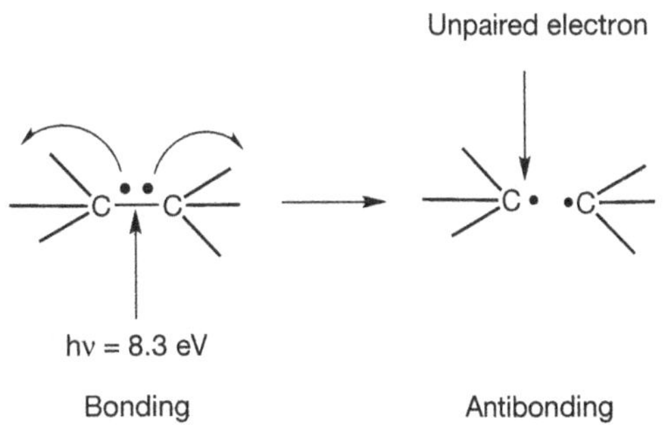

Figure 1.3 The effect of UV radiation on the electrons in a σ bond.

making the bond are moved apart. The use of curly arrows to represent movement of electrons is shown in more detail in Box 1.3. Because bonding energy is quantised, the energy required is an exact figure for a given bond. The anti-bonding state is unstable and short lived so either the bond will re-form or a new bond will form with some suitable chemical species in the environment.

Weaker bonds such as those found in DNA bases only require radiation around 260 nm (4.8 eV) to break them. This radiation is present in sunlight and hence the potentially damaging effects of overexposure to sunlight. A simple example of a weaker type of covalent bond is found in ethylene (Fig. 1.4). In this molecule the molecular orbitals have a more complex (hybrid) waveform than the simple 1S orbital of the hydrogen atom. The most important point to note is that the π bond in ethylene is formed by only partial overlap of the orbitals that form it. The stronger σ-bond in the molecule results from more complete overlap of the orbitals involved in it. Thus the energy required to excite the electrons in the π bond in ethylene to their excited (anti-bonding) state is lower than that required to excite those in the σ bond.

Table 1.2 shows the strength of some covalent bonds commonly found within drug molecules and within the biomolecules composing the human body, derived from calorimetric measurements.

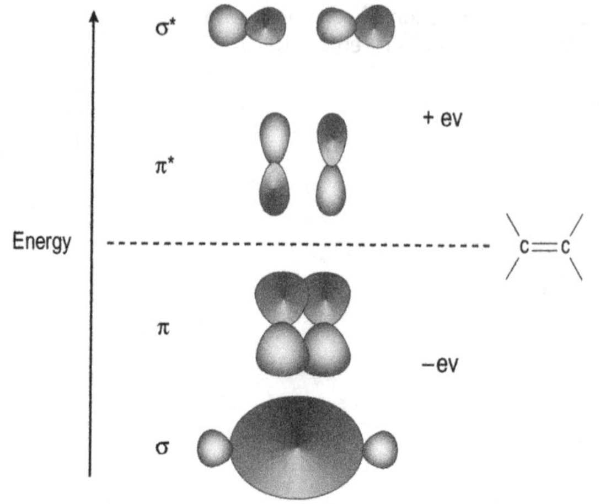

Figure 1.4 The carbon–carbon bonds in ethylene.

A method for estimating the strength of a bond is by using calorimetry, which measures the heat of a reaction. For example, the reaction between fluorine and hydrogen

Box 1.3 **Curly arrows**

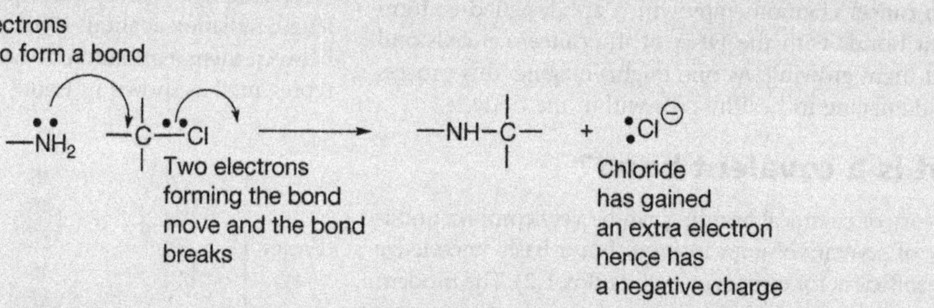

Throughout the book, extensive use is made of curly arrows to represent the movement of electrons. This convention is quite simple to understand.

1. Any bond is composed of two electrons.
2. A double-headed arrow indicates two electrons moving and can indicate the formation or the breaking of a bond.
3. A single-headed arrow indicates the movement of a single electron.

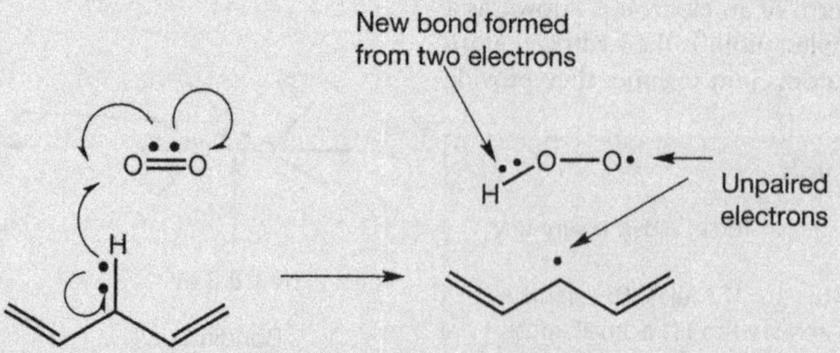

Unpaired electrons (free radicals) usually have a very short time of independence since they will rapidly pair with another electron to form a bond. This is why free radicals are very damaging to living tissues.

Table 1.2 The energy of some covalent bonds

Single bonds	Energy kJ mol^{-1}	Dipole $\longrightarrow$	Double bonds	Energy kJ/mol^{-1}	Dipole $\longrightarrow$
H–H	431				
H–O	455	1.51			
H–N	385				
H–S	367	0.68			
C–H	410	0.4			
C–O	330	0.74	C=O	170	2.3
C–C	330		C=C	146	
C–Cl	325				
C–N	275	0.22	C=N	147	3.5
C–S	235	0.9			
N–O	182				
P–O			P=O	120	

$$F_2 + H_2 \longrightarrow 2HF$$

shown above in theory generates 542 kJ mol^{-1} of heat. Using the values shown in Table 1.2, on the deficit side, the hydrogen–hydrogen bond (431 kJ mol^{-1}) and the fluorine–fluorine bond (155 kJ mol^{-1}) are broken but on the credit side two H–F bonds (2 × 564 kJ mol^{-1}) are formed. Thus the total energy derived from the reaction is 1128–586 = 542 kJ mol^{-1}. The heat given out by a reaction is called the enthalpy of reaction and given the symbol Δ H, it is also given a minus sign, indicating that heat is produced by the reaction; thus the theoretical Δ H for the above reaction is −542 kJ mol^{-1}. The heat of such a reaction can be measured using a calorimeter, which measures the amount of heat released by measuring the increase in temperature of water surrounding the sample being reacted. In this case, if 2 moles (40 g) of hydrogen fluoride were formed from hydrogen and fluorine the heat generated would be enough to raise the temperature of 1 litre of water from 0°C to beyond its boiling point (1 mole = 18 g of water requires 75.4 J to raise its temperature by 1°C). To break the bonds between H and F in 2 moles of HF, 1128 kJ of heat energy would be required. Thermal dissociation of bonds within molecules occurs, for example, when the analytical technique of inductively coupled plasma emission spectroscopy is used. In this technique temperatures of *ca.* 6000°C, provided by a heated plasma of argon gas, are used to disrupt the bonds in molecules so that the elements making them up can be analysed by exciting their electrons.

Dipole moments of bonds

The strengths of covalent bonds (Box 1.4) are less important in appreciating the relationship between drug structure and activity than the weaker interactions which occur between molecules as opposed to the forces within molecules. An example of a weak bonding force is that generated by the dipole moment of a bond. Linus Pauling produced a method for estimating the electronegativity of elements using equation 1 shown below.

$$|XA - XB| = \sqrt{D_{AB} - (D_{A2}D_{B2})^{1/2}} \qquad \textbf{1}$$

X is the electronegativity of elements A and B.

D_{AB}, D_{A2} and D_{B2} are the bond dissociation energies between AB, A_2 and B_2.

By arbitrarily defining the most electronegative element, fluorine, as having an electronegativity value of 4.0 the values for all the other elements can be defined and this led to the values shown in Table 1.1.

Many covalent bonds have dipoles and dipole moments within drug molecules are important for their interaction with the biomolecules within cells which transmit the drug's action. The larger the dipole, the stronger the dipolar interaction with proteins and receptors within the cell. In addition, the strength of the dipole moment gives an indication of how likely the drug is to be degraded by reactants with an affinity for positive or negative charge. As indicated above, in most cases drug action is not based on covalent bond formation. There

Box 1.4 How strong is a chemical bond?

Often, bond energy and the force holding two atoms together are used interchangeably. In fact, the energy is equal to force × distance since the force has to be applied in order to stretch the bond for a certain distance before it will break. Chemical bonds can be broken by applying a force in the same way as one might apply weights to a spring until it snapped. Of course, one cannot literally suspend a weight from a bond in order to break it but one can stretch it to snapping point using appropriate chemicals. If it were possible to stretch a bond by attaching a weight, it would require a weight of 5–10 micrograms to break a single covalent bond (a microgram is about the size of a speck of dust). This might not sound like much but one has to remember that 1 mole of a compound contains 6.022×10^{23} molecules.

Box 1.5 Covalent bond formation in drug therapy

Covalent bond formation is important in the action of the following classes of drugs:

1. Alkylating agents used in the treatment of cancer: covalent bond formation occurs with the bases in DNA and thus kills the cancer cells but also rapidly growing cells in the body such as white blood cells.
2. Penicillins and cephalosporins: covalent bond formation occurs with the growing bacterial cell wall.
3. Inhibitors of secretion of gastric acid secretion such as omeprazole: covalent bond formation occurs with the transporter in parietal cells.
4. Aspirin: acetylates COX enzymes inhibiting their activity.

are exceptions (see Box 1.5), and thus the importance of covalent bond strength in pharmaceutical chemistry relates mainly to the stability of drugs in formulations, although it usually relates to the lifetime of the drug *in vivo* as well. The likelihood of a drug degrading depends on a combination of bond strength and the ease with which it is attacked at either positive or negative centres of charge. Thus the carbon–carbon bond within biomolecules is one of the least susceptible to degradation, certainly *in vitro* and to some extent *in vivo*, since it does not have a large dipole despite the fact that it stores a large amount of energy.

In Table 1.2 above it can be seen that the carbon–carbon double bond is stronger than the carbon–carbon single bond but listing its additive strength in this way belies the fact that one of the carbon bonds, the π bond, within the double bond is relatively weak and thus is quite susceptible to chemical attack.

Some types of degradation reaction are more important with regard to drug molecules than others. Most often it is the polarised bonds within drug molecules which are most susceptible to chemical degradation, i.e. have the lowest activation energies in this respect. Figure 1.5 shows the partial charge distribution within aspirin and paracetamol.

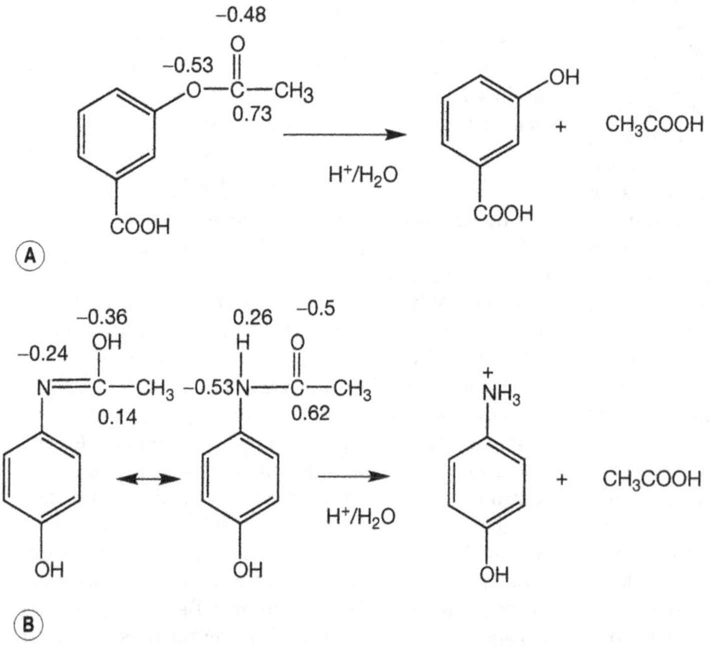

Figure 1.5 The hydrolysis of (**A**) aspirin and (**B**) paracetamol.

Under conditions of acidic hydrolysis of an ester or amide the positively charged protons in the acidic medium will attack the most negative point within the group undergoing hydrolysis. In the case of aspirin the greatest negative charge is on the two oxygens within the ester group and protonation can occur at either of these positions, thus promoting attack by water at the positively charged carbon, which results in the breakdown of aspirin into acetic acid and salicylic acid. The activation energy for this reaction is low and hydrolysis occurs slowly at room temperature. It can also be seen from the polarised distribution of charge that the ester bond in aspirin is also susceptible to attack by HO^- which will attach itself to the positively charged carbon and thus promote hydrolysis. The hydrolysis of esters is covered in Chapter 2. As pharmaceutical chemists, we are interested in what conditions are likely to cause our medicine to degrade. Obviously, aspirin should be kept dry.

The amide bond in paracetamol is also polarised and the charges on oxygen and carbon are not very different from those on the oxygens in the ester group in aspirin. However, amides hydrolyse much less readily than esters. One way of explaining this is that the carbonyl carbon is not as positively charged in the amide as in the ester and thus is less liable to attack by water or by the hydroxyl ion. However, calculation of charge distribution by chemical modelling software has its limitations and sometimes a less sophisticated view yields useful information. Without changing the charge on the amide group it is possible to write a resonance form for the amide where the proton is on the oxygen. The concept of resonance can be applied throughout organic chemistry and in simple terms all it means is that electron density is shared more evenly throughout a structure or group within a structure. As was discussed at the beginning of this section, the most stable bonds are those where electron density is distributed evenly and thus there is likelihood of degradative attack. If the charge distribution is calculated for the resonance form of paracetamol the charge distribution across the oxygen, carbon and nitrogen is evened out. Thus, activation energy required for hydrolysis of an amide is greater than that required for hydrolysis of an ester. It is important to note that once the activation energy for hydrolysis has been overcome the acidic hydrolysis of an amide proceeds rapidly and irreversibly, i.e. it is thermodynamically favourable and releases more energy than hydrolysis of the equivalent ester. In this case a non-polar molecule activation energy can be high but this is followed by a high release of energy (Box 1.6).

Box 1.6 Activation energy versus thermodynamic energy release

$$CH_3{-}CH_2{-}CH_3 + 35O_2 \longrightarrow 3CO_2 + 4H_2O$$

The absence of a dipole moment means that the activation energy required for degradation of a carbon–carbon bond to occur is high; for example, propane gas is a rich source of thermal energy (3671 kJ mol^{-1} is enough to boil several kettles of water when camping under the most arctic conditions). However, it has to be heated to a high temperature, e.g. with a match, gently warming it does not work, before it ignites and reacts with oxygen. Thermodynamically, this reaction lies far in the direction (to the right) of the formation of carbon dioxide from the carbon atoms and water from the hydrogen atoms in the propane. In contrast, the energy required to activate the degradation of an ester by acidic hydrolysis described below is minimal but the energy released by the reaction is small and thermodynamically the reaction lies only slightly in the direction of the reaction products.

Thus in chemical reactions we have two ideas: the ease with which the reaction can be triggered and the amount of energy released by the reaction.

Q Self Test 1.2

From the charge distribution in the following esters, arrange them in order of increasing rate of hydrolysis caused by HO^-.

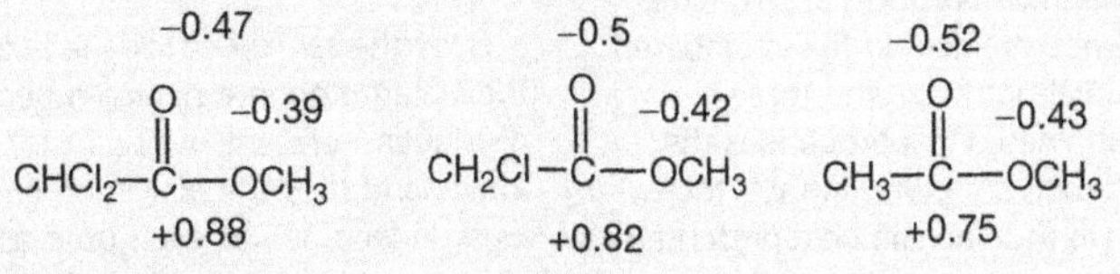

Dichloromethylacetate Chloromethylacetate Methylacetate

How much do you think the rate of acid hydrolysis might vary?

Under acidic conditions (pH 1) at room temperature, aspirin hydrolyses in a few hours whereas paracetamol can be stored at room temperature under acidic conditions (pH 1) for many days without much hydrolysis occurring. We will return to the properties of esters and amides in a little more detail in Chapters 3 and 4.

As can be seen in Figure 1.5 aspirin and paracetamol have many bonds in their structure but it is only the bonds where the charge distribution is polarised which are susceptible to hydrolytic attack. Ester bonds are among the most labile bonds which are found in drug molecules. Another type of bond which limits shelf life is found in the lactam ring of penicillins. This bond may look like an amide bond, and calculation of charge density on the C, N and O atoms in the bond does not reveal any great difference from the atoms in the amide bond of paracetamol. At this point an additional concept is required, which is that ring strain renders the lactam ring much more susceptible to nucleophilic attack (i.e. where a negative species attacks a positive) or electrophilic attack (where a positive species attacks a negative) and this is indeed also responsible for its biological activity (Ch. 22). Ring strain arises from the fact that carbon atoms have preferred angles between the bonds attached to them. The preferred angles for the four bonded carbons in the ring (A and B) is 109°28′ (Box 1.7) and for the three bonded carbonyl carbons 120°; in the lactam ring the carbons are forced to have angles approximating to 90°. The strained ring reduces the activation energy required for the hydrolysis reaction to proceed (Fig. 1.6).

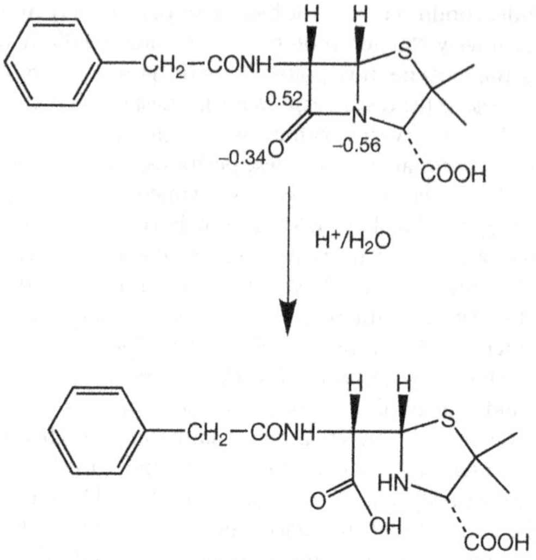

Figure 1.6 Hydrolysis of the lactam ring.

The distortion of the ring geometry is further reflected in the IR absorption of the carbonyl carbon within the lactam ring which is at high energy, *ca.* 1770 cm^{-1}. This is due to the lack of interaction between the nitrogen and the carbonyl oxygen, which normally occurs in amides, resulting from the distorted geometry. IR provides a simple method for examining bond strength (Box 1.8).

Box 1.7 **Ring strain**

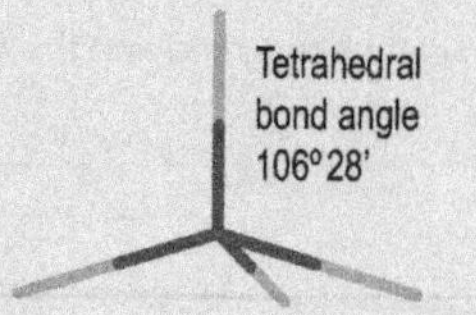

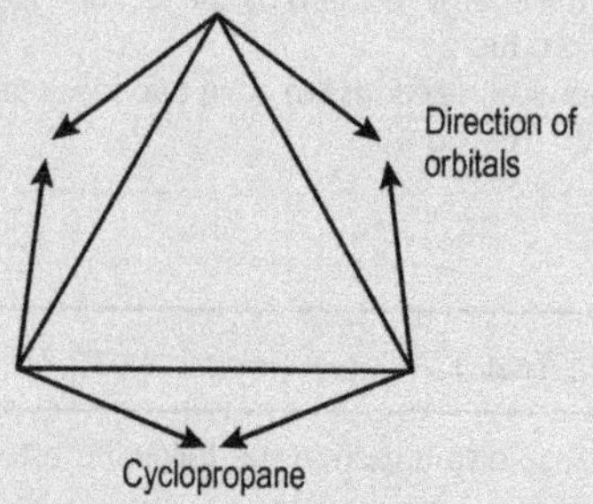

Four-bonded carbon prefers tetrahedral geometry. Any deviation from the preferred angle produces strain. Rings with six atoms or more are not strained. In five-membered rings the strain is fairly minimal but four- and three-membered rings are quite strained. Cyclopropane is the simplest three-membered carbon structure. In fact, the orbitals of the carbon atoms in this ring can be represented as being bent away from the ring with an angle of 9.4°, indicating that they do not overlap as extensively as in an unstrained structure.

Nevertheless, cyclopropane is quite stable compared to the lactam ring in a penicillin because its even charge distribution presents no point for nucleophilic or electrophilic attack and thus the activation energy for its reaction is high. Indeed, it was even used as a volatile anaesthetic, although it has fallen out of favour since a spark overcoming the activation energy for the molecular reaction results in a large thermodynamic change, i.e. an explosion.

Box 1.8 **Resonance and infrared spectrophotometry as a simple tool for observing bond strength**

The concept of resonance was first applied to the benzene ring where all the bonds were found to be identical. In the structure drawn on the left it looks as if there are two different types of bond and the structure is more correctly drawn as on the right with the electron density from the double bonds evenly distributed throughout the molecule.

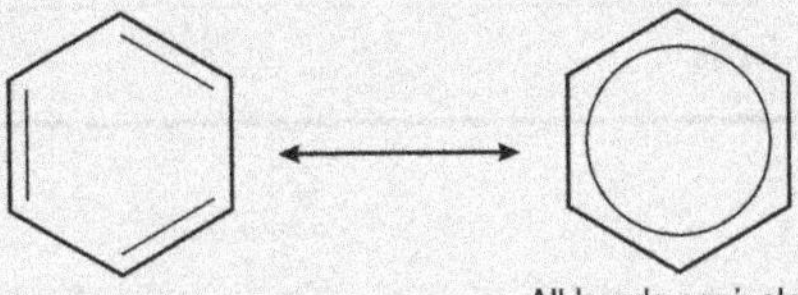

There are a number of ways of observing the electron density within double bonds. One simple method is infrared spectrophotometry (IR). IR observes interaction of IR radiation (heat radiation) with bonds in molecules. IR radiation causes bonds to stretch: the lower the wavenumber ($1/\lambda$) of the IR radiation required to stretch a bond the weaker a bond. The energy of the radiation used in IR is reported as 1/wavelength in centimetres. The higher the number, the higher the energy. Carbonyl groups absorb IR radiation between 1650 cm^{-1} and 1800 cm^{-1}. The carbonyl group of the ester in aspirin has an absorption at 1760 cm^{-1} whereas the carbonyl group in the amide of paracetamol absorbs at 1650 cm^{-1}. This indicates that the carbonyl in paracetamol has lost some of its electron density and thus some of its strength relative to the carbonyl in aspirin due to the resonance shown in Figure 1.5.

INTERMOLECULAR OR INTER-ATOMIC FORCES

Introduction

The actions of drugs on biological molecules involve intermolecular forces. There are a number of types of interactions between molecules, ranging from strong ionic interactions to weak but additively strong van der Waals interactions. The different strength of the different types of intermolecular force can be observed in the melting points of the series of compounds shown in Table 1.3, all of which have similar molecular weights but which exhibit different types of intermolecular interactions. The high degree of precision with which a naturally occurring ligand binds to its site of action depends on a delicate balance of the different intermolecular forces (see also Box 1.9). Drugs usually do not fit a given receptor with the same degree of precision as a natural ligand but have actions which originate in strong binding to parts of the receptor. With a knowledge of receptor structure, the intermolecular forces required for binding can be used to model ideal drug structures which will bind strongly.

Ionic bonds

When two atoms which are widely different in electronegativity are brought into contact, rather than a covalent bond forming, the more electronegative atom will take an electron or electrons from the less electronegative atom, thus becoming negatively charged while the less electronegative atom becomes positively charged. A simple example is the reaction between a sodium atom (a soft metal) and a chlorine atom (gas). Having gained positive and negative charges, the two atoms are now attracted to each other, and if they are considered to be point charges

Table 1.3 The effect of different intermolecular forces on melting point and boiling point

Substance	Mol. Wt.	M. P.	B. P.	Intermolecular forces
Argon (Ar)	40		−186°C	Dispersion forces
Carbon dioxide (CO_2)	44	−78.5°C sublimes		Increased dispersion forces due to larger number of bonds
Propane	42		−42°C	Further increase in dispersion forces due to more bonds
Methyl chloride CH_3Cl	50.5	−97°C	−23.7°C	Dispersion forces + weak dipole–dipole interaction
Nitrogen dioxide (NO_2)	42		21.2°C	Dispersion forces + dipole–dipole interaction
Ethanol C_2H_5OH	46	−114°C	78.5°C	Dispersion forces + hydrogen bonding
Sodium fluoride	42	993°C	1704°C	Ionic bonding

Box 1.9 A digression on the matter of force versus energy

It is quite easy to use the terms force and energy interchangeably. However, there is a difference. Intermolecular force decreases as the distance between two atoms or molecules increases. Thus, the spring analogy used to describe a bond is not strictly correct since the resistance produced by a spring when it is stretched beyond the point where it will spring back becomes high. Two better analogies are: moving two strong magnets apart, where the force decreases with distance until it is too weak to move them back together; or pulling a fence post out of some sticky mud where initially the resistance is high but, as it becomes less deeply buried, it moves more easily. In the two activities described, the energy required is the sum of the effort expended in overcoming the force of resistance (analogous to bond energy) which decreases with the distance moved from the starting point.

the magnitude of the energy of the attraction would be 694 kJ mol^{-1} if they were separated by a distance of 200 picometres in a vacuum. Such an energy is greater than the strength of most covalent bonds. However, in practice many ionic bonds can be readily broken using water as a solvent because of the strength of the bonds formed between the water and the positive and negative ions.

$$Na + Cl \longrightarrow Na^+ + Cl^-$$

When a salt is dissolved in a solvent, the force of attraction between its ions is governed largely by the dielectric constant of the medium in which it is dissolved and the distance of separation between the two ions. The force of attraction between two ions can be calculated according to equation 2.

$$\text{Force}(F) = \frac{Q1Q2}{\varepsilon r^2} \quad (2)$$

Where $Q1$ and $Q2$ are the charges on the ions, r is the distance of separation and ε is the dielectric constant of the medium.

The dielectric constant of water is defined as 80 relative to that of a vacuum. Thus energy of the bond between two point charges separated by two picometres in water would be 80 times less than the energy of the bond in a vacuum and have a value of *ca.* 8 kJ mol^{-1}. Water is the best solvent for ionic compounds because of its high dielectric constant. Table 1.4 shows the dielectric constants of some common solvents. Sodium chloride dissolves in water at 1 g in 2.8 mL and in glycerol, which has half the dielectric constant of water; 1 g dissolves in 10 mL. Sodium chloride is almost insoluble in ethanol; in this case the dielectric constant is too low for the inter-ionic attraction to be overcome.

In living systems, ionic associations take place in aqueous media and the energies involved in these types of interaction are between 4 and 40 kJ mol^{-1}. The reason for the wide range in energies of ionic interactions is that the strength of the interaction depends on the dielectric constant of the environment and on how closely the two ions approach. Strong interactions between ions may occur because within cell membranes and in the hydrophobic cavities of proteins the amounts of water present may be greatly reduced, resulting in a decrease in the dielectric constant of the environment. The binding of an ionic drug with hydrophobic groups attached may further reduce the water present in a binding site. Since the force of attraction between ions varies as the square of the distance of their separation ionic forces act over a greater distance than the other intermolecular forces described below. The long-range attraction of ions and the consequent speed of association between oppositely charged ions means that ionic forces are important in driving much of the mechanical work of the cell. Table 1.5 shows the principal ionic groups which are found in proteins, along with their pKa values and percentage ionisation of these groups at the physiological pH of 7.4. These charged groups within protein structures provide sites for the binding of ionic drugs through formation of ion pairs and non-ionic drugs through ion–dipole interactions.

Table 1.4 Dielectric constants of some common solvents

SOLVENT	DIELECTRIC CONSTANT ε
Water	78.5
Glycerol $C_3H_5(OH)_3$	42.5
Acetonitrile CH_3CN	36.2
Methanol CH_3OH	32.6
Ethanol $CH_3\ CH_2OH$	24.3
Benzene C_6H_6	4.6

Where ionic interaction is an important component in the interaction of a drug with a receptor or G-protein, other forces may come into play in reinforcing the ionic interaction and these include particularly dipole–dipole interactions, hydrogen bonding and van der Waals forces (as illustrated in Fig. 1.1 for adrenaline). Thus the thermodynamics of drug action is based on the interplay between several forces which are relatively weak compared to the covalent bonds which make up the scaffolding of living systems. That is not to say that these weaker forces do not result indirectly in the breaking or formation of covalent bonds, but this is a consequence of the initial interaction of the drug with its receptor, which may trigger off enzyme action which results the making or breaking of covalent bonds.

Table 1.5 Ionised groups found on proteins

Acidic groups	pKa	% Ionisation at pH 7.4
Terminal carboxyl (–COO^-)	1.8–2.4	100
Aspartic acid side chain (–$CH_2CH_2COO^-$)	3.7	99.98
Glutamic acid side chain (–$CH_2CH_2CH_2$ COO^-)	4.3	99.9
Basic Groups		
Terminal ammonium (–NH_3^+)	7.5–10.3	55.7–99.9
Arginine (–NH–(NH_2) C=NH_2^+)	12.5	100
Lysine (–$CH_2CH_2CH_2CH_2NH_3^+$)	10.5	99.9
Histidine	6.0	4
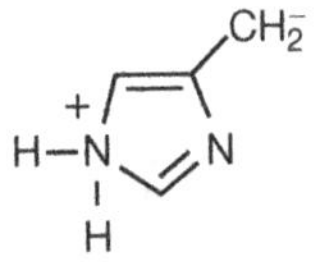		

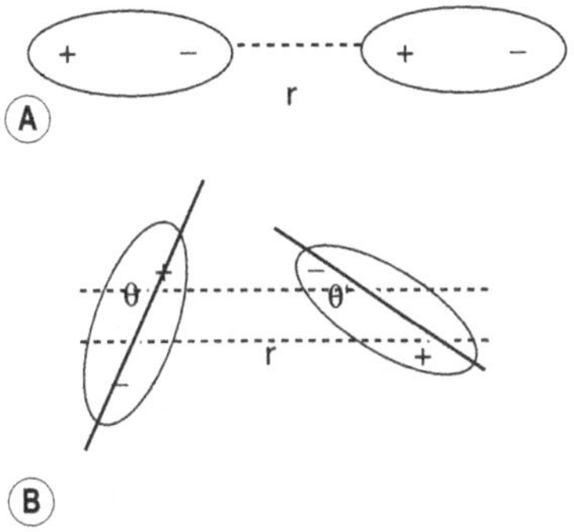

Figure 1.7 Dipole–dipole interactions.

Dipole–dipole interactions

The strength of a dipole (Fig 1.7) within a bond depends on the relative electronegativities of the atoms composing the bond. Where a molecule contains a dipole, it can interact with other molecules containing a dipole. The force between two dipoles is give by equation 3.

$$\text{Force}(F) = -\frac{2\mu_A\mu_B}{\varepsilon r^4} \quad (3)$$

Where μ_A and μ_B are the dipole moments of the molecules involved in the interaction, ε is the dielectric constant on the medium in which the interaction is taking place. r is the distance between the two dipoles.

Equation 3 holds if the dipoles interact in a linear fashion as shown in Figure 1.7A: in this case the interaction is maximal. Where the interaction is at an angle as in Figure 1.7B, the interaction is given by equation 4 (cos θ is <1).

$$\text{Force}(F) = -\frac{2\mu_A \cos\theta \mu_B \cos\theta'}{\varepsilon r^4} \quad (4)$$

Dipolar interactions are very dependent on temperature since an increase in temperature promotes random motion in molecules, which makes the linear orientation of the dipoles less likely. The interaction between dipoles falls off with the fourth power of distance and thus acts over a much smaller distance than ionic interactions, which are dependent of r^2. The strength of these interactions is within an energy range of 0.4–4 kJ mol^{-1}. When brought into close contact within a receptor, for example, ionic interactions, dipolar interactions with a drug become significant since contact is both close and at the optimum angle. If dipole–dipole interactions are important for activity at a receptor, any slight spatial adjustment in order to accommodate of a molecule could result in loss of activity.

Ion–dipole interactions

The interaction between an ion and a dipole (Fig. 1.8) depends on the cube of the distance between them (equation 5). Like dipole–dipole interactions, these interactions depend on the orientation of the dipole with respect to the ion.

Charged dipole interactions tend to be stronger than dipole–dipole interactions and have energies in the range 1–10 kJ mol^{-1}. These interactions are responsible for the solvation of ions in solution and are responsible for promoting the dissolution of ionic solids.

$$\text{Force}(F) = \frac{\mu q \cos\theta}{\varepsilon r^3} \quad (5)$$

Van der Waals forces

Van der Waals forces (or London dispersion forces) arise in molecules where the charge appears to be evenly distributed because vibrations within molecules cause transient dipoles. These transient dipoles induce transient attractive dipoles in

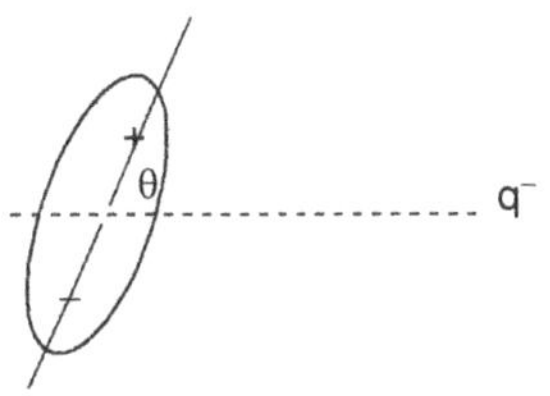

Figure 1.8 Ion–dipole interaction.

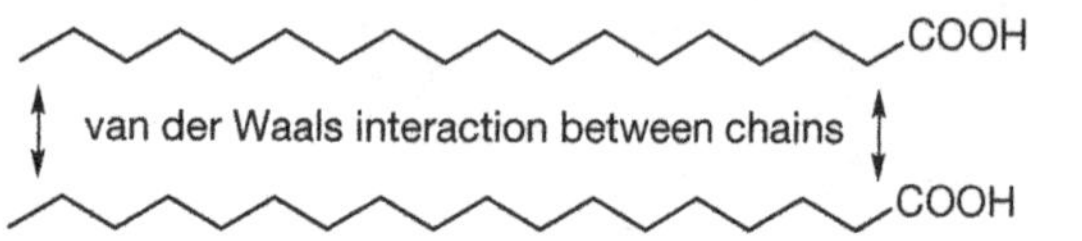

Figure 1.9 Van der Waals interaction between the chains of stearic acid.

adjacent molecules with energies in the range 0.3–1.9 kJ mol^{-1}. As can be seen from equation 6, these forces only operate at very close range and fall off at the rate of the seventh power of the separation of the interacting species.

$$\text{Force}(F) = \frac{3I\alpha^2}{4r^7} \quad 6$$

Where I is the first ionisation potential of the atom or molecule involved in the interaction, α is its polarisabliity and r is the separation distance.

However, at close range the additive effect of the interactions can be high and, for instance, it has been estimated that the additive effect of attraction between the atoms involved in the hydrocarbon chain of stearic acid is 33.5 kJ mol^{-1} (Fig. 1.9).

The strength of the forces involved depends on the polarisablility of the structural component in which the transient dipole is induced. The increased polarisability is related to increased molecular weight and large atoms within a structure increase the van der Waals interactions considerably because of their high polarisabilities. This can be seen in the case of C_2H_5Cl (B.P. 12°C), C_2H_5Br (B.P. 38°C) and C_2H_5I (B.P. 72°C). The dipole moment of these molecules increases from iodide to chloride but this is more than offset by the increasing van der Waals interactions from chloride to iodide.

CHARGE TRANSFER INTERACTIONS

Charge transfer interactions are also thought to be important in the interaction between drugs and proteins. These interactions are quite weak being <1 eV. A commonplace example is the complex formed between picric acid and creatinine (Fig. 1.10) in solution which is used as a

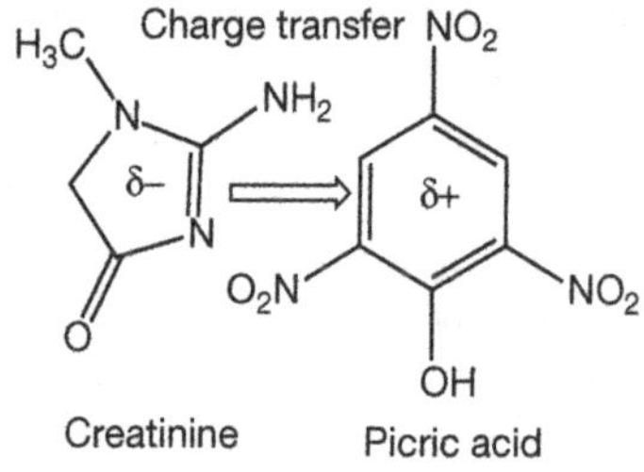

Figure 1.10 Charge transfer complex between creatinine and picric acid.

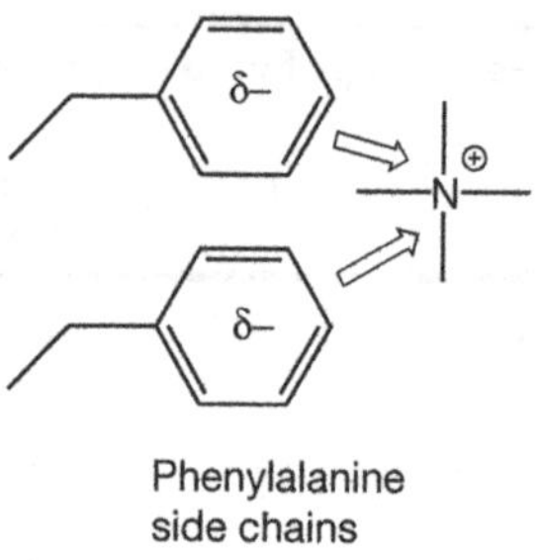

Figure 1.11 Interaction between aromatic amino acid residues and a quaternary ammonium ion.

clinical assay to normalise the concentration of urine samples. Charge transfer requires a π-base, in this case creatinine which is electron rich and a π-acid, in this case picric acid which is electron deficient due to electrons being withdrawn from the aromatic ring. The formation of the complex results in a shift in the ultraviolet spectrum, which can be quantitatively measured.

Such interactions are also possible between ions and electron-rich systems. In some cases, charge transfer interactions may be involved in receptor binding, e.g. interactions between a quaternary ammonium centre in a drug and phenylalanine side chains in a protein (Fig. 1.11).

THE HYDROGEN BOND, SOLVATION AND ENTROPY OF MIXING

The hydrogen bond occurs whenever hydrogen, which is bonded to an electronegative atom such as N or O, interacts with another electronegative atom. The most immediately familiar type of hydrogen bond is that which occurs between water molecules but the hydrogen bond is also very important in the structure of DNA and proteins. Compared to other hydrides of electronegative elements, the boiling point of water is high, e.g. compare water 100°C, HF 20°C and HCl −33°C. The boiling point of water is thus elevated above that which would be predicted on the basis of its molecular weight (MW). For instance H_2S has a boiling point of −61°C although its MW is 34 compared with a MW of 18 for water. The elevation of boiling point in the case of water is due to the strong hydrogen bonds between its molecules. Hydrogen bonds are specialised dipole–dipole interactions. The strength of the hydrogen bonds in water is partly due to the high electronegativity of oxygen and partly due to the favourable geometry of the water molecule that allows the formation of two hydrogen bonds per molecule and the formation of complex networks of water molecules. The hydrogen bond in water is expressed as shown in Figure 1.12.

The weaker hydrogen bond is represented by the dotted line. Hydrogen bond strength in water is around 20 kJ mol^{-1}. The bulk structure of water consists of cluster

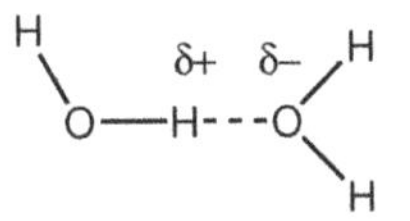

Figure 1.12 The hydrogen bond in water.

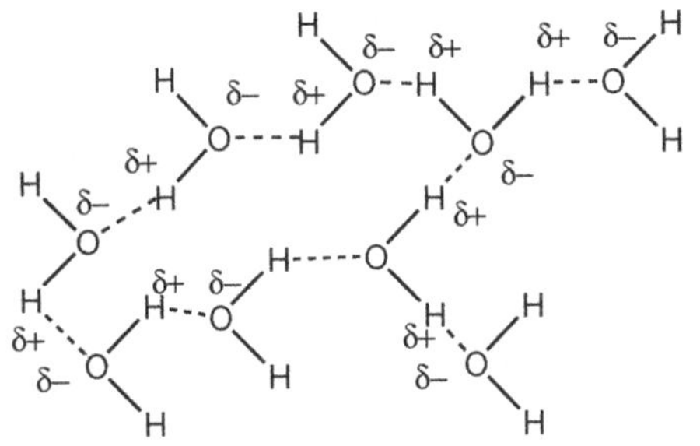

Figure 1.13 Formation of clusters of water molecules.

of hydrogen-bonded molecules (Fig. 1.13). If a water-soluble alcohol such as methanol is mixed with water, the temperature rises upon mixing. This is due to the thermodynamics of mixing.

We have touched on the ideas of thermodynamics in the process of discussing the release of energy when bonds are broken and reformed, e.g. propane burns in air, and because of the large release of energy resulting from the formation of H–O and C–O bonds. If we examine the preparation of a solution containing 20% w/w methanol in water by mixing the two liquids, it is not immediately apparent why the solution should get warmer.

On closer examination, it can be seen that the methanol can only hydrogen bond at one end of the molecule (Fig. 1.14) and thus it causes many of the hydrogen bonds between water molecules to break, and this process would be expected to require an investment of energy rather than generating heat. This simple, easily observable example necessitates the introduction of another concept into the generation of energy by chemical change. We have observed earlier when weaker bonds are replaced with stronger bonds energy is released. In the current example, it is the second law of thermodynamics that explains the warming of the methanol–water mixture. The change in energy during a process according to the second law of thermodynamics can be stated as follows:

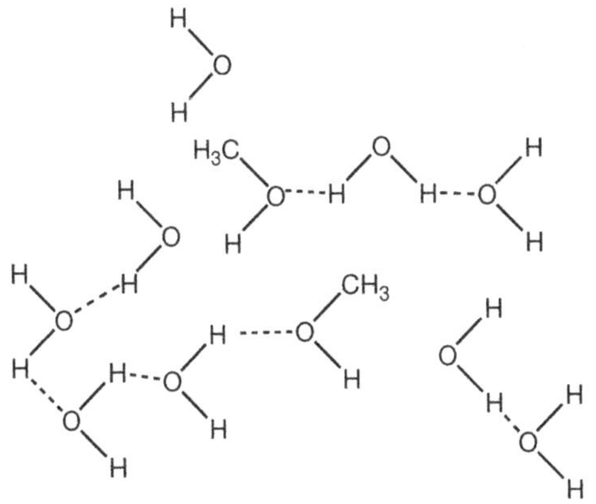

Figure 1.14 Disruption of hydrogen bonding in water by methanol.

$$\Delta G = \Delta H - T\Delta S$$

Where ΔG is the Gibbs free energy of a process, which is a measure of how thermodynamically favourable it is. We have already encountered ΔH in the form of the heat generated or by a chemical change, but heat alone does not fully describe a process. For instance, when ice melts the heat invested in breaking the bonds between the water molecules in the ice cannot be readily recovered in order to reverse the process; although the water remains at 0°C when it melts it does not spontaneously turn back into ice. The reason that processes are not readily reversible is because some of the energy generated or invested during the change takes the form of entropy, ΔS (Box 1.10). Entropy concerns the behaviour of molecules during a chemical or physical change. When ice melts, the molecules in the water produced have greater freedom to move about (kinetic energy) and greater freedom to vibrate and rotate (internal molecular energy) than they did in the ice. Such energy processes, which change the way in which molecules behave in space, are termed entropy and are not reversible without investing energy. For example, if we want to refreeze water to produce ice using a freezer we have to use electrical heating to evaporate the refrigerant in the freezer in order to produce the cooling required in the same way as eau de cologne cools the skin as it evaporates. The greater the freedom of molecules due to being able to move, and for complex molecules this includes vibration, rotation etc., as well as translational movement, the greater the entropy of a system. The heat generated when methanol is mixed with water indicates that mixing in this case is energetically favourable despite the loss of hydrogen bonding shown in Figure 1.14. The processes occurring during the mixing are complex but at least in part some of the energy emitted is due to a loss of vibrational energy in the methyl group, possibly due to compression by water molecules. This can be seen in the IR spectrum of the methyl group where the C–H stretching occurs at higher energy in methanol–water mixtures compared to pure methanol (Watson et al. unpublished). Such events at the molecular level may seem a little abstract but what we observe is that the methanol–water mixture emits heat radiation upon mixing. Indeed, our perception of the heat is due to transfer of some of the vibrational entropy to the molecules making up our skin surface from the warm molecules that our skin is in

Box 1.10 **Explanations of entropy**

Entropy is a troublesome concept, so it is worth trying to define it in a number of different ways.

- Increasing entropy is a tendency of molecules and atoms towards occupying increasingly diverse energy states. It is natural for matter to become disordered simply because there are many more ways in which molecules can be arranged in a disorderly fashion than an orderly fashion.
- A ball dropped onto a stone floor will continue bouncing until its kinetic energy has been dispersed. The original energy is transferred to the molecules of the ball and to those of its area of contact with the floor, which will slowly heat up (this is more easily seen in a squash ball after a few minutes' play) thus increasing the random movement of both the molecules within the floor and the molecules within the ball. To reverse the process and push the ball back to the height at which it started, an extremely unlikely event would have to occur. This would be that the molecules of the ball and the area of its contact with the floor would have to simultaneously move exactly in the opposite direction rather than randomly.
- It is important to distinguish entropy (disorder) at the molecular level from that at a macro level. Thus a tornado, which is a relatively ordered volume of air molecules, may cause chaos through devastating a town but the biggest change in entropy is undergone by the air molecules themselves which are seeking, and eventually find, a lower pressure, less ordered (warmer) volume of air with which they can mix. Only a very small proportion of the energy of the tornado is transferred to the things which it breaks in its path. With a wind turbine it is possible to harness such entropic changes and convert them into, for instance, heat.

contact with. The concept of entropy or energy change accompanying a change in the order of molecules is important in relation to the binding of drugs to their sites of action. The binding of a drug to a receptor can be extremely complex with regard to the effect on other molecules in solution since it can: displace bound water, displace ions which can have an effect both on the structure of the water surrounding the binding site, and change the position of hydrophobic or hydrophilic groups which can affect the structure of the protein to which it is binding and also the structure of the water in the environment. However, overall binding has to be thermodynamically favourable and for many drugs binding has to be more favourable than for the natural ligand at the binding site.

SOLVATION OF IONS

The medium for solvation of greatest interest in biological systems is water. As was seen in the case of hydrogen bonding, water, because of its strong dipole, has an affinity for both positive and negative centres of charge. This makes it an excellent solvent for ionic materials. For instance, sodium chloride will dissolve quite readily in water despite the high energy of the ionic bonds holding the ions together because when it dissolves there is a large gain in energy in the form of the dipolar bonds formed between water and the free ions in solution. Table 1.6 shows the hydration enthalpies and entropies for a number of ions. In water, ions are 'structure making' and the heat produced is due to favourable enthalpy where bonds are formed. The negative entropy values in the table indicate that entropy decreases when solvation occurs.

In general, the higher the charge density (charge/ionic radius) of an ion, the greater its enthalpy and entropy of hydration. When taking into account ionic radius, the degree of salvation of the ion has to be considered; thus, for instance, the sodium ion is too large for potassium ion channels since, although its ionic radius is smaller overall, it has a larger radius due to the fact that it is in association with more water molecules than potassium. Most organic cations have relatively low charge densities compared to inorganic cations and hence relatively low levels of hydration. As can be seen from Table 1.6, cations tend to be more extensively hydrated than anions. The mechanics of living systems are essentially driven by electrostatic interactions between ions and proteins and water.

Table 1.6 Solvation energy of some ions found in living systems

Ion	$-\Delta H^\circ_{hydr}$ (kJ mol^{-1})	$-\Delta S^\circ_{hydr}$ (J mol^{-1} K^{-1})	Ionic radius (A)
H^+	1089	109	
Li^+	509	119	0.6
Na^+	398	87	0.95
K^+	314	52	1.33
Mg^{2+}	1908	268	0.65
Ca^{2+}	1577	209	0.99
Cl^-	377	98	1.81
Br^-	343	83	1.95

A Self Test 1.1

Mimic: isoprenaline and terbutaline. Block: oxprenolol and propranolol.

The blocking agents will bind strongly to the carboxylic group via their amine groups and also interact where the side chain hydroxyl of adrenaline binds.

A Self Test 1.2

Methylacetate < chloromethylacetate < dichloromethylacetate.

Variation in the rate of acid hydrolysis is much less marked, as indicated by a lesser degree of variation in the negative partial charges on the oxygens.

Chapter 2

Hydrocarbons: alkanes, alkenes, aromatic and alkylhalides

David G Watson

CHAPTER CONTENTS

LIPOPHILICITY

The activity of a drug within the body depends on its pharmacokinetics and its pharmacodynamics. Pharmacodynamics describes how the drug affects the body, i.e. how quickly it diffuses into tissues and how strongly it binds to proteins and receptors. Pharmacokinetics describes how a drug is distributed by the body which tissues it accumulates in and how quickly it is eliminated from those tissues. Pharmacokinetics is a relatively slow process; when a drug reaches its site of action the process of binding to its receptor site is relatively rapid. One of the most important physicochemical properties governing drug distribution within the body is its lipophilicity/partition coefficient.

n-ALKANES

n-Alkanes are the simplest organic molecules. They are devoid of polarity and their physical properties are governed by van der Waals interactions between the molecules, which increase with the number of CH_2 atoms in the structure of the molecule (Table 2.1). Thus the boiling points of the hydrocarbons increase with the addition of each CH_2 group. The increments in b.p. for the addition of a CH_2 get less as the molecular weights of the hydrocarbons get larger.

Since boiling point gives an indication of the strength of van der Waals/lipophilic interactions from Table 2.1 it is evident that, when incorporated in a drug, the larger the alkyl group the more it is going to promote interactions with lipophilic structures in the body such as membranes and hydrophobic pockets within receptor proteins. If the alkene is branched, the boiling point is generally less than that of the straight-chain alkane since the molecules present a lower surface area to each other and hence van der Waals interactions are lower. This is exemplified by a series of octanes shown in Figure 2.1, all of which have a lower boiling point than octane. Thus, branching in an alkane substituent in a drug reduces van der Waals interactions as the shape of a molecule gets closer to that of a sphere, which has the lowest surface area to volume of any shape.

Table 2.1 Lower hydrocarbons

Hydrocarbon	Formula	b.p °C
Methane	CH_4	−162
Ethane	C_2H_6	−87
Propane	C_3H_8	−42
Octane	C_8H_{18}	126
Nonane	C_9H_{20}	150
Decane	$C_{10}H_{22}$	173

$CH_3CH_2CH_2CH_2CH_2CH_2CH_2CH_3$

n-octane

B.P. 126 °C
Surface area 1.772 nm²

$CH_3CH_2CH_2CH_2CH_2\overset{\overset{\displaystyle CH_3}{|}}{C}HCH_3$

2-methylheptane
B.P. 116 °C
Surface area 1.707 nm²

$CH_3CH_2CH_2\overset{\overset{\displaystyle CH_3}{|}}{C}HCH_2CH_2CH_3$

4-methylheptane
B.P. 118 °C
Surface area 1.704 nm²

$CH_2CH_3CH_2CH_2\overset{\overset{\displaystyle CH_3}{|}}{\underset{\underset{\displaystyle CH_3}{|}}{C}}CH_3$

2,2-dimethylhexane
B.P. 107 °C
Surface area 1.653 nm²

$CH_3CH_2\overset{\overset{\displaystyle CH_3}{|}}{\underset{\underset{\displaystyle CH_3}{|}}{C}}HCHCH_2CH_3$

3,4-dimethylhexane
B.P. 119 °C
Surface area 1.616 nm²

$CH_3\overset{\overset{\displaystyle CH_3}{|}}{\underset{\underset{\displaystyle CH_3}{|}}{C}}HCH_2\overset{\overset{\displaystyle CH_3}{|}}{\underset{\underset{\displaystyle CH_3}{|}}{C}}CH_3$

2,2,4-trimethylpentane
B.P. 99 °C
Surface area 1.588 nm²

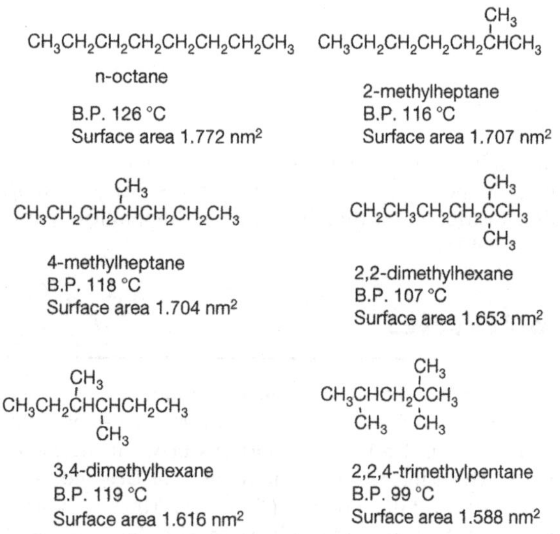

Figure 2.1 Isomeric octanes.

Alkanes are biologically fairly inert and are not readily metabolised by the body. For example, liquid paraffin, which is a mixture of long-chain alkanes and is used as a laxative, is not absorbed by the bowel and is excreted unchanged. Similarly, soft paraffins which are applied to the skin in greasy ointments are not appreciably absorbed by the skin. However, volatile hydrocarbons such as methane, which is present in natural gas, are readily absorbed into the bloodstream via the lungs. They thus become concentrated in lipophilic membranes and act as general anaesthetics, producing unconsciousness. Like all anaesthetics, the effects are reversible if an unconscious individual having accidently breathed in methane is found in time. Cyclopropane, a simple alkane, was actually used as a volatile anaesthetic. Although alkanes, particularly the higher boiling point hydrocarbons, are not readily absorbed by the body,

the small amounts that are absorbed by the body are hydroxylated via the action of cytochrome P450 (cyp450) in the liver.

STEREOCHEMICAL CONSIDERATIONS

As well as the surface area of hydrocarbons, another consideration is their stereochemistry, that is the shape that the molecules make in three dimensions. This is determined by the most favourable orientation of groups with respect to each other; in unfavourable orientations groups are brought too close and push against each other. One of the simplest examples for conformational analysis is butane. All bonds within a molecule can be rotated to give a higher or a lower energy arrangement of the atoms in space. The lowest energy state for butane is with the chain in the zigzag pattern where the central bond in the chain is rotated to give an anti or trans conformation (Fig. 2.2). Rotation about the central bond can give any number of conformational states with a range of energies between the lowest energy anti state and the highest energy eclipsed state which is at an energy level 6.1 Kcal/mole higher. At room temperature the thermal energy in the environment is great enough to allow the molecule to rotate freely about its central bond, passing through the higher energy state. The reason for the increase in energy in the eclipsed conformation can be viewed as being mainly due to steric repulsion between the two methyl groups. However, the total conformational energy includes tension within the bonds of the molecules which is either caused by them being stretched or twisted (torsional) and deformation of the tetrahedral angle of the bonds between the atoms of the molecule. When the groups involved in the eclipsed conformation are very large, free rotation about the bond under consideration is not possible. For example, the energy of the eclipsed conformation of 2,2 dimethyl pentane is 99 Kcal above the energy of the minimal energy trans configuration (see Fig. 2.2). As temperature increases even conformationally restricted hydrocarbon chains are freer to rotate and adopt a variety of conformations. This phenomenon is important in the behaviour of membrane lipids where the formation of kinks in the lipid chain, which at low temperatures exists in the completely zigzag form, causes the membrane to get thinner and spread out at the same time as temperature rises.

 Self Test 2.1

Draw the anti, anticlinal, gauche and eclipsed conformations about the number 3 bond of hexane. How do you think free rotation about this bond compares to free rotation about the central bond in butane?

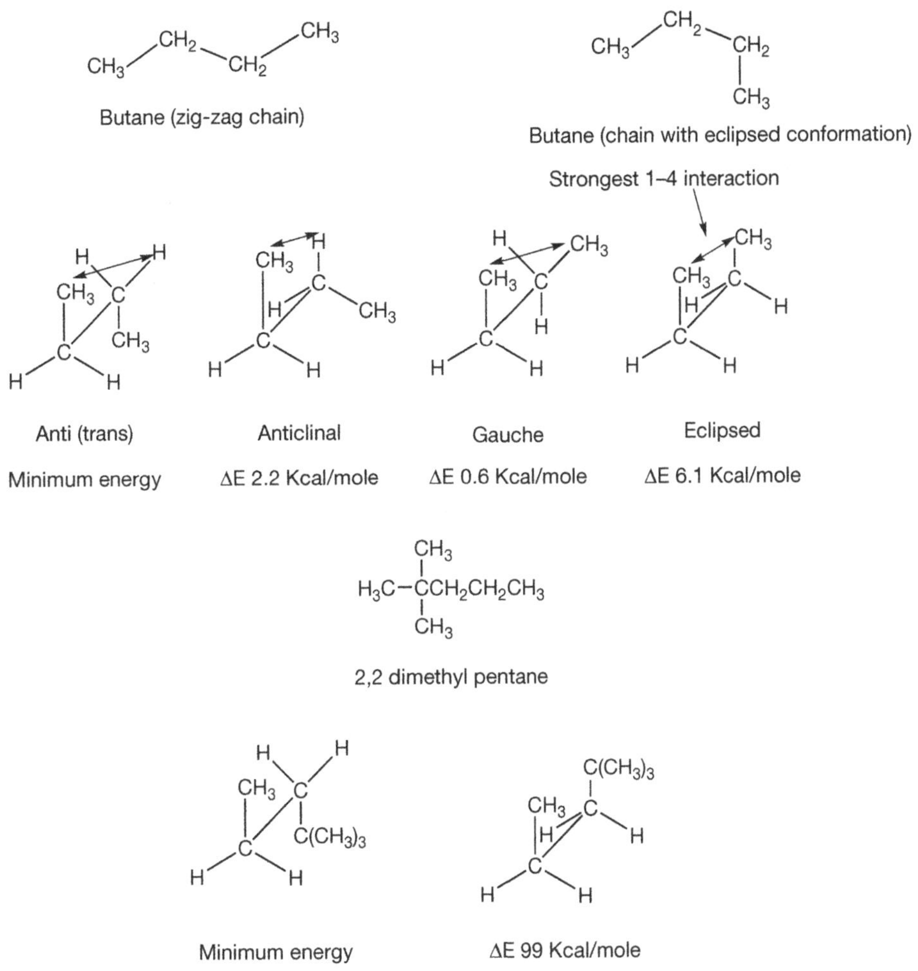

Figure 2.2 Different conformations of butane and dimethyl pentane.

CYCLOALKANES

The smallest cycloalkane is cyclopropane which has a very strained three-membered ring and the carbon bonds within the molecule are bent in order to compensate for the fact that they cannot adopt their natural tetrahedral structure. As the number of carbon atoms in the ring increases the rings become less strained. There is still considerable strain within cyclobutane but in cyclopentane the strain is minimal and cyclohexane is an unstrained ring. Apart from having been used as a volatile anaesthetic, the cyclopropyl ring has been used as an alkyl group in some drugs, e.g. ciprofloxacin (Fig 2.3), buprenorphine and prazepam.

Cyclohexane is free from strain since its ring is able to pucker, thus allowing the carbons to adopt their natural tetrahedral conformation (Fig. 2.4). The cyclohexane ring contains two types of protons, axial protons and equatorial protons, and the ring can flip between two forms so that the axial protons become equatorial and vice versa, e.g. protons a and b and c and d in the figure. The two forms of cyclohexane are indistinguishable but, since the axial positions are more sterically crowded, a large substituent on the ring will lock it into one configuration so that, for instance, tertiary butyl cyclohexane will exist almost completely in form A (Fig. 2.5).

Stereochemistry is very important in determining the biological activity of drugs and naturally occurring biologically active compounds. Among commonly used drug molecules the steroids are most prominent in having a rigidly defined polycyclic stereochemistry. A simple example of a drug with stereochemistry defined by bulky substituents in its ring is the haemostatic drug tranexamic acid.

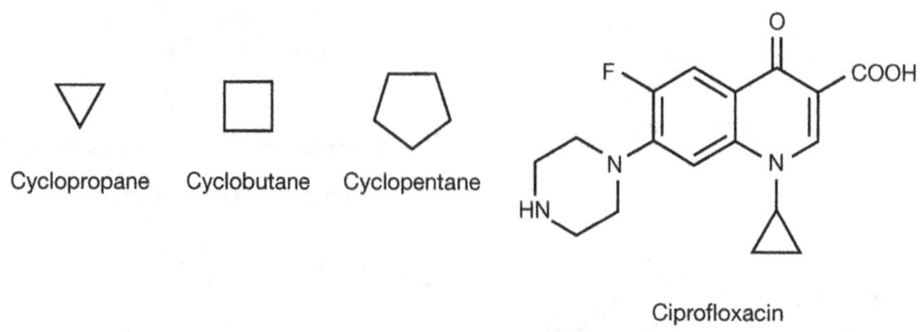

Figure 2.3 Cycloalkane groups.

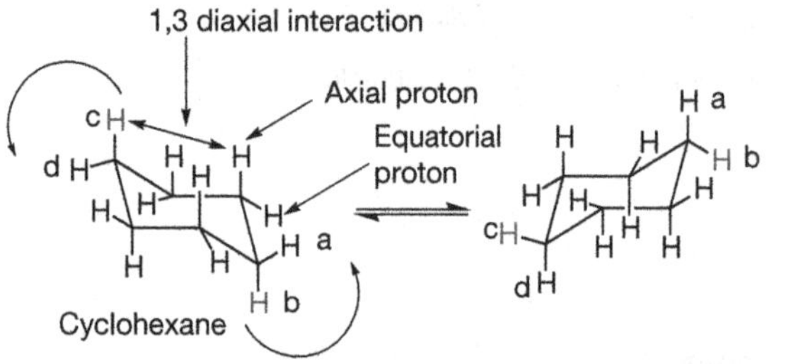

Figure 2.4 Cyclohexane and unstrained ring.

It can be drawn either viewed as a hexagon with substituents attached to it (Fig. 2.6A) or in a way indicating more directly that the substituents attached to it are in equatorial positions (Fig. 2.6B). When it is drawn in form A the wedge-shaped bonds indicate substituents which are closer to the observer relative to the substituents which are further away, which are indicated by dashed bonds. The substituents with the wedge-shaped bonds are said to be β and those with the dashed bonds are said to be α. When the structure is drawn in form B it is possible to see that the two substituents are equatorial, which is the least sterically strained form for the molecule, and that they are on opposite sides of the ring. Substituents on opposite sides of the ring are said to be trans to each other. Where the substituents are on the same side of the ring they are said to be cis.

For instance, if the methylamine group were substituted so that it was cis relative to the carboxylic acid group, a stereoisomer of tanexamic acid would be produced (Fig. 2.7). This molecule has a completely different shape from tanexamic acid and hence completely different biological properties.

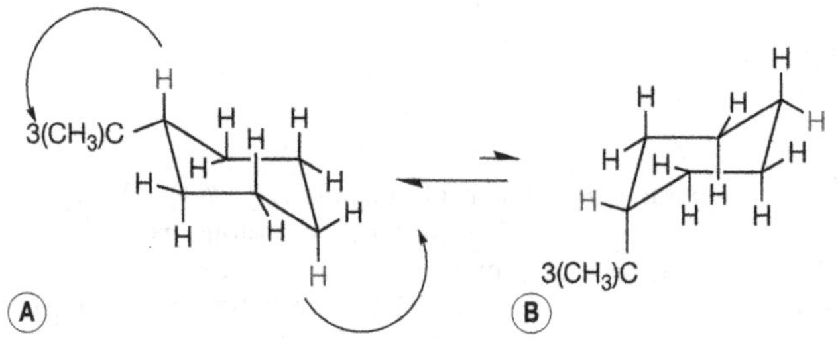

Figure 2.5 Tertiary butyl cyclohexane.

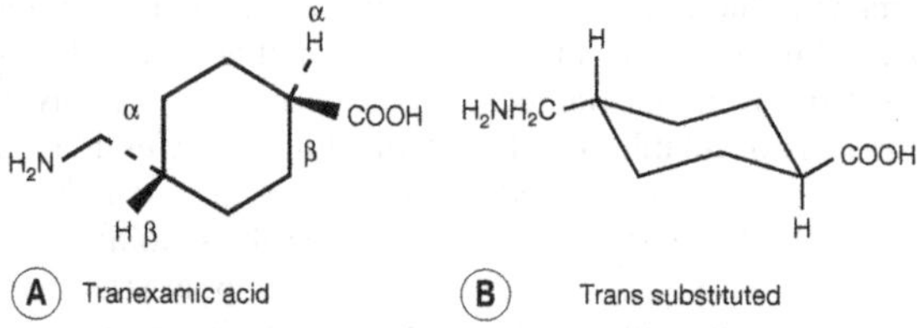

Figure 2.6 Tranexamic acid.

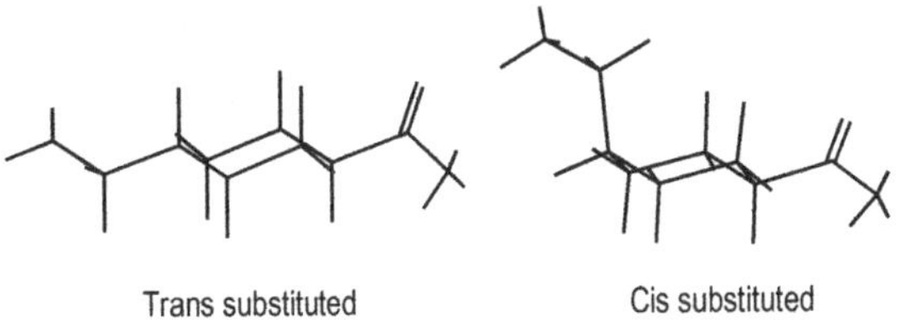

Figure 2.7 Tranexamic acid and one of its stereoisomers.

As the number of substituents on the ring increases, the number of possible isomers increases. Menthol, a commonly used pharmaceutical excipient, has three isomers. Menthol itself has all substituents in equatorial positions. Assignment of the stereochemistry of substitution is made relative to the hydroxyl group that, by convention, is given highest priority since the oxygen atom is the heaviest atom attached to the structure. Thus the methyl substituent is cis relative to the hydroxyl and the isopropyl group is trans. If all the possible permutations of this are taken into account three additional chemical compounds which are isomers are apparent. These are called isomenthol, neomenthol and neoisomenthol (Fig. 2.8). They have different properties from menthol, e.g. different melting points and boiling points, and it is possible to simply verify that they have different biological properties from menthol since, although all the isomers smell of mint, their exact smells are rather different.

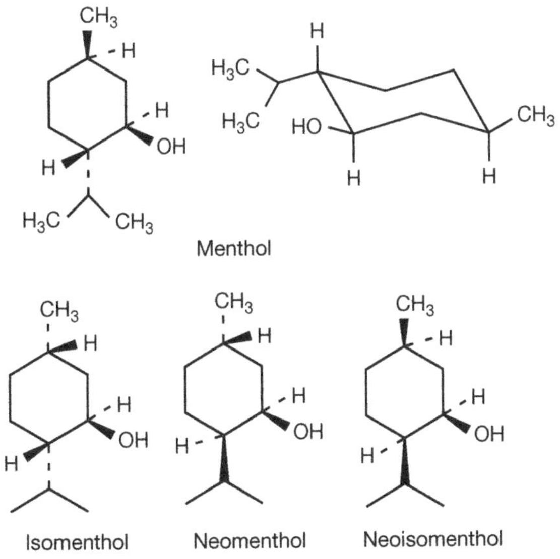

Figure 2.8 Stereoisomers of menthol.

Q Self Test 2.2

Draw the structures of the isomers of menthol, as shown in Figure 2.8, so that it is possible to see whether the substituents are axial or equatorial. Which of the structures which you have drawn do you think might rearrange to give less sterically strained forms?

OPTICAL ISOMERISM

In considering stereoisomerism above, we have ignored an additional form of isomerism which is of great importance in biologically active molecules. Optical isomerism is a specific form of stereoisomerism where the isomers do not differ in their physical properties such as melting point, boiling point or partition coefficient. There is only one physically measurable difference between them, which is that they tilt plane polarised light in opposite directions. Lactic acid, a by-product of glucose metabolism, can exist in two forms or enantiomers which are mirror images of each other (Fig. 2.9). This occurs when the groups attached to a central carbon atom, the chiral centre, are all different. The mirror images, like right and left hands, cannot be superimposed on each other.

Although enantiomers always have identical physical properties their biological properties can be quite different. The most notable example in pharmacy is thalidomide (Fig. 2.10), which was given as a sedative in the 1960s and was responsible for causing birth defects. The drug has a single chiral centre and is chemically synthesised as a 1:1 mixture of the two enantiomers (racemate). Because of their identical physical properties, enantiomers are difficult to separate and the drug was given as the racemate (1:1 mixture of the two enantiomers). It was presumed that both isomers had identical biological properties; however, subsequently it was found that the S-isomer was teratogenic. However, administration of the S-isomer alone would not necessarily

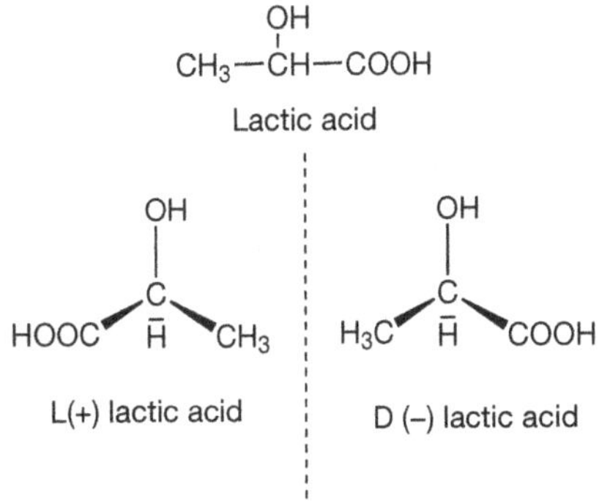

Figure 2.9 Enantiomers of lactic acid.

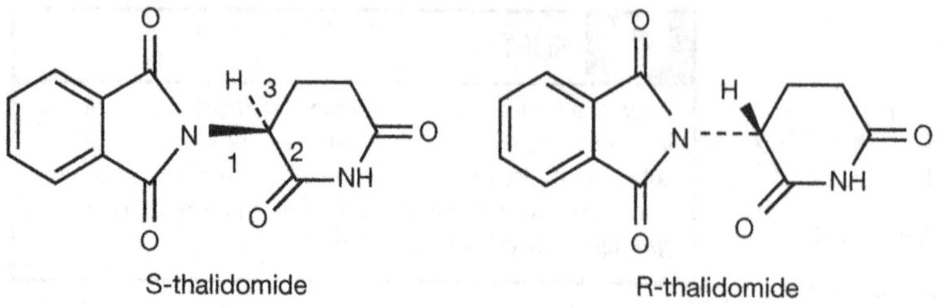

Figure 2.10 Enantiomers of thalidomide.

have improved matters since the two isomers interconvert *in vivo*. Thalidomide is still used as the racemic drug but for treating diseases that produce immunosuppression such as leprosy, in the absence of pregnancy.

The terms (+) and (−), L and D and R and S have been introduced without a complete explanation. The terms (+) and (−) simply refer to the direction in which a pure enantiomer rotates plane polarised light, i.e. to the right or to the left. In older literature (+) and (−) are often referred to as d and l where d stands for dextrorotatory and l for laevorotatory. This type of nomenclature persists where levodopa (LDOPA) is the (−) amino acid used to treat Parkinson's disease. Similarly, the terms D and L are the same as R and S that are the modern equivalents. R and S are a convention for describing the absolute configuration of a chiral centre. To assign the absolute configuration, the group of lowest priority, often a hydrogen atom, is placed behind the plane of the paper. Assignment of the configuration is then made on the basis of precedence rules based on the atomic weights of the atoms attached to the chiral carbon atom. For example, if C is the chiral carbon atom then the bonds attached would have the following precedence:

$$C-S > C-O > C-N > C-C-S > C-C-O > C-C-N > C-C-C_2 > C-C-CH > C-H$$

It is difficult to be comprehensive in the precedence order but this order will apply to the majority of drug molecules. If we examine S and R thalidomide we find for S thalidomide (as drawn) that the group of lowest priority is placed behind the plane of the paper and the precedence order for the groups attached to the chiral centre are N > C–O > C–C giving an anticlockwise, hence S, progression. Ignoring the fact that R thalidomide has the hydrogen above the plane of the paper we can make the same assignment as for S thalidomide but reverse it, giving us an R configuration. Alternatively, the figure could be redrawn with the hydrogen behind the plane of the paper. Some molecules have multiple chiral centres; an example we used earlier is menthol (Fig. 2.11). The fact that menthol has a mirror image was overlooked and thus menthol structure has a total of eight isomers (2^3) not four; however, these isomers are comprised of four enantiomeric pairs. Thus menthol, isomenthol, neomenthol and neoisomenthol all have mirror image isomers which have identical physical properties but all differ in

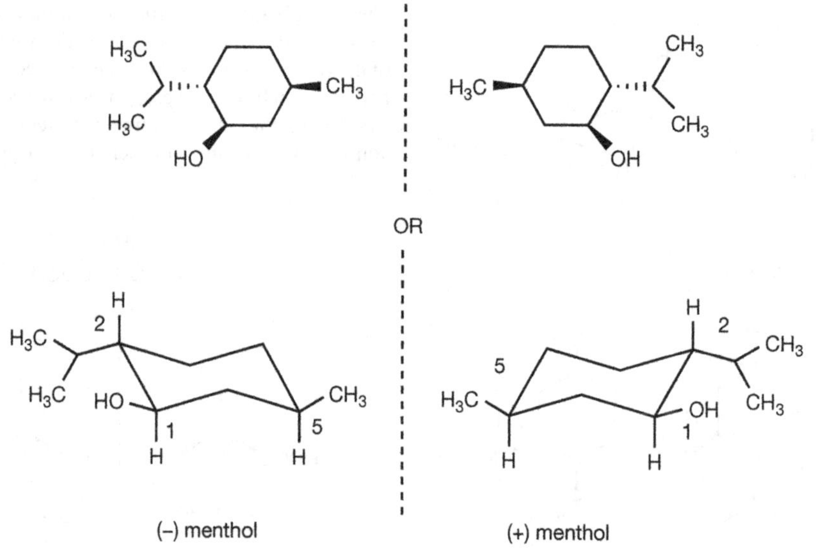

Figure 2.11 (−) Menthol and its enantiomer.

properties from the non-mirror image isomers. For example (−) neomenthol has the same physical properties as (+) neomenthol but different physical properties from both (+) and (−) isomenthol, which in turn have the same physical properties. The enantiomeric pairs all have different biological properties and thus (−) menthol has a slightly different smell from (+) menthol. The classic smell difference in this respect is between S (+) and R (−) carvone, the S (+) isomer smells of caraway and the R (−) isomer smells of dill. The (−) menthol has the following chiral centres: 1 (R), 2 (S), 5 (R) and it follows that (+) menthol has the configuration 1 (S), 2 (R), 5 (S). Although it is possible to draw the absolute configuration of a molecule on paper easily, it is only possible to relate this configuration to the direction in which a molecule will rotate plane polarised light by experiment. The principal method for determining the absolute configuration of a chiral centre or chiral centres within a molecule is single-crystal X-ray crystallography, which is a relatively complex technique. In contrast, polarimetry, which is the method used to determine relative configuration (whether a molecule is [+] or [−]) is an easy technique to use.

Care has to be taken in recognising a chiral centre; for example, pethidine (Fig. 2.12) may look as if it has a chiral centre at 1 but, in fact, it is symmetrically substituted by the heterocyclic ring. The isomer of ethambutol (see Fig. 2.11) is not a chiral molecule but is called a meso compound since it has a plane of symmetry running through its centre which means its mirror image is superimposable. Ethambutol itself, however, is a chiral molecule since its mirror image is not superimposable.

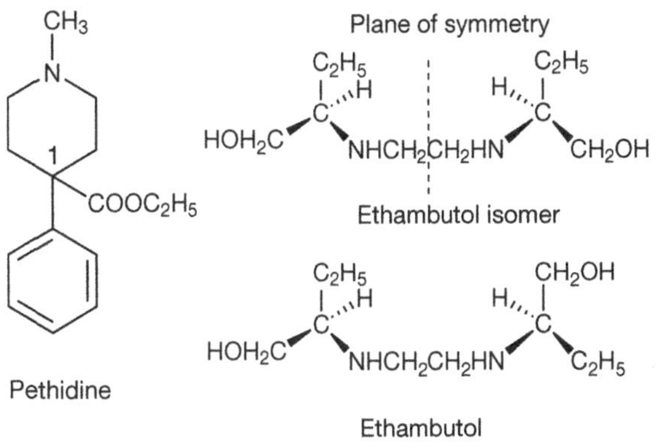

Figure 2.12 Stereochemistry of pethidine and ethambutol.

Many drug molecules contain several chiral centres and these types of drug molecules are generally derived from natural sources where they have been stereospecifically synthesised by plants or microorganisms. Examples include: penicillins, steroids, alkaloids, tetracyclines, aminoglycosides and amino acids. Where a drug has been wholly chemically synthesised it may often contain no chiral centres or have only a single chiral centre and be produced as a racemate.

Q Self Test 2.3

Assign the absolute configurations of the numbered centres in the following molecules and indicate how many isomers are possible for each structure.

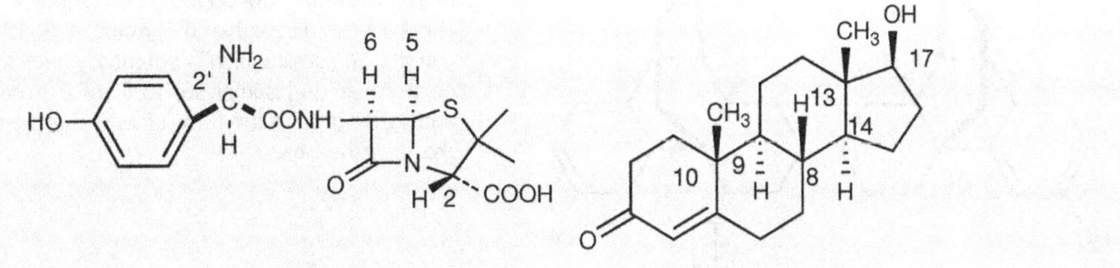

Amoxicillin Testosterone

Many drugs have a single chiral centre but are administered as a racemate. Table 2.2 shows some examples of drugs where the enantiomers of the drug have different biological properties.

There are a number of drugs such as dextrorophan and levorphan which are prefixed by dextro- or levo- to indicate that they rotate plane polarised light either in the (+) or the (−) direction, but remember that the prefixes L and D or levo- and dextro- only refer to the direction in which the compound rotates plane polarised light. It does not tell us whether the compound is R or S or, if it has more than one chiral centre, what the configurations of these centres are.

Table 2.2 Enantiomeric drugs and their biological properties

Drug	Properties
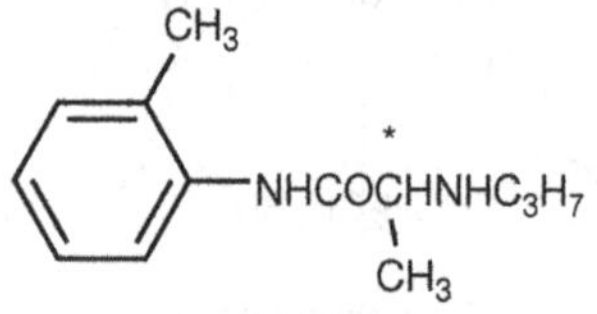 Prilocaine	Both isomers are local anaesthetics but the R isomer is enzymatically hydrolysed much more quickly than the S isomer. The hydrolysis product, toluidine, affects the oxygen-carrying capacity of red blood cells.
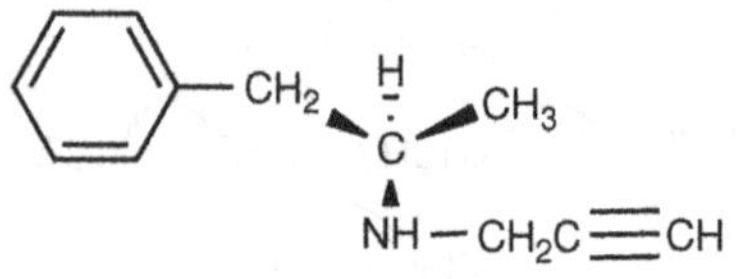 R(–) selegiline	Selegeline, a monoamine oxidase inhibitor, is dealkylated by metabolism to amfetamine. The R isomer forms R amfetamine which has little effect on the CNS whereas the S isomer forms S amfetamine which has strong CNS effects. The drug is given as the pure R isomer.
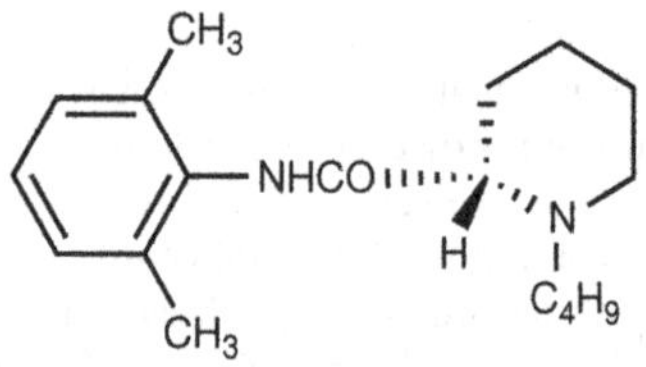 S(–) bupivacaine	Levobupivacaine (S (–)) has been recently introduced as an anaesthetic since there is some evidence that it is less cardiotoxic than racemic mixtures of bupivacaine.
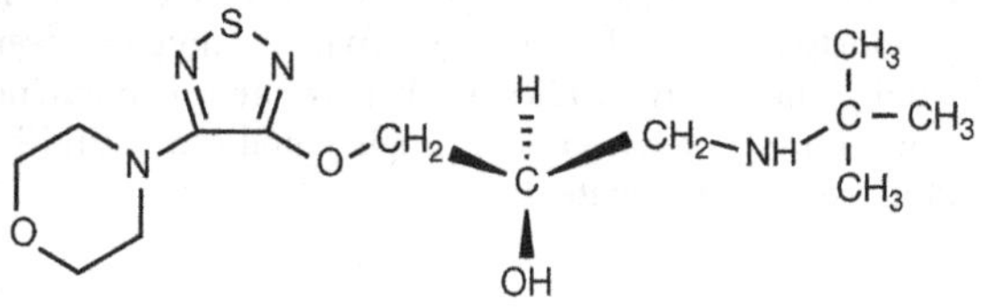 R(+) timolol	Timolol is used to treat both hypertension and glaucoma in the form of its S (–) isomer. However, there would be a reduction in side effects if the R(+) isomer were used to treat glaucoma since it is effective in treating glaucoma but has very weak β-adrenergic blocking activity.
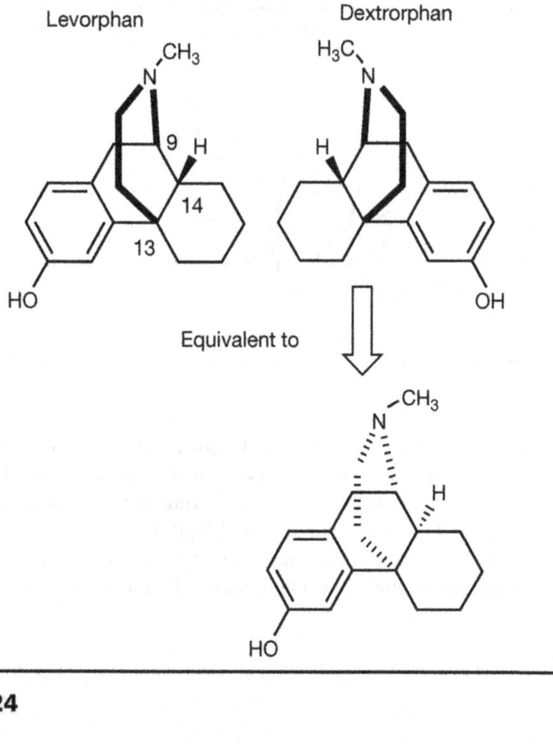	Most commonly, drugs which are administered as racemates have only one chiral centre. Levorphan and dextrorphan (based on the morphine structure) are unusual in that they have the opposite configurations at three chiral centres. Levorphan ([–] isomer 9 R, 13 R 14 R) is a narcotic analgesic which is potentially addictive whereas dextrorphan ([+] isomer 9S, 13 S, 14S) is used as an antitussive drug in the form of its O-methylether dextromethorphan.

Q Self Test 2.4

Assign the absolute configurations of the chiral centres of dextropropoxyphene and levopropoxyphene. These drugs are morphine analogues. Can you guess which is the antitussive and which is the narcotic analgesic? List all (+) (dextro-) and (−) (levo-) drugs which you can find in the BNF?

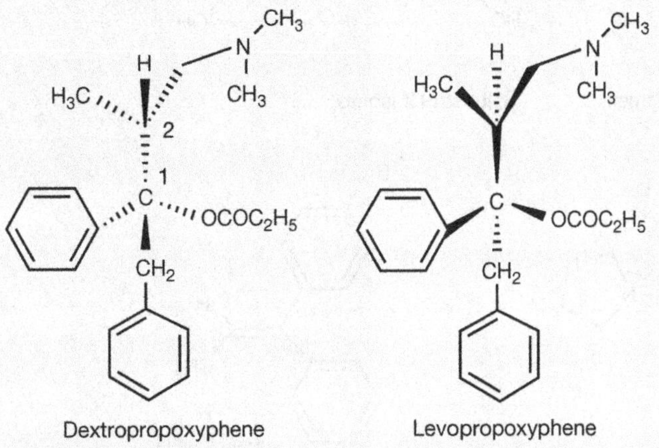

DOUBLE BONDS

Stereochemistry is most complex where carbon substitution is tetrahedral. Where double bonds are present in the molecule it is flattened and thus takes up less space. Ethylene is the simplest compound which contains a double bond. The σ bond is a strong bond produced by extensive overlap of orbitals whereas the π bond is produced by partial overlap of orbitals (Fig. 2.13) and hence is a weaker bond which is rich in electron density, which is available for sharing with a suitable reactive chemical species. Thus, in biological systems, reactive double bonds can prove problematical since they can form unwanted covalent bonds with biological structures.

The presence of a double bond, because of the lack of free rotation about the bond, within a molecule can give rise to a form of isomerism known as geometrical isomerism. There are not many drugs which exhibit geometrical

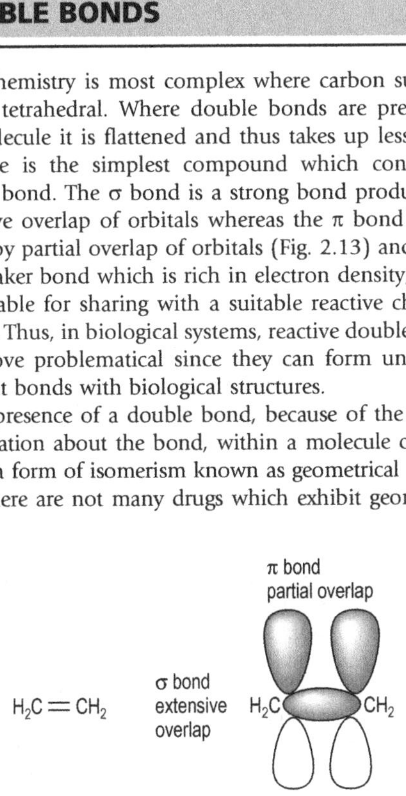

Figure 2.13 The bonds in ethylene.

isomerism since, unlike enantiomers, geometrical isomers can be more easily separated. One example is the E (trans) and Z (cis) isomers of the oestrogen analogue diethyl stilbestrol (Fig. 2.14). The E isomer is the therapeutic agent used and it is a much more potent oestrogen than the Z isomer. The letter E indicates that the highest priority substituents are on opposite ends of the double bond and are on opposite sides of the bond, whereas Z indicates that the highest priority substituents are on opposite ends of the bond and are on the same side of the bond. The priority rules are the same as those used in assigning absolute configurations. Thus the antihistamine triprolidine is used in the form of its E isomer since, working back from the point where they are attached to the bond, the two nitrogen-containing substituents have the highest priority. Similarly, the antidepressant zimelidine has the Z configuration.

When two or more double bonds are separated from each other by single bonds, a conjugated electronic system is produced where the electrons in the double bonds are delocalised onto all the atoms in the conjugated system. The simplest conjugated systems can be seen in butadiene (Fig. 2.15).

As a system of conjugated double bonds gets longer, the electrons become more loosely held within a molecule, producing a compound that can be excited by visible light and thus appears coloured. This is the case with beta-carotene (Fig. 2.16,) which occurs as an orange pigment in many plants, e.g. carrots, and may assist in the harvesting of light by plants. Beta-carotene can be converted by the human body into vitamin A, which is yellow in colour. Vitamin A is involved in the visual process as shown in

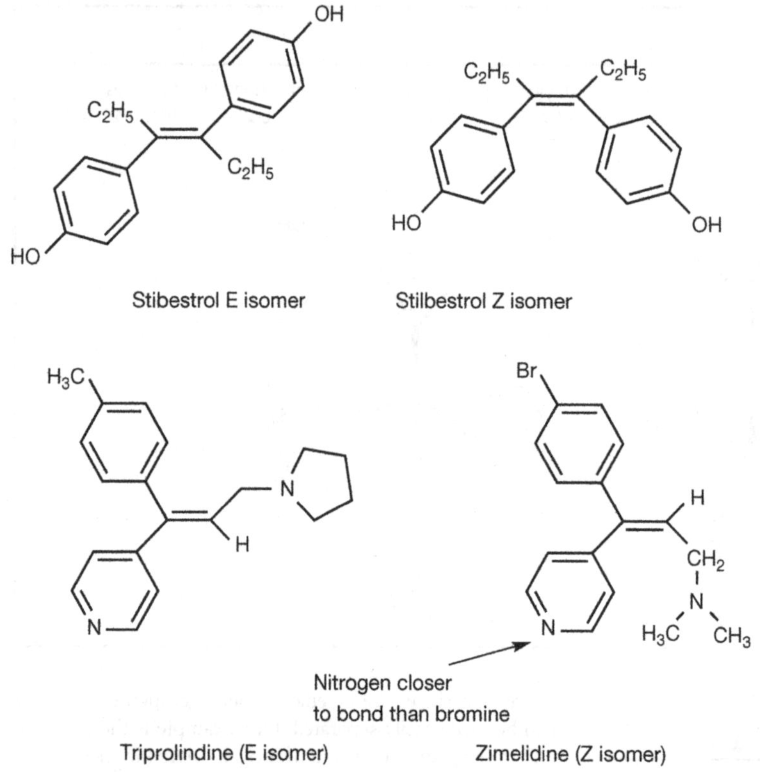

Figure 2.14 Diethylstilbestrol and triprolidine and their geometrical isomers.

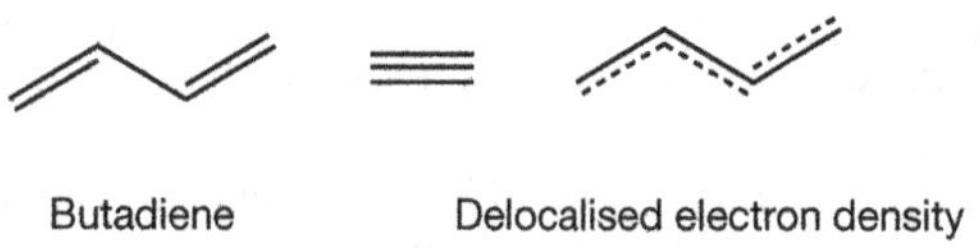

Figure 2.15 Butadiene the simplest conjugated double-bond system.

Figure 2.16 where it binds to the visual protein opsin in a form where one of its double bonds is Z (cis). Absorbance of light energy causes the bond to convert from Z to E (trans), thus altering the 3-D structure of the protein to which it is bound and triggering off events such as ion channel opening and formation of secondary messengers. The interconversion between cis and trans forms causes mechanical energy to be generated from light energy.

There are not many drugs which contain extended double-bond systems. Steroids such as testosterone and hydrocortisone (Fig. 2.17) have an enone double-bond system in their A ring. This is crucial for their biological activity and enzymatic reduction of the double bonds results in loss of the activity of the steroid. Tetrahydrocortisone is inactive and is the main urinary metabolite of hydrocortisone.

Nystatin (Fig. 2.18), a macrocyclic polyene antibiotic, is an example of a drug with an extended system of double bonds. The double bonds interact with membrane lipids, disrupting the cell membrane and thus killing the pathogen. Amphotericin B, another antifungal compound, works by a similar mechanism.

MEMBRANE LIPIDS

Double bonds are found in the lipids that compose cell membranes. Membranes are composed of complex mixtures of lipids and the complexity of the mixture enables membranes to produce their responsive properties. Membrane lipids are all amphiphilic and have a polar head group in combination with a lipophilic tail which causes in an aqueous medium the typical lipid double layer. Figure 2.19 shows some typical membrane lipids. The phospholipids are triesters of glycerol where R_1 may be a saturated or unsaturated fatty acid, R_2 is usually an unsaturated fatty acid and R_3 is one of a number of polar head groups. The lipophilic fatty acid tails of the molecules are composed of saturated and unsaturated hydrocarbon chains between 14 and 24 carbons long. Unsaturated lipids may contain cis or trans double bonds. Unsaturated lipids tend to orientate themselves as shown for the trans monounsaturated fatty acid shown in Figure 2.19.

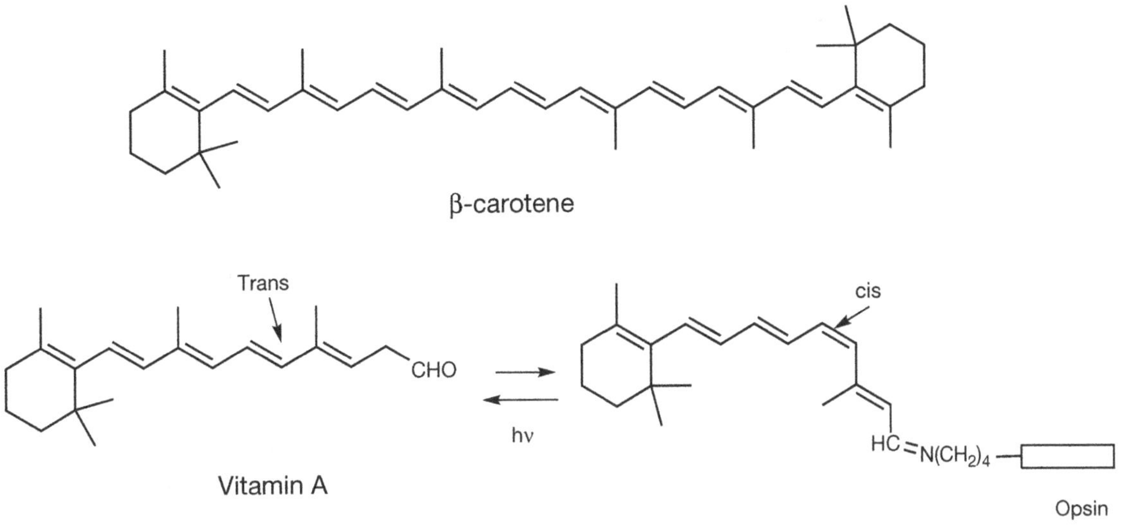

Figure 2.16 Carotene and the effect of light on vitamin A.

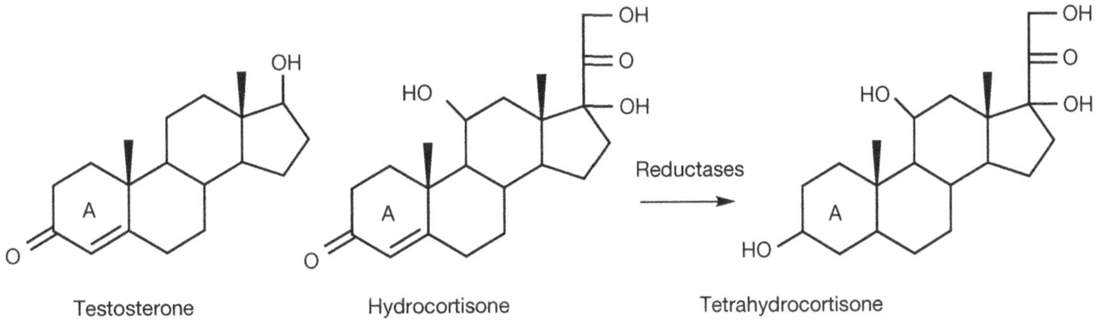

Figure 2.17 Enone systems in steroids.

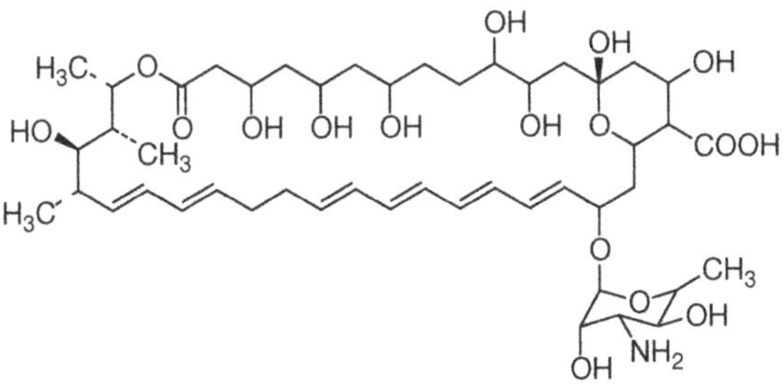

Figure 2.18 Extended conjugated system in nystatin.

Figure 2.20 shows a lipid bilayer. Such bilayers are regarded as being in a lyotropic liquid crystal form where they are highly ordered as in a crystal but the ordering of the molecules is very sensitive to temperature and other environmental factors. The bilayer is structured so that the polar head groups of the lipids are in contact with the surrounding water while the lipophilic chains are hidden inside the layer.

The composition of the fatty acids making up the membranes of cells varies from organ to organ and from species to species. The composition of the fatty acids making up the phosphatidylcholine lipid fraction from membranes of human red blood cells is shown in Table 2.3. As is the case with all membranes, the saturated fatty acid component predominates (in this case palmitic and stearic acids). The saturated fatty acids pack together closely in the membrane, producing a rigid membrane. The introduction of unsaturated fatty acids into the membrane (particularly cis fatty acids with their awkward shapes) prevents the membrane fatty acids from packing closely, thus producing a more fluid membrane. The fatty acid chains become increasingly bent as the number of cis double bonds in the hydrocarbon chain increases. The saturated fatty acids themselves can also adopt less linear

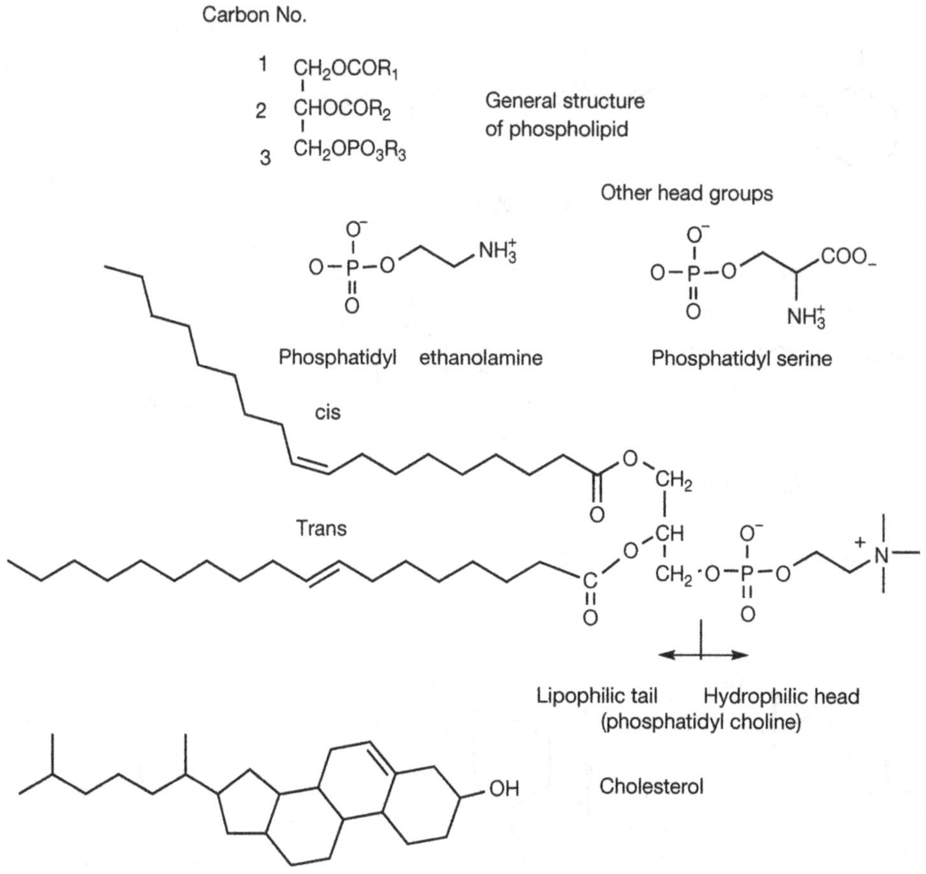

Figure 2.19 The structures of some phospholipids.

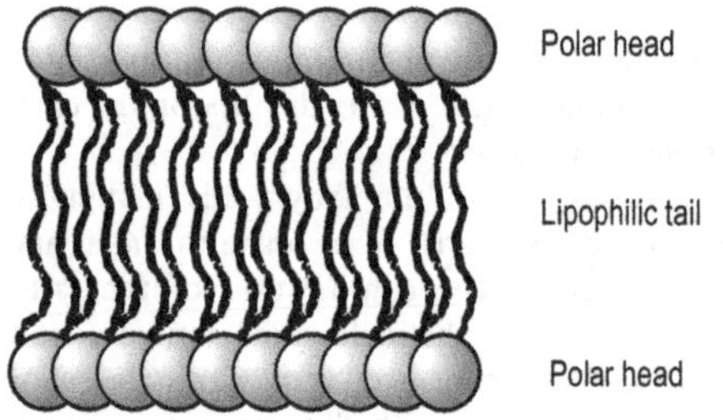

Figure 2.20 Lipid bilayer.

configurations, with kinks in their chains like the cis unsaturated fatty acids. In the liquid crystalline state the saturated fatty acids in lipids typically adopt a gauche configuration (Fig. 2.21) where the chain bends and thus shortens so that the membrane gets thinner but spreads out over a larger area.

LIPID OXIDATION

The presence of a double bond within a hydrocarbon chain increases its susceptibility to oxidation. The allylic position is particularly susceptible to attack by oxygen which can behave as a di-radical having two reactive unpaired electrons. The oxygen di-radical abstracts a hydrogen atom from an allylic position to form an allylic radical (Fig. 2.22), this process is favoured by the presence of the double bond which stabilises the allylic radical.

These types of radical are formed even more rapidly where more than one double bond is involved, e.g. in linoleic acid (Fig. 2.23).

The formation of a hydroperoxide generates another allylic radical so that a chain reaction occurs resulting in formation of further molecules of hydroperoxide. These hydroperoxides are unstable and decompose to give a mixture of degradation products which include a range of aldehydes, and hydroxyaldehydes such as

Table 2.3 The most abundant fatty acids within the phospholipids of red blood cells

Fatty acid	molar %	
Palmitic acid	33	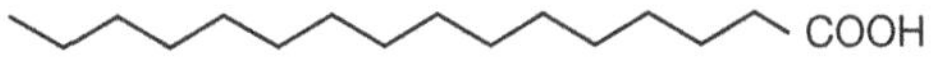
Palmitoleic acid	1	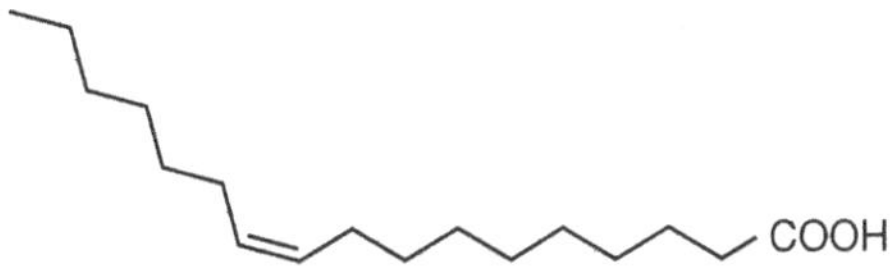
Stearic acid	11.7	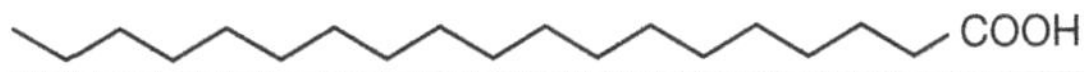
Oleic acid	20.6	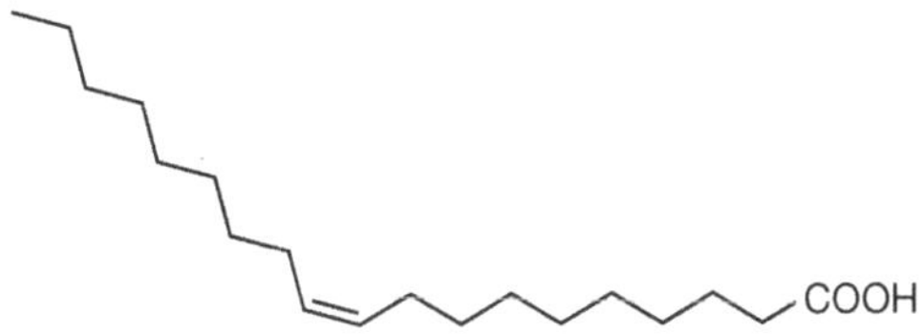
Linoleic acid	18.2	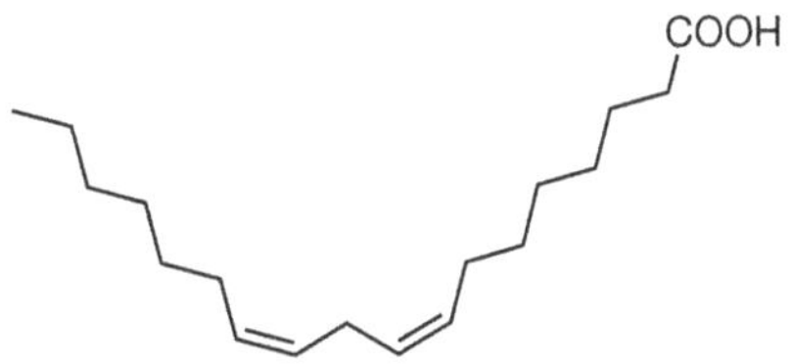
Eicosatetraenoic acid	5	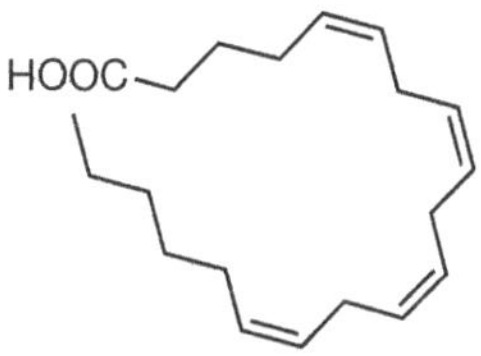
Docosapentenoic acid	5.4	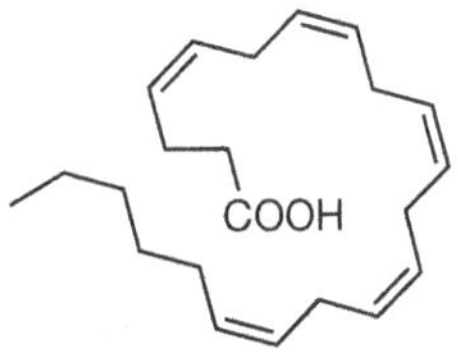

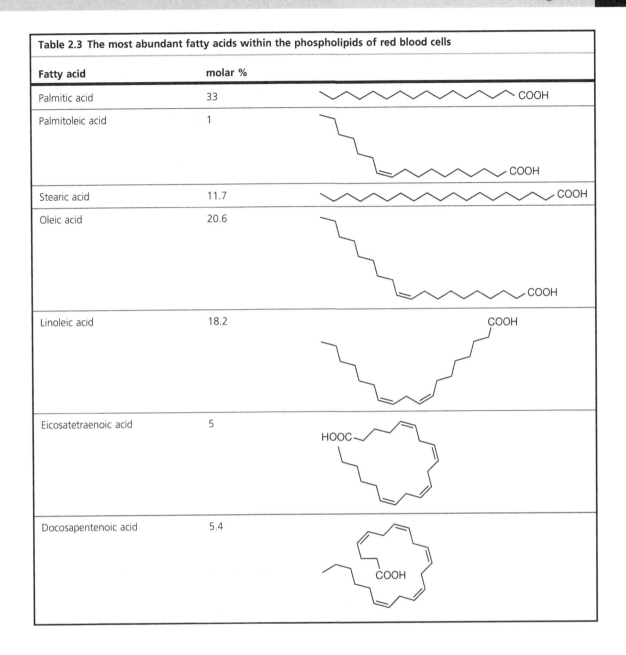

4-hydroxynonenal (4-HNE) which is a degradation product of arachidonic acid. Molecules such as 4-HNE may have a role in promoting apoptosis.

PROSTAGLANDINS

The susceptibility of unsaturated membrane lipids to oxidation by atmospheric oxygen is to an extent mirrored by the ease with which they can be oxidised via enzymatic action. Eicosatetraenoic acid (arachidonic acid, AA) provides the precursor for the prostanoid class of locally acting hormones (Fig. 2.24). Prostanoids are important mediators of inflammation and a wide range of other processes. The first step in the enzymatic conversion of AA to prostanoids involves enzymatic cleavage of the ester bond between AA and the glycerol backbone of a phospholipid into which it is incorporated and this reaction is carried out by phospholipase A_2. The next step is, probably, essentially the same as the allylic oxidation of polyunsaturated fatty acids carried out by atmospheric oxygen and

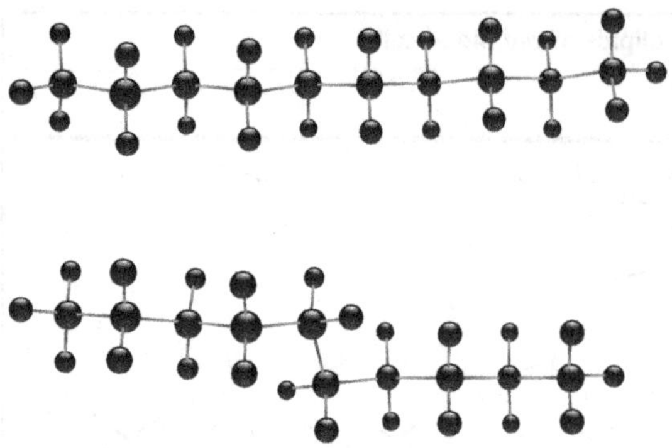

Figure 2.21 Conformational variation within a long hydrocarbon chain showing the effect of chain length.

this is followed by structural rearrangement within the molecule, giving rise to PGG_2. The main difference from a chemical process, of course, is that the stereochemistry of the reaction is enzymatically controlled and thus chiral centres are generated at positions 8 (R), 9 (R), 11 (S), 12 (R) and 15 (S). This would not occur with a purely chemical process. Nonetheless, lipid peroxidation may occur in cell membranes via reaction with reactive oxygen species forming prostaglandin-like structures and may be a component in autoimmune diseases. The oxygen bridge in PGG_2 can be simply modified to give rise to a range of prostanoids, the most important of which are: PGE_2, PGD_2, $PGF_{2\alpha}$, PGI_2 and TXA_2. AA also gives rise to another series of mediators called the leukotrienes which are also involved in inflammatory and immunological

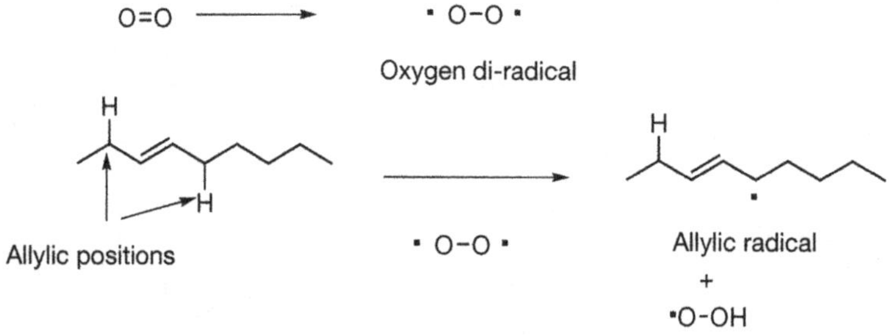

Figure 2.22 Formation of an allylic radical catalysed by oxygen.

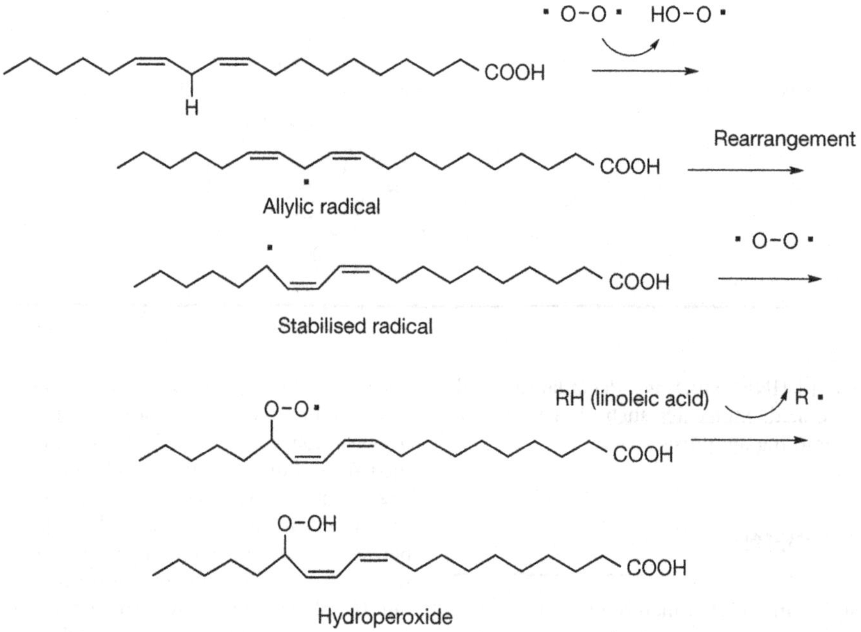

Figure 2.23 Reaction of linoleic acid with oxygen.

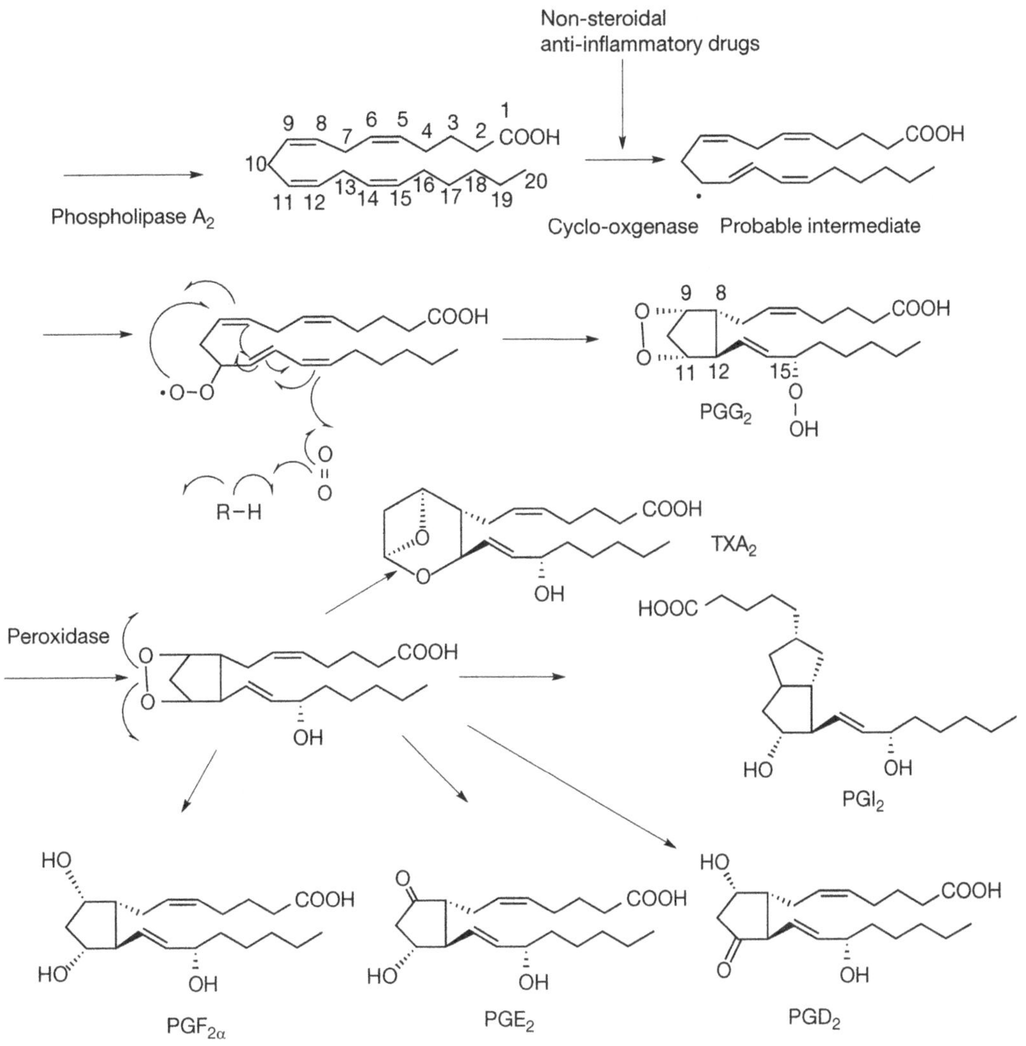

Figure 2.24 Biosynthesis of prostaglandins.

processes. Leukotrienes are also formed by peroxidation of the AA structure but lack the five-membered ring which gives rise to the hairpin structure of the prostaglandins.

MOLECULAR SHAPE AND STRUCTURE ACTIVITY RELATIONSHIPS

Drug action depends on the drug interacting effectively with its site of action which may be a receptor protein, an enzyme or DNA. The effectiveness of its interaction depends on how well the shape of the drug matches the shape of the target site. In the case of a receptor binding site there is usually a natural ligand which fits it and drugs are designed either to block the binding of the drug to the receptor without triggering of the receptor activity (antagonists) or to bind to the receptor more strongly than the natural ligand stimulating the same actions as the drug (agonists).

LIPOPHILIC GROUPS IN PROTEINS

The binding of a drug to a protein depends on the intermolecular forces described in Chapter 1. Thus electrostatic, dipole–dipole, hydrogen bonding, π–π interaction and van der Waals interactions, and even covalent bonding all play a part. The strength of van der Waals interaction depends on the availability of lipophilic groups within the protein. The amino acids with high

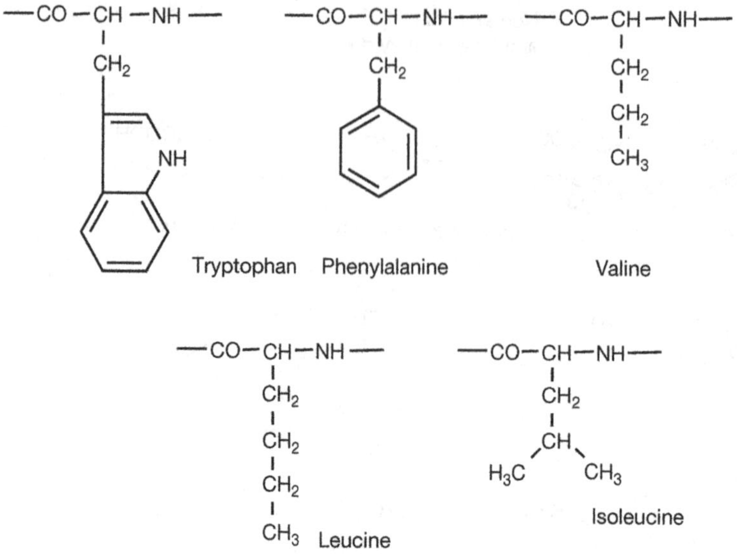

Figure 2.25 Lipophilic amino acid residues in proteins.

lipophilicity, and thus potential for van der Waals interaction, are shown in Figure 2.25.

Proteins with a high content of these amino acids are lipophilic; thus ApoE, a protein which is responsible for carrying lipids around the body, contains about 12.6% leucine residues where the average abundance of an amino acid is closer to 5%.

THE BENZENE RING

One or more benzene rings are found in a majority of drug molecules. Most of the time, it can be considered that it just contributes to the lipophilicity of a drug, although it does have chemical properties which are different from saturated hydrocarbons. The surface area of benzene is 1.01 nm^2 compared with 1.20 nm^2 for cyclohexane. Although the chemistry of cyclohexane and benzene is quite different, in most cases they can be regarded as being similar in biological terms so that dicycloverine and cyclopentolate, for example, are both anticholinergic drugs with similar structures (Fig. 2.26). The presence of the benzene ring in cyclopentolate does not dramatically alter its properties compared with dicycloverine. The benzene ring is often a convenient starting point for the synthesis of a drug molecule since it is chemically reactive and in addition it is found in many products which are either drugs or have been developed into drugs by chemical modification. Extensive discussion of the chemistry of the benzene ring can be found in organic chemistry textbooks.

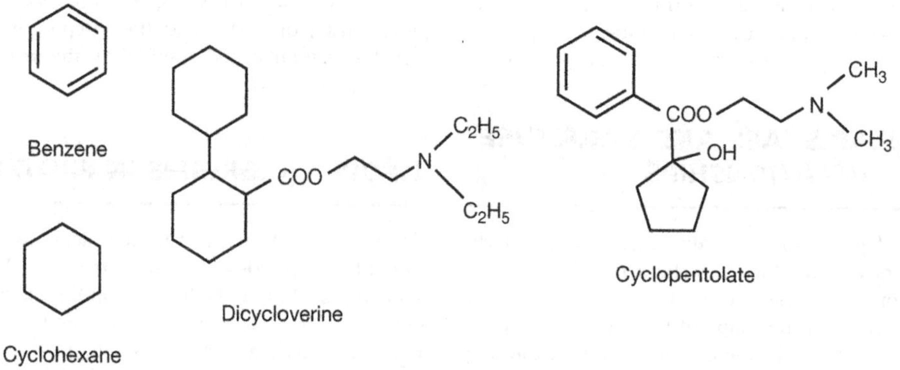

Figure 2.26 Two drugs with similar activities with and without an aromatic ring.

ALKYLHALIDES

Halogen atoms have been used extensively modify the activity of drug molecules. Often, the increase in the potency resulting from addition of a halogen atom to a drug molecule can be attributed to increased partition coefficient. Thus chlorpromazine (log P 3.4 at pH 7.4) is more potent than promazine (log P 2.5 at pH 7.4) as a tranquilliser (Fig. 2.27). The presence of the chlorine atom in its structure increases its lipophilicity and this means that it is more effective in crossing the blood–brain barrier. In the case of many drugs there is an optimum lipophilicity and, despite there being many analogues of chlorpromazine where the chlorine is replaced by another group, none of these offer significant advantages over chlorpromazine. There are a number of other examples where addition of a highly lipophilic chlorine to a structure increases the potency, e.g. pheniramine and chlorphenamine, mefenamic acid and diclofenac.

A Self Test 2.1

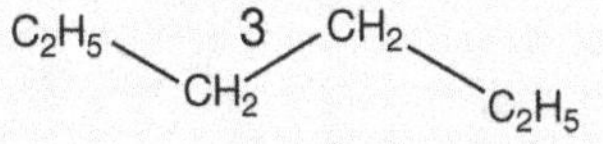

Hexane

Figure 2.27 Promazine and chlorpromazine.

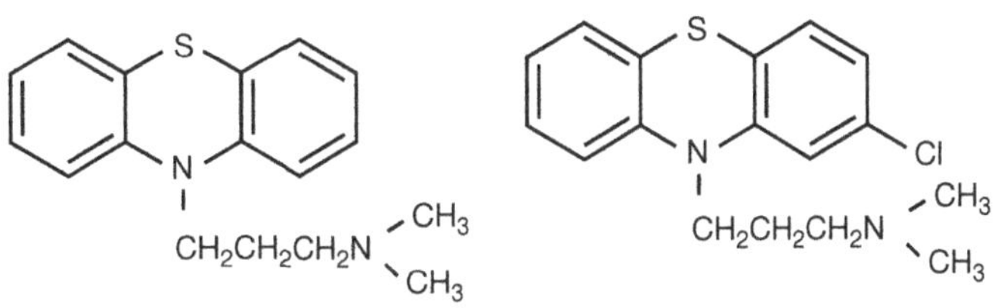

Promazine   Chlorpromazine

A Self Test 2.2

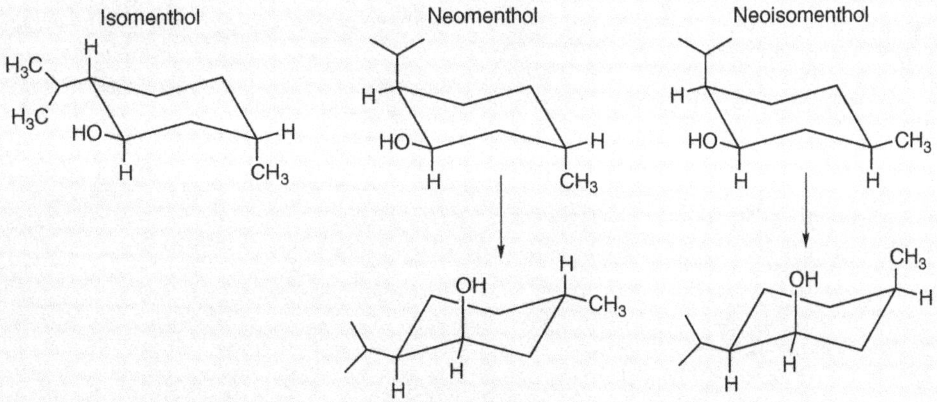

Neomenthol and neoisomenthol will approximate towards a configuration where the isopropyl group is equatorial.

A Self Test 2.3

Amoxicillin 16 isomers 2′R 6R 5R 2S. Testosterone 64 isomers 8R 9S 10R 13S 14S 17S.

A Self Test 2.4

Dextropropoxyphene 1S, 2R, levopropoxyphene 1R, 2S.

ALKYL HALIDES

Chapter | 3 |

Amines

David G Watson

CHAPTER CONTENTS

INTRODUCTION

The amine group can be considered as the single most important group for conferring pharmacological activity. This is because it is the principle group within organic molecules that bears a positive charge. When it is present in a drug molecule it can exert biological effects through electrostatic interactions with negatively charged groups within proteins and also compete with positively charged cations such as sodium, potassium and calcium ions in biological processes. Amines are derived from ammonia and have the structures shown in Figure 3.1 for mono-, di- and trisubstituted nitrogen.

The structures may look planar but, in fact, the structures of amines are more or less tetrahedral, like tetrasubstituted carbon, as shown for trimethylamine in Figure 3.2. In the case of nitrogen, the position that would be occupied by a fourth bond in tetrasubstituted carbon is occupied by a lone pair of electrons. Since nitrogen is less electronegative than oxygen the lone pair within an amine structure is more available than the lone pairs on an oxygen atom to interact with a proton. An approximate measure of the availability of lone pairs of electrons is given by the energy of the highest occupied molecular orbital (HOMO). The deeper the 'energy well' that the molecular orbital occupies the less available the electrons are for bond formation with a proton. Thus water has a HOMO of −12.5 eV while ammonia has a HOMO of −10.5 eV, and thus its electrons are more available and it protonates more readily than water. The energies of HOMOs are arrived at by complex calculation and do not always match the experimentally observed energy levels for bonds, but they can reveal trends. The availability of the lone pair of electrons on the nitrogen atom is increased by substitution with alkyl groups; thus the HOMO of trimethylamine has an energy of −9.18 eV, i.e. it does not lie in an energy well as deep as that of ammonia and is a stronger base.

A variety of factors contribute to the lone pair on the nitrogen being more or less available. The pKa value for a base is derived from the equilibrium between the forms of the base shown in Figure 3.3 for a secondary amine in water where *Kb* is the equilibrium constant. In water, the equilibrium for nitrogen-containing bases lies well to the left and, for instance, in ammonia solution ($Kb = 1.8 \times 10^{-5}$) in water only 0.0018% of the ammonia is protonated. Organic bases become increasingly water insoluble as the size of the

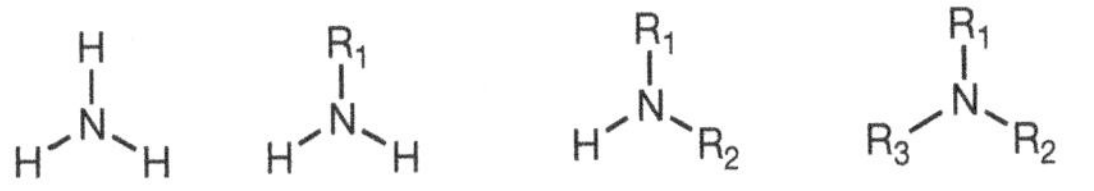

Figure 3.1 Amines.

Trimethylamine

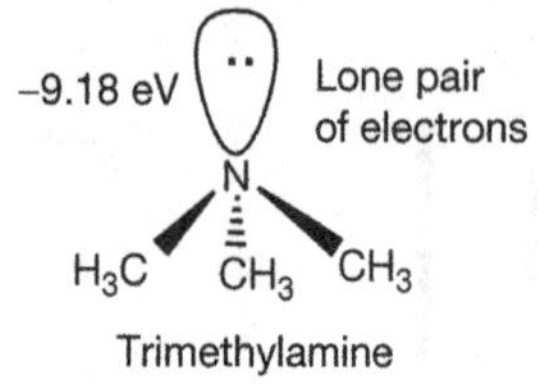

Figure 3.2 Tetrahedral nitrogen.

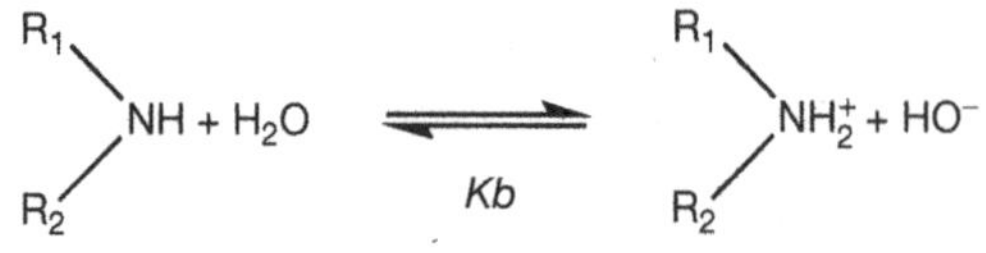

Figure 3.3 Equilibrium between free and protonated forms of a base in water.

R groups attached to them increases. However, in the case of a strong organic base the equilibrium shown in Figure 3.3 lies well to the right at physiological pH (7.4) and for most bases the equilibrium is almost entirely to the right at the pH of the stomach (1.0). The equilibrium constant Kb for the equilibrium shown in Figure 3.3 gives a measure of basic strength but more often the measure of basic strength given in tables is the pKa value, which describes the equilibrium shown in Figure 3.4 where B is a base.

For a strong base the equilibrium lies to the left at physiological pH since it does not readily give up its proton, thus behaving as a weak acid. The pKa value is $-\log Ka$ and the range of pKa values in water extends from 0 to 14. For a base, the higher its pKa value the stronger it is. At the pH of the stomach (*ca.* 1) the majority of amines are completely ionised but at physiological pH (pH 7.4) some basic drugs may contain an appreciable amount of un-ionised amine. The degree of ionisation of an amine drug has a bearing on its degree of protein binding and its degree of partitioning into tissues and hence the pharmacokinetics of a drug. The Henderson-Hasselbalch equation can be rearranged to calculate two important physicochemical properties for an ionisable

$$BH^+ \overset{H^+}{\underset{H^+}{\rightleftharpoons}} B + H^+$$

$$Ka$$

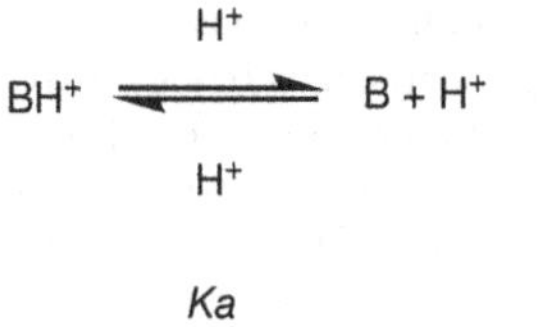

Where

$$Ka = \frac{[B][H^+]}{[BH^+]}$$

Figure 3.4 Equilibrium constant for a base in water.

drug. The percentage ionisation of a basic drug at a given pH may be determined from the following equation:

$$\% \text{ Ionisation} = \frac{10^{pKa-pH}}{1 + 10^{pKa-pH}} \times 100 \qquad \boxed{1}$$

The variation in partition coefficient with pH for a base may be given from the following equation:

$$Papp = \frac{P}{1 + 10^{pKa-pH}} \qquad \boxed{2}$$

where P is the partition coefficient of the un-ionised drug and Papp is its partition coefficient at a particular pH. From equation 2 it can be seen that the partition coefficient of a drug is halved when the pH = its pKa value.

CALCULATION EXAMPLE 3.1

Calculate the percentage ionisation and partition coefficient of procaine at pH 7.4. Partition coefficient of un-ionised procaine = 50, pKa = 9.0.

$$\% \text{ ionisation} = \frac{10^{9-7.4}}{1 + 10^{9-7.4}} \times 100 = \frac{39.8}{40.8} \times 100 = 97.5$$

$$Papp = \frac{50}{1 + 10^{9-7.4}} = \frac{50}{40.8} = 1.23$$

FACTORS AFFECTING THE pKa VALUE OF A BASE

Alkyl groups

In simple aliphatic amines the number of alkyl groups attached to the nitrogen has an effect on the basicity of the amine. Thus the order of basicity for amines is approximately: secondary > primary > ammonia > tertiary. The increased basicity of primary and secondary amines over ammonia is due to the inductive release of electron density from the alkyl groups which increases the electron density on the nitrogen atom. This can be seen for the methylamines in Figure 3.5.

In the case of tertiary amines there is a balance of two effects contributing to their basicity. Although the alkyl groups contribute to the electron density in tertiary amines the presence of three alkyl groups in the molecules reduces the ability of the protonated tertiary amine to hydrogen bond to water and thus increase its stability. In non-polar solvents, where hydrogen bonding does not occur, and thus does not contribute to the thermodynamics of protonation, tertiary amines are the strongest bases. The basicity also increases with increasing size of the alkyl group and this can override the unfavourable effects of trisubstitution on hydrogen bonding; thus tripropylamine (Pr_3N) is a strong base with a pKa value of 10.74 in water.

Self Test 3.1

Calculate the percentage ionisation and Papp for the following amine drugs at pH 1.0 and pH 7.4.

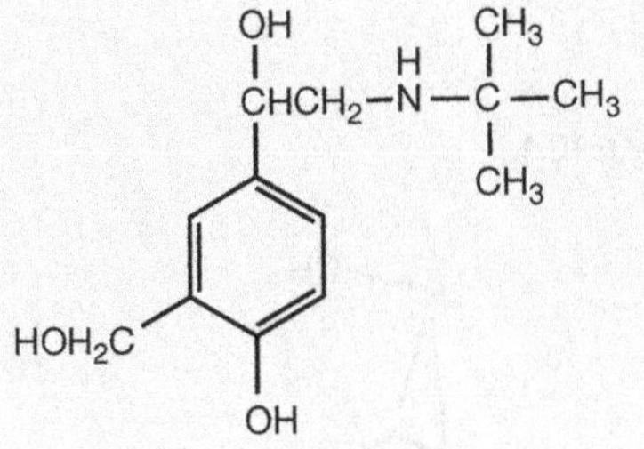

1. Salbutamol p*Ka* 9.3 P=9.3

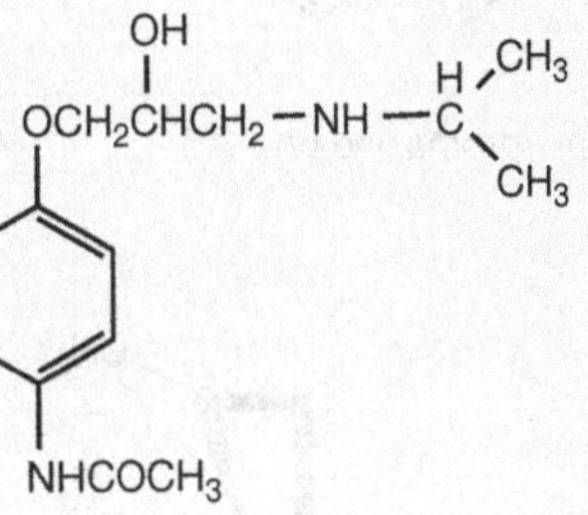

2. Practolol p*Ka* 9.6 P=15.8

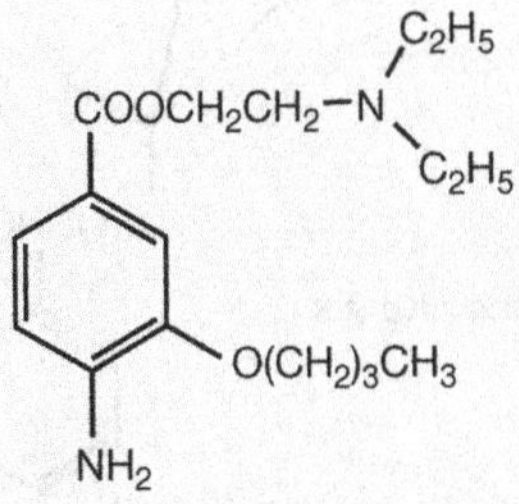

3. Oxybuprocaine p*Ka* 9.0 P=630

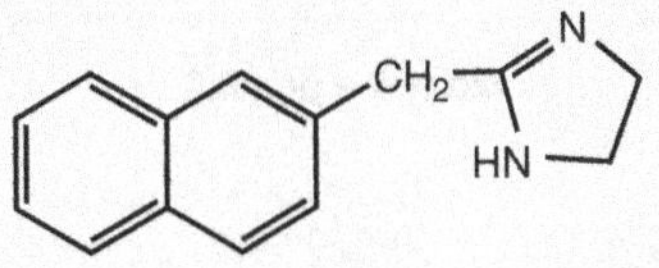

4. Napthazoline p*Ka* 10.9 P=126

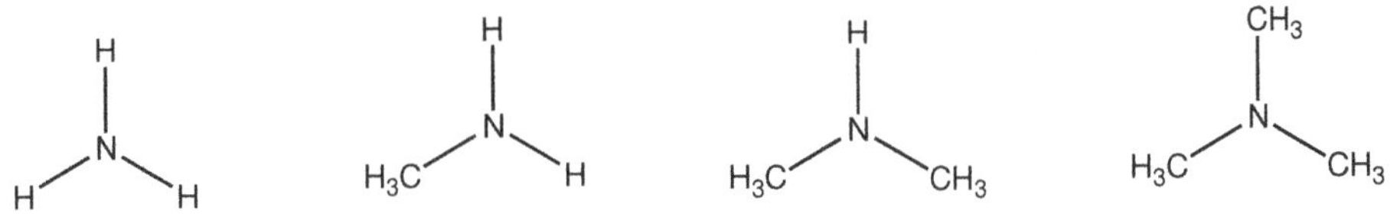

p*Ka* 9.3 HOMO −12.4 eV p*Ka* 10.6 HOMO −12 eV p*Ka* 10.7 HOMO −10.4 eV p*Ka* 9.72 HOMO −9.2 eV

Figure 3.5 Energy of highest occupied molecular orbitals (HOMOs) of amines.

Steric factors and basic strength in drug molecules

In practice, the reported p*Ka* values for tertiary amine groups within drugs vary widely. The main explanation for variation in basicity is that the degree of steric hindrance of the basic nitrogen is very variable in tertiary amines. Often, the effects of a polar group close to the basic centre has been invoked as the explanation; however, electron withdrawing groups only exert strong effects over one bond length, with weak effects over two bond lengths. In Figure 3.6 a selection of *N*-methyl tertiary amines is shown. The basic strength of these amines is determined by availability of the lone pair of electrons on the nitrogen for protonation. The lone pair in *N*-methylpiperidine is more favourably positioned than that in chlorpromazine for protonation since there is less conformational flexibility in the alkyl groups attached to the nitrogen in the latter. The effects of conformation can be seen most clearly when morphine and atropine are compared (Fig. 3.7). Both structures are composed of interlocking rings and hence are conformationally restricted. In morphine, the geometry of the six-membered ring is quite distorted. This can be seen if one observes the distances between the proton on the nitrogen atom and the nearest hydrogens which in an undistorted ring would be the same. In the case of morphine the distances between the proton and the nearest hydrogens are 2.09, 2.27 and 2.35 Å.

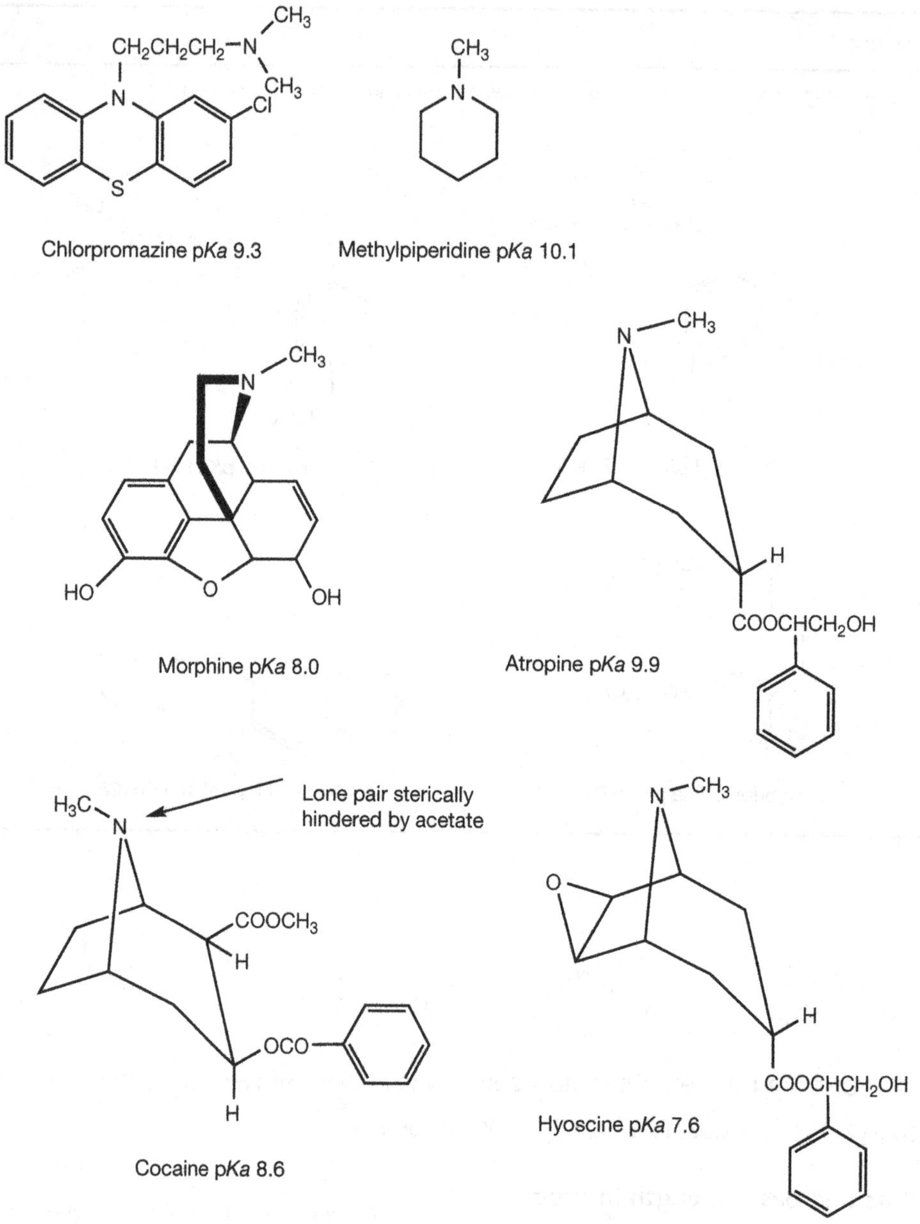

Figure 3.6 Tertiary amines.

The ring distortion results in a flattening of the ring which means that it is difficult for the protonated nitrogen to adopt its preferred tetrahedral conformation (the angles between the proton and adjacent alkyl groups are 103.5°, 103.7° and 103.9°). In atropine, the ring is more symmetrical and less flattened (measurements from nitrogen to the nearest hydrogens are 2.38, 2.39 and 2.4 Å). Thus the nitrogen is held closer to its preferred tetrahedral geometry, ready for protonation (angles between proton and adjacent alkyl groups 105.6°, 106.1° and 106.2°). This accounts for the large difference in p*Ka*: morphine 8.0 and atropine 9.9. This effect holds throughout the series of structural analogues. Thus codeine, dextromethorphan, diamorphine and nalorphine all have similar p*Ka* values to morphine and homatropine,while benzotropine and hyoscyamine have similar p*Ka* values to atropine. Cocaine is structurally related to atropine but its p*Ka* value is lower. This has been attributed to the electron withdrawing effect of the ester group, which

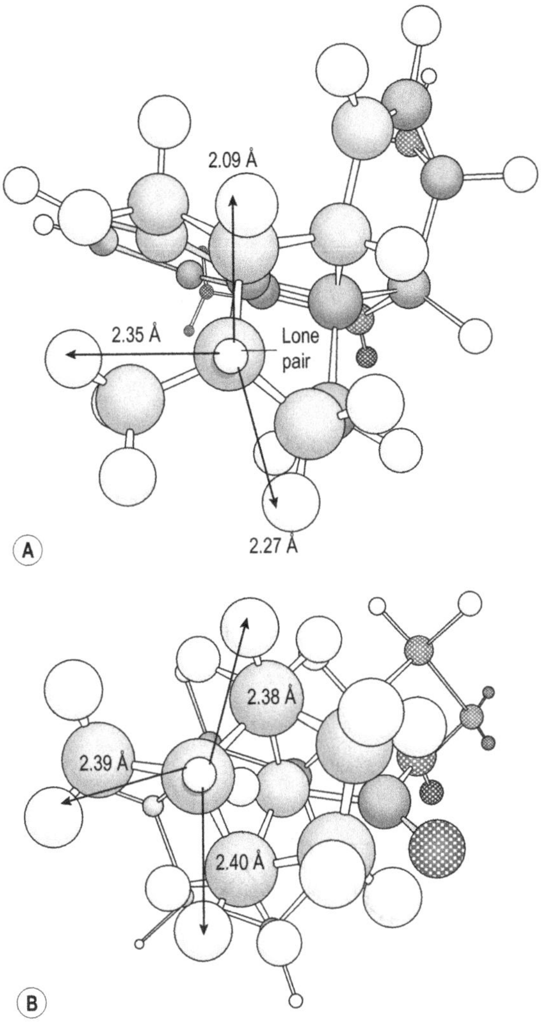

Figure 3.7 3-D structures of (**A**) morphine and (**B**) atropine showing distance of proton in the ionised basic centres from the nearest hydrogen atoms.

is two bonds removed from the nitrogen, but it is more likely that it is due to the proximity of the acetate ester group that sterically crowds the basic nitrogen. The acetate is forced into a close contact with the amine by the benzoic acid substituent that is next to it. A similar effect can be seen in hyoscine which has a p*Ka* value of 7.6. In this case, the epoxide ring pushes the methyl towards the six-membered ring causing the ring to appear more boatlike in conformation (see Ch. 2), thus sterically crowding the nitrogen.

Electron withdrawing groups

Tertiary amines

In some tertiary amines the proximity of electron withdrawing groups to the amine has an effect on basic strength. Thus diethazine has a p*Ka* of 9.1 while lidocaine has a p*Ka* of 7.9 (Fig. 3.8). In lidocaine the electron withdrawing amide group, separated by just one CH_2 group from the amine, has a base weakening effect.

Secondary amines

The basic strength of secondary amines is more predictable than that of tertiary amines. This is because one of the substituents is hydrogen and thus there are fewer problems with steric crowding, and hydrogen bonding to water is more favourable. This can be seen in the case of piperazine, ephedrine and sotalol (Fig. 3.9) which are quite different in structure but have similar p*Ka* values. If interaction with neighbouring groups is strong, then the basic strength of secondary amines is affected as in the case of piperazine where the basic strength of the second amine group is reduced due to the presence of a positive charge on the first basic centre which repels the approach of a second proton. Other examples include the morpholino ring where the presence of an oxygen atom, which is only two bond lengths away from the nitrogen, because of the puckering of the ring, withdraws electrons, thus reducing the p*Ka* of the secondary amine group to *ca.* 7.

Primary amines

Environmental factors have a strong influence on the basic strength primary amines. Thus amfetamine is strongly basic since there are no neighbouring electron withdrawing groups. The basic strength of phenylpropanolamine is lowered by the presence of a β-hydroxyl group which withdraws electrons from the amine group. In the case of DOPA the carboxyl group on the α-carbon withdraws electron density from the amine group, thus

Figure 3.8 The effect of an electron withdrawing group on basic strength.

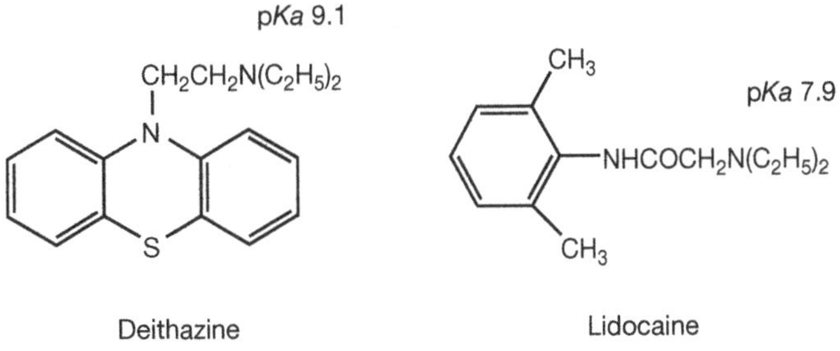

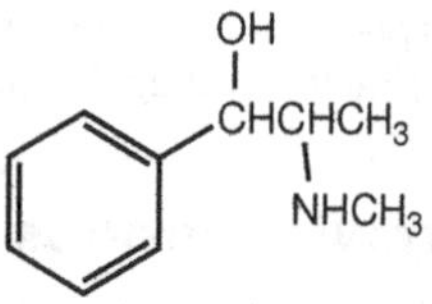

Ephedrine p*Ka* 9.6

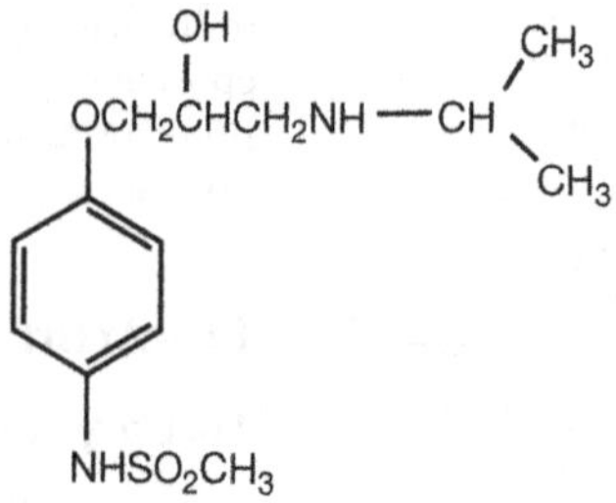

Sotalol p*Ka* 9.8

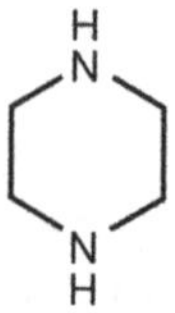

Piperazine p*Ka* 9.8

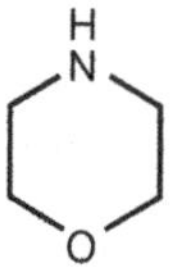

Morpholine p*Ka* 7.0

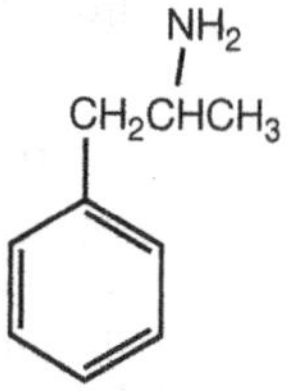

Amfetamine p*Ka* 10.0

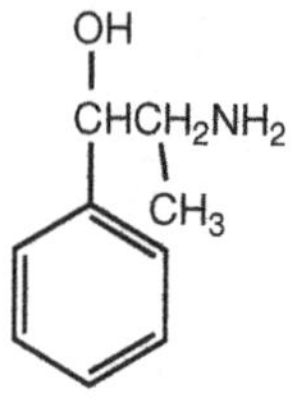

Phenylpropanolamine p*Ka* 9.1

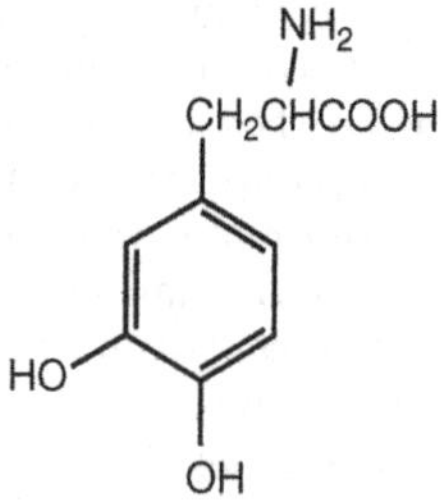

DOPA p*Ka* 8.7

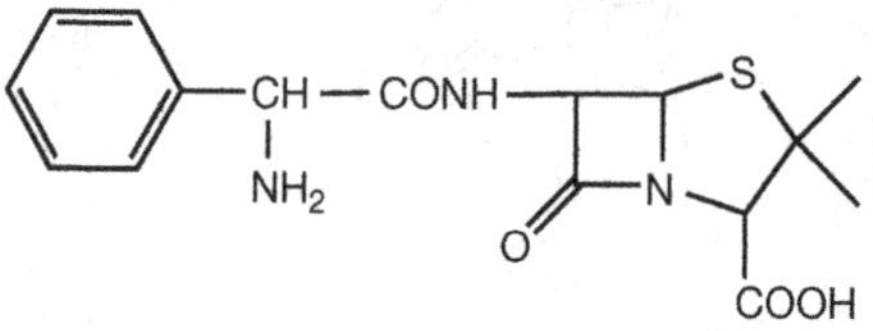

Ampicillin p*Ka* 7.3

Figure 3.9 Basic strength of secondary amines.

reducing its basic strength. In ampicillin the electron withdrawing effect of the amide and the benzyl group reduce the p*Ka* value of the primary amine to 7.3.

Aromatic amines

Aromatic amines are very weak due to the electron withdrawing effect of the benzene ring and aniline (Fig. 3.10) has a p*Ka* value of 4.6. The presence of a second aromatic ring as in diphenylamine (Fig. 3.10) reduces the p*Ka* value of the amine to 0.8. The presence of other electron withdrawing substituents in an aromatic ring either ortho or para to an aromatic amine group also reduces its p*Ka* value. The p*Ka* values of the aromatic amine groups found in sulphonamides such as sulfacetamide and some local anaesthetics such as procaine are *ca.* 2.

SUMMARY 3.1

- The lone pair electrons on an amine nitrogen is much more available for protonation than lone pairs on oxygen atoms.
- The higher the p*Ka* value of an amine the greater its basic strength. In a non-aqueous solvent the more alkyl groups that are attached to a nitrogen atom the greater the basic strength. Thus tertiary amines are the strongest bases under non-aqueous conditions.
- In water secondary amines tend to be the most strongly basic since solvation of the hydrophobic tertiary amine is unfavourable and thus its strength is reduced.
- The strength of tertiary amines is very influenced by steric factors and flattening of the basic centre reduces basic strength.

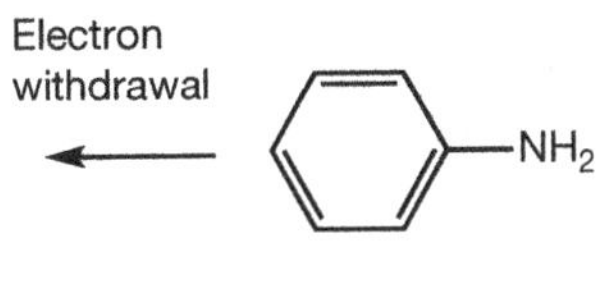

Aniline p*Ka* 4.6

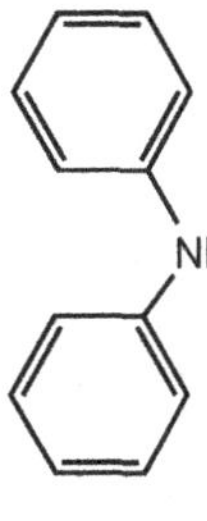

Diphenylamine p*Ka* 0.8

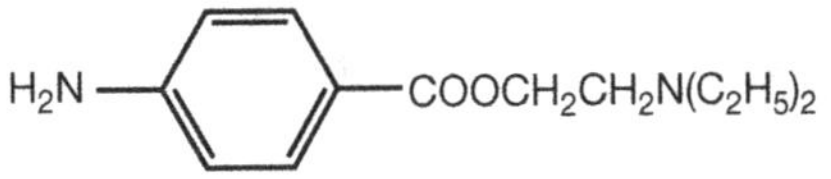

Procaine p*Ka* 2

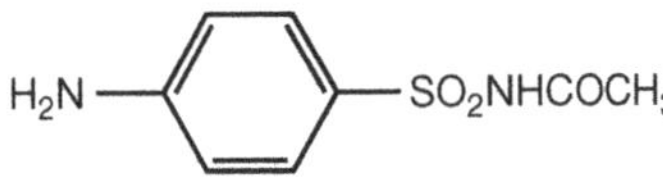

Sulfacetamide p*Ka* 2

Figure 3.10 Aromatic amines.

Q Self Test 3.2

Match the p*Ka* value to the basic centres in the amines below
p*Ka* values: 9.4, 9.6, 7.7, 0.5, 9.4 (N.B. amides are neutral).

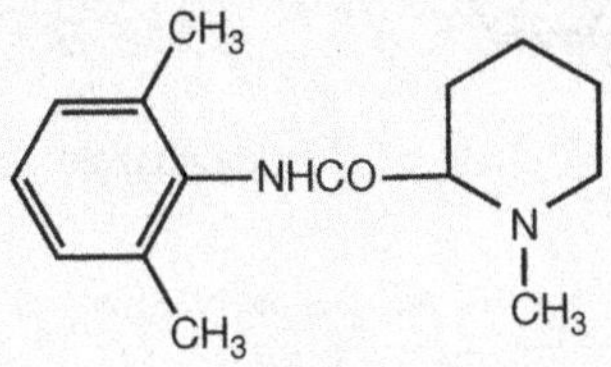

1 Mepivacaine

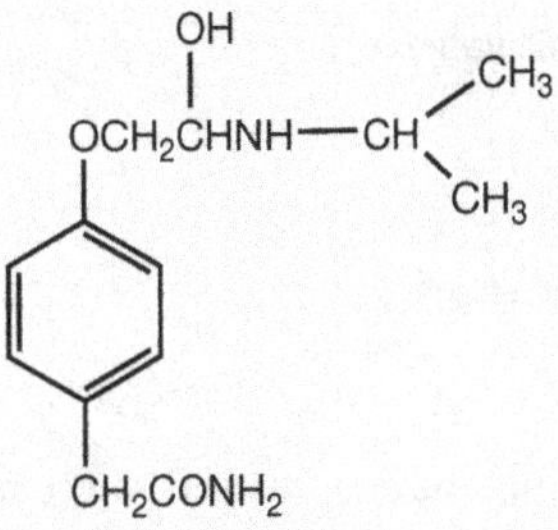

2 Atenolol

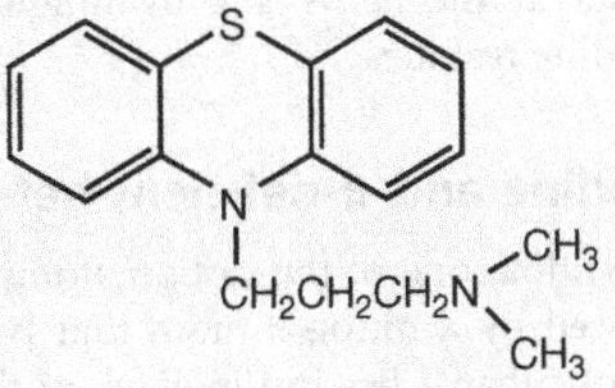

3 Promazine

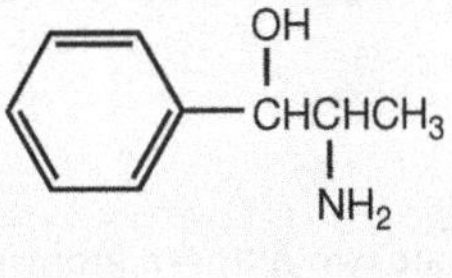

4 Cathine

Heterocyclic amines

Chapter 4 discusses heterocyclic compounds in more detail; in this chapter some of the heterocyclic amines are discussed. The basic properties of amines such as piperidine and azolidine are similar to those of open-chain amines. Thus piperidine has a p*Ka* of 11.1, that is similar to that of diethylamine that has a p*Ka* of 11.0 (Fig. 3.11). Introduction of double bonds into the ring containing the nitrogen atom affects its basicity. Introduction of a single double bond into the pyrrolidine ring, to

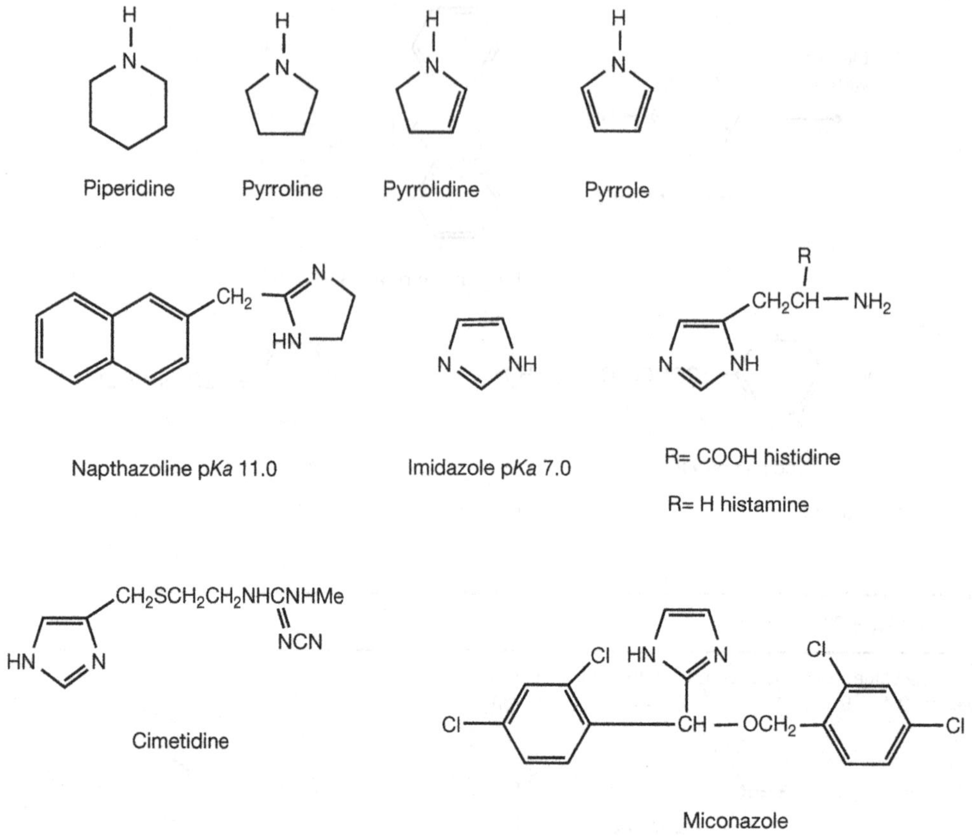

Figure 3.11 Heterocyclic amines.

form pyrroline, does not have a marked effect on the basicity of the nitrogen but the introduction of two double bonds in the case of the pyrrole ring produces a nitrogen atom that has lost its basic character and is essentially neutral. Pyrrole and other π-excessive compounds will be discussed in Chapter 4.

Imidazoles

In the case of imidazole there are two nitrogen atoms in a five-membered ring as well as two double bonds. Imidazoles are weakly basic having p*Ka* values in the range of 6–7. The basicity of the imidazole ring is weakened by the fact that the ring is very flat and thus the nitrogen cannot adopt its preferred tetrahedral stereochemistry when it is protonated. The imidazole ring occurs in histamine that is the natural ligand for histamine receptors. Histamine receptor antagonists such as cimetidine (Fig. 3.11) and omeprazole contain an imidazole ring. It is also found in the range of azole antifungal agents including clotrimazole, miconazole (Fig. 3.11) and ketoconazole. These agents all act as inhibitors of fungal P450 enzymes that are involved in the biosynthesis of ergosterol which is the major sterol of fungal membranes. The imidazole ring in these compounds in some way interferes with the binding of iron (II) at the active site of the enzyme; the iron is bound at the active site by imidazole ring containing histidine residues.

Pyridine and π-deficient heterocycles

In pyridine one of the carbon atoms in a benzene ring is replaced by a nitrogen atom that is in its sp^2 hybridised form so that it lies in the plane of the ring. The nitrogen lone pair is in one of the sp^2 orbitals and thus is less available for protonation because of the increased *s* character compared to the normal sp^3 hybridisation for nitrogen. In *s* orbitals electrons are held closer to the nucleus of the atom and are thus in a deeper energy well. The pyridine ring is quite distorted with C–N–C angle being 117° rather than the 120° angle that applies to the C–C–C bonds in benzene. This is an indication of increased *p*-character (with pure *p* the bond angles are 90°) in the bonding orbitals while the orbital containing the non-bonding lone pair has increased *s* character, i.e. the non-bonding orbital and the bonding orbitals are no longer completely equivalent. Thus pyridine is a much weaker base, p*Ka* 5.2, in comparison with piperidine, p*Ka* 11.1. When two nitrogens are introduced into a heteroaromatic ring the *s* character of the lone pairs on the nitrogen atoms is further increased and the dinitrogen heteroaromatics are all very weak bases. This may seem rather counterintuitive but if the values in Table 3.1 are examined it can be seen that, in particular, the C–N–C bond angle is indicative of increased *s* character in the lone pair of electrons, hence decreased basicity. This bond angle more or less reflects the relative basicities of the dinitrogen heteroaromatics. Quinazoline and pteridine are stronger bases than pyrimidine since the additional aromatic ring increases the rigidity of the pyrimidine ring, resulting in bond angles closer to 120°, and thus decreased

Table 3.1 p*Ka* values and bond angles for the heteroaromatic structures shown in Figure 3.12 (determined from molecular mechanical calculations)

Compound	p*Ka*	C–N–C bond angle(s)	C–C–N bond angles	C–C–C bond angles	N–C–N bond angles
Pyridine	5.2	117°	123.8° 123.8°	118.5° 118.3° 118.5°	
Pyrazine	0.6	115.5° 115.5°	122.2° 122.2° 122.2° 122.2°		
Pyrimidine	1.3	115.8° 115.8°	122.1° 122.1°	116.9°	127.3°
Pyridazine	2.3	119.3° 119.3°	124.5° 124.5°	116.2° 116.2°	
Sym-triazine		114.5° 114.5° 114.5°			125.5° 125.5° 125.5°
Quinoline	4.9	118.3°	124.2° 121.5°	119.2° 120.4° 120.3° 120.3° 120.2° 119.6° 118.9° 118.5° 118.6°	
Quinazoline	3.5	116.8° * 115.8°	122.2° 119.9°	119.3° 120.1° 120.5° 120.4° 119.9° 119.8° 117.5°	127.7°
Pteridine	4.1	117.1° * 115.9° 116.7° 116.5°	119.3° 119.6° 120.5° 122.4° 122.4° 122.5°	121.5°	127.6°

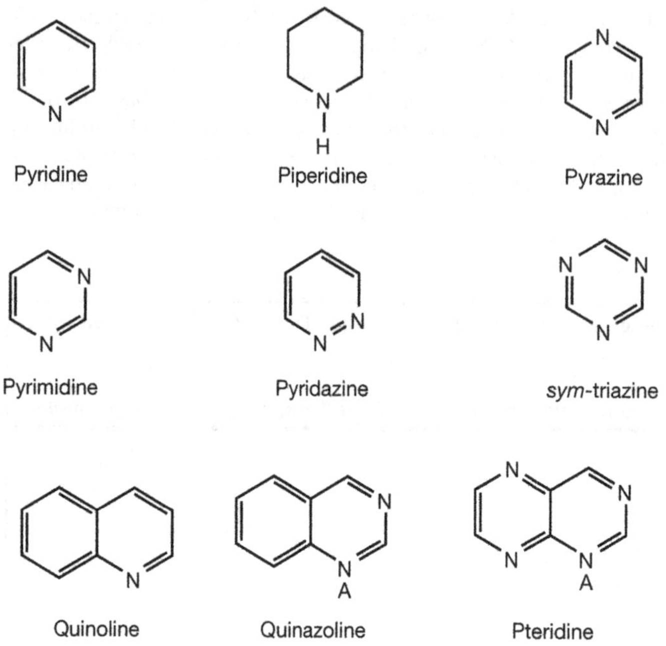

Figure 3.12 Some simple heteroaromatic compounds.

s character for the non-bonding lone pair at position A (Fig. 3.12).

π-Deficient heteroaromatic rings occur in many drug structures. The most consistent exploitation of their properties is in the sulphonamide drugs (Fig. 3.13) where the properties of the heterocyclic ring contribute to the acidity of the sulphonamide. The acidity of the sulphonamide is influenced by the electron withdrawing properties of the heterocyclic ring. This can again be viewed simply as electron withdrawal by the heterocyclic ring or it can be viewed in terms of increased *s* character of some of the carbon atoms within the ring. This can be seen

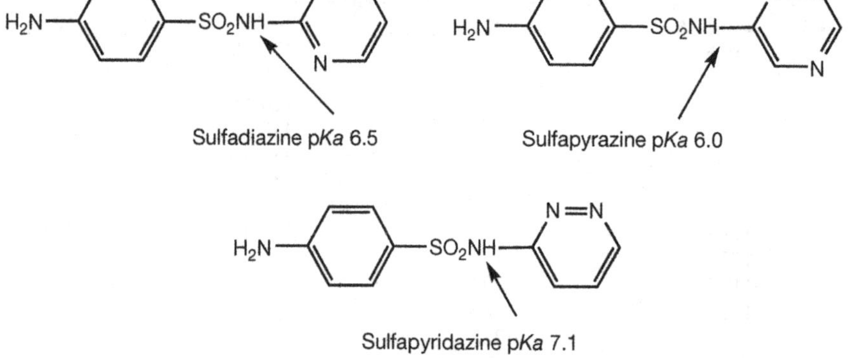

Figure 3.13 Some sulphonamides.

particularly where the bond angle is increased well above 120°, indicating movement towards the *sp* state where the bond angle is 180°. Thus, in comparison with sulfanilamide, sulfapyridine is a stronger acid and acid strength increases still further when two nitrogens are introduced into the heteroaromatic ring.

Substitution within the ring of nitrogen-containing heteroaromatic compounds can have a marked effect on their properties. Substitution with an amine or a hydroxyl causes the greatest effect on the p*Ka* values of the heteroatoms. Thus a hydroxyl adjacent to the nitrogen in pyridine almost eliminates its basicity due to electron withdrawal by the oxygen and the hydroxy pyridine can also exist in its pyridone form (Fig. 3.14). The compound 2,4-dihydroxypyrimidine is acidic rather than basic and exists largely in its pyrimidone form, which is commonly known as uracil. Uracil is one of the bases found in RNA but, in fact, it is a weak acid rather than a base and so is its methyl derivative thymine which is a DNA 'base'. 4-aminopyridine is a relatively strong base in comparison to aniline having a p*Ka* of 9.2. The compound 4-amino-2-hydroxypyrimidine is a weak base with a p*Ka* similar to that of aniline and is commonly known as cytosine, one of the DNA bases.

Guanidines

Guanidine is derived biosynthetically from urea. The ureides themselves will be discussed in Chapter 4. Guanidine is a very strong base with a p*Ka* value of 13.65; thus it can form salts even with very weak acids. The strength of the base arises from the resonance stabilisation of the charged base (Fig. 3.15). The high degree of symmetry of the guanidinium ion and its complete ionisation with the charge distributed over quite a large ion enables it to mimic inorganic ions to some extent. Thus it competes effectively with Mg^{2+} for binding sites on phosphate groups in phospholipids. This ability to mimic an inorganic ion may account for the ability of guanethidine to inhibit the Ca^{2+} promoted fusion of noradrenaline-containing vesicles with the membrane of a neuron and thus act as an anti-hypertensive agent.

Guanidino groups are also present in streptomycin, which was the first aminoglycoside antibiotic used in treating tuberculosis. Streptomycin and related antibiotics interfere in the translation of RNA into protein and this is probably due to their polycationic nature and ability to mimic both Mg^{2+} and polyamines that are involved in phosphate group stabilisation.

Figure 3.14 Substituted nitrogen containing heteroaromatic compounds.

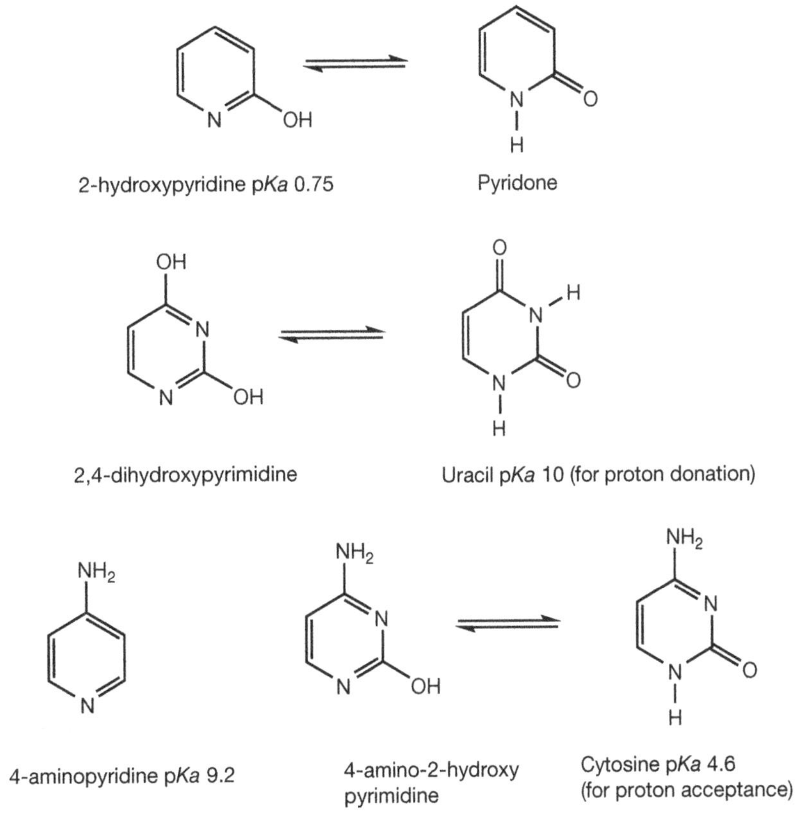

Q Self Test 3.3

a. Name the heterocyclic amine rings in the following drugs.
b. Select from the list the p*Ka* values that most closely correspond to the basic centres in the whole molecule. (p*Ka* values: 0.5, 1, 2, 5, 6, 7, 9, 11).

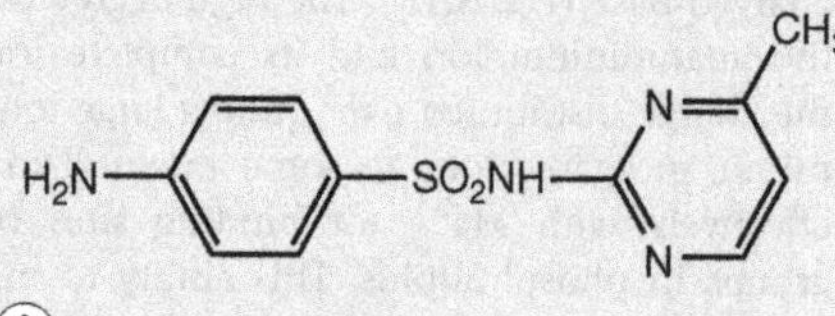

A

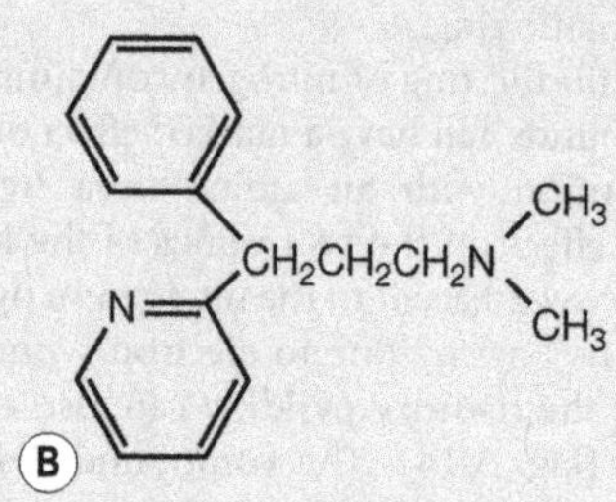

B

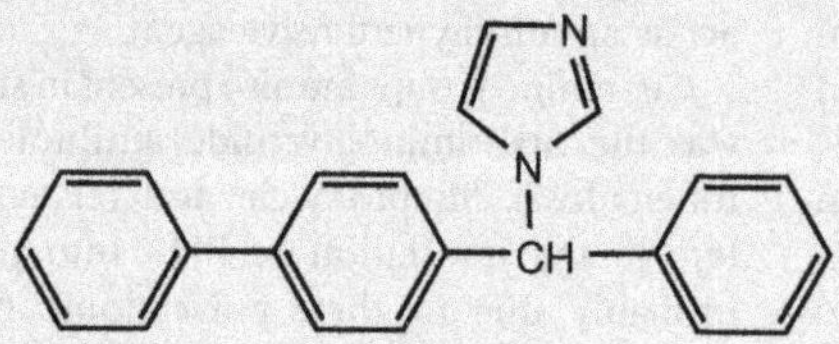

C

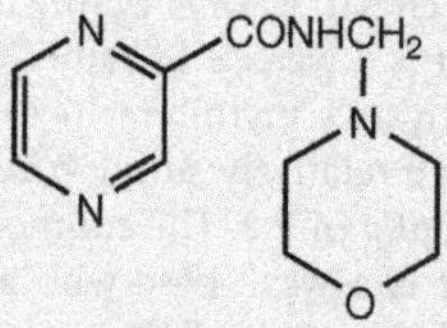

D

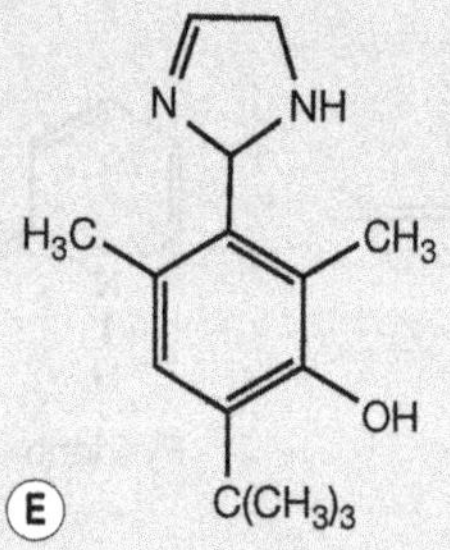

E

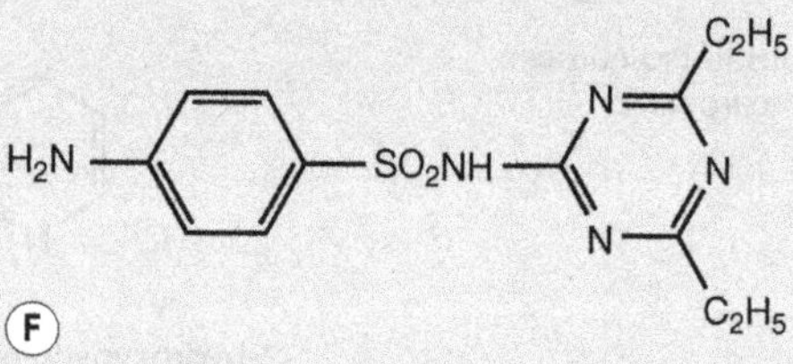

F

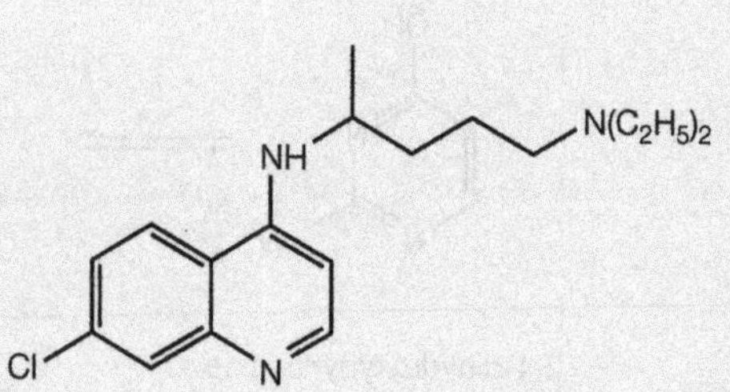

G

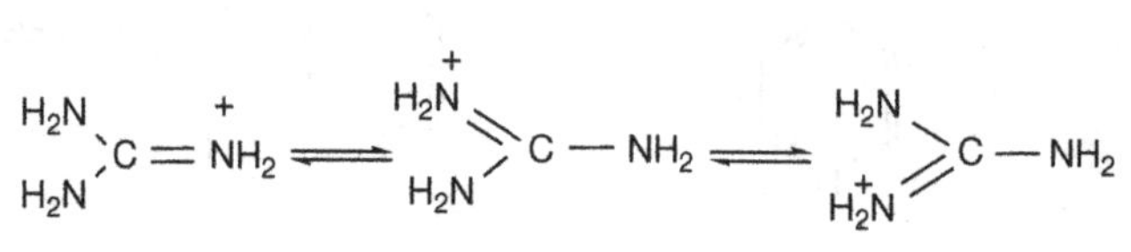

Figure 3.15 Resonance stabilisation of the guanidinium ion.

Biguanides

Biguanine, like guanine, is strongly basic, having a p*Ka* of 12.8. Biguanides occur in a number of therapeutic agents.

Proguanil (Fig. 3.16) was a relatively early antimalarial drug and it is still useful as a first line of defence against the erythrocytic stage of malaria. It is metabolised in the human body to an active metabolite which mimics the pteridine ring in folic acid and acts as a selective inhibitor of folate reductase in the parasite, thus inhibiting its DNA synthesis.

Phenformin (Fig. 3.16) is used as an antidiabetic drug and lowers plasma glucose levels in diabetics but has no effect on plasma glucose levels in non-diabetics. The mechanism of action of these drugs is not fully understood; however, they are believed to affect glucose metabolism. This might be linked to an ability to mimic magnesium that is involved as a co-factor in many of the enzymes of glucose catabolism.

The bisbiguanide chlorhexidine (Fig. 3.16) is a powerful antibacterial agent and its actions are related to those of other cationic surfactants that are effective antibacterial agents. The charged groups in the molecules bind to the bacterial membrane, thus disrupting the functioning of the cell.

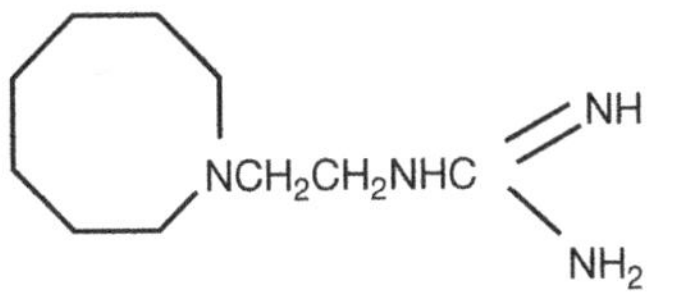

Guanethidine

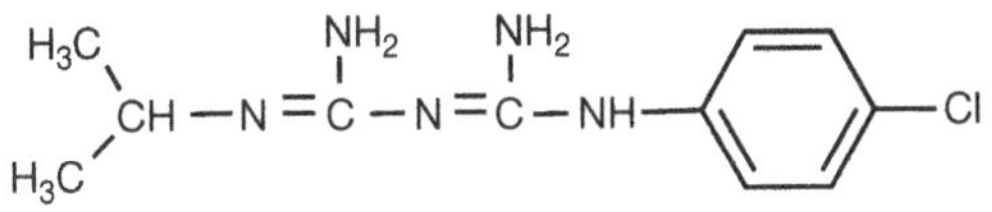

Proguanil

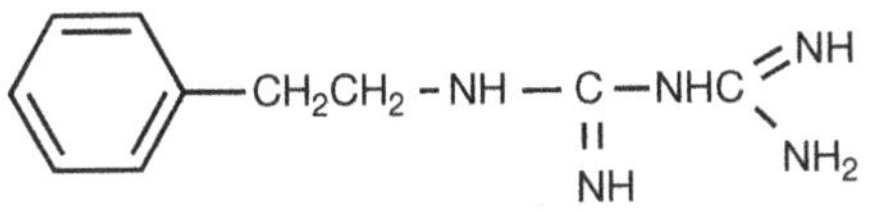

Phenformin

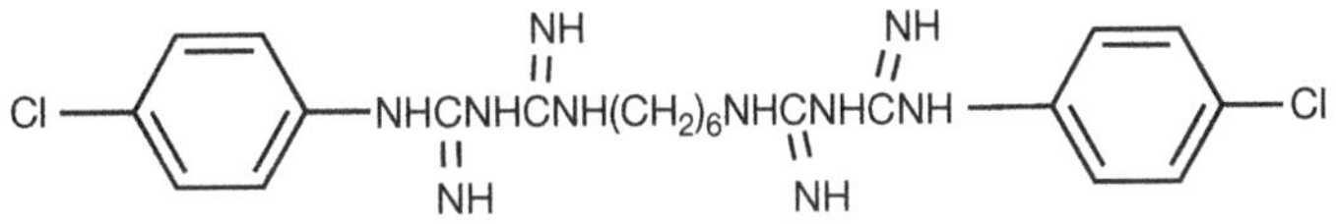

Chlorhexidine

Figure 3.16 Examples of drugs containing the guanidine group.

Q Self Test 3.4

Suggest therapeutic actions for the following guanidines and biguanides.

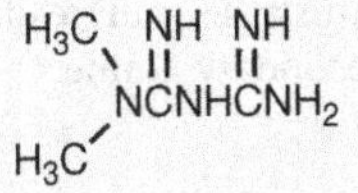

Metformin

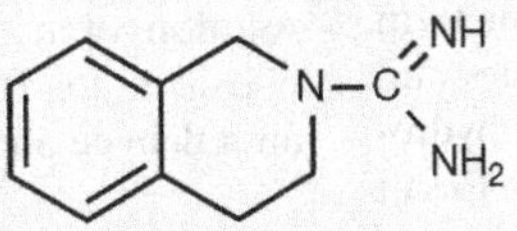

Debrisoquine

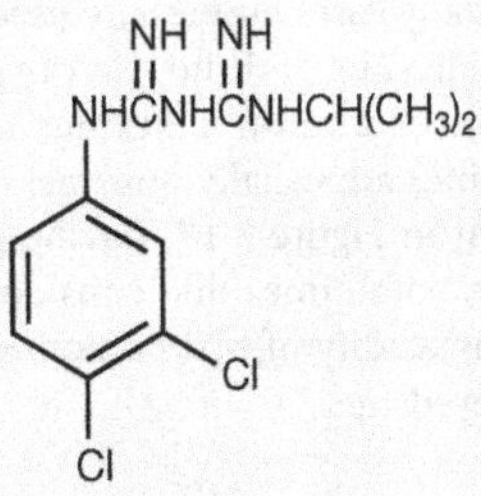

Chloroproguanil

SUMMARY 3.2

- Imidazoles are weakly basic having p*Ka* values in the range of 6–7. The basicity of the imidazole ring is weakened by the fact that the ring is very flat and thus the nitrogen cannot adopt its preferred tetrahedral stereochemistry when it is protonated. The imidazole ring occurs in histamine and is found in a number of drugs but particularly in H_2 receptor antagonists and azole antifungal compounds.
- Nitrogen in an aromatic ring system behaves as a weak base: the more nitrogen atoms present in the ring the less strongly basic they are. The base weakening effect can be explained by the distortion of the angles in the ring caused by the presence of the heteroatoms. This causes the lone pairs of electrons on the N atom(s) to have increased *s* orbital character and results in them being less available to accept a proton.
- In general, nitrogen-containing heteroaromatic systems withdraw electrons from their substituents and this effect has been utilised in the control of the relative acidity of sulphonamide drugs.
- The guanidine group is a strong base with a p*Ka* of 13.65 and it is thus completely ionised within the physiological pH range and behaves rather like an inorganic ion, e.g. Mg^{2+}.
- Mimicking of inorganic ions may account for the properties of drugs containing both guanidine and the biguanine group.

Salt formation

One of the fundamental reactions of amines is the formation of a salt that will generally occur by reaction with both inorganic and organic acids. Salt selection is an important step in pharmaceutical development. Most organic amines are water insoluble in the form of their free bases and for the purposes of convenience in their formulation they are usually used as a salt. The salts of amines can be purified by recrystallisation and are less susceptible to oxidative degradation than the free bases. They are also water soluble and thus readily formulated into injections. In many cases amines are used in the form of their hydrochloride salts and the use of sulphates and hydrobromides is also common. Solutions of the hydrochloride salts of amines are usually quite acidic due to salt hydrolysis, as shown in Figure 3.17, having pH values of *ca.* 4.0. Surprisingly, sometimes due consideration is not given to the irritating acidity of hydrochloride salts in formulations such as eyedrops.

$$BH^+Cl^- + H_2O \rightleftharpoons BOH + HCl$$

Figure 3.17 Hydrolysis of the hydrochloride salt of a base.

In some cases hydrochloride salts are not very water soluble due to the strength of association between the base and its counter ion, and other salts have to be used. For instance, salts may be prepared with di- or tricarboxylic acids, e.g. ergometrine tartrate, diethylcarbamazine citrate, sumatriptan succinate (Fig. 3.18) and lisuride maleate are all used because of the water insolubility of their hydrochlorides. Similarly strong monobasic organic acids such as mesilate are used to promote water solubility, as in the case of benzatropine mesilate (Fig. 3.18) and phentolamine mesilate. In some instances salts are too ready to absorb water from the atmosphere, for instance the muscle relaxant drug atracurium is formulated as its besilate salt to avoid the problems of water absorption experienced with its mesilate.

Sometimes, low water solubility is a desirable property and may be useful in the purification of a base after synthesis. It is also of therapeutic use in the formulation of some amines as depot injections, e.g. procaine penicillin (Fig. 3.18).

Salts are sometimes chosen with regard to their organoleptic properties and, for instance dextropropoxyphene napsylate (Fig. 3.18), is sometimes used because it is not as bitter as the hydrochloride.

REACTIONS OF AMINES IN RELATION TO STORAGE AND FORMULATION

Oxidation

All amines are prone to oxidation in air and aromatic amines are particularly unstable in this regard. Primary amines are susceptible to oxidation on the α-carbon, the reaction being catalysed by light (Fig. 3.19).

Secondary and tertiary amines behave in a similar manner (Fig. 3.20).

As well as being susceptible to oxidation on the α-carbon, tertiary amines readily form N-oxides. Traces of these compounds are usually formed when an aqueous solution of a tertiary amine is stored for a few days. N-oxides are fairly unstable and readily decompose to an aldehyde and a secondary amine.

Acylation

Primary and secondary amines can be chemically acylated with, for instance, an acid anhydride (Fig. 3.21) to give an amide, e.g. the acetylation of acetanilide, but this process can also occur with chemically incompatible ingredients in formulations. For example, aspirin is an acetylating reagent and can react with amines such a phenylephrine.

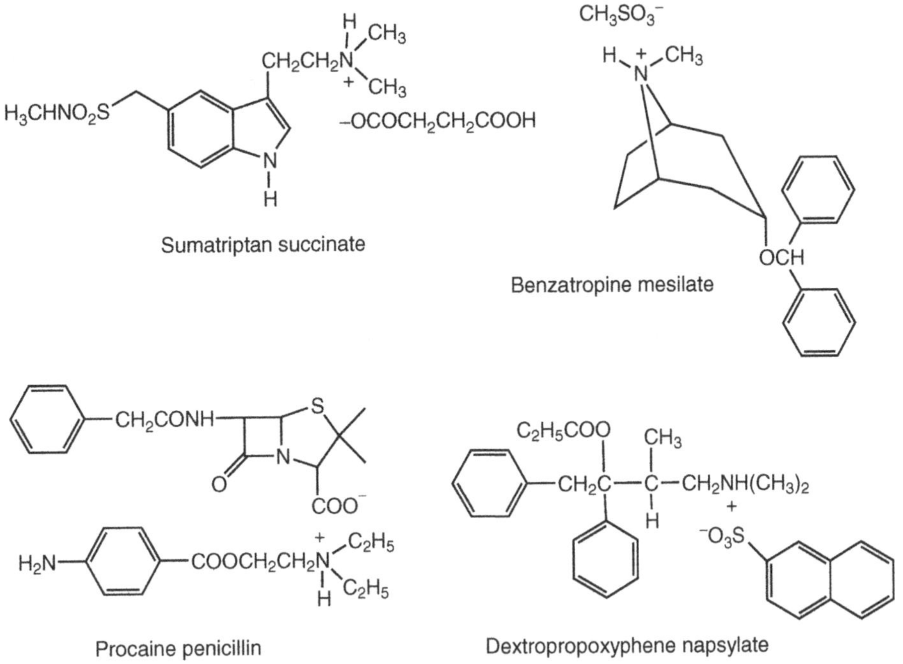

Figure 3.18 Some salts of amine drugs.

Figure 3.19 Oxidation of primary amines.

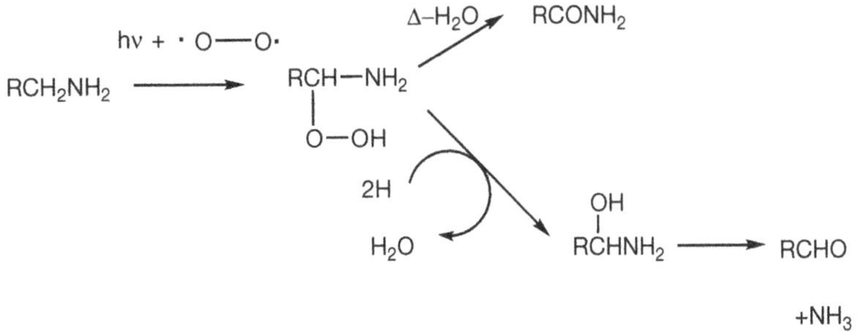

Both of these drugs are present in some proprietary formulations for treating colds and flu. Stearic acid is another possible acylating reagent since it is used as a releasing agent in some tablet formulations.

Acetylation of amines is an important route for the metabolism of primary aromatic amines such as the sulphonamide drugs or the antituberculosis drug isoniazid (Fig. 3.22). The co-factor involved in acetate transfer is acetyl co-enzyme A (acetyl CoA) and the reaction is catalysed by acetyl transferase, N-acetylation generally reduces toxicity.

Schiff's base formation

Primary and secondary amines can react readily with aldehydes and more slowly with ketones to give Schiff's bases or enamines, respectively. This reaction is particularly important with reducing sugars such as glucose, lactose and fructose that may be incorporated in formulations with amines. For instance, if LDOPA were formulated in a tablet with lactose as a filler, the reaction shown in Figure 3.23 could occur. Such reactions, leading to discolouration of lactose-containing tablets, have been

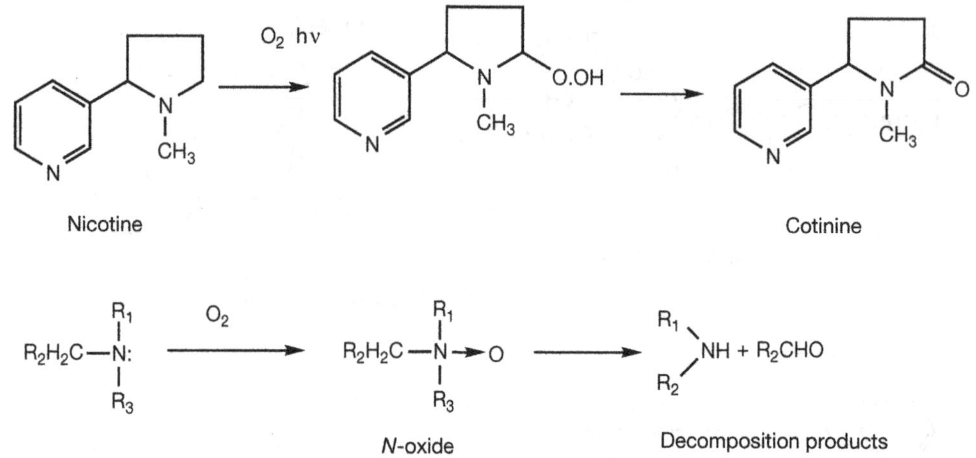

Figure 3.20 Oxidation of secondary and tertiary amines.

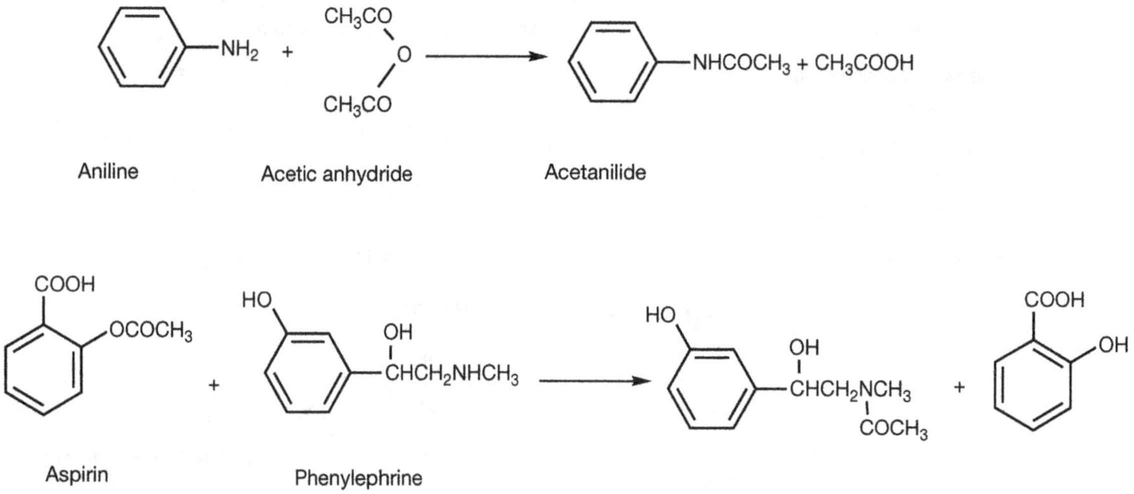

Figure 3.21 Acetylation of amines.

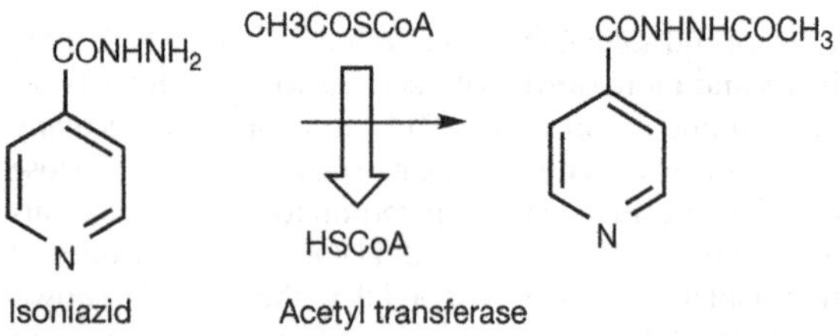

Figure 3.22 N-acetylation *in vivo*.

reported for the amines isoniazid and dextroamfetamine. During autoclaving of glucose or fructose, 2-hydroxymethylfurfuraldehyde is formed, which has been shown to react with sulphonamides and penicillins containing an amino group and aminoglycoside antibiotics, and this is potentially a problem in glucose-containing infusions. Glucose reacts with amino groups in proteins to form in the first instance Schiff's bases but then more complex, brown, rearrangement products are formed (the Maillard reaction, Fig. 3.24). This type of reaction is also

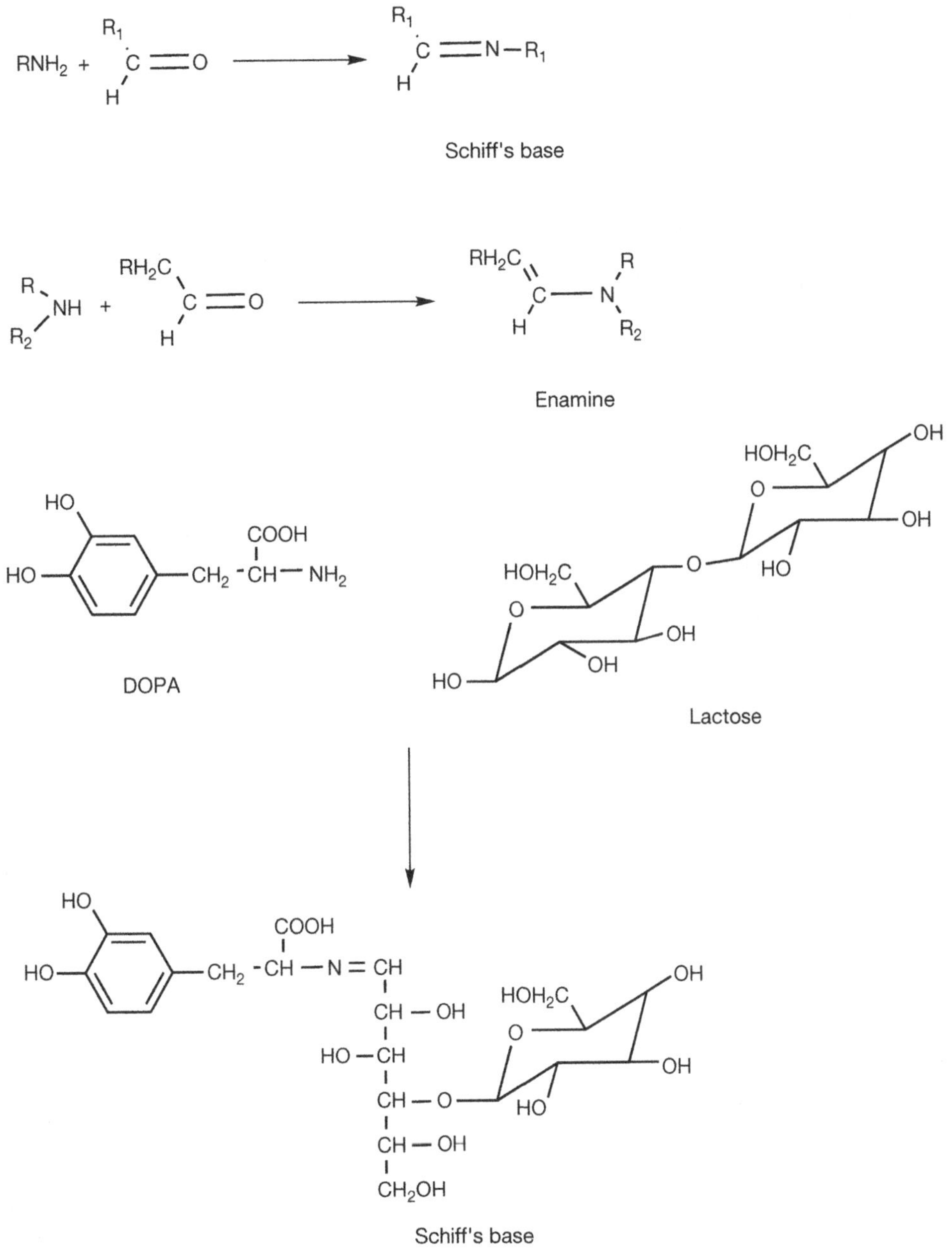

Figure 3.23 Schiff's base formation.

responsible for many of the complications of diabetes as such but also for some of the effects of ageing as well as being involved in the development of flavours during cooking of foodstuffs where nitrogen and oxygen heterocyclic compounds are generated from the type of 2 and 3 carbon intermediates shown in Figure 3.24. Cataracts in the eye arise from the reaction of glucose with the lens crystallin proteins, causing them to become opaque, and even wrinkles have been attributed to the cross-links that formed between protein chains as a

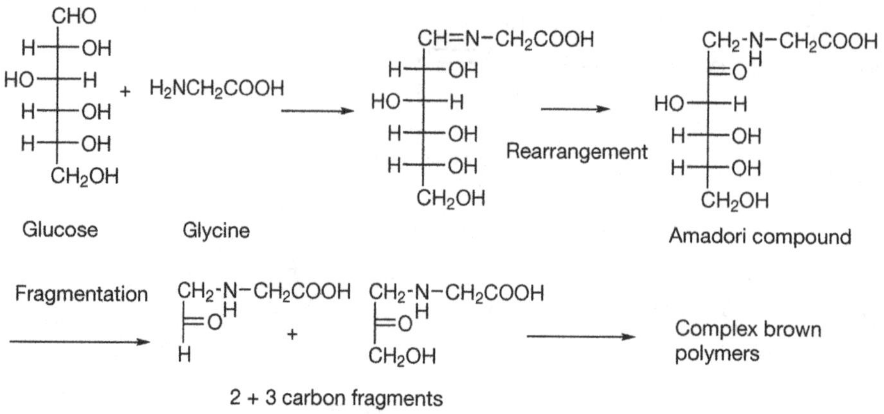

Figure 3.24 The Maillard reaction.

result of the Maillard reaction. Reactions of proteins with reducing sugars can also be a problem in the formulation of peptide drugs. If they are used as excipients, it is important to ensure that the peptide is efficiently freeze dried so that no traces of water remain that would favour the Maillard reaction.

SUMMARY 3.3

- Salts of amines can be used to alter their properties in relation to drug delivery e.g. for water solubility or solubility in oily injections.
- Primary and secondary amines are susceptible oxidation at the carbon alpha to the amine group. Tertiary amines readily form N-oxides.
- Acylation of amines to form amides can occur in combination with drugs such as aspirin and is also a route of metabolism for a number of drugs.
- Schiff's base formation occurs when a primary amine reacts with an aldehyde or ketone. An important example of this is in formulations containing reducing sugars such as glucose or lactose. In the case of proteins the products formed by reaction with reducing sugars rearrange to give complex products (the Maillard reaction).

Quaternary amines

Quaternary ammonium salts are formed by direct reaction of a tertiary amine with an alkyl halide. For example, trimethylamine can be reacted with cetyl bromide to produce the disinfectant agent cetrimide (Fig. 3.25).

In vivo, there are a number of important biologically active quaternary amines. The neurotransmitter acetyl choline is biosynthesised as shown in Figure 3.26.

Acetyl choline is a fixed non-pH dependent cation analogous to an inorganic cation such as K^+ or Na^+. Like all quaternary amines, it is charged at all pH values. Its positive charge attracts to negatively charged groups on proteins and it binds to such groups in the acetyl choline receptor that is a ligand-gated ion channel. Binding of acetyl choline causes the ion channel to open and allows the entry of Na^+ ions into the cell. Binding of acetyl choline requires both the charged and lipophilic portion of the molecule since its action is terminated by hydrolytic removal of the acetate portion of the molecule.

Quaternary ammonium salts with a single quaternary centre tend to be both water and fat soluble. Thus acetyl choline esterase inhibitor neostigmine bromide (Fig. 3.27) is both water soluble and moderately well absorbed from the GI tract, whereas polycationic quaternary amines such as gallamine triethiodide (Fig. 3.27) are much less lipophilic and have to be administered by injection. Apart from the role of long-chain quaternary amines as disinfectants, most quaternary amine drugs act on the cholinergic system either as acetyl choline esterase inhibitors or via direct actions on the acetyl choline receptor.

There is one important reaction of quaternary amines that has been exploited in drug design: the Hofmann elimination (Fig. 3.28). The reaction is promoted by strongly basic conditions and the more acidic a β-hydrogen atom the more readily the reaction occurs. Atracurium is based upon tubocurarine that was discovered as an arrow poison that paralyses muscles. Thus atracurium is used as a neuromuscular blocker that acts at the acetyl choline receptor and is used to relax muscles such as the abdominal muscles in preparation for surgery. The β-hydrogens in atracurium are particularly acidic and thus atracurium breaks down spontaneously at physiological pH and thus has a short duration of action and is less likely to produce cardiac side effects (see Ch. 16).

Q Self Test 3.5

Complete the reactions given below for various amine drugs.

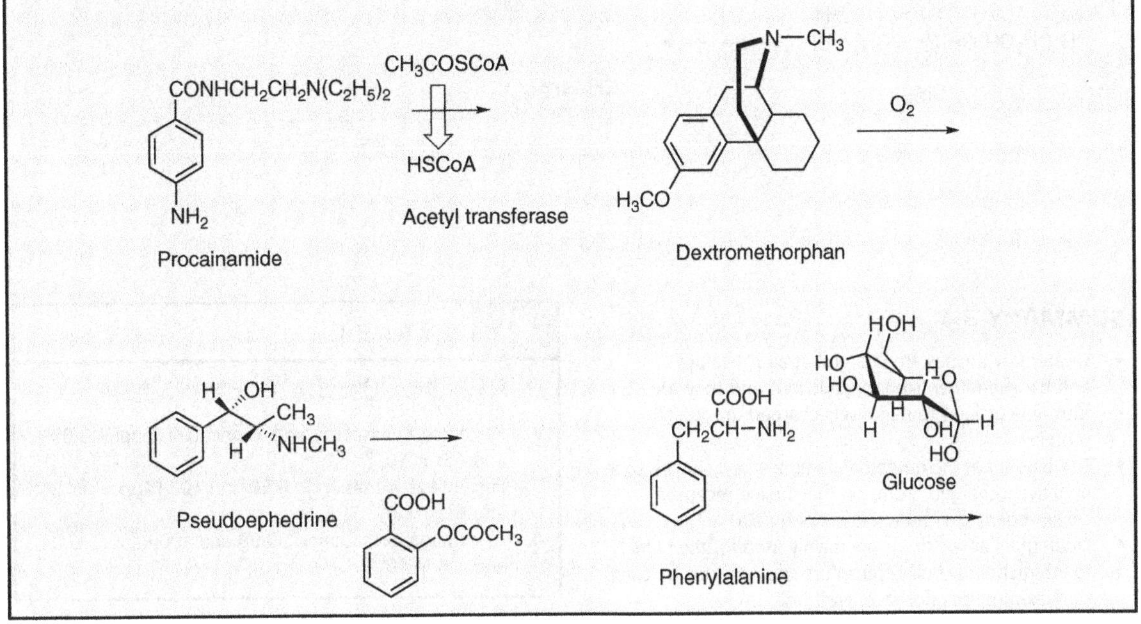

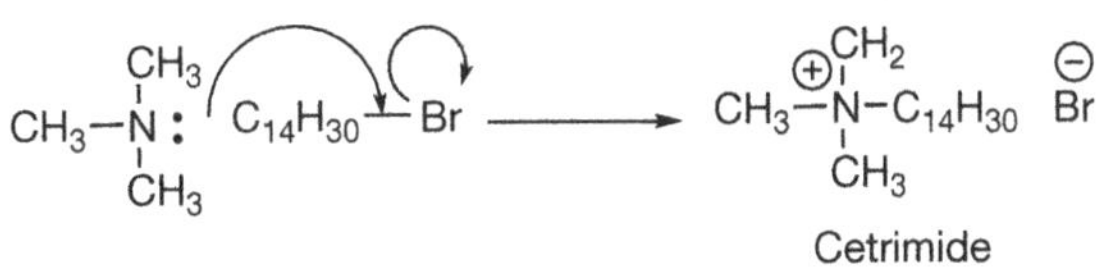

Figure 3.25 Quaternisation of a tertiary amine.

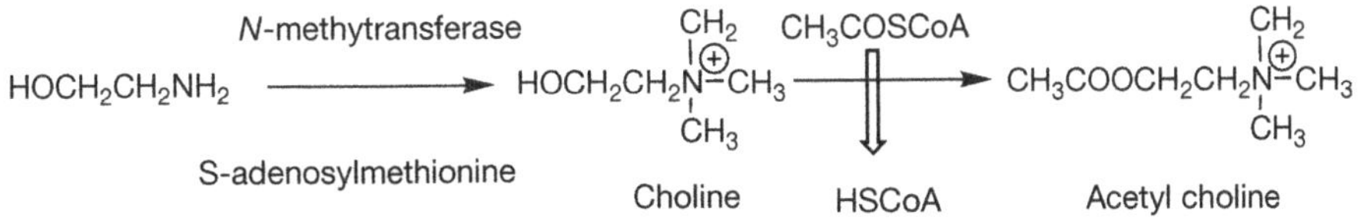

Figure 3.26 Biosynthesis of acetyl choline.

Figure 3.27 Drugs containing quaternary ammonium ions.

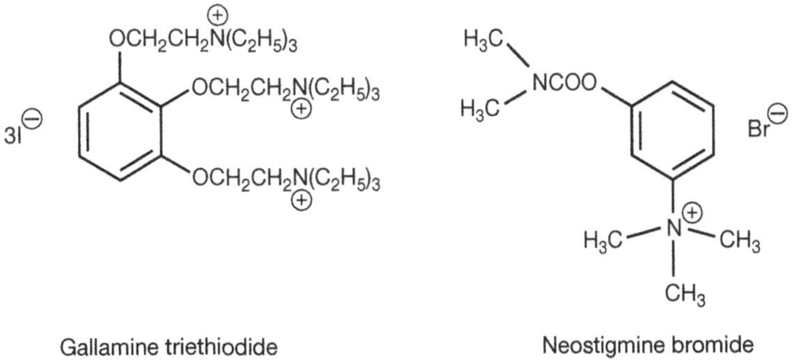

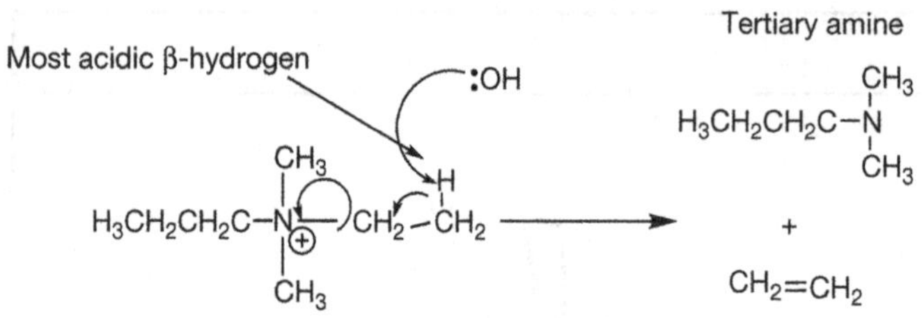

Figure 3.28 The Hofmann elimination.

SUMMARY 3.4

- Quaternary amines are charged at all pH values and behave rather like inorganic ions and they are thus able to bind to negatively charged groups on proteins.
- The binding of the quaternary amine acetyl choline to a negatively charged group on the choline receptor causes opening of an ion channel for Na^+.
- Quaternary amine drugs are mainly used for their ability to interact with choline receptors and can thus be used to relax muscles prior to operations.
- A particular reaction of quaternary amines, the Hofmann elimination, was used to determine the design of atracurium, a muscle relaxant which falls apart spontaneously and thus does not require metabolic elimination.

Q Self Test 3.6

Draw the mechanism for the Hofmann elimination for the atracurium analogue doxacurium chloride.

A Self Test 3.1

1. Percentage ionisation = 98.8 and 100 Papp = 0.12 and 4.6×10^{-8}
2. Percentage ionisation = 99.6 and 100 Papp = 0.099 and 4.0×10^{-8}
3. Percentage ionisation = 97.6 and 100 Papp = 15.8 and 6.3×10^{-5}.
4. Percentage ionisation = 99.98 and 100 Papp = 0.04 and 1.6×10^{-8}.

A Self Test 3.2

1. 7.4; 2. 9.6; 3. 0.5 and 9.4; 4. 9.4

A Self Test 3.3

a. A Pyrimidine, B Pyridine, C Imidazole, D Pyrazine, E Imidazoline, F *sym*-triazine, G Pyridine.
b. A 2, 6, 1. B 5, 9. C 7. D 0.5, 7. E 9. F 2, 6. G 9, 9.

A Self Test 3.4

Metformin – antidiabetic, debrisoquine – antihypertensive, chloroproguanil – antimalarial.

A Self Test 3.5

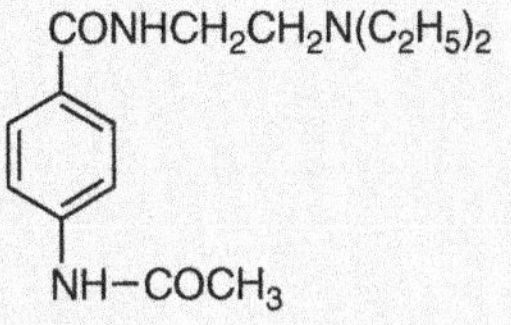

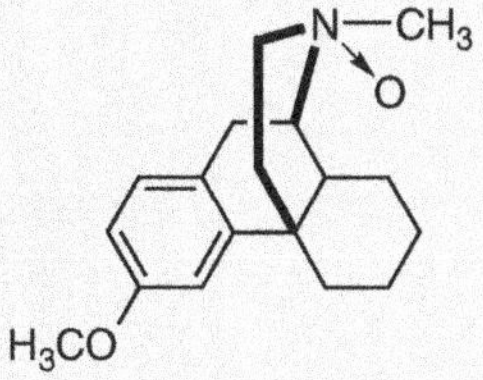

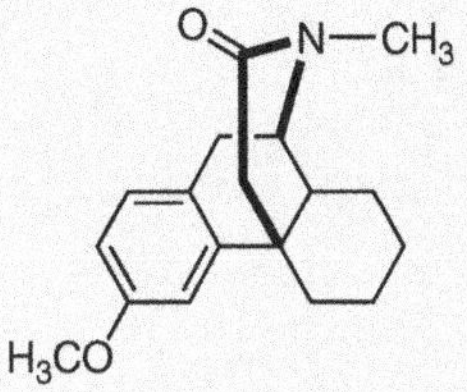

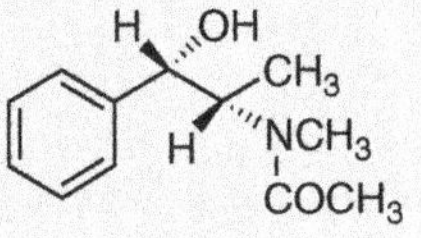

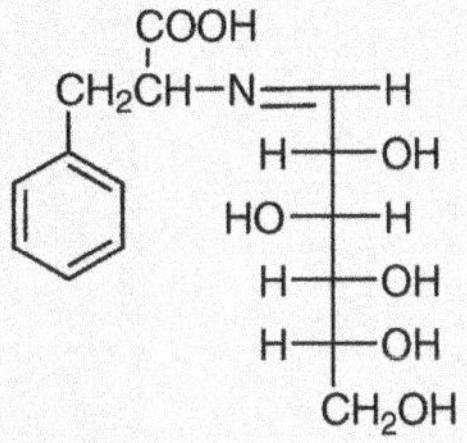

A Self Test 3.6

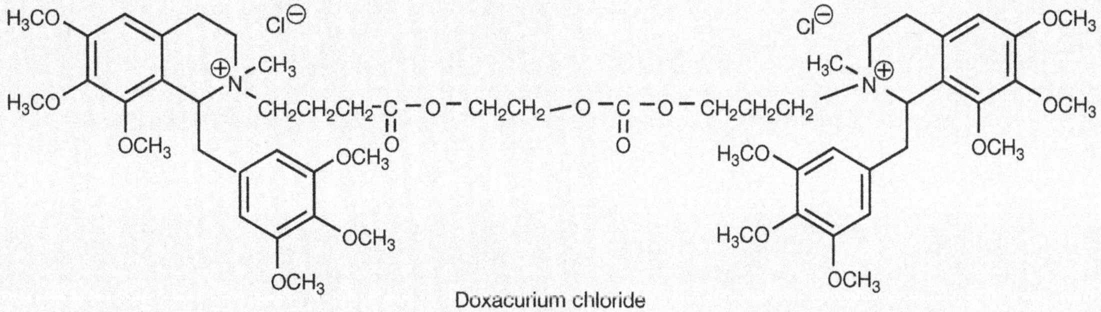

Doxacurium chloride

Chapter | 4 |

Neutral and acidic nitrogen compounds

Muhammed Hashem Alzweiri

CHAPTER CONTENTS

BARBITURATES

Introduction

The parent compound of barbiturates was firstly synthesised by Baeyer in 1864. The suffix (al) was added to the names because of the function similarity with the chloral hydrate and the latter is an aldehyde derivative. Most of the barbiturates have been largely replaced with benzodiazepines since the 1960s because of their addictive potential. Barbiturates bind with GABA-receptors. The 3-D structure of GABA-receptors has not been fully experimentally defined yet.

SUMMARY OF PHARMACOLOGY

- Gamma amino butyric acid (GABA) (Fig. 4.1) is an inhibitory neurotransmitter in the CNS. Its receptors can be activated by other chemicals e.g. barbiturates.
- Barbiturates bind with GABA-receptors and this prolongs the time of the chloride channel opening. Consequently the nerve polarisation is decreased.
- The inhibitory activity of barbiturates on the CNS is concentration dependent. At low doses, barbiturates are sedative (decreasing excitement), then hypnotic and anaesthetic. At high doses, barbiturates can block the respiratory centre in the brain and cause death.
- Generally, barbiturates were substituted with benzodiazepines because the latter have fewer side effects. However, phenobarbital is still used as an anticonvulsant drug and thiopental is used in general anaesthesia.
- Side effects: dependence and drug–drug interaction are the most serious side effects. Barbiturates can induce the Cyto P450 enzymes. This reduces the blood levels of the drugs via metabolism.

In the 1970s new types of GABA-receptors which could be stimulated by different drugs were discovered and named GABA-B receptors. Furthermore, GABA-C receptors were discovered as well. Hence, the GABA-receptor which was the first one discovered and which is stimulated by

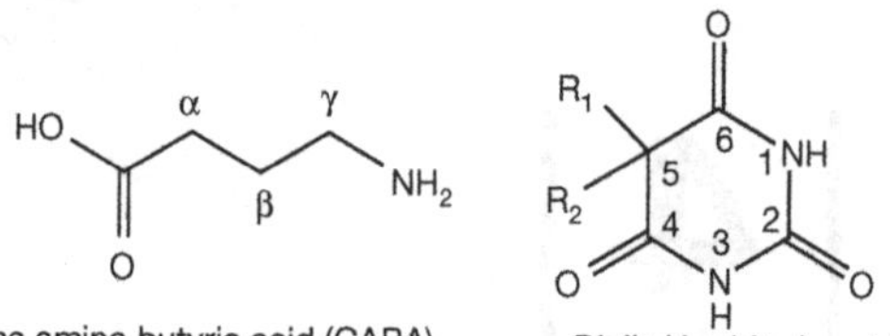

Gamma amino butyric acid (GABA)   Dialkyl barbituric acid

Figure 4.1 GABA and the general structure of barbiturates.

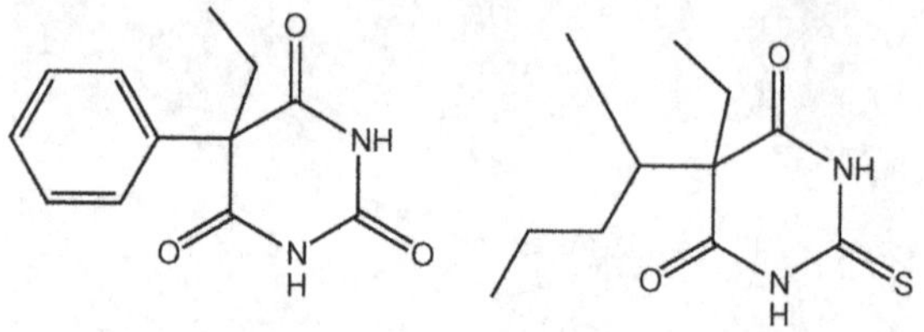

Phenobarbital
p*Ka* = 7.4
Log P = 1.47

Thiopental
p*Ka* = 7.4
Log P = 2.30

Figure 4.3 Examples of barbiturates.

barbiturates, and other agents like benzodiazepines, was distinguished by the name of the GABA-A receptor. In the 1980s GABA-receptors were firstly purified and the primary and secondary structures were determined. Barbiturates are derived from barbituric acid. They have a dialkyl barbituric acid form (see Fig. 4.1). They are dibasic acids (i.e. having two p*Ka* values). The first dissociation is the more significant one because it is stronger, p*Ka* = 7–8, while the second dissociation is extremely weak, p*Ka* = 11–12 (Fig. 4.2).

Phenobarbital and thiopental (Fig. 4.3) are still used in clinics. Phenobarbital is reserved for a serious type of epilepsy called status epilepticus, while thiopental is used in general anesthesia.

CALCULATION EXAMPLE 4.1

Phenobarbital has a p*Ka* = 7.4, calculate the ionised form ratio of it in the blood. (Physiological pH = 7.4.)

$$\text{pH} = \text{p}Ka + \text{Log}\frac{[\text{A}]}{[HA]} \rightarrow \text{Log}\frac{[\text{A}]}{[HA]} = 7.4 - 7.4 = zero$$

$$\frac{[A]}{[HA]} = 1 \rightarrow [A] = [HA]$$

So the ratio is 1:1.

Physiochemical properties

Barbiturates contain an imide group which has an acidic character because its conjugated base is stabilised by electron delocalisation (Fig. 4.4). The conjugation distributes the charge at different atoms in the structure and thus decreases the overall molecular energy. Unsubstituted barbiturates have a p*Ka* approximately 7 and for N-alkylated ones, the p*Ka* is around 8, because the alkyl group is an electron donating group and acidity is promoted by electron withdrawal. Thus barbiturates are weaker acids than acetic acid which has a p*Ka* = 4.8. However, their mid-range p*Ka* values enable barbiturates to be partially ionised at physiological pH (7.4). The ionised form is important to keep the drug soluble in the blood, while the non-ionised form facilitates the crossing of the blood–brain barrier.

Barbiturates can form sodium and potassium salts (Fig. 4.5). The negative charge is more stable on the large atoms like sulphur or oxygen.

Actually, barbituric acid and 5-alkyl barbituric acid are not pharmacologically active because they tautomerise to the more stable acid derivatives having a p*Ka* of approximately 4 and thus do not fit the receptor. The product is a trihydroxy pyrimidine derivative. It is more stable because the aromaticity of the ring formed is a strong driving force and this form is more thermodynamically favourable (Fig. 4.6).

Q Self Test 4.1

Calculate the non-ionised/ionised form ratio of trihydroxy pyrimide (p*Ka* = 4.0) in the physiological pH (7.4).

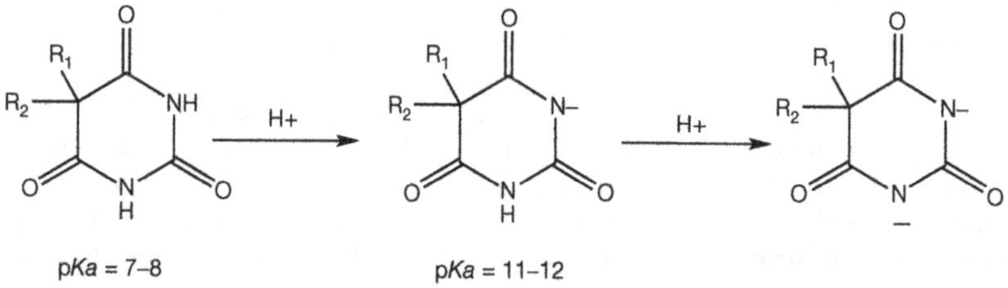

Figure 4.2 Ionisation of barbiturates.

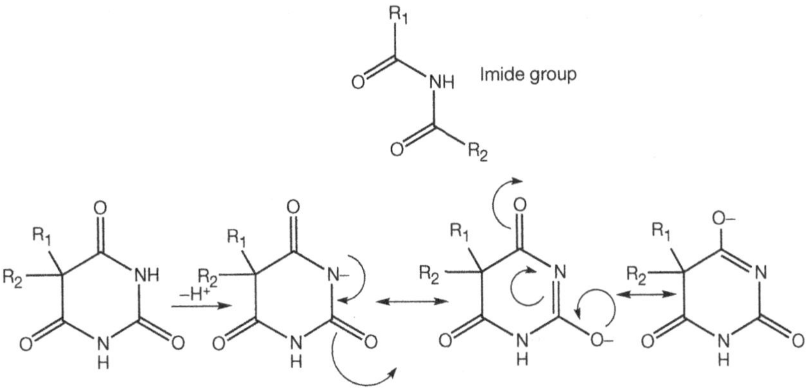

Figure 4.4 The imide group and resonance stabilisation of barbiturate anions.

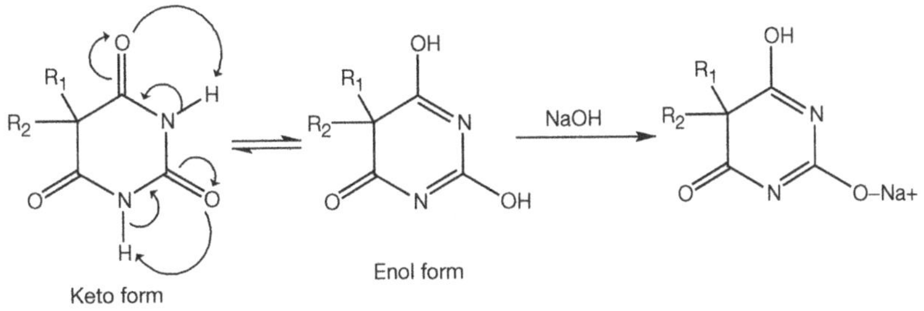

Figure 4.5 Formation of the sodium salt of a barbiturate.

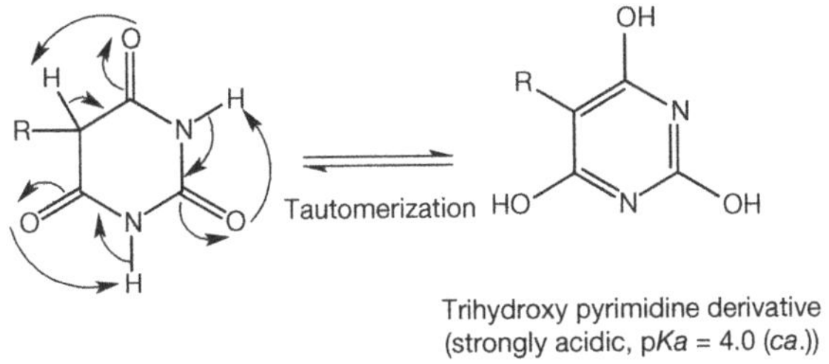

Figure 4.6 Barbituric acid and 5-alkyl barbituric acid tautomerisation.

GABA-A receptors

$GABA_A$ is a protein with a pentameric group of subunits (Fig. 4.7). Each subunit has approximately 200 amino acids. There are around four hydrophobic regions which enable the receptor to possess allosteric pockets for interactions, and the hydrophobic region is also important to anchor the protein into the cell membrane. Barbiturates bind with a site different from the site of binding of benzodiazepines, which bind at the active site rather than changing the receptor conformation via an allosteric interaction.

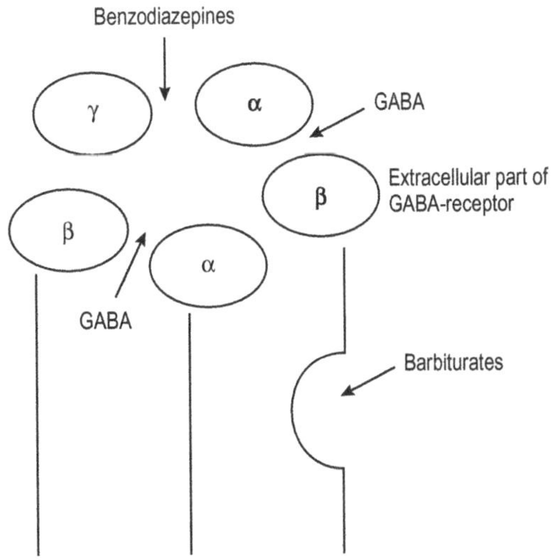

Figure 4.7 The GABA-A receptor.

Barbiturates structure–activity relationships

The barbiturate structure resembles that of hydantoins and dialkyl acetyl urea derivatives which are also neuroactive agents (Fig. 4.8). It is clear that the dialkyl substitution at position 5 of barbiturates is essential for their pharmacological activity. Also, if one or two hydrogens are left at position 5 of the barbiturate, the barbiturate will be converted to the trihydroxy pyrimidine derivative, as discussed earlier.

Substitution of carbonyl oxygen with sulphur atom increases the partition coefficient of the drug as in the case of thiopental. Increasing the lipophilicity of the drugs usually decreases their rate of elimination and prolongs their duration of action, but this is not the case for barbiturates. Long alkyl groups at position 5 of barbiturates increase the lipophilicity of barbiturates and this will increase the liver microsomal penetration of the drugs and consequently their metabolism. The lipophilic barbiturates also pass through the blood–brain barrier easily and this will achieve a rapid onset of action. Thiopental is quite lipophilic (log P = 2.3), so it is expected to have a short duration of action and it is used in general anaesthesia because of this character. Its pharmacological effect usually lasts to a maximum 30 minutes.

Metabolism of barbiturates

The main site of metabolism in the barbiturate structure is at the dialkyl substituents at position 5. They thus provide a good illustration of the types of metabolism which can occur to alkyl groups. Compounds containing a benzene ring, for example phenobarbital, are susceptible to epoxidation in phase I metabolism and to glutathione conjugation in phase II metabolism (Fig. 4.9).

Compounds containing an allyl group are susceptible to either olefinic or allylic oxidation (Figs 4.10, 4.11). Olefinic oxidation is mediated with an epoxidation step like the metabolism of secobarbital to secodiol. Allylic oxidation does not produce epoxide intermediates. The generated alcohol is conjugated with glucuronic acid in phase II metabolism in order to increase the compound hydrophilicity and consequently the urinary excretion. An example of

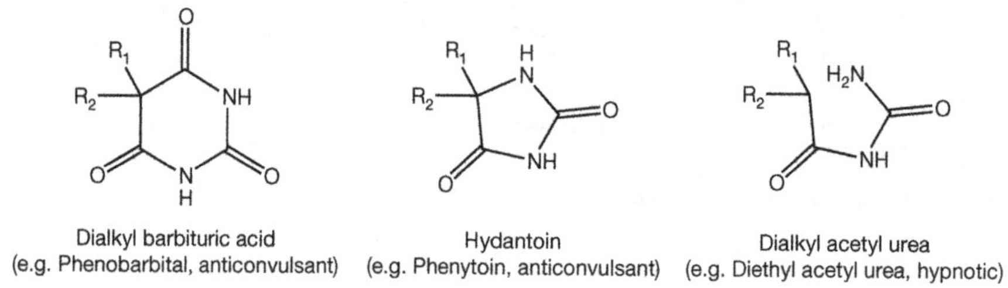

Figure 4.8 Barbiturate structure resembles that of the hydantoins and dialkyl acetyl urea derivatives.

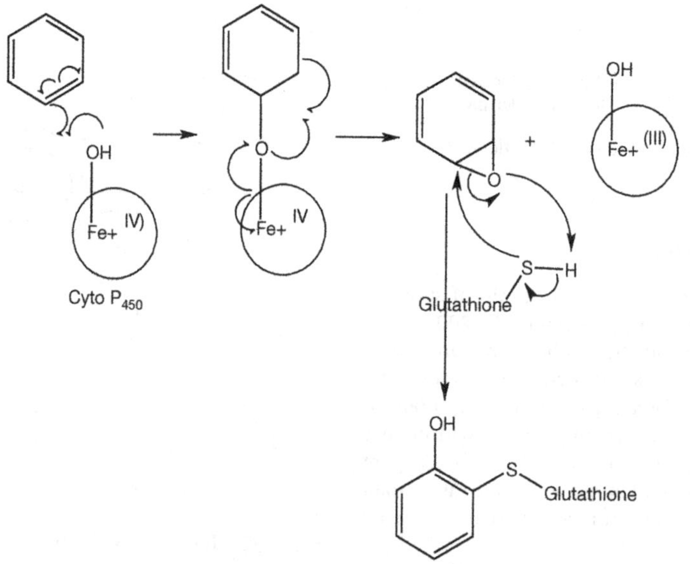

Figure 4.9 Aromatic ring metabolism in barbiturates.

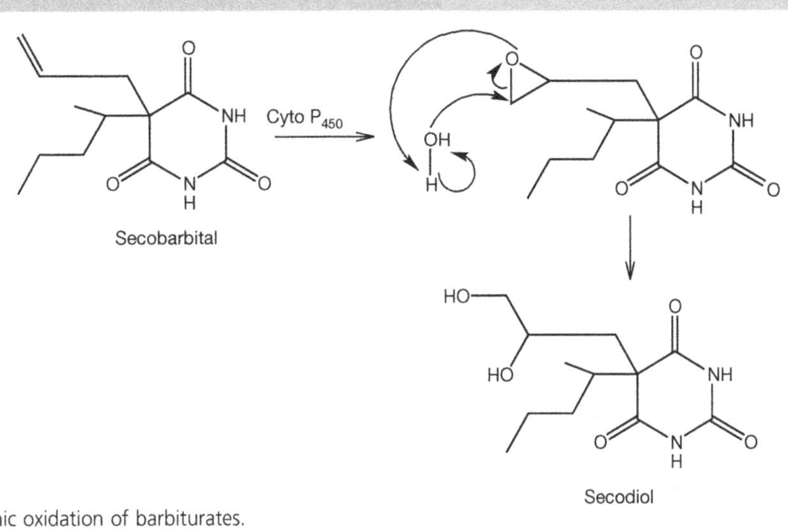

Figure 4.10 Olefinic oxidation of barbiturates.

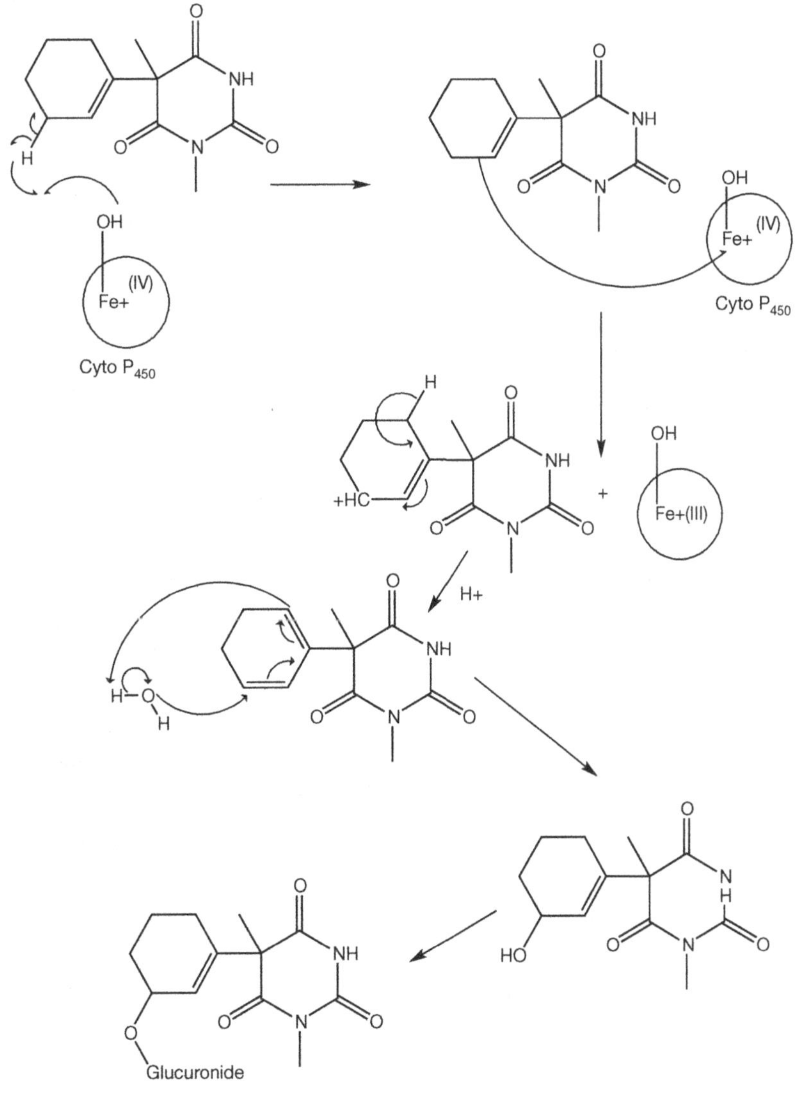

Figure 4.11 Allylic oxidation of barbiturates.

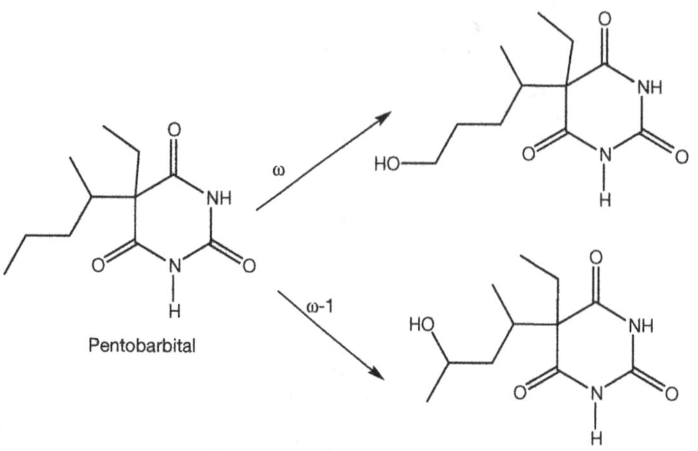

Figure 4.12 Oxidation of saturated alkyl groups of barbiturates.

this type of metabolism is the metabolism of hexobarbital. Saturated alkyl groups are also susceptible to the liver metabolism, mainly by ω oxidation (for the terminal carbon) or by ω-1 oxidation (for the carbon just before the terminal one). Pentobarbital is a good example of a barbiturate which undergoes this kind of oxidation (Fig. 4.12).

N-dealkylation is also possible. An example of this is the removal of the methyl at position 3 of hexobarbital. The heterocyclic ring of the barbiturates does not usually participate in their metabolism. However, cleavage of the (1–6) bond is possible and it produces malonyl urea derivatives.

Q Self Test 4.2

Predict two metabolic pathways by which the body can detoxify phenobarbital (Fig. 4.3).

SULPHONAMIDES

SUMMARY OF PHARMACOLOGY

- Folic acid is a vitamin essential for several biochemical pathways like DNA nucleotide synthesis.
- Humans take folic acid from dietary sources, while the majority of microbes synthesise it de novo.
- Sulphonamides block the pathway of folic acid synthesis and, consequently, the microbial proliferation.
- Other sulphonamides are used as hypoglycaemic agents. They increase the insulin secretion and inhibit the liver gluconeogenesis.
- Some sulphonamides can be used as diuretics since they are able to block carbonic anhydrase enzyme. This will increase the salt and the water retention in the urine.
- Side effects: crystalluria, haemolytic anaemia and hypersensitivity are the most serious side effects.

Introduction

The first reported use of sulphonamides was in 1933. Prontosil was the first agent of the sulphonamide family discovered. Domagk was awarded the Nobel Prize in 1938 because of his discovery of prontosil. Prontosil was active in vivo but not in vitro. This encouraged Trefouel to study this compound. He found that the compound is a prodrug requiring a reductive cleavage by the gut microflora in order to generate the active drug (sulfanilamide, Fig. 4.13). This discovery encouraged scientists to synthesise other sulphonamides. There were more than 4500 sulphonamides synthesised by 1948. However, many of them were not biologically active. Sulphonamides are analogues of para-amino benzoic acid (PABA). The latter is used in folic acid synthesis in microbes. Because of this similarity, sulphonamides block the pathway of the folic acid synthesis. Subsequently, they arrest DNA synthesis and exert a bacteriostatic effect (stopping cell proliferation). Sulphonamides are also used as oral hypoglycaemic agents (tolbutamide, Fig. 4.14) and diuretics (furosemide, Fig. 4.14).

Physiochemical properties

Sulphonamides contain the sulphamido group which has an acidic character because the sulphonyl part is electron withdrawing and the conjugated base is stabilised by electron delocalisation (Fig. 4.15). Substitution of the sulphamido nitrogen with an electron withdrawing group like acetyl or a heterocycle increases the acidity of the sulphamido group (Fig. 4.16). For example, acetyl substitution as in sulfacetamide (Fig. 4.17) produces four resonance forms instead of three, adding additional stability to the ionised form. This means that a further stabilisation of the ionised form occurs and sulfacetamide is one of the most acidic of the sulphonamides. Sulphonamides have also an aniline functionality which is considered as a very weak base (p*Ka* *ca.* 2) because the lone pair of electrons is involved in the resonance of the aromatic system (Fig. 4.18).

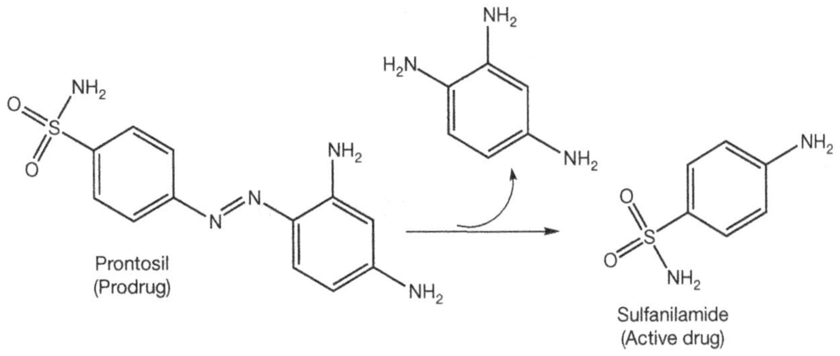

Figure 4.13 Reductive cleavage of Prontosil by gut microflora.

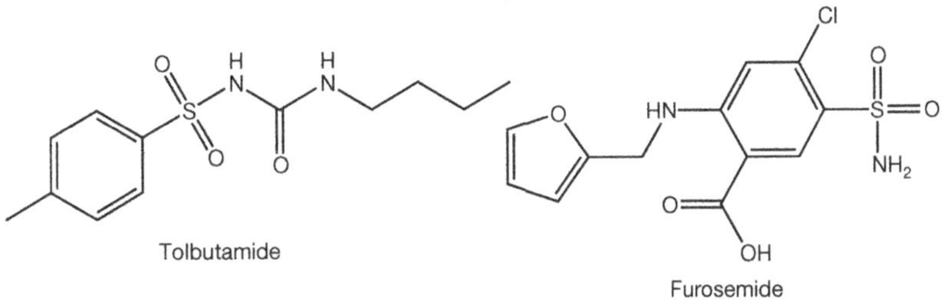

Figure 4.14 Sulphonamides used as hypoglycaemic and diuretic agents.

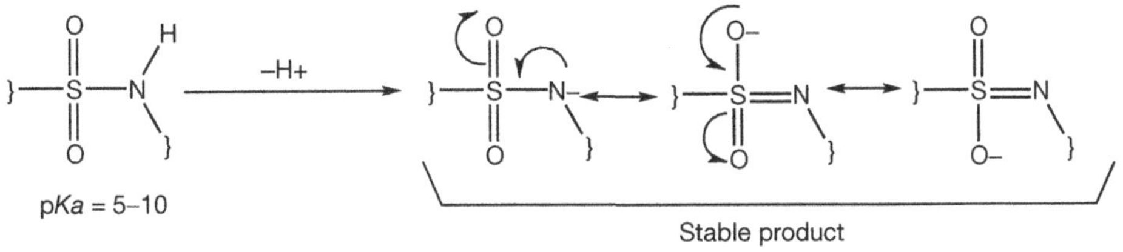

Figure 4.15 Acidity of sulphonamides.

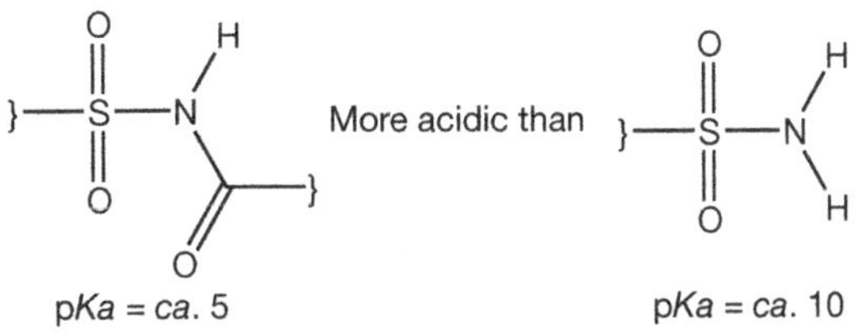

Figure 4.16 Acetyl substitution of sulphonamide group increase the sulphonamide acidity.

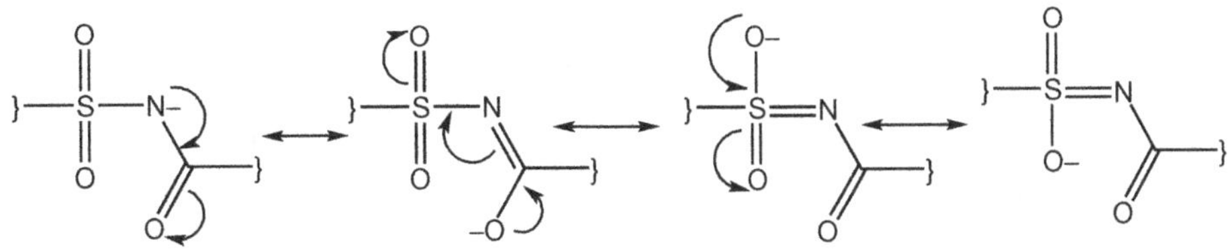

Figure 4.17 Resonance stabilisation of conjugate base of acetyl sulphamido group.

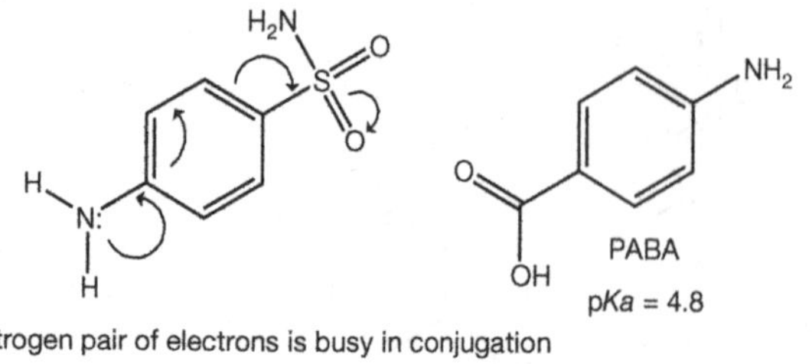

Figure 4.18 Structure similarity between sulphonamides and PABA.

Sulphonamides have to be partially un-ionised to enable penetration of the cell membrane of the microbial cell. Thus the antimicrobial activity is increased with an increase in the p*Ka* value of the drug up to the point where the degree of penetration into the microbial cells is hindered by the extent of low ionisation of the drug in physiological fluids. It was found that the ionised form of a sulphonamide has the antimicrobial activity because of its ability to accumulate inside the microbial cell and its close similarity to PABA (Fig. 4.18) which has an acidic p*Ka* = 4.8 and is totally ionised at the physiological pH. In addition, low p*Ka* sulphonamides (e.g. sulfisoxazole, p*Ka* = 5.0, Fig. 4.19) are fully ionised at physiological pH and are consequently excreted rapidly in the urine. Thus these agents can be used for the urinary tract infections.

Most sulphonamides are well absorbed orally except for a few of them, e.g. sulphadiazine. Such agents are reserved for gastrointestinal tract infections or for skin infections. Silver sulphadiazine (Fig. 4.20) is poorly absorbed through the skin so it is used as a topical antimicrobial. Sulphonamides with relatively high p*Ka* values are quite lipophilic at the physiological pH. This increases their binding with plasma protein and also facilitates their accumulation in adipose tissue. Consequently, this prolongs the duration of action of these agents.

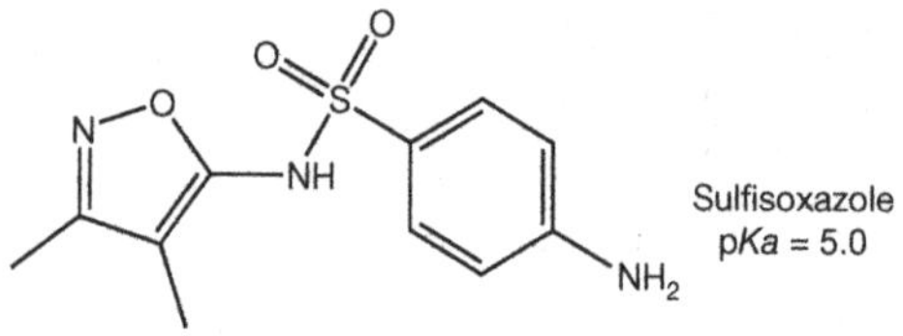

Figure 4.19 Sulfisoxazole structure.

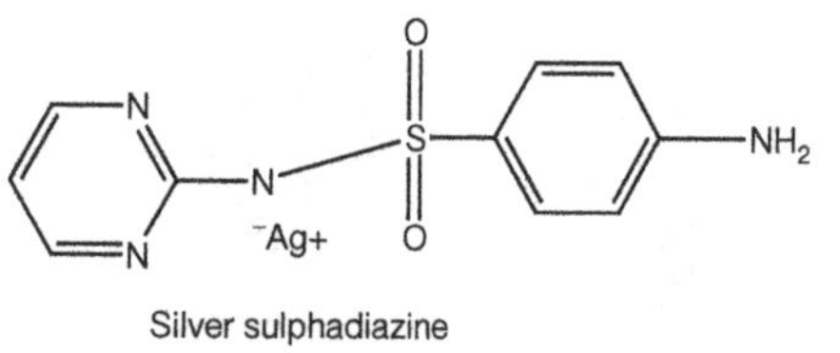

Figure 4.20 Silver sulphadiazine structure.

Q Self Test 4.3

Justify Prontosil antimicrobial activity *in vivo* but not *in vitro*.

Mechanism of action

In mammalian cells, folic acid can not be synthesised de novo but it should be taken from dietary sources. While most microbes are not able to take folic acid from the surrounding environment, they instead synthesise it de novo. Folic acid produces derivatives of tetrahydrofolate (FAH_4), playing an essential role in the biochemical reactions involving a one carbon transfer process such as methylation of uracil (Fig. 4.21). Lack of folic acid disturbs many pathways, such as nucleic acid synthesis and amino acid synthesis. Impairing the synthesis of DNA stops cell division and consequently cell multiplication.

Sulphonamides resemble PABA, so they block dihydropteroate synthase (Fig. 4.22), which is an important enzyme in the folic acid synthesis pathway inside the microbial cell. Microbes can resist sulphonamides by increasing the synthesis of PABA, decreasing the permeability of their membranes to sulphonamides or by promoting active efflux of sulphonamides out of the microbial cell. For resistant species, sulphonamides might be mixed with other antimicrobial agents such as trimethoprim. The combination of sulfamethoxazole and trimethoprim produces a synergism (the antimicrobial activity of the combination is more than the additional activity of two independent antimicrobials). Trimethoprim can block the dihydrofolate reductase enzyme in the folic acid pathway which catalyses the conversion of dihydrofolate (FAH_2) to tetrahydrofolate (FAH_4) while sulfamethoxazole competes with PABA. The combination therapy is suitable for more resistant microbes.

Q Self Test 4.4

Justify the ability of sulphonamides in inhibiting the folic acid synthesis.

Some of the sulphonamides can be used as diuretics. The mechanism of their action relates to carbonic acid excretion. Carbon dioxide generated from catabolic processes is carried to the lung and then removed by exhalation. However, part of the carbon dioxide is still dissolved in the blood. The dissolved carbon dioxide produces carbonic acid and its conjugated base (i.e. bicarbonate). This mixture of the weak acid and its conjugate base is one of the important buffer systems in the blood. The dissolved carbon dioxide is excreted in the urine. The processes of the conversion of carbon dioxide to carbonic acid and then

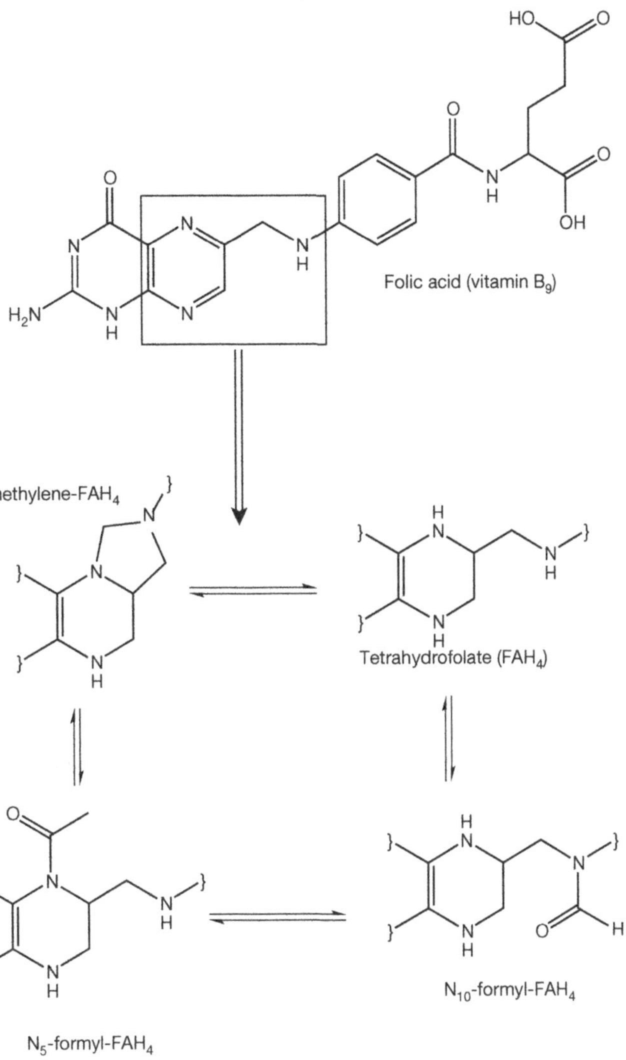

Figure 4.21 Biologically active forms of folic acid.

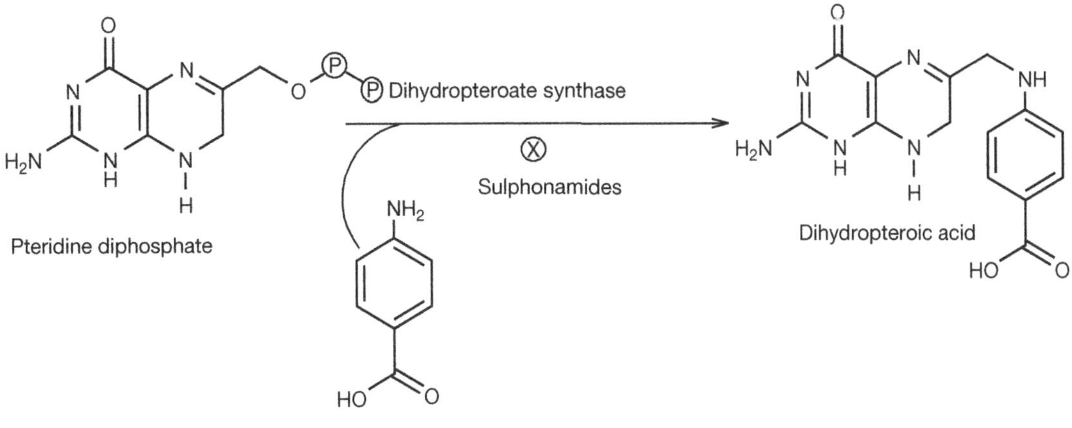

Figure 4.22 Sulphonamides block folic acid synthesis by inhibiting dihydropteroate synthase enzyme.

$$CO_2 + H_2O \longleftrightarrow \underset{\substack{\text{Carbonic anhydrase} \\ \text{(X) by Acetazolamide}}}{} H_2CO_3 \longleftrightarrow H^+ + HCO_3^-$$

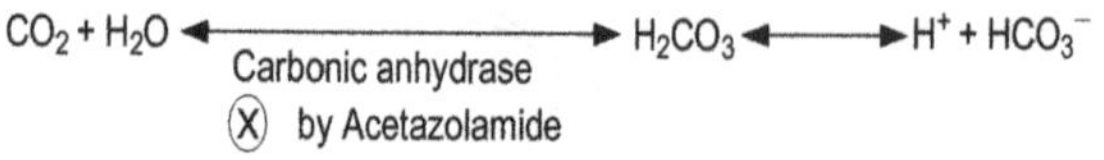

Figure 4.23 Diuretic mechanism of acetazolamide by inhibition of carbonic anhydrase enzyme.

to bicarbonate are reversible processes, so there is no big thermodynamic favouritism for one of them over the others (Fig. 4.23). These conversions occur normally with a reasonable speed if no catalytic enzyme is available. However, the carbonic anhydrase enzyme speeds up the conversion process. Carbonic anhydrase is abundant in the epithelial tissue of the proximal part of the renal filtration units (i.e. the tubules). The activity of the enzyme increases the concentration of the ionised species (bicarbonate and protons). This process increases the osmotic pressure of the urine filtrate and the urine volume if there is no secretion and reabsorption processes in the proximal tubules counteract this effect. There is electrical voltage across the urinary tubules because the difference in the electrolyte distribution. Differences in the electrolyte distribution generate an electrical field force for negative ions such as bicarbonate to be reabsorbed by the body and for protons to be secreted in the urine (Fig. 4.24). If carbonic anhydrase is inhibited, then most of the dissolved carbon dioxide can reach the distal tubules without being converted into carbonic acid. In the distal tubules there is no significant absorption and secretion except for sodium and water. So the dissolved carbon dioxide slowly becomes hydrated and produces bicarbonate and protons. This increases the osmotic pressure of the urine in the distal tubules and decreases water reabsorption by the body. Consequently, the volume of the urine is increased and diuretic action is established. Carbonic anhydrase forms carbonic acid with a help of a metal which can be considered a co-factor (Fig. 4.25). Sulphonamide can block the carbonic anhydrase enzyme by the reaction between the sulphamido group and the enzyme amine functionality (Fig. 4.26). Acetazolamide (Fig. 4.27) is an example of sulphonamide having a diuretic effect.

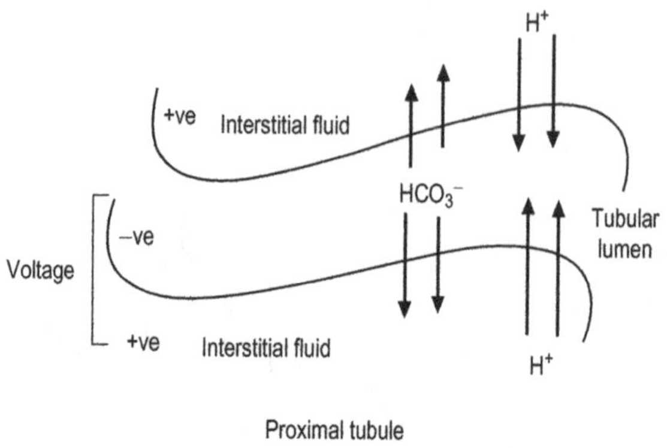

Figure 4.24 Proximal tubules are the site of carbonic anhydrase inhibition by acetazolamide.

The mechanism of action of hypoglycaemic sulphonamides is not fully understood. They have several targets. Maybe the most important ones are in decreasing liver gluconeogenesis and promoting insulin secretion from β-cells in the pancreas. It is proposed that a shortage of insulin decreases the glucose level inside the body's cells, including the β-cells. The shortage of glucose inside the β-cells decreases energy metabolites so the ATP/ADP ratio is decreased. This closes potassium efflux channels and changes the electrical polarisation of β-cells. This electrical change stimulates calcium channels, allowing calcium influx into the β-cells. Accumulation of calcium in the cell is considered as an internal messenger and induces the exocytosis of insulin vesicles and thus insulin secretion.

Sulphonamides structure–activity relationships

The optimum antimicrobial activity of sulphonamides is obtained wherever the sulphonamide group is in a para position relative to the amino group. The amino group (at N4 position, Fig. 4.28) should remain primary to be

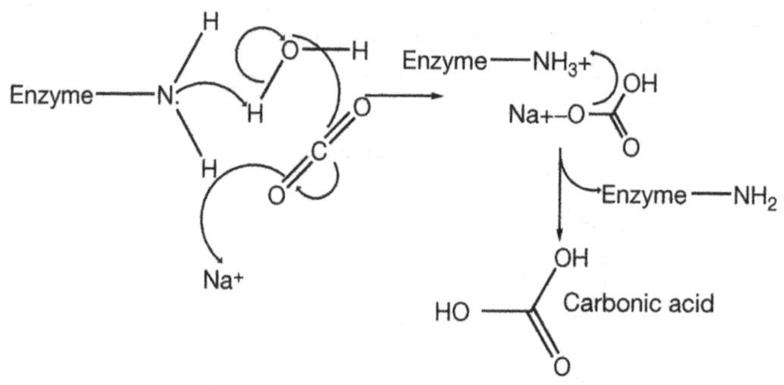

Figure 4.25 Catalytic mechanism of carbonic enzyme in producing carbonic acid from water and carbon dioxide.

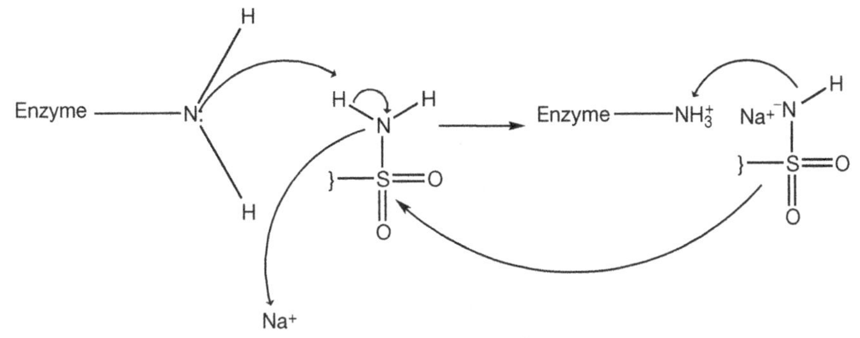

Figure 4.26 Mechanism of inhibition of carbonic anhydrase enzyme by diuretic sulphonamides.

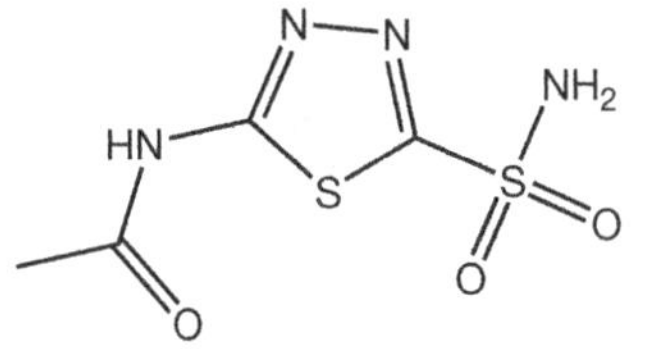

Acetazolamide

Figure 4.27 Acetazolamide structure.

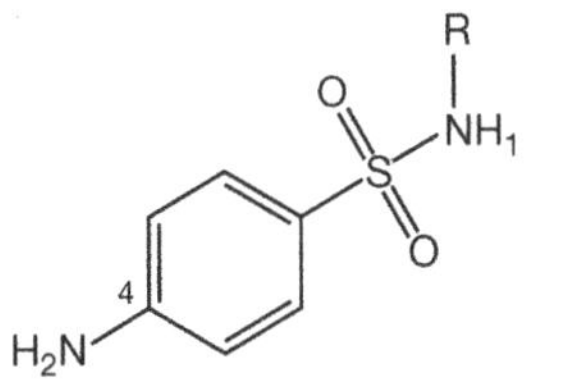

Figure 4.28 N4 nitrogen should remain free for obtaining optimum antimicrobial activity of sulphonamides.

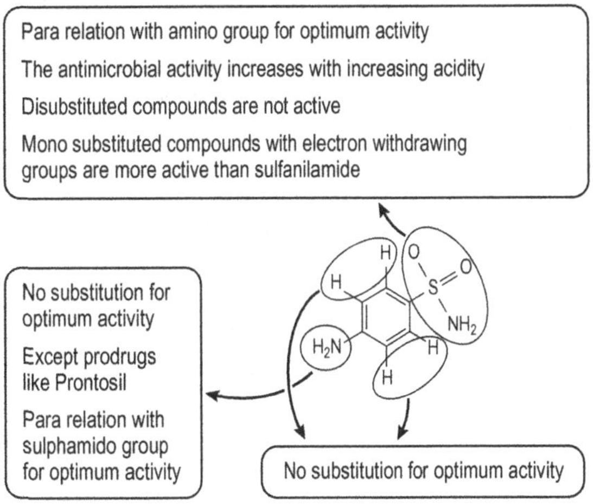

Figure 4.29 Structure–activity relationship of antimicrobial sulphonamides.

active enough for the nucleophilic attack on the pteridin diphosphate.

Sulphonamides with unsubstituted ortho and meta positions are more active than ones substituted on these positions because the unsubstituted sulphonamides resemble PABA. The substitution of the sulphamido group at N^1 position with an electron withdrawing group such as a heterocycle increases the antimicrobial activity because this increases the acidity of the drug (until p$Ka \approx 5.0$) and consequently the similarity to PABA in terms of acidity. This information is summarised in Figure 4.29. Sulphonamides which are used as oral hypoglycaemic agents (Fig. 4.30) do not require the substitution at position 4 to be a primary amine. It can be any small group such as methyl or chlorine. However, substitution of large groups at this position decreases the hypoglycaemic activity. It was found that the modification of the first-generation sulphonamides by introducing the carbonyl amido part to obtain a derivative of urea (called sulphonylurea) increased the hypoglycaemic activity. Reserving the distance between

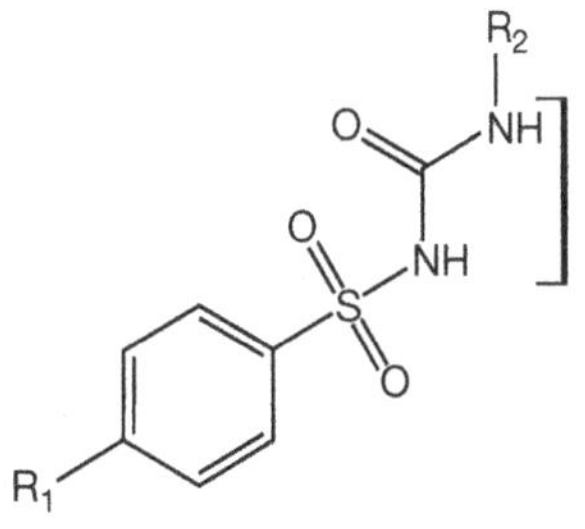

Figure 4.30 Sulfonylurea derivative of sulphonamides used as hypoglycaemic agents.

two nitrogens of urea gives optimum activity. Activity is greatest if the R_2 group is quite lipophilic and larger than R_1 (e.g. a propyl or butyl group), e.g. the group is propyl in chlorpropamide (Fig. 4.31). The optimal diuretic action of sulphonamides requires an unsubstituted sulphamido group at the N^1 position, e.g. acetazolamide and furosemide (Fig. 4.32).

Metabolism of sulphonamides

The amino group at position 4 of sulphonamide is a nucleophile and this reactivity can lead to toxicity in the human body. However, the body protects itself by blocking this group with an acetyl group (Fig. 4.33). The acetyl group is produced in the body from catabolic processes such as fat burning. There is a common interindividual variability among people with respect to rate at which they acetylate such groups. There are fast acetylators who detoxify sulphonamides quickly and slow acetylators who are more at risk of sulphonamide toxicity. Acetylation is not like the majority of phase II conjugation reactions since it decreases the water solubility of the compound instead of increasing it because it is a lipophilic group and it converts the polar amine to a less polar amide. This can lead to drug crystallisation in the urine and generates a side effect called crystalluria. This problem can be solved by using sulphonamides with a p*Ka* equal to or less than the urine pH (approximately 6.0) such as sulfisoxazole (p*Ka* = 5.0) or sulfamethoxazole (p*Ka* = 6.1, Fig. 4.34). This means that the acetylated metabolite is significantly ionised at the pH values of urine. For weakly acidic sulphonamides such as sulfanilamide (p*Ka* = 10.4), alkalisation of the urine is required. This can be achieved by administering sodium bicarbonate or another safe alkalising agent.

If the amino group is modified by an alkyl group such as methyl in the case of oral hypoglycaemic agents, the alkyl group undergoes ω-oxidation. An example of this is in tolbutamide metabolism (Fig. 4.35). However, substituting the alkyl group at position 4 with a halogen increases the duration of action because it is less susceptible to the liver metabolism. Tolbutamide has a plasma half life of *ca.* 7 hours whereas chlorpropamide (see Fig. 4.31) has a plasma half life of *ca.* 35 hours.

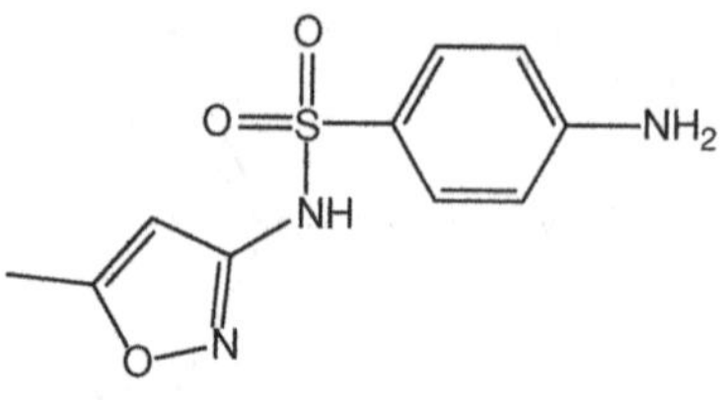
Sulfamethoxazole
p*Ka* = 6.1

Figure 4.34 Sulfamethoxazole structure.

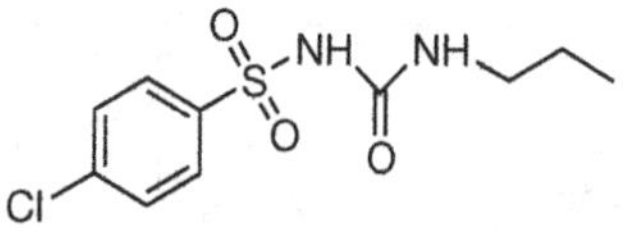
Chlorpropamide

Figure 4.31 Example of hypoglycaemic sulphonamide.

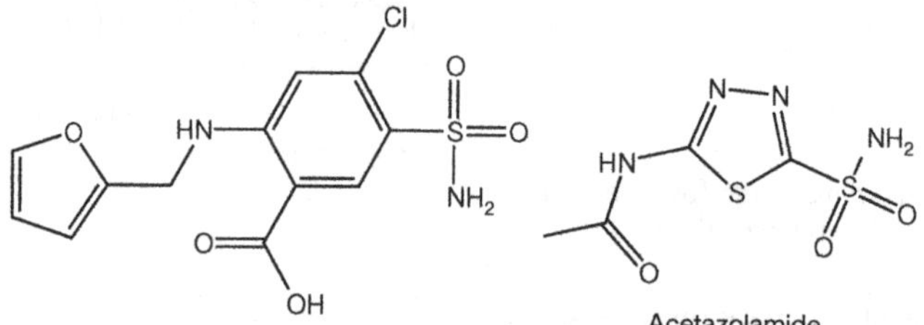
Furosemide
Acetazolamide

Figure 4.32 Examples of diuretic sulphonamides.

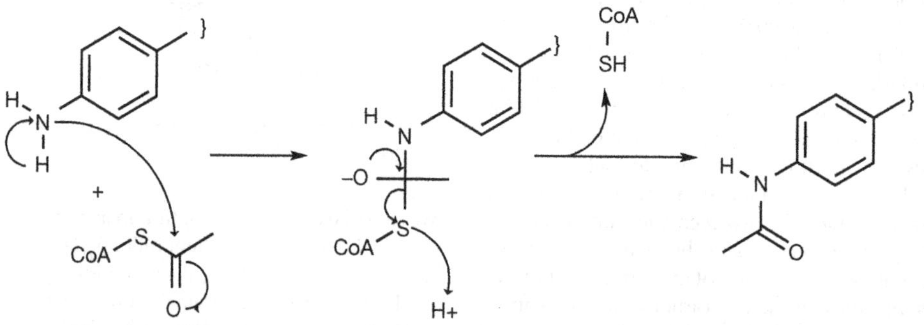

Figure 4.33 Acetylation metabolism of reactive N4 group of sulphonamides.

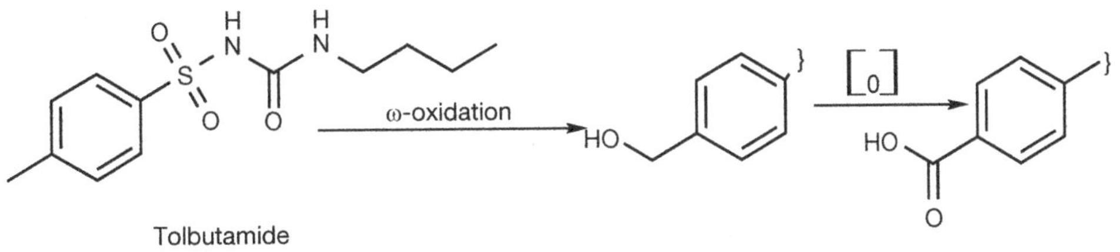

Figure 4.35 Metabolic oxidation of tolbutamide.

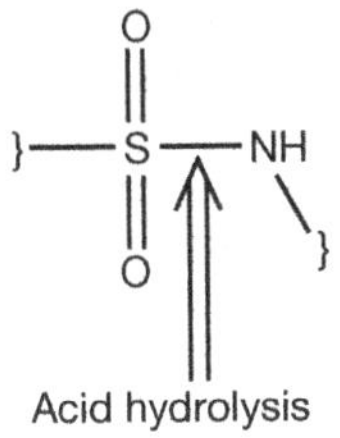

Figure 4.36 Sulphamido group is susceptible to acid hydrolysis.

Chemical stability of sulphonamides

Breakdown of the sulphamido group does not occur in alkaline solutions, but strong acids can degrade it (Fig. 4.36). Sulphonamides are generally photosensitive because of the reactivity of the primary amine at position 4. This group is oxidised under the catalytic action of light to produce diazo dimers.

However, the diazo dimer is still susceptible to further oxidation. This leads to the oxidation of the benzene ring (Fig. 4.37). Protecting the sulphonamide solution from exposure to the light is essential; addition of antioxidant as sodium metabisulfite is also important. Sulphonamides undergo a hydrolysis reaction at the amide bond at high temperatures, so sulphonamide aqueous products are not autoclavable unless they are dissolved in other solvents such as propylene glycol. Sterile products of sulphonamides can also be dissolved in previously sterilised water. In addition, aqueous solutions of sulphonamides should be free from carbon dioxide because the dissolved carbon dioxide produces carbonic acid which catalyses the hydrolytic degradation of sulphonamides.

METHYL XANTHINES

SUMMARY OF PHARMACOLOGY

- Methyl xanthenes such as caffeine have several mechanisms of actions. One of the most important of them is the inhibition of phosphodiesterase enzyme and inhibition of adenosine receptors.

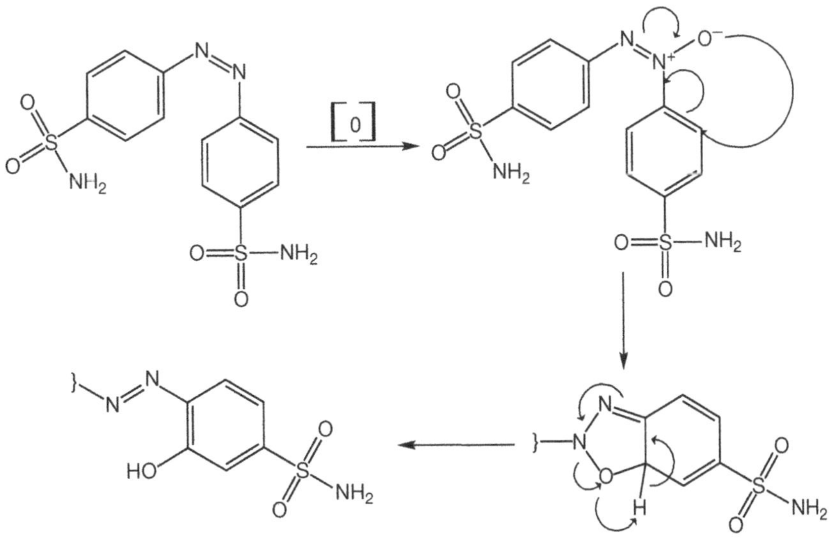

Figure 4.37 Diazo oxidation of sulphonamides.

- They have stimulant effect on the CNS, they increase the heart rate, they have a mild diuretic action, they dilate the lung bronchi and they increase the gastric hydrochloric acid secretion.
- They pass the blood–brain barrier and the placenta. They are also secreted in breast milk.
- Side effects: insomnia (lack of sleeping) and cardiac arrhythmias are the most serious side effects.

Introduction

The history of the xanthine alkaloids (Fig. 4.38) goes back to ancient times when their plant sources were discovered. Caffeine was extracted from tea, coffee and cocoa; theophylline was mainly found in tea extract, while theobromine was found in cocoa extract. Methyl xanthines are considered as very weak bases with p*Ka* values <1. They are classified as alkaloids (alkali-like compounds) although they are not really classical alkaloids. For example, theophylline (Fig. 4.39) is a strong enough acid (p*Ka* = 8.8) to be dissociated in a weak base such as ammonia (p*Ka* of ammonia = 9.25). Theobromine (Fig. 4.40) is weaker acid than theophylline and thus it requires stronger bases, such as sodium hydroxide, for it to be ionised. However, caffeine (Fig. 4.41) lacks acidic character because it has no exchangeable protons, so it is not soluble even in sodium hydroxide solution. This makes caffeine more lipophilic than theophylline and thus it has greater action on the CNS, whereas theophylline is used mainly in the peripheral system as a bronchodilator. Caffeine and the other methyl xanthines are much more soluble in hot water than cold water.

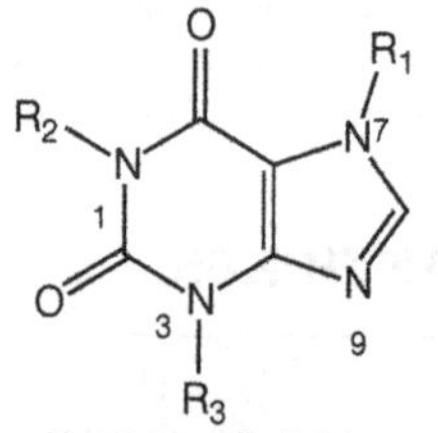

Figure 4.38 Xanthine alkaloid structure.

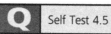

Self Test 4.5

Imidazole ring in theophylline has sp2 and sp3 nitrogen, which of them is basic and why?

Physiochemical properties

Methyl xanthines are derivatives of pyrrole and pyridine (Fig. 4.42).

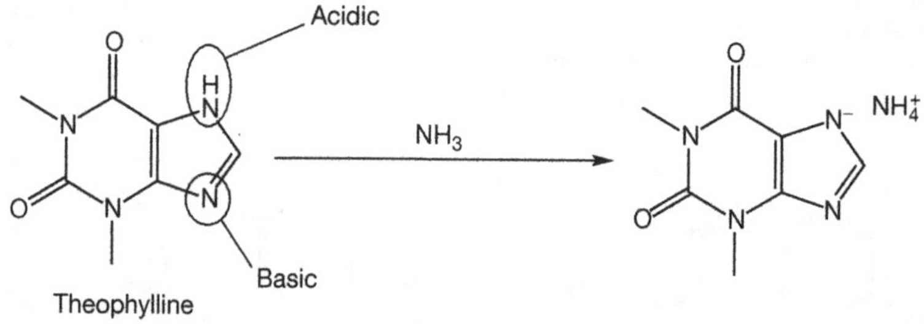

Figure 4.39 Theophylline acidic character.

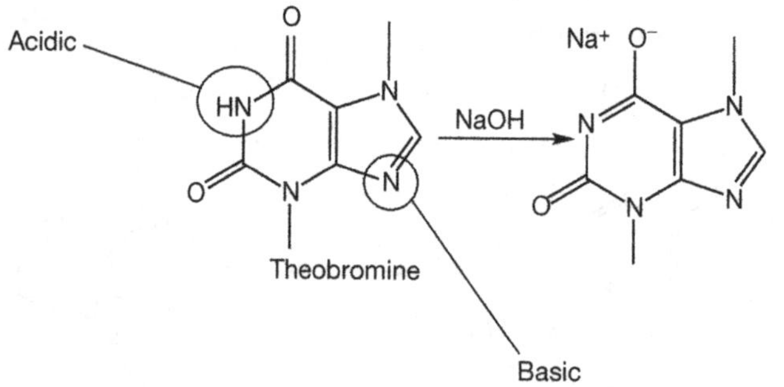

Figure 4.40 Theobromine is a weak acid.

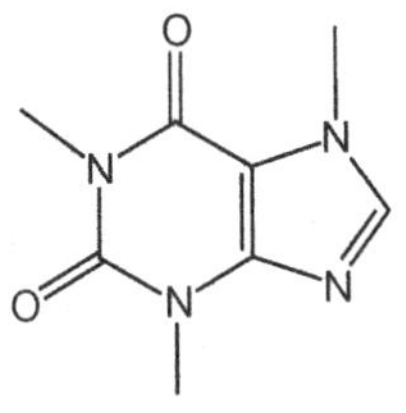

Figure 4.41 Caffeine structure.

Pyridine is a weakly basic compound (pKa = 5.2). Huckel theory defines an aromatic ring as having (4n+2) pi-electrons where n is 0,1,2,3.... Thus aromatic rings have two pi-electrons but not three also they have six electrons but not five and so on. Pyridine has three pi-bonds so it has six electrons. Consequently, the lone pair of electrons on the nitrogen is not part of the ring sextet (the six pi-electrons). However, pyrrole obviously has two double bonds (4 pi-electrons) so it is impossible to have (n = 0) in the Huckel rule, also if n = 2 then pyrrole should have 10 pi-electrons and these are too much for a small ring. Thus the only possibility is when n = 1 (equivalent to 6 pi-electrons), but pyrrole has only two double bonds so the lone pair of electrons on the nitrogen is part of the ring sextet and it is not available to bond with protons. From this point of view, pyrrole has no basic character. Pyrrole can be considered neutral or a very weak acid because the conjugated base is stabilised by resonance (Fig. 4.43).

Pyrrole acidity is quite weak and is almost equivalent to the acidity of acetylene. It requires a strongly basic alkali, stronger than sodium hydroxide such as sodamide to be ionised (Fig. 4.44).

Mechanism of action

There are several targets for the methylxanthines in the human body. The most common two are phosphodiesterase enzyme inhibition and adenosine receptor inhibition.

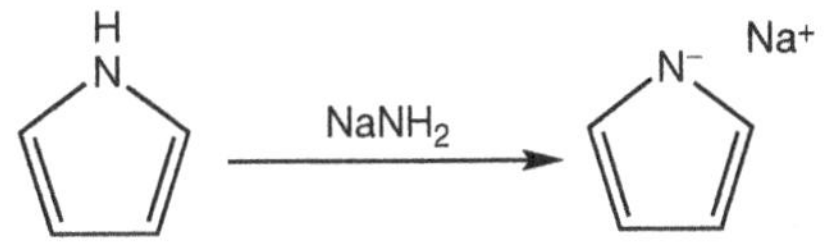

Figure 4.44 Pyrrole reacts with strong bases such as sodamide.

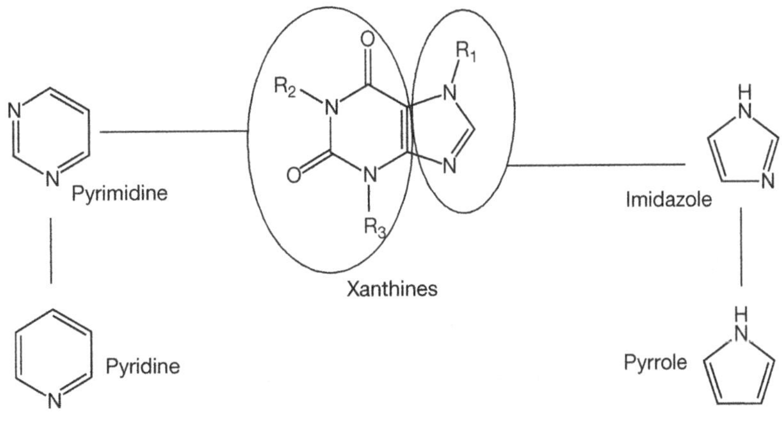

Figure 4.42 Methyl xanthines are derivatives of pyrrole and pyridine.

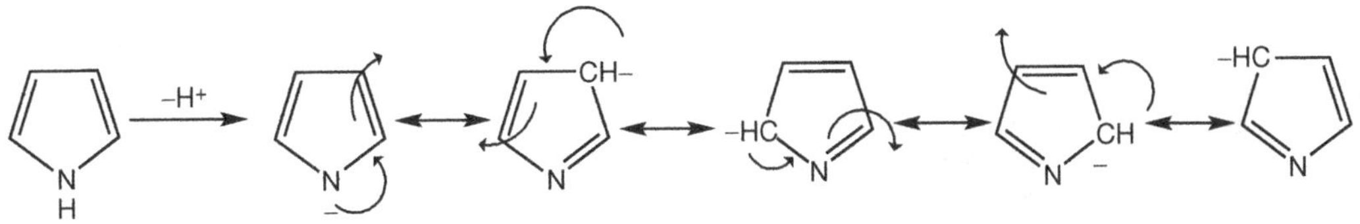

Figure 4.43 Pyrrole is a very weak acid.

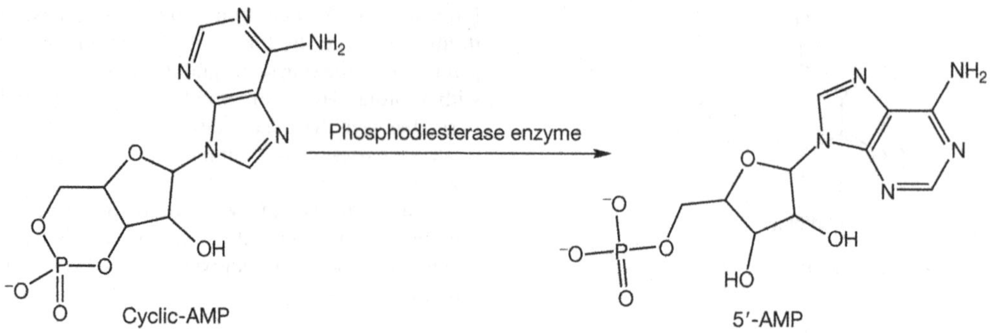

Figure 4.45 cAMP is deactivated by phosphodiesterase enzyme.

Some endogenous metabolites and some drugs such as sympathomimetics (e.g. adrenaline) trigger the secretion of intracellular second messengers such as cyclic-AMP in order to complete their pharmacodynamic action with no need for them to enter the cell. Subsequently, cAMP is deactivated by phosphodiesterase (Fig. 4.45) in order to terminate the pharmacological action of the sympathomimetics. Methylxanthines inhibit phosphodiesterase enzyme and consequently prolong the action of cAMP. This explains some of the sympathomimetic-like actions of methylxanthines such as increasing the heart rate. Methylxanthines can also increase cGMP, which is used by the body as a second messenger as well. This is also due to the inhibition of the family of phosphodiesterase enzymes. A second important mechanism of action is the inhibition of adenosine receptors which are found in the brain.

Neutral and acidic heterocycle-containing compounds

Heterocycles such as pyrrole and pyridine derivatives are found commonly in drugs. The main reason for this is their similarity to the benzene ring which enables them to be quite lipophilic, and consequently they are able to penetrate the cell lipid membrane and to pass the blood–brain barrier; this also makes them suitable to be absorbed passively and quickly. They also take some of the characteristics of bases, which gives them some hydrophilicity and enables them to interact with the receptors, to accumulate inside microbial cells, to be distributed well in the blood stream and to be metabolised quickly and easily.

The most important heterocycles are the five- and six-membered rings. The six-membered rings are the derivatives of pyridine which is considered as a basic compound, and its derivatives are basic unless strongly electron withdrawing groups are added to the ring. Pyrrole, as discussed above, is considered either a neutral compound or a very weak acid. It was also mentioned that pyrrole has six pi-electrons according to the Huckel theory. These electrons are distributed to the carbon atoms of the small ring of the pyrrole, so the carbon atoms of pyrrole have greater electron density than those in a benzene ring since there are only five atoms in the ring. Because of this, the pyrrole derivatives are called pi-excessive compounds. This explains the susceptibility of pyrrole to the electrophilic substitution (Fig. 4.46) which is greater than that of benzene.

Pyrrole under acidic conditions has a tendency to polymerise instead of forming salts (Fig. 4.47).

Indole, which is a fusion between pyrrole and benzene, also has the same acidic properties as the pyrrole ring. An example of an indole-containing drug is psilocin (Fig. 4.48).

Replacement of the pyrrole nitrogen with oxygen results in the formation of a furan, which is a neutral compound. Furan polymerises in acidic conditions as does pyrrole. Nitrofurantoin and dantrolene are examples of furan-containing compounds (Fig. 4.49).

The substitution of the pyrrole nitrogen with a sulphur atom produces thiophene. Thiophene is stable in acidic solution (not polymerised) and is also a neutral compound. Ketotifen is an example of a drug containing thiophene (Fig. 4.49).

Addition of a nitrogen at the 3 position of the pyrrole results in formation of imidazole (Fig. 4.50). Examples of compounds containing this ring include the imidazole

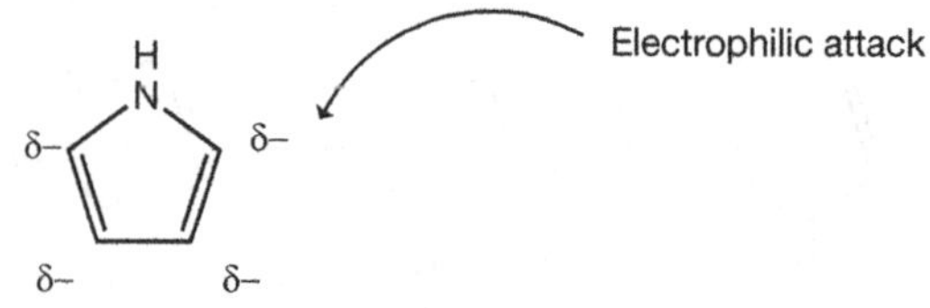

Figure 4.46 Pyrrole is an electron-rich ring.

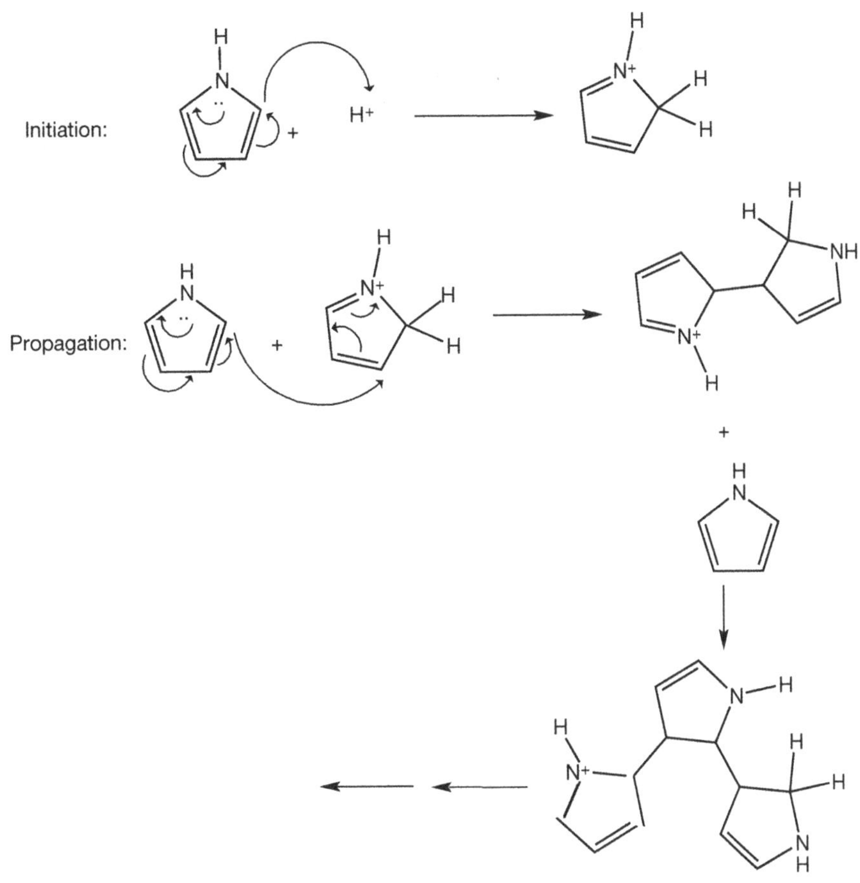

Figure 4.47 Polymerisation of pyrrole under acidic conditions.

family of antifungal agents, e.g. clotrimazole (Fig. 4.50, see Ch. 24). Substitution of the 3 carbon of thiophene with a nitrogen produces thiazole (Fig. 4.51). The nitrogen of thiazole is still weakly basic (p*Ka* 2.5), weaker than sp2 nitrogen in imidazole because the sulphur is a large atom and thus less effective than nitrogen at committing its lone pair as part of the aromatic sextet. An example of thiazole-containing compound is nizatidine (Fig. 4.51).

Substitution of the 3 carbon of a furan with a nitrogen produces oxazole (Fig. 4.52). The nitrogen is a very weak base (p*Ka* = 0.8) because of the high value of the oxygen electronegativity. Moreover, the substitution of the 2 position of pyrrole with nitrogen forms pyrazole. One nitrogen is considered neutral, while the other nitrogen is considered as a weak base, weaker than imidazole because of the close proximity of the electronegative. Its sp2 nitrogen has a p*Ka* = 2.5.

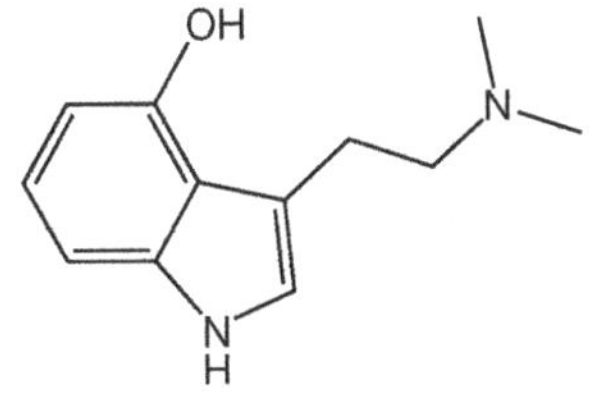

Psilocin

Figure 4.48 Psilocin contains indole ring.

An example of a pyrazole-containing compound is allopurinol (Fig. 4.53). On the other hand, the ortho substitution of furan with nitrogen gives isoxazole, which is considered neutral and found in sulfisoxazole (Fig. 4.53). Isothiazole (Fig. 4.53) is also a neutral compound. Addition of electronegative atoms to imidazole, thiazole, oxazole, isoxazole, pyrazole and isothiazole make them neutral or acidic rings. Figure 4.54 shows drugs containing this type of ring.

Q Self Test 4.6

Heterocycles are commonly found in the drug structure. Justify.

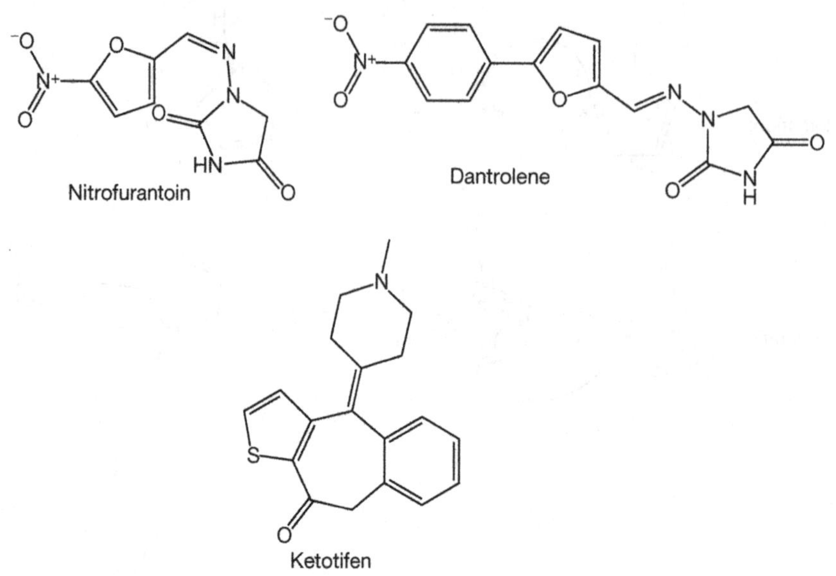

Figure 4.49 Drugs contain furan and thyophene rings.

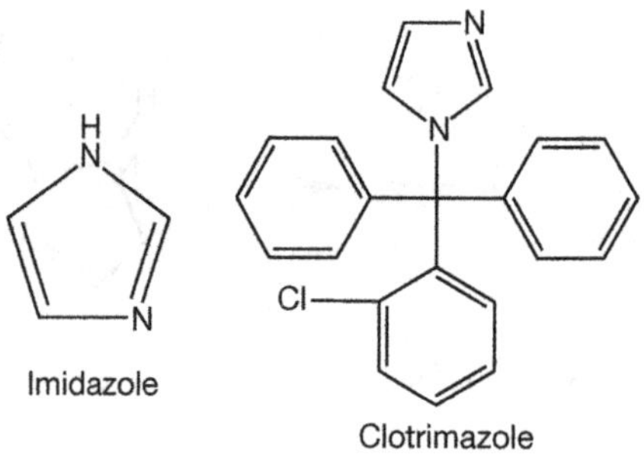

Figure 4.50 Imidazole ring.

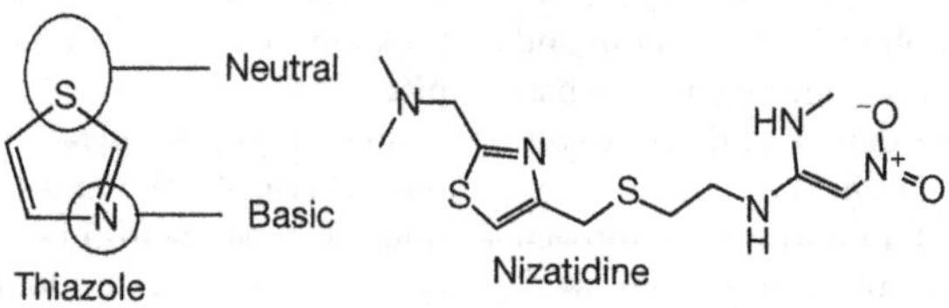

Figure 4.51 Thiazole ring.

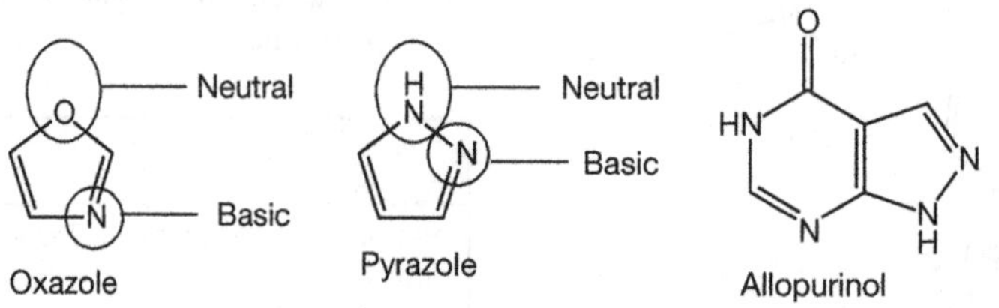

Figure 4.52 Oxazole and pyrazole rings.

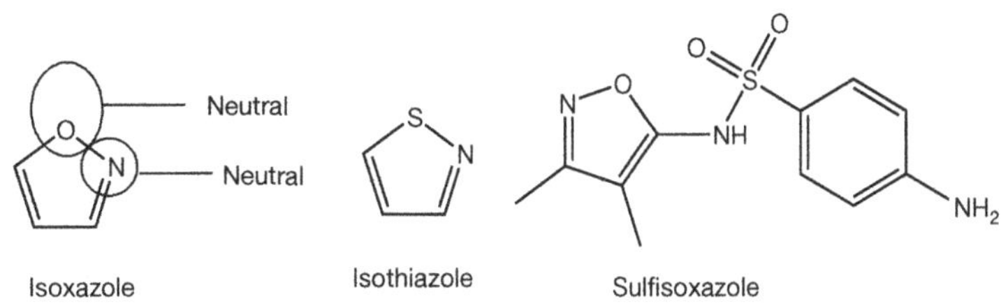

Figure 4.53 Isoxazole and isothiazole rings.

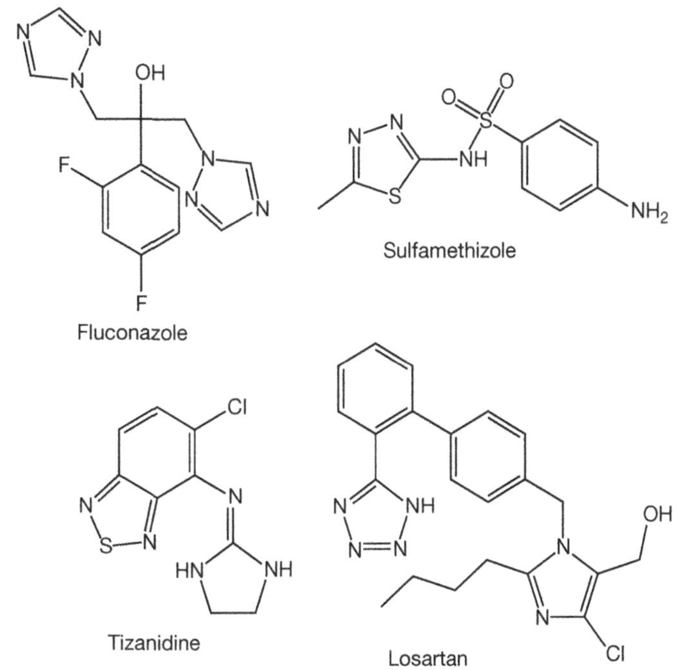

Figure 4.54 Drugs contain five member rings with more than two hetero atoms.

A — Self Test 4.1

Answer = 1/2500.

A — Self Test 4.2

Oxidation of benzene ring to phenol and omega-oxidation of the 5-alkyl group.

A — Self Test 4.3

Prontosil has no free N4 group unless reduced by the gut bacteria.

A — Self Test 4.4

Sulphonamides and PABA are isosters; they have very close structures.

A — Self Test 4.5

sp2 is basic because the lone pair of electrons is available for attacking the proton, while sp3 electrons are busy in the ring aromaticity.

A — Self Test 4.6

They have the lipophilicity of benzene and hydrophilicity of hetro atoms. Consequently this helps in drug distribution in the blood and the drug action through the lipid barrier of the cells.

Chapter | 5 |

Oxygen- and sulphur-containing functional groups

David G Watson

CHAPTER CONTENTS

INTRODUCTION

Oxygen in the most electronegative element found in biomolecules since fluorine does not occur naturally in biological compounds. Its high affinity for electrons means that unlike nitrogen it does not share its lone pairs with protons readily. Thus oxygen-containing groups tend to be less potent in conferring pharmacological activity. For example, dopamine differs from noradrenaline by lacking a hydroxyl group but they both have potent effects on the heart: remove the amine group and activity is totally abolished. This is really a generalisation, it is probably truer to say that where oxygen-containing groups play an important role in conferring pharmacological activity they have a very specifically targeted function. In contrast, the charged nitrogen atom exerts a more general effect and may affect a number of targets. This theme will be expanded later in the chapter. Water is the fundamental oxygen-containing biologically active substance and some of its unique properties have been discussed in Chapter 1.

The 3-D structure of water is shown in Figure 5.1. The geometry is more or less tetrahedral with the lone pairs occupying two of the corners of the tetrahedron and the

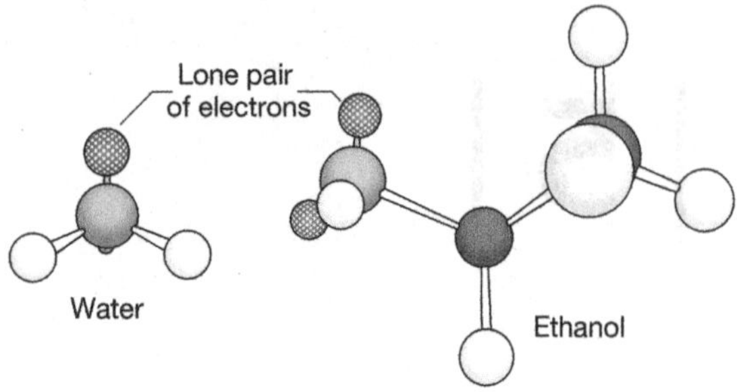

Figure 5.1 3-D structure of water and ethanol.

$$H_2O \underset{-H^+}{\overset{+H^+}{\rightleftharpoons}} H_3O^+$$

$$H_2O \underset{+H^+}{\overset{-H^+}{\rightleftharpoons}} HO^-$$

Figure 5.2 Ionisation of water.

two protons the other two. The lone pairs in water lie in a deeper energy well (highest occupied molecular orbital [HOMO] −12.4 eV) than the lone pair in ammonia (HOMO −10.4 eV). In the case of ethanol, the energy well occupied by the most accessible lone pair is slightly shallower at −11.2 eV, indicating that alcohols are slightly more basic than water and conversely water is a stronger acid than alcohols. Water can function both as a weak acid and a weak base as indicated in Figure 5.2.

MONOHYDRIC ALCOHOLS

The lower alcohols are liquids with low boiling points. Methanol, ethanol and propanol are all miscible with water but n-butanol is only soluble 1 part in 10 in water and amyl alcohol is immiscible with water. If the surface area of the hydrocarbon chain of the alcohol is decreased, then water solubility will increase. Thus the order of water solubility for the primary, secondary and tertiary butyl alcohols is: t-butanol > butanol-2-ol > n-butanol (Fig. 5.3); t-butanol is freely soluble in water. The properties of some alcohols are shown in Table 5.1.

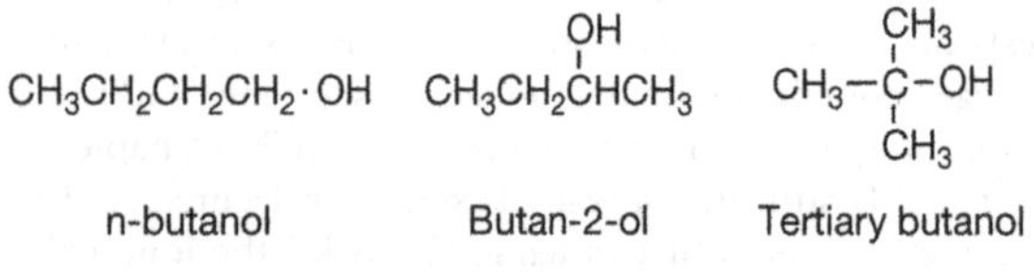

Figure 5.3 Primary, secondary and tertiary alcohols.

Table 5.1 Some monohydric alcohols

Formula	Name	b.p. °C
CH_3OH	Methanol	64.5
CH_3CH_2OH	Ethanol	78.5
$CH_3CH_2CH_2OH$	n-propanol	97.8
$(CH_3)_2CHOH$	propan-2-ol (isopropyl alcohol)	82.3
$CH_3CH_2CH_2CH_2OH$	n-butanol	118
$CH_3CHOHCH_2CH_3$	butan-2-ol	99.3
$(CH_3)_3COH$	t-butyl alcohol	83
		m.p. °C
$CH_3(CH_2)_{14}CH_2OH$	cetyl alcohol	49
$CH_3(CH_2)_{16}CH_2OH$	stearyl alcohol	59.5

Ethanol

Simple alcohols are useful as pharmaceutical aids for their solvent and emulsifying properties. Methanol is too toxic to be useful, as its toxicity arises from its oxidation by the body to formaldehyde, which is a highly reactive chemical compound which causes damage to tissues. Solutions of formaldehyde are, of course, useful in preserving biological specimens, and formaldehyde gels and lotions are used in the removal of warts; these preparations contain <1% of formaldehyde. Methanol itself is used as a denaturant, being added to industrial ethanol to discourage drinking of it. Ethanol is a useful solvent and is used in many preparations as such solutions of disinfectant, mouthwashes and surgical spirit. Ethanol itself has disinfectant properties which are due to its ability to interact with biological membranes, which also explains its physiological effects as a sedative. The interaction of ethanol and other alcohols with membranes is non-specific and based on a general affinity for lipophilic materials. Affinity for membranes accounts for the action of ethanol as an antimicrobial compound since it can disrupt microbial membranes and also disrupts protein structure. Concentrations of >20% inhibit microbial action, and ethanol is most effective at concentrations of >70%.

Ethanol is a useful solvent for topical application of therapeutic agents; for instance, topical antibiotics and disinfectants are often formulated in ethanol. The volatility of ethanol is useful in topical applications since it evaporates rapidly, allowing the product to dry out on the surface of the skin. The recreational use of ethanol is discussed in Chapter 29.

Other aliphatic alcohols

Isopropyl alcohol is often used instead of ethanol in topical formulations; however, it is not suitable for internal use because it is more toxic than ethanol. It has greater antimicrobial effects than ethanol. The antimicrobial strength of alcohols increases up to a chain length of eight and falls off thereafter as a result of decreasing water solubility. However, only ethanol and isopropyl alcohol are used as antiseptic agents. Long-chain alcohols such cetyl and stearyl alcohol are used as emulsifying agents (a 40:60 mixture of the two alcohols is called cetostearyl alcohol) since they concentrate at the interface between oil and water.

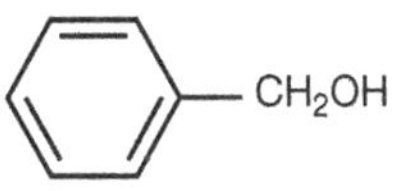

Benzyl alcohol

Figure 5.4 Benzyl alcohol.

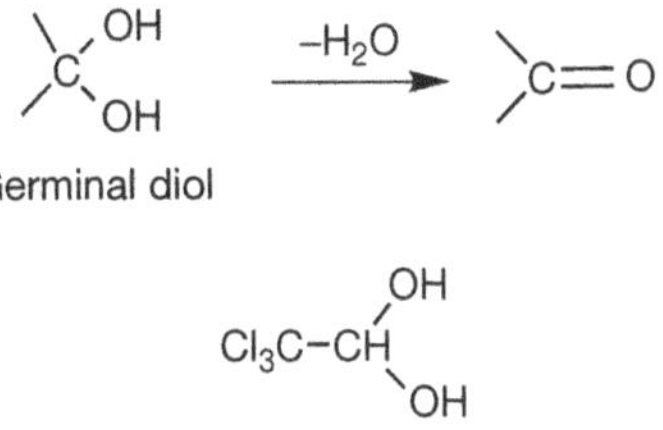

Germinal diol

Chloral hydrate

Figure 5.5 Germinal diols.

Benzyl alcohol

Benzyl alcohol (Fig. 5.4) has both antiseptic and mild local anaesthetic properties and is used in lotions and ointments for topical application. It is also used as a preservative in injection solutions.

Diols and triols

Dihydroxy alcohols (diols) and trihydroxy alcohols (triols) are viscous, hygroscopic, high boiling point liquids with a sweetish taste. Some of them are useful as solvents for pharmaceutical use. In the case of diols the two hydroxyl groups are usually attached to different carbon atoms. If the hydroxyl groups are attached to the same carbon an atom of water is eliminated to give a carbonyl compound (Fig. 5.5). There are exceptions to this; for example, in the case of chloral hydrate the diol is stabilised by the electron-withdrawing chlorine atoms.

Where the hydroxyl groups are on adjacent carbon atoms the diols are called glycols. The simplest glycol is ethylene glycol (Fig. 5.6) which is too toxic for pharmaceutical use, although, because of its sweet taste, it has been used illegally as a sweetener with disastrous consequences (a recent example was as an additive in wines), since it is oxidised to the toxic acid, oxalic acid. Propylene glycol is used as a formulation aid since it is non-toxic and is a water-miscible organic solvent. It is a common excipient in injections containing poorly water-soluble drugs and also in creams.

Triols have three hydroxy groups in their structure and the simplest triol glycerol is widely distributed in nature, being present in esterified form in triglycerides which make up fats and in the phospholipids which make up cell membranes. Glycerol is also useful as a water-miscible organic solvent, it has a sweet taste and is useful in the formulation of syrups. There are a number of instances of glycerol being substituted with the toxic but closely related diethylene glycol (Fig. 5.6) in elixirs which have resulted in fatalities. Thus quality control checks that can distinguish between the members of this group of excipients are particularly important.

Both propylene glycol and glycerol are not entirely suitable as solvents in formulations used for instillation of drugs into the eye and nose because of their potential for causing irritation. Despite this, glycerol is used in some nasal preparations.

Examples of formulations containing propylene glycol or glycerol

Phenobarbital sodium injection: 200 mg/mL in propylene glycol/water (90:10).
Phenytoin sodium injection: 50 mg/mL in propylene glycol/ethanol/water (40:10:50).
Chloramphenicol ear drops: 5% w/v chloramphenicol in propylene glycol.
Propylene glycol: is used as a solvent in most creams for topical application of corticosteroids and antifungal agents.
Glycerol: is used in osmotic laxatives because its hygroscopic (water absorbing) nature promotes peristalsis and in some cream formulations.

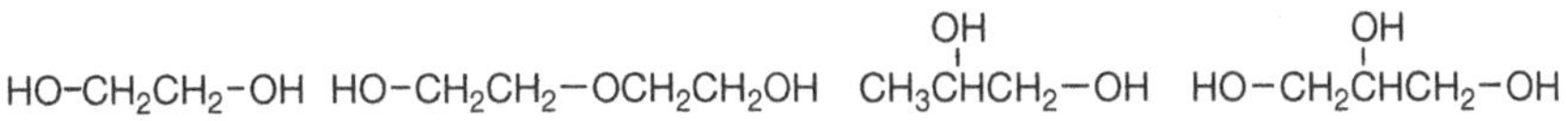

Ethylene glycol   Diethylene glycol (toxic)   Propylene glycol   Glycerol

Figure 5.6 Diols and triols.

Q Self Test 5.1

Indicate whether the alcohol groups in these drugs are primary, secondary, tertiary or benzyl.

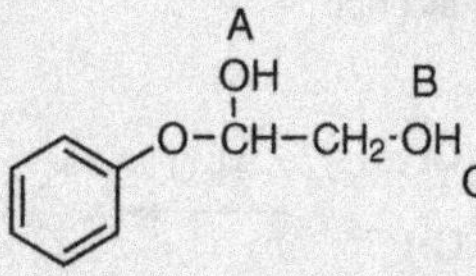

Guaifenesin

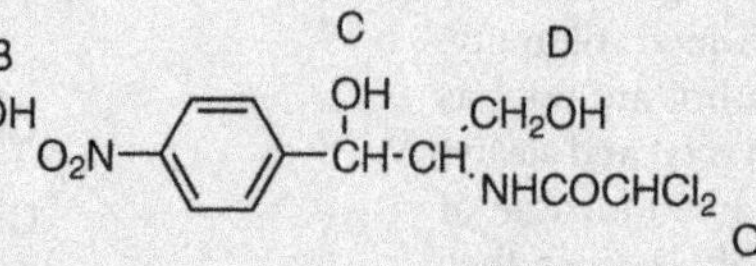

Chloramphenicol

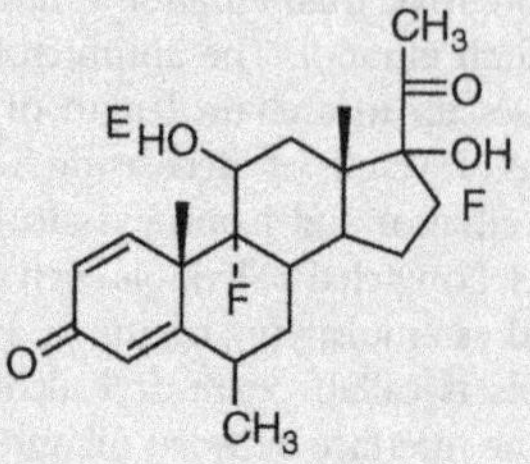

Fluorometholone

POLYOLS

Tetritols, pentitols and hexitols are largely known according to the names of the sugar molecules from which they derive. Thus the pentitol, xylitol (see Fig. 5), derives from xylose and mannitol from mannose; sorbitol derives from glucose. Such reduced sugars may be used as sweetening agents without promoting the growth of bacterial plaque. Sorbitol (Fig. 5.7) is commonly used as a diluent in lozenge formulations and has a useful property in that it has a positive enthalpy of solution (absorbs heat from the environment) and thus has a cooling effect on the mouth. It has *ca.* 60% of the sweetness of glucose and most of it is metabolised without contributing to glucose levels in the blood and thus it is a useful diabetic sweetener.

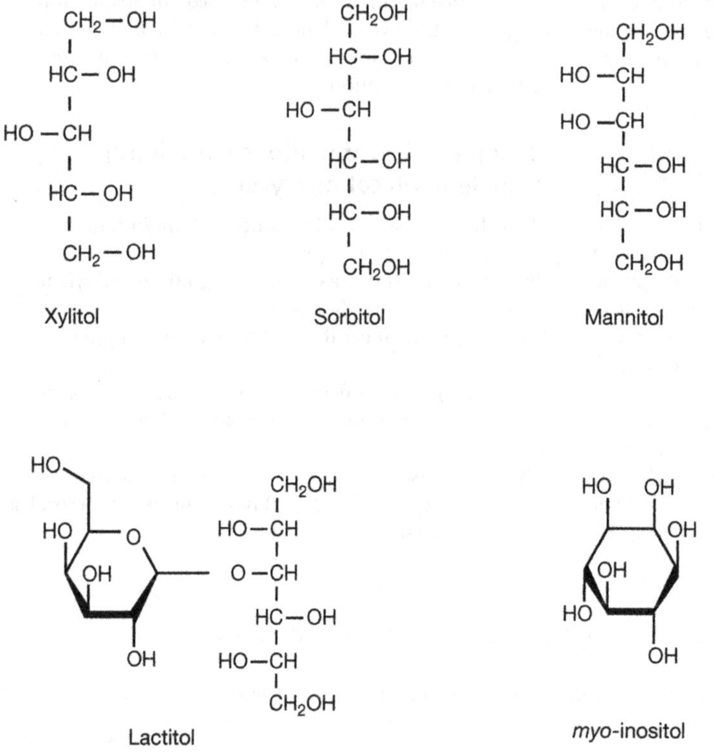

Figure 5.7 Some polyols.

The hygroscopic nature of polyols makes them effective osmotic laxatives since they retain water in the bowel thus softening faeces. The polyol, lactitol (Fig. 5.7), is even more effective for this purpose since it is not absorbed by the intestine and passes straight through to the bowel. Mannitol is used in infusions in order to treat cerebral oedema by drawing water away from brain tissue, e.g. due to the effects of high altitude.

Inositol is hexahydroxy cyclohexane. Its particular importance is as a constituent of membrane lipids and it is important biochemically in the form of its phosphate esters, which have a role in cell-signalling.

SOME CHEMICAL PROPERTIES OF ALCOHOLS

Loss of water

Alcohols are slightly more basic than water because the release of electrons by the alkyl group attached to the oxygen increases its electron density. Protonation of the hydroxyl group decreases the stability of the C–O bond and water can be eliminated. For instance, ethanol is dehydrated to form ethylene (Fig. 5.8) under strongly acidic conditions. The ease of dehydration is tertiary > secondary > primary alcohols, which reflects the relative stability of the intermediate carbonium ion (Fig. 5.8). Thus corticosteroids such as prednisolone can readily dehydrate at the tertiary 17 position under acidic conditions and this is a consideration in their storage in solution. Polyols are equally likely to dehydrate; thus acidic conditions convert ethylene glycol to acetaldehyde and glycerol is converted to acrolein (Fig. 5.8).

Oxidation

Alcohols are not particularly readily oxidised under normal conditions of storage, e.g. in a sealed container at room temperature. Primary alcohols such as ethanol are oxidised to aldehydes and then if oxidation is allowed to proceed further they form carboxylic acids. Secondary alcohols such as propan-2-ol are oxidised to ketones (Fig. 5.9) and oxidation does not proceed easily beyond this stage. Benzyl alcohol and other benzylic alcohols are more readily oxidised than aliphatic alcohols such as ethanol and the B.P. includes a limit test for benzaldehyde in benzyl alcohol.

Phenols

Where the OH group is attached directly to an aromatic ring it becomes acidic. The simplest phenol is phenol (Fig. 5.10) itself which was originally isolated from coal tar and was used as an early antiseptic in the nineteenth century. Phenol is a weak acid having a p*Ka* value 10.0 and is soluble 1 in 20 in water. It is still used occasionally in the form of an oily injection, because of its caustic nature, to promote sclerosis in the treatment of haemorrhoids.

When additional hydroxyl groups are attached to the benzene ring a range of fairly reactive compounds, e.g. catechol, hydroquinone and pyrogallol (Fig. 5.10) results. These compounds, unlike ordinary alcohols, are all readily oxidised and the oxidation products (quinones) are also highly reactive with biological structures and certainly not desirable as the products of drug metabolism. The phenolic hydroxyl group is widely found in natural products such as tyramine, dopamine which is used therapeutically, and in phenolic pigments such as quercetin which is a dietary antioxidant compound (Fig. 5.10). Phenolic acids occur widely in the diet; for example, the rich content of phenolic acids in cranberry juice is the basis for its mild antibacterial action in treating cystitis. Phenolic groups can have a strong effect on biological activity. The presence of a catechol group is critical for biological activity in noradrenaline; *p*-octopamine lacks the *m*-hydroxyl group found in noradrenaline (Fig 5.11) and has little activity at noradrenergic receptors. However, by a quirk of nature it fulfils the role of noradrenaline in the nervous systems of insects.

Phenol acidity and antibacterial action

Unlike alcohols, which are neutral, phenols are weakly acidic. The acidity of the hydroxyl group results from the electron withdrawing effect of the aromatic ring which weakens the OH bond. The acidic strength of the phenol increases with the strength of electron withdrawal. Thus electron withdrawing substituents such as nitro or chloro groups increase the acidity of the phenol (Fig. 5.12). The effects of such substituents are greatest in the ortho and para positions. The amphiphilic nature of phenols means that they are surface active and can absorb on membrane surfaces such as bacterial membranes. The more acidic phenols have stronger antibacterial action and chloroxylenol is commonly used in disinfectants, ethylparaben is used as a preservative in liquid formulations and triclosan (Fig. 5.12) is used as an antibacterial compound in toothpaste and household detergents.

Oxidation of phenols

An important property of phenols, both in pharmacy and in biology, is their susceptibility to oxidation. Unlike ionisation of the phenolic group, which can be said to be heterolytic, oxidation produces homolytic cleavage of the OH bond and produces a free radical with an unpaired electron (Fig. 5.13). The free radical is resonance stabilised by the presence of the aromatic ring.

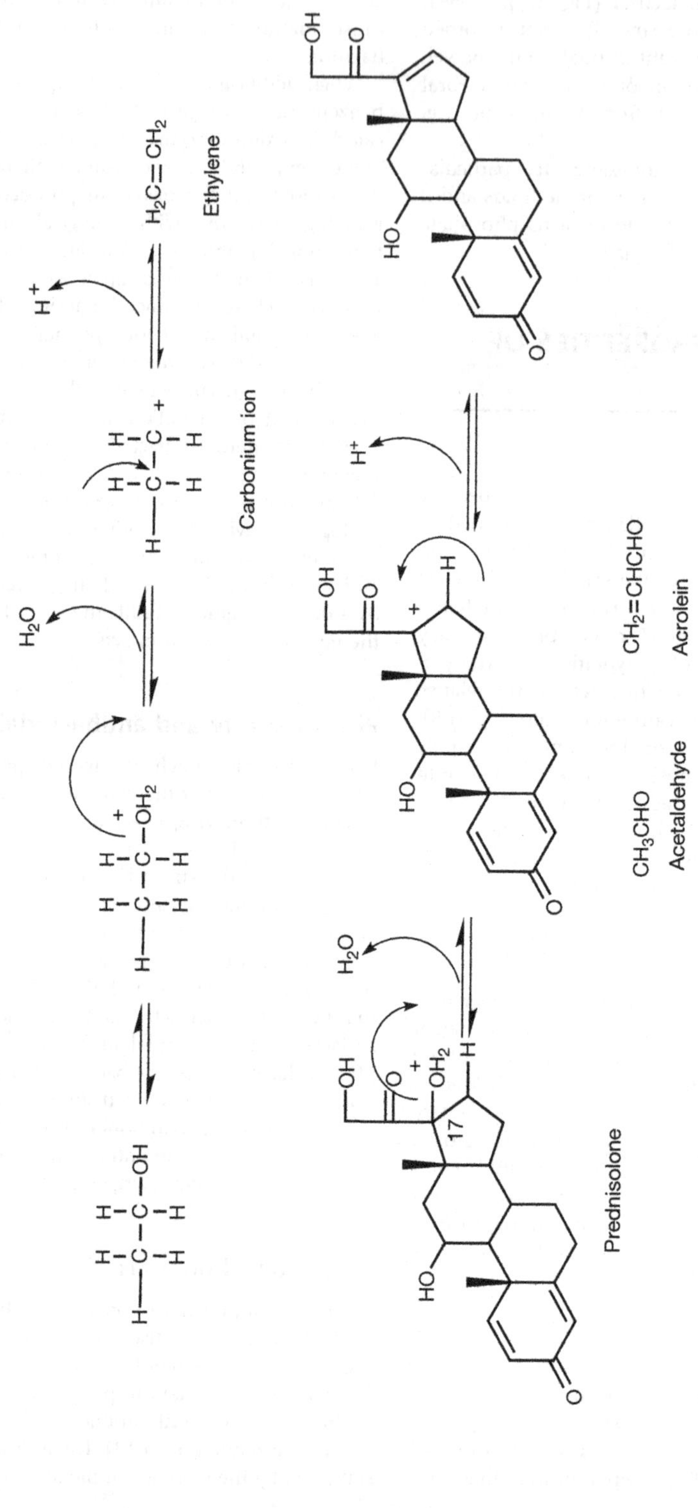

Figure 5.8 Alcohol dehydration.

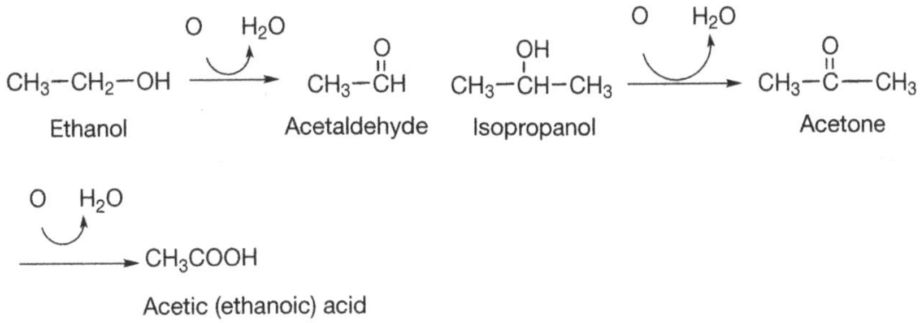

Figure 5.9 Alcohol oxidation.

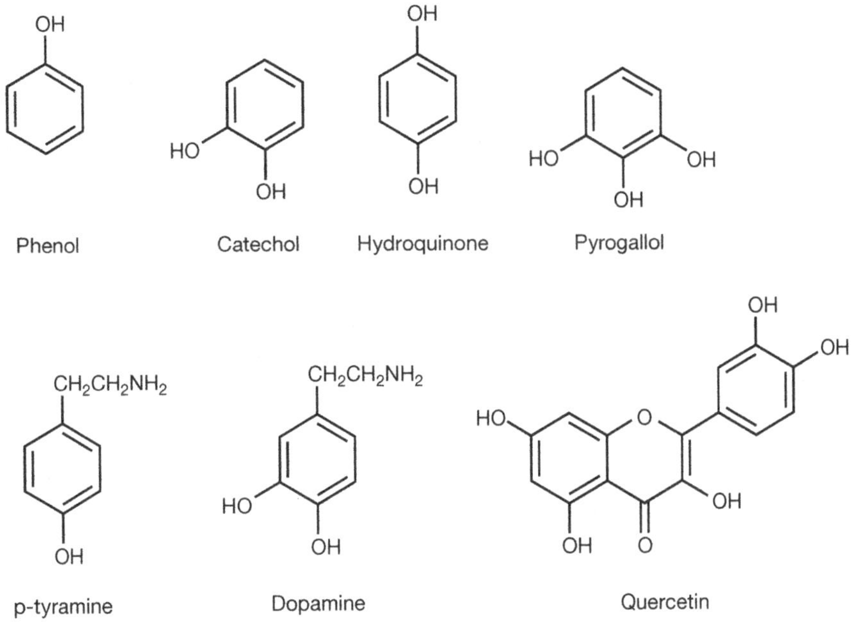

Figure 5.10 Phenols.

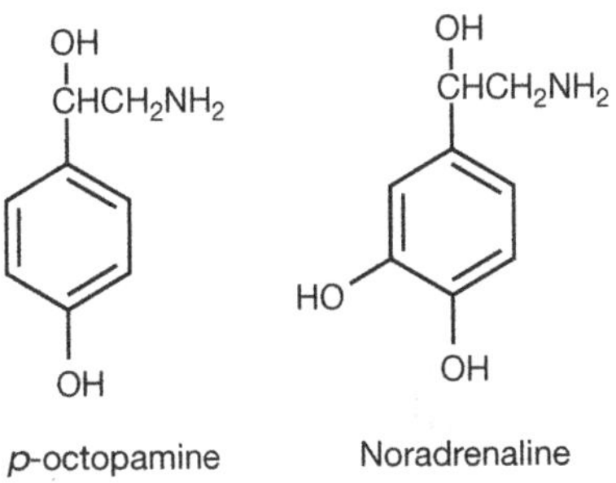

Figure 5.11 Biologically active phenols.

Some phenolic drugs produce breakdown products resulting from this type of oxidation, the classic example being morphine which oxidises to produce the dimer pseudomorphine (Fig. 5.14). The radical intermediate is stabilised by the presence of the aromatic ring. This property makes phenols useful as antioxidants. For example, thymol is a naturally occurring antioxidant and it acts to protect against oxidation as shown in Figure 5.15.

Thymol oxidises in preference to the substance it is protecting from oxidation, the alkyl groups attached to the aromatic ring help to stabilise the radical, and the end-point of the oxidation is the coupling of two thymol radicals to produce a dimer (Fig. 5.15). Other commonly used phenolic antioxidants include butylated hydroxyanisole and butylated hydroxy toluene, which work via a similar mechanism.

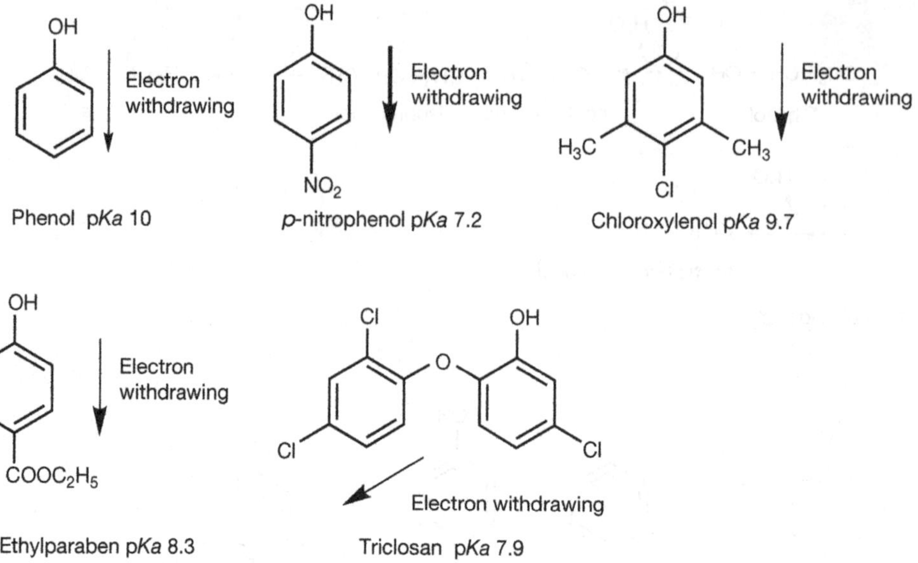

Figure 5.12 Phenol acidity.

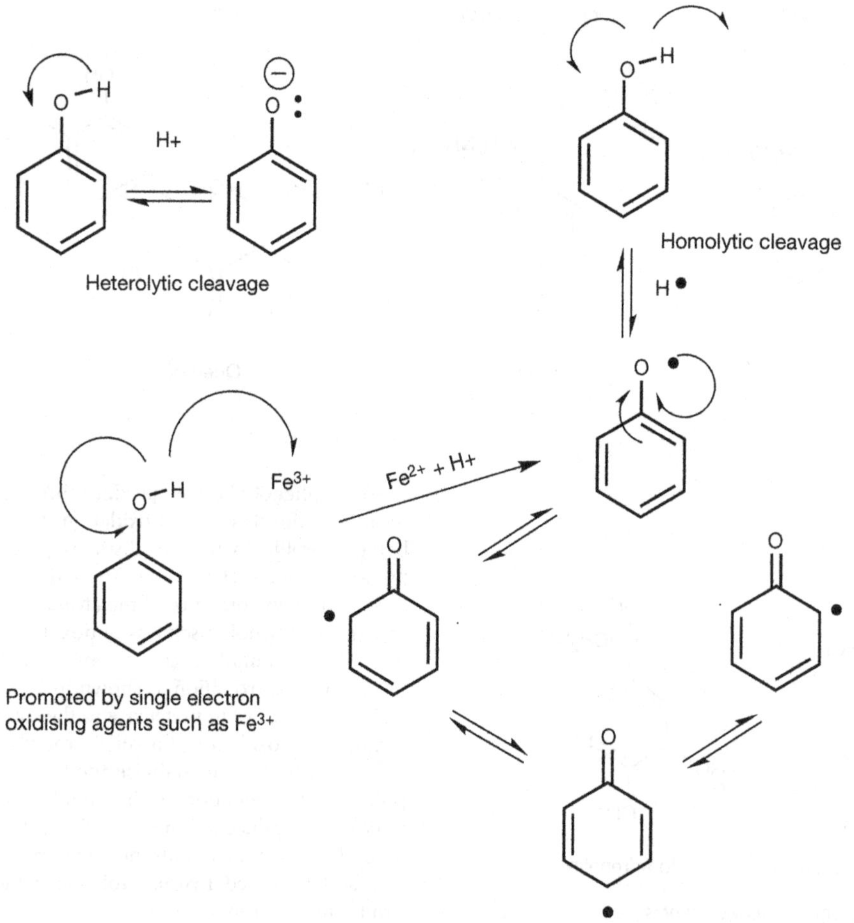

Figure 5.13 Oxidation of phenol.

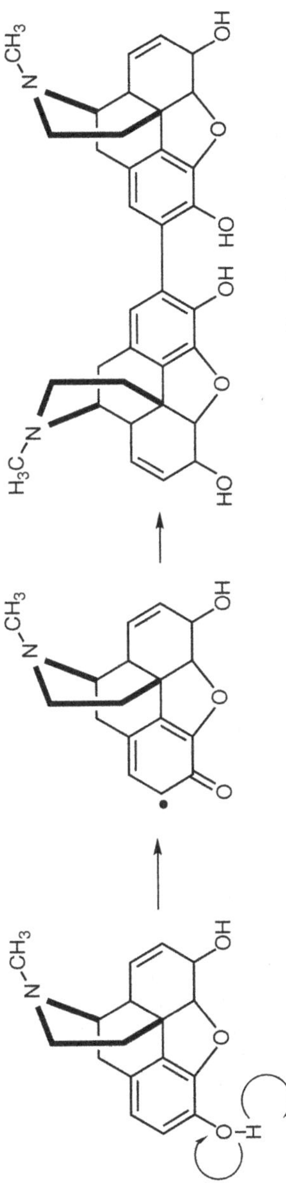

Pseudomorphine

Morphine

Figure 5.14 Oxidation of morphine to the dimer pseudomorphine.

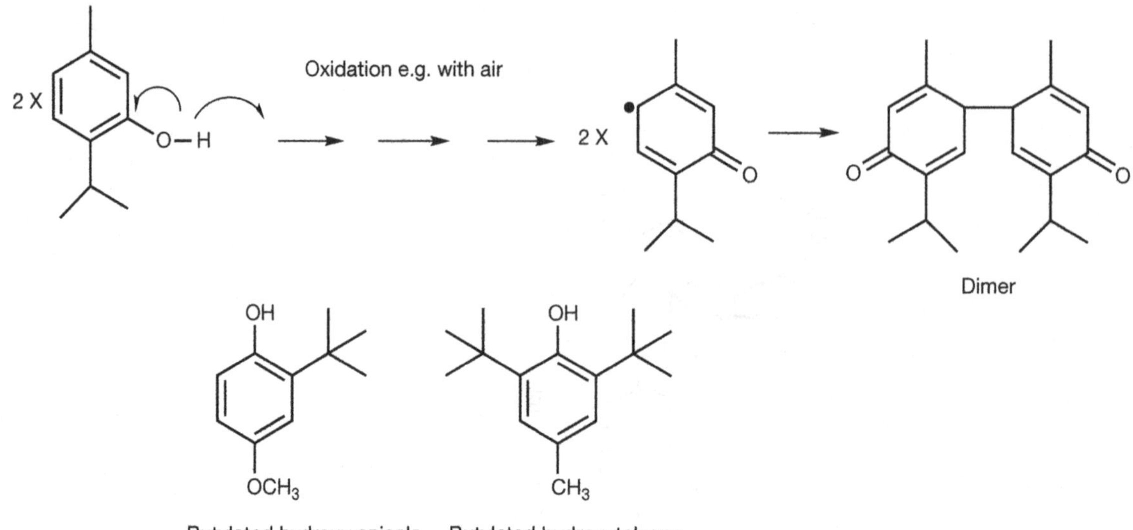

Figure 5.15 The mechanism of thymol as an inhibitor of oxidation and typical phenolic antioxidants.

Q Self Test 5.2

Draw a dimer which could be formed as a result of the antioxidant action of butylated hydroxy anisole.

Di- and trihydroxy benzenes are even more prone to oxidation than monohydroxy compounds. Thus drugs such as adrenaline or the amino acid LDOPA, which is used to treat Parkinson's disease, are very susceptible to discolouration caused by oxidation when in contact with air. The polymerisation of DOPA is also a natural process which takes place in the body to produce dark melanin skin pigments which protect against ultraviolet radiation and also protect the eye against UV radiation. Incorporation of the amino acid cysteine into these structures results in the red and yellow pigments that, in conjunction with the simpler DOPA eumelanin polymers, are responsible for hair colour. Figure 5.16 shows a trimer formed from DOPA via the same type of coupling reaction observed above for thymol. Adrenaline and noradrenaline form similar coloured products upon exposure to oxygen, particularly in solution at high pH. Similar types of polymerisation reactions are responsible for the formation on the hard exoskeleton of insects and the formation of hardwoods. In another role as a reactive intermediate, the quinone type of structure can be found in co-factors such as ubiquinone (CoEnzyme Q) (Fig. 5.17) which is involved in the electron transport chain and is an essential co-factor in energy metabolism.

On the other hand, the occurrence of quinone structures as a result of drug metabolism can be unwelcome. For instance, paracetamol in overdose is converted to a quinone imine structure (Fig. 5.18) which is highly reactive and can react with proteins within the liver, thus causing irreversible tissue damage. Such damage occurs when the stores of glutathione, which has a protective role against chemically reactive species, become depleted.

There are a number of drugs which undergo such potentially damaging metabolic activation. The most recent example was the antidiabetic drug troglitazone which had to be withdrawn from the market because of idiosyncratic liver toxicity. The toxicity can be attributed to the formation of a reactive quinine, although the variation between individuals is not fully explained.

ESTERIFICATION

One of the most important properties of alcohols is their ability to form esters. The ester group has a number of important roles in both natural ligands such as acetyl choline and the glycerol esters and also in drugs such as the corticosteroid esters which are used for topical delivery of these drugs. In view of the broad importance of the ester group, esters are discussed in a separate section. Esters are formed by reaction between an alcohol and either an organic or an inorganic acid (Fig. 5.19). The reaction is catalysed by acidic conditions which promote the loss of hydroxyl as water from the acid and its replacement by the alkoxy group. The reaction is readily reversible if the ester is attacked by protonated water or the hydroxyl group and thus esters are unstable to aqueous acidic or basic conditions. Ester formation does not occur readily between acids and tertiary alcohols; thus, for instance, ester formation at the hindered 17 position of steroids does not take place via a simple esterification reaction.

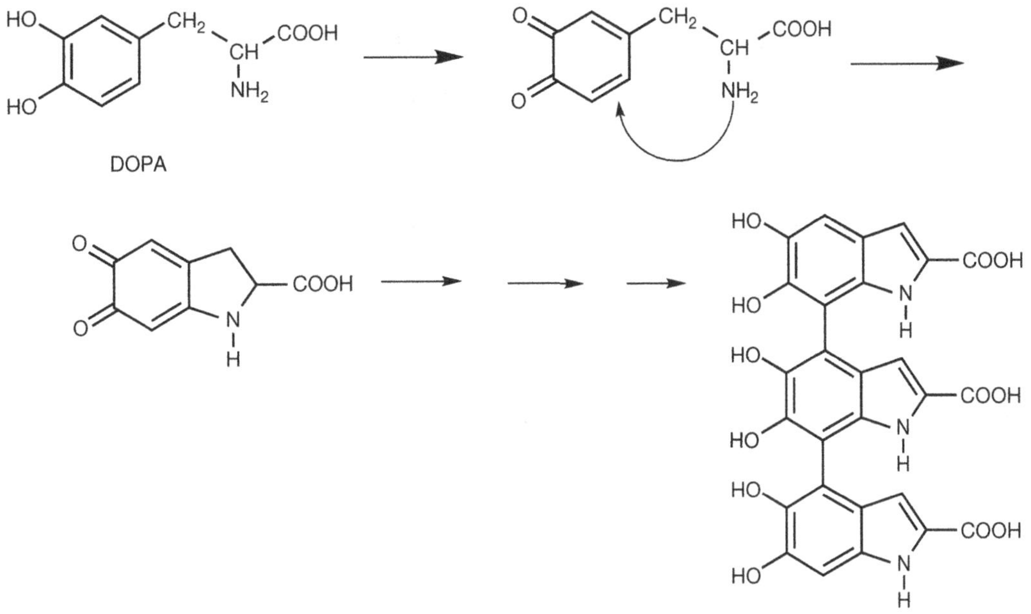

DOPA

Eumelanin trimer

Figure 5.16 A trimer formed from DOPA.

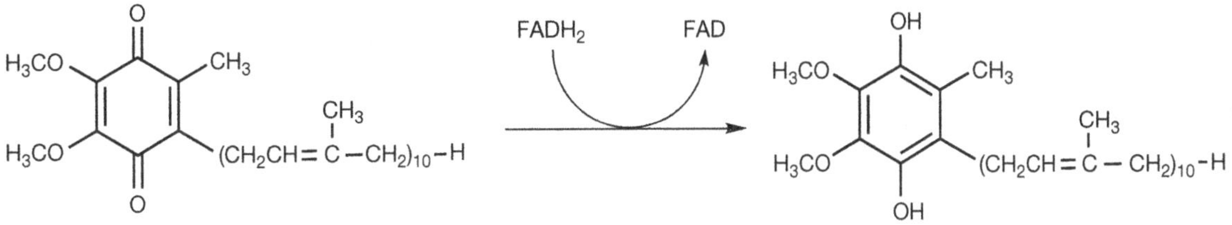

Co Enzyme Q oxidised

Co Enzyme Q reduced

Figure 5.17 Quinones as oxidising reagents.

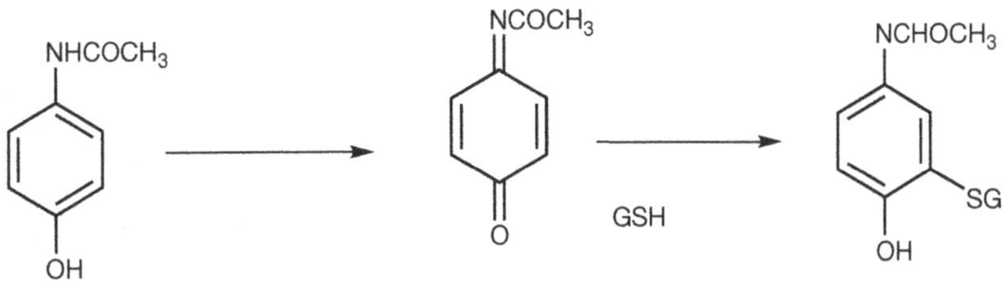

Paracetamol

Quinone imine

Paracetamol glutathione conjugate

GSH = glutathione

Figure 5.18 Formation of a quinone imine from paracetamol.

$$CH_3COOH + C_2H_5OH \overset{H^+}{\rightleftharpoons} CH_3COOC_2H_5 + H_2O$$

Acetic acid Ethanol Ethyl acetate

Detailed mechanism

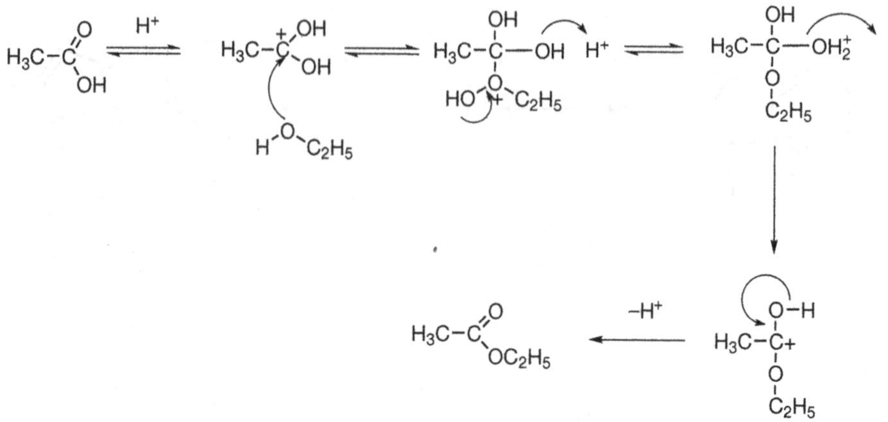

Figure 5.19 The mechanism of esterification.

> **Q Self Test 5.3**
>
> Draw the original acids and alcohols from which the esters below were formed.
>
> 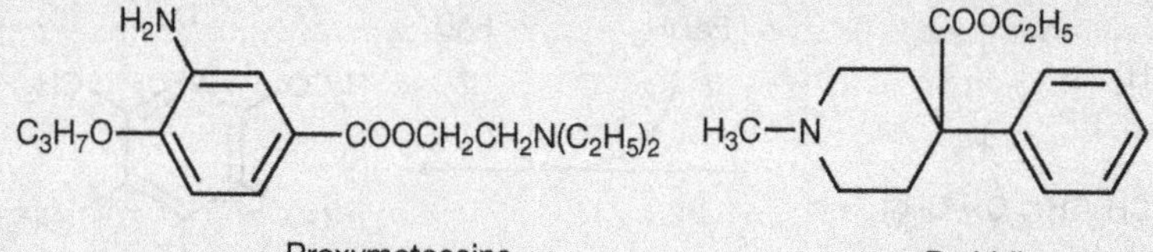
>
>
> Proxymetacaine Pethidine

ETHERS

Ethers are less significant than esters in biological systems. Like esters with organic acids ethers are much less polar than the parent alcohol, and ether formation may be used as a metabolic deactivation reaction such as in the metabolism of adrenaline to metanephrine (Fig. 5.20) which removes its biological activity.

The early members of the homologous series of ethers are low boiling, flammable liquids. Diethylether was an early anaesthetic but it is little used now, having been replaced with non-flammable inhalation anaesthetics such as enflurane, which is a halogenated ether (Fig. 5.21). Such anaesthetics act via a non-specific mechanism where they dissolve in lipid membranes and, in the case of anaesthesia, they dissolve in neurological membranes, thus preventing them from functioning properly.

In general, cyclic ethers have similar properties to their open chain counterparts; however, one exception is epoxides where the three-membered ring is sterically strained and thus quite reactive. Ethylene oxide (Fig. 5.22) is the simplest epoxide and as a result of its reactivity it may be used as a cold sterilising gas, e.g. for sterilising syringes. When it is used in this manner the sterilised samples are carefully checked for residues of ethylene oxide. Ethylene oxide is used in the preparation of various formulation aids such as diethylene glycol monoethyl ether, which is prepared as shown in Figure 5.22, and hydroxyethyl cellulose, which is prepared in a similar manner.

Under conditions of high temperature, pressure and basic catalysis ethylene oxide will form polyethylene glycols (Fig. 5.23). The chain lengths of these polymers varies from a few to several hundred units, and they may include a lipophilic group such as is present in the macrogols. Again, these agents are important components in formulations.

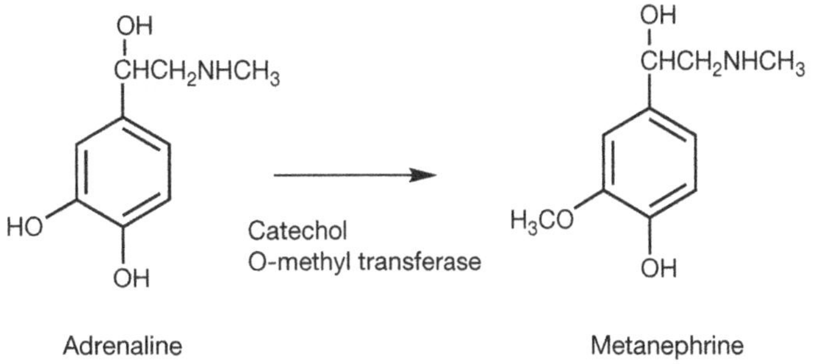

Figure 5.20 Route for metabolic deactivation of noradrenaline.

$C_2H_5OC_2H_5$ — Diethylether B.P. 34.5°C

CHF_2OCF_2CHFCl — Enflurane B.P. 56.5°C

Figure 5.21 Ethers as anaesthetics.

Epoxides also occur as metabolic intermediates, e.g. in metabolism of aromatic rings (see Ch. 4).

ALDEHYDES AND KETONES

Alcohols can be oxidised if the reaction conditions are relatively strong. Primary alcohols are oxidised to aldehydes and secondary alcohols to ketones. Primary alcohols may be oxidised via an aldehyde to the final product a carboxylic acid.

Ketonic groups are found in a number of drug molecules, for example corticosteroids such as hydrocortisone, and they form an important part of the pharmacophore in these molecules. Reduction of the keto group removes the pharmacological activity. In contrast, aldehydic groups are not widely found in drugs and this is because they are relatively reactive and form covalent bonds with nucleophilic groups such as primary amine groups and thiol groups in proteins (Fig. 5.24). Aldehydes also react with alcohols to form hemiacetals and acetals. A common example of the hemiacetal structure is seen in sugars such as glucose where the acetal is formed internally between the sugar aldehyde group and the 5-alcohol group. When glucose is attached to another alcohol such as in the case of sucrose an acetal is formed. Hemiacetals retain the properties of the aldehyde although they are somewhat less reactive, whereas the acetals such as sucrose do not behave like aldehydes. Acetals can be found in a number of drug structures, whereas hemiacetals are less common. The mineralocorticoid aldosterone is a rare example of a hemiacetal structure which has been used as a drug (Fig. 5.25), although synthetic alternatives to it are preferred (see Ch. 20). Examples of acetals include budesonide which is an acetal of butyraldehyde and a range of structures with glycosidic bonds in them such as aminoglycoside antibiotics and the cardiac glycoside digoxin (Fig. 5.25).

The reactivity of aldehydes themselves is not a desirable property and aldehydes are naturally fairly cytotoxic. This is particularly true of small reactive aldehydes such as formaldehyde and glutaraldehyde (Fig. 5.26), which are used in solutions to remove warts by destroying the tissue making up the wart. Glutaraldehyde is also used in sterilising solutions. Malondialdehyde is a naturally occurring aldehyde which is formed from the oxidation of unsaturated fatty acids and is one of a number of such reactive metabolites which may be involved in the aging of cells. Another ubiquitous aldehyde is glucose, which is usually

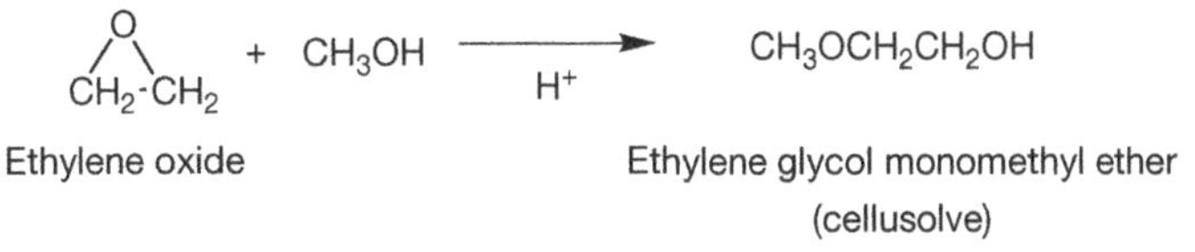

Figure 5.22 Epoxide ring opening.

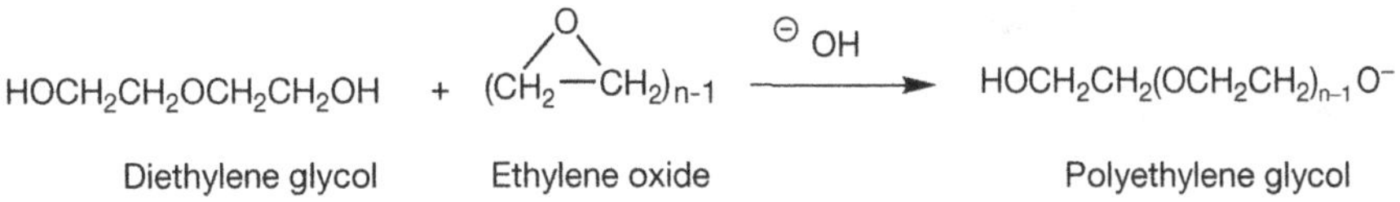

Figure 5.23 Epoxidation.

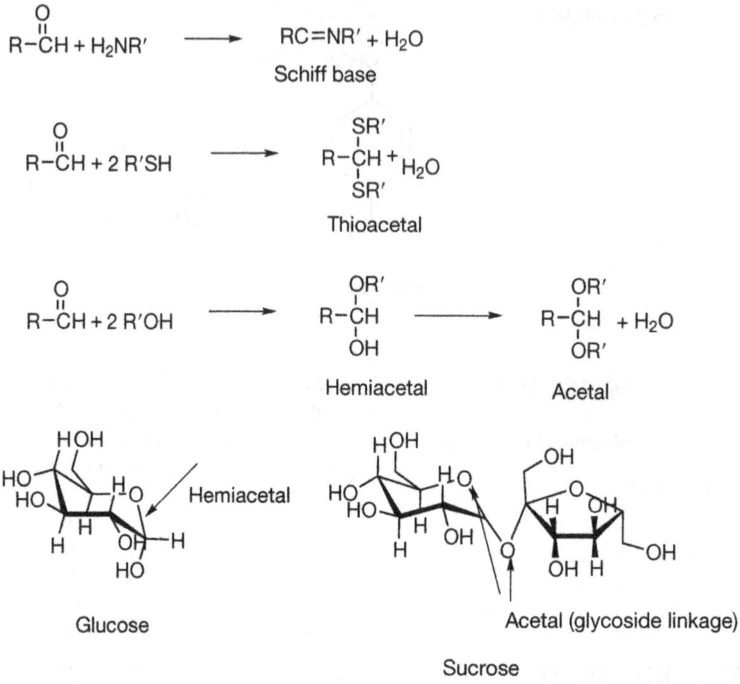

Figure 5.24 Reactions of aldehydes with primary amine and thiol groups.

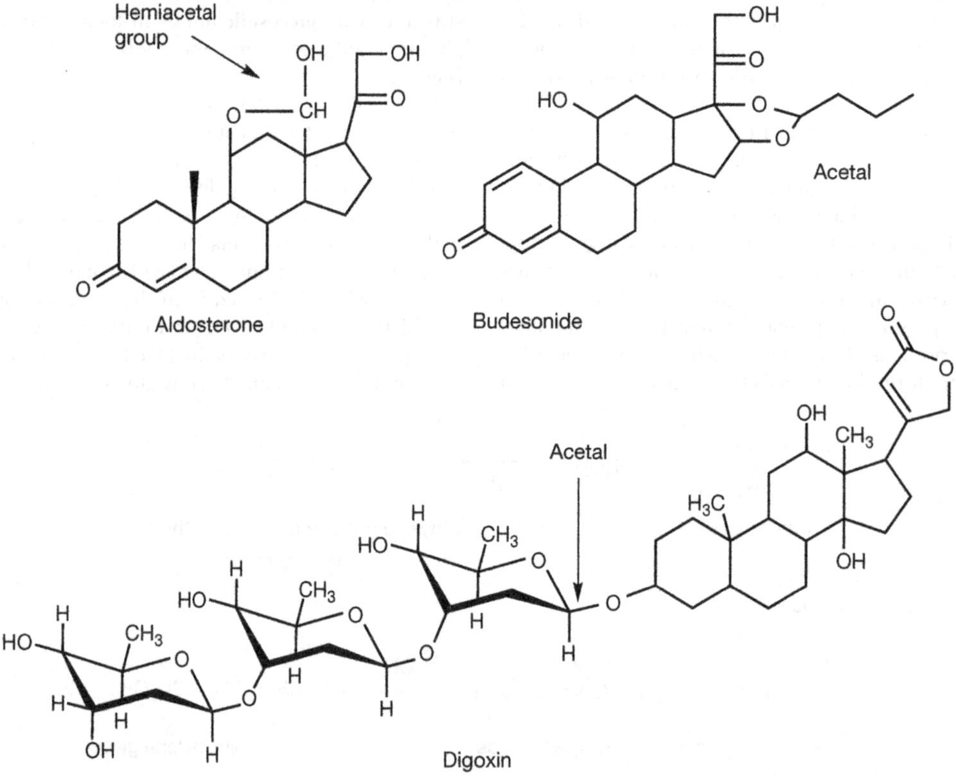

Figure 5.25 Hemiacetals and acetals in drug molecules.

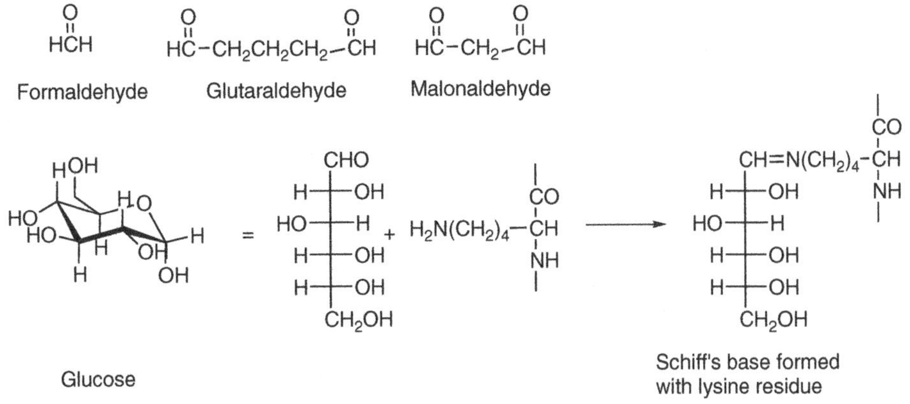

Figure 5.26 Schiff's base formation.

written in the form of its hemiacetal but chemically it behaves as an aldehyde. The reaction of glucose with lysine or terminal amino groups in haemoglobin is used to monitor the variation of glucose levels in diabetics over time. In general, the reaction of glucose with proteins (non-enzymatic glycation) has been offered as an explanation for some of the manifestations of the aging process such as cataract formation and the formation of wrinkles. Sometimes, the Schiff's base linkage is used as part of a biochemical process and a Schiff's base linkage is used to bind the aldehyde form of vitamin A to the opsin protein as part of the visual process (see Ch. 26). Schiff's base formation is also involved in the actions of vitamin B_6 (see Ch. 26).

CARBOXYLIC ACIDS

As the bond between O and H becomes weaker the OH group becomes more ready to donate a proton to a suitable recipient, i.e. a base. As was seen in the case of phenols, the weakening of the bond in the OH group arises from electrons being withdrawn by an adjacent chemical structure. In a carboxylic acid this electron withdrawing group is C=O. The ionisation of a carboxylic acid is shown in Figure 5.27. The proton separates from the hydroxyl group, leaving a negative charge on the oxygen group. The charged form of the acid is further stabilised by the ability of the negative charge to delocalise over both C–O bonds.

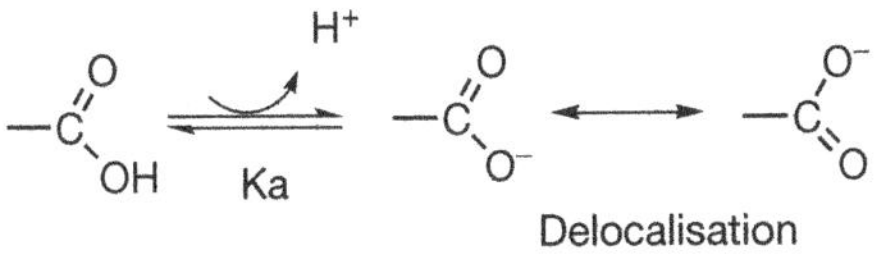

Figure 5.27 Ionisation of a carboxylic acid group.

The tendency of the acid to lose a proton is indicated by the equilibrium constant *Ka* where:

$$Ka = \frac{[COO^-][H^+]}{[-COOH]}$$

The term $-\log Ka$ is known as the p*Ka* value and the smaller the value of p*Ka*, the stronger the acid. The Henderson-Hasselbalch equation for an acid can be written as follows:

$$pH = pKa + \log\frac{[A^-]}{[HA]}$$

The groups attached to the carbonyl have an additional effect on acid strength. Thus the simplest carboxylic acid formic acid has a p*Ka* value of 3.77 while acetic acid is a weaker acid with a p*Ka* value of 4.76 due to the inductive release of electrons by the methyl group which strengthens the O–H bond. In contrast, trichloroacetic acid has a p*Ka* value of 0.65 due to the withdrawal of electrons from the O–H bond by the electronegative chlorine atoms (Fig. 5.28). The amino acids are all relatively strong acids with p*Ka* values of *ca.* 2.5 which result from the positive charge on the alpha amino group (the amino group being completely ionised below *ca.* pH 7) exerting an electron withdrawing effect. Benzoic acid is also a stronger acid than acetic acid because of the electron withdrawing effect of the benzene ring.

The carboxyl group of substituted benzoic acids is greatly affected by whether or not the substituents in the ring are electron withdrawing or electron donating. Substituents in ortho, meta and para positions have an effect, the most marked usually being produced by ortho substituents. Electron donating groups such as the amino group or the phenolic group generally reduce acidic strength (Fig. 5.29).

Acidic strength can also be affected by hydrogen bonding to adjacent groups. Thus salicylic acid (p*Ka* 2.8) is a stronger acid than aspirin (p*Ka* 3.5) (Fig. 5.30). Where the substituted hydroxyl group is unable to increase acid strength through hydrogen bonding, the meta- and para-hydroxy benzoic acids are much weaker acids. The strong

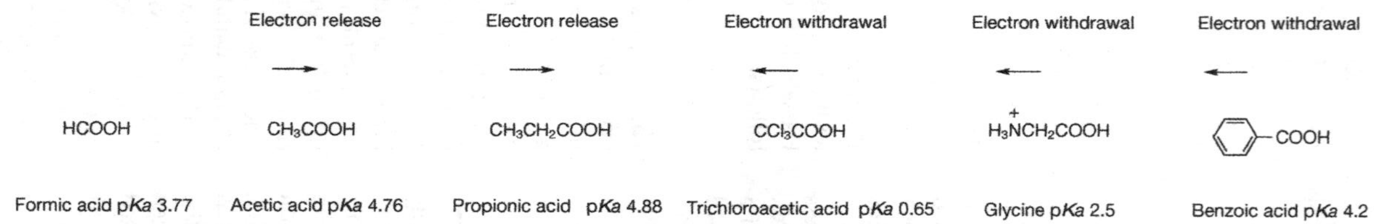

Figure 5.28 The strength of various carboxylic acids.

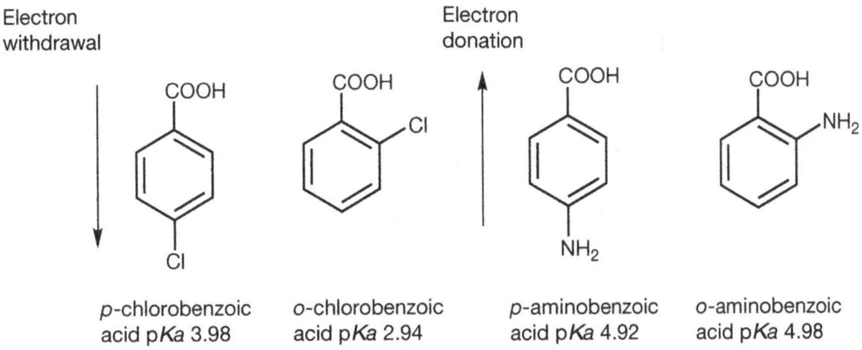

Figure 5.29 The strength of aromatic carboxylic acids.

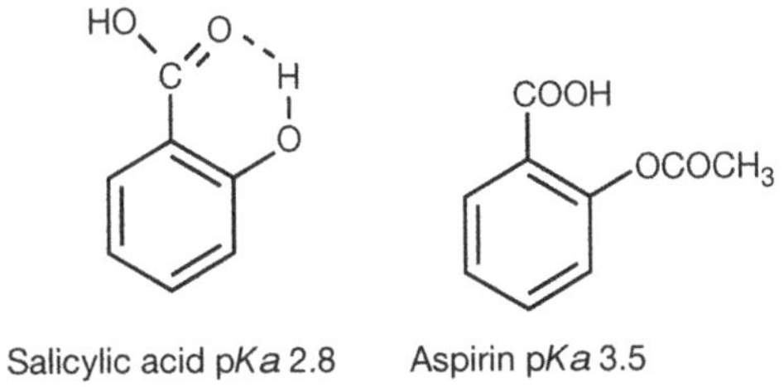

Figure 5.30 The effect of hydrogen bonding on acidic strength.

acidity of salicylic acid makes it useful as a keratolytic agent for use in the removal of warts and corns.

Salts of carboxylic acids

Carboxylic acids form salts with alkalis and this provides a method for obtaining water-soluble forms of acidic drugs since organic acids containing more than five carbon atoms are poorly water soluble. Thus, for example, the antiepileptic drug valproic acid is formulated as its sodium salt and non-steroidal anti-inflammatory drugs such as diclofenac and naproxen may be formulated as sodium salts (Fig. 5.31). Acidic drugs in the form of their water-soluble sodium salts are released more rapidly from tablets even into the acidic medium of the stomach contents. The water-soluble sodium salt of diclofenac is used in water based anti-inflammatory eye drops.

As the number of carbon atoms in organic acids increases, even their sodium salts begin to have limited water solubility. However, salts of long-chain fatty acids such as sodium stearate are fairly water soluble (*ca.* 1 in 20) and form soaps which have both a degree of water solubility and the ability to dissolve organic compounds. These reduce the surface tension of water, thus acting as wetting agents. The soap molecules form ionic micelles, as shown in Figure 5.32, which have the ability to improve the solubility of organic molecules in water. They also have a basic antibacterial action because their amphiphilic nature means that they can disrupt cell membranes. Simple soaps derived from fatty acids have a disadvantage compared to detergents in that their water solubility is relatively low and at pH values below *ca.* 4.0 they will be largely in

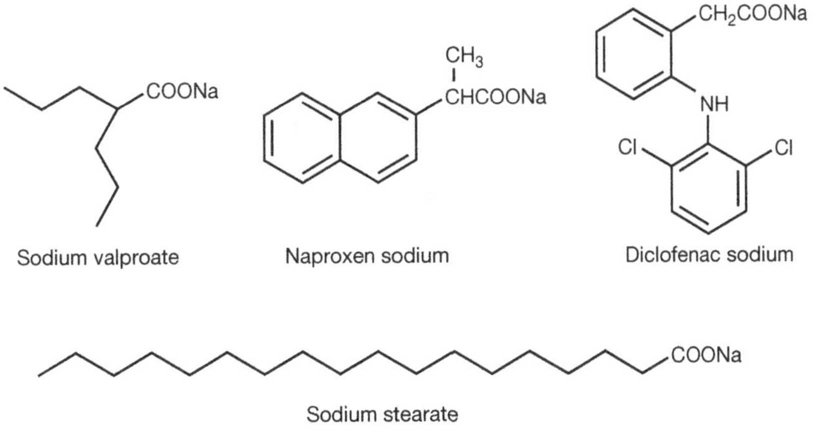

Figure 5.31 Sodium salts of water otherwise water-insoluble drugs.

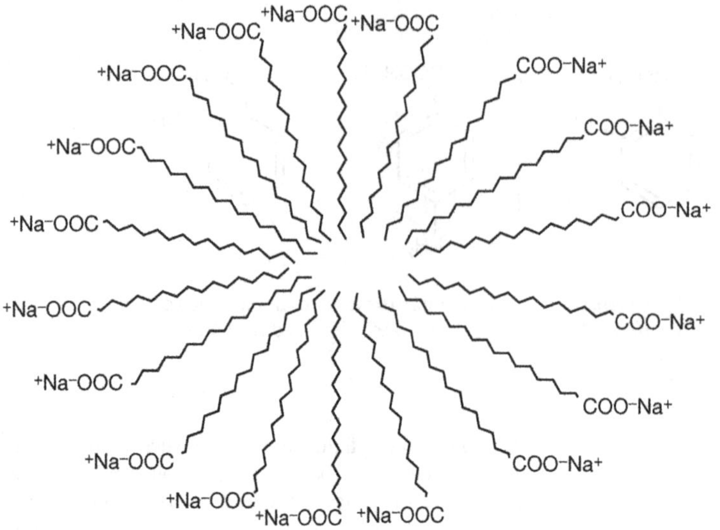

Figure 5.32 Micelle with highly ionised surface and hydrophobic core.

the form of water-insoluble fatty acids. Although the sodium and potassium salts of soaps are quite soluble, the calcium and magnesium salts are much less so. However, these salts are still waxy and are used as lubricants in tablet compression and also have soothing effects when incorporated into talcum powders. Zinc salts of fatty acids such as zinc stearate are also used for their mild astringent and antimicrobial properties in topical preparations.

Salts formed between amines and carboxylic acids

When an amine drug is formulated, the choice of carboxylic acid used as a counter-ion is important with regard to the properties desired for the salt. For instance, erythromycin is formulated as its lactobionate salt (Fig. 5.33) for use in injections since this salt is freely water soluble, whereas it is formulated as its lipophilic stearate salt in order to improve its oral bioavailability. The use of salts in the formulation of amines is discussed further in Chapter 3.

ESTERS

Carboxylic acids react with alcohols to form esters. The reaction is catalysed by the presence of acid and the equilibrium is driven to the right by the removal of water. Esters formed with many organic acids are much less water soluble than the parent alcohol and acid. However, esters formed between alcohols and inorganic acids such as phosphate or sulphate or with dicarboxylic acids such as succinic acid are often used in order to increase the water solubility of alcohols. Inorganic esters such as phosphate and particularly sulphate are more susceptible to hydrolysis than those

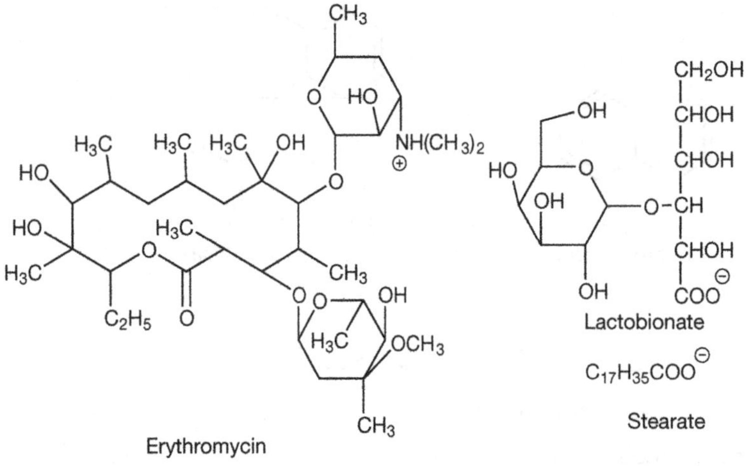

Figure 5.33 Erythromycin with lactobionate and stearate counterions.

of carboxylic acids. Thus esters can be used either to render a drug molecule more lipophilic or to improve its water solubility, depending on the type of ester formed.

Chemical stability

Esters are unstable at extremes of pH. Their rate of hydrolysis in alkaline solution is greater than their rate of hydrolysis in acidic solution, thus within the pH range in water esters are most stable at around pH 4.5. Acidic and basic hydrolysis of the ester group of procaine is shown in Figure 5.34. This reaction was one of the factors which led to procaine being less frequently used in local anaesthesia, since the hydrolysis reaction was promoted by the heating required to sterilise injections containing it. The stability of ester drugs is a consideration when drugs containing esters groups are stored. Aspirin is the usual example used to illustrate problems of storage since it is readily hydrolysed to acetic acid and salicylic acid; however, it is an ester of a phenol and is thus less stable than aliphatic esters such as procaine or hydrocortisone acetate.

The rate of ester hydrolysis is affected by the substituents which are present within the structure of the ester. This is more of an important consideration in the case of basic hydrolysis, as rates of acid hydrolysis are less affected by substituents. Electron withdrawing substituents increase the rate of hydrolysis since they increase the susceptibility of the carbonyl carbon to attack and, conversely, bulky electron releasing substituents decrease the rate of hydrolysis. The detailed mechanisms of acid and base catalysed ester hydrolysis are shown in Figures 5.35 and 5.36. In both cases the positively charged carbonyl carbon is attacked by a base; in the case of acid hydrolysis the attacking base is water, whereas under alkaline conditions the base is the hydroxyl group.

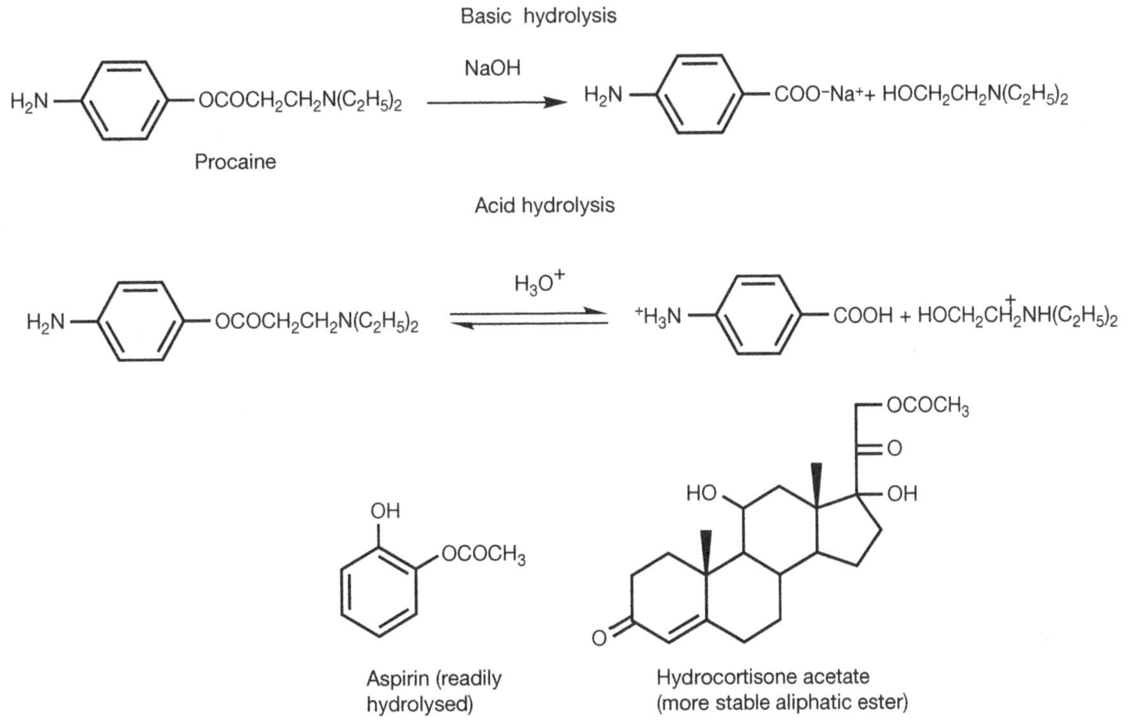

Figure 5.34 Ester hydrolysis.

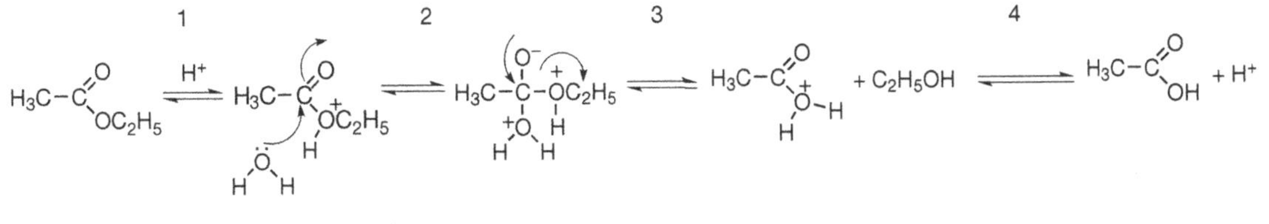

Figure 5.35 Acid catalysed hydrolysis of an ester.

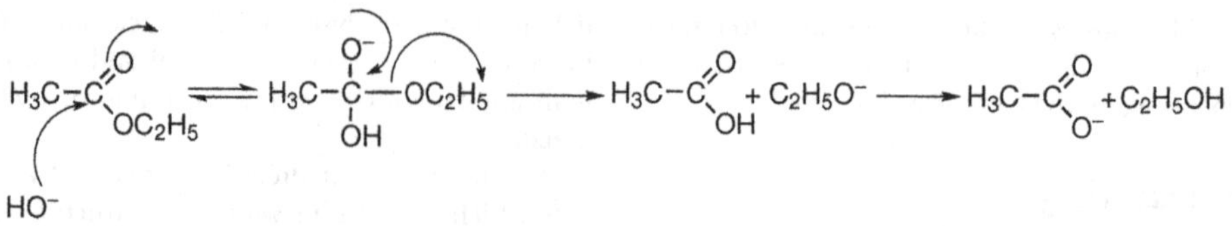

Figure 5.36 Base catalysed hydrolysis of an ester.

The effect of substituents on hydrolysis rates can be seen clearly for a series of esters of nicotinic acid shown in Table 5.2.[1] The rate of hydrolysis is greatly increased where the substituent is electron withdrawing. Increased bulk of the alkyl group results in a decreasing rate of hydrolysis and if the alkyl chain is branched at a point close to the oxygen to which it is attached the rate of hydrolysis declines even more.

As can be seen for the nicotinic esters, esters of aromatic acids are strongly affected by substituents. Substituents within an aromatic ring also have an effect. Electron releasing substituents such as an amine of aromatic ether in the ortho or para positions reduce the rates of hydrolysis of ester groups in comparison with H in these positions (opposite to their effect in the aliphatic alcohol chains shown in Table 5.2). Electron withdrawing groups such as halogen or nitro in the ortho- or para- positions increase the rate of hydrolysis in comparison with H in these positions. Substitutions in the ortho- positions have less marked effect in increasing the rate of hydrolysis because the bulky group in the ortho- position hinders the hydrolysis (Fig. 5.37).

The rate of acid hydrolysis of esters is relatively little affected by the substituents within aliphatic ester chains. The strongest effects are in the case of halogenated alkyl groups where esters such as trifluoroacetate and trichloroacetate are much more susceptible to acid hydrolysis than acetate esters.

Q Self Test 5.4

List the following steroid esters in order of increasing rate of hydrolysis in solution at pH 7.4 and 37°C.

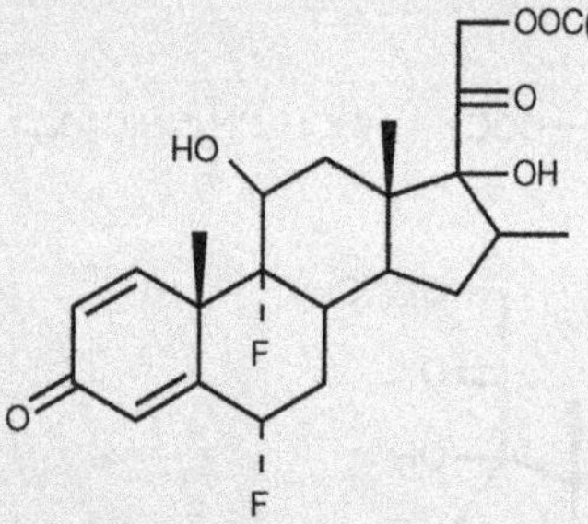

1. Flumetasone pivalate

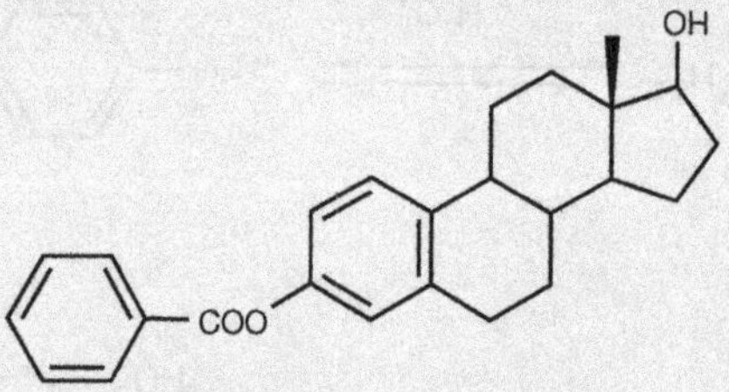

2. Estradiol benzoate

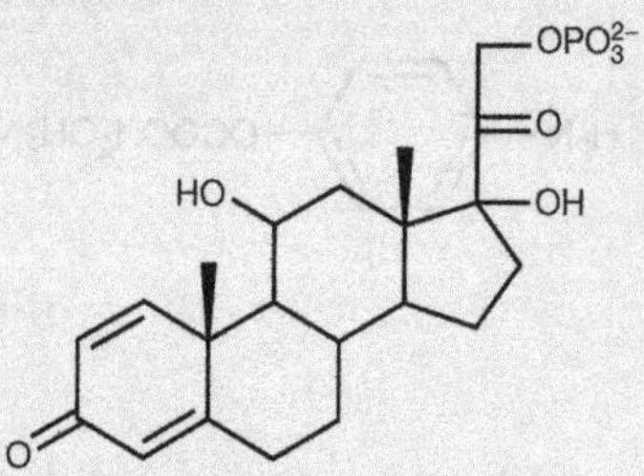

3. Prednisolone phosphate

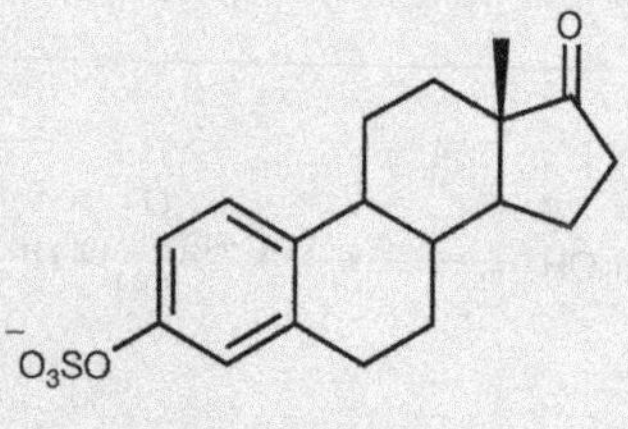

4. Estrone sulphate

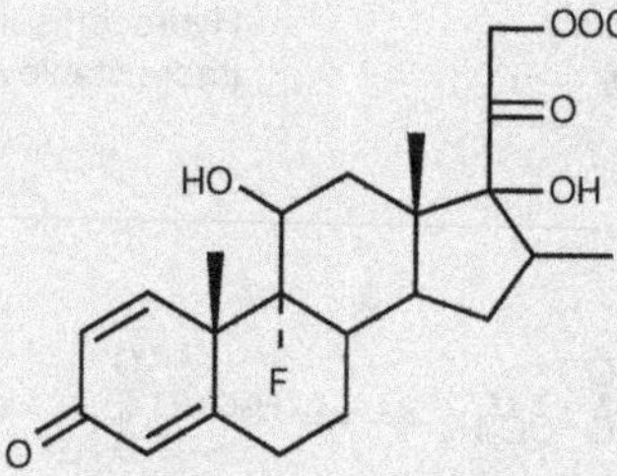

5. Betamethasone acetate

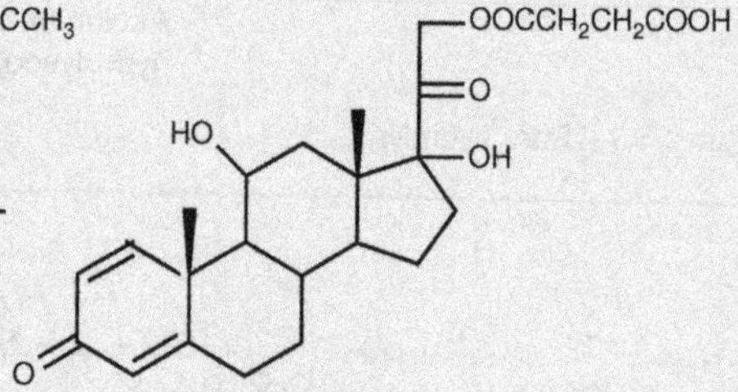

6. Prednisolone hemisuccinate

Table 5.2 Hydrolysis of nicotinate esters at pH 7.4, 37° C

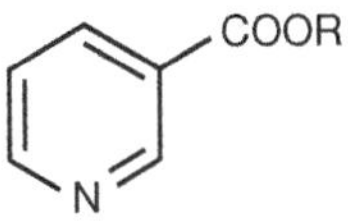

R	Relative rate of hydrolysis	Half life days	Comments
CH_3-	1	12.3	
C_2H_5-	0.39	30.7	Hydrolysis slower with increasing bulk of R
C_3H_7-	0.40	30.7	Hydrolysis slower with increasing bulk of R
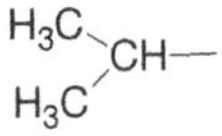	0.21	58	Branching of chain hinders hydrolysis
C_6H_{13}-	Too low to measure	Years	Group very hydrophobic and slow to hydrolyse
$ClCH_2CH_2-$	1.6	7.7	Electron withdrawing Cl increases rate of hydrolysis
$H_3\overset{+}{N}CH_2CH_2CH_2-$	3.1	3.9	Amino group positively charged at this pH, withdraws electrons
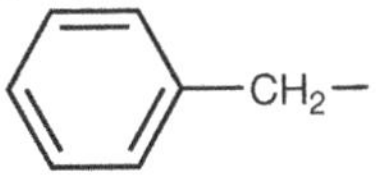	1.3	9.3	Benzyl group slightly electron withdrawing
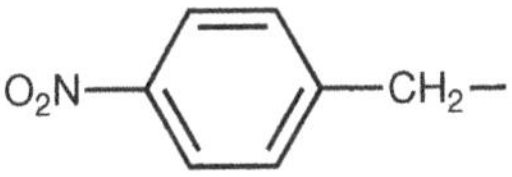	100	0.12	Nitro group very strongly electron withdrawing and greatly increases rate of hydrolysis
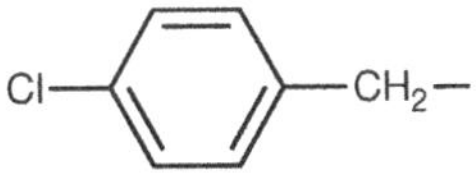	17	0.71	Chlorine atom withdraws electrons increasing rate of hydrolysis

Transesterification

A variation on the basic hydrolysis process is transesterification which is a widespread process in biological systems (c.f. the action of aspirin, choline esterase inhibitors and phosphorylation of proteins) but can also occur in vitro. In this case, the ester transfers the acyl group to the base carrying out the hydrolysis. Thus, for instance, if the base is paracetamol, as has been observed in mixtures of aspirin and paracetamol, acetylated paracetamol is produced (Fig. 5.38).

Aspirin has been shown to acetylate a number of alcohols and phenols when combined in formulations.

Enzymatic hydrolysis of esters

Esterases within the body hydrolyse esters at varying rates. From a physiological point of view it is important that lipophilic ester groups are removed from a drug molecule so that the free alcohol group can be conjugated to a polar glucuronide or sulphate moiety in order to improve water solubility and thus aid in its elimination from the body. The rate of hydrolysis of esters by enzymes is an important area of study since the susceptibility of esters to hydrolysis has a bearing on several aspects of drug action. It is difficult to generalise about what structural factors affect enzyme hydrolysis of esters but it is clear

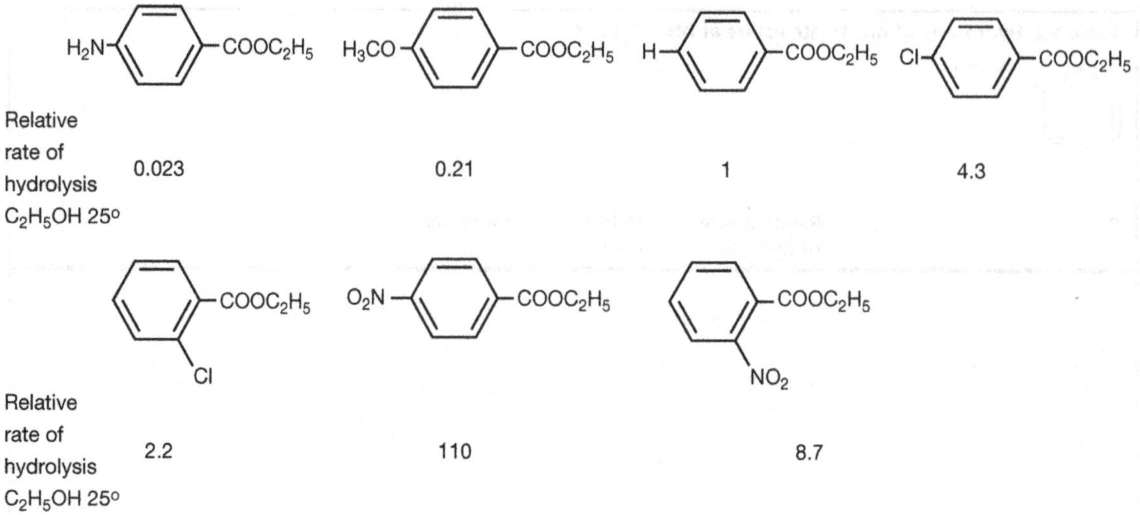

Figure 5.37 Effect of ortho and para substitution on ester hydrolysis rate.

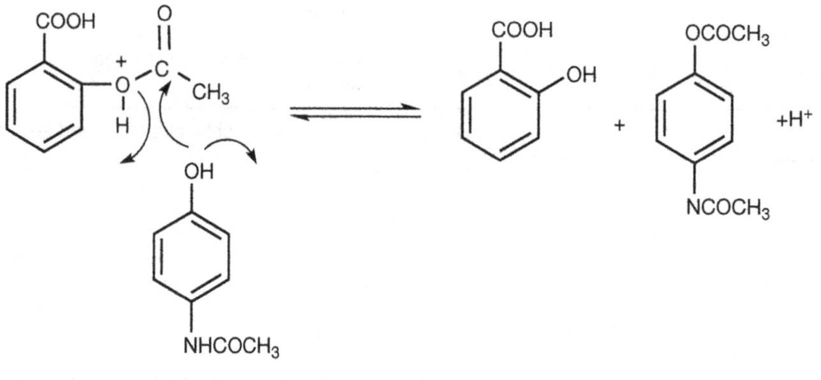

Figure 5.38 Transesterification resulting in acetylation of paracetamol by aspirin.

that, like chemical hydrolysis, the rates of hydrolysis are strongly influenced by electronic and steric factors. However, another parameter which is important is how strongly the ester binds to the esterase and how well it fits into its active site. Hydrolysis of the series of nicotinic acid esters described above was studied in microsomes from rat liver.[1] Nicotinic acid itself can be used as a lipid-lowering drug but has a very short lifetime in the body and esterification prolongs its lifetime. Of the straight chain esters, the most rapid rate of hydrolysis was for the ethyl ester (Table 5.3). With longer chains, the strength of binding to the enzyme does not increase but the rate of hydrolysis falls, indicating that the substrate does not fit into the active site as well. The fastest rate of hydrolysis is for the phenolic ester, which reflects the chemical instability of these esters, despite the fact that the phenyl group is bulky and a poor fit into the active site.

In an attempt to design ester prodrugs, more complex esters may be formed. Tables 5.4 and 5.5 show the rates of hydrolysis of some esters of paracetamol and *p*-acetamidobenzoic acid (PAABA) by different esterases.[2] The rate of hydrolysis of the phenolic hexyl ester is more rapid than that of the propyl ester although the rate of hydrolysis of this ester in buffer alone is very slow. The cationic (diethylamino) and anionic esters are hydrolysed very slowly, reflecting their weak binding to the esterase due to low lipophilicity and poor fit of the active site. The carboxyethyl ester is hydrolysed relatively slowly by all but the plasma esterases, reflecting its relatively low lipophilicity.

The esters of PAABA reflect the pattern observed for the esters of paracetamol but the hydrolysis rates are much lower, apart from the alkyl esters which have similar rates of hydrolysis to the paracetamol esters in plasma and liver.

Table 5.3 Enzymatic binding strength and rate of hydrolysis for nicotinic acid esters

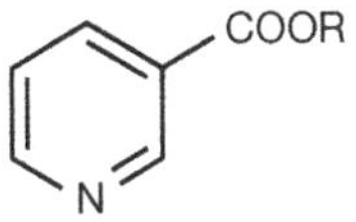

R	Relative rate of hydrolysis in microsomes	Relative strength of binding to enzyme	Comments
CH_3–	1	1	
C_2H_5–	1.3	1.5	Optimum chain length for chemical hydrolysis
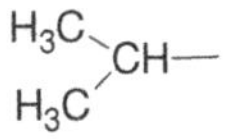	0.14	9.6	Steric hindrance slows hydrolysis
C_4H_9–	0.56	30	Rate of hydrolysis still quite high
C_6H_{13}-	0.14	96	Rate of hydrolysis much higher than in buffer alone
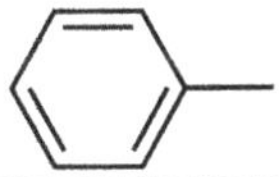	3.3	9.4	Phenolic esters very labile despite bulky group
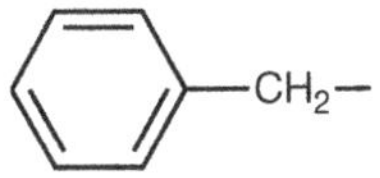	0.72	28	Hydrolysis rate high despite bulky group

Table 5.4 Rates of hydrolysis of esters of paracetamol

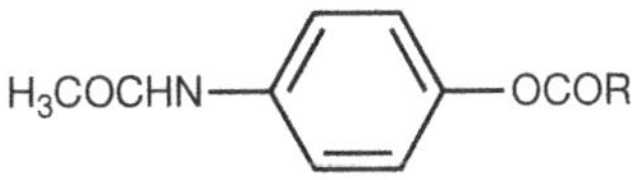

R	Half life pH 7.0, 37°C days	Relative rate of hydrolysis intestine	Relative rate of hydrolysis liver	Relative rate of hydrolysis plasma
C_3H_7–	3.5	1	1	1
C_6H_{13}-	Not measurable	8	8	9
$(C_2H_5)_2N(CH_2)_2$—diethylamino	ND	0.0009	0.0007	0.08
$HOOC(CH_3)_3$—glutaryl	ND	0.006	0.05	0.008
C_2H_5OCOO—carboxyethyl	ND	0.35	0.35	1

ND = not determined.

Table 5.5 Rates of hydrolysis of esters of *p*-acetamido benzoic acid

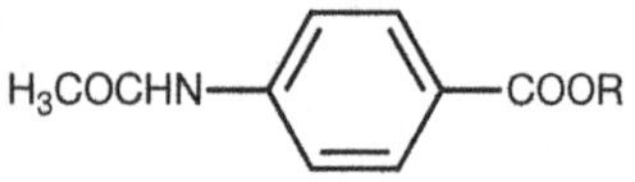

R	Half life pH 7.0, 37°C days	Relative* rate of hydrolysis intestine	Relative* rate of hydrolysis liver	Relative* rate of hydrolysis plasma
C_3H_7–	Not measurable	0.002	0.3	0.9
C_4H_9–	Not measurable	0.007	0.2	1
$(C_2H_5)_2N(CH_2)_2$—	6.7	0.0001	0.003	0.01
$HOOC(CH_3)_3$—	Not measurable	<0.001	<0.001	<0.001

*Rates relative to the hydrolysis rate of paracetamol propionate.

Table 5.6 Rates of hydrolysis of esters of R and S propranolol

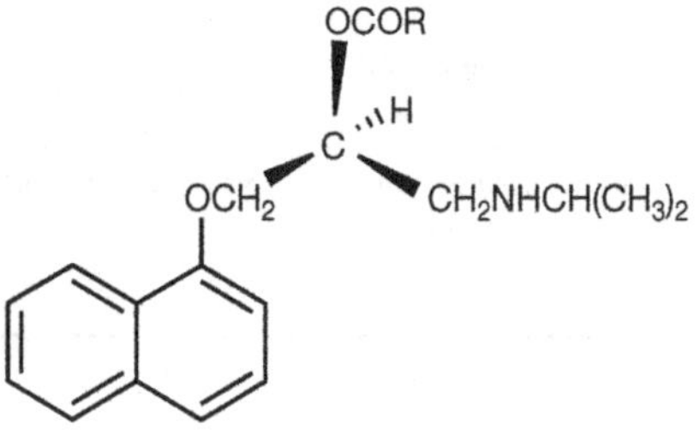

S propranolol ester

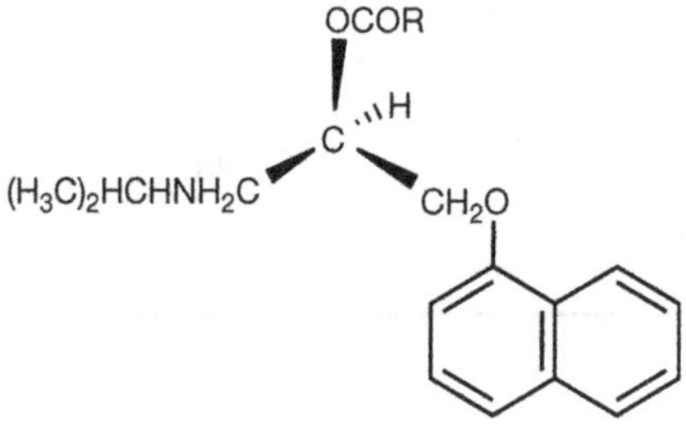

R propranolol ester

R	*Plasma	*Intestine	*Liver
CH_3–R	1	0.031	0.007
CH_3–*S*	0.18	0.064	0.021
C_3H_7–*R*	1.4	0.31	0.056
C_3H_7–*S*	0.18	0.51	0.16
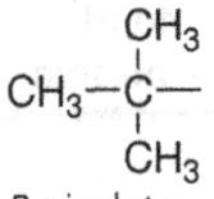 CH_3–C(CH_3)(CH_3)— *R* pivalate	0.13	0.014	0.011
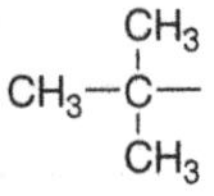 CH_3–C(CH_3)(CH_3)— *S* pivalate	0.075	0.018	0.011

*Rates of hydrolysis relative to the *R* acetate in plasma, based on rates min^{-1} per mg of protein.

For a series of esters of propranolol, esterases from different tissues displayed varying rates of hydrolysis towards esters of the R and S forms of the drug. Plasma esterases hydrolysed the *R* esters at about ten times the rate of the *S* esters, where the rate of hydrolysis was rapid (Table 5.6). In the case of the hindered pivalate ester the rate of hydrolysis was much slower and the chiral discrimination was much reduced. Chiral discrimination by liver and intestinal esterases favoured hydrolysis of the *S* esters but was less marked, reflecting the less rapid hydrolysis of the esters by extracts from these tissues.[3]

As in the case of base catalysed hydrolysis, substituents in the aromatic ring influence the rate of hydrolysis of benzoyl esters. Halogens in the ortho- or meta- positions promote rapid hydrolysis while an amino group para to the ester results in relatively slow hydrolysis. Thus, for example, chloroprocaine is a shorter-acting version of procaine since its rate of hydrolysis by plasma esterases is about four times that of procaine.

Q Self Test 5.5

Place the following esters in order of increasing rate of hydrolysis by plasma esterases.

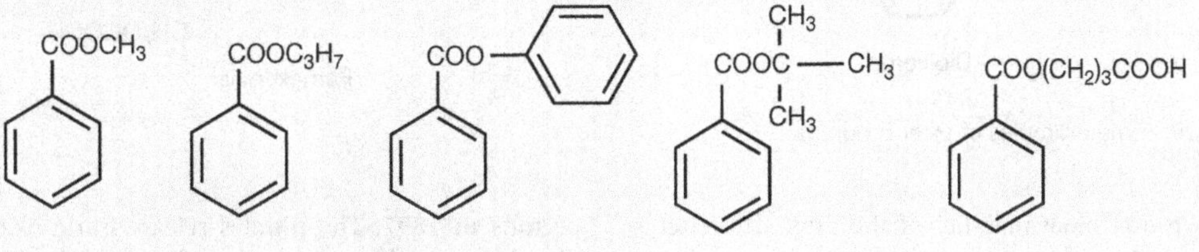

1 2 3 4 5

Q Self Test 5.6

Place the following esters in order of increasing rate of hydrolysis by plasma esterases.

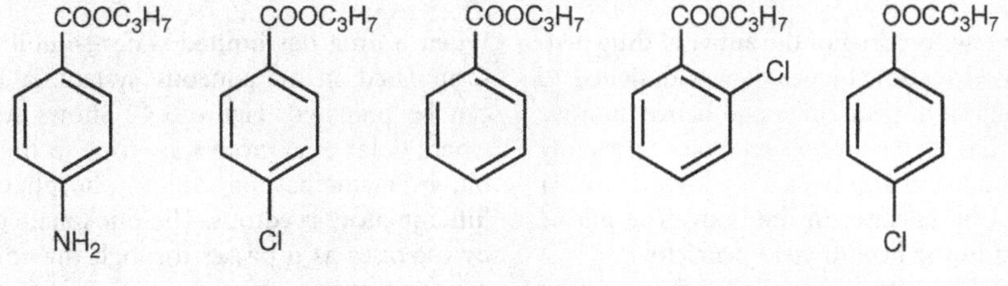

1 2 3 4 5

The role of esters in modifying physicochemical properties of drugs

Esters can be used in a number of situations to improve the delivery of drugs. However, to be effective, the ester group must be enzymatically removed so that the drug is converted into its active form in the body. Thus the ester must have good stability in vitro but be a good substrate in vivo, and ideally the half-life conversion of the ester in vivo into the active drug should be about 10 minutes. In contrast, the half-life in formulations should be >10 years.

Esters for improving drug absorption

Figure 5.39 shows some ester prodrugs. Esters of corticosteroids such as betamethasone 17-valerate are used in topical anti-inflammatory creams. The presence of the lipophilic ester group increases the penetration of the corticosteroid into the skin which itself is lipophilic. The ester group is rapidly removed by esterases in the tissues to yield the corticosteroid; thus the ester functions as prodrug with improved skin penetration.

Diloxanide furoate is an ester prodrug of the amoebicide diloxanide and was produced to be more lipophilic

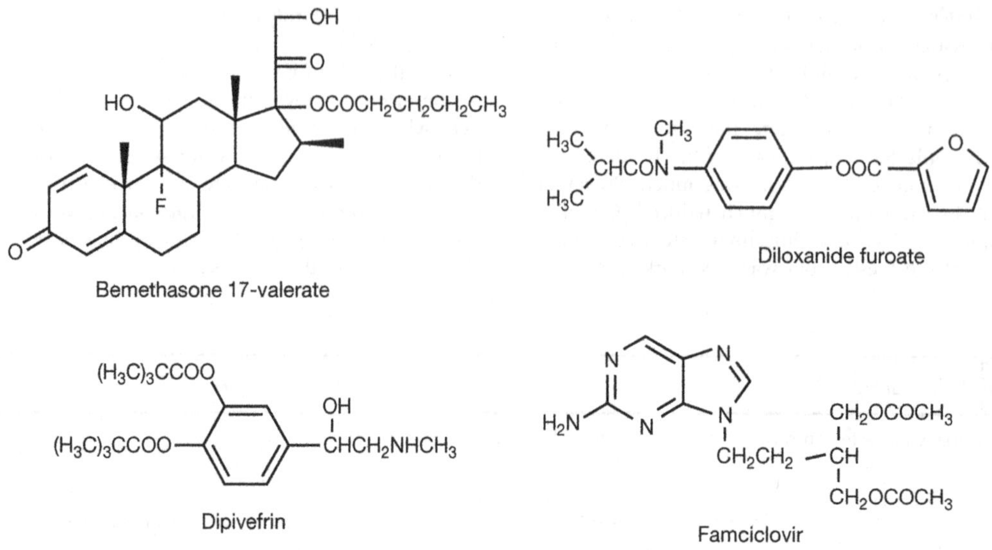

Figure 5.39 Some examples of ester prodrugs.

to improve oral bioavailability of the drug. The ester is rapidly hydrolysed by esterases in the liver and plasma to yield the free drug.

Dipivefrin is a prodrug of adrenaline which can be used to lower intraocular pressure in the treatment of glaucoma. Drugs with a balance of lipophilic and hydrophilic properties are best absorbed by the eye. Dipiverfrin is more lipophilic than adrenaline and penetrates the eye efficiently, being converted to free adrenaline by esterases in the cornea.

Famciclovir is an ester prodrug of the antiviral drug penciclovir which is used to treat herpes. It was designed to increase the lipophilicity of penciclovir and hence improve oral absorption. It has to be administered less frequently than less lipophilic antiviral agents such aciclovir. The ester groups are removed by esterases in the body. The purine ring is also oxidised in the liver to yield penciclovir.

Pivampicillin (see Ch. 22) was designed to improve the oral bioavailability of ampicillin, which is poorly absorbed. The ester group increases its lipophilicity, resulting in better absorption in the stomach. It is not a simple ester since there is a spacer group in the molecule derived from formaldehyde and pivalic acid. Such esters are known as acyloxy esters. Free ampicillin is rapidly released in two stages: first, the pivalate group is hydrolysed by esterases and then is followed by spontaneous release of the formaldehyde used in the spacer group. The second step may account for the reluctance to use the drug in humans since formaldehyde is a toxic compound; however, the prodrug is widely used in veterinary medicine (Fig. 5.40).

A specific group of ester prodrugs are the esters of nitrous acid and nitric acid which are used in treatment of angina. Amyl nitrate was first used to treat angina pectoris in 1897. The nitrates release nitric oxide (NO) directly when the ester is hydrolysed in the body. The alkyl nitrates have been replaced by the volatile nitrate esters such as glycerol trinitrate and isosorbide dinitrate. These compounds are also believed to act via the generation of nitric oxide, and glutathione is involved in their metabolic activation (Fig. 5.41).

Esters for improving water solubility

When a drug has limited water solubility and has to be formulated in an aqueous system, a hydrophilic ester can be prepared. Figure 5.42 shows some examples of where polar ester groups are used to improve water solubility. Betamethasone sodium phosphate is used in anti-inflammatory eyedrops. The phosphate group is removed by esterases as it passes through the cornea. Betamethasone phosphate is also used in injections as is the water-soluble hydrocortisone sodium succinate which is formulated in high-dose injections used to treat septic shock. Clindamycin phosphate provides better water-solubility characteristics for the drug so that it can be formulated into injections. In the case of diethylstilbestrol diphosphate (fosfestrol sodium), the addition of phosphate ester groups is not designed to improve water solubility but rather to improve site-directed therapy. Tumour cells contain elevated levels of phosphatases in comparison with the rest of the tissues in the body and the removal of the phosphate groups converts it to its active form at its site of action. Water-soluble esters also feature in drug metabolism where the body converts alcohol or phenol groups into sulphate esters, e.g. estrone and paracetamol sulphates.

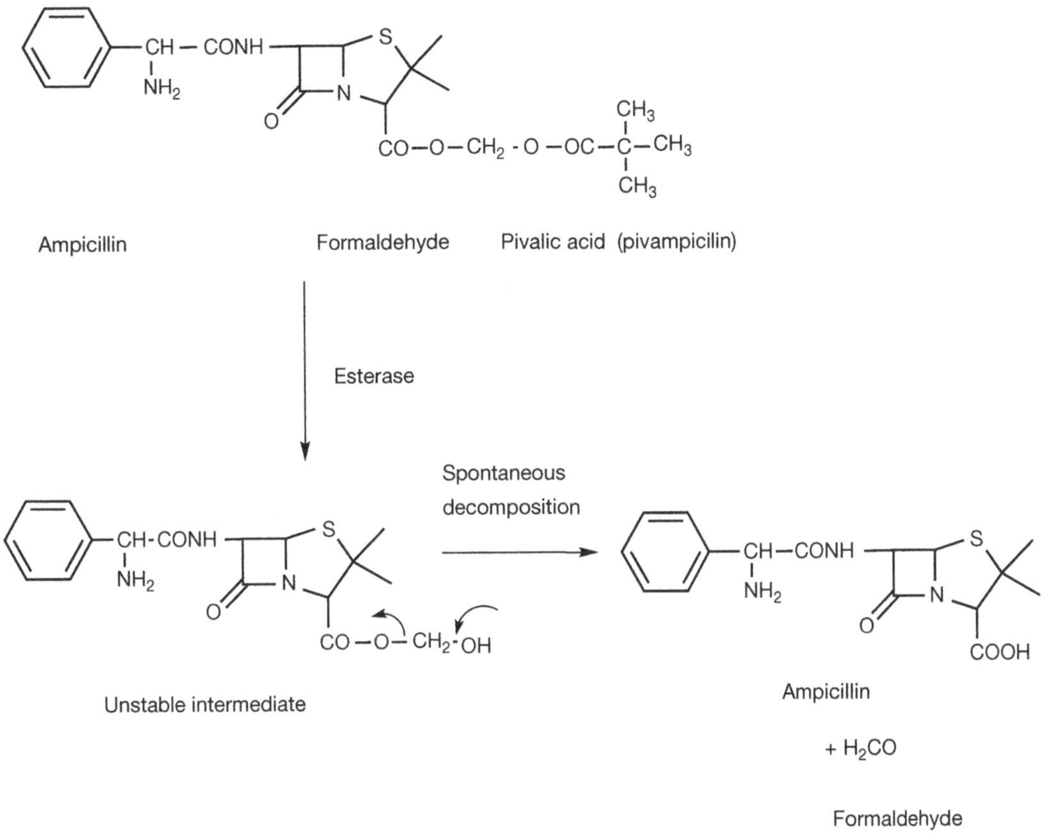

Figure 5.40 Ester prodrug of pivampicillin.

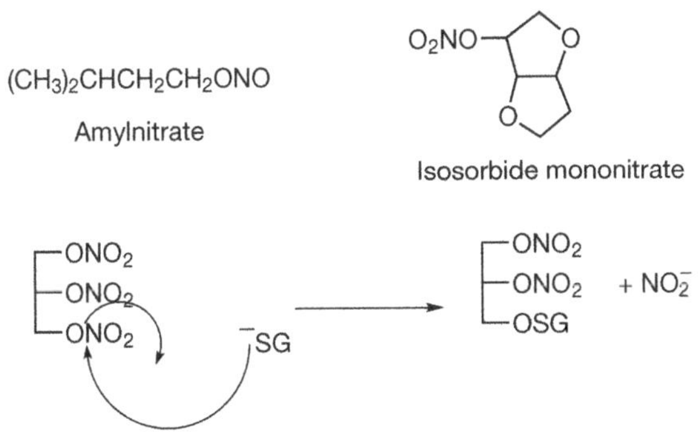

Figure 5.41 Nitrate esters used in the treatment of angina.

Esters used for sustained drug delivery

Testosterone is used in the form of esters such as its enanthate in hormone replacement therapy. The drug is given in an oily injection and, because of its high degree of lipophilicity, it forms a depot in fatty tissue and thus dosing may only be required once a month. Other steroid hormone esters are used in a similar manner, e.g. hydroxyprogesterone caproate and nandrolone decanoate. The same approach is used in the treatment of psychosis with haloperidol decanoate. The drug is given in an oily injection once a month and forms a slow-release depot, being hydrolysed to the free drug by plasma esterases (see Ch. 20). A number of other antipsychotic drugs are also used in the form of esters with long-chain fatty acids (Fig. 5.43).

Esters for improving drug acceptability and reducing side effects

Esters have been studied in relation to the reduction of some drug side effects. Of particular interest has been the reduction of the gastric irritation produced by non-steroidal anti-inflammatory drugs (NSAIDs). An example of this is acemetacin (Fig. 5.44), which is an ester prodrug of indometacin which, since it requires conversion via an esterase to the active form of the drug, is reported to have reduced potential for producing gastric irritation.

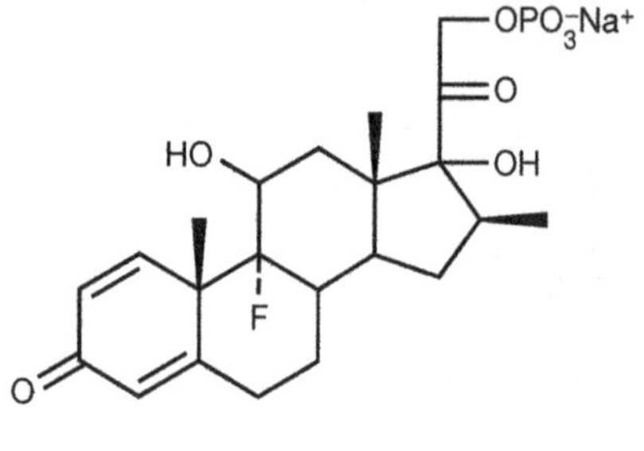

Betamethasone 21-sodium phosphate

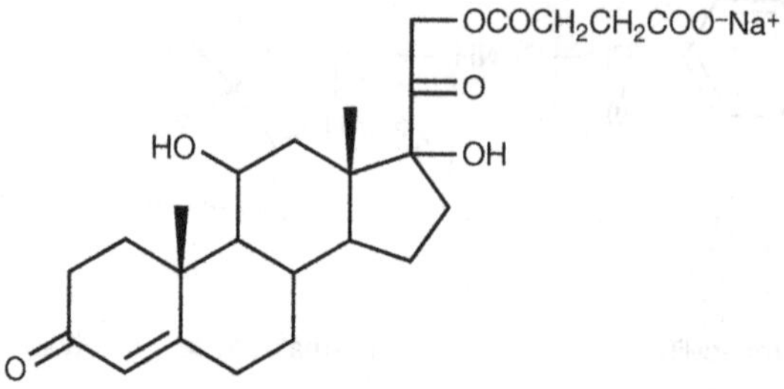

Hydrocortisone 21-sodium succinate

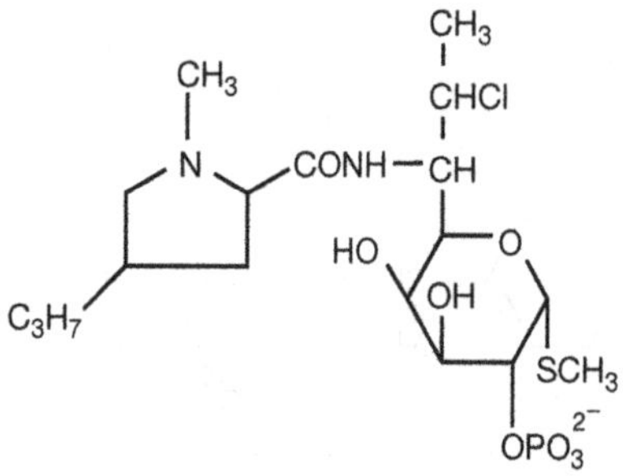

Clindamycin phosphate

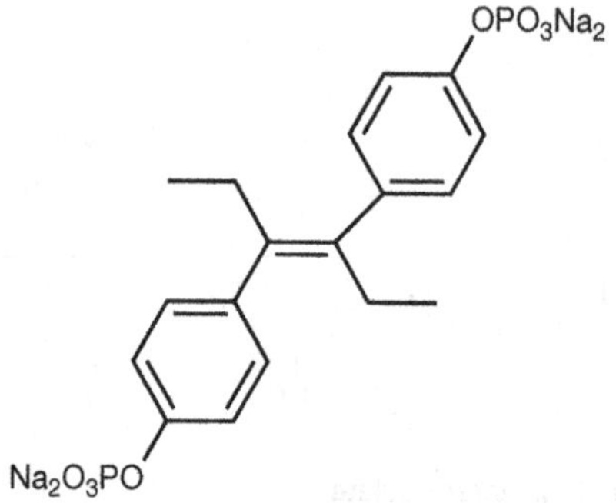

Fosfestrol sodium

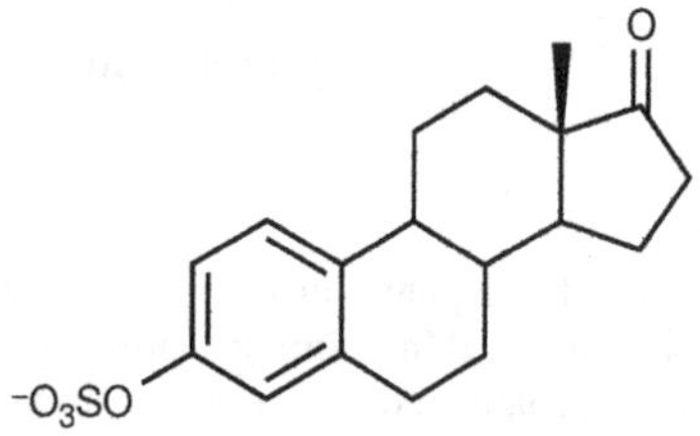

Estrone sulphate

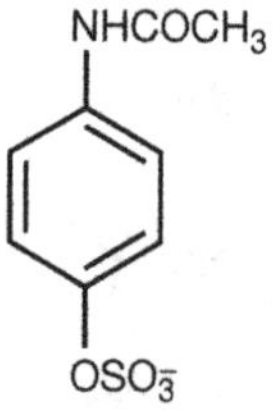

Paracetamol sulphate

Figure 5.42 Esters used to increase water solubility of lipophilic drugs.

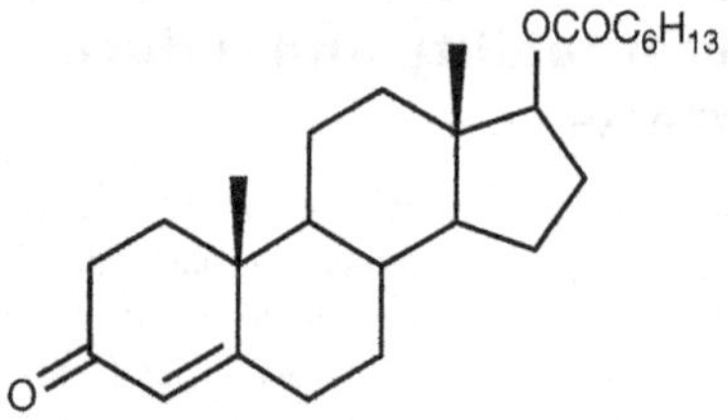

Testosterone enanthate

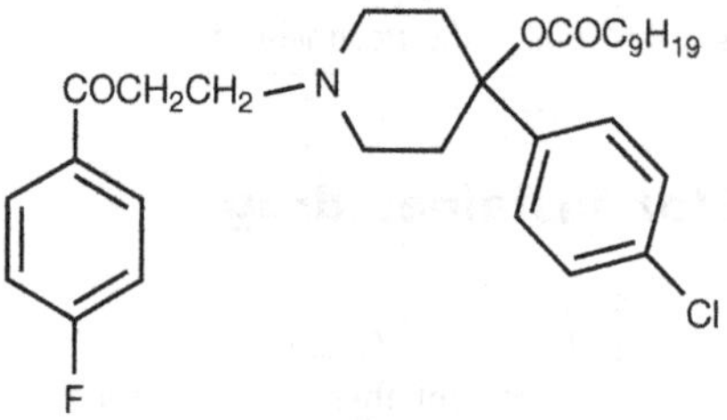

Haloperidol decanoate

Figure 5.43 Esters used to promote increased drug half-life.

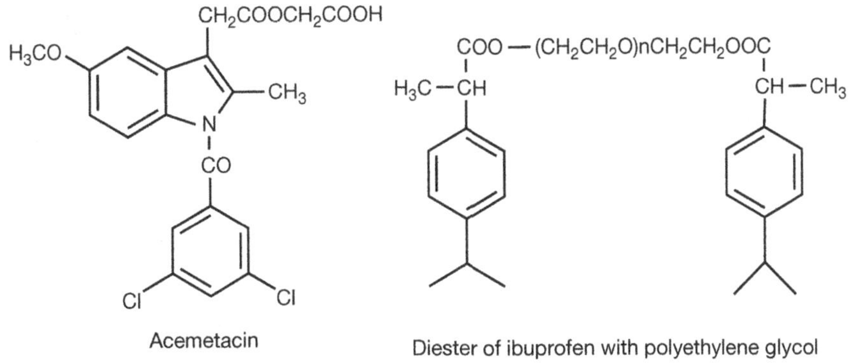

Figure 5.44 Esters used to reduce drug side effects.

In an experimental drug, the NSAID ibuprofen was esterified to a polyethylene glycol (Fig. 5.44) in order to reduce gastric irritation and to produce a sustained-release form of the drug having a longer plasma half-life.

Esters have also been used in a number of instances to mask unpleasant tastes. Examples include chloramphenicol palmitate, clindamycin palmitate and erythromycin ethyl succinate where in each case the free drug tastes extremely unpleasant but its esterified form is tasteless.

The role of esters in terminating drug action

Ester prodrugs such as those described above can be converted to their active form by esterases within the body but the esterases responsible for such conversions are naturally present in order to deactivate biologically active molecules such as acetylcholine. Figure 5.45 shows some examples. The neurotransmitter acetylcholine has its action terminated via the action of acetylcholine esterase which reduces its lipophilicity so that it no longer binds to its receptor (see Ch. 16). Many of the drugs which are agonists of acetylcholine may also have a hydrolysable ester group built into their structure which governs duration of action. Loss of the ester function results in loss of activity. For instance, cyclopentolate is an acetylcholine and antagonist which is deactivated by hydrolysis of its ester function and is used as a short-acting mydriatic. Atropine is also an acetylcholine antagonist which contains a hindered ester function which is only hydrolysed very slowly and is thus a longer-acting mydriatic than cyclopentolate.

Local anaesthetics are predominantly of two types, one containing an ester group and the other containing an amide group. Ester-containing anaesthetics such as procaine have a short duration of action because they are rapidly inactivated via hydrolysis of the ester group. Chloroprocaine (no longer used) was used as a short-duration anaesthetic; the presence of the chlorine weakens the ester bond and promotes rapid hydrolysis by esterases. Oxybuprocaine is moderately stable to esterase activity and is useful in anaesthesia of the eye where a long duration of action is often not desirable.

Suxamethonium is used as a muscle relaxant and its activity is terminated by hydrolysis of one of its ester linkages.

Participation of the ester group in drug action

The acyl group from an ester can be transferred to another alcohol group via the process of transesterification. Aspirin is the most widely used drug in which the ester group is partly responsible for its mechanism of action. In common with the acetylcholine esterase inhibitors discussed below, the target is a serine residue in the enzyme cyclooxygenase 1 (COX-1). However, in the case of aspirin the covalent modification of the enzyme is irreversible. Acetylation of COX-1 prevents the production of prostaglandin inflammatory mediators. The salicylate portion of the molecule also possesses anti-inflammatory action (Fig. 5.46).

Acetylcholine esterase acts very rapidly on acetyl choline removing the acetate group by a base-catalysed mechanism where a histidine residue in the protein accepts a proton from a serine residue which then attacks the carbonyl carbon of the acetate group on the acetylcholine. This results in the production of an acetylated serine residue which hydrolyses rapidly to restore the enzyme to its active state. Choline esterase inhibitors participate in the same enzymic reaction as acetylcholine but the group that they transfer during transesterification (or transcarbamoylation) is hydrolysed much more slowly. For example, neostigmine transfers a dimethylcarbamoyl group (the properties of the carbamoyl group and the ester group are similar) to the serine residue in the active site of acetylcholine esterase. The carbamate formed is hydrolysed much more slowly than the acetyl group (Fig. 5.47) formed under normal circumstances and thus the enzyme undergoes prolonged inhibition (for a more detailed discussion see Ch. 16).

Another class of acetylcholine esterase inhibitors causes irreversible inhibition of the enzyme through the transfer of an organophosphate ester group to the serine residue in the active site. This class of inhibitors has largely been used as either insecticides or nerve gases such as dyflos and parathion (see Ch. 16).

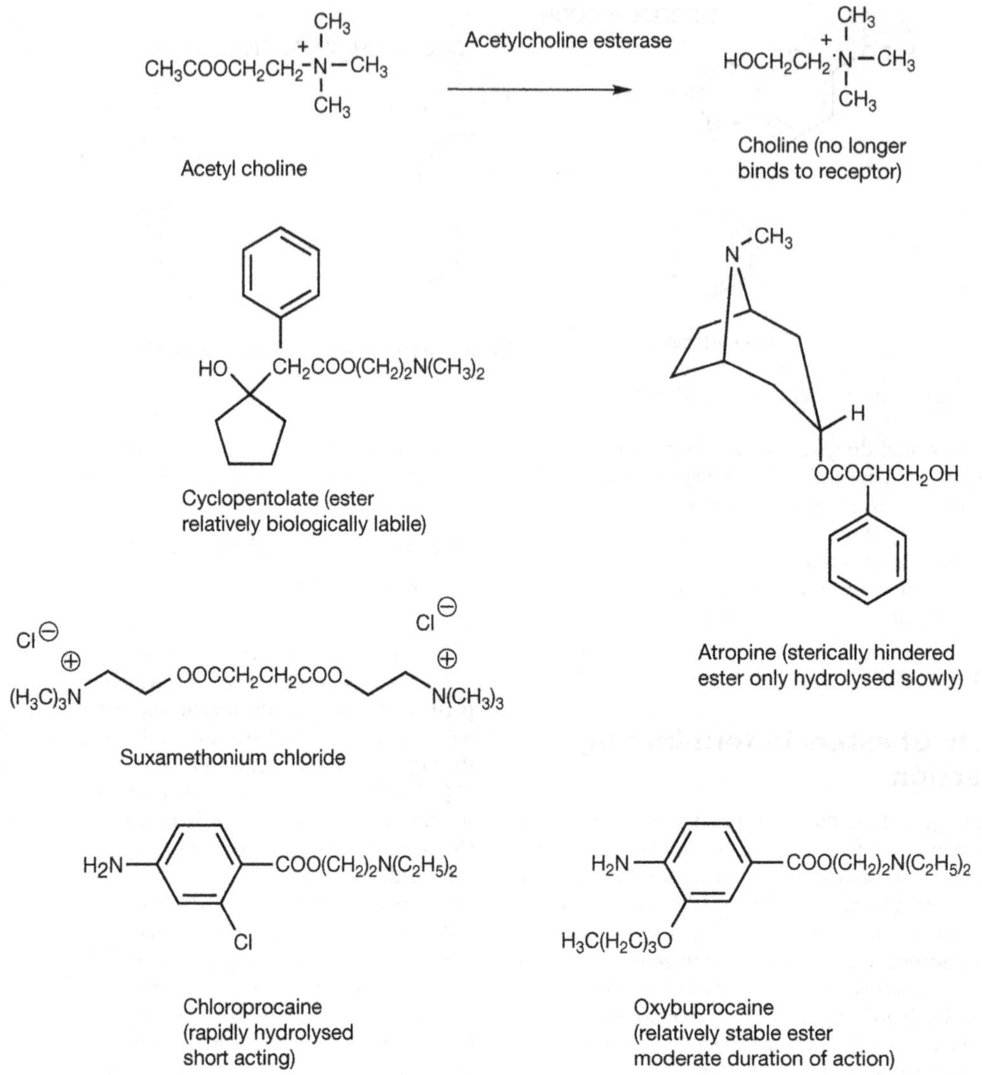

Figure 5.45 The role of the ester group in the termination of drug action.

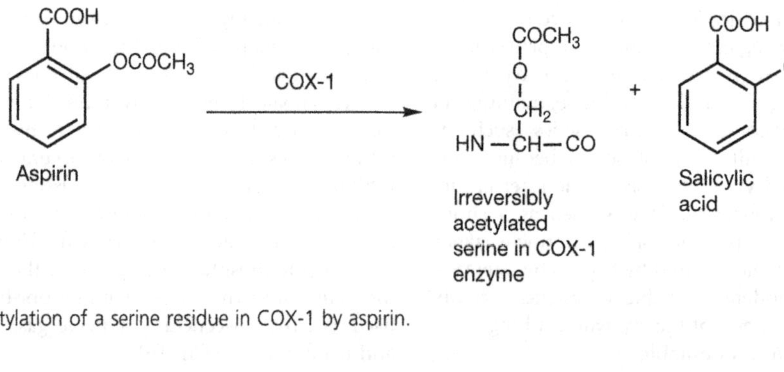

Figure 5.46 Acetylation of a serine residue in COX-1 by aspirin.

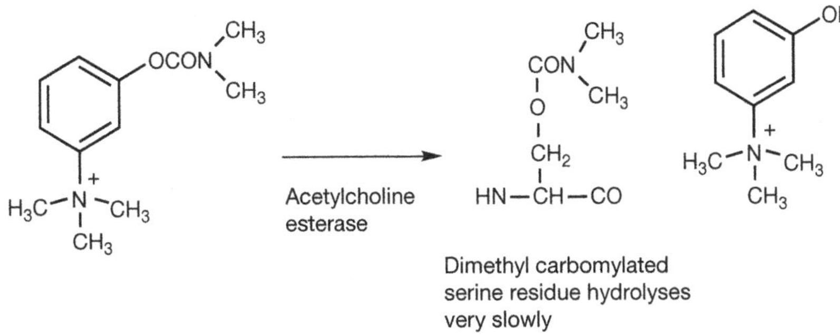

Figure 5.47 Inhibition of choline esterase by carbomylation.

Self Test 5.7

a. Draw the hydrolysis products of the following ester drugs

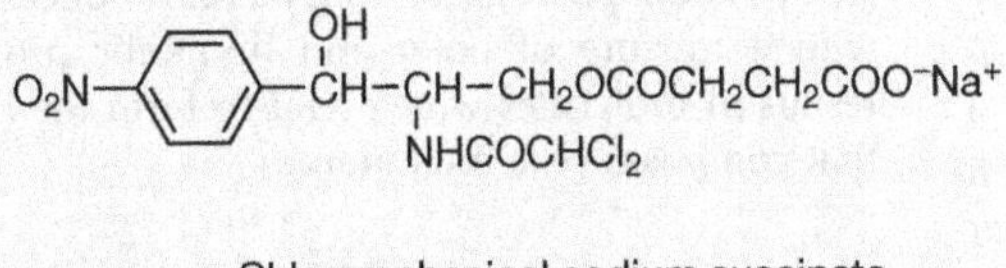

Chloramphenicol sodium succinate

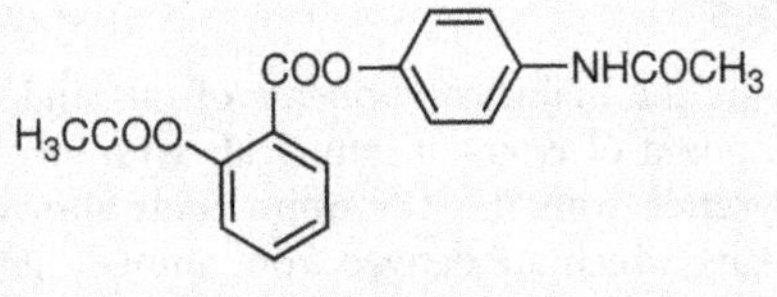

Benorilate

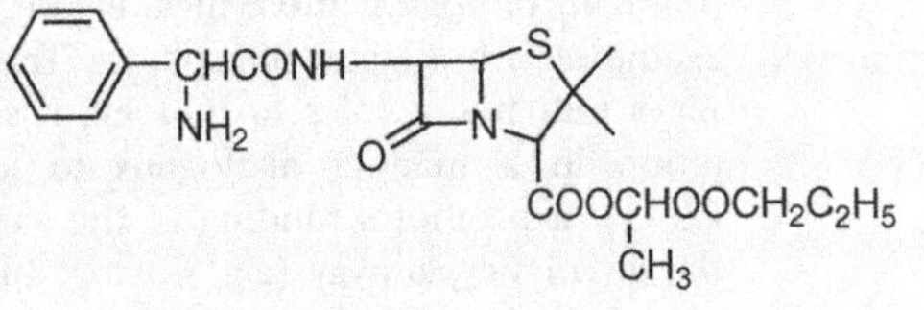

Bacampicillin

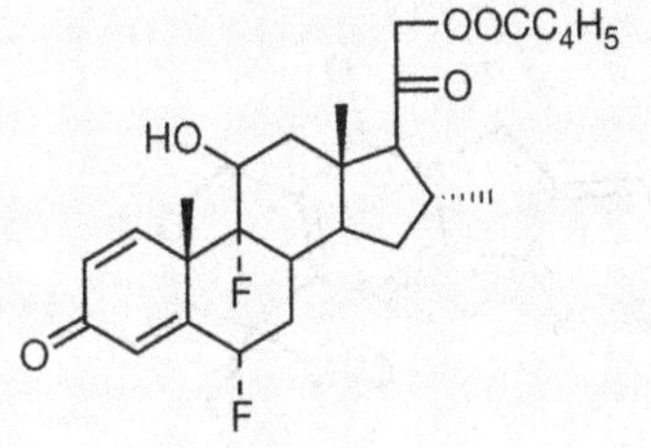

Diflucortolone valerate

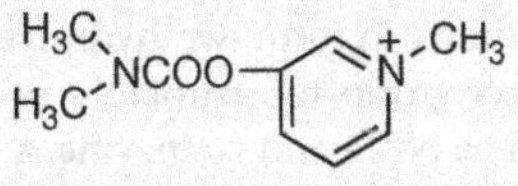

Pyridostigmine

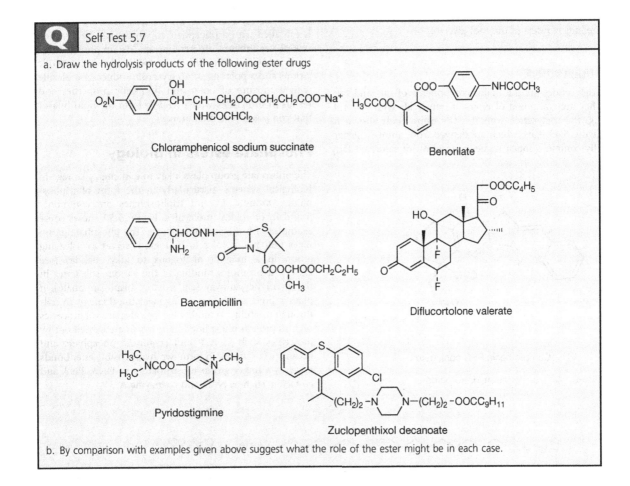

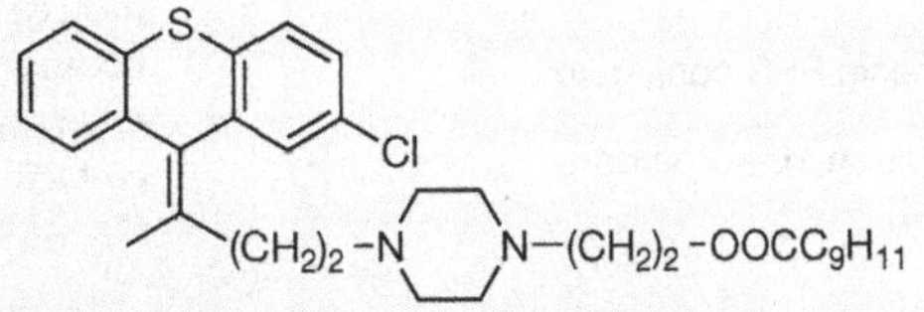

Zuclopenthixol decanoate

b. By comparison with examples given above suggest what the role of the ester might be in each case.

The ester linkage in polymeric drugs

The ester linkage provides a useful labile linkage to attach drugs to polymeric drug delivery systems. The production of drug polymer conjugates is increasing rapidly. As it becomes more difficult to register new chemical entities, companies are investing money in optimising the effectiveness of currently used drugs through improved pharmacokinetics and targeting. Also, linkage to polymers has a role in the delivery of peptide-based drugs. The most widely used polymer is polyethylene glycol (PEG). A number of PEG-conjugated proteins have received regulatory approval and there is a number of lower molecular weight PEG-conjugated drugs which are in clinical trials. The most developed to these is Prothecan® which is a PEG conjugate of the anti-tumour drug camptothecin (Fig. 5.48). The polyethylene glycol chain is linked via the amino acid alanine. This form of the drug affords improved toxicity and pharmacokinetic profiles.

Esters in biological systems

The ester linkage is one of the most important in biological systems because of its relative ease of both formation and degradation. It is involved in driving many of the processes within cells. The most ubiquitous ester groups are those found in various types of lipid which are largely esters of the triol glycerol.

Triglycerides

Triglycerides are the major components of oils and fats. They are composed of esters of fatty acids with glycerol, e.g. the triglyceride with the 18-carbon acids shown in Figure 5.49. Fats, which are derived from animals, generally contain a much higher proportion of saturated fatty acids in their triglycerides, whereas oils which are derived largely from plant seeds or fish contain largely unsaturated fatty acids. Triglycerides in the body are largely a storage form of fatty acids and, since they are water insoluble, they are transported around the body bound to lipid-carrying proteins. Triglycerides provide a reserve store of energy and are stored in adipose cells in the form of oil droplets. As with all esters, they are readily hydrolysed by plasma esterases and thus, when they are used in formulation vehicles such as oily injections, their metabolism presents no problems for the body.

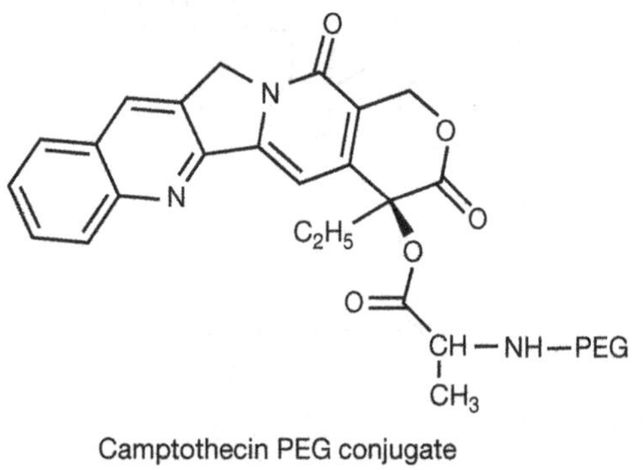

Figure 5.48 Camptothecin PEG prodrug.

Phospholipids

Phospholipids are only esterified with organic acids on two of the glycerol hydroxyl groups. The third position is esterified with a phosphate to which may be attached one of a number of different groups, e.g. in phosphatidyl cholines (Fig. 5.49). The attachment of two lipophilic groups and a polar group to glycerol produces a molecule with a mixture of polar and lipophilic properties and results in molecules which tend to form the lipid bilayer that composes cells membranes.

Phosphate esters in biology

The phosphate group plays a key role in energy storage in biological systems, particularly in the form of triphosphates. Mono-, di- and triphosphates are commonly found in biological molecules. Figure 5.50 shows some examples of biological phosphates. The phosphate group plays four major roles in biology: it serves as a leaving group in a manner analogous to alkyl halides (see Ch. 1), it promotes binding of the various substrates in the glycolytic pathway (e.g. fructose bisphosphonate), it plays a direct role in generating mechanical energy in cells through its ability to modify biological space via processes such as protein phosphorylation which are carried out by molecules such as ATP and creatinine phosphate, and because of its ability to form two hydrolysable ester bonds it serves a linker group most notably in DNA, RNA and co-factors such as NAD and coenzyme A.

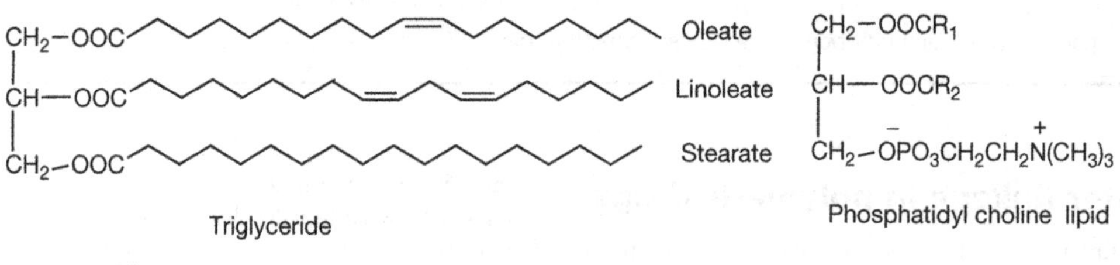

Figure 5.49 Fatty acid esters.

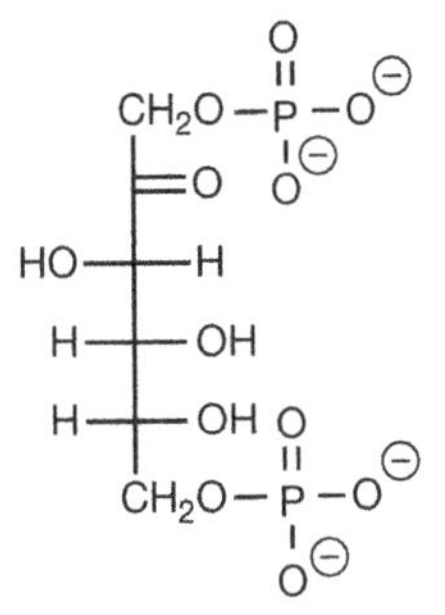

Fructose bisphosphonate

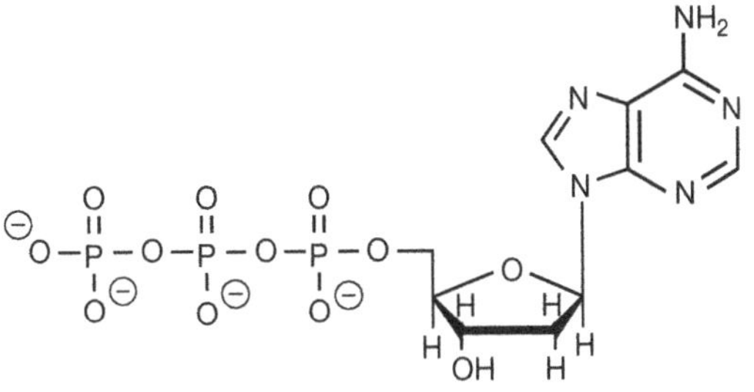

Adenosine-5′-triphosphate

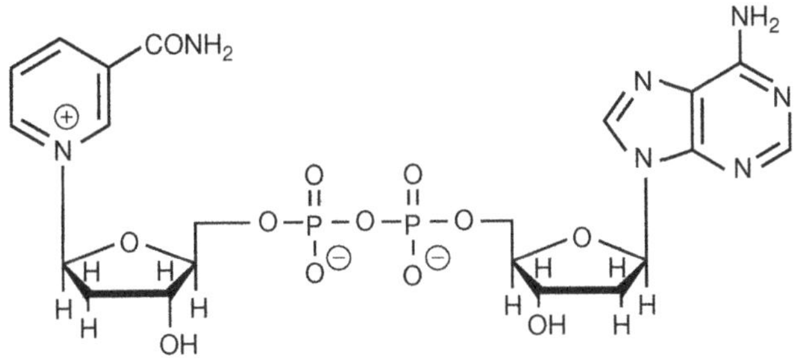

Nicotinamined adenosine dinucleotide

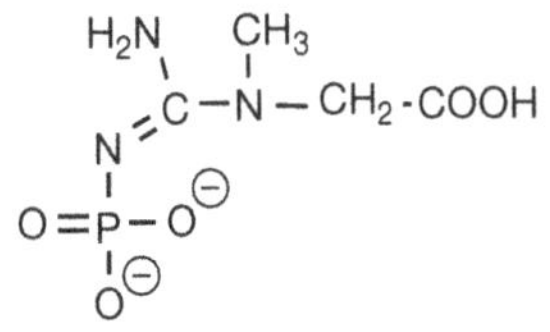

Creatine phosphate

Figure 5.50 Some biologically important phosphates.

Its role as a leaving group can be seen in the biosynthesis of terpenoid compounds which include the steroids. In Figure 5.51 the decarboxylation of the precursor to isopentenyl pyrophosphate and the formation of a carbon–carbon bond between dimethyl allyl pyrophosphate and isopentyl pyrophosphate are promoted by the properties of phosphate and pyrophosphate as leaving groups. Repetition of this process leads to the biosynthesis of steroids. It is also an important leaving group in uridine diphosphate glucose (UDP-glucose) which is used in glycogen biosynthesis. UDP-glucuronic acid is also involved in this type of transfer reaction where a glucuronic acid moiety is transferred to a drug molecule in order to promote its elimination from the body by increasing its water solubility. Figure 5.52 shows the glucuronidation of paracetamol with UDP-glucuronic acid as the co-factor, the reaction is catalysed by the enzyme UDP-glucuronyl transferase.

The phosphate group can also form cyclic esters and this is observed in the case of the biosynthesis of cyclic adenosine monophosphate (cAMP) (Fig. 5.53), which is an important intracellular messenger formed within cells, for instance, in response to the binding of adrenaline to its receptor on the cell surface. The cAMP goes on to stimulate events within the cell such as protein phosphorylation.

The phosphate bond and energy metabolism

The phosphate bond is used for energy storage in cells. Table 5.7 shows the standard free energies for the hydrolysis of some phosphate compounds at pH 7. All the ΔG values are negative, indicating that these are spontaneous processes which occur with liberation of energy. It can be seen that ATP, which is the most important energy storage molecule, has an intermediate ΔG value. If its value was too high, biological processes involving it would occur too quickly; with a lower energy, they would be too slow. The basis for reactions involving phosphate transfer relates to the relative energies produced by breaking the phosphate bond. Thus, for instance, the first step in glycolysis is the phosphorylation of glucose to produce glucose 6-phosphate. This reaction is coupled to the hydrolysis of ATP to ADP and, consulting Table 5.7, it is apparent that the reaction is favourable to the extent

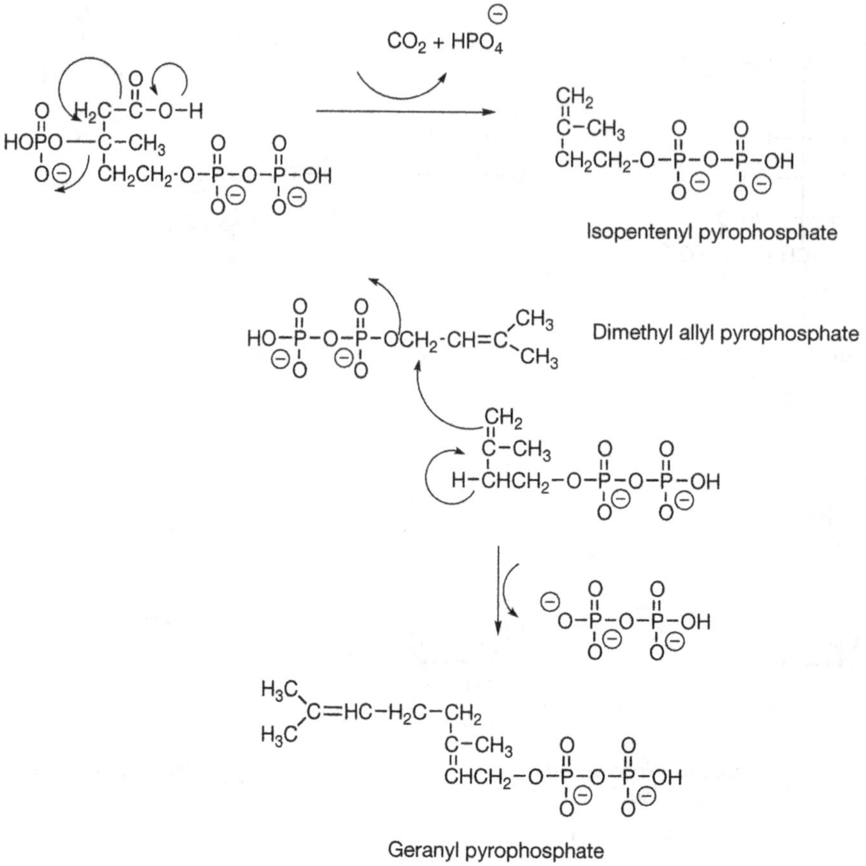

Figure 5.51 Phosphate and pyrophosphate as leaving groups.

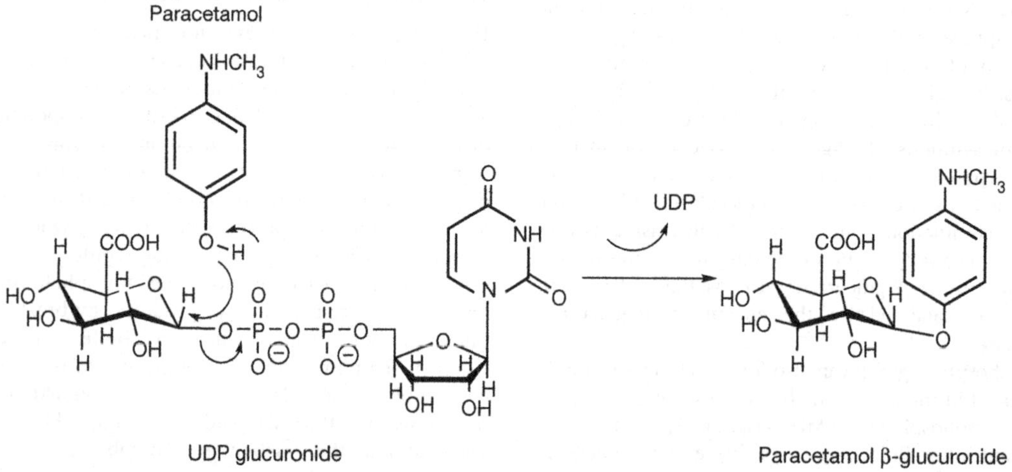

Figure 5.52 Glucuronidation of paracetamol with UDP glucuronyl transferase.

Figure 5.53 cAMP formation.

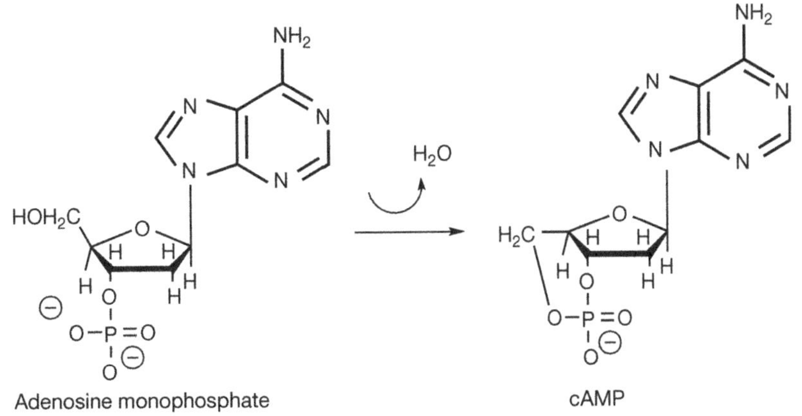

Table 5.7 Standard free energies for the hydrolysis of some biologically important phosphates at pH 7.0	
Phosphate	**ΔG° (kJ mol^{-1})**
Phosphoenyl pyruvate	−61.9
Acetyl phosphate	−43.1
Creatine phosphate	−43.1
Pyrophosphate	−33.5
ATP	−30.5
Glucose 1-phosphate	−20.9
Glucose 6-phosphate	−13.8
Glycerol 1-phosphate	−9.2

of −30.5 to −13.8 = −16.7 kJ mol^{-1}. Phosphates with higher bond energies can be coupled to the conversion of ADP back into ATP. For instance, phosphocreatine, which has a very high phosphate bond energy, is present in muscle tissue and is used to catalyse rapid conversion of ADP into ATP following intense muscular effort. Phosphoenol pyruvate is also used to generate ATP from ADP during glycolysis.

Protein phosphorylation

Phosphates such as ATP and guanine triphosphate (GTP) are used to phosphorylate proteins. This is one of the fundamental mechanisms where chemical energy is converted into mechanical energy, since transfer of the bulky phosphate group causes proteins to change shape and thus produces mechanical effects. The effects of phosphate produce medium-term effects on protein conformation; rapid effects are produced by electrostatic interactions most often with calcium ions. Figure 5.54 shows the phosphorylation of a tyrosine residue within a protein by ATP. The other sites of phosphorylation in proteins are at serine and threonine residues. The effects of conformation change due to phosphorylation include: opening or closing of ion channels in cell membranes, opening or closing of the active sites of enzymes and conformational changes allowing separate proteins to associate with each other.

Sulphur compounds

Unlike oxygen, sulphur has three oxidation states: 2, 4 and 6. Thus the divalent state can be readily oxidised to the 4 and 6 states. The divalent state is the most biologically important.

Thiols and thiophenols

Thiol compounds are more acidic than alcohols so that while ethanol has a p*Ka* value of *ca.* 17 ethanthiol has a p*Ka* value of 11. This is because sulphur is a larger atom than oxygen and is better able to accommodate the negative charge resulting from loss of a proton. The thiol group has a strong affinity for heavy metal ions and thus dimercaprol (Fig. 5.55) is used to treat heavy metal poisoning with metals such as mercury and arsenic since it complexes with them, preventing them from reacting with thiol groups in proteins, and complexes are sufficiently water soluble to be excreted from the body. Penicillamine is used on a similar basis to treat lead poisoning. A complex formed between gold and the thiol of butanedioic acid, aurothiomalate, is used in therapy of rheumatoid arthritis.

The most common biological thiol is the amino acid cysteine which is responsible for cross-linking within or between protein chains (e.g. the linking of the A and B

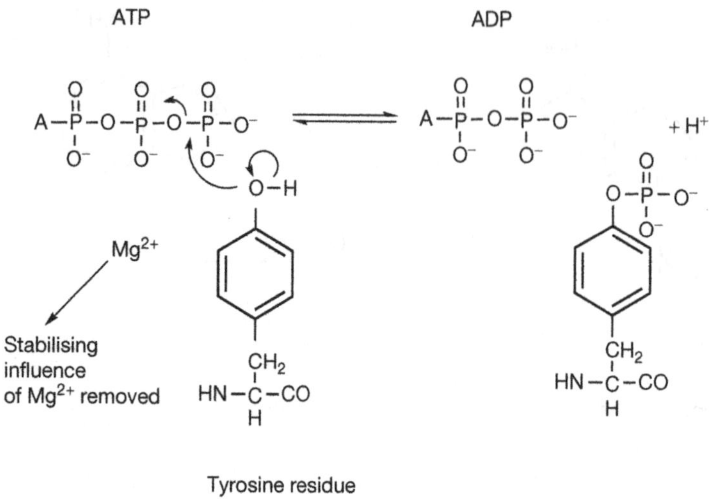

Figure 5.54 Protein phosphorylation at a tyrosine residue.

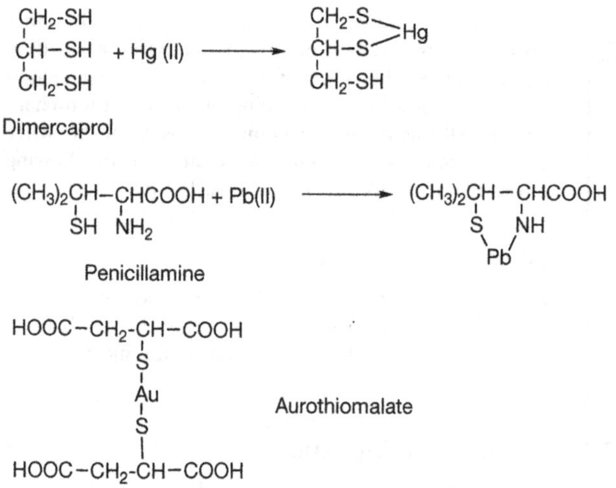

Figure 5.55 Thiols used in metal detoxification.

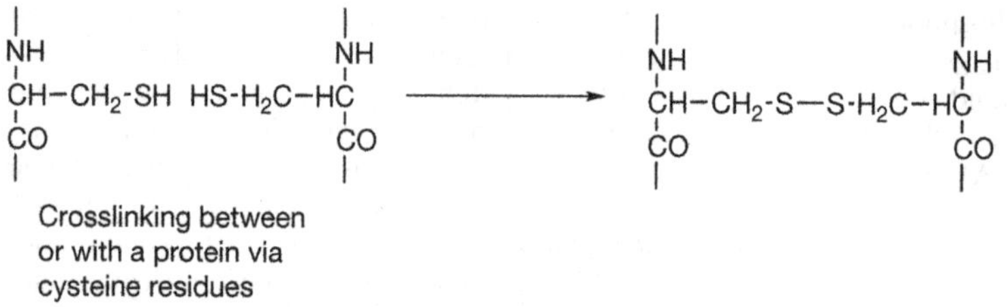

Figure 5.56 Formation of an S–S bridge between cysteine residues.

chains of insulin) through formation of S–S bridges and it is also part of glutathione which is an important natural detoxifying molecule (Fig. 5.56). The reaction of glutathione (GSH) in detoxifying the reactive metabolite of paracetamol is shown in Figure 5.57. Liver toxicity is produced by paracetamol in overdose when the GSH levels in the liver become depleted and the reactive metabolite reacts with SH groups in liver proteins instead. N-acetyl cysteine (Fig. 5.57) is used to reduce the effects of toxicity in paracetamol overdose through replacing GSH.

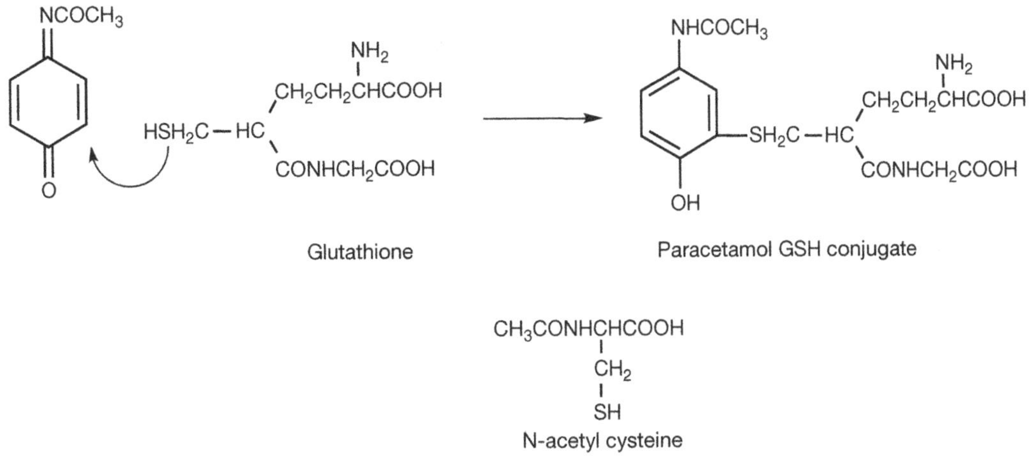

Figure 5.57 Detoxification of reactive quinone imine metabolite of paracetamol.

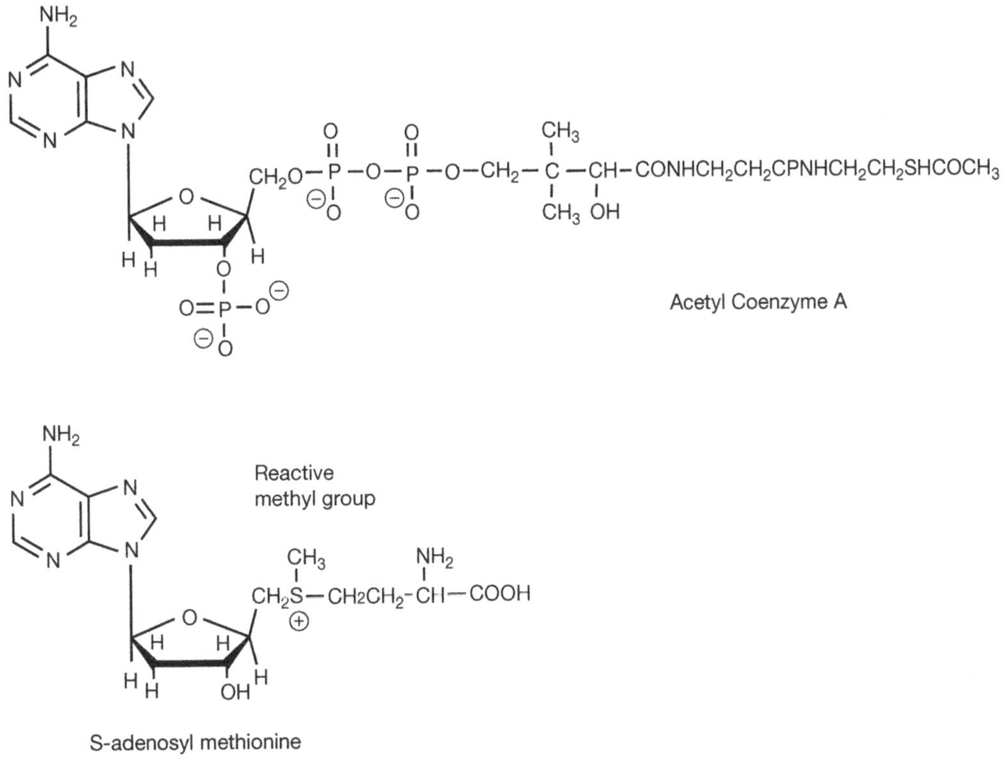

Figure 5.58 Two important sulphur containing co-factors.

Another important thiol in biological systems is Co-enzyme A (Fig. 5.58) which is a key co-factor involved in fatty acid biosynthesis. The acetyl group attached to Co-enzyme A becomes incorporated into the fatty acid chain. The transfer of carbon units is an important function of sulphur-containing compounds and the amino acid methionine, which is a thioether, forms the co-factor S-adenosyl methione (Fig. 5.58), which acts as a methyl group donor in a number of biochemical pathways including: lipid, nucleic acid and protein biosynthesis.

Methimazole and the related thiouracils are used to treat hyperthyroidism and it is believed that the thiol

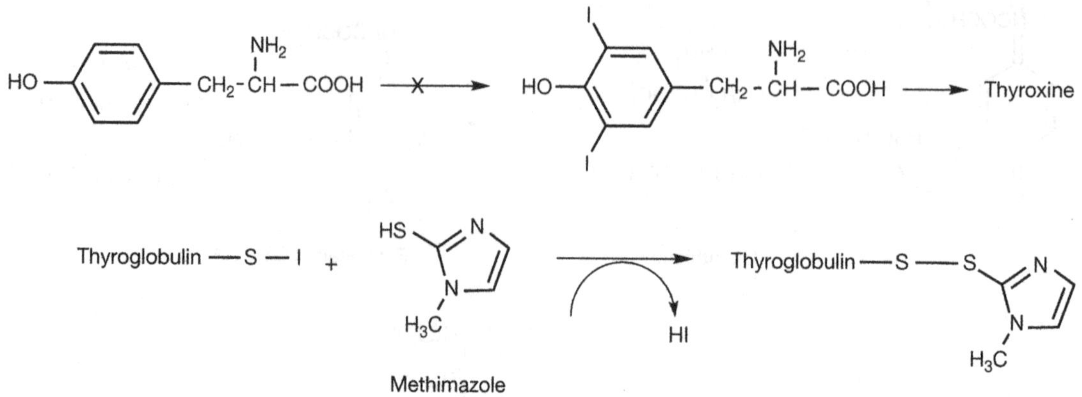

Figure 5.59 Inhibition of thyroxine formation by reaction of methimazole with thyroglobulin sulphenyl iodide.

group in the structure interferes with the introduction of iodine into tyrosine which is required for the synthesis of the thyroid hormone thyroxine. The protein thyroglobulin binds an iodine atom by forming a sulphenyl iodide. This intermediate is very reactive and it has been proposed that methimazole reacts with the SH group in thyroglobulin displacing the iodine and thus inhibiting production of thyroxine (Fig. 5.59).

Omeprazole and other benzimidazole antiulcer drugs are converted via a series of rearrangements catalysed by the strongly acidic conditions in the gastric secretory cells to a reactive intermediate (Fig. 5.60) which functions much like a thiol group. The intermediate then reacts with a thiol group present in the proton pump enzyme H^+, K^+ ATPase which is responsible for secretion of gastric acid. This stops the secretion of gastric acid, giving an ulcer a chance to heal.

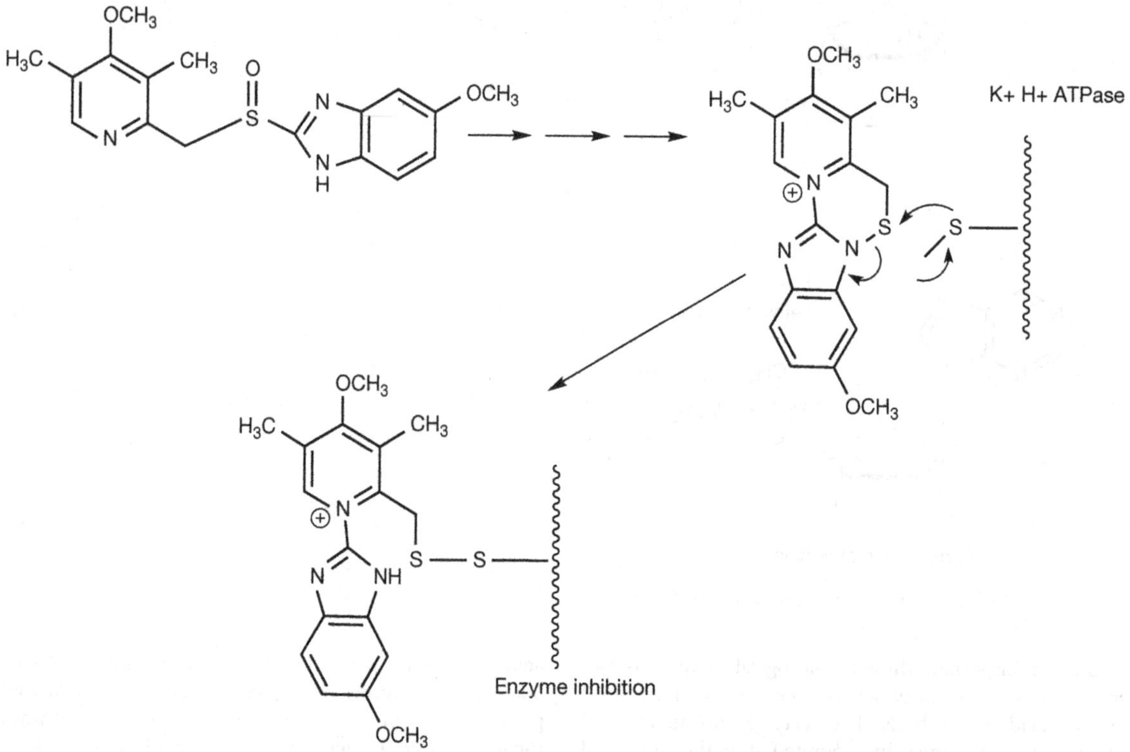

Figure 5.60 Formation of a covalent bond between omeprazole and a proton pump enzyme.

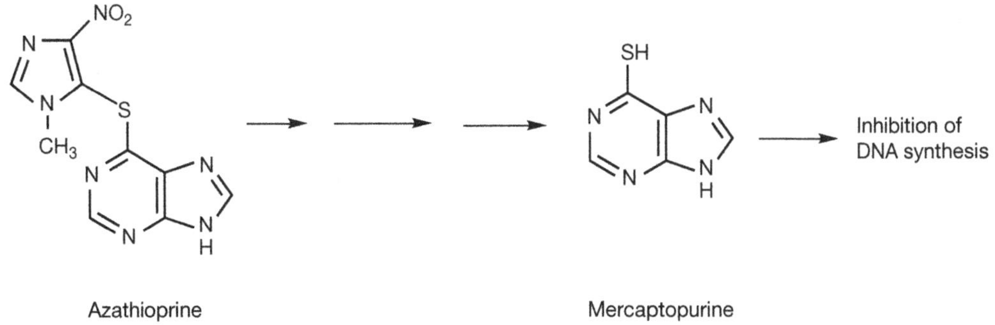

Figure 5.61 Azathioprine thioether prodrug.

Thioethers

Thioethers are found in quite a number of drugs but often the role of sulphur in the biological activity of the drug is not known. However, slight structural changes in which the sulphur is removed can alter the biological activity of a drug. Thus while chlorpromazine has antipsychotic and tranquilliser activity, imipramine, where the sulphur has been replaced with two methylene groups, is antidepressant and does not have tranquilliser activity (see Ch. 18). The largest series of compounds containing a thioether group is the series of penicillin and cephalosporin antibiotics (see Ch. 22). There are some examples where thioethers are converted in the body to the active form of a drug. For example, azathioprine is a less toxic prodrug for mercaptopurine (Fig. 5.61), which is sometimes used as an immunosuppressant in the prevention of organ rejection or in the treatment of rheumatoid arthritis.

A Self Test 5.1

Answer A, secondary; B, primary; C, benzyl; D, primary; E, secondary; F, tertiary.

A Self Test 5.2

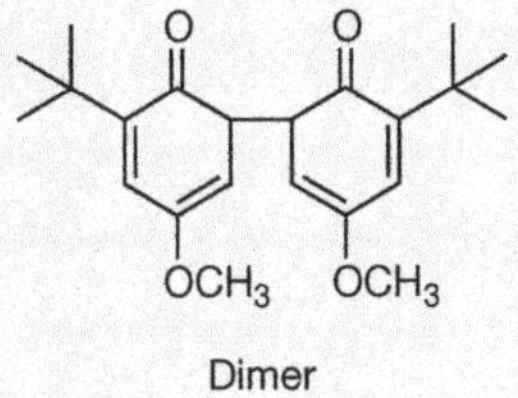

A Self Test 5.3

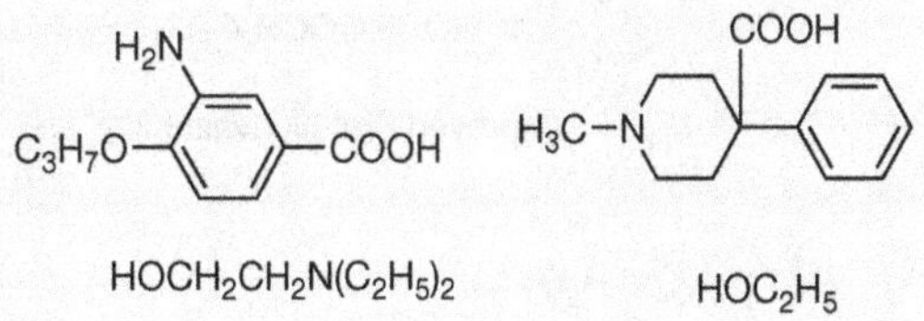

A Self Test 5.4

1, 5, 6, 2, 3, 4.

A Self Test 5.5

4, 5, 1, 2, 3.

A Self Test 5.6

1, 3, 4, 2, 5.

A Self Test 5.7

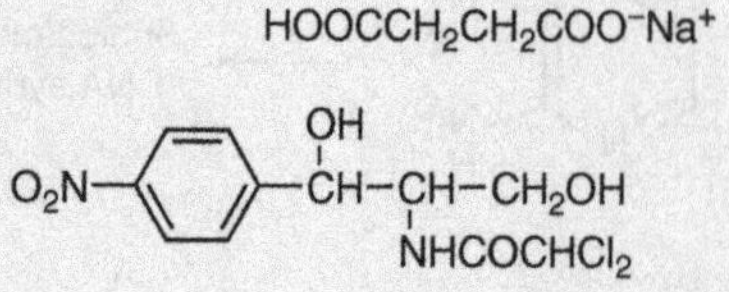

Improved water solubility

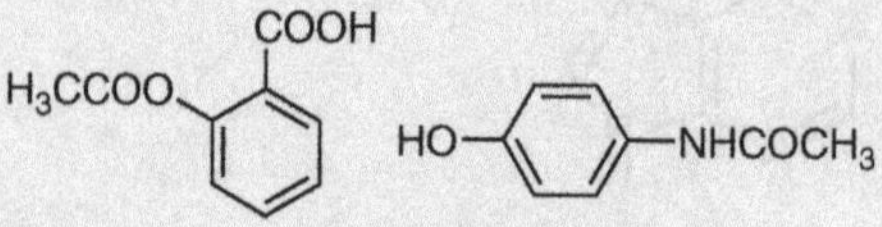

Reduced gastric irritation

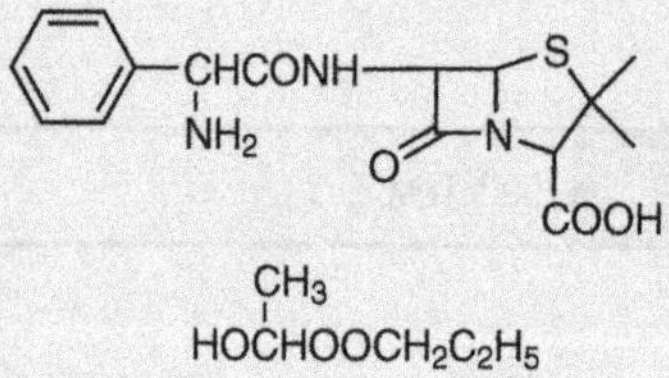

Improved oral bioavailability

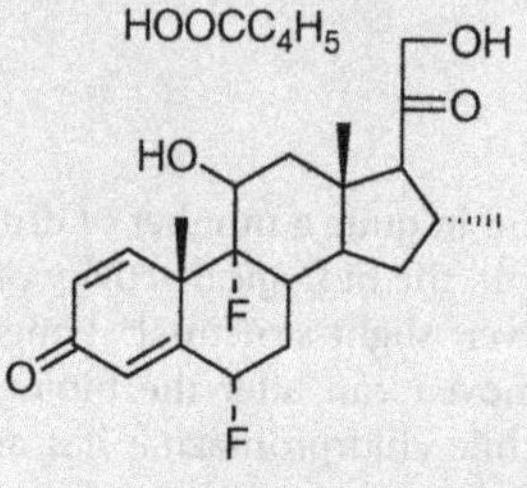

Improved dermal absorption

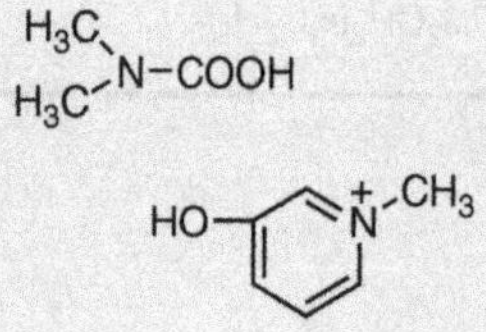

Carbomylation of choline esterase

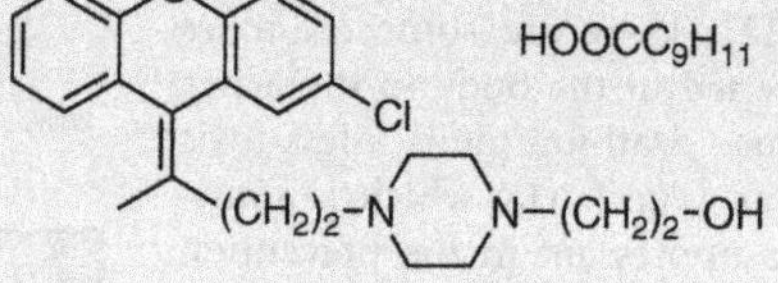

Preparation of oily injection for slow release

REFERENCES

1. Durrer A, Walther B, Racciati A, Boss G, Testa B. Structure-metabolism relationships in the hydrolysis of nicotinate esters by rat liver and brain. *Pharm Res*. 1991;8:832–839.
2. Seki H, et al. Specificity of esterases and structure of prodrug esters. Reactivity of various acylated acetominophen compounds and acetylaminobenzoated compounds. *J Pharm Sci*. 1988;77:855–860.
3. Takahashi K, et al. Effects of the ester moiety on the stereoselective hydrolysis of several propranolol prodrugs in rat tissues. *Biol Pharm Bull*. 1995;18:1401–1404.

Chapter | 6 |

Protein structure and its relevance to drug action

David G Watson

CHAPTER CONTENTS

AMINO ACIDS

The basic building blocks which make up proteins are the 20 amino acids. The simplest amino acid is glycine (Fig. 6.1) which has a carboxylic acid group (p*Ka* 2.5) and a primary amine group (p*Ka* 9.7). Like all amino acids in its free state, when not part of a protein chain, it can carry both positive and negative charges depending on the pH of the solution it is dissolved in, and there is no pH at which it is not charged. A molecule which carries both positive and negative charges in solution is known as a zwitterion, and in the case of a simple amino acid like glycine, the charges are equal and opposite at a pH halfway between the two p*Ka* values, i.e. at pH 5.1. This point is known as the isoelectric point and its value is known as the p*I* of the molecule. As shown in Figure 6.1, an amino acid is completely positively charged only at low pH and completely negatively charged only at high pH. In the case of glycine, the side chain of the amino acid represented by R=H but the other 19 amino acids occurring in proteins have various R groups (Fig. 6.2).

There are various ways of classifying the amino acids but perhaps the most useful in terms of protein function is classification into hydrophobic, polar and charged. Glycine can be classified on its own since it does not fall into any of these categories, although lack of a side chain gives it flexibility and it has an important role in protein structure for this reason. The importance of the different classes of amino acids will be discussed in more detail as we build up protein structures but the different categories are briefly considered below.

Hydrophobic amino acids

Hydrophobic amino acids exhibit varying degrees of hydrophobicity depending on how large the hydrophobic side chain is. Alanine is the least hydrophobic and tryptophan is the most hydrophobic even though it contains a weakly polar indole nitrogen. These amino acids are quite water soluble at extremes of pH but if the pH is adjusted to around their p*I* then they are effectively neutral and their hydrophobicity will cause them to come out of solution. This class of amino acid is found buried inside proteins avoiding contact with water and thus form the protein core. If the protein has a helical portion which passes through a lipophilic cell membrane this portion of the protein will be found to be rich in hydrophobic/lipophilic amino acids.

Charged amino acids

Charged amino acids are found predominantly on the surface of proteins in contact with the surrounding solution. Thus they are responsible for the solution stability of the protein and if they lose their charge the protein will become unstable and precipitate out of solution. A standard

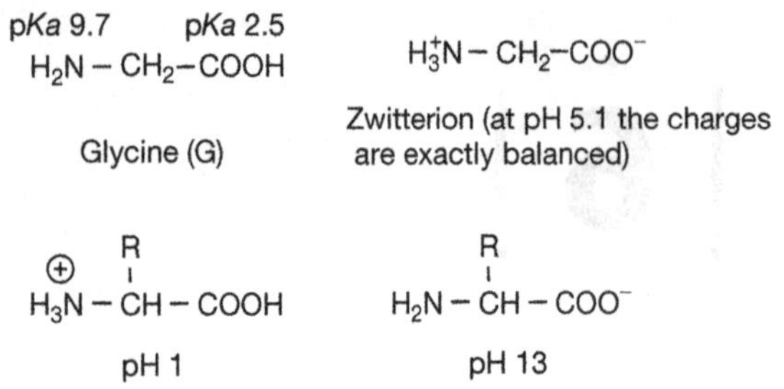

Figure 6.1 The effect of pH on the charge state of amino acids.

method for removing a protein from a solution is to adjust it so that it is strongly acidic so that the negatively charged side chains of the protein become uncharged, thus destabilising its structure in solution. Often, proteins cannot be re-dissolved after such treatment. A more gentle method of removing proteins from solution is to salt them out with concentrated ammonium sulphate, which effectively competes with the protein groups for the solvating water molecules required to keep the protein in solution, thus destabilising it. The charged residues in proteins are important in the action of many drug molecules, as many drugs

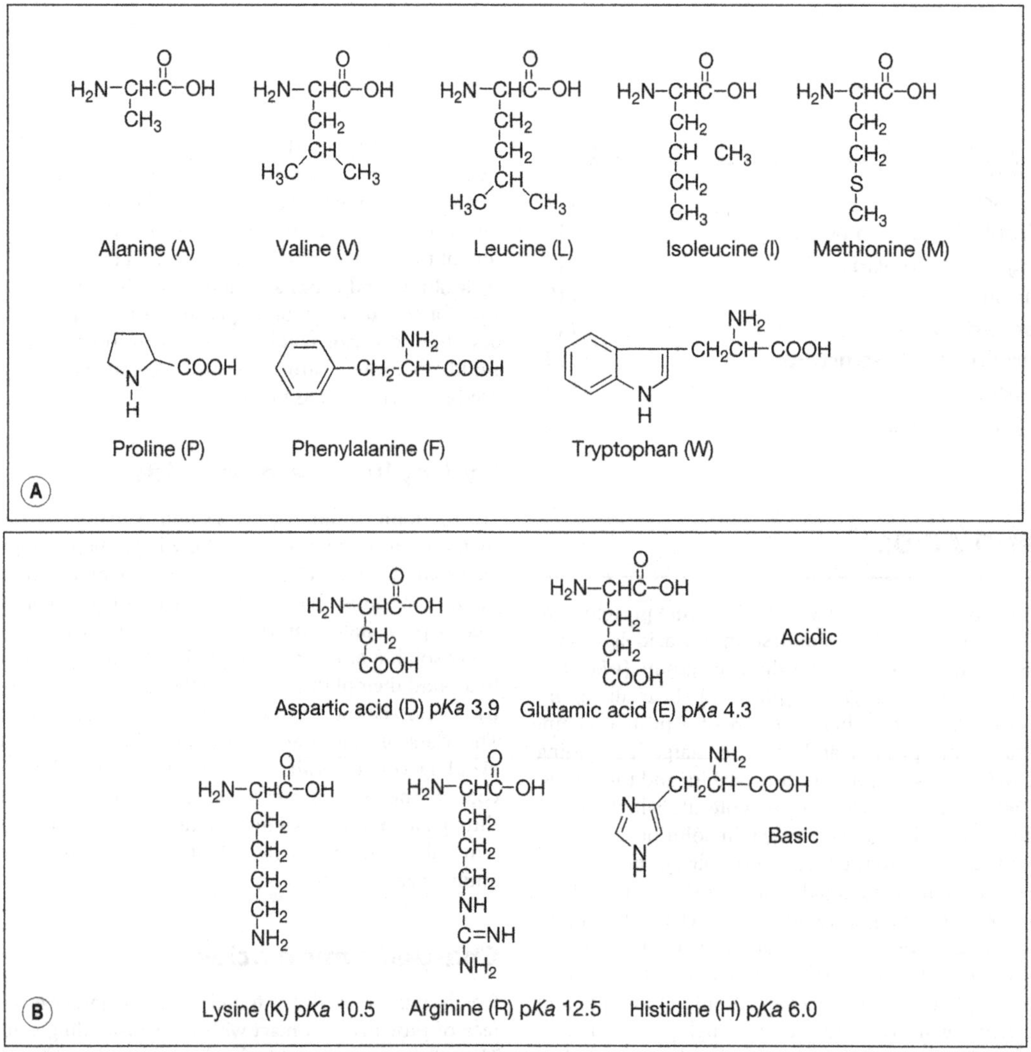

Figure 6.2 The 19 amino acids in addition to glycine occurring in proteins. (**A**) Hydrophobic amino acids. (**B**) Charged amino acids.

Continued

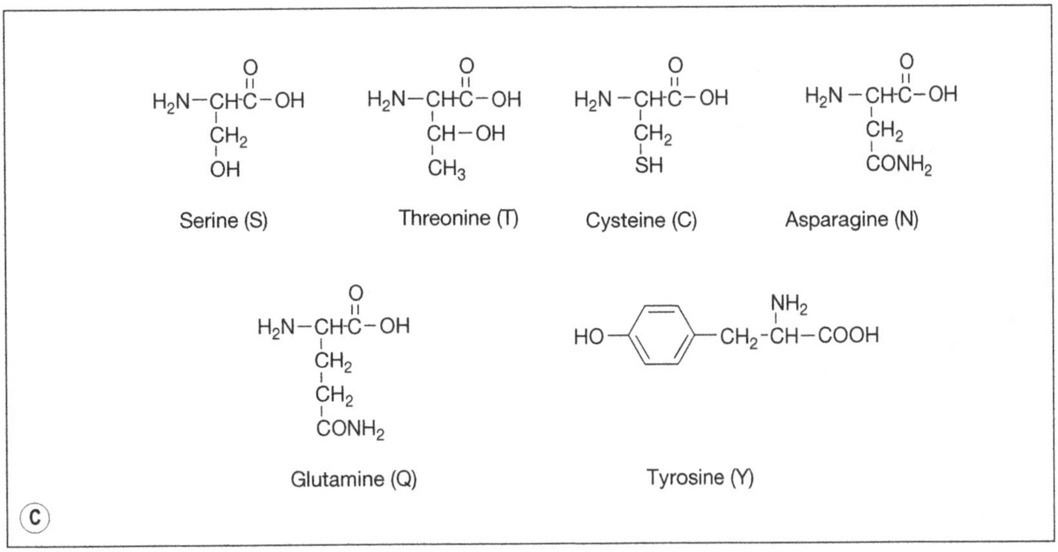

Figure 6.2—cont'd (C) Neutral hydrophilic amino acids.

are bases and they bind to the negatively charged aspartate or glutamate side chains in proteins. Histidine can be classified as a polar neutral amino acid residue since it is only about 4% ionised at physiological pH. However its charge state is important since its p*Ka* value of 6 provides buffering in the pH range where many proteins exert their functions. The p*I* values of the charged amino acids are either higher or lower than those of neutral amino acids such as glycine. Figure 6.3 shows the ionisation states of glutamic acid, the p*I* is at the average of the p*Ka* values for the two acids in the structure at pH 3.0.

Polar amino acids

Polar amino acids have a diverse range of functions. Serine residues are important in enzyme-catalysed reactions, cysteine is important in determining the 3-D structure of proteins because of its ability to form S–S bridges with another cysteine residue, and tyrosine and serine are important because they form phosphate esters which cause an alteration of protein conformation, thus triggering other cellular events. Asparagine and glutamine are important sites for hydrogen bonding within proteins and with ligands binding to proteins. In addition, cysteine is important for its ability to bond to metal ions, which are often present at the active sites of enzymes.

THE PEPTIDE BOND

The amino group of one amino acid reacts with the carboxylic acid of another amino acid to form an amide – the peptide bond. In the process of production of the peptide the DNA sequence coding for a particular amino acid is transcribed to produce the RNA sequence corresponding to a particular amino acid. The RNA sequence then binds

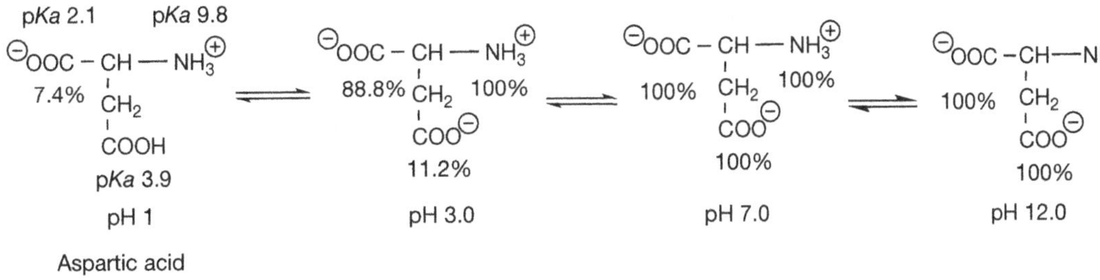

Figure 6.3 The variation of the charge on aspartic acid with pH.

to a sequence in a tRNA molecule (see Ch. 7) corresponding to a particular amino acid. The tRNA is largely a single-stranded molecule but at the 5′ end of the main chain there is a short sequence of seven DNA bases. The final base at the 3′ end of this short chain is unpaired and is adenine monophosphate. The amino acid to be attached to the tRNA is first converted to its aminoacyl AMP (equation 1) and then this reactive form of the amino acid is transferred to the 3′ terminal AMP group of the acceptor sequence in the tRNA (equation 2). The amino-acyl-AMP at the 3′ then undergoes nucleophilic attack by the terminal amino group of the growing peptide (Fig. 6.4). This process occurs in the cellular ribosomes which contain a binding site which specifies the next amino acid to be added to the growing peptide and recruits the appropriate aminoacyl-tRNA to be added to the growing peptide chain which is held in another binding site within the ribosome. Thus the ribosomal RNA can be described as having ribozyme activity, indicating that it functions like an enzyme. The sequence of amino acids in a peptide constitutes its primary structure. By convention, the amino terminal (N-terminal) of a peptide is at the left-hand end of a sequence of amino acids and the carboxyl (C-terminal) of a peptide is at the right-hand end.

$$\text{amino acid} + \text{ATP} \rightarrow \text{aminoacyl} - \text{AMP} + \text{pyrophophosphate} \quad \boxed{1}$$

$$\text{aminoacyl} - \text{AMP} + \text{tRNA} \rightarrow \text{aminoacyl} - \text{tRNA} + \text{AMP} \quad \boxed{2}$$

The structure of a pentapeptide (having five amino acid residues) leucine encephalin is shown in Figure 6.5. Proteins such as enzymes have many more amino acids, but there are many small peptides which have important biological activities. The encephalins are endogenous pain regulation molecules which act at opioid receptors in the body. The abbreviated version of the sequence for leucine encephalin is also shown in Figure 6.5. As instrumental methods have advanced it has become easier to determine the structure of unknown proteins. Protein molecular weights and sequences can now be rapidly determined by using mass spectrometry. The protein sequence is most often determined by carrying out a tryptic digest which

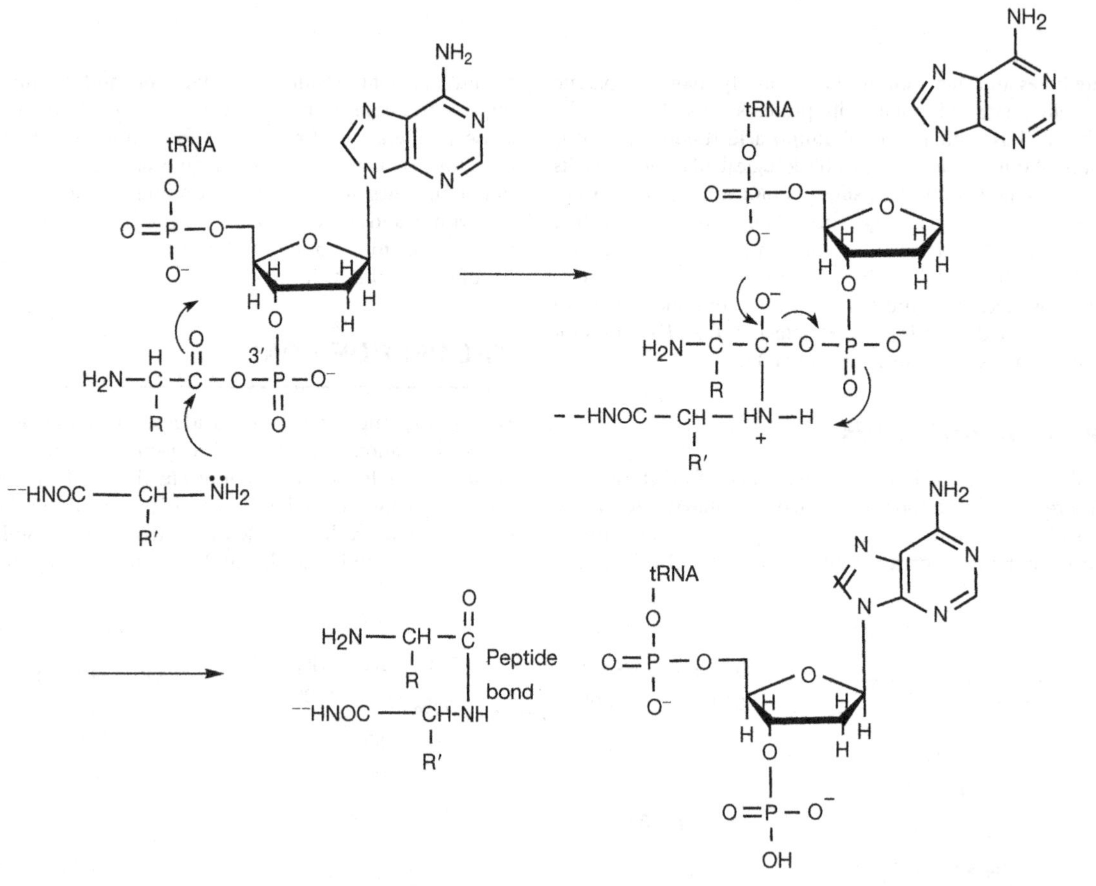

Figure 6.4 Formation of peptide bond via the action of aminoacyl t-RNA.

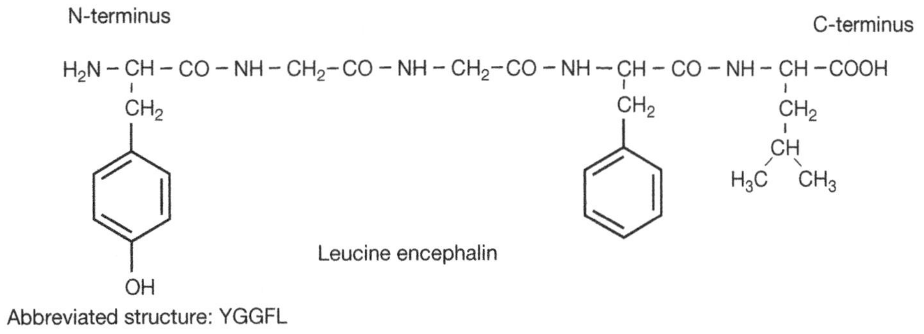

Figure 6.5 Structure of leucine encephalin.

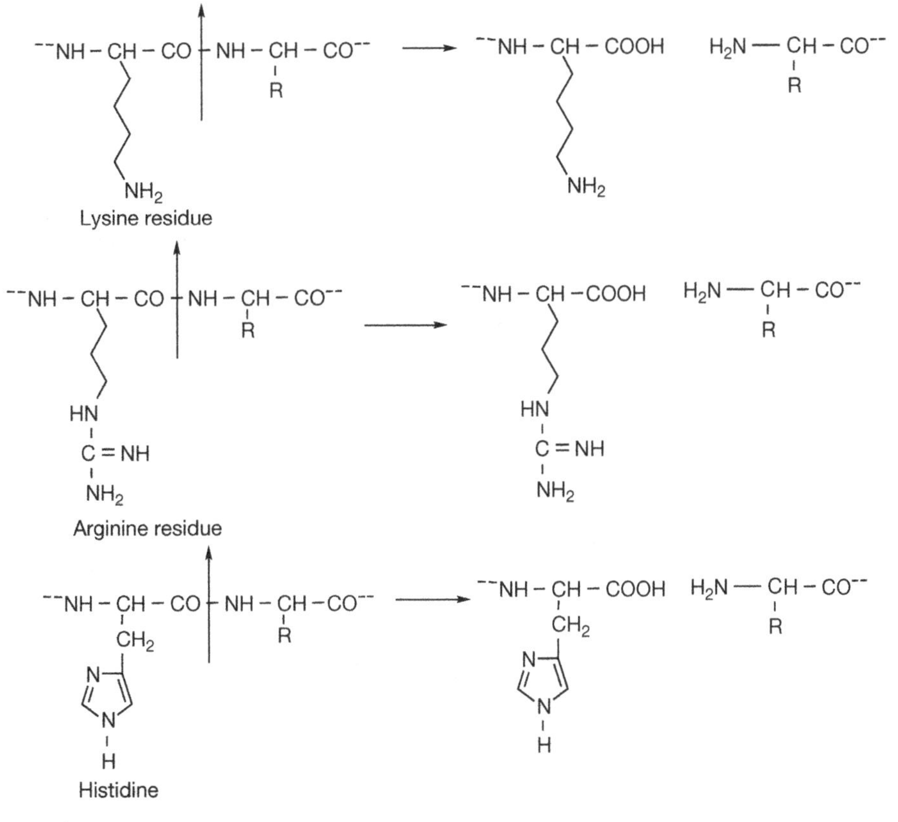

Figure 6.6 Trypsin cleavage points.

cleaves proteins at the C-terminus side of one of the basic amino acid residues (Fig. 6.6) except when they are followed by a proline residue.

This results in a limited number of peptides which are generally in the range of 500–3000 amu and are thus amenable to analysis by mass spectrometry. Tandem mass spectrometry produces a series of fragments arising from cleavage of the peptide bonds within the molecule and the sequences for each peptide can thus be determined and the molecular structure thus determined. Considering the peptide hormone glucagon, which is involved in glucose regulation, it is possible to predict that the sequence of peptides shown in Figure 6.7 would be formed following tryptic digest. Cleavage next to the histidine, lysine and two arginine residues should, in theory, yield the five peptides and amino acid residues shown in Figure 6.7. These small peptides can then be fragmented to yield their amino acid sequence. The sequences of short peptide

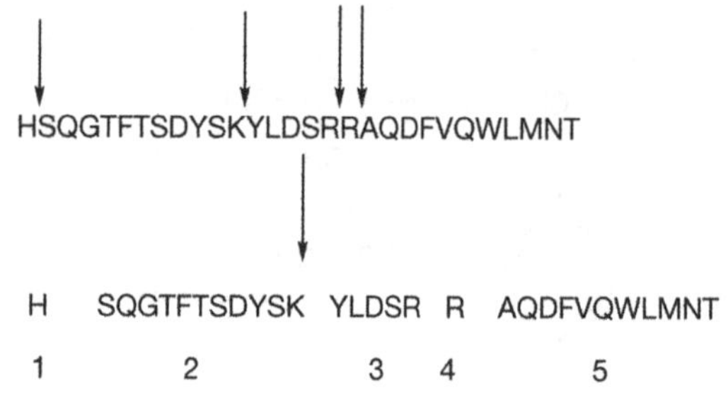

Figure 6.7 Peptide fragments resulting from tryptic digestion of glucagon.

fragments are often sufficiently unique to yield an identity for the full peptide. Thus if the sequence of peptide 2 shown in Figure 6.7 is submitted to the Uniprot database (http://services.uniprot.org) then a series of glucogen peptides or glucogen peptide precursors is returned as containing this short sequence of amino acids. Thus the primary amino acid sequence of this undecapeptide is sufficiently unique to indicate that it originates from glucagon.

> **Q Self Test 6.1**
>
> Predict the fragments which result from the tryptic digestion of salmon calcitonin.
>
> 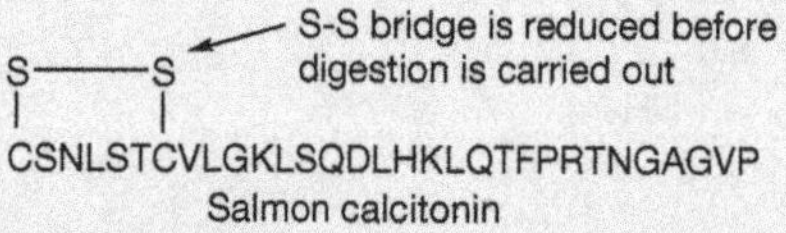
>
>
> Answer: CSNLSTCVLGK LSQDLDLH K LQTFPR NGAGVP

> **Q Self Test 6.2**
>
> Use the blast search facility at http://services.uniprot.org in order to determine which proteins the following sequences are found in. Type the sequence into the blast search form.
> a. GIVEQCCTSICSLYQLENYCN
> b. TSLLLAFGLLCLPWLQEGSAFPTIPLSR

PROTEIN SECONDARY STRUCTURE

The sequence of amino acids making up a protein assumes a particular three-dimensional (secondary) structure. It is possible to predict the secondary structure to some extent from the sequence of amino acids making up the primary structure. There are two fundamental structural motifs which can occur in proteins, α-helices and β-sheets, and particular protein functions tend to be associated with these motifs.

α-Helices

Alpha-helices are pharmacologically important since they are the main structural element in membrane-spanning helices which are present in many receptors, and also ion channels are formed from groups of transmembrane helices. Figure 6.8 shows a schematic diagram of an α-helix, the helix is stabilised by H-bonding between the NH and CO groups of the protein backbone and has a regular structure with 3.6 amino acids per turn.

α-helices have a number of important functions and perhaps the most significant role in relation to drug action is that they form ion channels and membrane receptor binding sites. The general view of many membrane receptors is shown in Figure 6.9 where the α-helices are shown as cylinders connected by loops of peptide chain. There are usually seven membrane-spanning α-helices in receptor proteins although there may be many more in ion channel proteins. Membrane-spanning receptors are coupled to G-proteins which initiate a chain of events including binding of GTP followed by activation of adenylate cyclase, resulting in the formation of cAMP which functions as a

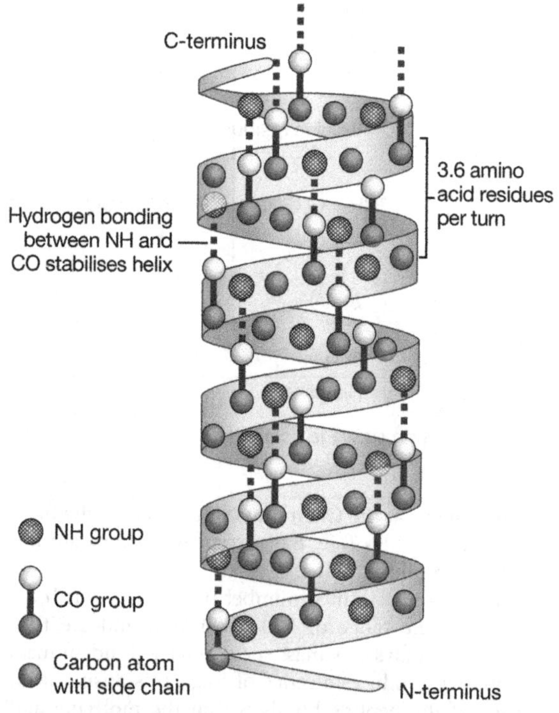

Figure 6.8 α-helix.

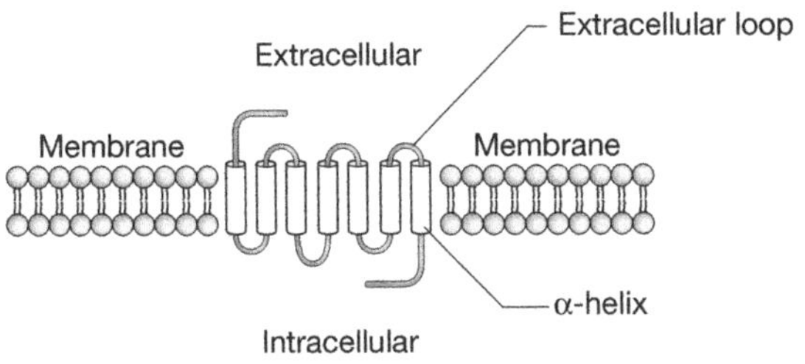

Figure 6.9 Membrane-spanning helix.

second messenger and initiates further cellular events such as opening of ion channels in the cell membrane. Many disease states can be linked to the activity of G-proteins coupled to membrane-spanning receptors. G-protein coupled receptors include: light and olfactory receptors, receptors for adenosine, adrenaline, dopamine, bradykinin, opioids, GABA, acetylcholine, prostaglandins, glucagon, calcitonin, oxytocin, histamine, serotonin and many more. G-protein coupled receptors are also involved in drug resistance. Thus they present essentially the most important target for drugs. In addition, another mechanism of drug action is exerted via direct effects on ion channels which are also composed of membrane-spanning α-helices. There are many cases where a gene coding G-protein coupled receptors has been identified but the function of the receptor remains unknown.

The first G-protein coupled receptor to be investigated was the adrenergic receptor.[1,2] Figure 6.10 shows the primary amino acid sequence of the β_2-adrenergic receptor. A major goal in biological sciences is to be able to predict how primary amino acid sequences can lead to specific types of secondary protein structure, but despite some general rules this is still very difficult and where protein structures are well known this has been arrived at by crystallising them and then being able to locate the positions of the atoms in space, making up the protein using X-ray crystallography. The best way to determine the way in which a ligand binds to its receptor is to co-crystallise the ligand with the receptor protein. Again, this is technically difficult but has been achieved for a number of important receptors. In retrospect, once the protein secondary structure is known, there are often some well-established features in the primary amino acid sequence that indicate the secondary structure of the protein. The structure of the adrenoreceptor contains seven membrane-spanning helices and even if the structure of the receptor was unknown it might be possible to characterise these as areas which are rich in amino acids with lipophilic side chains which have an affinity for the hydrophobic environment of the core of the cell membrane which the helices span. The helices in the receptor are very regular with helices 1, 2, 4, 5, 6 and 7 having 24 amino acids, and helix 3 which has 22 amino acids. The helices have between 63% and 75% of lipophilic amino acid content (except for helix 7 which has 50%). In contrast, loop regions 1 and 2, which are in contact with the aqueous extra- and intra-cellular environments, have 53% and 40%, respectively. However, this is quite a crude predictive tool. The binding sites for adrenaline occur within the membrane in the helix regions. The charged amine group binds via electrostatic interaction to a glutamic acid residue in helix 3, the catechol group hydrogen bonds with the first and third serine residues in helix 5, the lipophilic portion of the benzene rings undergoes van der Waals interaction and possibly charge transfer interaction with the phenylalanine residues in helix 6, and the benzyl alcohol group hydrogen bonds with a tyrosine residue to helix 7. These interactions can be

N terminus ExC 35 Helix 1 58
MGQPGNGSAFLLAPNRSHAPDHDVTQQRDEVWVV**GMGIVMSLIVLAIVFGNVLVITAI**AKF

InC 72 Helix 2 95 ExC 107 Helix 3
ERLQTVTNYF**ITSLACADLVMGLAVVPFGAAHIL**MKMWTFGNFWCE**FWTSIDVLCVT**

129 InC 151 Helix 4 174
ASIETLCVIAVDRYFAITSPFKYQSLLTKNKAR**VIILMVWIVSGLTSFLPIQMHWY**RATH

ExC 197 Helix 5 220
EAINCYANETCCDFFTNQ**AYAIASSIVSFYVPLVIMVFVYSR**VFQEAKRQLQKIDKSEGRF

InC G-protein binding region 275 Helix 6 298
HVQNLSQVEQDGRTGHGLRRSSKFCLKEHKALKTL**GIIMGTFTLCWLPFFIVNIVHVIQ**D

ExC 306 Helix 7 329 InC
NLIRKE**VYILLNWIGYVNSGFNPLIYCRSP**DFRIAFQELLCLRRSSLKAYGNGYSSNGNT

C-terminus
GEQSGYHVEQEKENKLLCEDLPGTEDFVGHQGTVPSDNIDSQGRNCSTNDSLL

Figure 6.10 The amino acid sequence of the human β_2 adrenergic receptor (ExC, extracellular; InC, intracellular). Membrane-spanning helices in bold, adrenaline binding sites in red, and serine phosphorylation sites in blue.

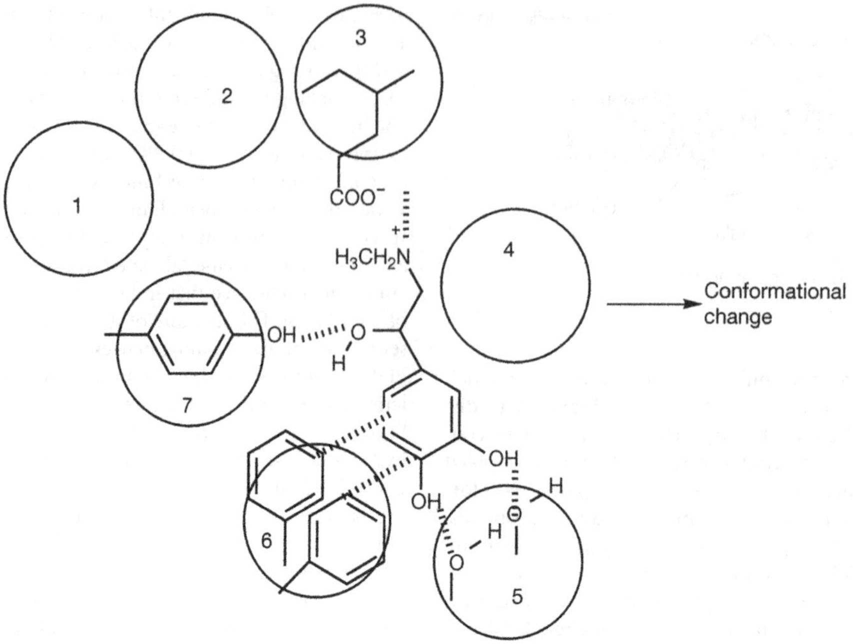

Figure 6.11 Interaction of adrenaline with the α-helices in the β_2-adrenaline receptor which lead to a conformational change and activation of the coupled G-protein.

visualised as shown in Figure 6.11 and they lead to a change in the conformation of the receptor, which in turn affects the conformation of the coupled G-protein, which is bound to the long intracellular loop between residues 220 and 275, leading to the cascade of events outlined briefly above. As described in Chapter 10, only R (−) adrenaline can contact all the points of interaction within the receptor and thus the S (+) isomer is much less biologically active. The β_2 agonists reinforce the reaction with the receptor. One aspect of this may be that they have higher partition coefficients than adrenaline, which encourages them to enter the lipophilic region within the transmembrane-spanning helices.

Another feature relating to the activity of the receptor can be observed in the primary structure of the final intracellular sequence at the C-terminus of the receptor. If receptors are stimulated for a long period with a ligand then they become desensitised and their action is terminated. In the adrenoreceptor, the activity of the receptor is terminated by phosphorylation of serine residues which are abundant at the C-terminus end of the receptor.

Figure 6.12 shows the primary sequence of the β_1-adrenergic receptor. Like the β_2-adrenergic receptor it has seven transmembrane helices which are extensively composed of lipophilic amino acids. However, there are many differences in the structure, e.g. the first extracellular loop in the β_1 receptor is much longer than that in the β_2 receptor. The sequences of amino acids in the helix regions of the β_1 receptor are not the same as in the β_2 receptor and thus the binding of noradrenaline, which is the ligand for the receptor, is not the same as adrenaline in the β_2 receptor. In fact, much more is known about the β_2 receptor than the β_1 receptor and the binding sites in the β_1 receptor are not completely elucidated, although the second and seventh helices are known to contain important binding sites.

First extracellular loop
MGAGVLVLGASEPGNLSSAAPLPDGAATAARLLVPASPPASLLPPASESPEPLSQQWTA**GM**
GLLMALIVLLIVAGNVLVIVAIAKTPRLQTLTNLFI**MSLASADLVMGLLVVPFGATIVV**
WGRWEYGSFFC**ELWTSVDVLCVTASIETLCVIALD**RYLAITSPFR**YQSLLTRARARGLVC**
TVWAISALVSFLPILMHWWRAESDEARRCYN**DPKCCDFVTNRAYAIASSVVSFYV**PLCIM
AFVYLRVFREAQKQVKKIDSCERRFLGGPARPPSPSPSPVPAPAPPPGPPRPAAAAATAPLA
NGRAGKRRPSRLVALREQKALKT**LGIIMGVFTLCWLPFFLANVVKAF** HRELVPD**RLFVFFN**
WLGYANSAFNPIIYCRSPDFRKAFQRLLCCARRAARRRHATHGDRPRASGCLARPGPPPS
PGAASDDDDDDVVGATPPARLLEPWAG CNGGAAADSDSSLDEPCRPGFASESKV

Figure 6.12 Primary sequence of the β_1-adrenergic receptor showing helix regions in bold.

Q Self Test 6.3

The primary amino acid sequence of the HT1 receptor,[3] which binds the neurotransmitter serotonin, is shown below. Answer the following questions.

1. How long are the transmembrane spanning regions (shown in bold)?
2. What is the % of lipophilic amino acids in the first helix?
3. Identify the position of the aspartic acid residue in helix 3 which interacts with the amine group in serotonin and the serine and threonine residues in helix 5 which interact with the phenolic hydroxyl group in serotonin.
4. Identify the long intracellular loop region which binds the coupled G-protein.

MDFLNSSDQN LTSEELLNRM PSKILVSLT **LSGLALMTTTINSLVIAAIIV**TRKLHHPANY

LICS**LAVTDFLVAVLVMPFSIVYIV** RESWI MGQVVCD**IWLSVDITCCTCSILHLSAIA**LD

RYRAITDAVE YARKRTPKHA **GIMITIVWIISVFISMPPLFW**RHQGTSRDD ECIIKHDH

IVSTIYSTFGAFYIPLALILILYYKIYRAAKTLYHKRQASRIAKEEVNGQVL LESGEKSTKS

VSTSYVLEKSLSDPSTDFDKIHSTVRSLRSEFKHEKSWRRQKISGTRERK**AATTLGLILG**

AFVICWLPFFVKELVVNVCDKCKISEEMS**NFLAWLGYLNSLINPLIYTIF**NEDFKKAFQK

LVRCRC

Another major category of α-helix rich proteins which is important in drug action is the ion channel proteins. These proteins are much larger than the receptor-coupled G-proteins and have many transmembrane-spanning helices. For example, the sodium ion channel protein associated with the action of local anaesthetics in nerve blockade has 1988 amino acid residues which form 24 transmembrane helices connected by intracellular and extracellular loops.

The β-sheet motif

The other major structural element found in proteins is the β-sheet. In this case, the primary sequence folds so that strands of the backbone are arranged parallel to each other to form a pleated sheet. Unlike the α-helix, the strands making up the sheet are not part of one continuous sequence of amino acids but have intervening loop regions. There are two ways of arranging the strands, either parallel or antiparallel, as shown in Figure 6.13. The sheets are held together by hydrogen bonding between the amide nitrogens and the carbonyls of the peptide backbone. The strands in a β-sheet can be represented by an arrow which points towards the C-terminus of the peptide. This enables parallel and antiparallel sheet motifs to be drawn, as shown in Figure 6.14. Where the ends of the strands are joined by loops of peptide, the length of the loops is greater in the case of the parallel arrangement of strands. Although the strands can be drawn in such a two-dimensional representation they have a three-dimensional structure, and a common way for a β-sheet to fold is into a barrel shape where enzymatic activity occurs within the barrel, much like the receptor binding that takes place amongst a group of α-helices. Many enzymes have a mixture of β-sheet and α-helix motifs.

Retinol-binding protein provides an example of a protein that is largely composed of β-sheets. Retinol (vitamin A) is one of the fat-soluble vitamins and is important in a number of physiological functions, including vision (see Ch. 26). Since it has to be transported from the intestine where it is absorbed to its site of action it requires a carrier protein since, unlike a water-soluble vitamin such as ascorbic acid, it does not dissolve in physiological fluids. Retinol-binding protein has eight antiparallel strands which form a β-sheet which arranges itself into a barrel-like structure. Its primary sequence is shown in Figure 6.15, with the strands making up the β-sheet shown in bold. It can be viewed as having its β-sheet

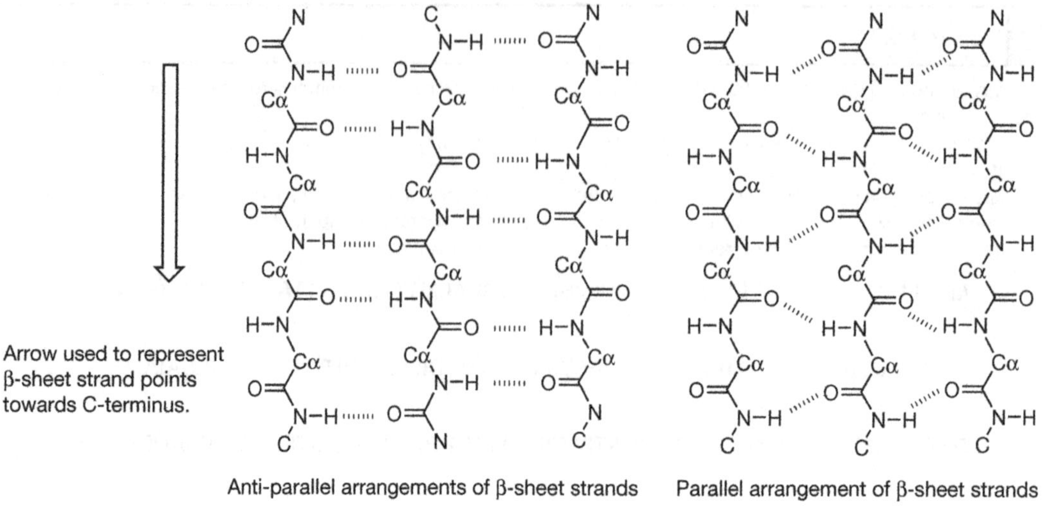

Figure 6.13 Parallel and antiparallel arrangements of the peptide backbone to form β-sheets.

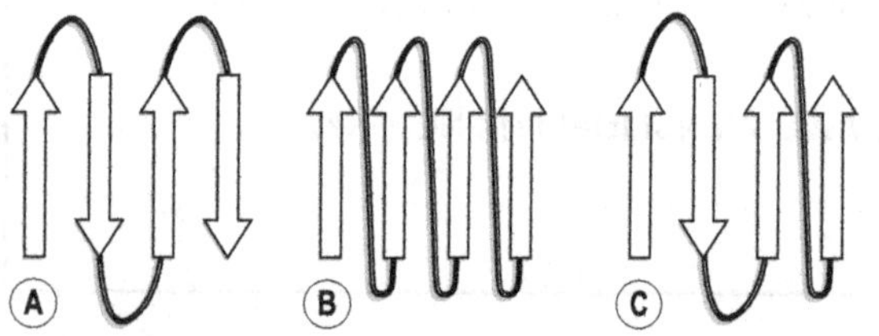

Figure 6.14 (**A**) Antiparallel, (**B**) parallel and (**C**) mixed parallel and antiparallel arrangement of peptide strands in β-sheets.

folded into a barrel arrangement, as shown in Figure 6.16. As can be seen from the amino acid sequences of the strands, they contain a mixture of polar and non-polar residues. The polar residues orientate themselves outwards into the hydrophilic environment while the hydrophobic residues due to amino acids such as valine, leucine and phenylalanine which occur in the residues lining the interior of the barrel and bind the hydrophobic retinol molecule (Fig. 6.17). The amino acids at the N-terminus and C-terminus ends of the molecule are partly in the form of α-helices and fold over to close the barrel so that the retinol is protected from the hydrophilic environment. These types of proteins are classed as lipocalins and they have a widespread role in binding lipophilic molecules such as essential fatty acids, pheromones and olfactory molecules. They all have the barrel-like structure shown in Figure 6.16.

Many proteins have a mixture of α-helix and β-sheet domains. Neuraminidase is a large protein composed of β-sheet domains arranged in a propeller-like conformation surrounded by α-helices. It is a target in chemotherapy against influenza (see Ch. 23).[4,5] The active site of the enzyme is located within the β-sheet domains. Once crystal structure information on the enzyme became available, it became possible to see that certain residues within the binding pocket of the enzyme were conserved between different strains of the virus and, using modelling software, that these residues would be likely to interact favourably with the substrate. Compounds with inhibitory activity were designed and the formation of crystals of the inhibitor enzyme complexes enabled refinement of the design of the inhibitor. The interactions of the

N-terminus 1 2
MKWVWALLLLAALGSGRAERDCRVSSFRVKENFDKARFS**GTWYAMAKK**DPEGLF**LQDNIV**

3 4 5 6
AEFSVDETGQ**MSATAKGRVRLLNNWDVCADMVGTFT**DTEDPA**KFKMKYWGVA**SFLQK**GN**

7 8
DDHWIVDTDYDTYAVQYSCRLLNLDG**TCADSYSFVFSRD**PNGLPPEAQKIVRQRQEELCLA

RQYRLIVHNGYCDGRSERNLL C-terminus

Figure 6.15 Primary sequence of retinol binding protein. The eight β-sheet regions which form the barrel are shown in bold.

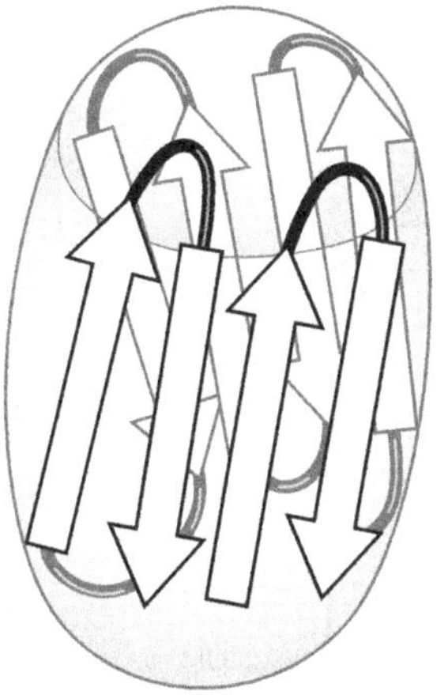

Figure 6.16 Barrel-like conformation adopted by retinol-binding protein β-sheets in order to shield retinol from a hydrophilic environment.

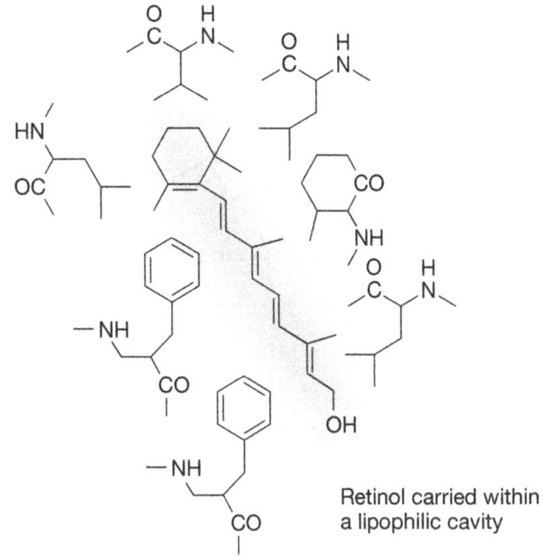

Figure 6.17 Lipophilic interaction between retinol and the groups lining the barrel formed by the β-sheet.

substrate with the active site are shown in Figure 6.18. The substrate is strongly bound into place by the interaction of three arginine residues with its carboxyl group. The actual hydrolysis of the glycosidic bond is most probably catalysed by an aspartate or a glutamate residue (Fig. 6.19). The substrate binds very strongly to the active site and its conformation becomes distorted from a chair to a boat form. The boat form is very strained and the relief of steric strain upon hydrolysis helps to promote it. Once the rest of the sugar chain has been removed, a transition state oxonium ion is formed which instantaneously reacts with water (this is called a transition state analogue but in fact the true transition state is at the point

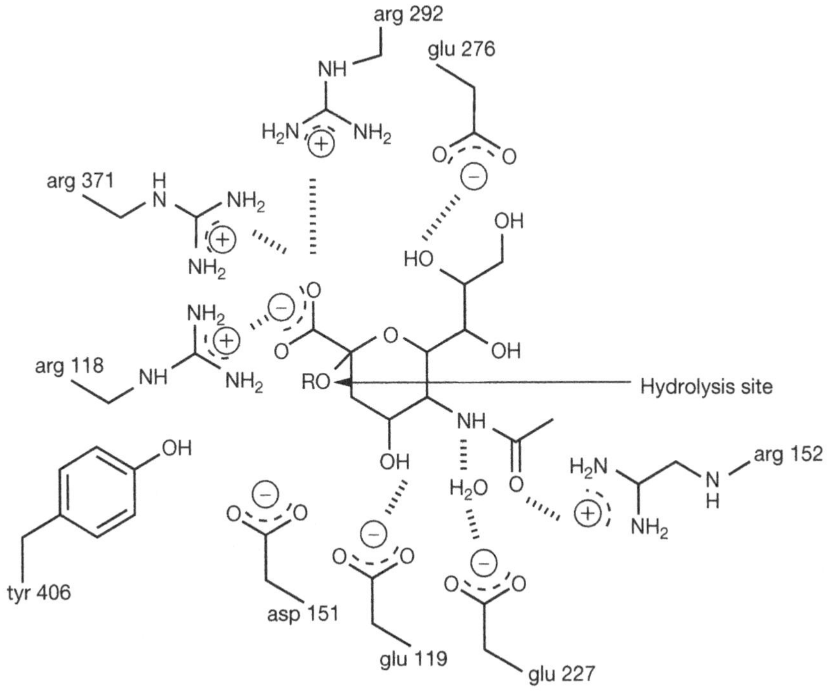

Figure 6.18 The binding pocket of viral neuraminidase.

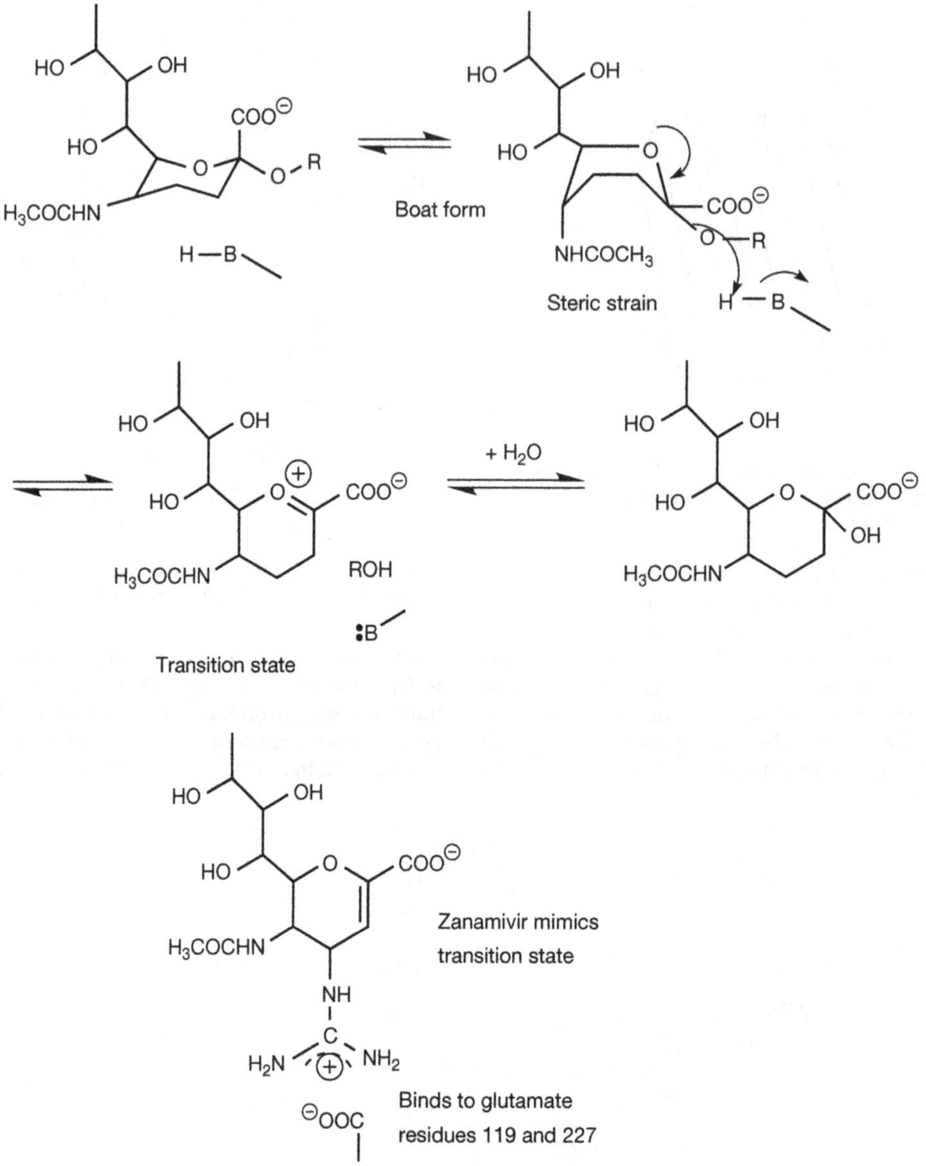

Figure 6.19 Mechanism of hydrolysis of neuraminidase and zanamivir as a transition-state analogue.

where RO is just leaving the molecule). Zanamivir mimics the structure of the intermediate formed during hydrolysis and at the same time is strongly bound to the enzyme via interaction between its positively charged guanidine group and negatively charged aspartate residues at the active site of the enzyme.

The design of selective cyclooxygenase (COX) inhibitors has attracted much interest over the last few years because of the side effects associated with the existing non-steroidal anti-inflammatory drugs (NSAIDs) which inhibit both COX-1 and COX-2.[6,7] COX-1 is generally found in cells without being induced and, for instance, exerts a protective effect on the GI tract whereas COX-2 is up-regulated in response to, for instance, infection, and drives inflammatory processes and is the target of drugs used to treat inflammation. COX-1 and COX-2 have very similar primary amino acid sequences and thus drugs such as NSAIDs affect COX-1 potentially causing damage to the GI tract as well as affecting COX-2 to reduce inflammation. COX-2 is largely composed of helical regions, and

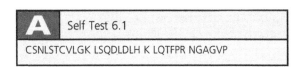

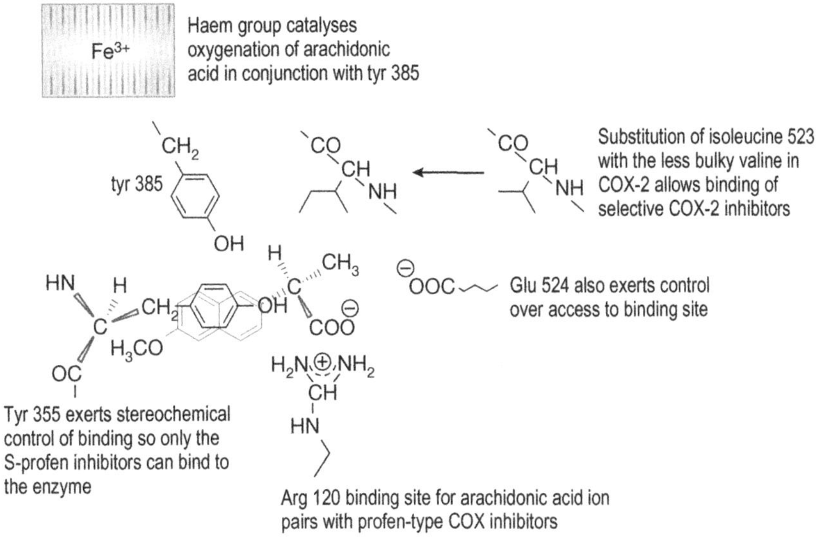

Figure 6.20 The binding site in COX enzymes.

the binding of substrate and the regions of catalytic activity are found largely in the loops joining the helices together. The binding site residues in COX-1 are shown in Figure 6.20. The arginine group at position 120 in the protein strongly binds to the carboxyl group of the enzyme substrate arachidonic acid or to the carboxyl group of a profen-type NSAID. The entry of the substrate to the active site is stereochemically controlled and there are a number of other key residues at the binding site, including a tyrosine at position 355 which exerts a steric hindrance effect restricting the compounds, which can enter the binding site, and a glutamate residue at position 524 which also exerts stereochemical control. The stereochemical control explains why the S-isomers of profen-type NSAIDs are active. COX-2 inhibitors were largely found by random screening and they bind specifically to COX-2 due to stereochemical effects in the region around a valine residue at position 523 which is replaced by a more bulky isoleucine group in COX-1.

A Self Test 6.1

CSNLSTCVLGK LSQDLDLH K LQTFPR NGAGVP

A Self Test 6.2

a. Insulin b. Human growth hormone.

A Self Test 6.3

1. Seven helices all with 21 amino acids.
2. 67%.
3. D 5 residue in the 3rd helix.
4. Between the 5th and 6th helix starting with L and ending with K.

REFERENCES

1. Isogaya M, Sugimoto Y, Tanimura R, et al. Binding pockets of the β1- and β2-adrenergic receptors for subtype-selective agonists. *Mol Pharmacol.* 1999;56:875–885.
2. Behr B, Hoffman C, Ottolina G, Klotz K-N. Novel mutants of the human β1-adrenergic receptor reveal amino acids relevant for receptor activation. *J Biol Chem.* 2006;281:18120–18125.
3. Lopez-Rodriguez ML, Vicente B, Deupi X, et al. Design, synthesis and pharmacological evaluation of 5-hydroxytryptamine 1a receptor ligands to explore the three-dimensional structure of the receptor. *Mol Pharmacol.* 2002;62:15–21.
4. von Itzstein M. The war against influenza discovery and development of sialidase inhibitors. *Nature Drug Discovery Rev.* 2007;6:967–974.
5. Magesh S, Suzuki T, Miyagi T, Ishida H, Kiso M. Homology modeling of human sialidase enzymes NEU1, NEU3 and NEU4 based on the crystal structure of NEU2: Hints for the design of selective NEU3 inhibitors. *J Mol Graph Model.* 2006;25:196–207.
6. Kiefer JR, Pawlitz JL, Moreland KT, et al. Structural insights into the stereochemistry of the cyclooxygenase reaction. *Nature.* 1999;405:97–101.
7. Marnett LJ, Kalgutkar AS. Cyclooxygenase 2 inhibitors: discovery, selectivity and the future. *TIPS.* 1999;20: 465–469.

Chapter | 7 |

DNA structure and its importance to drug action

Simon P Mackay

CHAPTER CONTENTS

INTRODUCTION

The elucidation of the structure of deoxyribonucleic acid (DNA) in 1953 by James Watson and Frances Crick was one of the major scientific events of the last century. The recent unravelling of the human genome would not have been possible today without Watson and Crick's fundamental descriptions of the role of complementary base pairing and the organisation of the component deoxynucleotides into a double helical structure. Since Rosalind Franklin's groundbreaking research using X-ray crystallography to define two general forms of helical DNA, a whole variety of experimental techniques have shown that the structure of DNA is far more complex than originally proposed. Not only are there different morphological states (e.g. A, B, Z), the structure is also sequence dependent, where the order of the nucleotides can influence the three-dimensional shape in different regions of the helix. Such variations in structure according to sequence are fundamental to the function of DNA and its interactions with the many different proteins that seek to influence its role in cellular biochemistry. It is not the purpose of this chapter to discuss in depth the minutiae of DNA structural variations; there is already a wealth of literature available which describes these phenomena. Here, we provide the basics of DNA structure and function in order to lay foundations for later chapters where DNA plays a part in the pharmacological action of specific drugs. These work through a variety of chemical mechanisms including DNA cleavage and cross-linking, or by reversible association, usually by intercalation or binding in one of the DNA grooves. It is fair to say that a number of drugs whose cellular target is DNA were in use before the structure of DNA had been solved, or even before it was recognised as the repository of the genetic code, e.g. the nitrogen mustards in the treatment of cancer. However, this does not detract from the fact that in the design of new drugs which target DNA, and to grasp the mechanisms of action of current DNA-targeting drugs already in the clinic, an understanding of the target's structure, function and chemistry is necessary.

DNA is a polymeric molecule composed of subunits called deoxynucleotides in whose sequence is stored our genetic code. The information necessary for a cell to function and replicate in a programmed manner is ultimately determined by this code, and which parts of it are turned on or off. Essentially, the specific order of the deoxynucleotides within the DNA sequence, codes for specific proteins, which when synthesised, perform explicit functions of a cell's biochemistry. Sometimes the code is continually turned on (expressed) to produce proteins which are in constant demand, whereas for proteins which are required in response to a particular signal, their code will be turned off until such a time as that signal in question is initiated, e.g. release of a hormone such as oestrogen in puberty. Considering that it is the DNA sequence that holds the code for proteins to be synthesised, and that it is the interactions of specific proteins with particular code sequences that turn on and off these sequences, we can already appreciate the highly complex role of DNA within cellular function and replication. In fact, with DNA and proteins it is the proverbial chicken and egg problem; without DNA, proteins cannot be synthesised, yet without proteins, our genetic code cannot be expressed. Ultimately, drugs that exert their pharmacological effect at the DNA level act by altering the interactions between these two classes of biological macromolecule. So how is this code stored and how is it translated?

THE STRUCTURAL COMPONENTS OF DNA – DNA PRIMARY STRUCTURE

The structure of DNA is like a long piece of string, composed of two strands wound around each other like strands in a rope. Each strand consists of subunits or monomers linked together like beads, and each subunit is called a deoxynucleotide. DNA is therefore a biological polymer, and it is the order of the deoxynucleotide monomers and their chemical nature and linkage that is responsible for the genetic code, and is referred to as the primary structure of DNA.

The deoxynucleotide monomers in DNA are made up of the same chemical moieties, namely a phosphate group, a deoxyribose sugar and a heteroaromatic base. The latter moiety can be one of four different bases and it is this chemical diversity that enables a code to be constructed. The sugar and the phosphate groups of the deoxynucleotides form the backbone of each polymeric strand, being linked together through phosphodiester bonds.

DNA bases

The DNA bases, as their name suggests, are mainly basic molecules, and fall into two categories of aromatic heterocycle: the pyrimidines and purines. Although some of the DNA bases are bases, none of them is a strong enough base or acid to carry a charge at physiological pH (7.4) and their p*Ka* values are at least 2 units above or below physiological pH.[1]

Pyrimidine bases

The bases thymine and cytosine are derivatives of the heterocycle pyrimidine. Thymine and cytosine are examples of tautomers, and the structures shown in Figure 7.1 are the major, stable tautomeric forms of these bases. Those stable forms have an amino substituent in the amino form as opposed to the imino form, and the oxygen atoms prefer to exist as the keto rather than the enol form at physiological pH. However, since the nitrogens in the molecule are weakly acidic at very high pH the oxygen atoms can bear a negative charge (see Ch. 4). The fact that the major tautomeric form is found in DNA is crucial to the existence of DNA as a double-stranded, self-replicating structure.

Thymine is a very weak base p*Ka* *ca.* 4.5 and cytosine is not a base at all, being a very weak acid.

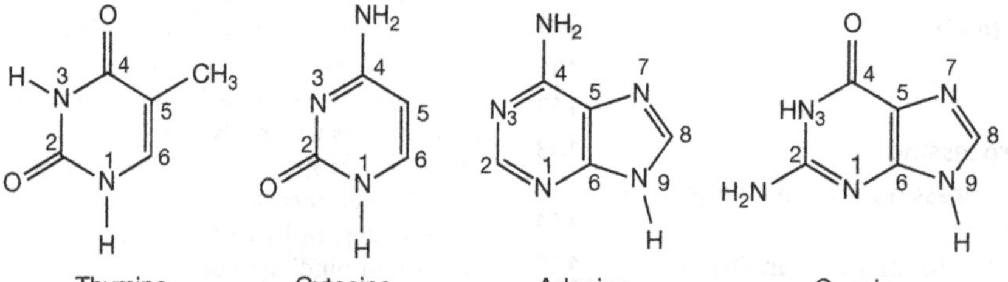

Figure 7.1 The pyrimidine and purine bases of DNA.

Purine bases

The bases adenine and guanine are heterocyclic purine derivatives. Again, they are the major tautomers that are present in DNA (Fig. 7.1), and are weak bases, having their p*Ka* values around 5.

Deoxynucleosides

The sugar unit found in the backbone linkages of DNA is the furanose, deoxyribose (Fig. 7.2), which differs from its parent sugar ribose at the 2 position; the hydroxyl group has been replaced by a hydrogen and, in other words, has lost an oxygen, hence the prefix *deoxy*ribose. Attachment of the pyrimidine or purine bases via the 1 or 9 position, respectively, to the 1 position of deoxyribose (through the loss of water) yields the four deoxynucleosides. The bond linking the base to the sugar is called a β-glycosidic link, β because the base is above the plane of the sugar, in common with the carbon at the 5′ position (if the base were below the sugar plane, it would be an α-glycoside). Note how the numbering system changes for the sugar in the deoxynucleoside, with each number having a 'prime' associated with it to distinguish it from the positions in the covalently attached base. In nomenclature terms, because the deoxyribose sugars are associated with these molecules, they are given the *deoxy* prefix in their names. The suffix to the base name also changes, to indicate that it is part of a base-sugar conjugate, hence we have deoxythymidine, deoxycytidine, deoxyadenosine and deoxyguanosine (Fig. 7.3).

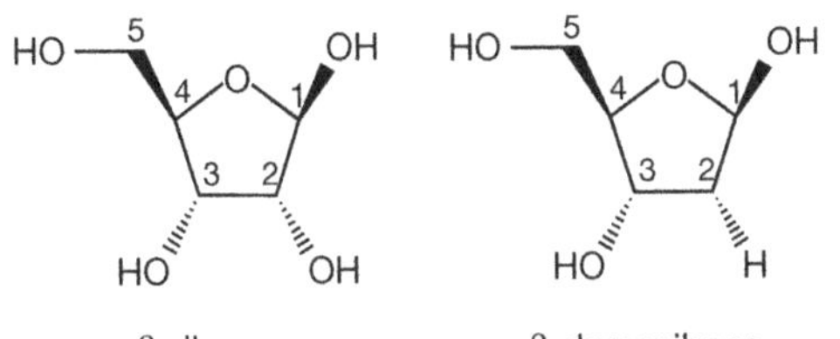

Figure 7.2 Sugars found in nucleic acids.

Q	Self Test 7.1
	Draw the structure of the corresponding α-glycoside of deoxythymidine.

Deoxynucleotides

Deoxynucleotides are the phosphate esters of the deoxynucleosides. Just as a carboxylic ester can be considered as the product of a carboxylic acid and alcohol, then a phosphate ester is the product of phosphoric acid and an alcohol, where the alcohol, in this instance, is the sugar moiety of the deoxynucleoside. As there are two alcoholic functionalities on the deoxynucleoside sugar at the 5′ and 3′ positions, the corresponding deoxynucleotides can be 5′-monophosphates, 3′-monophosphates, or

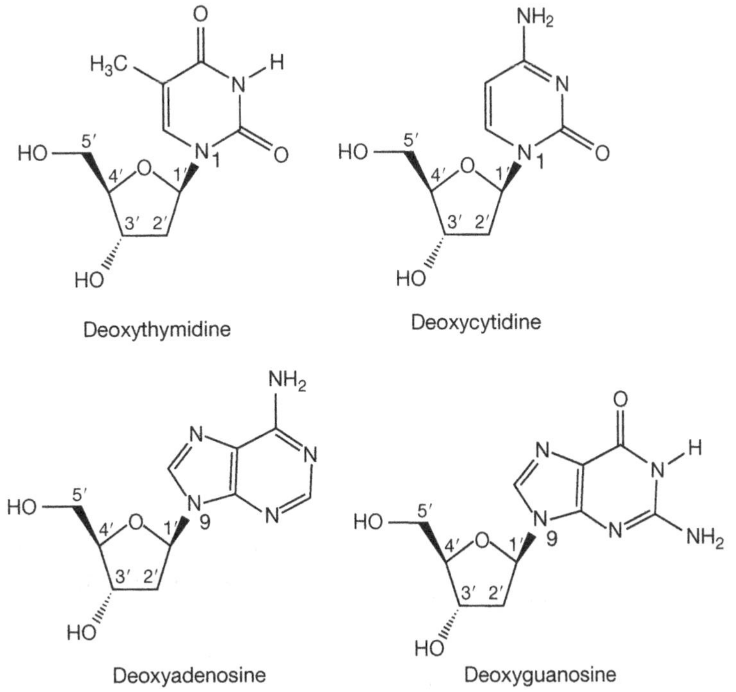

Figure 7.3 The deoxynucleosides of DNA.

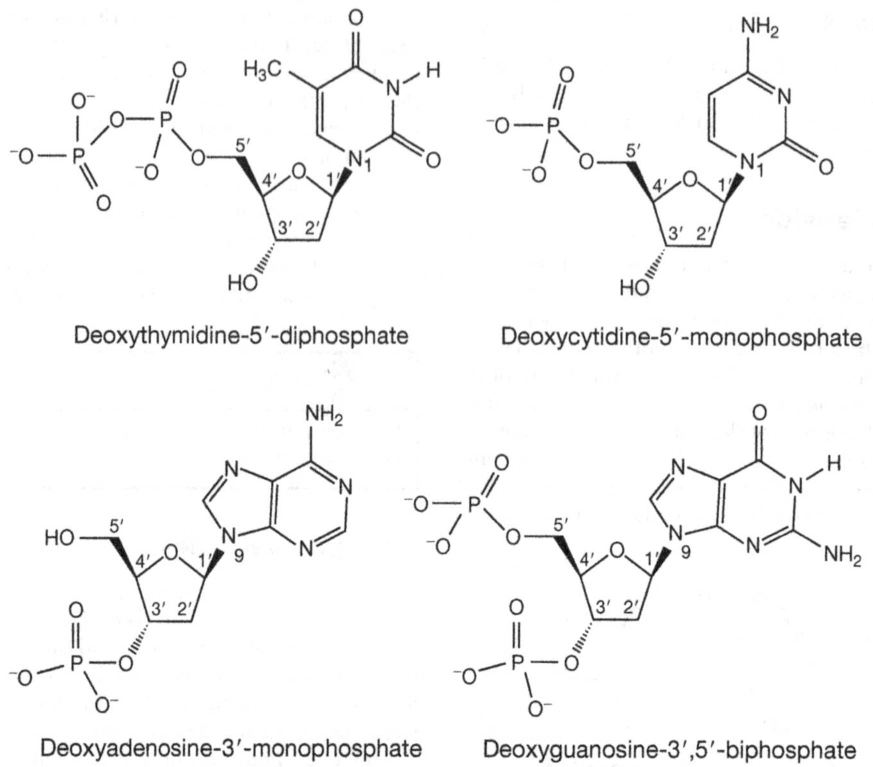

Figure 7.4 Examples of deoxynucleotide structures.

even 3′,5′-biphosphates (Fig. 7.4). If two or three phosphate groups were attached via the 5′ hydroxyl, the deoxynucleotide would be given the 5′-di- or triphosphate respectively, e.g. deoxythymidine-5′-diphosphate.

> **Q** Self Test 7.2
>
> The universal energy cofactor ATP is an abbreviation of adenosine-5′-triphosphate – draw the structure.
>
> Cyclic AMP is a secondary messenger in cellular biochemistry and is an abbreviation for cyclic adenosine-3′,5′-monophosphate – draw the structure (hint: one phosphate group is bonded to two positions).

If the deoxynucleotides are the monomeric units that compose DNA and their order along its backbone is the foundation of the genetic code, how are they linked together? Phosphoric acid is a tribasic acid and therefore has the capacity to form more than one ester linkage with alcohols. There are two alcoholic groups on each deoxyribose, so a phosphodiester linkage between two separate deoxynucleosides is possible. Within DNA, there is an order to such linkages, with a phosphodiester bond only forming between the 5′ and 3′ hydroxyl groups of different monomers in a contiguous fashion. Formation of phosphodiester groups from phosphoric acid leaves one free acidic oxygen on the phosphate which is fully ionised at physiological pH. Consequently, DNA strand backbones will have an overall net negative charge. We can now see the route of the name for unabbreviated deoxyribonucleic acid; deoxyribose is the sugar present in each of the linked deoxyribonucleotides, and the acid arises from the acidity of the phosphodiester backbone.

Examination of the four deoxynucleotides linked together by phosphodiester bonds shown in Figure 7.5 reveals that DNA strands have directionality, i.e. we can move in a 5′ to 3′ direction along the strand, or in a 3′ to 5′ direction. Such directionality features in the secondary structure of DNA, and is vital to the replicatory and decoding process of the genetic code.

Complementary hydrogen bonding between DNA strands

Within the cell nucleus, DNA is present not as a single polymeric strand, but as a double strand, where two chains of deoxynucleotides are bound together. The

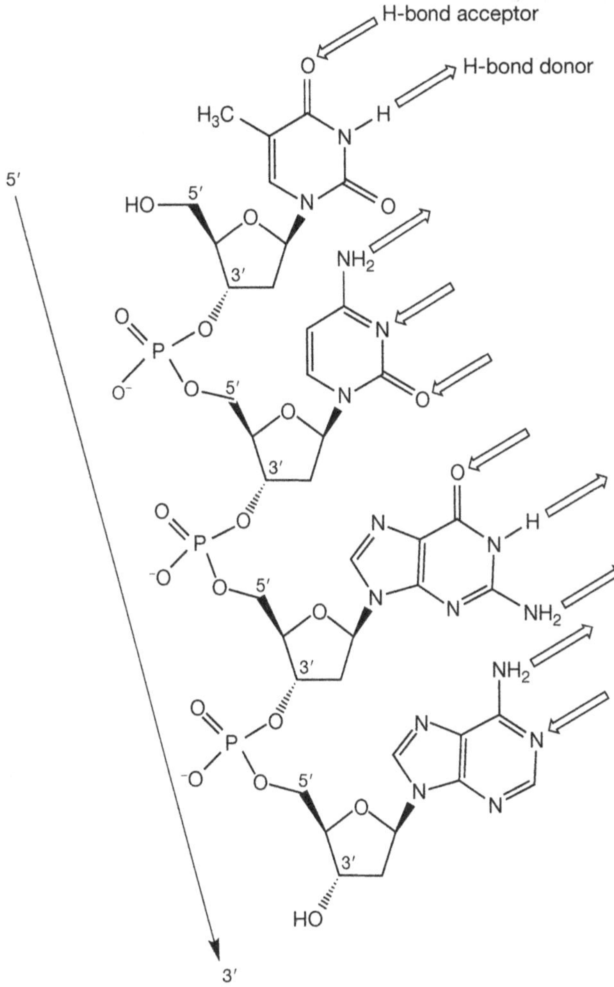

Figure 7.5 A schematic section of a DNA single strand illustrating directionality and the hydrogen bond donor and acceptor groups of the bases.

binding interaction between the strands is not covalent in nature, but involves weaker forces that can be overcome by thermal heating. Raising the temperature of a solution of double-stranded DNA results in strand separation at about 100°C. If such a solution is then cooled, the strands anneal to the same original, double-stranded structure, which indicates that the forces that bind the strands together are highly specific and discriminatory. Inspection of the single-stranded structure shown in Figure 7.5 reveals the presence of hydrogen-bonding functional groups on the bases which project away from the sugar–phosphate backbone. It is these hydrogen bond donors and acceptors that are instrumental in holding the two strands together in a highly specific manner.

The hydrogen-bonding compatibilities between deoxyadenosine (dA) and deoxythymidine (dT) ensures that these two bases pair with each other in a complementary fashion via two hydrogen bonds. For deoxycytidine (dC) and deoxyguanosine (dG), three hydrogen bonds between compatible hydrogen bond donors and acceptors give rise to the second type of base pair. The arrangement of the respective hydrogen bond donor and acceptor groups on each base means that under normal conditions, dA will only bind with dT, and dC with dG. The nature and positions of the hydrogen bonds ensures that each base pair is planar. In Figure 7.6, position 1 of the pyrimidine deoxynucleotides (dC and dT) and position 9 of the purines (dA and dG) are the points of attachment of each base to the deoxyribose sugar in the strand backbone. Significantly, the distance between these attachment points for each base pair is practically the same because each base pair consists of a purine and pyrimidine base. The consequent effect of such an arrangement ensures that the backbone of each strand remains more or less equidistant along the whole double-stranded structure, thus imparting a degree of regularity which is irrespective of the sequence of the bases within that structure.

Q Self Test 7.3

You have two separate solutions of double-stranded DNA: one solution contains DNA composed only of dG and dC as self-complementary strands, and the other only of dA and dT (shown below). Heating the solutions will result in strand separation. Which strands will separate at the lower temperature, and why?

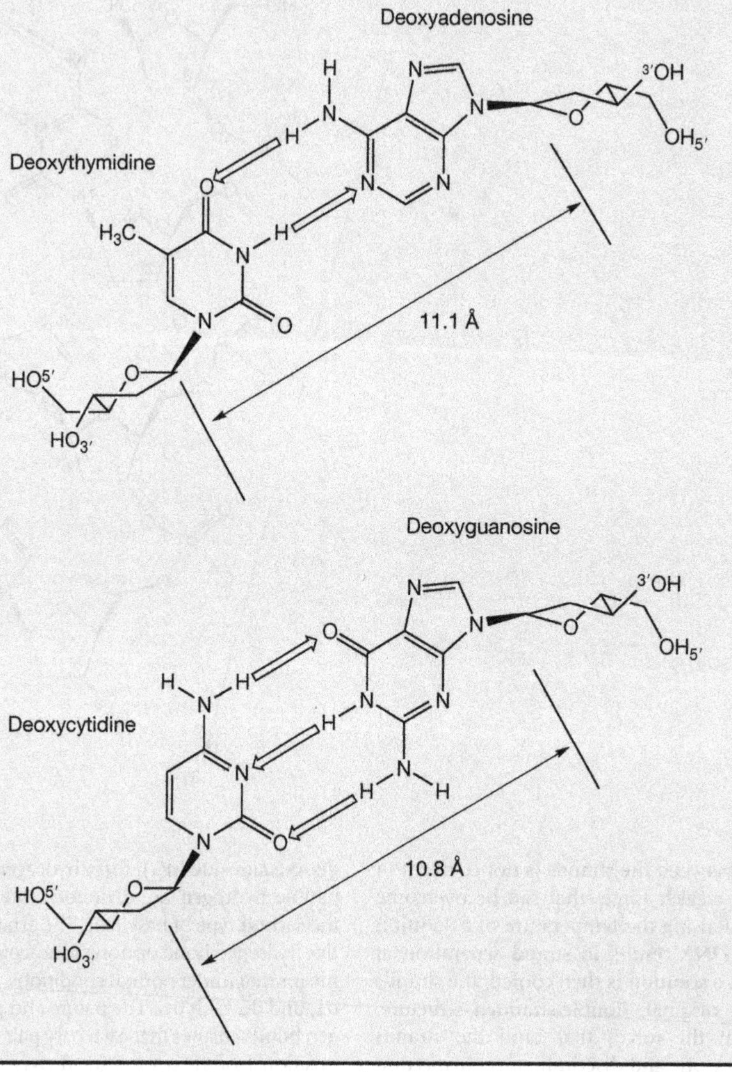

For the base pairs to hydrogen bond in the manner shown in Figure 7.6, one base from each pair must be rotated by 180° to ensure that the hydrogen bonding groups are directed towards each other. Because the opposing complementary bases are not isolated, but linked together in a strand, in order to rotate the opposite base to ensure complementarity, the whole strand must have a directionality that is opposite to the strand with which it is bound (Fig. 7.6). Two strands having opposing directionality are said to be antiparallel, where direction is defined by the phosphodiester links in the sugar–phosphate backbone i.e. 5′ to 3′ versus 3′ to 5′ (Fig 7.7).

Before discussing the three-dimensional secondary structure of double-stranded DNA, it is worth making

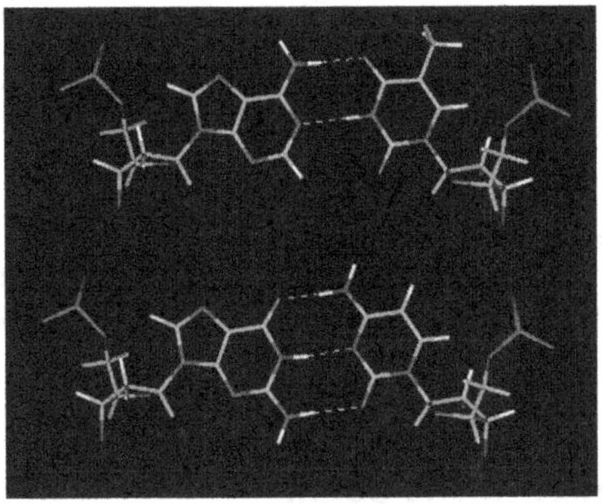

Figure 7.6 Molecular models of the DNA base pairs illustrating 'Watson–Crick' hydrogen bonding complementarity.

a few observations of the two-dimensional representation of the primary structure illustrated in Figure 7.7.

- The two strands have opposing directionality, i.e. they are antiparallel.
- The two strand backbones are essentially equidistant from each other irrespective of base sequence.
- The phosphate and sugar moieties are essentially equidistant from each other within each antiparallel strand.
- The negatively charged phosphate containing backbone will produce a polar, hydrophilic exterior in any three-dimensional structure.
- The bases are projected towards each other to enable complementary hydrogen bonding, and thereby form a hydrophobic 'inner core' within the structure.

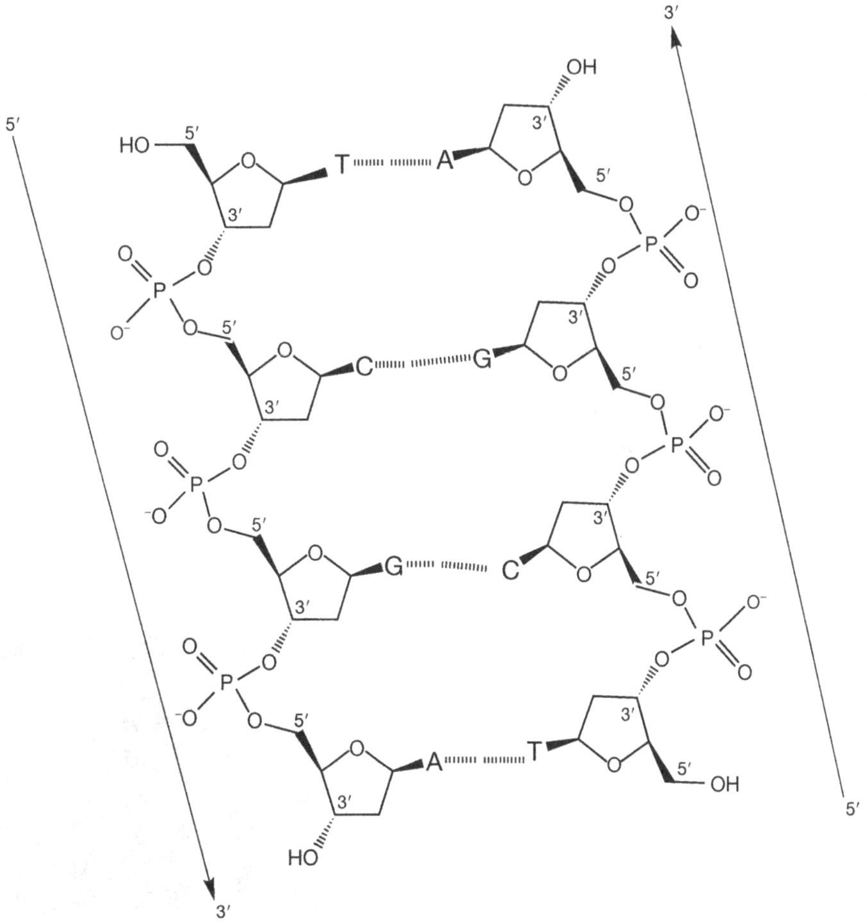

Figure 7.7 A schematic section of a DNA double strand illustrating antiparallel directionality and interstrand hydrogen bonding.

DNA SECONDARY STRUCTURE – THE DOUBLE HELIX

The three-dimensional secondary structure of DNA is determined by the conformational preferences and restrictions of the relatively rigid individual deoxynucleotides which are linked together in each of the strands, which are, in turn, influenced by the properties of the DNA primary structure listed above. Thus, the inspection of some of the factors that influence deoxynucleotide conformation can help in the extrapolation to the more complex three-dimensional nature of the double-stranded polymer itself.

Conformation of the deoxyribose sugar

The pentagonal representations of the deoxyribose sugar moieties have so far been as a 'plan' view. However, they are saturated rings (as illustrated by the stereochemical centres at the 1′, 3′ and 4′ positions) and will be twisted out of plane to reduce the non-bonded repulsions between the ring substituents in order to adopt low energy conformations. Two low energy structures for free deoxynucleotides in solution are the $C^{2'}$ *endo* and $C^{3'}$ *endo* conformations, *endo* referring to the position of the carbon atom most distorted from planarity in the ring structure and on the same side of the ring as the attached base (Fig. 7.8). The two different conformations will influence the relative spatial positions of phosphate groups attached at the 5′ and 3′ hydroxyls (Fig. 7.8). $C^{2'}$ *endo* sugar pucker produces an interphosphorus distance of 7.0 Å, whilst the $C^{3'}$ *endo* conformation results in an equivalent distance of 5.9 Å. If these conformations were adopted within the deoxynucleotide strand, then an exclusively $C^{2'}$ *endo* backbone would be more elongated than a corresponding $C^{3'}$ *endo* chain.

Conformation of the base with respect to the sugar

Low energy structures of the base with respect to the deoxyribose sugar are achieved when the base plane is perpendicular to the sugar plane and bisects the C2′-O-O4′ angle to produce a *syn* or *anti* conformation. *Syn or anti* refers to the base with respect to this angle at the β-glycosidic bond (Fig. 7.9). Of the two, the *anti* conformation is more stable because of lower steric repulsion between the base substituents and the sugar ring. The pyrimidine bases have an oxygen atom in position 2 which, in an *anti* conformation, is projected away from the sugar. In the corresponding *syn* conformation, this oxygen is in direct conflict with the sugar ring and 5′-phosphate atoms (Fig 7.9). The effect is more pronounced with the purine bases, where the *syn*

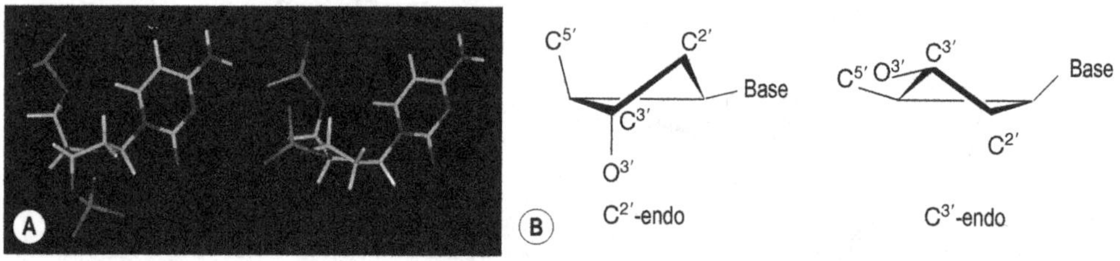

Figure 7.8 Deoxyribose sugar pucker conformations commonly found in DNA.

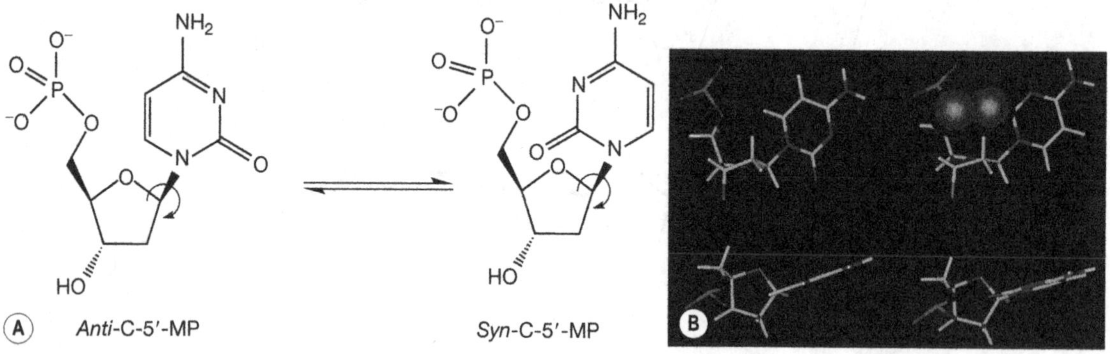

Figure 7.9 The possible *anti* and *syn* conformations of cytosine with respect to the deoxyribose sugar unit in a cytidine deoxynucleotide.

conformation places an aromatic ring directly over the sugar. The net effect of the deoxynucleotides preferring an *anti* conformation is to direct the hydrogen bond donor and acceptor groups of the bases away from the backbone and into a position where complementary hydrogen bonding with an antiparallel strand is favoured.

The *anti* conformations of the bases are stabilised further by a weak electrostatic interaction between the electron-deficient acidic hydrogen in position 6 (pyrimidines)/ position 8 (purines) and the O5′ oxygen of the deoxyribose sugar. These hydrogens are electron deficient (acidic) because of their proximity to the electronegative nitrogen and oxygen atoms within the heteroaromatic bases. Such an interaction helps ensure that the hydrogen bonding functions of the bases are directed away from the backbone in the DNA structure.

The phosphodiester bonds

The P–O bonds in the phosphodiester backbone are the positions of greatest flexibility within the DNA strands, and are the main pivots affecting polydeoxynucleotide structure and allow for some degree of flexibility. If a degree of strain is introduced into the double stranded structure, it will more than likely be relieved at these bonds initially (Fig. 7.10). The phosphodiester P–O bonds are also orientated so that the negatively charged oxygens are removed from the hydrophobic core interior where the bases lie, and project out into the water which surrounds the exterior, where they can interact with hydrophilic cationic counter-ions and water molecules.

Base pair stacking

The complementary base pairs in the centre of the double-stranded DNA structure are planar yet perpendicular to the plane of the sugars in the backbone. The optimum orientation relative to each other is therefore for them to stack on top of each other, subject to the restrictions of the sugar–phosphate backbone to which they are joined on opposite strands (Fig. 7.11). In fact, single deoxynucleotides will aggregate in aqueous solution by stacking their planar, heteroaromatic bases on top of each other. Van der Waals forces and charge transfer interactions between π-electron systems of the bases drive the hydrophobic stacking process, and such self-stacking of the rings into aggregates removes them from the hydrophilic aqueous environment. The optimum balance between the attractive and repulsive forces between the base pairs in this stacking environment is achieved at a distance of 3.4 Å between the respective planes.

Taking into account the conformational preferences and restrictions of the individual deoxynucleotides in both strands, hydrogen bonding between the bases of opposite strands, the equidistance between those strands, the stacking of the base pairs within the hydrophobic interior, and the flexible P–O bonds directing the negatively charged oxygens towards the structural exterior, the most stable conformation for DNA is a right-handed double helix (Fig. 7.11). The 3.4 Å optimum distance between the base pair planes is determined by the sugar pucker of the deoxyribose in the backbone to which the bases are attached, which in turn is dependent on the degree of hydration by water molecules and the salt content of the solution in which the DNA is present. The backbone of the DNA helix is negatively charged, and the mutual repulsion between the anionic oxygens to a distance of 7 Å, promotes the $C^{2'}$-endo sugar conformation within the deoxynucleotides, which subsequently enables an optimum base pair separation of 3.4 Å. Water molecules and cations such as sodium ions, which are attracted towards the sugar–phosphate backbone, mask the interanionic repulsive forces and stabilise the helical structure by forming a hydration sheath.

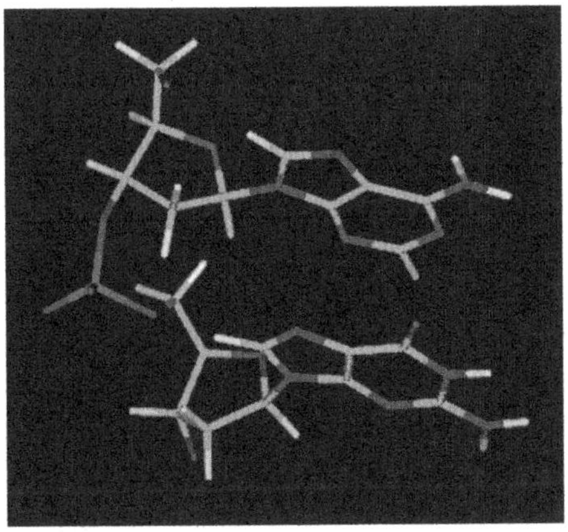

Figure 7.10 Molecular model of a dAdG dinucleotide linked via flexible P–O bonds.

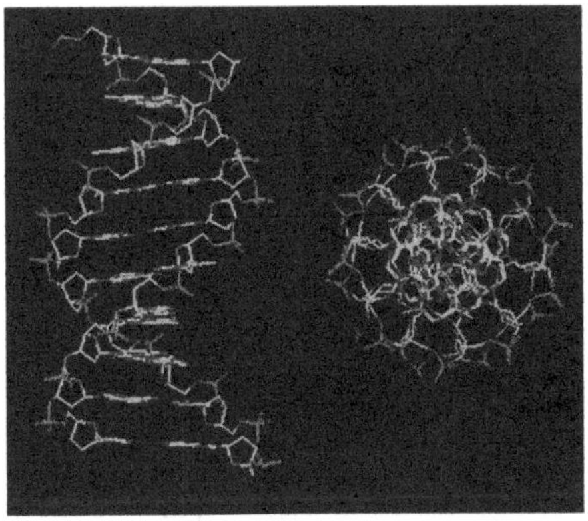

Figure 7.11 Molecular model of double-stranded DNA illustrating base pair stacking from the side and above the helix.

Why a helix, not a ladder?

It is apparent that planar base pairs stacked on top of each other and attached at each side to the sugar–phosphate backbones could adopt a structure akin to a ladder, as opposed to the spiral staircase dimensions of a double helix. Here the analogy is appropriate, considering that DNA contains millions of base pairs, so in terms of simple packing, more base pairs can be stacked on top of each other in a helical form. To adopt a ladder, the sugar–phosphate backbones would have to be extended, pulling the base pairs further apart to a distance approaching 7.0 Å, which would also reduce the attractive stacking interactions between the bases. Because the sugar–phosphate backbones twist around each other, the long base pair axes are rotated with respect to each other's long axis by an angle of 36° for each step up the staircase (Fig 7.12). This is referred to as the helix twist or winding angle, and is an average value for the whole helix. There will be small variations of this angle, depending on the base pair sequence, within specific regions of the helix.

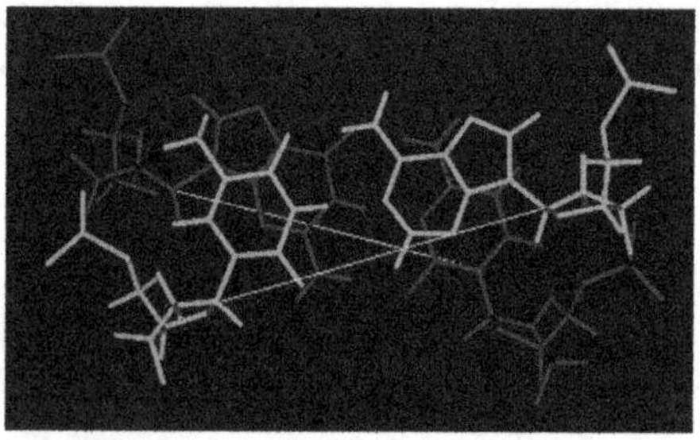

Figure 7.12 Top section from a DNA model illustrating the twist of the base pair long axis through the helix.

HELICAL GROOVES – MAJOR AND MINOR

One of the most significant structural properties of the double-stranded DNA is the presence of two differently sized grooves that plough furrows along and around the double helix. It is these grooves that provide access to the genetic code, and form the basis of recognition with the proteins that bind and process the DNA during the various cellular events in which it is involved. The presence of two grooves of different sizes can be explained by inspecting the positions of attachment of the base pairs to the sugar–phosphate backbone. In Figure 7.13, the sugars from opposite backbones are not attached to the bases directly opposite each other, but displaced from the central helical axis. If the backbones were attached at the 6 position of the pyrimidine bases whilst still at the 9 position of the purines, i.e. opposite each other, then the two grooves between the backbones would be the same size, width and depth. The fact that they are attached off-centre means that there are two different-sized grooves, one wide, known as the major groove, and one narrow, referred to as the minor groove. When viewed from the side of the helix (Fig. 7.14), the edges of the base pairs can be seen on the groove floors. It is here

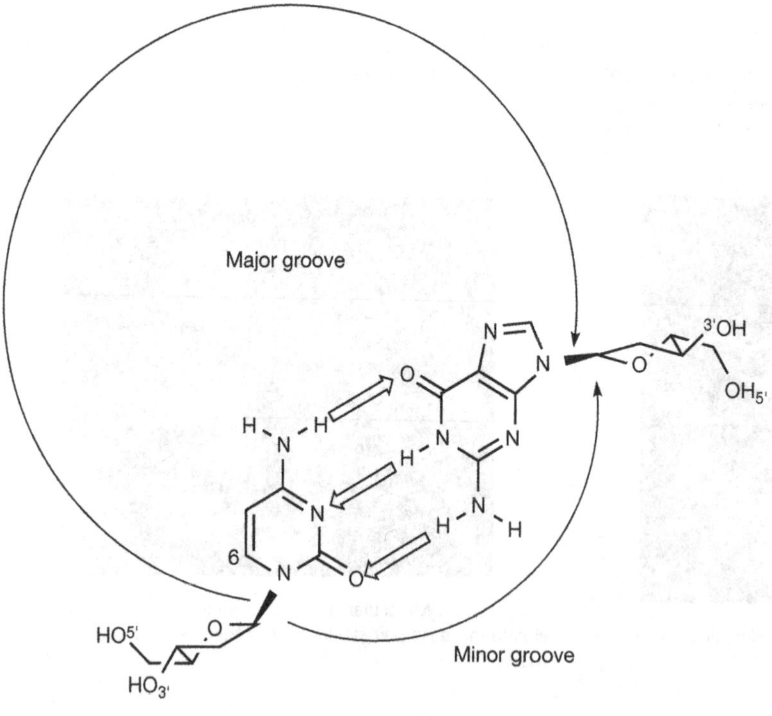

Figure 7.13 Schematic representation of a dc:dG base pair from above the helix illustrating that off-centre points of attachment between the backbones and the bases produce different-sized grooves.

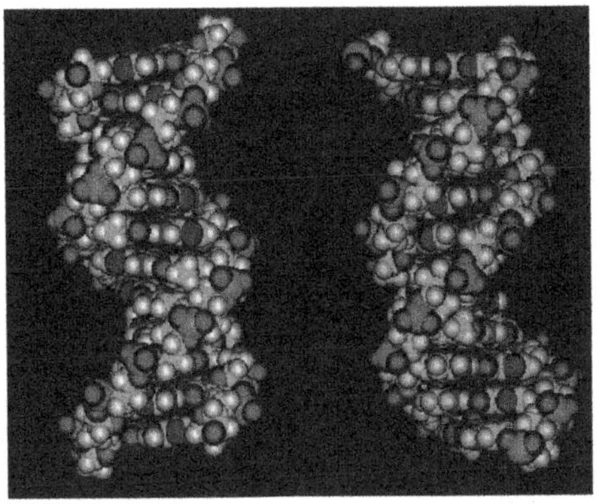

Figure 7.14 CPK models of the same DNA segments viewed from two 180° extremes to illustrate the two grooves ploughed around the helix.

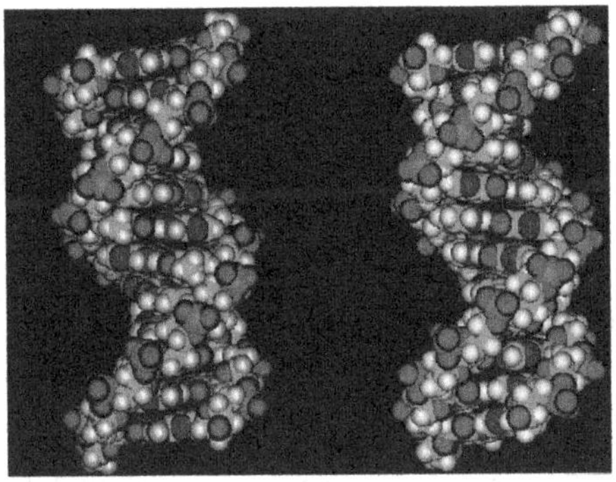

Figure 7.15 CPK models of two different DNA sequences illustrating the individual functional groove patterns expressed in the groove floors according to base pair sequence (blue, nitrogen; red, oxygen; white, hydrogen).

that the genetic code can be accessed, because the functional groups exposed on the groove floor are totally dependent upon the base sequence/code (Fig. 7.15). Both grooves also have water molecules associated with them, hydrogen bonded to the base pairs and sugar–phosphate backbone, which form spines of hydration along the groove floors.

HELICAL REPEAT/PITCH

The dimensions and parameters described above for double-helix DNA are associated with one particular polymorph or conformation of DNA known as B-DNA. In this form, one turn, or repeat of the helix contains ten base pairs, and the length of that turn is 34 Å (Fig. 7.16). To define a helical repeat, we can use the spiral staircase analogy again: if you stand on the bottom stair (base pair) and climb upwards until you reach the stair that is directly above the starting position, you have moved through one helical repeat, having climbed ten base pairs. B-DNA is the most common form of DNA, the structure of which was elucidated by Watson and Crick, and is generally associated with the physiological conditions of the cell. It must be stressed, however, that during cellular processing, DNA is a dynamic structure, and can morph between different structural motifs, depending upon the environment to which it is being subjected. Additionally, the dimensions and parameters so far discussed are considered as average values, because structural variations in the helical parameters are sequence dependent. New polymorphs of DNA are continually being discovered, and it is not in the remit of this chapter to discuss all of these forms. However, to illustrate the flexibility of the structure, a brief description of A-DNA is appropriate.

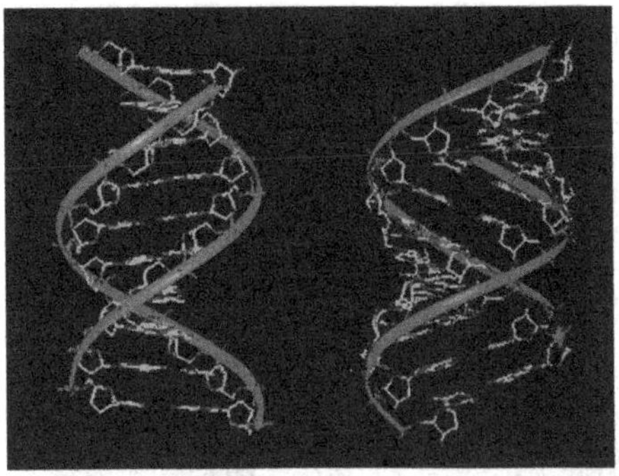

Figure 7.16 One helical turn of B-DNA contains 10 base pairs (left), whilst the equivalent for A-DNA incorporates 11 base pairs.

A-DNA

Low levels of hydration and higher salt concentrations will convert B-DNA to its A form by increasing the screening of the repulsive forces between the anionic oxygens in the phosphate backbone. Consequently, the deoxyribose sugars tend to adopt a $C^{3'}$-*endo* pucker which reduces the interatomic distance between the phosphorus atoms of the phosphate groups in the backbone to 5.9 Å, thus compressing the structure compared with B-DNA. Drawing the phosphate groups closer together along the backbone forces the base pairs into closer proximity from 3.4 Å to 2.6 Å, which increases their ring stacking net repulsive forces. Whilst the helical twist angle remains around 36°, a parameter, known as base pair tilt, becomes predominant within the structure. In order to reduce the repulsion between the base pairs, they become tilted through 20° with respect to each other's planarity: in other words, the stairs in the spiral staircase are no longer even, but are tilted as you climb them (Fig. 7.17). The overall effect on the structure is to compress the helix, giving it a smaller helical pitch of 2.8 Å in comparison with B-DNA, with eleven base pairs in each turn (Fig. 7.16). Within A-DNA, the groove sizes are different from those of B-DNA: the major groove is deeper while the minor groove is more shallow.

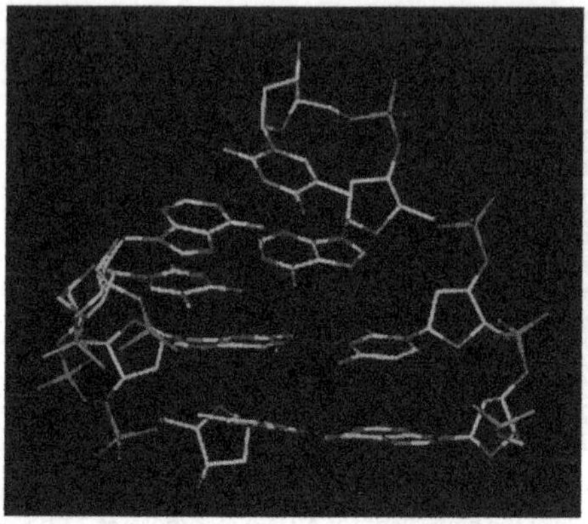

Figure 7.17 Model of a 5′-d(ATGT)-3′ section of A-DNA (with complementary strand) illustrating base pair tilt.

RNA

Another class of nucleic acid which is important in gene expression is RNA. Chemically, RNA and DNA are very closely related, but with two significant differences, one of which can be deduced from the expansion of the abbreviated name of RNA: ribonucleic acid. As the name suggests, RNA contains a different sugar within its subunits, namely ribose as opposed to deoxyribose. The 2′ position is no longer 'deoxy', but has a hydroxyl group oriented in the same way as the 3′ hydroxyl, below the plane of the sugar ring. Consequently, all subunits found in RNA drop the 'deoxy' prefix, and are referred to as nucleosides/nucleotides, or alternatively as ribonucleosides/ribonucleotides. The other essential chemical difference with DNA is the replacement of the thymine base within the structure by the equivalent pyrimidine base, uracil. Uracil has the same properties as thymine, forming two hydrogen bonds in a complementary base pair with adenine, but does not have a methyl group in the 5 position of the pyrimidine ring (Fig. 7.18).

> **Q** Self Test 7.4
>
> Draw the structure of the uridine:adenosine base pair.

Whilst the chemical distinctions between the nucleic acids may be small, their structural and functional differences are more significant. Whilst DNA may be responsible for storing the genetic code, in order to turn the genetic information into a protein two steps are required: transcription and translation. During transcription the template of the DNA is used to produce messenger RNA (mRNA) and the mRNA template is used to assemble a protein using transfer RNA (tRNA) which literally fetches the amino acids coded for by the mRNA. These are then used to assemble the peptide chain (see Ch. 6). Table 7.1 shows the genetic code triplets in RNA corresponding to the different amino acids used to assemble peptides.

Table 7.1 shows 61 codons used to code for 20 amino acids. As can be seen, some amino acids have several different codes. In addition to the codons shown in the table there are three more codes from the permuations of four bases: UAA, UGA and UAG. These codons are stop signals indicating where the ribosome should stop translating the RNA since the C-terminus of the protein has been reached. Methionine is one of two amino acids which have only one codon. In addition, it shares this codon with a start signal indicating where the N-terminus of a protein is; thus all proteins in eucaryotes (organisms with complex cell structures) have methionine at their N-terminus. The methionine is usually removed post-translationally.

RNA generally does not form a double-stranded structure with a complementary strand of RNA, although its polymeric nature does allow for complementary base pairing within its single-stranded structure, i.e. it can fold back on itself. Messenger RNA (mRNA) can form double-stranded helices with the region of DNA being transcribed, where the two strands of the DNA have become separated for transcription, and the dimensions of the DNA–RNA helix in these regions are reminiscent of A-DNA. The presence of the 2′-hydroxyl group of the ribose in RNA hinders the formation of a B-type helix. Once released from the DNA, mRNA is a particularly flexible polymer, but can form transient single-stranded helices and complementary hairpins and loops in particular regions (Fig. 7.19), in order to aid recognition with the various biological macromolecules involved in the translation of the code into the amino acid sequence of the new protein.

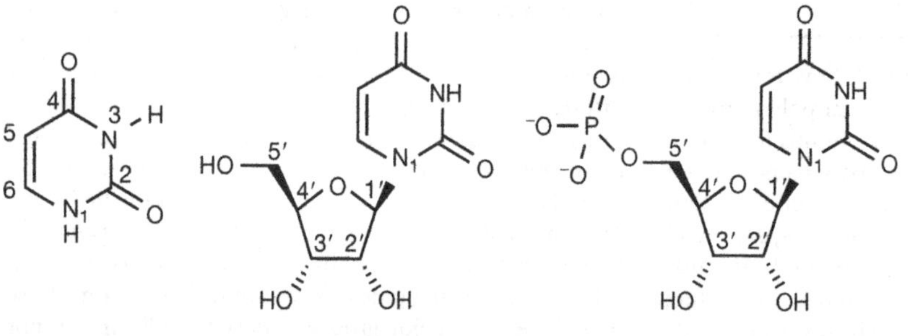

Uracil Uridine Uridine-5'-monophosphate

Figure 7.18 The pyrimidine base, uracil, and its associated nucleoside and nucleotide.

Table 7.1 Three base codons used to code for the 20 amino acids found in proteins

Amino acid	Codes
Glycine	GGU, GGC, GGA, GGG
Alanine	GCU, GCC, GCA, GCG
Serine	UCU, UCC, UCA, UCG, AGU, AGC
Proline	CCU, CCC, CCA, CCG
Valine	GUU, GUC, GUA, GUG
Threonine	ACU, ACC, ACA, ACG
Cysteine	UGU, UGC
Leucine	CUU, CUC, CUA, CUG, UUA, UUG
Isoleucine	AUU, AUC, AUA
Aspargine	AAU, AAC
Aspartic acid	GAU, GAC
Glutamine	CAA, CAG
Lysine	AAA, AAG
Glutamic acid	GAA, GAG
Methionine	AUG
Histidine	CAU, CAC
Phenylalanine	UUU, UUC
Tyrosine	UAU, UAC
Arginine	GCU, CGC, CGA, CGG, AGA, AGG
Tryptophan	UGG

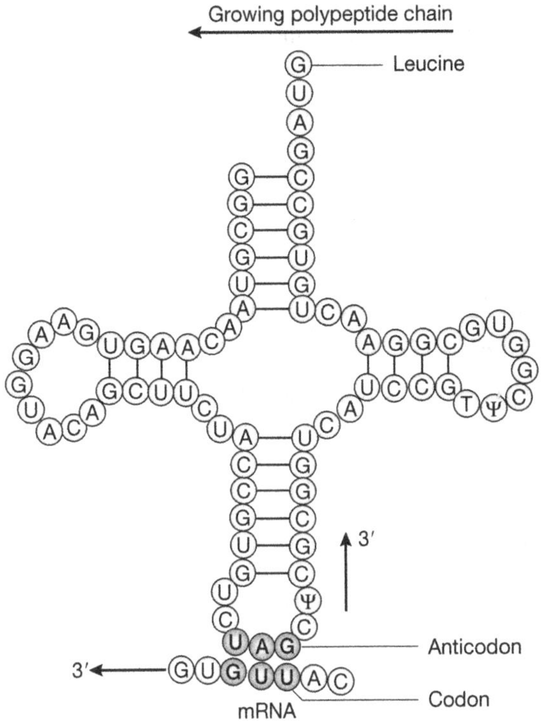

Figure 7.19 tRNA, showing the characteristic cloverleaf structure formed through base pairing within complementary regions within the one strand. N.B. uridine can pair with guanidine as well as adenine in tRNA.

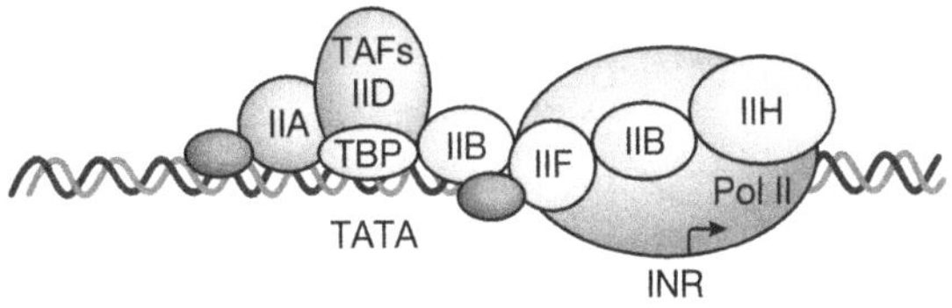

Figure 7.20 Example of a protein–DNA complex which associates in order to initiate transcription by RNA polymerase.

tRNA has a characteristic three-dimensional 'cloverleaf' motif associated (Fig. 7.19). Such structures are held in place by base pairing (C with G and U with A) formed by hydrogen bonding between regions of the polymer that have complementary sequences when folded. There are certain nucleotide sequences which are highly conserved between different tRNAs and form the characteristic 'double-stranded' regions which stabilise the three-dimensional structures of the tRNA molecules. Figure 7.20 illustrates the role of tRNA in translating the mRNA originally transcribed from the DNA genetic template. The tRNA has an anticodon which recognises the codon in mRNA and then adds the corresponding amino acid to the growing polypeptide chain. The recognition process by the anticodon during translation is more flexible than the recognition during transcription, and this means that it is not necessary to have 61 different tRNA molecules to recognise the 61 codons for 20 amino acids. In the example shown, the anticodon shown will also recognise UUA in the mRNA which codes for leucine. The bases in tRNA may be modified post-translationally, e.g. T= thymidine and ψ = pseudouridine.

NUCLEIC ACID PROCESSING

The biochemical mechanisms for converting DNA into RNA into protein, and the processes of DNA replication, are covered in more detail in undergraduate biochemistry textbooks, and do not require detailed examination here. We make the assumption that the reader is aware of the role of enzymes such as DNA polymerase and RNA polymerase in the overall schemes of these processes. There are, however, specific chemical mechanisms performed by certain enzymes in DNA replication, repair, transcription and translation, which are fundamental to the chemical modes of action of specific classes of drugs, which necessitate a closer inspection. Such mechanisms will now be discussed within the context of these processes, without a detailed examination of the overall biochemical processes themselves.

Nucleic acid processing enzyme targets for drug action

Nucleic acid polymerase enzymes

When DNA is replicated during cell division, or complementary mRNA is transcribed from a DNA sequence for protein synthesis, or viral RNA or DNA is replicated in order to promote cellular invasion and viral regeneration, a new nucleic acid is synthesised. A polymerase enzyme such as DNA polymerase, RNA polymerase, or RNA directed DNA polymerase (viral reverse transcriptase) performs the actual elongation process, all are basically involving the same chemical mechanism. In order to synthesise a new nucleic acid polymer, a complementary DNA template within the genome has to be exposed on which the new polymer is to be based. This template may be a gene that is to be expressed, a region of a chromosome to be replicated, or viral or bacterial RNA or DNA. The processes which initiate the process of template preparation are extremely complex, but generally involve the association of proteins such as recognition factors which bind to specific DNA sequences, e.g. a promoter sequence upstream from the sequence to be transcribed. These sequences are recognised within the major groove of the DNA and the complex formed acts as a signal for the polymerase to bind to the sequence to be transcribed (Fig. 7.20) and begin either transcription (RNA production) or DNA replication (as part of the cell division process). Polymerisation is a unidirectional procedure, meaning that the new nucleic acid can only be synthesised in one direction, and that is 5′ to 3′.

The polymerase enzymes require two substrates for chain elongation: the template and the new nucleotides (RNA) or deoxynucleotides (DNA) from which they synthesise the new polymer in a complementary and antiparallel manner. For example, if the template sequence were as follows:

3′-ATGGTTCCGACTACTCG-5′

then a new DNA sequence would be synthesised as follows:

3′-AGCTGTTCCGACTACTCG-5′

5′-TCGA →

or 5′-UCGA → for mRNA

The enzyme catalyses nucleophilic attack by the terminal free 3′ hydroxyl of the growing strand at the electrophilic phosphorus of the triphosphate group directly bonded to the 5′ hydroxyl (Fig. 7.21). The leaving group in the reaction is a diphosphate group, because the substrates the enzymes use for chain elongation are the 5′-triphosphate nucleotides. The triphosphate group is very reactive if Mg^{2+} which is used to stabilise it is removed and this is often a component

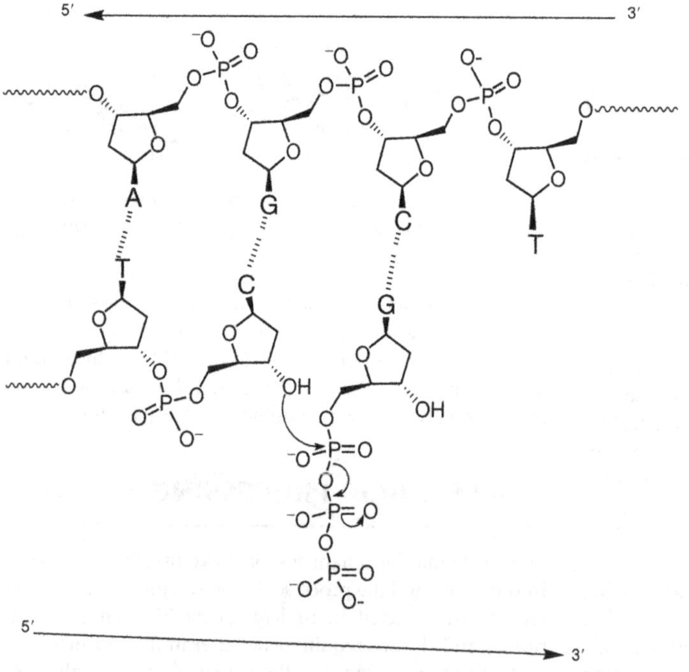

Figure 7.21 Mechanism of action of DNA polymerase in chain elongation, an enzyme which catalyses nucleophilic attack by the free 3′ hydroxyl of the new chain on the first phosphate group of the next deoxynucleotide substrate to be added, in this case, deoxyguanosine 5′-triphosphate.

in the mechanism of phosphorylating enzymes (see Ch. 26). The active sites of these polymerase enzymes can only bind 5′-triphosphate (deoxy) nucleotides and the 3′-terminal hydroxyl group of the growing chain and hence will only synthesise the new polymer in a 5′→3′ direction.

DNA topoisomerase enzymes

DNA topoisomerases are essential enzymes that play a role in virtually every cellular DNA process; they solve the topological problems in DNA that are generated by nuclear processes such as DNA replication, transcription, recombination, repair, chromosome segregation and chromatin assembly by introducing transient breaks in the sugar–phosphate backbone of the helix. Strand cleavage by all topoisomerase enzymes involves nucleophilic attack by a catalytic tyrosine residue in the active site of the enzyme on a phosphodiester bond in the helix backbone, resulting in a covalent linkage between the enzyme and one end of the broken strand. The essential difference between the two main types of topoisomerase is that topoisomerase I breaks one strand of duplex DNA, whilst topoisomerase II breaks both strands of the backbone to generate a gate through which another region of DNA can be passed. The latter enzyme requires the energy cofactor ATP to perform its function, whilst the former does not. During transcription and replication, DNA topoisomerase I acts to reduce the torsional stress which arises within the DNA helix during these processes. DNA topoisomerase II, on the other hand, by virtue of its double-stranded DNA passage reaction, is able to regulate DNA over- and underwinding, and can resolve knots and tangles in the genetic material.

THE ORIGINS OF TORSIONAL STRAIN IN DNA

In the preceding sections that describe the structure of DNA, the associated figures show short sections of DNA. DNA within cells is, in fact, millions of base pairs long and is bound up within chromosomes to a variety of storage proteins such as histones. Such proteins are rich in positively charged lysine and arginine amino acid residues which, by electrostatic interactions with the negatively charged backbones of the DNA, fold it into an ordered compact form known as chromatin. In human somatic cells, a single DNA duplex of about 4 cm in length is found in each of the 46 chromosomes. During replication and transcription, only short sequences of DNA are exposed for the processing enzymes to act upon, so essentially, the ends of the DNA of the exposed section are fixed. Replication and transcription require strand separation in order to expose the template for the polymerases to work with. One way of aiding strand separation is to increase the strain within the helix so that the strands will overcome the hydrogen-bond attractive forces between the complementary base pairs, and naturally move apart. Such strain must be significantly greater than can be relieved by rotation around the flexible P–O bonds in the sugar–phosphate backbone. Topoisomerase II, by breaking both strands in the exposed regions, generates a gate, and passes another section of the exposed DNA through it. The more times the DNA is passed through the gate, the more 'wound up' the exposed DNA becomes because the tension cannot be relieved at the fixed ends. The resultant effect of this increase in strain into the helix forces it to adopt a new tertiary structure, known as supercoiled DNA, which is a higher-energy structure than relaxed, double-helical DNA. The hydrolysis of ATP by the topoisomerase II enzyme provides the energy input for this process. Because supercoiled DNA is a high-energy structure, the strands will separate more easily for the polymerase enzymes to replicate or transcribe the exposed DNA. Topoisomerase II performs other DNA processing functions, but the above description serves to illustrate its essential role in transcription and replication.

Supercoiling by topoisomerase II and the action of the various replication and transcription proteins and enzymes on the exposed DNA can result in strand knotting which will hinder process progression. Topoisomerase I, by breaking one of the sugar–phosphate backbones in the knotted region, can relieve the excess strain by allowing the second strand to unravel, driven by its own high, inherent energy. The conversion of the superhelical DNA back to its relaxed form after processing has taken place is also catalysed by topoisomerase I by the same mechanism. DNA replication and transcription is therefore controlled, in part, by a balance of the actions of topoisomerases I and II. Interference with these enzyme mechanisms would have implications for nucleic acid processing and this is the basis for the action of a number of drugs including the anticancer drugs camptothecin and etoposide (Ch. 21) and the isoquinolone antibiotics (Ch. 22).

The mechanism of action of both the topoisomerase enzymes involves a tyrosine residue in the active site of the enzyme which, by nucleophilic attack, becomes covalently linked to the sugar–phosphate backbone via a phosphotyrosyl bond, releasing the sugar hydroxyl to generate a nick. Topoisomerase II attacks both strands, from opposite sides with two tyrosine residues, to generate two 5′-phosphotyrosyl links with each strand, and two free 3′ ends in the nicked strands. After another region of the DNA has been passed through the gate, the strands are resealed by the reverse action of nucleophilic attack by the free 3′ hydroxyls on the phosphotyrosyl groups to release the enzyme from the complex (Fig. 7.22). Topoisomerase I produces a single-stranded break by the action of one tyrosine residue, but generates a single 3′-phosphotyrosyl link between the enzyme and the DNA, and produces a free 5′ end in the cleaved strand. After release of torsional strain by passing the intact single strand through the gap, resealing follows by reversing the nucleophilic attack (Fig. 7.23). For the topoisomerase enzymes to perform their function, they need to bind double-stranded DNA around the phosphate backbone to perform the strand-cleavage reactions. Figure 7.24 shows schematically how topoisomerase I approaches and binds to a segment of DNA.

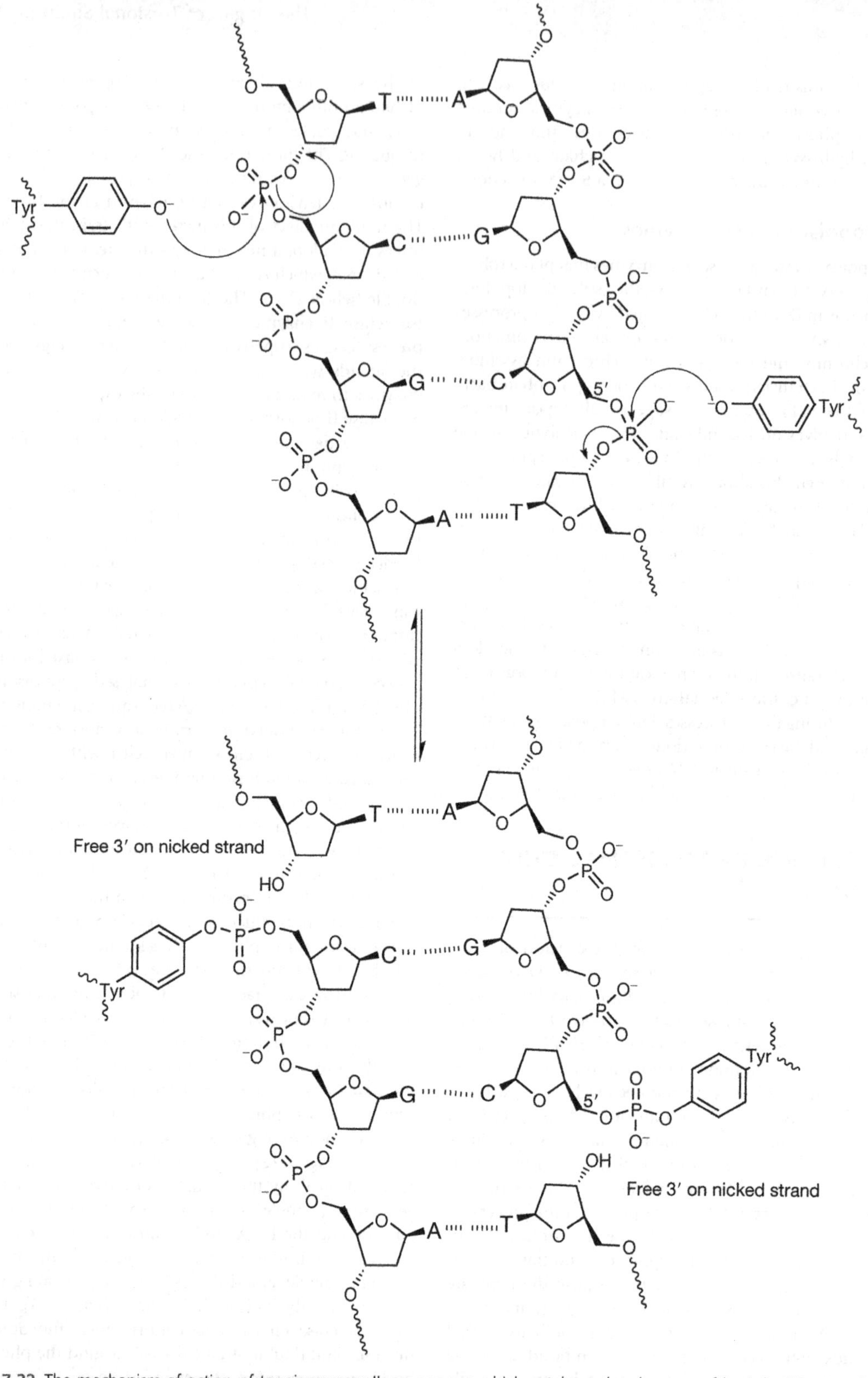

Figure 7.22 The mechanism of action of topoisomerase II, an enzyme which catalyses the cleavage of both backbones of DNA four bases apart to generate a staggered gate within the helix for double strand passage. The DNA strands are covalently linked via a 5′-phosphotyrosyl to the enzyme, generating two free 3′-termini on the scissile strands.

Figure 7.23 The mechanism of action of topoisomerase I. Cleavage of the phosphate backbone occurs when one DNA strand is covalently linked via a 3′-phosphotyrosyl to the enzyme, generating a free 5′-termini on the scissile strand.

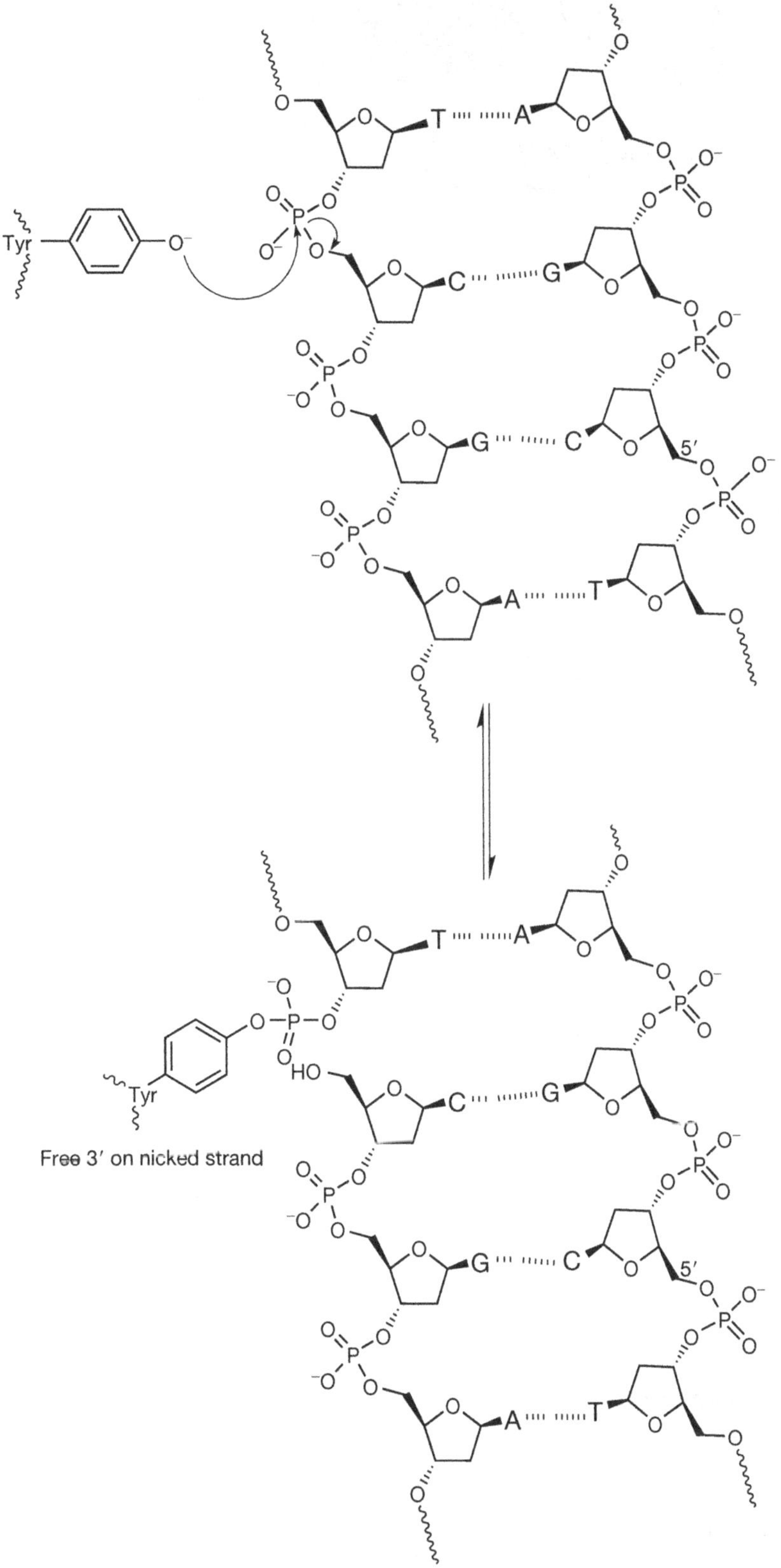

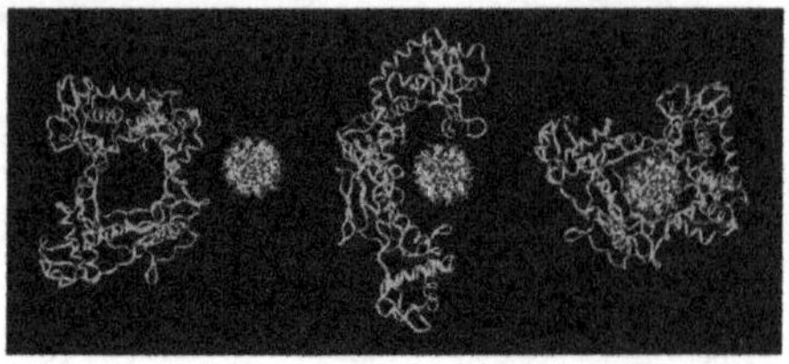

Figure 7.24 Molecular models illustrating how topoisomerase I, which contains a central pore of the same dimensions as the DNA helix, unfolds in order to bind prior to strand cleavage.

A Self Test 7.1

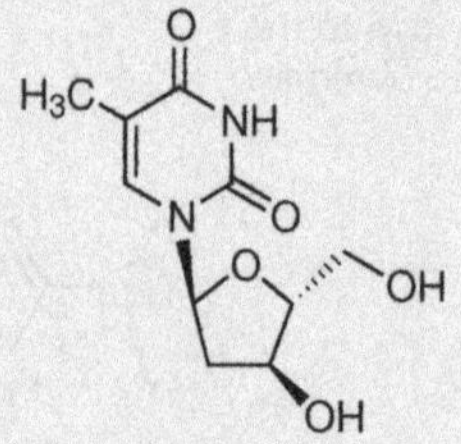

α-Glycoside of deoxythymidine

A Self Test 7.2

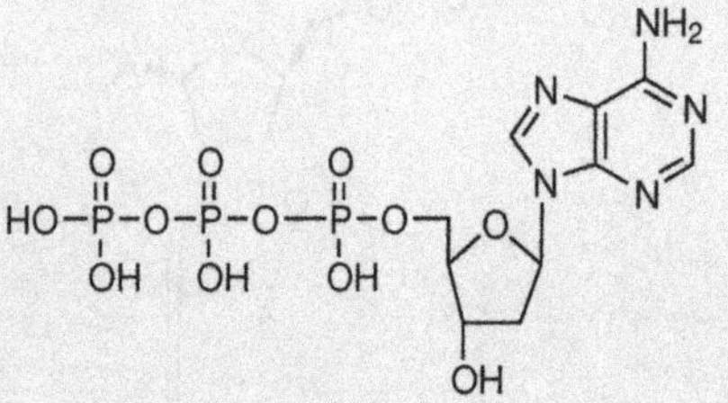

ATP

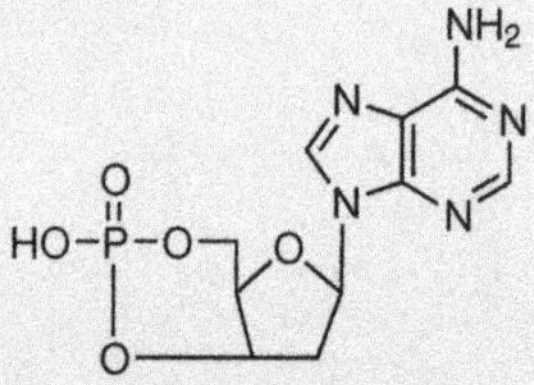

Cyclic AMP

A Self Test 7.3

The AT strands will separate at a lower temperature than the GC strands because they are only held together by two hydrogen bonds per base pair compared with three hydrogen bonds per base pair for the GC strands.

A Self Test 7.4

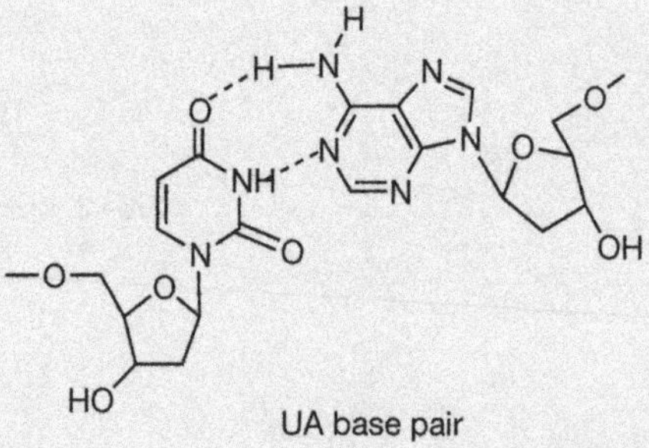

UA base pair

REFERENCE

1. Jang YH, Goddard WA, Noyes KT, et al. p*Ka* values of guanine in water: Density functional theory calculations combined with Poisson-Boltzmann continuum-solvation model. *J Phys Chem B*. 2003;107:344–357.

Chapter | 8 |

Drug absorption, distribution, metabolism and excretion

Simon P Mackay, Clive G Wilson

CHAPTER CONTENTS

INTRODUCTION

For pharmaceutical chemists to understand the principles of drug administration, distribution, metabolism, excretion (ADME) and therapeutic action, they must have a complete understanding of the medicinal chemistry of those drugs. In other words, the chemistry and physical properties of molecules fundamentally affect everything they do to the body (pharmacodynamics), and what the body does to them (pharmacokinetics). Indeed, how a drug is formulated to get it into the body in the first place, for example as a tablet, injection or suppository, depends on its inherent molecular properties.

Consider the drug dose–response profile shown in Figure 8.1.

The pharmacokinetic response of the body to the drug delineated in Figure 8.1 is due significantly to the medicinal chemistry of the drug in question. If one changes its medicinal chemistry, the dose–response curve will change.

The dose–response of a drug is also determined by the physiological responses of the body to its introduction, which are summarised in Figure 8.2, and the physiological responses are determined by the medicinal chemistry of the drug.

The main medicinal chemistry properties of drugs that influence pharmacokinetics are:

- partition coefficient
- dissociation constant (ionisation state)
- solubility
- chemical stability.

If we consider Figure 8.1, and the physiological responses shown in Figure 8.2, how do we assess the relevance of these parameters to pharmaceutical considerations?

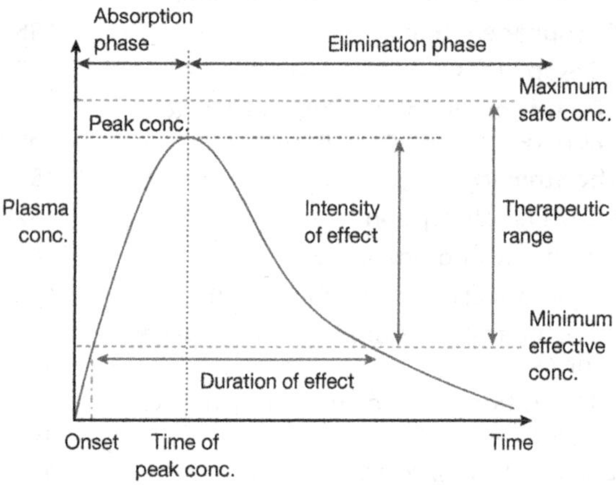

Figure 8.1 Drug dose response profile for a hypothetical drug, showing the absorption and elimination phases following administration.

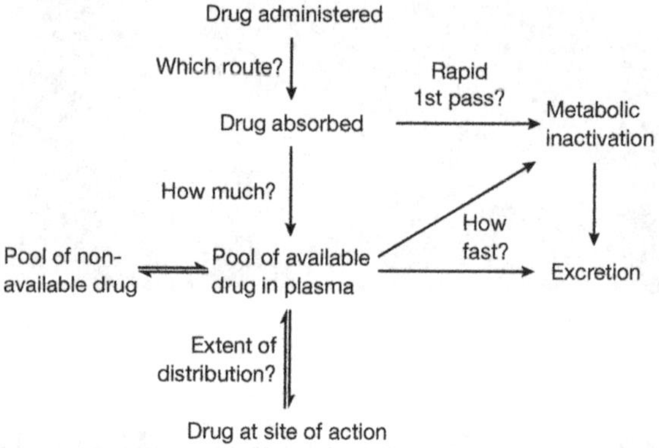

Figure 8.2 The route of a drug into the body.

- Drug administration: How is the drug to be formulated? If as an injection, is it soluble in aqueous solution? If as a tablet, will it dissolve when released in the gut? If as a cream or ointment, is it soluble in the basis?
- Drug absorption: Can the drug pass through the barrier membranes in the gastrointestinal tract? Can it pass through the skin barriers? These barriers are made up in large part by lipids, so the drug must be sufficiently fat-soluble to diffuse through them.
- Drug metabolism: Metabolism increases the water solubility of drugs by enzymatically introducing polar functional groups so that they can be excreted: what is the chemistry of the drug? How fast is it inactivated? Is it converted into more active or even toxic components?
- Drug excretion: The kidney excretes water-soluble metabolites. If the drug is very water soluble, it will be excreted more rapidly.
- Drug action: The shape of the drug, its chemistry and its compatibility with the target receptor/enzyme determines the extent of the response.

In addition to the above considerations, there is the nature of the ailment or disease being treated. The pharmacokinetic processes also need to be accounted for and can even be taken advantage of in order to optimise medical treatment.

Despite the oral route being the preferred means of drug administration, problems arise because most drugs are discovered by testing on animals using routes of administration such as peritoneal, subcutaneous or intramuscular injection. This does not guarantee that the drugs are suitable for oral administration. A drug developed for one specific therapeutic application may not be ideal for another. For example, a long-acting hypnotic would be useless as an intravenous anaesthetic since the patient could remain anaesthetised for some considerable time after the operation has ended. Yet a simple molecular manipulation may convert the hypnotic into a short-acting agent suitable for inducing anaesthesia. Or a drug may act on the whole body and produce side effects on the central nervous system (CNS) if the dose is increased. However, a polar analogue which does not cross the blood–brain barrier may be more appropriate in a different disease involving only the peripheral nervous system.

THE CHEMICAL DEVELOPMENT OF PHARMACEUTICALS

Existing or newly discovered drugs are not always ideal for every therapeutic application for which they need to be administered. In some cases the formulation scientist may overcome deficiencies, but in others it is the medicinal chemist who is successful.

Most drugs are administered by mouth, but to achieve this, considerable work will have been done by both medicinal chemists and formulation scientists. It is essential that the latter be aware of the chemical approaches, for much time and effort will be wasted if extensive formulation studies are carried out on a compound about to be superseded by one with superior properties. The formulation scientist must recognise what scope the chemist has for overcoming problems with a candidate compound that is difficult to formulate or which has, say, poor oral bioavailability.

A variety of case studies are discussed below for the purpose of illustrating these issues. The case studies will examine, for example, how chemists have addressed problems of poor oral bioavailability resulting from the following common causes:

- excessive first-pass metabolism
- inadequate intestinal absorption
- acid instability in the stomach.

The case studies will also consider situations where chemists have addressed the problem of irritancy to the gastrointestinal tract by making appropriate analogues. As a pharmaceutical chemist, because one will be able to relate the medicinal chemistry to the drug's pharmacokinetics and pharmacodynamics, one will not only be able to understand why a patient needs a particular drug, but what the best way to administrate it is, what dose and duration of action to expect (and why this is so), and why it elicits its effect. By understanding the medicinal chemistry of drugs, from a pharmacokinetics perspective, one will be able to explain:

- why diamorphine is more potent than morphine,
- why benzylpenicillin cannot be taken orally,
- why a paracetamol overdose does not kill immediately,
- why some steroids can be administered as creams, and others as injections or orally,
- why crack cocaine has a rapid onset of action,
- why drinking large volumes of Coca-Cola can prevent a drug overdose,
- why spraying a drug under the tongue can rapidly alleviate a cardiovascular angina attack,
- and many more pharmaceutical conundrums!

To help in our understanding, we need to review some of the chemical properties of drugs that are fundamental to ADME processes.

Partitioning

The chemical structure of a drug will determine whether it prefers to dissolve in water or in oil.

- Affinity for water: HYDROPHILIC (water loving) or LIPOPHOBIC (lipid hating).
- Affinity for oil: LIPOPHILIC (lipid loving) or HYDROPHOBIC (water hating).

Why is consideration of whether a drug is lipophilic or hydrophilic important? For drugs to get into the body, and thereafter move around the body, they must pass through biological membranes as shown in Figure 8.3.

In addition to there being a diffusion gradient for the drug to move down, the drug must have lipophilic properties so that it can partition into the membrane in order to move across it. If the drug is very hydrophilic, it will not partition into the membrane, and will not be absorbed into the body. Drugs must therefore partition between aqueous and lipid media – and here is the really confusing part: for a drug to move into the body, it must be fat soluble to get across membranes. For a drug to move around the body, or be administered, it must be soluble in the aqueous environment of the blood or the gut contents. How can a drug be soluble in both? Understanding medicinal chemistry will hopefully enable us to understand how this dichotomy works.

So if we are to know how fat- or water-soluble a drug is, we need a means of measuring the property. How readily does a drug partition between the two media?

$$\frac{\{\text{concentration}\}\text{hexane}}{\{\text{concentration}\}\text{water}} = \text{constant}$$

The constant is usually called P and is known as the partition coefficient. It is usual to divide the concentration in

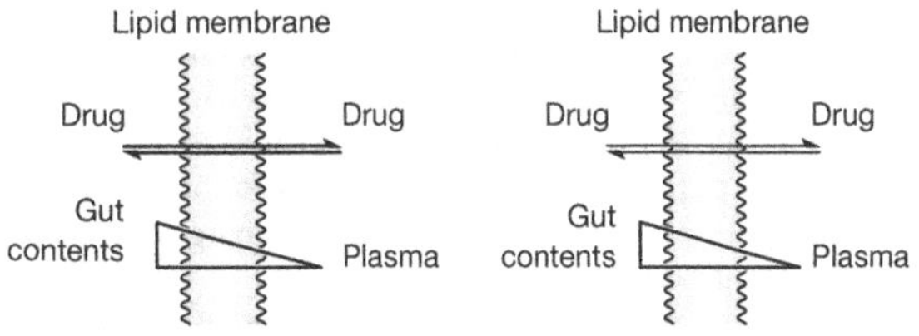

Figure 8.3 Passage of a drug through the biological membranes of the gut and of a cell.

the organic solvent by the concentration in the water, so that if P>1 the solute favours the organic solvent. Since P varies for common compounds over at least 10 orders of magnitude it is normal to use log P, which thus can range from +5 to −5 and occasionally more. The value of log P, which is an equilibrium constant, gives valuable insight into the properties of the molecule and has been used in drug design for many years as a descriptive parameter. Drugs with low values of log P, for example, will not penetrate the blood–brain barrier and so will not produce direct effects on the central nervous system.

Although broad observations on the different partitioning behaviour of compounds such as naphthalene and glucose have been made since the later years of the nineteenth century, it was only in the 1960s that careful quantitative measurements allowed more confident predictions of partition coefficients to be made for compounds for which they were previously unknown. Log P for benzene between octanol and water (the most commonly quoted solvent pair, as described above) is 2.13. The value for toluene (methylbenzene) is 2.79, so the extra -CH2- contributes 0.66. The value of log P for ethylbenzene is 3.45, so the extra -CH2- again contributes 0.66. With some provisos, it is found that the contribution of a specific molecular fragment to log P is more or less constant. This is discussed in more detail in Chapter 9.

The acidity and basicity of functional groups

To complicate drug partitioning, most drugs are weak acids or bases and they can dissociate and ionise (see Chs 3 and 5).

In general:

- The ionised/charged forms of drugs (salts) tend to dissolve in water and they will not cross lipid membranes.
- The un-ionised/uncharged forms (free acids or bases) tend to dissolve in organic solvents and will cross lipid membranes.

This important molecular property means that because an equilibrium exists between the charged and the uncharged form, drugs can have both water-soluble and fat-soluble properties, which means they can be formulated so that they can get into the body.

- For a drug to be administered, it needs to dissolve in an aqueous medium if it is to be given orally or by injection (it needs to be ionised/charged).
- For a drug to be absorbed through a lipid membrane, it needs to partition from the aqueous to the lipid medium (it needs to be un-ionised/uncharged and lipophilic).
- For a drug to be transported around the body, it needs to dissolve in the aqueous plasma (it needs to be ionised/charged) (Fig. 8.4).

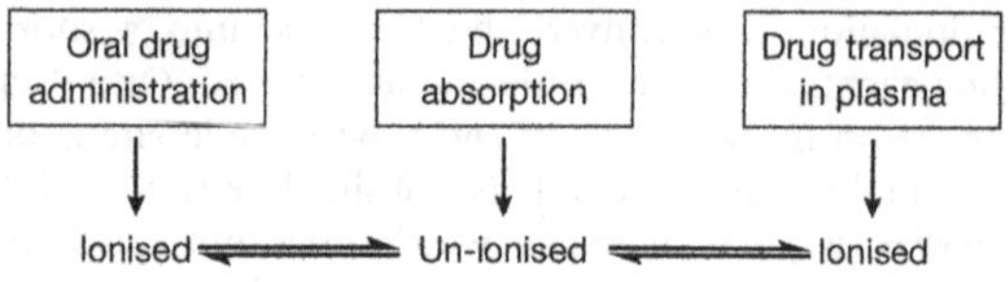

Figure 8.4 Effect of ionisation on drug absorption and transport.

What determines the ratio of the ionised to the un-ionised forms for a given drug?

- the dissociation constant, p*Ka* (which is fixed for a given drug)
- the pH of the solution which the drug is in (which is variable).

Consequently, we cannot change the ratio of the ionised to un-ionised species by changing the p*Ka* of the drug (unless we change its structure, and therefore its activity), but we can formulate at different pHs, and we need to take into account how pH in the body compartments change. For example, the pH in the stomach is 1–2, the small intestine pH varies from 6 to 8, whilst the plasma pH is 7.4.

Consider aspirin, which is a weak acid with a p*Ka* of 3.5. Figure 8.5 shows the variation in the percentage ionisation in different compartments in the body.

This has implications for aspirin's movement around the body: aspirin is undissociated/un-ionised in the stomach, and will therefore be absorbed through the stomach's barrier membranes. It is dissociated/ionised in the small

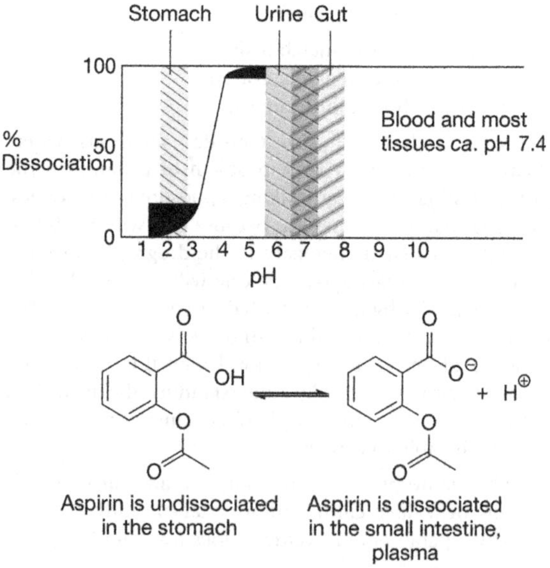

Figure 8.5 Variation in the percentage ionisation of aspirin in the body.

intestine, so cannot be absorbed from here. However, in its ionised state at pH 7.4, it can be transported in solution in the plasma.

Partitioning of acids and bases

We already know that organic compounds tend to partition between immiscible solvents so that the ratio of concentrations in the two solvents is constant (the partition coefficient). We also know that organic acids and bases tend to associate with or dissociate from hydrogen ions according to pH, as described by the Henderson-Hasselbalch (H-H) equation. We can therefore picture a situation in which the two solvents may each contain both ionised and un-ionised material (Fig. 8.6).

In practice, the concentration of ionised material in the organic layer is often very small and can conveniently be neglected. We can therefore draw a simpler diagram (Fig. 8.7).

The equilibrium in the aqueous layer is determined by the p*Ka* of the compound in question, and the pH of the solution, so why is this important for pharmaceutical scientists?

- Only the un-ionised form of the drug can pass through biological membranes (providing the un-ionised form is lipophilic) which is required for drug absorption into the body.
- Usually, only the ionised form of the drug is water-soluble, which is required for drug administration and its distribution in plasma.

The pH of solutions will therefore influence the partitioning and solubility properties of acidic or basic drugs. The pH of the gastrointestinal tract varies considerably, and will therefore affect significantly the equilibrium between the ionised and un-ionised forms of the species in question, which has important implications for drug absorption.

Consider drugs that are acids, for example RCOOH, which has a p*Ka* of 4.0 (Fig. 8.8).

- If the pH shifts the balance towards the un-ionised/undissociated form, the drug will be absorbed.
- If the pH shifts the balance towards the ionised/dissociated form, the drug will not be absorbed.

Assume the pH of the stomach is 2.0 and the pH of the small intestine is 8.0. Where would one expect absorption to take place from?

Now consider a drug that is basic, with a p*Ka* of 7.0 (Fig. 8.9). Where in the gut would you expect absorption to take place from?

Using the above two examples, consider the problem from a drug formulation point of view. We wish to administer orally as an aqueous solution, which means the drug in question needs to be in its ionised form to be soluble. Ideally, we would not want the solution to be too acidic or basic, as this would harm the gut, so would a solution of pH 6–8 produce around 100% ionisation for the acidic drug to enable formulation? Would the same apply for the basic drug?

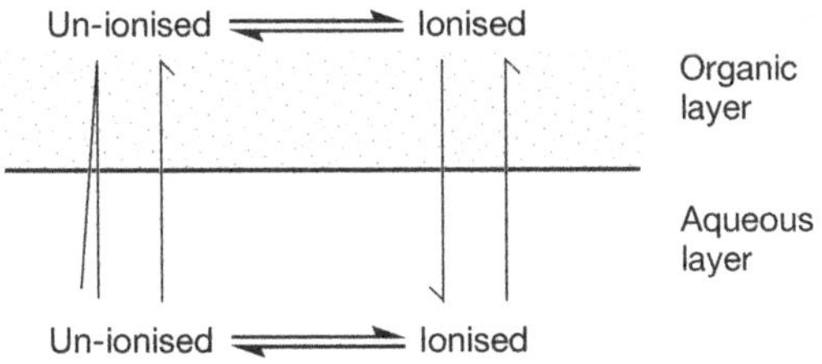

Figure 8.6 Ionised and un-ionised drug in aqueous and organic phases.

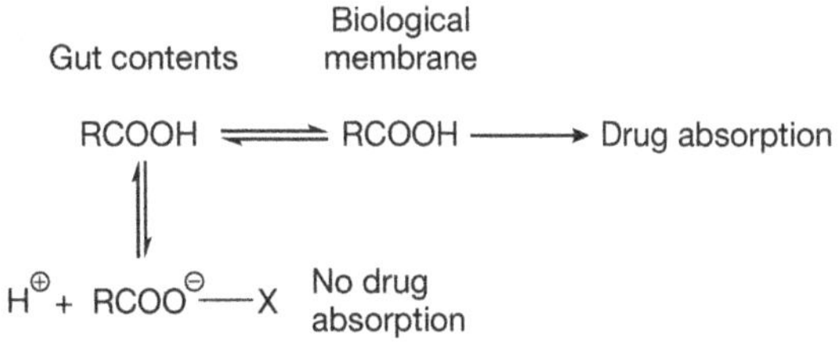

Figure 8.8 The effect of pH on the absorption of an organic acid.

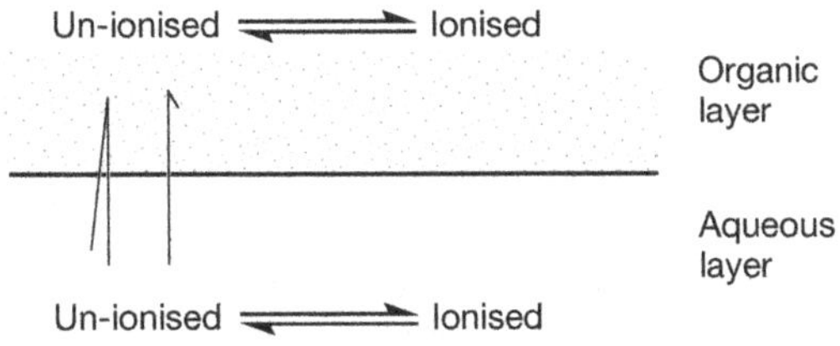

Figure 8.7 Un-ionised drug in an organic layer in equilibrium with un-ionised and ionised drug in an aqueous layer.

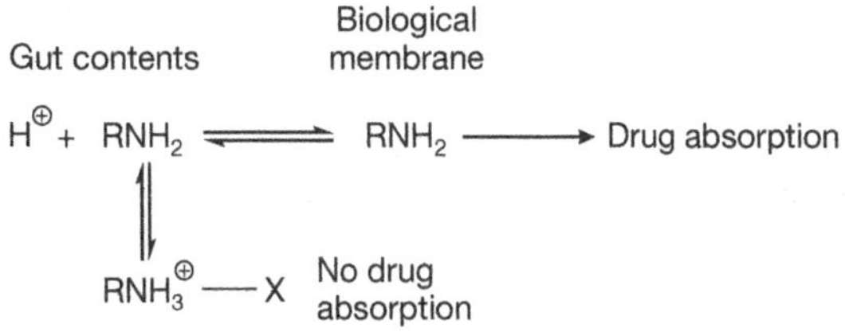

Figure 8.9 The effect of pH on the absorption of an organic base.

The effect of the partition coefficient on drug distribution

Going back to the equilibrium model we have defined for the movement of a drug between an organic and aqueous phase (see Fig. 8.7), there is one further parameter to consider: the partition coefficient. When we were calculating where we would expect our acidic or basic drug to be absorbed from, we were assuming that the un-ionised form of the drug would partition into the lipid membrane. However, this may not be the case: the un-ionised form of a drug may still be hydrophilic owing to properties conveyed upon it by polar functional groups. An un-ionised hydrophilic drug would therefore not partition very readily into the body. We therefore have to account for the partitioning properties of our un-ionised drug when determining whether we expect absorption to occur. Various symbols have been used to describe this relationship, and the most common are D, for Distribution coefficient, or P_{app}, for apparent Partition coefficient. It is possible to derive from the Henderson-Hasselbalch equation expressions for the variation in the partitioning of organic acids and bases into organic solvent with respect to the pH of the solution that they are dissolved in.

From the Henderson-Hasselbalch equation, for an acid substance:

$$P_{app} = \frac{P}{1 + 10^{pH-pKa}}$$

P_{app} is the apparent partition coefficient, which varies with pH, because it is taking account of the distribution of the drug. Remember, P is a constant because it refers to the partition coefficient of only the un-ionised form.

This is the mathematical definition of P_{app} that we can use to predict the behaviour of a compound at all pH values, as long as we know P and p*Ka*.

For acids, at pH values well below their p*Ka* value, for all intents and purposes $P_{app} = P$, since ionisation is suppressed and we are dealing with only the un-ionised form of the species. At pH values above the p*Ka*, the value of P_{app} decreases because the species is ionising and moving into the aqueous layer. This approximate relationship is very simple and allows us to predict the distribution of the drug at all pH values, provided that we know p*Ka* and log P, for any given compound. The same applies to bases as discussed in Chapter 3.

Consider RCOOH, which has a p*Ka* of 4.0, and a partition coefficient of 200. If the pH shifts the balance towards the un-ionised/undissociated form, the drug would be absorbed, providing the P_{app} was favourable. Using the equation above, P_{app} becomes 198 in the stomach, suggesting that absorption will take place, whilst at pH 8.0 in the small intestine, the calculated P_{app} suggests no absorption. This equation allows us to predict that an acidic drug whose un-ionised form has a very low partition coefficient would not be absorbed.

Drug stability

The major stability issues when considering the pharmacokinetic profiles of drugs is chemical hydrolysis in the gastrointestinal tract prior to absorption into the body, and metabolic stability once absorbed. If absorbed from the intestine, transport via the hepatic portal vein directly to the liver will reduce effective drug concentrations rapidly if they possess functional groups prone to metabolism. There are also enzymes in the plasma (non-specific esterases and amidases that hydrolyse esters and amides, respectively) that can alter drug structures. Changes in drug structure prior to absorption via chemical hydrolysis can reduce absorption, and therefore lower therapeutic effect, whilst changes in drug structure via metabolism can change pharmacodynamic activity and enhance excretion, both of which can lower therapeutic effect. However, medicinal chemists can make use of these processes to alter pharmacokinetic profiles to their advantage, and examples of such will be discussed in more detail in later sections.

Drug hydrolysis

By far the most important chemical reaction when considering drug absorption is hydrolysis. Exposure of esters to strongly acidic conditions such as those found in the stomach for prolonged periods of time will result in hydrolysis to the component carboxylic acid and alcohol (see Ch. 5). Amides tend to be more stable to hydrolysis in the gastrointestinal tract and generally require catalysis by metabolic enzymes in order to be hydrolysed. The acid-catalysed hydrolysis in the stomach converts an essentially non-polar, non-ionic system into one which can potentially ionise, given that the p*Ka* of the carboxylic acid produced is generally in the region of 4. As soon as the released acid reaches an environment where the pH is 6.0 or above (e.g. in the intestine), 99% will be converted to the ionised form, which will not pass through the lipid barrier membrane, thus lowering the amount absorbed. Most esters and amides are stable in the acidic environment of the stomach because they are not in contact with the contents for long enough for a significant amount of degradation to take place. There are a few case examples where there is a problem, and this usually applies to esters or amides that are particularly labile, and this is covered in a later section.

Once absorption has taken place from the gastrointestinal tract into the plasma, non-specific plasma esterases tend to be the main source of ester hydrolysis and drug degradation. In terms of the hydrolytic mechanism, the esterase facilitates the protonation of the ester to generate the strongly electrophilic species. If the ester is the pharmacodynamically active species of the drug, then this could be a problem; however, if the released acid (or alcohol) is the active form, then medicinal chemists can make use of this process from a drug delivery and drug-targeting perspective.

DRUG ABSORPTION

Now that we have reminded ourselves of some of the molecular properties that are fundamental to pharmacokinetic processes, let us return to the dose–response curve we initially introduced in Figure 8.1. The shape of the curve is determined by the rate of drug absorption into the body, how extensively it is distributed around the body, and how quickly it is eliminated. These processes can be illustrated using the flowchart shown in Figure 8.2. The movement of drugs around the body that follows the flowchart shown in Figure 8.3 inevitably involves the transport of drugs across biological membranes. Whether it is gastrointestinal mucosa, hepatic cell membranes, muscular tissue or the lining of the lung, drugs must move across them in order to transport around the body. Suffice to say, bulk movement is associated with passive diffusion, and the rate of transfer follows the general principles of Fick's diffusion equation:

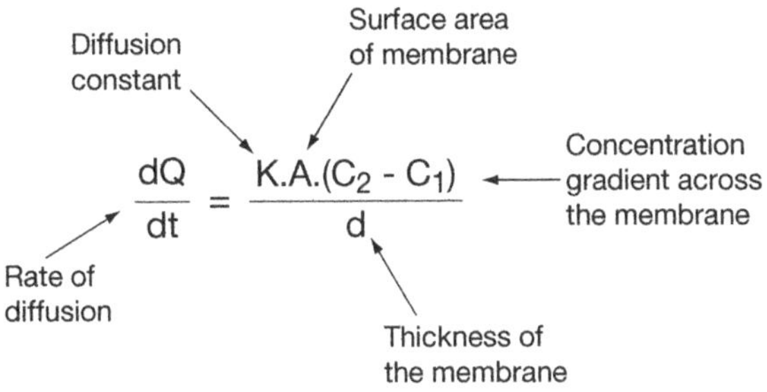

The diffusion constant, K, is a function of:

- aqueous solubility of the drug i.e. hydrophilic character
- lipid solubility of the drug i.e. o/w partition coefficient
- molecular size, i.e. RMM
- molecular shape
- p*Ka* of the drug
- pH of the environment.

Only the more lipid-soluble un-ionised form of the drug traverses biological membranes by passive diffusion. A log P value of about 2 appears to be optimal for gastrointestinal absorption if dissolution phenomena are not rate-limiting.

Oral administration and absorption

Although oral administration is the preferred delivery route for the majority of drugs, the complexity of the gastrointestinal (GI) tract needs to be considered. Figure 8.10 shows the GI tract with the processes that can occur which affect a drug at various stages during transit.

As drug transits the GI tract the pH of its environment changes (Table 8.1).

If a drug is to be absorbed through the mucosal membranes that line the gut, then it must be in its lipophilic, un-ionised form in order to partition out of the aqueous medium. Consequently, acidic drugs tend to be absorbed more rapidly from the stomach, whilst basic drugs must pass through to the small intestine before absorption and the associated onset of action. The partition coefficient of the un-ionised form will also determine how much is absorbed. The absorption phase of the dose–response curve is therefore heavily influenced by the p*Ka* and log P of a drug.

Other factors that need to be taken into account when considering the oral route are discussed below.

Chemical stability

The GI tract is a hostile environment that contains strong acids and enzymes which can cause degradation. Compounds susceptible to hydrolysis, such as esters or lactams, may not survive this environment intact.

Desired onset of action

It takes time for a drug to reach the small intestine where bulk absorption occurs, which is not suitable if a rapid onset is required, such as in cases of acute pain.

Systemic or local effect

Oral absorption is associated with systemic action and associated side effects. Local administration may be considered more appropriate.

Incompatible physicochemical properties

Non-ionic, highly lipophilic drugs are not water soluble, and will not dissolve in the aqueous media of the gut. Drugs with low partition coefficients may not penetrate the mucosal membranes of the GI tract, e.g. gentamycin (Fig. 8.11).

Irritability

Some drugs may prove unacceptably irritating to the gut, and may require an alternative route of administration such as via a suppository or chemical modification to overcome the irritancy.

Food incompatibility

Bioavailability and absorption problems may occur through interactions between the drug and particular foodstuffs that can hinder (or promote) absorption. Enhancing absorption also needs to be considered because if plasma concentrations are higher than expected, then the therapeutic index of the drug may be exceeded with resultant toxic effects. The most commonly cited example of

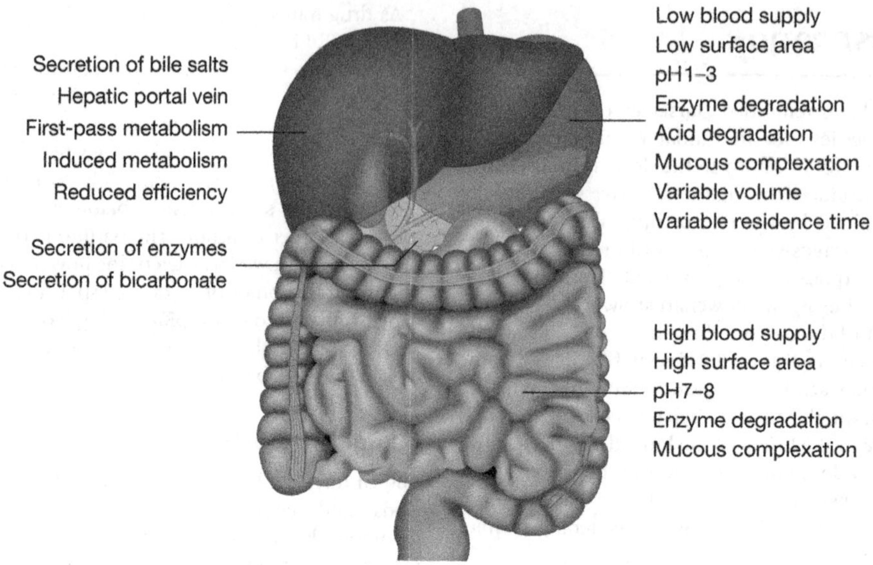

Figure 8.10 Gastrointestinal tract with processes affecting drug absorption efficiency.

Table 8.1 Variation in pH in the GI tract

Compartment	pH
Buccal cavity	6.2–7.2
Stomach	1.0–3.0
Duodenum	4.8–8.2
Jejunum & ileum	7.5–8.0
Colon	7.0–7.5

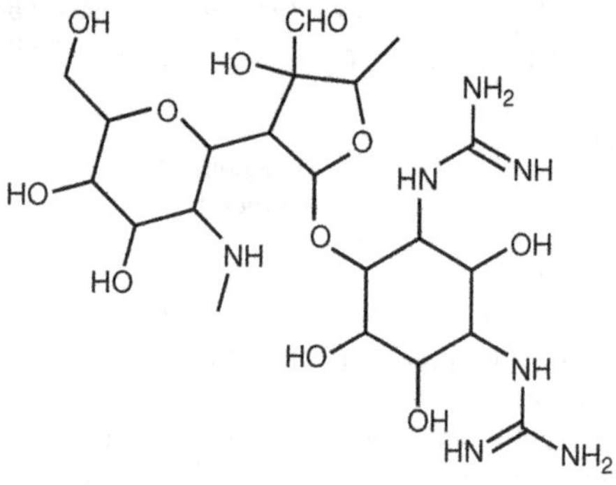

Figure 8.11

drug–food interactions is between the tetracyclines and foodstuffs containing calcium ions such as dairy products. Complexation between the tetracycline and the calcium ion results in the formation of an insoluble complex that cannot be absorbed from the gut (Fig. 8.12). The antibiotic ciprofloxacin demonstrates similar problems.

First-pass effect

Drugs absorbed from the small intestine are transported by the hepatic portal vein to the liver, the key site of metabolism (Fig. 8.13). Drugs that are rapidly metabolised in this 'first pass' are not suitable for oral administration.

If the oral administration route is not appropriate, the other routes of administration are:

- Rectal: Local administration, and an alternative systemic route that avoids degrading pH and enzymes.
- Vaginal: Local administration
- Topical: Local administration and systemic delivery of lipophilic drugs by transdermal patches.
- Buccal: Fast onset of action that avoids first-pass metabolism.

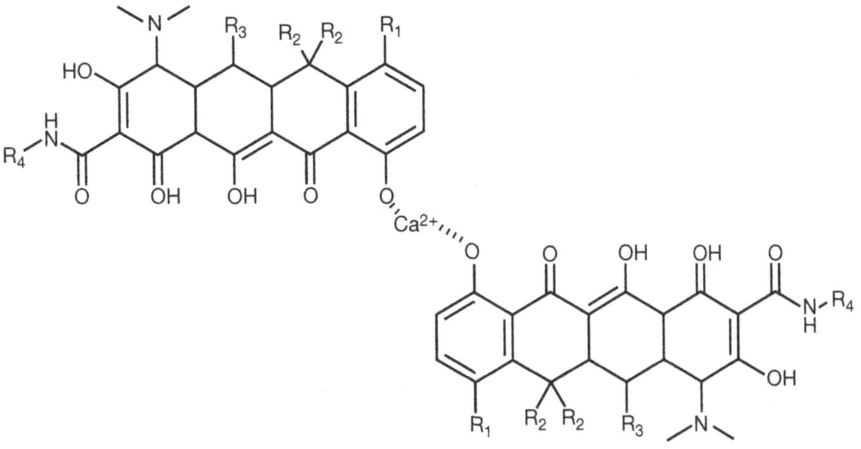

Tetracycline calcium complex

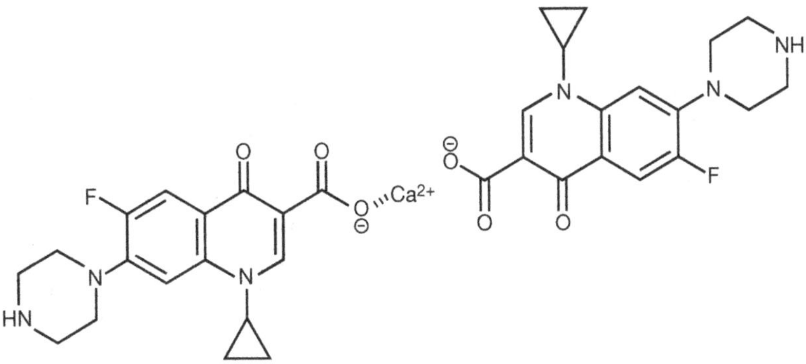

Ciprofloxacin calcium complex

Figure 8.12 Complex formation between tetracycline and ciprofloxacin with calcium ions.

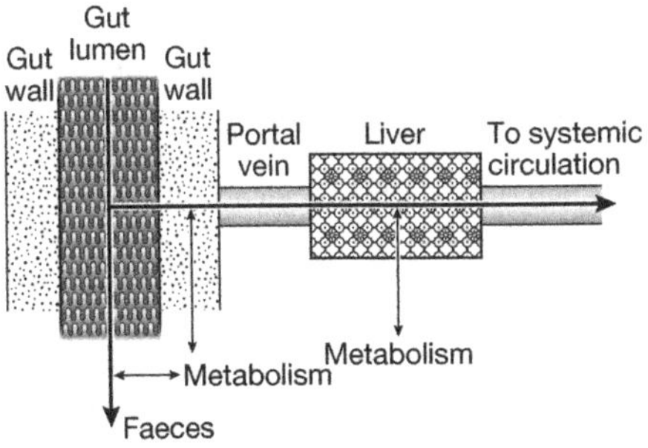

Figure 8.13 The liver and sites of first-pass metabolism of oral drug administration.

- Parenteral injection: i.v. for rapid onset, requires water-soluble forms; i.m for depot injections.
- Respiratory: Local administration by aerosols to the lungs.

Prodrug design and drug latentiation

A common term encountered in the chemical development of pharmaceuticals is prodrug design and drug latentiation. Prodrug design comprises an area of drug research concerned with the optimisation of drug delivery that can circumvent pharmaceutical formulation problems. Optimisation of drug delivery, and consequent improvement in drug efficacy and reduction in toxicity and unwanted effects of drugs, implies an efficient and

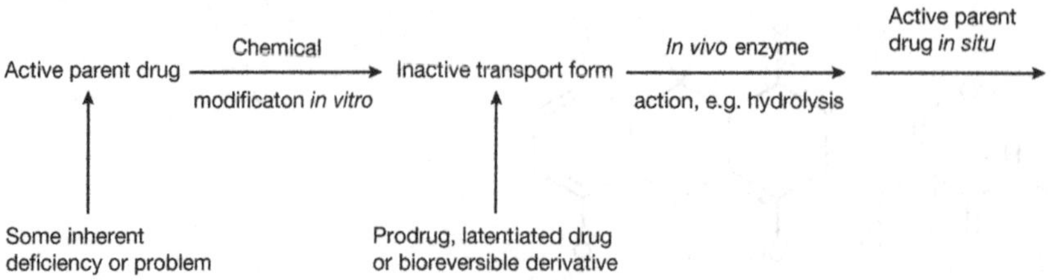

Figure 8.14 Prodrug activity.

selective delivery and transport of the drug from its site of administration to its site of action. The term prodrug was originally introduced to describe compounds which undergo metabolic transformation prior to exhibiting their pharmacological action. The term drug latentiation was introduced to describe the chemical modification of drugs to overcome pharmaceutical problems. It involves the chemical modification of a pharmacologically active parent compound to form a pharmacologically inactive derivative which, upon in vivo enzymatic attack, will liberate the parent compound. The chemical modification is such that a change in physicochemical properties will alter or eliminate undesirable characteristics of the parent drug by modifying its absorption, distribution, metabolism and excretion. The definition of drug latentiation has now been extended to include non-enzymatic regeneration of the parent drug, e.g. by spontaneous hydrolysis. This is summarised in Figure 8.14.

Chemical development can be contrasted with the pharmaceutical formulation and drug delivery which involves the presentation of a pharmacologically active compound with a stable, non-irritant, relatively non-toxic, easily administrable form, which is clinically acceptable and has the desired specific activity by modification of the physical properties of the compound. No chemical modification is involved. However, the two approaches are not independent or mutually exclusive, and should be viewed as complementary methodologies for optimising therapeutic activity.

The rational design of prodrugs can be divided into three basic steps:

1. identification of the drug delivery problem
2. identification of the physicochemical properties required for maximum efficacy or delivery, and
3. selection of an appropriate derivative that has the desired physicochemical properties and which will be cleaved efficiently in the desired biological compartment to liberate the parent drug.

Several criteria have to be considered in the design of a prodrug, including:

1. the functional group(s) in the parent drug molecule which are amenable to chemical derivatisation
2. the mechanism(s) available in the body for bioactivation of the prodrug
3. ease of synthesis and purification of the prodrug, i.e. economic considerations
4. stability of the prodrug per se and its compatibility with other components of a pharmaceutical formulation
5. the rate and extent of regeneration of the parent drug from the prodrug in vivo, i.e. biochemical considerations
6. toxicity of the prodrug and also of its transport group.

The main application of the prodrug approach is to design new drugs principally with the aim of overcoming some problem(s) associated with the parent compound. Examples of such problems include the following:

1. The duration of the action of a drug is too short and prolonged or sustained release is desired. Some advantages of sustained or prolonged release are:
   - A. reduces the number and frequency of dosage administered,
   - B. eliminates 'peak and valley' effects associated with fast release formulations,
   - C. reduces the incidence of peak blood levels rising above toxic blood levels,
   - D. often reduces the total amount of drug needed to achieve a desired effect,
   - E. eliminates the problem of night-time administration of drugs,
   - F. helps to minimise the problem of patient non-compliance by decreasing the number of times needed to remember to take medication,
   - G. often reduces the incidence of gastrointestinal side effects.
2. Incomplete systemic bioavailability due to pre-systemic (first pass) metabolism.
3. Formulation problems – attributable to a bitter taste, unpleasant odour or volatility of the parent compound.
4. Instability of the parent compound.
5. Low aqueous solubility. Some advantages of increasing the water solubility of a drug are:

A. allows rapid attainment of therapeutic blood levels to be attained – especially useful in emergency treatment,
B. permits efficient delivery of the drug, especially for drug-testing,
C. overcomes limited oral bioavailability due to poor aqueous solubility,
D. facilitates parenteral administration of the drug (i.v. or i.m.),
E. allows delivery of a drug when oral therapy is not feasible, e.g. in an unconscious patient,
F. ophthalmic use.

6. Toxicity and adverse reactions of the parent compound – gastric irritation or irritation at the site of injection; diarrhoea; ulceration.
7. Bioavailability problems due to poor/incomplete absorption associated with poor membrane permeability – from gastrointestinal tract, through the blood–brain barrier or through the skin due to high polarity or ionisation.
8. Lack of clinical specificity – need for localisation in order to increase the site-specificity of the drug.
9. Poor doctor or nurse acceptance – due to pragmatic reasons.
10. Poor patient acceptance – due to a variety of reasons including unpleasant odour or taste or to intolerable side effects.

The many examples of prodrugs may fall into several categories. For example, the poor bioavailability of an orally administered drug may be due to many different factors including:

1. lipophilicity too low (7),
2. water solubility too low (5),
3. low acid-stability (4),
4. extensive first-pass metabolism (2).

Prodrug drug conversion may take place (1) before absorption, e.g. in the GI tract, (2) drug absorption, e.g. on passage through the GI mucosa, (3) after absorption, e.g. in the plasma or (4) at the specific site of action in the body. Ideally, prodrug to drug conversion should occur as soon as the goal is reached. For example, prodrugs designed to overcome stability problems in formulating i.v. solutions should preferably be converted to the parent drug rapidly following injection. Conversely, if the objective of the prodrugs is prolongation of duration of action, the rate of conversion should be relatively slow. By far the most common prodrug is based on the ester linkage (see Ch. 5). The popularity of using esters as prodrugs stems primarily from the fact that enzymes which catalyse hydrolysis (esterases) have a ubiquitous distribution, several types being found in the blood, liver, kidneys and other organs and tissues. However, there are some examples of other groups introduced into drugs in order to form a prodrug. Examples of different types of prodrugs are given below and also in Chapter 5 and the chapters covering different therapeutic categories.

ORAL DELIVERY

Solving a problem of low oral bioavailability due to instability

Erythromycins

Erythromycin is a macrolide antibiotic isolated from *Streptomyces erythraeus*. It has a similar spectrum of activity to that of the early penicillins and was therefore often used as a substitute in patients who displayed life-threatening penicillin allergies. Erythromycin is a base, where the aliphatic tertiary amino group has a p*Ka* of 8.8. Despite this, oral preparations are difficult to formulate because the tertiary alcohols at the 6 and 12 positions cause instability in stomach acid. As with many tertiary alcohols in strong acid, the C–OH bond can break to form highly reactive carbonium ions, in this case at either the 6 or 12 positions. An intramolecular cyclisation via the carbonyl oxygen at C-10 with the electrophilic carbonium ions results in formation of the inactive erythralosamine (Fig. 8.15).

Simplifying the structure helps to clarify the mechanism, which is initiated by the loss of water through protonation of the tertiary alcohol as shown in Figure 8.16.

For administration of solid doses of erythromycin, enteric-coated tablets or acid-resistant capsules are used, which can pass through the acidic environment of the stomach and this avoids degradation. For liquid formulations, it is necessary to use salts which are insoluble in the stomach but then dissociate in the small intestine, e.g. erythromycin stearate or erythromycin estolate. The salts are formed by formulating the tertiary amine as the sulphate salt of a long chain lipophilic sulphate such as lauryl sulphate (Fig. 8.17). Such salts, which are only soluble 1 part in 40 000 of water, are formulated as suspensions for oral delivery that pass through the stomach and dissociate in the higher pH of the upper intestine. Erythromycin estolate, in addition to being the sulphate salt, is also in the form of apropanoate ester in order to raise the partition coefficient and aid absorption. Once the ester is released in the higher pH of the small intestine, it is then absorbed and enters the circulation where it is exposed to esterases and free erythromycin is released.

Clarithromycin (Fig. 8.18) was specifically designed to be more stable in acid by converting the alcohol at the 6 position to an ether, thus preventing carbonium ion formation. The enhanced oral bioavailability is reflected in a halving of the typical dose when compared to erythromycin. It also turned out serendipitously to have improved activity against *Haemophilis influenzae*.

In azithromycin, the ring was altered to remove the 9-carbonyl, which in acid conditions is required for

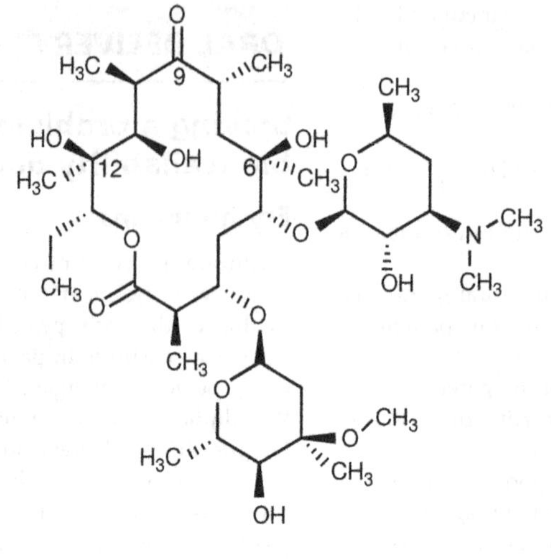

Erythromycin

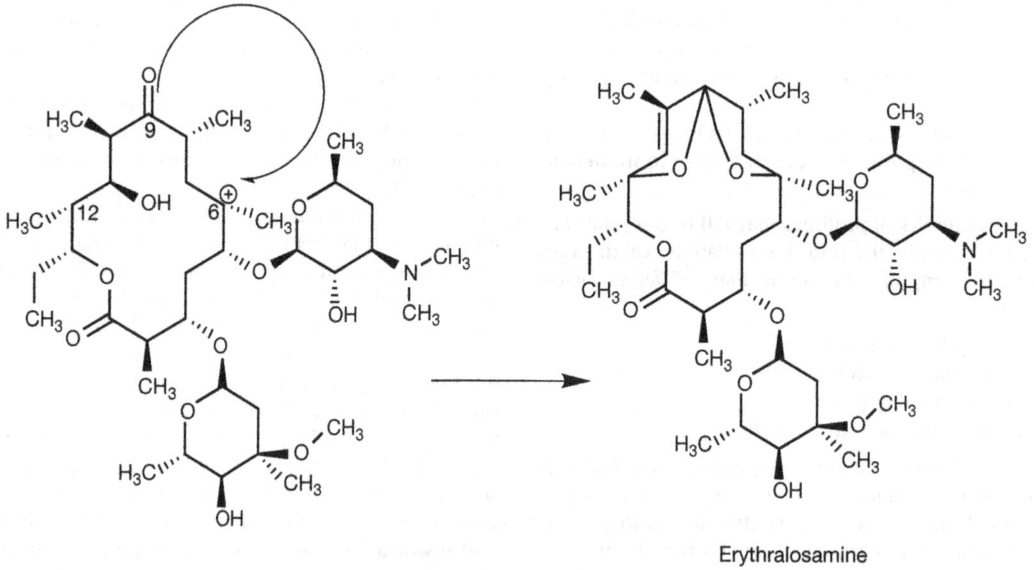

Erythralosamine

Figure 8.15 The mechanism responsible for the instability of erythromycin to stomach acid.

intramolecular cyclisation with the carbonium ions formed at the 6 and 12 positions. Consequently, it has enhanced acid stability. This modification produced improved activity against certain Gram-negative organisms, but somewhat reduced activity against Gram-positive bacteria.

Penicillins

The first penicillins, e.g. benzylpenicillin, were excellent antibiotics but had very poor oral bioavailability due to their instability in gastric acid. The chemical modifications made in order to improve penicillin stability are discussed in Chapter 22.

Low oral bioavailability due to poor absorption

Some drugs are poorly orally bioavailable. A common strategy is to convert such a drug to an ester to increase its lipophilicity. Examples of this approach in relation to penicillins are discussed in Chapter 22. The design features of this approach to improved oral absorption are indicated in Figure 8.19. Simple aliphatic or aromatic esters are insufficiently labile in vivo to function as prodrugs because the environment around the carbonyl group attached to the heterocyclic ring is highly sterically hindered and cannot be accessed by esterase enzymes. However, the double ester used in

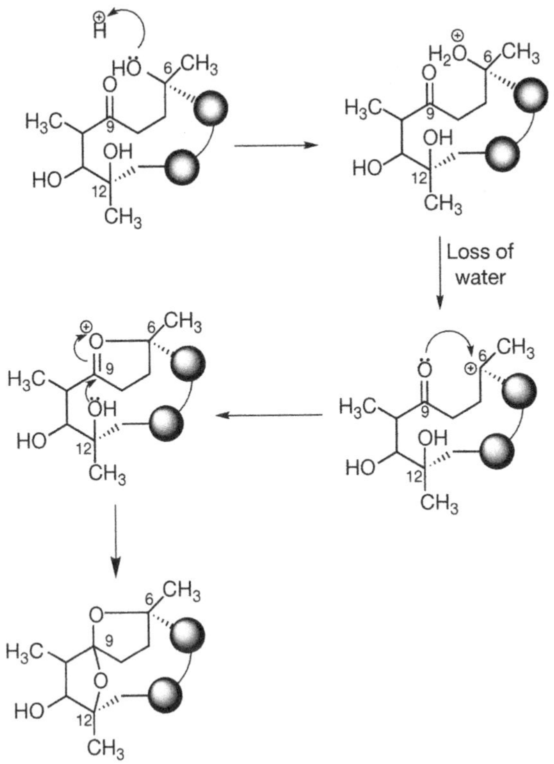

Figure 8.16 Acid-catalysed rearrangement of erythromycin in more detail.

pivampicillin undergoes enzymatic cleavage of the least sterically hindered terminal bond after absorption. This is followed by spontaneous decomposition of the product to the parent drug, ampicillin, and an aldehyde (Fig. 8.19).

The chemical hydrolysis of esters is discussed in Chapter 5. Esters are not normally chemically hydrolysed particularly quickly under physiological conditions, primarily because chemically catalysed hydrolysis is relatively inefficient when compared with the enzymatically catalysed process. Enzymes are more efficient because they can perform acid- and base-catalysed hydrolysis simultaneously within the local environment of their active site. Figure 8.20 shows the enzyme catalysed hydrolysis of an ester.

1. A histidine base donates a proton to the carbonyl group in the ester; histidine is the least basic of the amino acids thus is more ready to give up a proton at physiological pH (acid catalysis step).
2. The carboxylate group of an aspartic acid residue on the protein acts as a base by accepting a proton from water, thus increasing its ability to make a nucleophilic attack on the carbonyl carbon (base catalysis step).
3. The dihydroxylated species in 4 is unstable and the histidine residue removes a proton from it while the aspartic acid residue donates a proton to the alcoholic portion of the ester resulting in an alcohol and an acid 6.

α-methyl dopa

α-methyl dopa is a hypertensive agent used in the treatment of high blood pressure but, being amphoteric, it suffers from poor absorption from the gastrointestinal tract (25%). Preparation of the drug as the double-ester prodrug produces superior absorption characteristics (65%), and the active drug is released by non-specific plasma esterases once absorbed (Fig. 8.21).

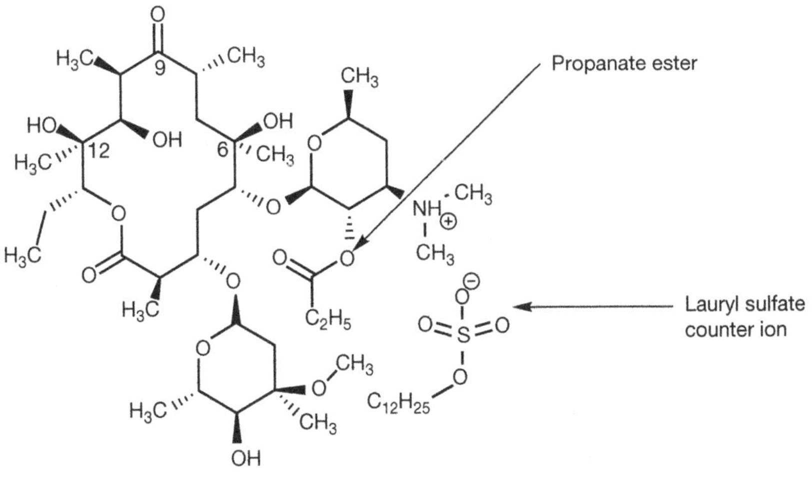

Erythromycin estolate

Figure 8.17 Erythromycin estolate.

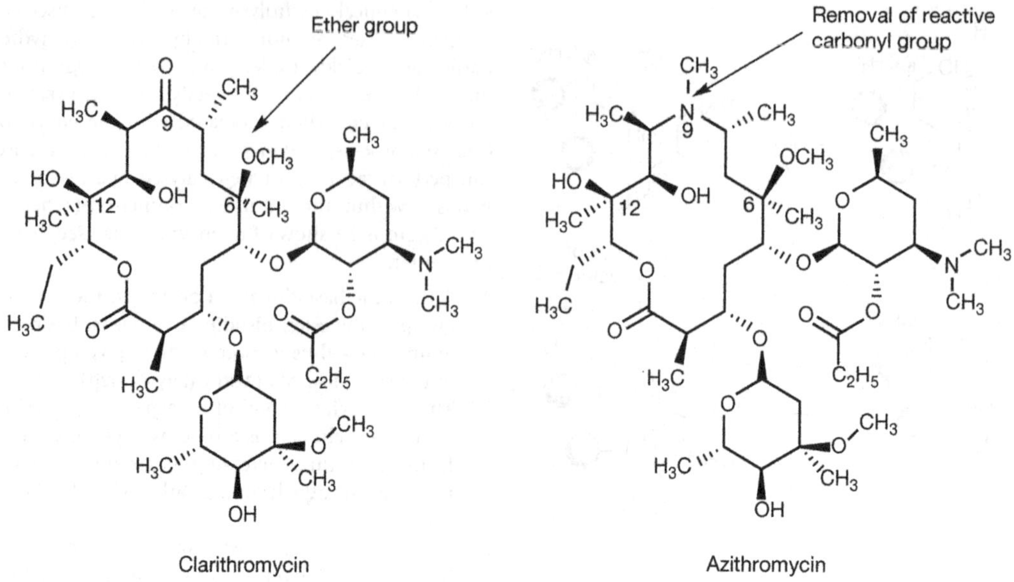

Figure 8.18 Clarithromycin and azithromycin.

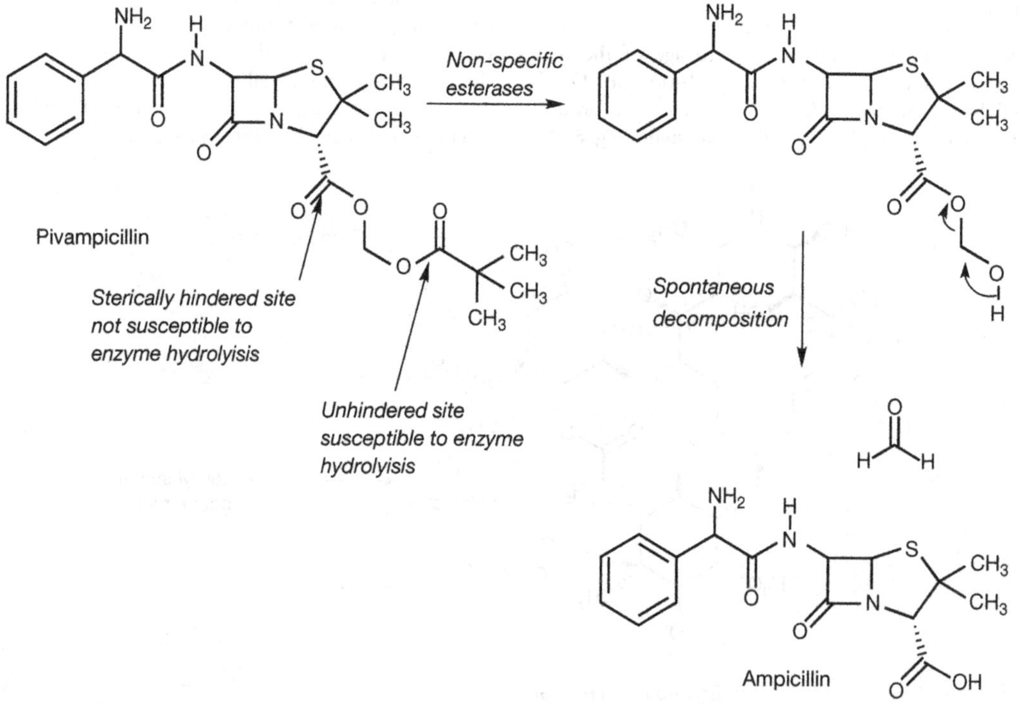

Figure 8.19 Conversion of pivampicillin into ampicillin by esterase activity followed by spontaneous decomposition.

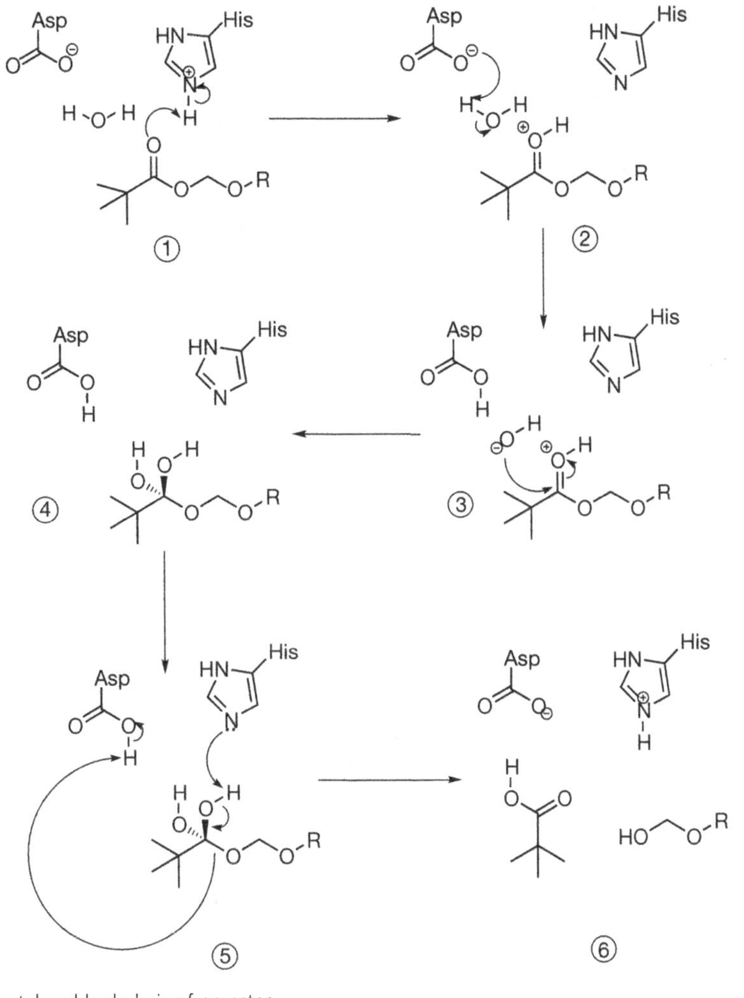

Figure 8.20 Esterase-catalysed hydrolysis of an ester.

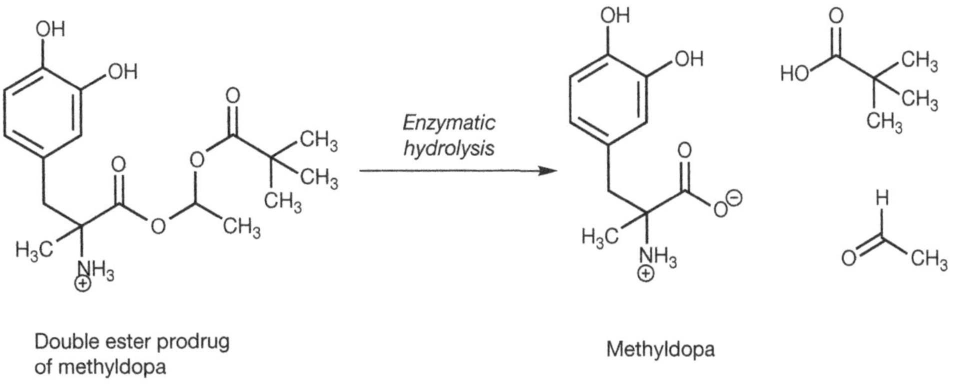

Figure 8.21 Methyl dopa as its ester prodrug.

Unacceptable irritancy via the oral route

Non-steroidal anti-inflammatory drugs

Gastric irritation, ulceration and bleeding is a recognised problem in patients treated with non-steroidal anti-inflammatory drugs (NSAIDs), and is associated with the local inhibition of protective prostaglandin synthesis in the stomach lining that normally serves as a protective mechanism against the strong acid produced by the parietal cells. NSAIDs are often administered in tablet formulations that prevent release of the drug in the stomach environment, e.g. enteric-coated tablets, but prodrug chemistry has also produced an alternative successful approach. Esters of ibuprofen (Fig. 8.22) are pharmacologically inactive and therefore do not adversely affect the stomach lining, whereas once absorbed, hydrolysis by plasma esterases releases the parent drugs, which can then achieve their anti-inflammatory effect systemically.

Opiates

The original concept behind the preparation of diamorphine (Heroin®) from morphine in the late nineteenth century was to protect the stomach from the irritancy presumed to be caused by the presence of phenolic groups by preparing acetate ester prodrug. It was also believed that such an approach would also overcome the dependency side effects associated with morphine. However, the pharmacological properties were altered in an unanticipated manner; not only was the diamorphine (Fig. 8.23) a more potent antitussive (for which it had originally been prescribed), but a more potent analgesic with greater dependency associations. With the benefit of hindsight, we can now attribute this to the enhanced penetration rate through the blood–brain barrier by the more lipophilic diacetate form of the drug. In addition the salts of diamrophine, perhaps surprisingly, have better solubility in water and thus are more suitable for preparation of infusions.

Non-oral drug delivery

One of the main challenges for the medicinal chemist to enable the parenteral delivery of drugs is to alter their solubility profile, and often involves the preparation of prodrugs to facilitate delivery.

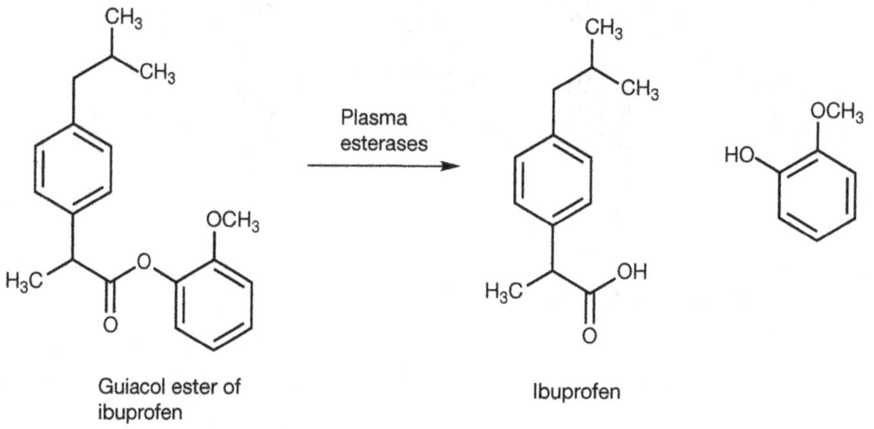

Figure 8.22 Prodrug esters of ibuprofen designed to reduce gastric irritation.

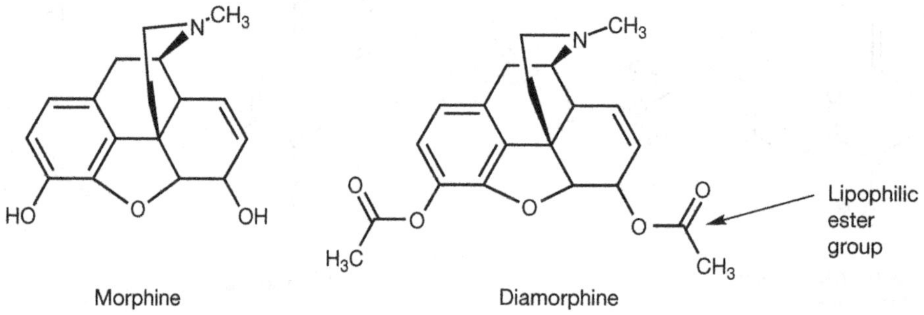

Figure 8.23 Diamorphine – a lipophilic prodrug of morphine.

Chloramphenicol esters

Increasing the aqueous solubility of drugs containing a hydroxyl group for intravenous or ophthalmic use is probably the greatest utility of the prodrug approach in solving pharmaceutical formulation problems. This can be accomplished by introducing an ionic or ionisable functional group which can be converted into a water-soluble sodium salt.

Chloramphenicol (Fig. 8.24) is an antibacterial agent that is used topically to treat infections of the eye and ear, but systemic treatment is reserved for treatment of life-threatening diseases such as those caused by *Haemophilus influenzae* and typhoid fever. Systemic administration through oral or parenteral delivery poses several problems: chloramphenicol has a very bitter taste that cannot be masked effectively by conventional flavouring agents, which means there are therefore formulation problems that are needed to overcome poor patient acceptance. Additionally, poor water solubility makes formulation as an aqueous solution for parenteral administration difficult. Formation of the palmitate ester renders the compound virtually tasteless, and, whilst it remains relatively insoluble in water, it can be formulated as an oral suspension to enable good patient acceptance. Enzymatic hydrolysis in the small intestine releases the non-polar parent drug that can be absorbed into the systemic circulation from the gut.

Chloramphenicol sodium succinate (Fig. 8.24) is an ester that contains an anionic group that can be formulated as the sodium salt. Salts are water soluble and can therefore be formulated as a solution for parenteral administration, such as in eye drops. Plasma esterases release the parent drug once it is in the systemic circulation.

Metronidazole

Metronidazole is an antimicrobial agent used for treating anaerobic bacterial and protozoal infections. It is administered in tablet form or as a suppository, but has low aqueous solubility, rendering it unsuitable for parenteral administration in life-threatening cases. It is weakly basic with a p*Ka* of 2.5 (the electron-withdrawing effect of the aromatic nitro-group renders the lone pair on the imidazole-nitrogen much less available for proton acceptance compared with unsubstituted imidazoles), which means that water soluble chloride salts are not particularly stable for parenteral administration, readily

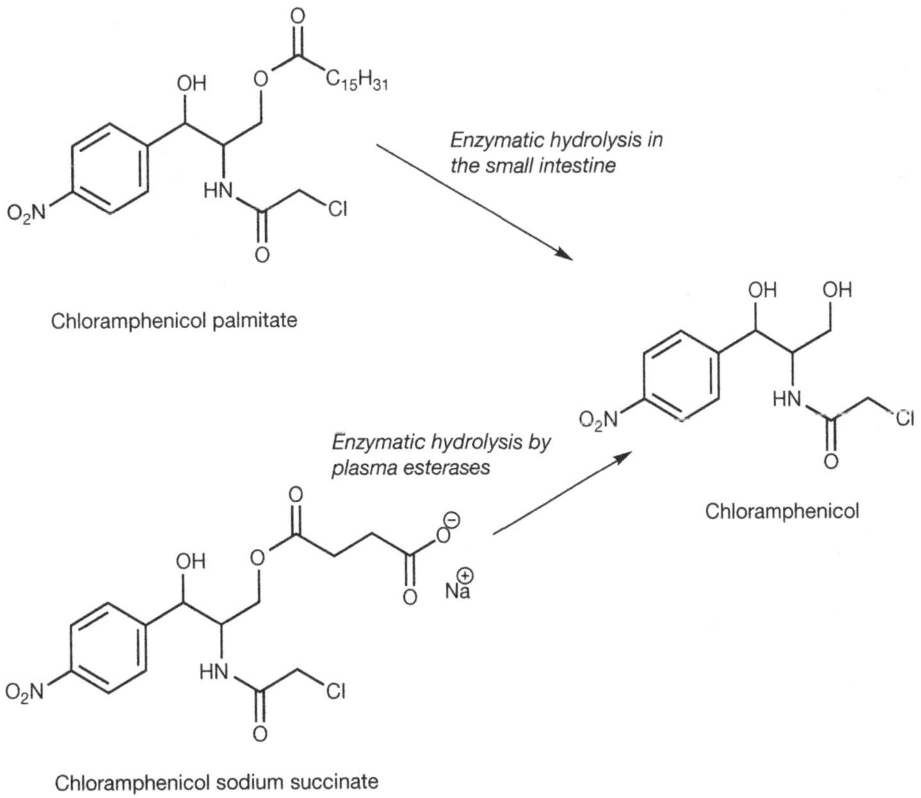

Figure 8.24 Chloramphenicol ester prodrugs.

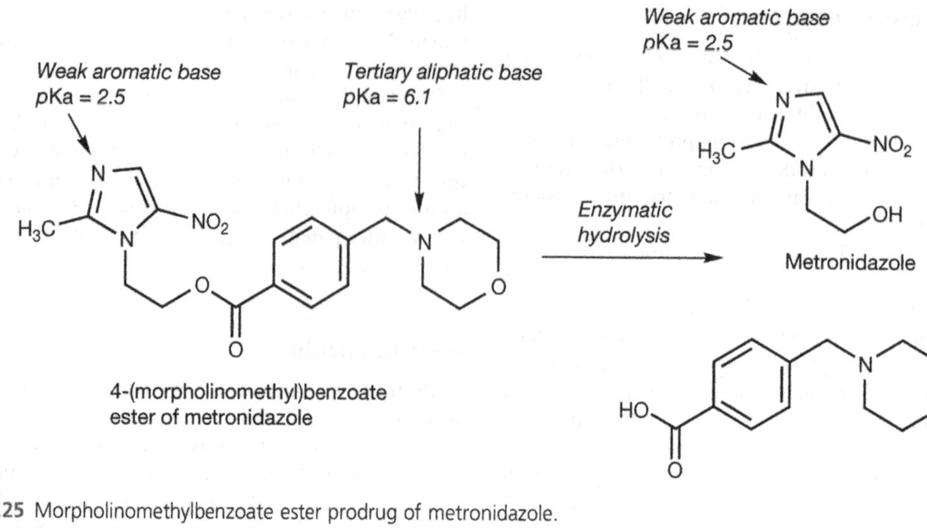

Figure 8.25 Morpholinomethylbenzoate ester prodrug of metronidazole.

converting to the free base water-insoluble form on standing. The 4-(morpholinomethyl)benzoate ester of metronidazole (Fig. 8.25) contains an aliphatic tertiary amine, which is a stronger base ($pKa = 6.1$) that forms stable water-soluble chloride salts suitable for parenteral injection. The half-life of the ester in human plasma is 0.5 minutes due to facile enzymatic hydrolysis by plasma esterases, which release the parent drug systemically.

Adrenaline

Improvement of ocular absorption of polar drugs can be achieved by the prodrug approach, the major problem being the attainment of an optimal drug concentration at the site of action within the eye due to poor absorption through the cornea. Adrenaline lowers intraocular pressure in glaucoma cases, but is poorly absorbed because it is highly polar. It also has a short duration of action due to metabolic inactivation through methylation of the catechol groups. Dipivefrine (Fig. 8.26), the di-tert-butylcarboxy ester, significantly enhances the lipophilic character of the un-ionised form, which enhances corneal absorption. The duration of action is enhanced by approximately 20 times through protection of the catechol against methylation.

It is often clinically advantageous to prolong the duration of action of drugs, which is most frequently applied to antibiotics, hormones, antipsychotics and neuroleptics. The main objective in the case of antibiotics is to maintain high plasma levels, and in the case of hormones and neuroleptics to maintain adequate plasma levels of the drug for prolonged periods of time without having to resort to frequent administration, and therefore improve patient compliance. This objective can be achieved by reducing the solubility of the drug in water and/or by delaying its metabolism.

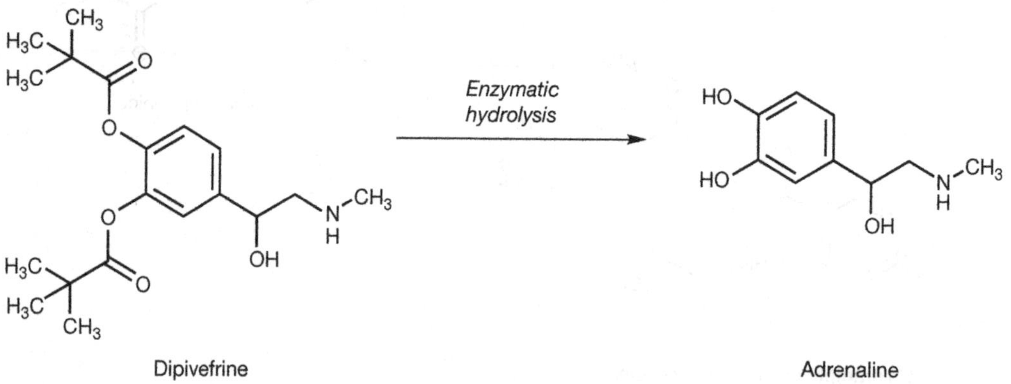

Figure 8.26 Conversion of dipivefrine prodrug into its active form, adrenaline.

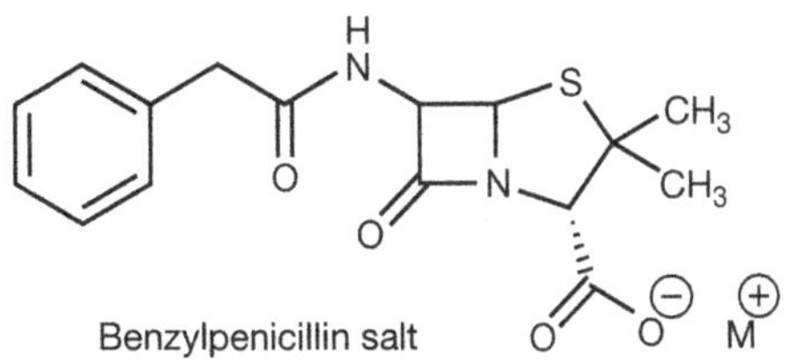

M^+	Name	Solubility in water
Na^+ or K^+	Benzylpenicillin or Penicillin G	Very soluble
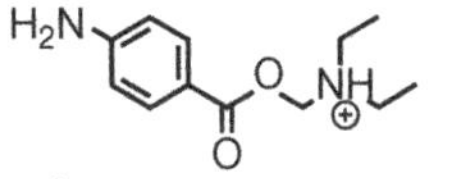	Procaine penicillin	1 in 200
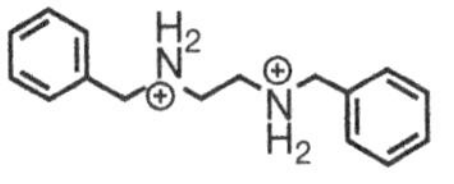	Benzathine penicillin	1 in 6000

Figure 8.27 Lipophilic ion pairs formed between benzyl penicillin and procaine and benzathine.

Penicillins

In contrast to the sodium or potassium salt of benzylpenicillin, which is very water soluble and has a short duration of action, the procaine and benzathine salts (or more accurately, the 'ion-pair' complexes) shown in Figure 8.27 are only sparingly soluble in water and very lipophilic. They are dissolved in an oily vehicle, such as ethyl oleate or sesame oil, and administered by intramuscular injection to create a depot from which the penicillin anion is slowly released into the bloodstream, achieving a sustained-release profile. An added advantage of these depot penicillins is their superior stability compared to benzylpenicillin.

An ion-pair complex is an externally neutral complex formed by electrostatic attraction between a large cation and a large anion, in which the charges are buried deep within the complex. This interaction is accompanied by a change in physicochemical properties compared to the isolated ions, such as a significant decrease in hydrophilic properties and a marked increase in lipophilic properties. These complexes are therefore appreciably soluble in non-polar organic solvents and lipids.

Phenytoin

Intramuscular injection can often induce adverse side effects or local toxicity in the form of tissue irritation or pain, particularly with drugs having a low aqueous solubility and that are formulated in water-miscible cosolvent systems such as aqueous propylene glycol solutions of diazepam, digoxin or phenytoin. This may be partially attributable to precipitation of the drugs at the site of injection, which is often accompanied by erratic and incomplete absorption. These problems may be overcome by converting the drugs into water-soluble prodrugs. Preparation of the sodium salt of the phosphate ester of the hydroxymethyl analogue of the anticonvulsant phenytoin (Fig. 8.28) produces a very water-soluble prodrug that is stable in aqueous solution, and is rapidly hydrolysed systemically by phosphatase enzymes. The hydroxymethylphenytoin spontaneously decomposes to phenytoin and formaldehyde once released by the enzyme.

DRUG ELIMINATION

Competing against drug absorption into the body is its removal from the body. Drugs are viewed as toxins and the body has evolved mechanisms for their removal: *metabolism and excretion*. Figure 8.1 shows the absorption and elimination phases for a drug. The shape of this curve is influenced by the properties of a drug and thus is an important consideration in drug design.

DRUG METABOLISM

Metabolism refers to enzyme-mediated biotransformations that alter the pharmacological activity of both endogenous and exogenous compounds. Metabolism and elimination can be considered to be intrinsically linked since numerous biotransformations increase hydrophilic character and the metabolite is rendered water soluble which, in turn, aids urinary excretion.

Biotransformation may render a drug:

- pharmacologically inactive,
- pharmacologically active,
- change the pharmacological activity.

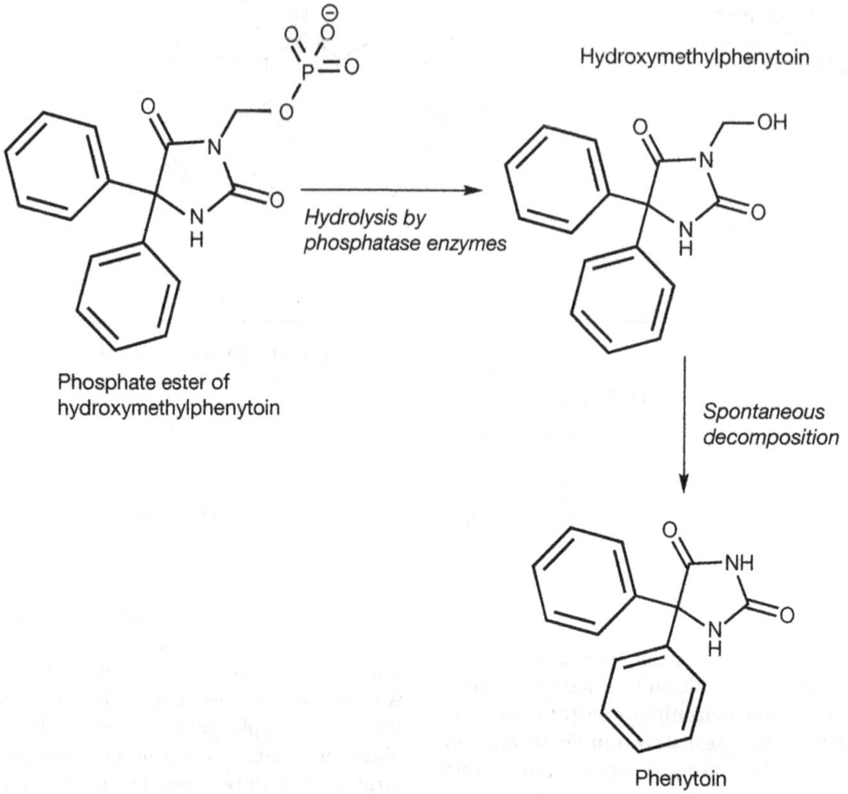

Figure 8.28 Water-soluble phosphate ester prodrug of phenytoin.

The latter two transformations may have undesirable consequences as toxic metabolites may be produced.

Metabolism of drugs can be divided into two distinct categories (Fig. 8.29):

- Phase I reactions: which introduce or unmask hydrophilic groups in the drug (functionalisations).

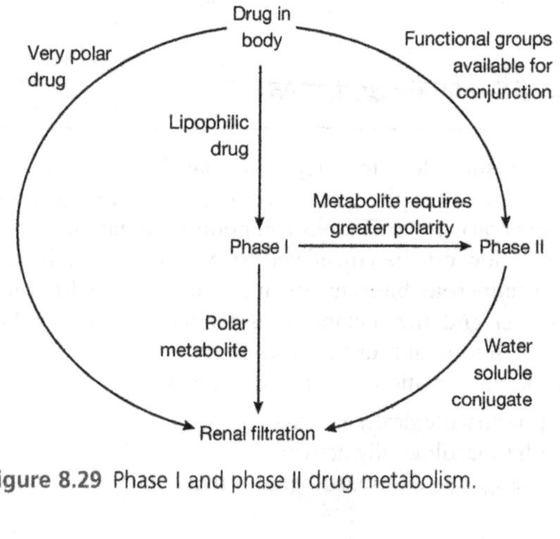

Figure 8.29 Phase I and phase II drug metabolism.

- Phase II reactions: which conjugate the drug or its phase I metabolite with a hydrophilic, endogenous species (conjugation reactions)

Both pathways aim to produce more water soluble species

Phase 1 reactions (functionalisations)

Phase I reactions include:

- aliphatic hydroxylation
- dealkylation
- deamination
- N- and S-oxidation
- alcohol/aldehyde dehydrogenase
- reduction
- hydrolytic reactions.

In general these reactions introduce or expose hydrophilic groups. Two mono-oxygenase systems have been characterised:

- Cytochrome P450 (cyp450) dependent mono-oxygenase. This system is associated with the endoplasmic reticulum and catalyses a wide variety of oxidations at carbon, nitrogen and sulphur. It requires NADPH and O_2 as co-factors. There are a number of different P450 enzymes with different specificities.

- Flavin mono-oxygenase (FMO) which is also a microsomal enzyme and requires NADPH and O_2 as co-factors but only catalyses oxygenation at nitrogen and sulphur.

Oxidative phase I transformations involving cytochrome P450

Cyp450 enzymes have iron at their catalytic sites. As in haemoglobin, the iron can carry an oxygen atom and in this case the haem unit in the cyp450 enzyme donates an oxygen on the hydrocarbon. Examples of cyp450 oxidations of hydrocarbon groups are given in Chapter 4, where the metabolism of barbiturates provides a number of different examples. Two very important cyp450 transformations are O-dealkylation (Fig. 8.30) and N-dealkylation (Fig. 8.31). N-dealkylation in particular is an important deactivating step for many biologically active amines.

Monoamine oxidase (MAO), which is related to cyp450, is used to catalyse the oxidation of amine groups in drugs. There are two forms of this enzyme; the enzyme present in plasma contains iron at its active site whereas the enzyme present in the nervous system has copper at its active site. Figure 8.32 shows the metabolism of propranolol, which can either undergo N-dealkylation via cyp450 or oxidation to an aldehyde via the action of MAO.

Reductive phase I transformations

Reductive metabolism is a relatively uncommon route of drug metabolism. The beta-blocking drug levobunolol is converted into its active form via reduction (Fig. 8.33), the co-factor in such reductions is NADPH. A number of steroids are inactivated via reduction either of carbonyl groups or carbon–carbon double bonds.

Reduction of nitro compounds occurs via the action of cyp450 in conjunction with NADPH in higher organisms, e.g. the inactivation of nitrazepam (Fig. 8.34) but an important pathway which is exploited in antibacterial compounds is the reduction of antibacterial compounds such as metronidazole (Fig. 8.34) and nitrofurantoin to their active forms by bacterial nitroreductases.

Hydrolytic phase I transformations

The activation of ester prodrugs via the action of esterases is described above and in various other chapters, e.g. Chapter 5 and Chapter 22. Esterases are also employed to inactivate drugs or to prepare them for phase II conjugation. For example, the local anaesthetic lidocaine is rapidly hydrolysed to p-aminobenzoic acid deactivating it (Fig. 8.35). The closely related antiarrythmic compound procainamide is not readily hydrolysed and its major deactivated metabolite is desethyl procainamide (Fig. 8.35), although much of the drug is excreted unchanged. Hydrolysis of esters occurs much more readily than the hydrolysis of amides

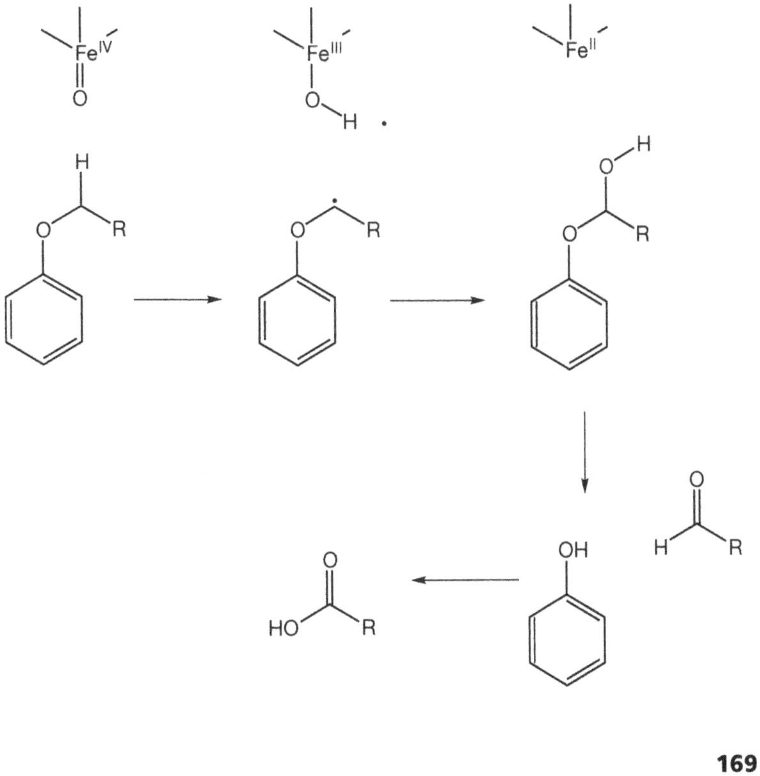

Figure 8.30 O-dealkylation by cyp450.

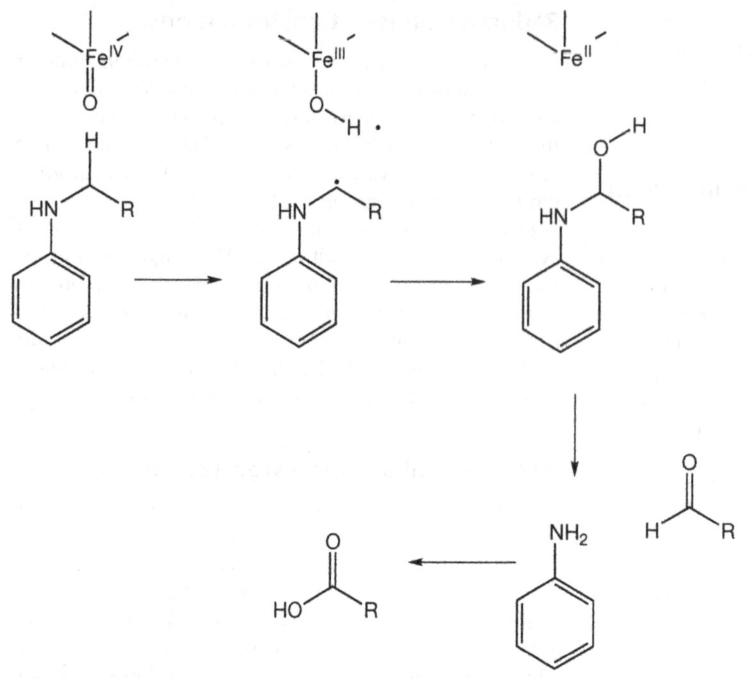

Figure 8.31 N-dealkylation by cyp450.

and for most drugs containing amide groups the amide is not the major site of metabolism. The liver is the major site of oxidative drug metabolism and the blood contains amidases and esterases. Metabolism does occur at other sites such as the kidney, skin, lung and gastrointestinal tract. Enzymes are also secreted by bacteria that colonise the gut.

Phase II reactions (conjugation reactions)

Phase II conjugation reactions include:

- glucuronidation
- glycosylation

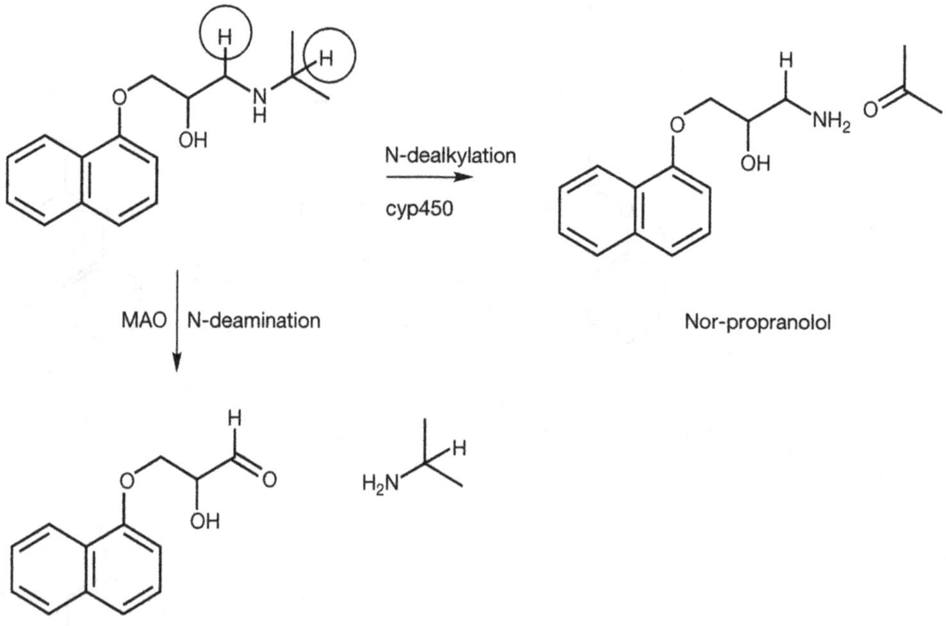

Figure 8.32 Metabolism of propranolol via the action of MAO or cyp450.

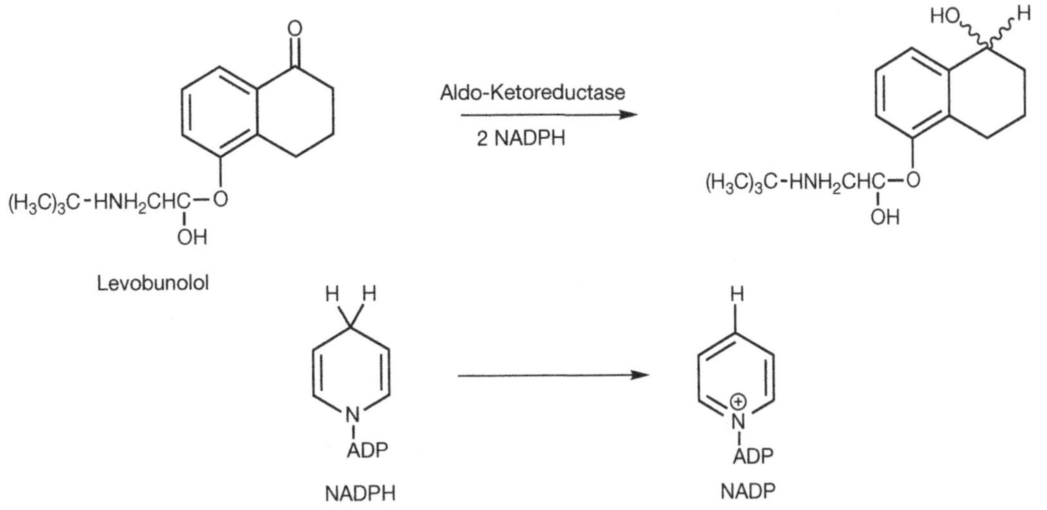

Figure 8.33 Carbonyl reduction by aldo-keto reductase.

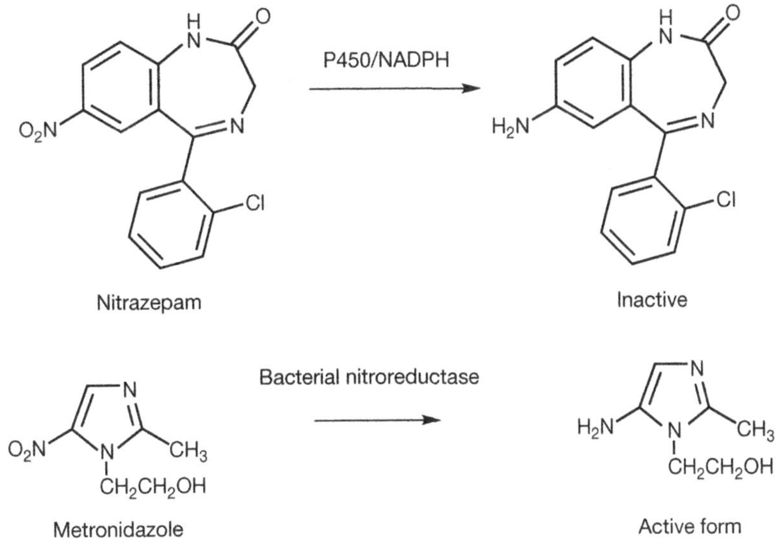

Figure 8.34 Nitro reduction.

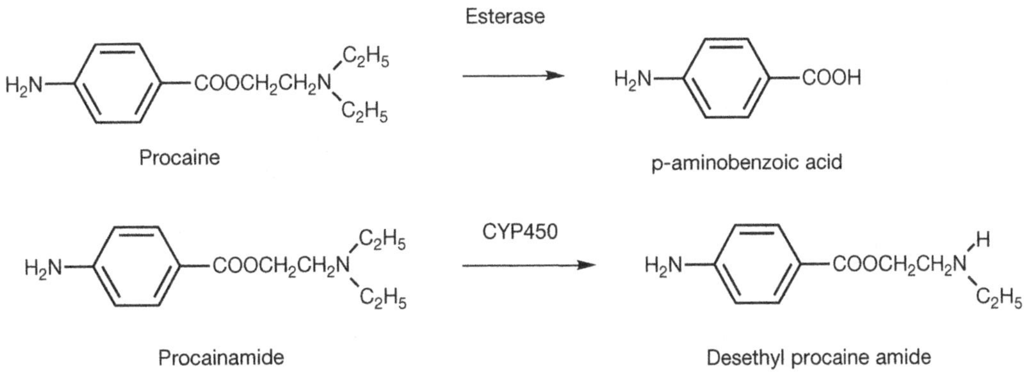

Figure 8.35 Hydrolysis of procaine by plasma esterases and the metabolism of procainamide.

- sulphation
- amino acid conjugation.

Nucleophilic metabolites

O-glucuronidation is catalysed by glucuronyl transferase that transfers a glucuronic acid moiety from uridine diphosphate glucuronide to an alcohol, phenol or carboxylic acid group (Fig. 8.36). This is the most important conjugation reaction for hydroxylated drugs or hydroxylated metabolites in man. Figure 8.37 shows the glucuronidation of estradiol which is converted by this process from a very lipophilic compound to a very hydrophilic compound. O-glucuronidation of carboxylic acid groups can also occur as in the case of indometacin (Fig. 8.38). Primary aromatic amines may undergo N-glucuronidation as shown for dapsone in Figure 8.39. However, this is generally not the preferred route of metabolism, as

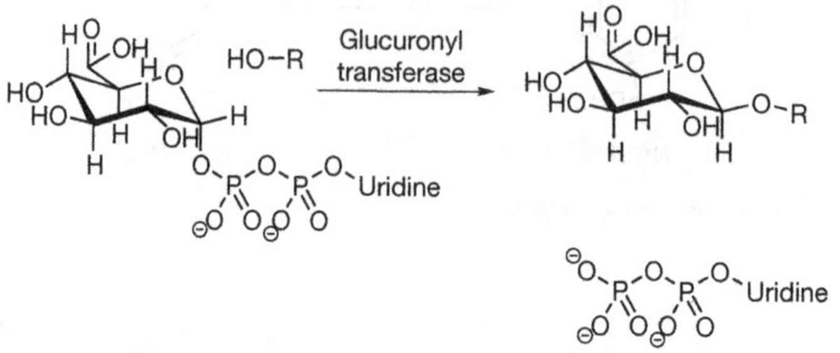

Figure 8.36 Glucuronidation of a hydroxylated compound by UDP-glucuronyl transferase with uridine diphosphate glucuronide (UDPG) as the co-factor.

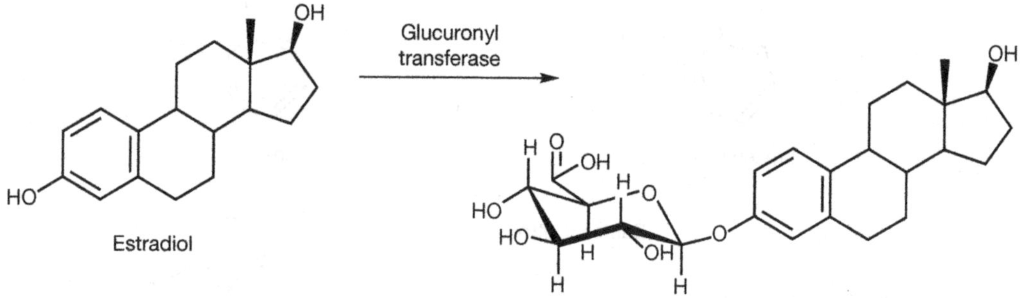

Figure 8.37 Glucuronidation of estradiol.

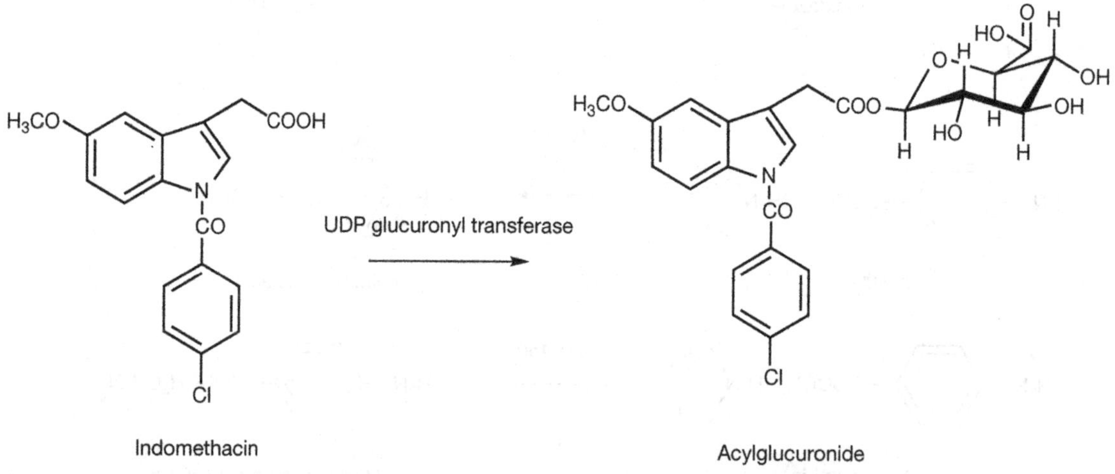

Figure 8.38 Formation of acylglucuronide from indometacin.

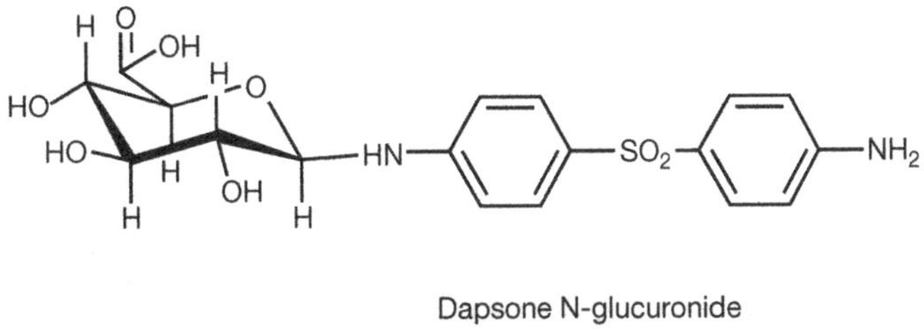

Figure 8.39 N-glucuronide of dapsone.

usually hydroxylation would occur and this would be followed by O-glucuronidation.

The other common conjugation reaction for hydroxyl groups in drugs is sulphation. The sulphate group is transferred from 3′-phosphoadenosine-5′-phosphosulfate (PAPS) via the action of sulphotransferase. Figure 8.40 shows the formation of the sulphate of salbutamol which is the main urinary metabolite of the drug.

Electrophilic metabolites

Electrophilic drugs are generally not welcome unless, of course, they are created deliberately to be electrophilic, as in the case of the DNA alkylating reagents which are used to treat cancer. Electrophilic compounds tend to react with biomolecules such as proteins and DNA. The main defensive compound against electrophilic compounds is the tripeptide glutathione. Figure 8.41 shows

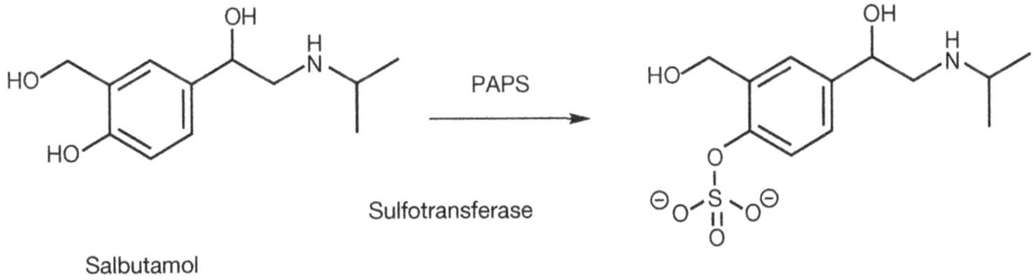

Figure 8.40 Formation of the sulfate metabolite of salbutamol.

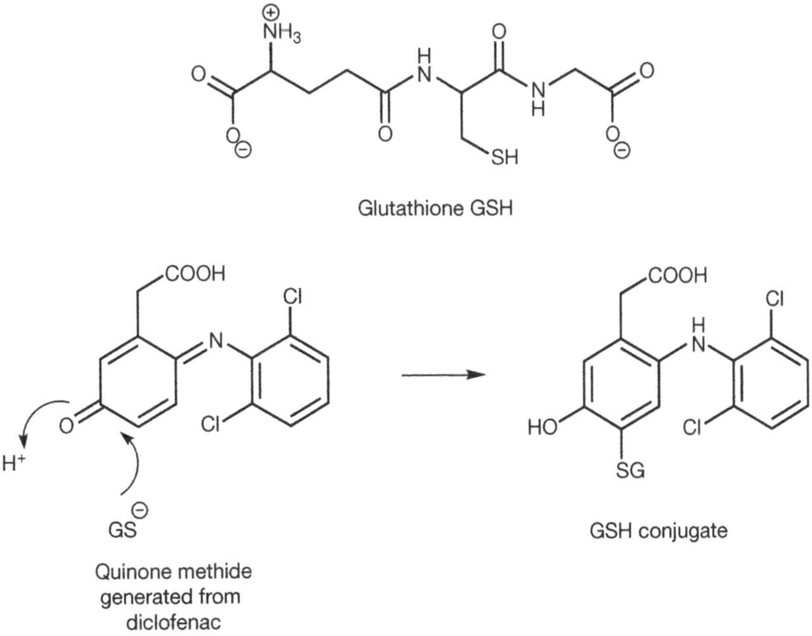

Figure 8.41 Gluathione conjugation.

the structure of glutathione and its reaction with an electrophilic (quinone methide) of diclofenac. If glutathione stores are depleted, then electrophilic species can react with proteins as is the case in paracetamol overdosing where a reactive quinone metabolite formed from paracetamol causes damage to the liver.

MODIFYING DRUG METABOLISM AND EXCRETION

The end products of drug metabolism are usually excreted via the kidneys in the urine. Hence, most phase I & II reactions are designed to increase the hydrophilicity of the drug molecule and render it more water soluble. This is important when one considers the functioning of the kidneys. Blood flows into the kidneys and is filtered at the glomerulus. The filtrate produced in a healthy adult amounts to around 120 mL per minute. The glomerular filtrate passes down the kidney tubules and most of this volume is actively reabsorbed as water. The filtrate is concentrated about 100 times and the net production of urine is only 1 or 2 mL per minute - thankfully! An ionic water-soluble conjugate, e.g. a glucuronide, will remain in solution and be excreted in the urine. More lipophilic drugs will tend to be passively reabsorbed as the concentration gradient in the filtrate increases. Drugs with molecular weights above 300 may be excreted via the bile. Bile is collected in the gall bladder and the ingestion of fatty foods stimulates contraction of the gall bladder. The bile is expelled into the top of the small intestine and serves to emulsify the contents of the gut and aids digestion prior to absorption. Conjugated drug metabolites, e.g. glucuronides, may be broken down by bacterial β-glucuronidases and the parent drug reabsorbed through the gut wall, along the portal vein and back to the liver. This process is called 'enterohepatic circulation' and can significantly increase the elimination half-life of certain drugs. Let us now consider some case examples of chemical modifications of drugs performed to alter their elimination profiles. Many drugs are efficiently absorbed from the gastrointestinal tract but show limited systemic bioavailability due to first-pass metabolism. Extensive first-pass metabolism requires careful monitoring of plasma levels, especially for those drugs that have narrow therapeutic indices. While first-pass metabolism can be avoided through administration of susceptible drugs by routes that avoid absorption into the hepatic portal vein, such as sublingual, inhalation or transdermal, the oral route is generally preferred.

Drugs containing phenolic groups

A major class of drugs known to undergo extensive first-pass metabolism are those containing phenolic hydroxyl groups, such as morphine, propranolol, dopamine and naloxone. The traditional approach has been to mask the metabolically vulnerable phenolic group by ester formation, but a refinement of this approach involves selecting an ester with a built-in esterase inhibiting functional group to enable the prodrug to slow down its own rate of hydrolysis. This permits the prodrug to move intact through the small intestine and liver into the systemic circulation without extensive metabolism by intestinal or hepatic esterases. Bambuterol is an example of this strategy, and is the bis-N,N-dimethylcarbamate of terbutaline, a β_2-agonist and bronchodilator used to treat severe acute asthma (Ch. 10). Carbamate groups are relatively stable against chemical and enzymatic hydrolysis compared with esters owing to resonance stabilisation of the carbonyl group from the lone pair in the amido moiety. When bambuterol passes into the liver on first pass, the metabolising complex cyp450 oxidises one of the tertiary carbamate methyl groups to the corresponding aliphatic alcohol, which spontaneously degrades to the secondary carbamate (Fig. 8.42). Systemic pseudocholinesterase enzymes in the lung are then able to hydrolyse the secondary carbamate in order to release the bronchodilator at its site of action. Side effects such as muscle tremor are reduced, and bioavailability is enhanced because the terbutaline phenolic groups are protected from drug inactivation via conjugation reactions. Bambuterol consequently has a longer duration of action than terbutaline.

Alkyl nitrates

The main effect of the alkyl nitrates is venodilation (although arteriodilation also occurs and some dilation of coronary arteries) and this results in a reduction on heart preload in the treatment of angina. The alkyl nitrates are esters formed between alcohols and nitric acid. They contain a nitroxy group. This functional group is distinguished from nitrites which are esters formed from nitrous acid and from nitro compounds in which carbon and nitrogen are directly bonded. Over the years, a large number of alkyl nitrates have been shown to be therapeutically active, but the currently prescribed ones are limited to glyceryl trinitrate (GTN), isosorbide dinitrate (ISDN) and isosorbide mononitrate (IS-5-MN) (Fig. 8.43).

The generation of nitrite ion in the presence of reducing thiols is a key event in the metabolic activation of the alkyl nitrates. Alkyl nitrates are among the earliest examples of prodrugs, although this did not become apparent until recently. The lipophilic alkyl nitrate partitions into vascular smooth muscle and undergoes reductive hydrolysis to release nitric oxide (NO). NO then reacts with specific thiol groups to form the S-nitrosothiol which is believed to activate guanylate cyclase with a corresponding increase in the concentration of cyclic GMP and a concomitant reduction in intracellular calcium concentration. Calcium mediates muscle contraction and a reduction in calcium concentration results in relaxation, i.e. vasodilation.

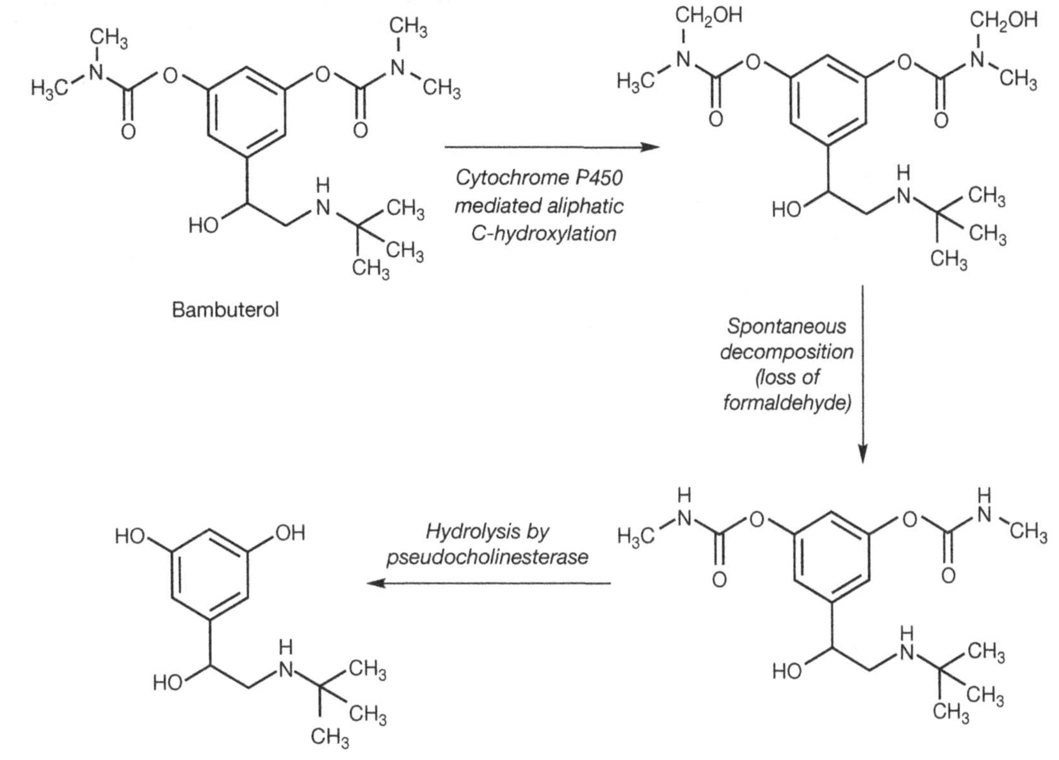

Terbutaline

Figure 8.42 Protection of phenolic hydroxyl groups in terbutaline by use of bambuterol prodrug.

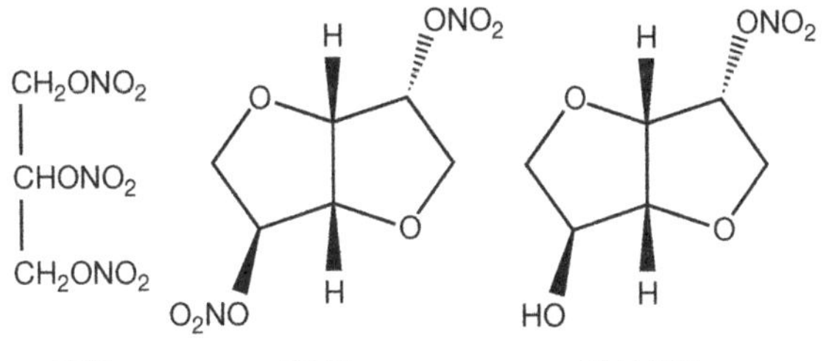

GTN ISDN IS-5-MN

Figure 8.43 Alkyl nitrates.

For the alkyl nitrates to exert the desired venodilation they must reach the systemic circulation intact. Large-scale denitration and release of nitrite ion outside the vascular endothelial cells renders these drugs ineffective as the polar nitrite ion does not readily partition through lipid barriers. Orally ingested drugs, after adsorption from the small intestine, are carried by the hepatic portal vein to the liver. The liver contains an enzyme that catalyses the reductive hydrolysis of alkyl nitrates. Organic nitrate reductase (ONR), in the presence of glutathione, speeds up the denitration of the alkyl nitrates.

GTN undergoes very rapid (and near complete) denitration on passing through the liver. Hence it is said that GTN undergoes extensive first-pass metabolism. In comparison, the metabolism of ISDN by the same enzyme system is much slower (Table 8.2).

The oral bioavailability of GTN is only 6% while the sublingual bioavailability is 80% and the percutaneous bioavailability is also high. These data are not surprising when we consider that sublingual and percutaneous routes of absorption avoid first-pass metabolism and offer

Table 8.2 Rates of metabolism of different alkyl nitrates

Alkyl nitrate	ONR V_{max} mmoles/kg protein/min
GTN	120.0
ISDN	21.5
1,2-GDN	5.0
1-GMN	0.7

significant advantages over the oral route in the case of GTN. The high potency and lipophilicity of GTN make it the drug of choice (sublingually) for the treatment of an anginal attack. GTN may be administered sublingually by tablet or aerosol spray and relief of the anginal pain may be achieved within a minute. The prophylactic use of GTN necessitates the use of transdermal patches which maintain a steady therapeutic plasma concentration. After a single intravenous dose of GTN the elimination half-life has been measured at 4 minutes. The rapid clearance is the result of high tissue extraction and liver metabolism.

As with all the alkyl nitrates, GTN accumulates in the venous side of the circulation more than the arterial side. This phenomenon probably explains why these drugs reduce ventricular preload more than afterload (unlike the calcium channel blockers). GTN is excreted via the kidneys as a mixture of mono- and dinitrates, probably as their glucuronides.

The oral bioavailability of ISDN is 25%, and this increases to 60% by the sublingual route. The higher oral bioavailability compared to GTN can be understood in relation to ONR catalysed metabolism. The decreased sublingual bioavailability compared to GTN is probably related to the differences in lipophilicity, the log P values quoted for GTN and ISDN are 0.98 and 0.04, respectively. Log P is a significant parameter when comparing rates of sublingual absorption as the drug will only remain in the mouth until the swallowing reflex removes it. No unchanged ISDN is excreted; denitration occurs in the following proportions: IS-5-MN (60%), IS (10–20%), IS-2-MN (20%).

A closer inspection of the chemical structure of ISDN (Fig. 8.44) helps to rationalise this pattern of metabolism. The two five-membered rings in ISDN are cis-fused and as a result they form a V-shaped molecule. The nitroxy group in the 5 position is concealed inside the V while the nitroxy group in the 2 position projects towards the outside of the V. Denitration of the exposed 2-nitroxy group by ONR therefore proceeds more readily than denitration of the 5-nitroxy group.

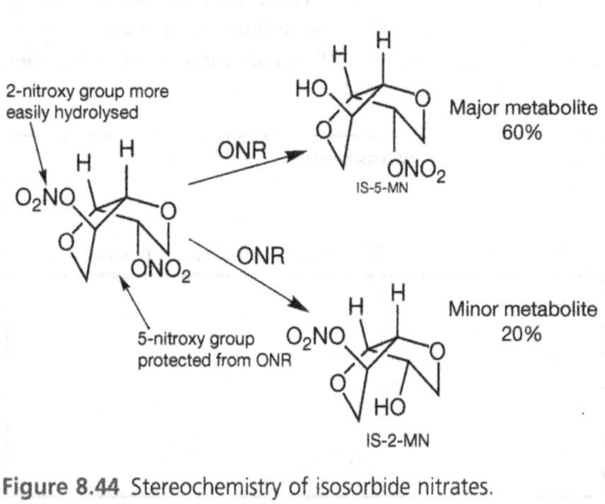

Figure 8.44 Stereochemistry of isosorbide nitrates.

Table 8.3 Elimination half lives of nitro isosorbides

Isosorbide analogue	Elimination half-life (hr)
ISDN	1
IS-2-MN	2
IS-5-MN	5

The oral bioavailability of IS-5-MN is nearly 100%. No data are available for the sublingual route because its lower lipophilicity (log P: −0.4) in comparison with ISDN prevents sufficiently rapid absorption via the mouth to achieve a therapeutically effective systemic concentration. Clearly IS-5-MN is a poor substrate for ONR and no significant metabolism occurs on the first pass through the liver (Table 8.3).

Thus IS-5-MN has been developed as an antianginal drug because of its longer elimination half-life and the reduced incidence of interpatient variability.

Steroids

Elimination of steroid hormones occurs mainly by metabolism in the liver followed by excretion via the kidneys. The metabolic profile of hydrocortisone shows the transformations common to most steroid hormones (Fig. 8.45). Reduction of the 4,5 double bond and then the C-3 keto group, in most cases, destroys the biological activity of the hormone. The C-11 hydroxyl group undergoes reversible oxidation/reduction, while reduction of the C-20 keto group is irreversible and precedes cleavage of the C-17 side chain. In order to aid urinary excretion the metabolites usually undergo conjugation to form their glucuronides or sulphates. Oestrogenic conjugates are known to be excreted in the bile and there may be significant enterohepatic recycling of natural and synthetic oestrogens. Assuming intimate attachment of the steroid with a hormonal receptor is required a priori to elicit a biological effect. It can be appreciated that the overall shape and functionality of the molecule will determine binding affinity and hence response. Consequently, altering structure in order to modify the elimination rate must take this into account. Numerous examples testify to this hypothesis and none better than the development of the oral contraceptives. Combined oral contraceptives (COC) contain a progestational and an oestrogenic component; the natural hormones progesterone and estradiol (Fig. 8.46) both suffer extensive first-pass metabolism when taken orally and for this reason synthetic analogues were developed.

The male sex hormone, testosterone, when chemically modified by removal of the C-19 methyl group followed by ethinylation at the C-17α position becomes transformed into the progestationally active norethisterone,

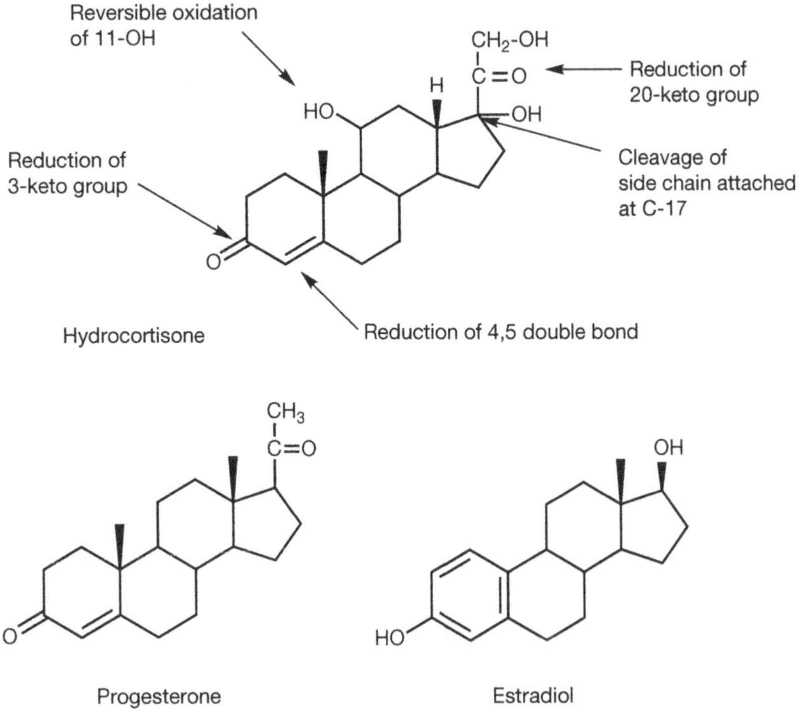

Figure 8.45 Metabolism of hydrocortisone.

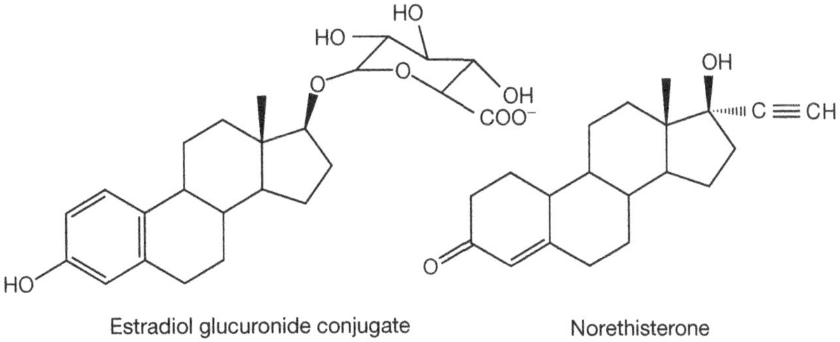

Figure 8.46 Steric hindrance of the C-17α position of estradiol as in norethisterone prevents glucuronidation.

which is orally active, and is one of the common progestational components of the COC. First-pass metabolism is reduced through steric hindrance of the hydroxyl at the 17 position which prevents attachment of the glucuronide moiety (Fig. 8.46).

Simvastatin

Statins are given to lower cholesterol levels in patients with hypercholesterolaemia. They also decrease low-density lipoprotein (LDL) levels and raise high-density lipoprotein (HDL) levels. This helps to prevent cardiovascular disease since high levels of LDL promote atherosclerosis, whereas HDL retards it.

Lovastatin (Fig. 8.47) is a metabolite isolated from the fungus *Aspergillus terreus*. On screening, it was found to inhibit the key enzyme which regulates hepatic synthesis of cholesterol, viz. 3-hydroxy-3-methylglutaryl co-enzyme A reductase (HMG-CoA reductase).

Cholesterol is a steroid which stabilises cell membranes and is also a biosynthetic precursor of steroid hormones and bile salts. The accumulation of plaques on the walls of coronary and carotid arteries which have a high cholesterol content results in a condition

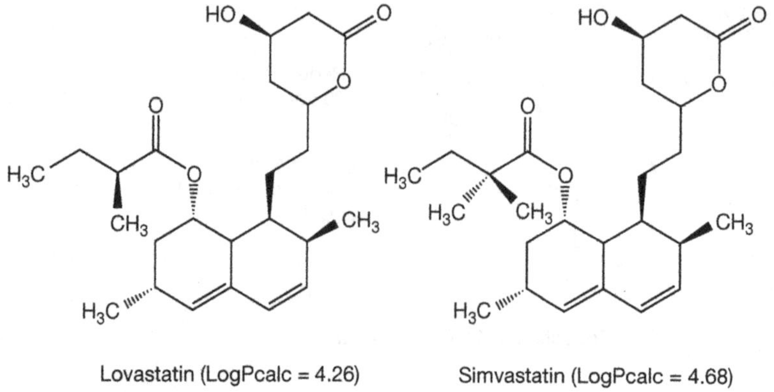

Figure 8.47 Lovastatin and simvastatin.

known as atherosclerosis where the heart has to pump more strongly to circulate the blood, and this is associated with increased risk of cardiovascular disease. Since at least 60% of the cholesterol in the body is synthesised in the liver, the ability to inhibit HMG-CoA reductase was considered to be a potential target if cholesterol levels in patients at risk were to be reduced.

Lovastatin is rapidly metabolised, which is undesirable for any drug likely to be chronically administered. In order to achieve once-daily dosing, steric hindrance around the ester carbonyl was increased by the introduction of an extra methyl group close to the ester bond in order to reduce the rate of esterase hydrolysis. This resulted in formation of simvastatin, a highly successful lipid-lowering agent. Simvastatin (like lovastatin) is inactive until metabolised in the liver to form its active metabolite mevinolinic acid (Fig. 8.48). Part of mevinolinic acid is structurally similar to the HMG portion of HMG-CoA, the substrate for HMG-CoA reductase, and hence competes with it for the active site of the enzyme. This reduces the amount of mevalonic acid which is produced. Mevalonic acid is a precursor of cholesterol.

Sulphonylurea hypoglycaemics

During a clinical trial in 1954 of the sulphonylurea antibacterial sulphonamide known as carbutamide (Fig. 8.49), patients experienced severe side effects. A physician in charge tested the drug on himself and realised it produced hypoglycaemia. After further clinical investigations, carbutamide was marketed in Europe as an oral hypoglycaemic in patients with mild diabetes, even though it had many side effects.

Tolbutamide (Fig. 8.49) is a safer analogue that can be taken by mouth three times a day. It has now been in use for over 40 years, but has been eclipsed by newer long-acting agents. These, however, can accumulate and produce hypoglycaemia in elderly patients whose liver function is impaired. For them, the short-acting tolbutamide is often preferred. The major metabolite is the carboxylic acid (Fig. 8.49), which is formed through oxidation of the metabolically sensitive methyl group, initially via aliphatic hydroxylation.

Longer-acting sulphonylureas were obtained by replacing the metabolically sensitive methyl group. The first of these was chlorpropamide, which is twice as potent as tolbutamide and is taken once daily. Unfortunately, it is

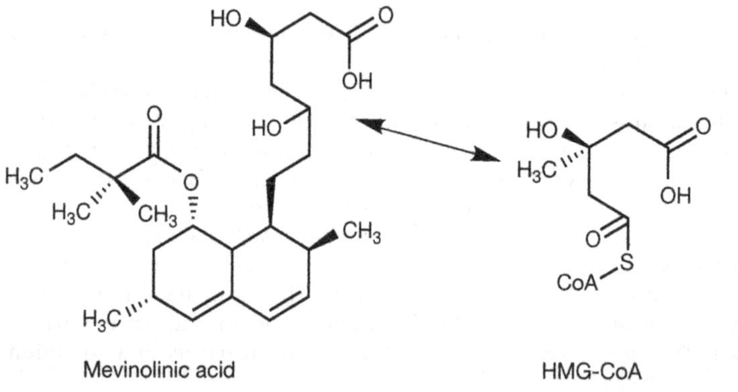

Figure 8.48 Structural similarity between mevinolinic acid and HMG-CoA.

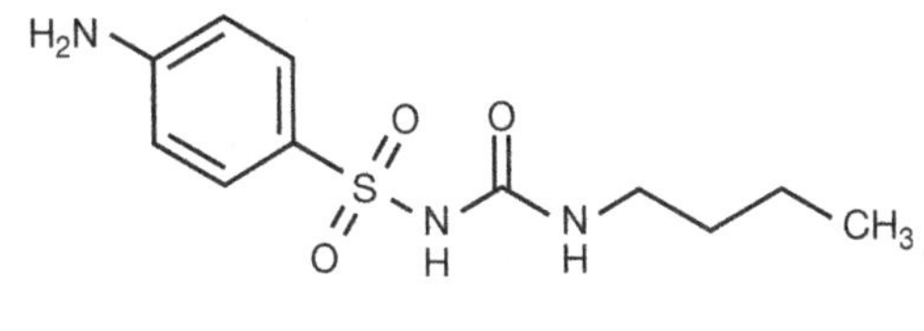

Carbutamide (Log Pcalc = 1.01)

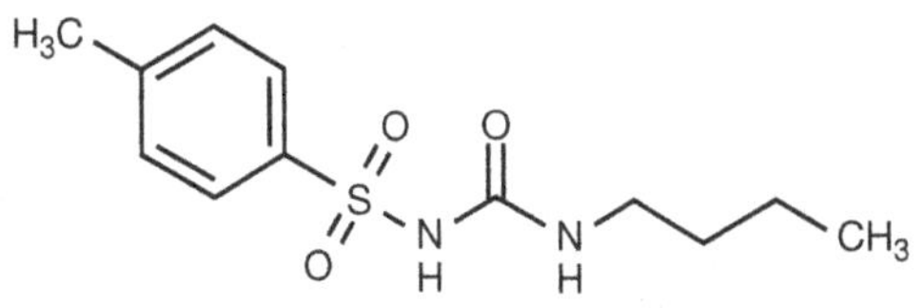

Tolbutamide (Log Pcalc = 2.34)

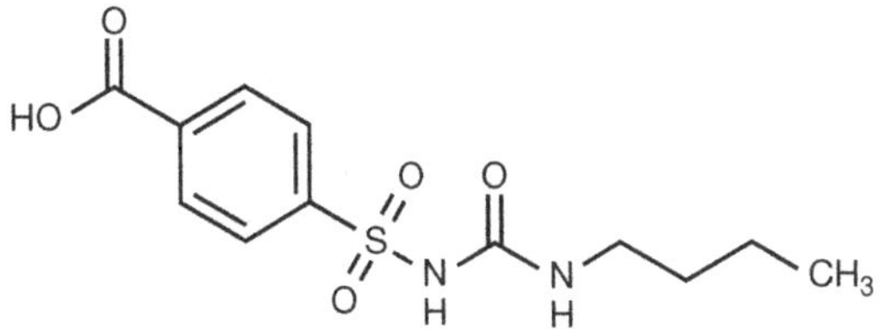

Tolbutamide carboxylic acid metabolite

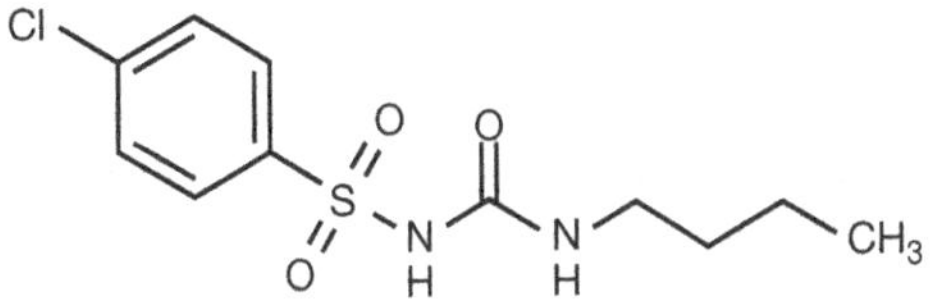

Chlorpropamide (Log Pcalc = 2.27)

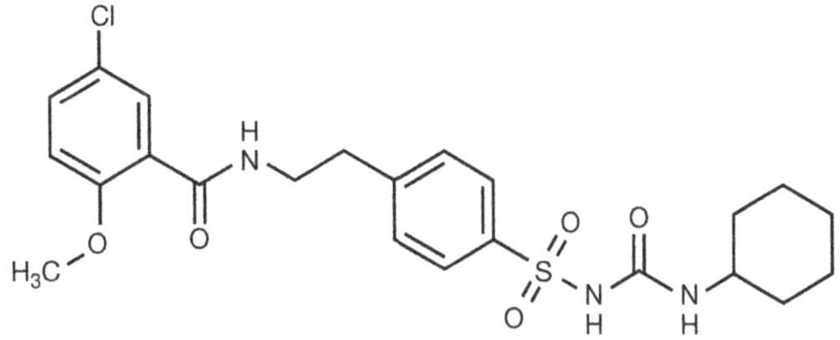

Glibenclamide (Log Pcalc = 4.79)

Figure 8.49 Sulphonyl urea hypoglycaemics.

perhaps too successful insofar as it can accumulate in the body and cause hypoglycaemia.

Several not quite so long-acting agents such as have appeared on the market over the years since there are good financial returns on drugs taken for years by large numbers of patients. One of the first was glibenclamide, although the BNF is scathing about these developments:

'There are several sulphonylureas but there is no evidence for any difference in their effectiveness. Only chlorpropamide has appreciably more side effects, mainly because of its prolonged duration of action and the consequent hazard of hypoglycaemia (but also as a result of the common and unpleasant chlorpropamide-alcohol flush phenomenon).'

In conclusion, lengthening the duration of action is not always beneficial and has to be carefully considered in drugs likely to be used by elderly patients in whom renal and hepatic function is compromised. A safer approach in some cases is for pharmaceutical scientists to formulate a short-acting preparation in a manner that will lengthen duration of action as a result of controlled release rather than altered metabolism.

TARGETED DRUG DELIVERY

Most successes of targeted drug delivery have been through localised drug delivery to an external organ such as the skin, the eye or the ear where the drug input is direct to the target organ, such as the antiglaucoma agent dipivefrine (see Fig. 8.27). Systemic drug delivery to a specific internal organ is much more difficult to achieve because the drug has to cross various barriers to get from its site of administration to its site of action. Despite this difficulty, some degree of success has been achieved using chemical development and/or formulation design, and we shall concentrate on the former here. The latter approach is covered in textbooks on pharmaceutics. One of the best examples of a prodrug showing a high degree of site-specific bioactivation is omeprazole, which is an effective inhibitor of gastric acid secretion used in the treatment of ulcers. The mode of action of this drug is described in Chapter 12.

Another interesting example involves site-specific delivery of drugs to the brain. This involves coupling the drug through an amide or an ester bond to a quaternary carrier such as N-methylnicotinic acid. The resulting quaternary complex can be reduced chemically in vitro to the neutral lipophilic dihydro form and oral administration of this form results in its distribution throughout the body, where it is systemically oxidised enzymatically back to the original quaternary complex. The ionic, hydrophilic character of the oxidised quaternary complex ensures that it is eliminated rapidly from the body, except from the brain because the quaternary ion cannot pass back out through the blood–brain barrier, and is therefore retained at the site of action (Fig. 8.50). Slow, enzymatic cleavage of the quaternary complex in the brain results in the steady release of the drug in situ, and because the drug tends to be hydrophilic in nature (the reason for using the delivery system in the first place) on release in the brain it is retained at the site of action. This dihydropyridine-pyridinium salt redox delivery system has been applied successfully for the brain-specific or brain-enhanced delivery of drugs including dopamine, phenytoin and penicillins.

Anticancer agents

The problem of localisation of drug action has also been extensively studied in the field of cancer chemotherapy. A problem arises because the vast majority of drugs used to treat cancer are highly reactive but unselective in their action, i.e. they attack all fast-growing cells indiscriminately, including healthy cells of the tongue, intestine, bone marrow and hair. Their anticancer activity cannot be separated from numerous toxic side effects such as severe nausea, vomiting, alopecia and suppression of the production of blood cells by the bone marrow, so transport to and localisation at the site of action are of vital importance. Quite often, this approach requires the existence of exploitable metabolic differences between cancerous cells and the healthy cells essential to the integrity of

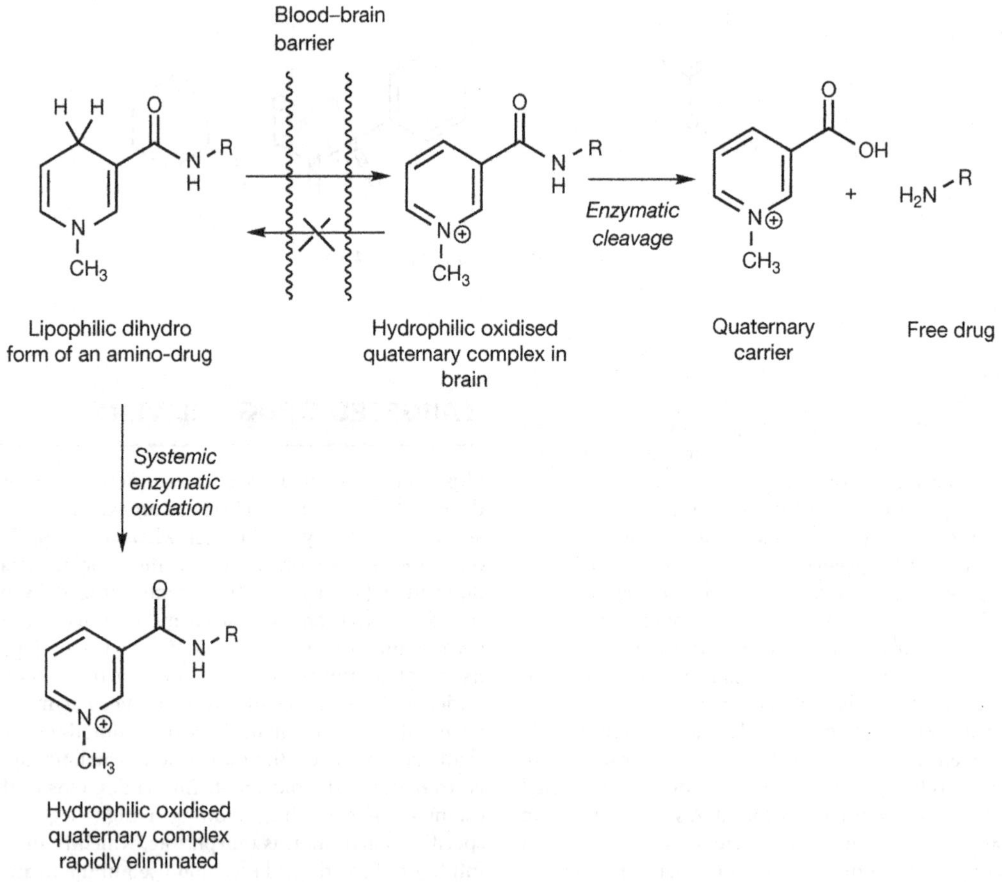

Figure 8.50 Oxidation of a dihydropyridinium prodrug which causes it to be retained in the brain.

the organism. Examples of the targeting of anticancer drugs are given in Chapter 21.

PARENTERAL DRUG DELIVERY

The term parenteral drug delivery covers a number of administration routes which have little in common other than the fact that they generally involve the use of a hypodermic needle to inject the drug into the body. This route of administration bypasses a number of physiological barriers. The constraints on the composition and formulation of the medicine are much more rigorous than for less invasive routes such as oral or transdermal delivery. Despite this, a surprising range of materials can be injected into various tissues if the appropriate precautions are taken.

Direct introduction into the systemic circulation is usually employed for the rapid attainment of a pharmacological effect or when the drug is too hydrophilic to cross the gastrointestinal tract. In most cases, the rate at which the drug in the plasma compartment achieves an equilibrium with other tissues is a function of blood flow. The compartmentalisation of a drug following parenteral administration is shown in Figure 8.51. Only un-ionised, non-bound drug can traverse cellular membranes although, since protein-binding is readily reversible, it is not per se an important determinant of flux. The extent of binding to the receptor will be affected since protein binding provides a high-capacity, low-affinity alternative.

Protein binding

One of the underlying principles of clinical pharmacology is that only the unbound, free drug is pharmacologically active and that only in this form can a drug cross a biological membrane or interact with a receptor. Interaction with the receptor results in a biochemical change leading to a physiological response. Drugs bind to a number of plasma proteins including albumin, lipoproteins, α_1-acid glycoprotein and gamma globulins, and the more extensively the drug is bound, the lower will be the drug activity available to exert a pharmacological effect. Since the concentrations of these proteins change in disease, and as a function of nutrition, the effect of the drug may be significantly and unpredictably modulated. For example, most antimicrobials bind primarily to albumin, while basic drugs including erythromycin, clindamycin, and trimethoprim bind to the 'acute-phase' serum protein, α_1-acid glycoprotein. Moreover, binding is not limited to proteins in the serum. Because albumin is the principal protein in interstitial fluid, substantial binding to this protein and to other tissue constituents takes place. Differential concentrations of these proteins, and cell debris, leads to marked alterations in peripheral concentrations around an inflamed area such as a wound or abscess.

The role of the blood supply

When the oxygen demands of tissue increase, the blood flow is adjusted appropriately. One competing demand for a homeothermic animal is the loss of heat which necessitates wasteful catabolism and blood flow is thus under autonomic nervous control. The large arteries, starting from the aorta, take blood to all parts of the body. In order to reach the tissues, the surface area for exchange must be large. This is brought about by the division of vessels into a capillary network which eventually drains into larger venules and ultimately into capillary veins.

The blood transports the drug to the tissues; however, the drug concentration in the tissues is usually not equal to that in the blood. A number of factors influence the

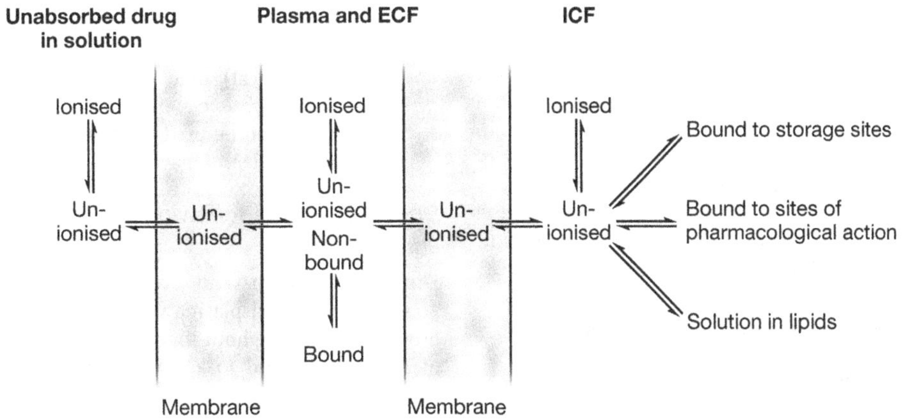

Figure 8.51 Compartmentalisation of a drug administered by the parenteral route.

Table 8.4 Rates of blood perfusion through different tissues

Tissue	Blood flow (litres min^{-1})	Tissue mass as % of body weight
Blood	5.4	8.0
Poorly perfused		
Skeleton	0.2	17
Adipose tissue	0.25	14–20
Adequately perfused		
Skin	0.4	7
Muscle	0.8	48
Well perfused		
Kidneys	1.2	0.5
Heart	0.25	0.5
Liver	1.55	3.5
Brain	0.75	2.0

drug concentration in tissues, one of the most important being the blood flow per unit mass of the tissue. Tissues can be broadly classified as poorly perfused, adequately perfused and well perfused on the basis of blood flow as shown in Table 8.4. Note how organs with a relatively small mass, such as the heart and brain, only require a modest blood flow to perfuse them well. The blood flow to the heart musculature (not to be confused with the flow *through* the heart) is equal to that through the adipose tissue, but the heart has a much smaller mass and so is thus correspondingly better perfused.

The blood flow controls the rate at which the drug is supplied to the particular tissue, and will be reflected in the drug concentration profile in that tissue. If the tissue is well perfused, the tissue pharmacokinetics will reach a maximum value at a similar time to that in the blood. However, if the tissue is less well perfused, the supply of drug to the tissue will be rate-limiting and so the concentration in the tissue will increasingly lag behind that in the blood, as shown in Figure 8.52, so that the tissue fails to achieve the same level as that present in the blood.

Routes for drug administration

Parenteral administration

The main route of parenteral administration is intravenous administration, the injection usually given into a large, convenient vein and infused slowly. The drug is

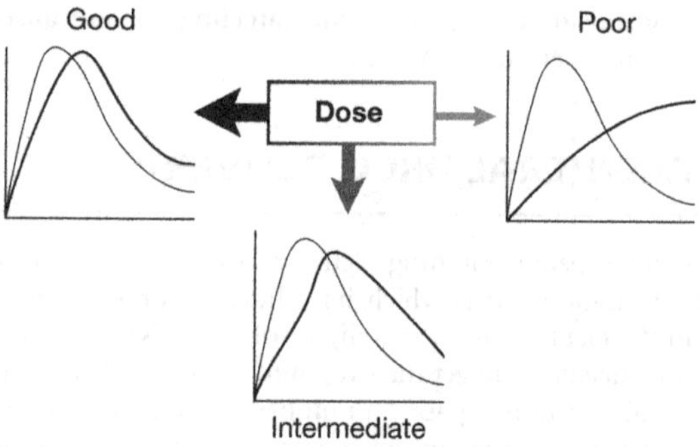

Figure 8.52 Pharmacokinetic profiles of drugs in tissues of varying perfusion. The curve to the left is the central compartment and that on the right represents peripheral supply.

administered in a solution or an emulsion and there is a requirement therefore that the solution be particle free, sterile and non-pyrogenic. Often, the drug may be placed in a drip-set, assuming that changes in drug-infusion solution such as precipitation of the drug do not occur with time. Although intravenous administration is well known, there are many other methods of parenteral administration, including:

- *Intralymphatic*: used to place tracer or drug into peripheral lymph nodes.
- *Subcutaneous*: for the administration of test substances (e.g. pentagastrin to elicit a maximum secretory response from the stomach when testing for achlorhydria).
- *Intramuscular*: into a large muscle mass for sustained delivery.
- *Intralipomatous*: into fat. A short needle used to deliver drug to arm or thigh will often be intralipomatous in females and intramuscular in males. Less injury results from tissue response as the agent is delivered more slowly.
- *Epidural*: used in childbirth to provide regional pain relief.
- *Spinal* (intrathecal): used in treatment of brain-threatening disease, e.g. meningitis.
- *Microdialysis*: can be used when a local increase in tissue pressure is to be avoided.

Drug distribution following parenteral administration

Drugs distribute unevenly between red cells, white cells, plasma protein and plasma water. Once in the blood, a drug diffuses throughout the various body fluid compartments at a rate and to an extent which depends on its physicochemical characteristics. The relative volumes of the fluid compartments into which the drug can diffuse are shown in Figure 8.53. Total body water comprises 40% intracellular and 20% extracellular fluid (ICF and

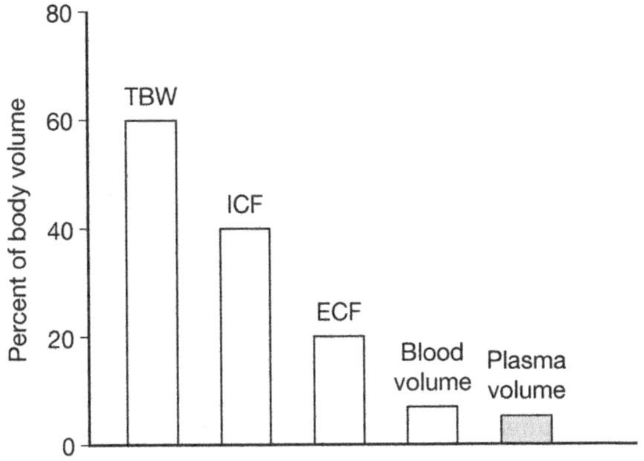

Figure 8.53 Distribution of fluid within the body. TBW, total body weight; ICF, intracellular fluid; ECF, extracellular fluid.

ECF, respectively). The ECF comprises interstitial fluid (15%) and plasma (5%). The total blood volume (TBV) is 8% of body water, the 3% of the body water associated with red cells being counted as part of the intracellular fluid volume. The localisation of a drug into blood cells is often studied since it provides a measure of how the compound will distribute into other tissues. Apart from water, the overall body composition is made up (approximately!) as follows: water 60%, protein 18%, fat 15% and minerals 7%.

Most substances in the blood distribute rapidly throughout the ECF. The extent of penetration into the ICF depends on whether or not they can traverse the cell membranes and specialised barriers including the blood–brain barrier, the blood–CSF barrier and the placenta. Localisation within these tissues depends on specific binding to proteins and the lipid content of the cell. The majority of tissue membranes behave as typical lipid barriers. Because the body can be thought of as a closed compartment, the amount of drug available is a feature of weight, and calculations are often made on a mg/kg basis. This can produce problems if age and body fat are not taken into account. There is a risk that an obese person treated with a water-soluble drug will have transient concentrations higher than expected, whereas a highly lipid soluble drug will be cleared faster than expected from plasma due to partitioning into fat. This leads to uncertainty is setting an optimal dosage regimen.

Equilibrium drug concentration ratios are maintained by diffusion of drugs into and out of tissues, across membranes which are selective for relatively lipid soluble materials. Less commonly, active transport is involved in the movement of drug molecules across tissue membranes.

Lipid solubility and drug action

There is good evidence that the majority of the central nervous system is surrounded by a specialised barrier which behaves as an extreme form of lipid membrane. This membrane is highly selective for lipid-soluble foreign molecules (xenobiotics) which are transferred rapidly by simple diffusion. The lipidic nature of the blood–brain barrier often leads to drug molecules being freely exchanged between brain cells and plasma water, while metabolites of the same compound do not penetrate the brain. Lipid-soluble molecules generally leave the brain by the route by which they arrived, by diffusion back through the blood–brain barrier. This diffusion process is driven by the need to maintain a constant ratio of drug concentration in brain and plasma water in the face of falling plasma drug levels resulting from metabolism and excretion.

Some examples of drug distribution

Tissue distribution of thiopental

Thiopental is a barbiturate drug with extremely high lipid solubility. It is used as a general anaesthetic. The effect of thiopental is very short-lived, and the effect wears off as the result of loss of the drug from plasma, brain, liver and other highly vascularised tissues, to muscle and fat. The drug is not metabolised or excreted particularly rapidly and sufficient additional doses can be given to achieve a long-lasting anaesthesia. Localisation of this drug in tissues occurs entirely by passive diffusion. The concentration of the drug in fat, which is negligible at first, rises continuously with each dose and thus each successive dose exerts a duration of action longer than the previous dose, until an excessively long-lasting effect occurs even when administration ceases. It was suggested that this was due to saturation of tissues (muscle and fat) so that an excessive amount of the drug remained in circulation after dosing had ceased. Anaesthesia wears off during the distribution phase following the first dose. Subsequent doses then exert their effects as before, superimposing on the elimination phases of the earlier doses. The rapid succession of administered does not allow complete distribution of the drug to occur, the concentration in fat (which is not saturable) maintains plasma concentrations above the threshold required for an anaesthetic effect.

Tissue distribution of guanethidine

Guanethidine depletes catecholamine stores and is thus useful in the treatment of hypertension. This compound shows interesting distribution kinetics. Concentrations of guanethidine were measured in four tissues and in the plasma of rats over a 24-hour period following intravenous doses of 28 mg/kg. For liver kidney and plasma a constant equilibrium concentration ratio was achieved instantaneously which was maintained for as long as the drug was detectable in plasma. The heart, however, showed a difference because guanethidine is maintained at a high concentration in this tissue by an active transport process.

Tissue distribution of diazepam and N-desmethyldiazepam

Diazepam is converted metabolically to N-desmethyldiazepam. A study of the relationship between blood, brain and adipose tissue has been carried out for the two compounds in mice. Blood and brain concentrations of diazepam decreased from the time of administration, whereas adipose tissue concentrations reached a maximum at 30 minutes. The metabolite (N-desmethyldiazepam) showed a growth and decay pattern in blood with a peak at 60 minutes. The brain concentration followed a similar time course, but the adipose tissue concentration reached its peak considerably later. This peak was also later than that of diazepam, and the tissue-to-plasma concentration ratios were less for the metabolite in comparison with those for diazepam. Note that the peak drug concentration is achieved within 1 hour, whereas the peak concentrations of the metabolite occur at 8–10 hours post dosing.

Since the N-desmethyldiazepam is also active pharmacologically, the period of response (the pharmacodynamic profile of the drug) does not follow the blood level of the parent substance.

There are three general principles applicable to tissue localisation:

- The degree of localisation will depend on the lipophilicity and binding properties of the drug.
- An equilibrium concentration ratio will eventually be reached, after which the tissue and plasma concentrations will change in a similar fashion.
- The speed with which this equilibrium is reached will be governed by the blood supply to the tissues.

BUCCAL DRUG DELIVERY

The epithelial lining of the oral mucosa is composed of squamous cells with a characteristic layered structure formed by the process of cell maturation. The composition of this layer varies according to the tissue functions; the hard palate and tongue, for example, are composed of keratinised epithelium whilst the lining of the cheek is distensible and non-keratinised. The thickness of the epithelium also varies in the buccal cavity (Table 8.5). The buccal cavity, like the entire alimentary canal, behaves as a lipoidal barrier to the passage of drugs. Only small lipophilic drugs with a favourable partition coefficient at the pH of the saliva (6.2–7.4) will be absorbed (Log P of 1.5–3.5).

Since blood supply to and from the face enters the circulation near to the heart, the liver does not have the opportunity of removing the material prior to entry into circulation. As a consequence, drugs which are unstable in the stomach and intestine may be reasonably well absorbed in the buccal cavity. Examples include the nitrates and formulations such as Temgesic® which delivers buprenorphine sublingually and Buccastem® which delivers the antinausea drug prochlorperazine via the buccal route. The lining under the tongue is thin and drugs placed sublingually are absorbed rapidly. The site is, however, unsuitable for long-term delivery as the tongue would flick it away. The buccal pouch – between gum and cheek – is more suitable and is used for delivery of drugs prophylactically. Anything which isn't swallowed is easy to retrieve, which forms the focus of attention for the use of this site to deliver potent pain-controlling agents such as morphine.

Examples of buccal delivery systems

There are many different formulations:

- *Sublingual tablets* Use: Relief of anginal pain (nitrates), buprenorphine, prochlorperazine. Advantage: Fast onset of action. Issues: Taste, potency.
- *Lozenges* Use: Palliative for sore throats, drug delivery, e.g. fentanyl. Advantage: Nice taste. Issues: Tooth decay, effectiveness, coverage.
- *Adhesive tablets* Use: Delivery of many materials. Advantage: Can be used for long treatment duration. Issues: Loss of drug in swallowed saliva, potency.

Table 8.5 Different types and thickness of epithelia in the buccal cavity

Tissue	Location	Thickness (μm)	Keratinisation	Polarity of lipids
Buccal	Cheek Upper and lower lip	500–600	No	Polar
Sublingual	Frenulum Floor of mouth	100–200	No	Polar
Gingival	Gums	200	Yes	Non-polar
Palatal	Roof of mouth	250	Yes	Non-polar

- *Chewing gums* Use: delivery of nicotine. Advantage: moderately fast onset of action, discourages eating. Issues: Taste, addiction.
- *Buccal patches* Use: Delivery of potent agents. Advantage: can occlude surface avoiding loss, tissue permeation enhancers. Issues: Cost, potency.
- *Mouth rinses and sprays* Use: Delivery of panaesthetics, antimicrobials, antifungals, fluoride. Advantage: patient acceptability and coverage of buccal cavity, easy for patients. Issues: Residence time, potency.

Bioadhesion

In order to hold a drug delivery device in place, it may be necessary for the formulation to be adhesive or to be formulated with adhesive excipient. The interaction of glue and glycocalyx occurs due to pressure or to water being withdrawn from the buccal epithelium. Treatment advantages were first noted by dental surgeons treating persistent infections. The oral cavity contains a diversity of microorganisms and over 300 different species of bacteria have been identified in the mouth. The density of microorganisms is high and saliva which contains 10^7–10^8 bacteria per millilitre. Most bacteria in the mouth are commensals and may have a protective role against pathogenic bacteria. Oral infections are categorised as primary bacteria-associated diseases where bacteria cause diseases such as caries, chronic gingivitis, and inflammatory periodontal disease and secondary disease. Secondary infections are characterised by aggravation of existing damage associated with contaminated tissue. Antibacterial agents are used in the treatment of chronic gingivitis and effective agents, such as chlorhexidine, can persist for many hours. However, most topical drugs delivered into the mouth tend to be rapidly dislodged or diluted. The role of a vehicle is to sustain retention and maintain a high concentration gradient; this may give sufficient time for the material to be absorbed onto plaque. Antimicrobial plaque inhibitors are effective in preventing formation rather than destroying established plaque and most formulations are based on toothpaste, gels and mouthwashes. Chewing gum and varnishes have been used in order to achieve medium-term delivery. Such agents are of no value in the treatment of chronic peridontitis unless delivered directly into the pocket by irrigation or sustained delivery vehicles. Treatment of buccal infections with penicillins was improved by the incorporation of sodium carboxymethylcellulose into white paraffin. Squibb developed further hydrocolloids including pectin and gelatin in polyethylene oxide/mineral oil as delivery systems for treatment of mucosal infections with triamcinolone acetonide and hydrocortisone. Later developments moved towards the employment of single components such as xanthan gum as non-ointment bases.

The surface of the gut epithelia is covered with a glycolcalyx. The mucus gel adhering to mucosal surfaces is composed of polydisperse high molecular weight glycoproteins with molecular weights in excess of 1.8×10^6. The protein spine of mucus consists of around 800 amino acid residues to which sugar chains are attached (*ca.* every three residues) to yield approx 200 side chains with the main linkage through serine and threonine. Glycoproteins adsorb well on practically all surfaces and interact with other macromolecules. The salient rules are as follows:

- The higher the molecular weight, the better the adsorption.
- A polymer of higher molecular weight and the same chemistry displaces the same polymer of lower molecular weight.
- Macromolecules are good glues because they stick to each other with ease using multiple contacts. Even when present at low concentration, they saturate binding sites.
- Macromolecular adhesion layers are viscoelastic. They can both carry and distribute stress.

OESOPHAGEAL TRANSIT

Oesophagus

The oesophagus is a 25-cm long, 2-cm diameter muscular tube which joins the pharynx to the cardiac orifice of the stomach. The stratified squamous epithelium lining the buccal cavity continues through the pharynx and down the oesophagus. The lowest 2 cm or so of the oesophagus, which lies within the abdominal cavity, is normally lined with gastric mucosa and covered by peritoneum. The stratified squamous epithelium provides a tough impermeable lining resisting the abrasive nature of food boluses, whilst the gastric mucosal lining resists damage by gastric acid. The lumen of the oesophagus is highly folded in the relaxed state. The pH of the normal oesophageal lumen is usually between 6 and 7.

The functions of the oesophagus are to facilitate the delivery of boluses of liquids, food and medication from the oropharynx to the cardia of the stomach and to prevent the reflux of acid contents into the oropharynx. The environment of the oesophagus is wet rather than moist and the walls are lined with squamous epithelium with few secretory glands. The liquid that bathes the oesophagus therefore comes from swallowed saliva or liquid taken in with the diet.

Oesophageal tissue resembles that seen in the buccal cavity: stratified squamous epithelium. Due to the contact with the food, the cells near to the lumen are dead. Liquid is only provided by swallowed saliva – note the absence of secretory cells. Oesophageal retention of a formulation containing an irritant drug can lead to damage to the mucosa, ulceration and even stricture or perforation. Damage is produced by a prolonged contact of the drug at high concentrations with the mucosa. Oesophageal ulceration has been reported for many drugs including emepronium bromide, some antibiotics especially tetracycline, theophylline and non-steroidal anti-inflammatory drugs. Tablets tend to stick about two-thirds of the way down the oesophagus. If the heart is enlarged, the ventricle tends to push against the oesophagus.

Factors predisposing formulations to adhere, in order of importance

In general, there are several factors which predispose a formulation to adhere:

- shape of dosage form
- size of dosage form
- position of subject
- volume of water with which the dosage form is administered
- surface characteristics of the dosage form.

When a dose form gets lodged, either a large volume of water or intake of food is required to shift the adhered tablet since water flows over the non-contact surface, and does not dislodge the zone of bioadhesion.

THE STOMACH

The major function of the stomach is to temporarily store food and release it slowly into the duodenum. It processes the food to a semi-solid chyme which enables a better contact with the mucous membrane of the intestine, thereby facilitating absorption of nutrients. The stomach reduces the risk of noxious agents reaching the small intestine, first by a bacteristatic action of the gastric juice and secondly (if all else fails!) by stimulation of the vomiting reflex.

Contrary to popular belief, very little drug absorption occurs in the stomach; more significantly, it provides a barrier to the delivery and hence absorption of drugs by the small intestine. The motility patterns which are responsible for gastric emptying depend on the nature and frequency of food intake and are therefore extremely variable within and between individuals. The stomach is located below the diaphragm, but its exact position varies with the volume of food ingested, posture, skeletal build and the tone of the abdominal muscles

The human stomach secretes between 1.0 and 1.5 litres of gastric juice per day. This juice is highly acidic because of its hydrochloric acid content, and it is rich in enzymes. Gastric juice provides a medium for soluble food particles to dissolve and it initiates digestion, particularly for proteins. Gastric pH is primarily influenced by two factors: acid secretion and gastric content. In a 24-hour period, the median daytime pH for eight subjects was 2.7 (range 1.8–4.5) in the body and 1.9 (range 1.6–2.6) in the antrum of the stomach. Food buffers and neutralises gastric acid, producing an increase in pH. The pH is not uniform in the stomach, due to the differences in the distribution of parietal cells, and the different patterns of motility in various regions of the stomach. By measuring stomach pH it was found that a meal raised the pH in the fundus to approximately 4.5, but this rapidly began to decline, returning to baseline after 2.5 h. The pH in the body of the stomach was slower to respond, again increasing to about 4.5, 15 min later than the fundus. This region returned to basal pH 3.5 h after meal ingestion.

Acid secretion is increased after hot or cold meals even though temperature of the meal per se does not alter gastric emptying. It takes significantly longer for cold meals to be brought to body temperature than hot meals. Content of the meal also affects gastric pH; for example, a pure carbohydrate meal given as a pancake has no detectable effect on acidity, while a protein meal of similar calorific value has a significant buffering effect. A liquid meal, rather than a mixed-phase meal, with a balance of carbohydrate and protein, has a strong buffering effect but the pH rapidly returns to basal levels as the liquid is emptied. The situation is complicated by feedback effects; for example, pepsin normally hydrolyses proteins to peptides and amino acids, which are potent secretagogues, and increase the acidification of gastric contents. However, pepsin is inactivated above pH 5, so a large meal which raises the pH above this value will prevent the production of these substances, and peak gastric acid secretion will be reduced. Changes in gastric pH occur after a light meal. Normal people produce a basal secretion of up to 60 mL hr^{-1} with approximately 4 mmol of H^+ per hour, which rises to more than 200 mL and 15 to 50 mmol H^+ when maximally stimulated. In both sexes, the basal acid output does not change significantly with age, but the maximal acid output decreases progressively but not significantly. After the intake of food, the buffering action of the proteins and the dilution of hydrogen ions provided by the acid bulk cause the pH to rise. Gastric juice can be produced at 200 mL per hour with a hydrogen ion concentration of 150 mM. Resting pH is usually around 1.8 and not 1.0 as suggested in some textbooks!

The surface of the mucosa is always covered by a layer of thick, tenacious mucus that is secreted by the columnar cells of the epithelium. Gastric mucus is a glycoprotein which lubricates food masses, facilitating movement within the stomach, and forms a protective layer over the lining epithelium of the stomach cavity. Mucus is secreted by cells which are concentrated at the neck of the gastric gland. The mean thickness in man is about 140 μm. It provides the important function of protection from autodigestion by the pepsin and acid of the lumen. The production of bicarbonate under the mucus blanket and the inability of strong acid to penetrate mucus (acid interacts with mucus to surround itself with precipitated mucin, preventing back diffusion), combine to provide protection.

Gastric emptying occurs even during fasting. After a meal, the indigestible remnants need to be evacuated – this occurs about 2 hours after the duodenum receives no more calories – and the housekeeper sequence or migrating myoelectric potentials are triggered.

In the fed state, the duodenum receives substrates which cause a feedback inhibition. This is mediated by a rise in the wall tension which opposes the flow of liquid from the stomach.

Liquids and solids empty at different rates – this is due to the differential functions of the fundal and pyloric regions of the stomach. The intake of calories may be associated with a significant lag phase before gastric emptying occurs. This can cause a change in the rate of emptying of pelleted dose forms according to whether they are given before or after a meal.

Heavy meals decrease the rate of gastric emptying of tablets. Enteric coated or enteric matrix tablets may not empty readily from the stomach on a heavy feeding regimen. This effect is very large if the formulation is taken in the morning with a heavy breakfast as the continual intake of food suppresses the housekeeper sequence. The discrimination between the emptying of dosage forms in the presence of food is very evident when the tablet size exceeds the diameter of the pylorus.

INTESTINAL ABSORPTION

Anatomy and physiology

The small intestine is between 5 and 6 metres in length and its main functions are to mix food with enzymes to facilitate digestion, to mix the intestinal contents with the intestinal secretions to enable absorption to occur, and to propel the unabsorbed materials in an aboral direction. The small intestinal epithelium has the highest capacity for nutrient and drug absorption within the gastrointestinal tract, due to the large surface area provided by epithelial folding and the villous structures of the absorptive cells. The small intestine is the longest section of the digestive tube and it is arbitrarily divided into three parts. The first 20 to 30 cm is termed the duodenum, the second 2.5 metres the jejunum and the final 3.5 metres the ileum. This tissue has the highest capacity for nutrient and drug absorption within the gastrointestinal tract due to the large surface area provided by epithelial folding and the villous structures of the absorptive cells. The small bowel is arbitrarily divided into three parts, the first 20 to 30 cm is termed the duodenum, the second 2.5 metres the jejunum and the final 3.5 metres the ileum. These regions are not anatomically distinct, although there are differences in absorptive capability and secretion. The small intestine consists of the serosa, the muscularis, the submucosa and the mucosa. The serosa is an extension of the peritoneum, and consists of a single layer of flattened mesothelial cells overlying some loose connective tissue. The muscularis has an outer longitudinal layer and an inner circular layer of muscle. The submucosa consists largely of dense connective tissue sparsely infiltrated by lymphocytes, fibroblasts, macrophages, eosinophils, mast and plasma cells. The submucosa contains an extensive lymphatic network. The mucosa of the small intestine has a surface area which is greatly increased by the folds of Kerckring, villi and microvilli (brush border) and is about 200 m^2 in an adult. The surface of the mucous membrane of the small intestine possesses about five million villi, each about 0.5–1 mm long. Although the villi are often described as 'finger-like', their shape changes along the gut, and duodenal villi are shorter and broader than those found in the jejunum. Further down the gut the villus height decreases. Diet and environment markedly affect mucosal morphology.

The epithelium which covers the intestinal villi is composed of absorptive cells, goblet cells, a few endocrine cells and tuft or calveolated cells. The absorptive cells or enterocytes, are tall, columnar cells, with their nuclei located close to their base.

The principal permeability barrier is represented by the luminal surface of the brush border. Most drugs are absorbed by passive diffusion in their un-ionised state. The pH of the small intestine determines the degree of ionisation and hence controls the efficiency of absorption; this is the basis of the pH-partition theory of drug absorption. Protein binding at the serosal side of the epithelium helps maintain a concentration gradient by binding the absorbed drug, which is then removed by blood flow from the absorption site.

Between cells, epithelial brush borders come into close contact and under the electron microscope it appears as if the membrane is fused. However, functionally, the tight junctions are not sealed but are permeable to water, electrolytes and other charged or uncharged molecules up to a certain size. The size of the 'pore' varies along the length of the gastrointestinal tract and can be calculated from recoveries of polyethylene glycols of various molecular weights. Intercellular transport may be important for oligosaccharides and small peptides, which is an area of considerable current interest.

There is a special mode of permeation across the intestinal wall in which the cell membranes are not involved. Intestinal cells are continuously produced in the crypts of Lieberkühn and migrate towards the tip of the villus. During digestion, the cells are sloughed off, leaving a temporary gap at the cell apex and through this gap large particles can slip into the circulation. This has been termed 'persorption'. The observation that large objects such as starch grains can be found in the blood after a meal of potatoes or corn is often quoted as the prima facie evidence of persorption or phagocytosis.

Although the absorption of most drugs can be explained by passive diffusion, some compounds have specific transport mechanisms. An example is the absorption in the intestine of some penicillin derivatives, e.g. cyclacillin (1 aminocyclohexylpenicillin). This process is saturable, proceeds against an unfavourable concentration gradient and shows temperature dependence. Transport of amoxicillin is also carrier mediated but it is not an active process. Since these materials are xenobiotics, the transport mechanism is probably one which serves some other function in the body. The two penicillins probably share the same carrier since they are mutually competitive. Digitalis and other cardioselective glycosides also demonstrate behaviour not compatible with simple partition theory which suggests carrier-mediated transport.

Food effects on drug absorption

As shown in previous sections, food markedly alters the delivery of drug taken with a meal. The presence of food may influence the absorption of several drugs and can either enhance, delay or reduce absorption. Food can adsorb or absorb drug, and the metal ions present in food such as milk can chelate drug or the drug can bind to dietary proteins, thus changing its bioavailability. The presence of viscous chyme can act as a physical barrier reducing drug access to the absorbing surface. The absorption of drugs such as penicillin V and G, theophylline and erythromycin is reduced by the presence of food, but food delays absorption of such drug as cimetidine, metronidazole and digoxin. Certain components of food, notably fibre, have a particularly important effect on drug absorption. Fibre is known to inhibit the absorption of digoxin and entrap steroids. It is well accepted that foods with a high content of polyvalent metals such as calcium, magnesium, iron, aluminium and zinc, such as milk products, inhibit the absorption of tetracycline and reduce availability. Doxycycline has a slightly lesser tendency to form chelates, thus milk reduces its bioavailability somewhat less than other tetracyclines.

Small intestinal transit time of dosage forms

During fasting, both monolithic and multiparticulate dosage forms will be swept rapidly through the small bowel by the migrating myoelectric complex.

The action is propulsive and not mixing in nature, thus a capsule containing pellets given on an empty stomach may leave the stomach and pass down the small intestine as a bolus with minimal dispersal. The increased dispersal of pelleted formulations within the small intestine when the formulations are taken with a meal occurs because the pellets become dispersed in the food mass within the stomach. As their particle size is small, pellets will continue to be emptied from the stomach as part of the chyme, thus prolonging their delivery to the small intestine. Monolithic tablets, on the other hand, depending upon their size, will empty erratically from the stomach after food and as the single unit traverses the small bowel. Hence, the presentation of the drug to the small intestinal mucosa will depend solely upon its dissolution characteristics in each area. The degree of spread of a formulation within the small intestine is particularly important for drugs with poor solubility or for drugs which are slowly transported across the epithelium. Microparticulate dosage forms show longer and more reproducible median transit times compared with single-unit tablets, giving rise to more predictable and uniform blood levels and reducing the risk of enlodgement and mucosal damage. A review of data suggests that the small intestinal transit is around 4 hours for solutions, pellets and single-unit formulations. Small intestinal transit of dosage forms is not affected by their physical state, size or the presence or absence of food, but high calorific loads may slow it slightly, although the majority of the effect is on gastric emptying.

Fat has a marked inhibitory effect on small intestinal transport. This effect has been used experimentally to increase the absorption of moderately absorbed drugs such as riboflavin.

Once material has entered the small intestine, transit through to the ileocaecal junction appears to be remarkably consistent, irrespective of particle size, shape or viscosity. The mean intestinal transit time in humans is between 3 and 4 hours, though faster transit in vegetarians has been noted.

Absorption of drugs from mesenteric lymphatic vessels

Absorption of the fat-soluble vitamins A, D, E and K all exhibit significant, if not total, absorption via the lymphatic route. Some lipophilic drugs also enter by this route, at a rate dependent on the availability of lipid. Note that the lymphatic system avoids the first-pass effect. The lymph vessels, in contrast to the blood vessels (where arteries and veins form a circuit), begin from blind vessels from the central lacteals of the villi.

In the GI tract, the lymph is drained at a rate of the order of a few cubic centimetres per minute. The lymph plexuses of the entire GI tract are collected into the mesenteric lymph duct and enter the circulation near to the heart through the subclavian vein. The total flow rate of the lymph in the thoracic duct is approximately 100–200 mL/h.

Factors that increase drug transport into the systemic circulation via the lymph vessels

Entry of a drug molecule in the lymph is normally associated with the transport of triglycerides in the lymph vessels. Fats, taken up from the GI fluids in the form of fatty acids and monoglycerides are reconverted in the enterocyte to triglycerides. Within the cytoplasm these are packaged into lipoprotein structures, of which the most important are the chylomicrons. The concentration of chylomicrons in the lymph generally ranges between 1% and 2%. The anabolic process of simple lipids is complicated. Most drugs enter the lymph vessels bound to the triglyceride part of the chylomicrons and of the very low density lipoproteins (VLDL).

After arrival in the systemic circulation the drug is released from the chylomicrons, either due to hydrolysis of the triglycerides (by the lipoproteinic lipases of the blood), or by diffusion of the drug from an intact chylomicron to the water of the plasma. For these reasons, the possibility of a drug being transported via the lymph depends on the physicochemical properties of the administered drug, as well as the quantity and the properties of the co-administered lipid carrier which is used to induce the intracellular production of chylomicrons.

COLONIC DRUG ABSORPTION

Table 8.6 shows the conditions in different parts of the gastrointestinal tract. The large intestine is responsible for the conservation of water and electrolytes, the formation of a solid stool and storage until a convenient time for defecation. Unlike the small intestine, the residence time in the large bowel can be highly variable, ranging from as little as a few hours to as long as 1 week. In most individuals, dietary and social habits condition the time of defecation. The majority of adults defecate once a day, although frequencies from 2 per day to once every 2 days are considered normal.

For the purposes of drug delivery, the colon has to be considered as two regions; the distal colon, which can be reached from the anus, and the proximal colon, which is only accessible via the oral route. The splenic flexure limits the area of exposure of drugs administered by the anal route to the descending and sigmoid colon, rectum and anus.

The colonic mucosa is devoid of villi and therefore the colonic surface area is very much reduced compared with the small intestine. The other noticeable feature is the many goblet cells, which increase the thickness of the mucous layer to 300 μm in the distal small intestine.

After the hepatic flexure, the consolidation of faecal matter gradually increases the viscosity of the luminal contents with a resulting difficulty of diffusion of drug to the absorbing membrane. Therefore only in the ascending colon are conditions favourable for drug absorption. Limited work has been carried out on investigating the behaviour of pharmaceutical preparations in the colon, but present knowledge suggests that it is possible to optimise delivery systems for topical release of drugs to the colon, taking into account the predictable and nutritionally independent nature of small intestinal transit. The major problems are reduced surface area, wider lumen, sluggish movement, low volume of available dissolution fluid and the reduced permeability of the colonic epithelium to polar compounds. Thus it would be expected that the absorption of most drugs from the colon is slower than from the small intestine, but this is balanced by the longer residence time in this part of the gastrointestinal tract. There is considerable variability in the colonic transit times. Work in the USA has shown marked differences between males and females, indicating that the colonic musculature may be influenced hormonally. The ingestion of food causes large increases in propulsive activity (mass movements). This increased activity may terminate the action of a drug in the colon by movement of the lumenal contents to the descending colon, where the viscosity and mucus forms a significant diffusional barrier.

The colonic microflora contain up to 400 different species of both aerobic and anaerobic bacteria. The most prevalent anaerobes are *Bacteroides* sp. and Bifidobacterium whilst the most numerous aerobes are *Escherichia coli*, enterococci and *Lactobacillus*.

Table 8.6 Comparison of the environment in different parts of the gastrointestinal tract

Region	Length (m)	Surface area (m^2)	pH	Residence time	Microorganisms
Oesophagus	0.3	0.02	6.8	>30 seconds	unknown
Stomach	0.2	0.2	1.8–2.5	1–5 hours	$\leq 10^2$
Duodenum	0.3	0.02	5–6.5	>5 minutes	$\leq 10^2$
Jejunum	3	100	6.9	1–2 hours	$\leq 10^2$
Ileum	4	100	7.6	2–3 hours	$\leq 10^7$
Colon	1.5	3	5.5–7.8	15–48 hours	$\leq 10^{11}$

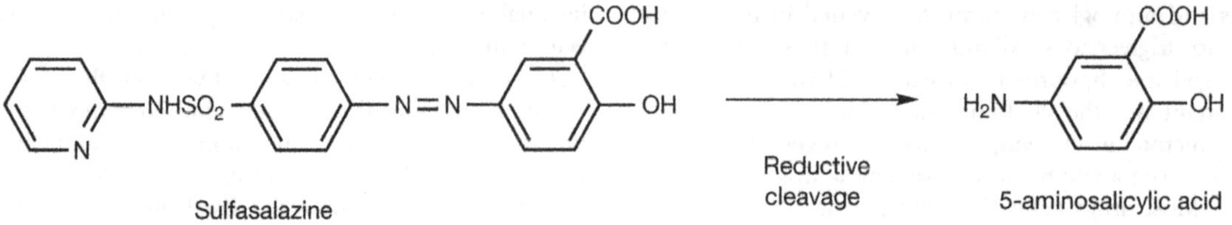

Figure 8.54 Cleavage of sulfasalazine by bacterial azo-reductase.

The major site of bacterial activity is the caecum where the anaerobic bacteria ferment substrates (e.g. soluble fibre) in a liquid mixture. The fermentation in the caecum produces a marked drop in the pH of the luminal contents. The low oxygen tension in the colonic lumen encourages reductive conditions and this principle has been used to deliver drugs specifically to the colon in the treatment of ulcerative colitis. pH studies using a pH-sensitive radiotelemetry capsule in normal, ambulatory volunteers have shown that the mean pH in the colonic lumen is 6.4±0.6 in the ascending colon, 6.6±0.8 in the transverse colon and 7.0±0.7 in the descending colon. The azo-bond of sulfasalazine is cleaved by bacterial azo-reductase activity to release the active component 5-aminosalicylic acid (Fig. 8.54).

Drugs are not necessarily absorbed as well in the large bowel as in more proximal tissues. This appears to be due to the tighter intercellular junctions in the epithelial cells. Triggered release of drugs in a radiofrequency-fired pill monitored by X-ray has shown that more polar drugs including furosemide and atenolol are poorly absorbed in the colon; thus sustained release formulation of such compounds are not practical.

Rectal administration of drugs

The rectal route is often used when administration of dosage forms by mouth is inappropriate, for example in the presence of nausea and vomiting, unconscious patients, if upper gastrointestinal disease is present which could affect the absorption of the drug, if an unpleasant tasting drug is used, and for gastro-labile drugs. It has been argued that a significant advantage of the rectal route might be the avoidance of first-pass metabolism. Venous return from the colon and upper rectum is via the portal vein to the liver. If a drug is delivered to the upper part of the rectum, it is transported into the portal system, and therefore does not escape metabolism in the liver. The only way of avoiding first-pass metabolism therefore is to deliver the drug to the lower part of the rectum. This simple principle is complicated by the presence of anastomoses which do not allow a precise definition of the areas which drain to the portal and systemic circulation. The presence of portal hypertension (as in cirrhosis) causes a redirection of blood flow which would favour avoidance of first pass.

Gut diseases and drug absorption

Diarrhoea causes changes in the electrolyte content of the colonic lumen which therefore alters luminal pH, resulting in changes in the rate of absorption of drugs from the lumen. Diarrhoeal diseases cause decreased gut transit time and cause incomplete metabolism of prodrugs such as sulfasalazine. The increased rate of transit would also be responsible for the premature voiding of sustained-release formulations before complete drug release.

Patients with Crohn's disease are subject to gastrointestinal strictures where a controlled-release matrix may lodge and cause epithelial damage due to the release of concentrated drug at one site over a prolonged period of time. A similar iatrogenic condition arose in the treatment of arthritic patients with indometacin in a non-disintegrating dosage form (Osmosin). In a few patients with clinically silent diverticular disease, the units fell into the small intestinal pouches, causing perforation into the peritoneal cavity.

Chapter | 9 |

Structure, activity and drug design

David G Watson

CHAPTER CONTENTS

INTRODUCTION

Much of modern drug discovery took place between 1930 and 1980 before there was a comprehensive understanding of how drugs can be specifically designed to work in a particular way. For example, the non-steroidal anti-inflammatory drug indomethacin (Fig. 9.1) was produced since there was a theory that serotonin was involved in inflammatory processes.[1] However, although there are links between serotonin and inflammation, it acts at specific transmembrane-spanning receptors, whereas indomethacin is an inhibitor of cyclooxygenase enzymes. Alternatively, bioactive lead compounds, bearing no direct resemblance to the biomolecule of interest, have often been found by random testing. For example, compound 929 F (Fig. 9.1) was tested for its activity in blocking the action of histamine and most subsequent antihistamine compounds bear some resemblance to it although it does not closely resemble histamine itself.

The additional tranquillising effects shown by antihistamines then gave rise to antipsychotic agents such as chlorpromazine. Thus, to some extent, the formulation of the rules governing structure activity relationships of drugs has been carried out retrospectively. As outlined in Chapter 1, there are several types of intramolecular bonding involved in drug action, ranging from covalent bonds through to hydrogen bonds and van der Waals forces. All of these forces are utilised in the modification of a lead compound into a successful drug. Since the focus of this book is on pharmaceutical, rather than medicinal, chemistry, this chapter will concentrate more on explaining relationships between existing drugs rather than focusing on how to discover new ones.

ISOSTERES

Isosteres are structural elements that are deemed to have more or less equivalent chemical or physical properties, and they have been used extensively in modification of lead compounds in order to enhance drug action. Table 9.1 shows some classical isosteres. The definition of an isostere is an atom or a group in which the peripheral layers of electrons are identical.[2] However, this definition is not adhered to and, for instance, F is often considered as a substitute for H although it has three lone pairs of electrons in its peripheral layer whereas H does not have any. Thus the strict definition of isosteres quite quickly breaks down and, for instance, benzene can be substituted for by a number of ring types and carbonyl and carboxylate substituted by groups which are not that close to them in structure. Thus isosteric substitution is not an exact science.

Substitution of isosteric components can alter the activity of a compound. For example, one of the first non-steroidal anti-inflammatory (NSAID) compounds produced was mefenamic acid. Its structure derives from that of salicylic acid, the first non-steroidal anti-inflammatory drug. First there is an isosteric substitution of NH_2 for OH in salicylic acid (Fig. 9.2), which causes loss of anti-inflammatory activity. Then a dimethylbenzene group is added to the NH_2 group as a substituent to produce the

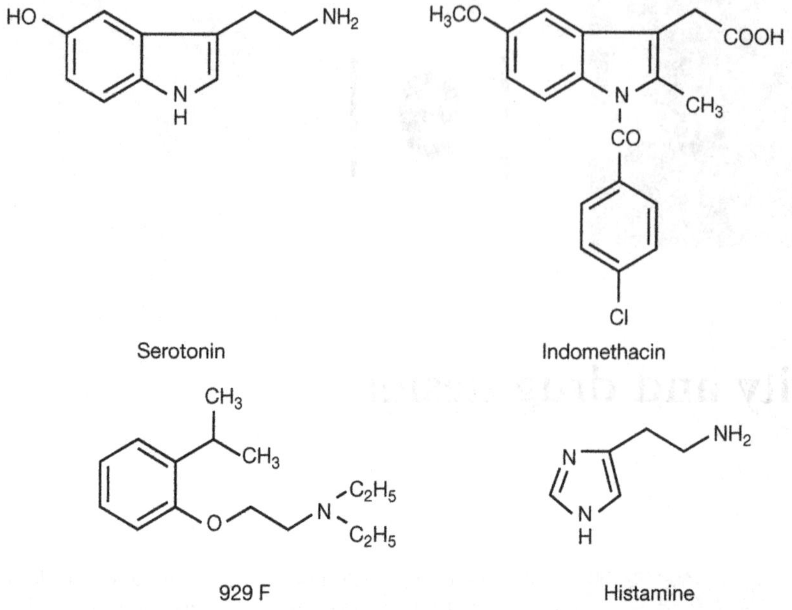

Figure 9.1 Serotonin, indomethacin, 929 F, histamine.

Table 9.1 Classical isosteres

Type of group	Isosteres
Univalent	H, F, Cl
Univalent	CH_3, NH_2, OH, F, SH, Cl, CF_3,
Univalent	Br, i-Pr
Univalent	I, t-Bu
Bivalent	$-CH_2-$, -NH-, -O-, -S-.
Trivalent	-CH=, -N=
Rings	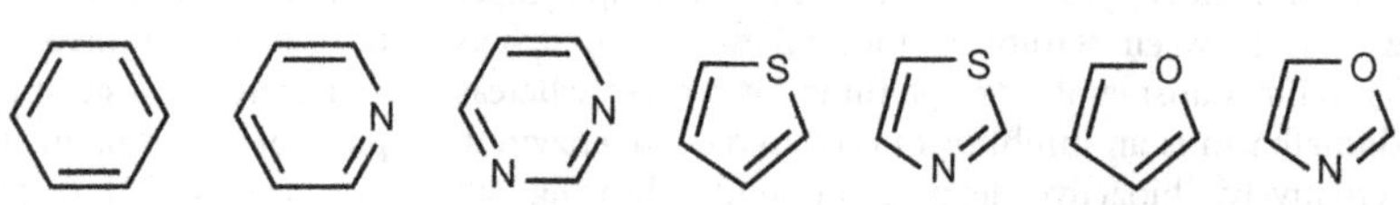
Carbonyl CO	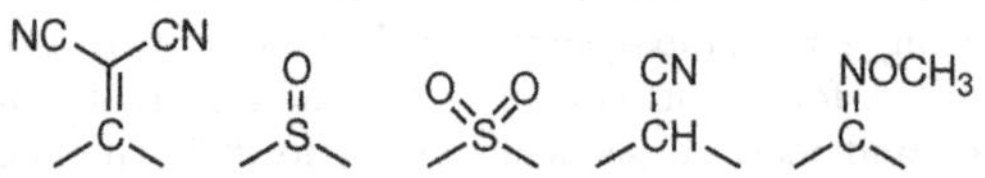
Carboxyl COOH	CONHR SO_2NH_2 SO_2NHR SO_3 CONHCN

NSAID mefenamic acid (Fig 9.2). This has the effect of making the resultant NH group into a very weak base so it is hardly charged at stomach pH and not at all at plasma pH. In diclofenac (Fig. 9.2) an isosteric substitution of chlorine for the methyl groups in mefenamic acid is made and the carboxyl group is separated from the ring by a CH_2 group. These small alterations cause increase in potency, with diclofenac having about five times the potency of mefenamic acid. The exact reasons for the increased potency cannot be defined although one site of metabolism is removed in substituting Cl for methyl since in mefenamic acid the 3′-methyl group is a

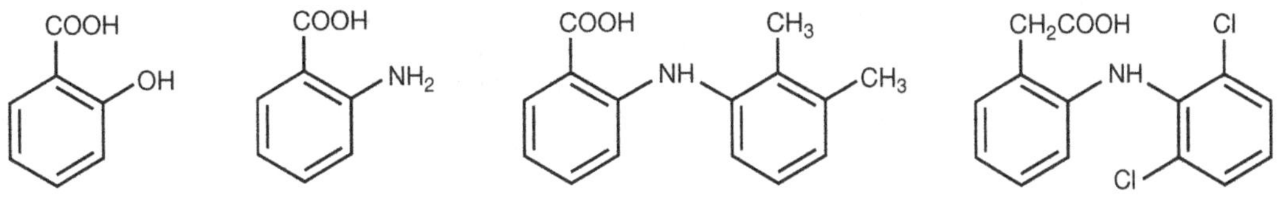

Salycylic acid — Anthranilic acid — Mefenamic acid — Diclofenac

Figure 9.2 Isosteric substitution on non-steroidal anti-inflammatory agents.

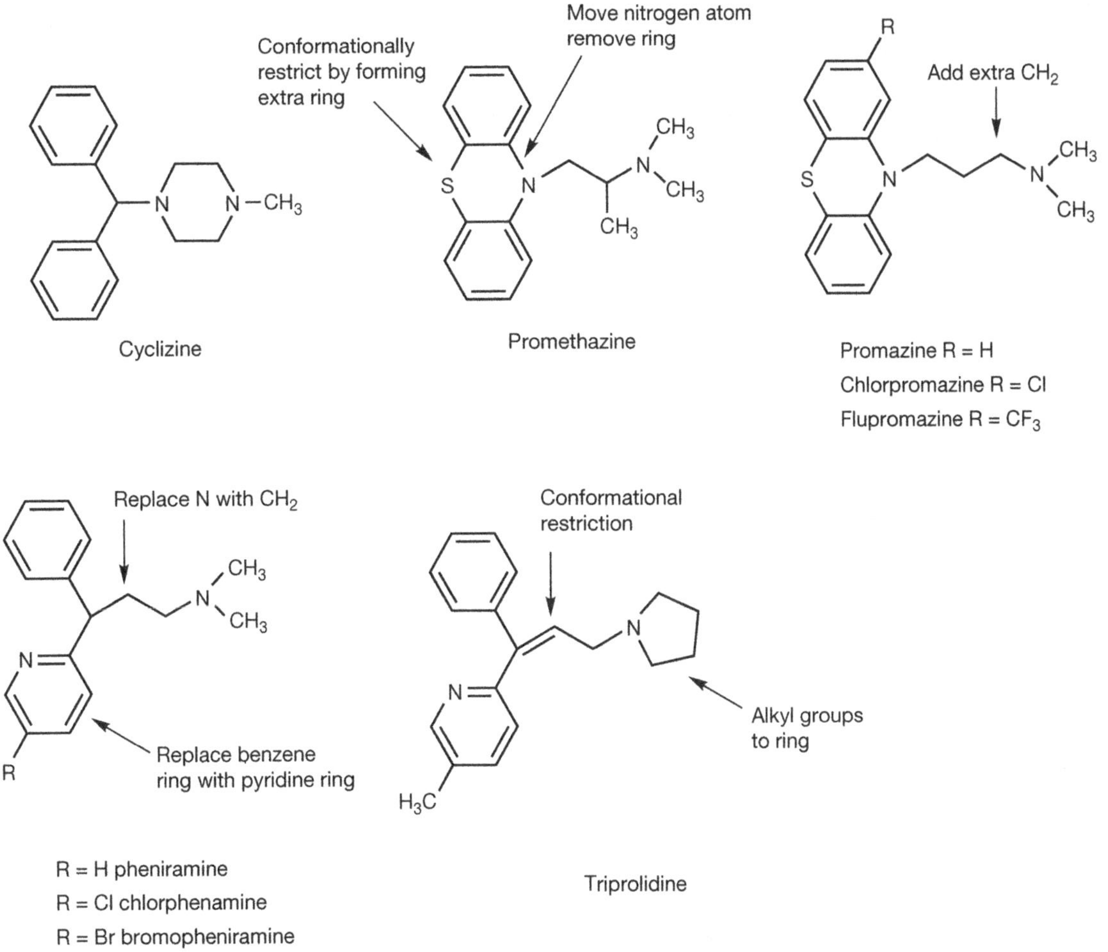

Figure 9.3 Isosteric changes in antihistamine compounds.

site of metabolism being converted to a carboxylic acid (*cf.* chlorpropamide and tolbutamide, Ch. 4) and moving the carboxyl group away from the aromatic ring weakens the acidic group slightly.

Similar types of isosteric substitution can be seen in the evolution of antihistamines with the addition of ring to chain transformations and ring formation. The conversion between rings and chains is a common modification in the evolution of a drug structure. The introduction of a ring restricts the stereochemical conformations that a drug can take, which can potentially increase potency. Cyclizine (Fig. 9.3) was one of the first antihistamines. Its structure was evolved in a number of different directions. Isosteric substitution of nitrogen for carbon, conversion of the ring to an open chain and locking of the two benzene rings together with a sulphur atom led to promethazine which is somewhat more potent than cyclizine. Both drugs are currently used to treat nausea. Addition of an extra methylene unit into the side chain of promethazine and removal of the methyl group substituted onto the side chain led to its isomer, promazine. The small structural change led to the development of a series of antipsychotic agents based on promazine, which is still used as an antipsychotic. The simplest modifications were isosteric substitutions of hydrogen by chlorine and by trifluoromethyl, producing chlorpromazine and flupromazine which have higher partition coefficients than promazine and thus greater CNS penetration and higher potency.

The replacement of the nitrogen atom in the side chain of cyclizine by carbon and isosteric replacement of one of the benzene rings by a pyridine ring led to pheniramine which was further elaborated by replacement of a hydrogen atom by chlorine or bromine thus increasing potency. In triprolidine conformational restriction is introduced into the side chain via a double bond and the methyl groups attached to the nitrogen in the side chain are changed into a ring, increasing potency further.

During the golden era of drug discovery between 1930 and 1980 there was often no clear awareness of isosteres in drug design, but retrospectively it is possible to see a pharmacore evolving through a series of compounds, often starting with one type of biological activity and finishing with another. For example, the biological effects of atropine (Fig. 9.4) which occurs in some members of the solanaceous plants, e.g. deadly nightshade, was known for centuries due to its effects as an antagonist of cholinergic receptors. Thus plant extracts containing atropine were

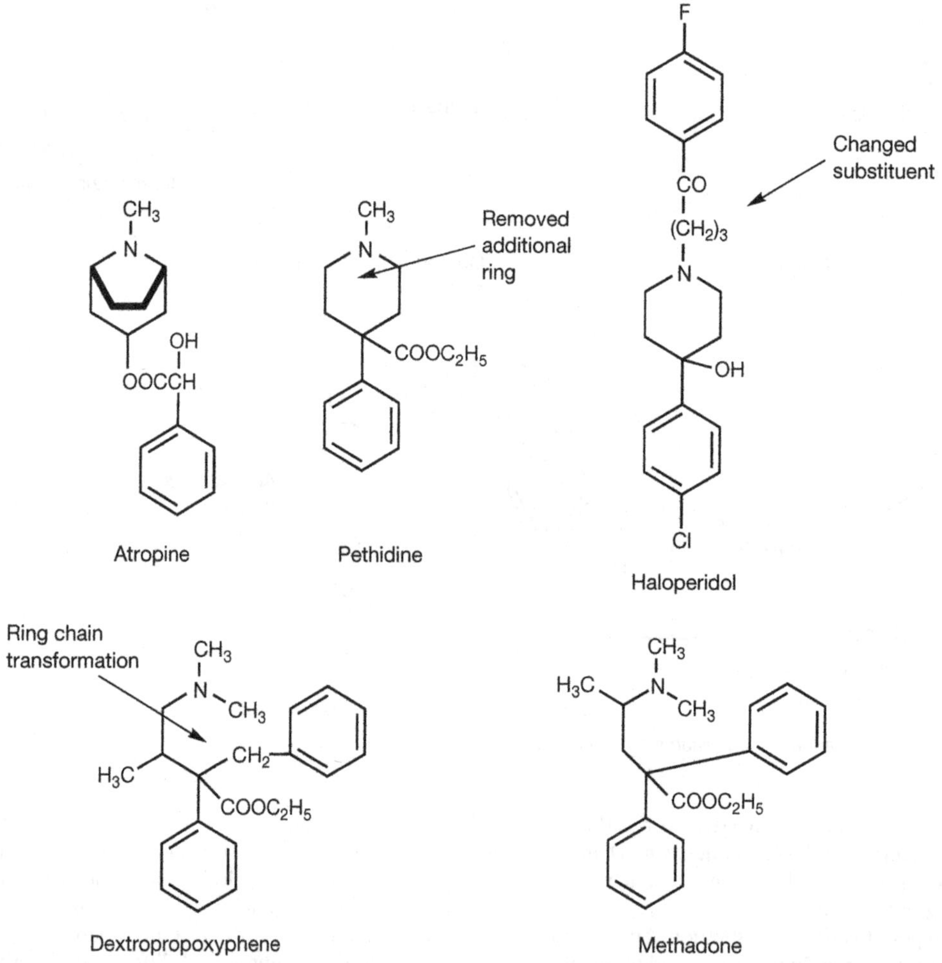

Figure 9.4 Development of the atropine pharmacophore.

used to treat colic by relaxing the smooth muscle of the gut and for pain relief in neuralgia. The structure of atropine is close to that of the synthetic analogue pethidine, which is used in analgesia, and the basic pharmacophore is also retained in haloperidol, which is used as a sedative to control hyperactive psychotic states. In moving to dextropropoxyphene, the piperidine ring was converted into a chain producing an analgesic which does not have the addictive potential of pethidine. The structure of methadone is also based on this basic pharmacophore and again has analgesic properties and is used as a morphine substitute since it is orally bioavailable.

Q Self Test 9.1

Indicate obvious isosteric changes in the evolution of the diuretics shown below from hydrochlorthiazide. Outline the structural element which is the most important pharmacophore.

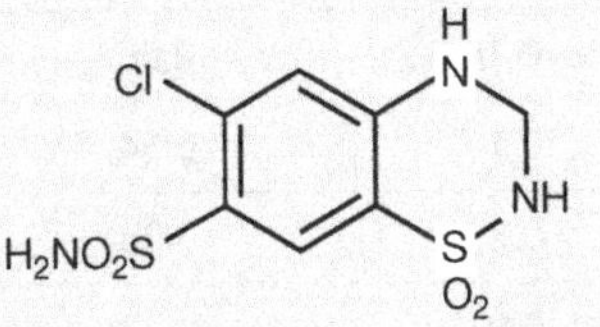

Hydrochlorthiazide

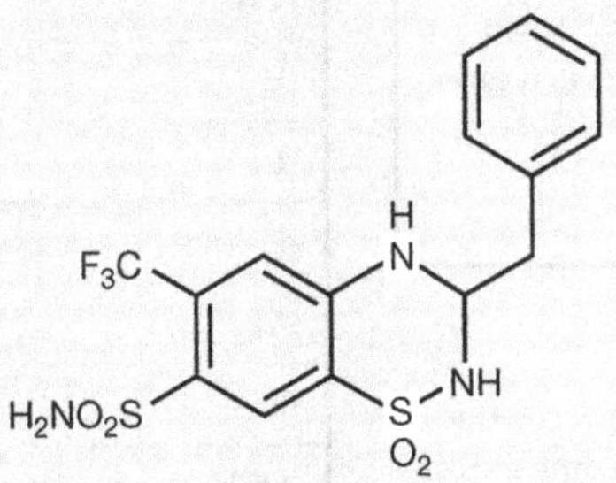

Bendrofluazide

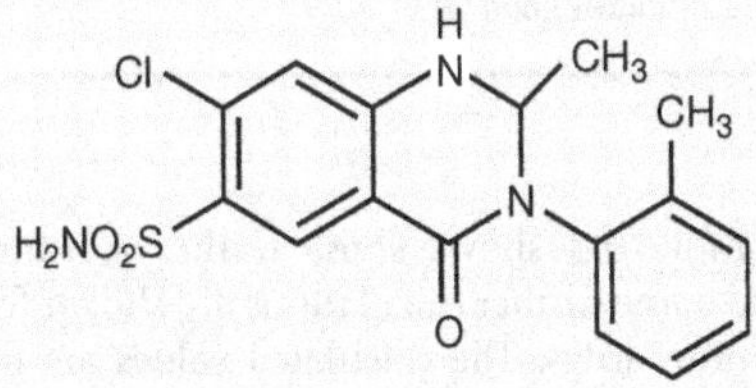

Metolazone

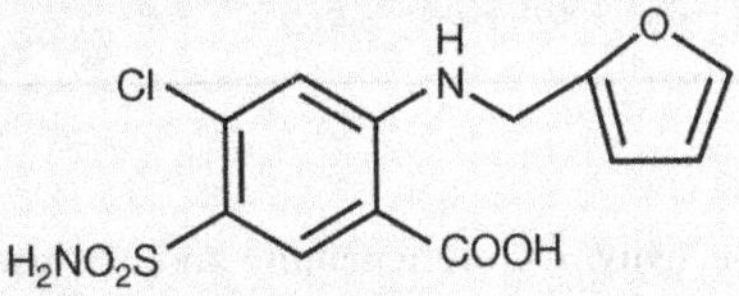

Furosemide

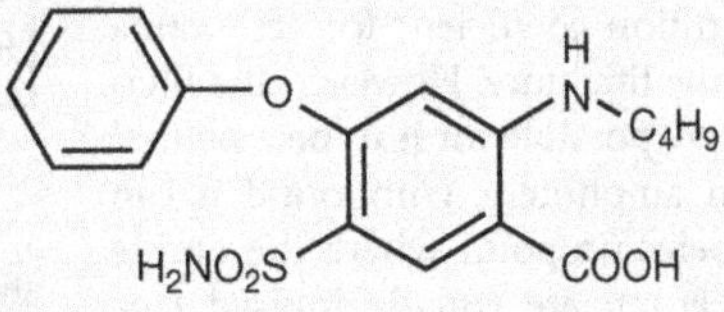

Bumetanide

INTRAMOLECULAR FORCES GOVERNING DRUG ACTION

Lipophilicity

The importance of lipophilicity in the interaction of drugs with membranes has been discussed in Chapter 2. Lipophilicity is governed by van der Waals forces and these have been discussed in Chapter 1. It is difficult to focus on one type interaction within a drug since the overall interaction of the drugs with proteins and membranes depends on all the forces outlined in Chapter 1. Thus the overall interaction may involve covalent bonding, ionic bonding, dipole–dipole interaction, hydrogen bonding, charge transfer or van der Waals interaction. However, it is simplest to consider one factor at a time. The simplest type of structure activity relationships can be viewed when one factor is varied while everything else is held constant. A classical series for illustrating how substituent groups affect partition coefficient is provided by the barbiturates, which are rarely used because of their addictive potential. The Hansch approach to estimating partition coefficients (log P values) uses substituent coefficients (π). Table 9.2 gives some Hansch substituent coefficients. The values can be applied in the calculation of theoretical partition coefficients for the barbiturates shown in Figure 9.5. The higher the partition coefficient the greater the penetration into the CNS and thus the higher the sedative potency. The larger the lipophilic subsituent the higher the partition coefficient. Many compounds do not fall into such a convenient series for the calculation of log P.

Table 9.2 Hansch π-values

Group/residue	π
barbiturate ring	−1.35
N-methyl barbiturate ring	−1.07
-CH-/-CH_2-/CH_3-/-C=	0.50
C_6H_5-(phenyl)	1.96
Cyclohexen-1-yl	2.21
-CH_2-(ring residue)	0.40

The following increments are deducted if the alkyl group is either branched or contains a double bond or both:
Each branch (π) = −0.2
Each double bond (π) = −0.3

Table 9.3 Some examples of Hansch π and σ constants

Substituent	π	ρσ
-COOH	−0.32	0.41
-COO-	−4.36	−0.1
-OH	−1.12	−0.38
>N—	−1.23	−0.66
-CN	−0.57	0.5
-H	0	0
-Cl	0.71	0.23
-F	0.14	0.06
-CF_3	0.1	0.54
-Br	0.86	0.23
-OCH_3	−0.02	−0.27
Pyridine ring	0.5	0.44
CONH	−1.49	0.36
$Log\ 1/C = -a\pi^2 + b\pi + \rho\sigma + cE_s + dS + e$		

Table 9.3 shows some further substituent constants, and some further calculations are shown for some antihistamine drugs. The calculated values are not in complete agreement with the literature; however, calculated values are never perfect and the π-constants vary within the literature. Comprehensive lists of these are available.[3] The calculated octanol/water partition coefficient for acrivastine does not agree well with the literature. However, the literature is reported as if it were possible for it to be a neutral species but since it is an amphoteric compound it can only be neutral at its isoelectric point where the amine group and the carboxyl group are equally ionised (see Ch. 7 for discussion of isoelectric points). Taking a naive approach and putting all the charge on the carboxyl group produces a partition coefficient which is too low. An important point is made by the examples shown in Figure 9.6, which is that partition coefficient alone does not predict activity. Chlorphenamine and acrivastine are of a similar potency as antihistamines but differ in their partition coefficients. The Hansch approach has been refined over the years and an example of the Hansch equation is shown below:

$$Log\ 1/C = -a\pi^2 + b\pi + \rho\sigma + cE_s + dS + e$$

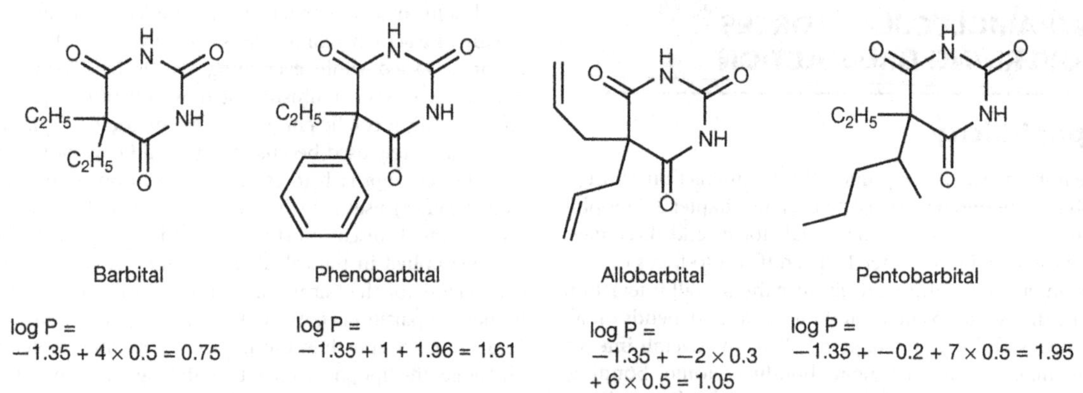

Figure 9.5 Calculation of partition coefficients for barbiturates.

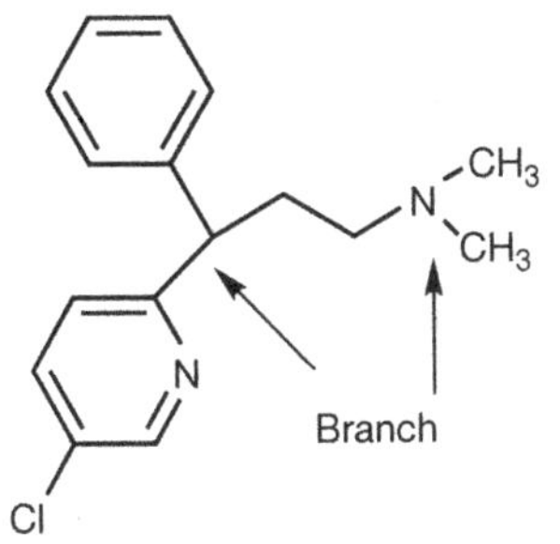

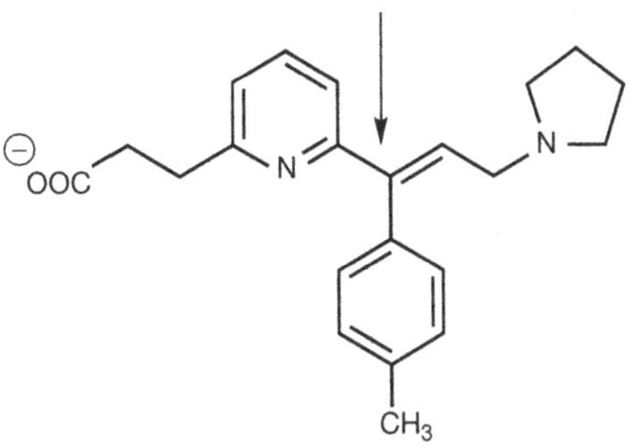

1.96 (Ph) + 0.5 (pyridine) + 0.71 (Cl)
+ 5 × 0.5 (CH/CH_2/CH_3)
− 2 × 0.2 (branches)
− 1.23 (amine)
= 4.04 (Literature 3.38)

1.96 (Ph) + 0.5 (pyridine) 6 × 0.5 (CH/CH_2CH_3)
+ 5 × 0.4 (ring CH_2) − 1.23 (amine) − 4.36 (COO−) − 0.2 (branch) = 1.67
(Literature 2.83)

Figure 9.6 Hansch calculations for two antihistamines.

The terms in the equation can be explained as follows:

Log1/*C* gives an indication of the potency of the drug and is the molar concentration which gives 50% of maximal response, whether this is enzyme inhibition (IC_{50}) or receptor agonism/antagonism (LD_{50}). The lower the value of this term, the lower the potency of the drug.

The term $-a\pi^2$ relates to the substituent constants that we have already considered. It takes account of the fact that for any drug there is an optimum partition coefficient and thus a plot of potency against partition coefficient is a parabola. The term a is experimentally derived from the observation of how large the partition coefficient has to be before potency starts to reduce. The $b\pi$ reflects the positive contribution of partition coefficient to activity and obviously the constant b has a much larger value than a. The term $\rho\sigma$ gives an indication of the contribution of the electronic nature of functional groups to the activity of the molecule; in simple terms it indicates which groups can be substituted for each other in optimising structure activity. Of course, not all groups in the molecule are critical to its activity. Table 9.2 shows some σ constants; negative values indicate that the substituent donates electrons to the structure and positive values indicate electron withdrawal. The values given in the table only apply to substituents attached to benzene ring and this is a weakness of the Hansch approach. The terms E_s and dS relate to the shape of the molecule. The complexity of the parameters within the Hansch equation means that complex computer models have to be set up in order to predict activity from structure. Still, the vast majority of drugs on the market have not been designed in a particularly rational way. One modern approach which will be considered throughout this book is drug optimisation based on a better understanding of the structures of the proteins which are the targets of drugs. The availability of protein crystal structures and sometimes the structures of co-crystals with a ligand bound to a protein assist in getting a better understanding of what governs the binding of a drug to an enzyme or a receptor. Where the structure of a co-crystal of the drug with its target is available, it is possible to see directly what the important interactions between the drug and amino acids in the protein are. In the absence of a co-crystal, molecular docking studies can be carried out where computer simulation of the interaction of the drug with its binding site is carried out in order to determine the likely mode of binding and how binding might be optimised in order to design more potent analogues of the drug.

A Self Test 9.1

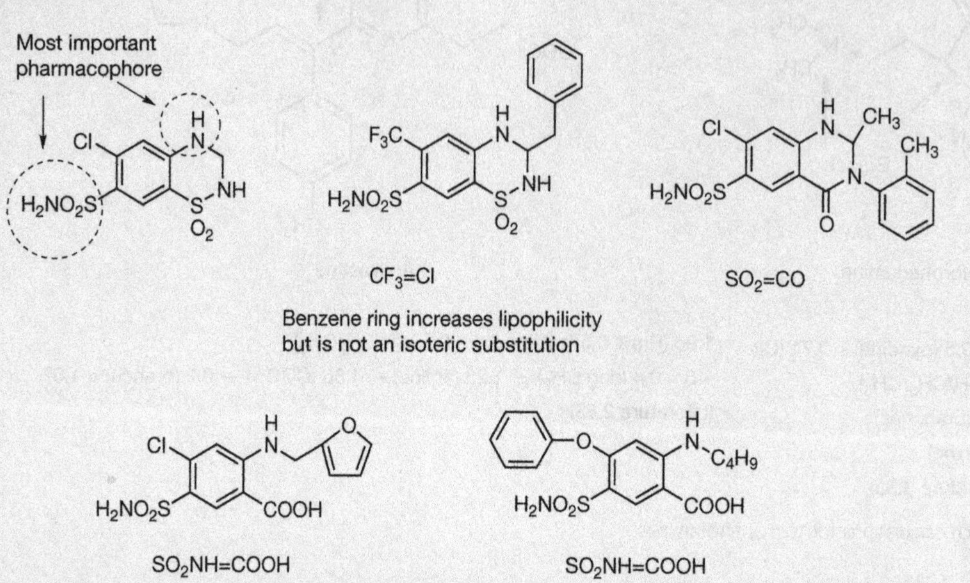

REFERENCES

1. Sneader W. *Drug Disovery. A History*. John Wiley and Sons; 2005.
2. Silverman RB. *The Organic Chemistry of Drug Design*. 2nd ed. Elsevier Academic Press; 2004.
3. Hansch C, Leo A, Hoekman D. *Exploring QSAR. Hydrophobic, Electronic and Steric Constants*. American Chemical Society; 1995.

Chapter | 10 |

Drugs affecting the adrenergic system

David G Watson

CHAPTER CONTENTS

SUMMARY OF PHARMACOLOGY

- The pharmacology of the adrenergic system is complex. There are four main types of receptor: β_1 and β_2 receptors and α_1 and α_2 receptors.
- The main effects of the receptors are:
  - β_1 increases heart rate and force of contraction.
  - β_2 receptors dilate bronchioles and blood vessels.
  - α_1 constricts blood vessels, bronchioles and bladder sphincter; increases blood sugar.
  - α_2 receptors constrict blood vessels.
- Noradrenaline is the neurotransmitter involved in regulating the adrenergic system; it acts at α and β receptors but is most potent at α receptors.
- Adrenaline is a methylated metabolite of noradrenaline and functions as a circulating hormone. It is released from the adrenal gland and acts at both α and β receptors but is most potent at β receptors.
- Drugs can act in this system at several points (Fig. 10.1)
  - Stimulate or block β_1, β_2, α_1 or α_2 receptors.
  - Reduce noradrenaline reuptake into the neuron and function as false neurotransmitters.
  - Reduce noradrenaline synthesis.
  - Reduce noradrenaline release from vesicles.

INTRODUCTION

The vasoconstricting effects of adrenaline were first observed in 1897 in extracts from adrenal glands and the drug was first synthesised in 1904. Adrenaline has one chiral centre and it was observed early on that synthetic adrenaline had half the potency of adrenaline isolated from adrenal glands since it consists of a racemic mixture of (−) biologically active R(−) adrenaline and the weakly active (+) adrenaline. Pure (−) adrenaline was isolated from the synthetic mixture produced by preparation of a diastereomeric tartrate salt (Fig. 10.2). The tartrate of R(−) adrenaline had a much lower solubility in methanol than the tartrate of S(+) adrenaline and thus it could be selectively crystallised while leaving the unwanted S(+) adrenaline tartrate in solution.

ADRENERGIC RECEPTORS

Adrenaline functions as a hormone being released from the adrenal gland in response to stress and acts most strongly at β receptors. Although noradrenaline (Fig. 10.3) has a very similar structure to adrenaline, its mode of release is

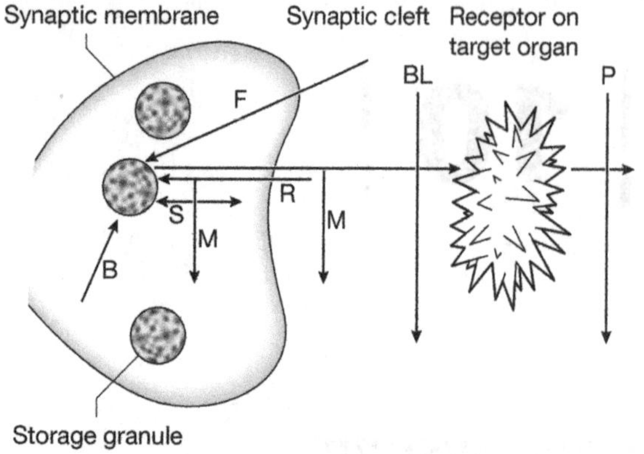

Figure 10.1 Targets for drug action in modulating noradrenergic neurotransmission B, biosythesis; S, storage; M, metabolism; D, depolarisation; R, reuptake; F, false neurotransmitter storage; BL, receptor blockade; P, post-receptor inhibition.

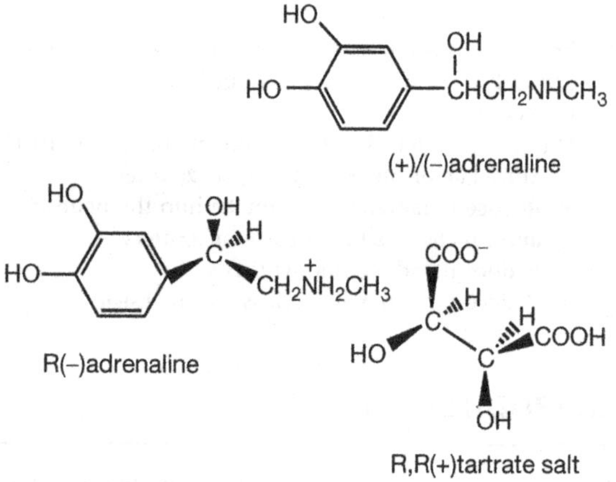

Figure 10.2 Racemic adrenaline and the (+) tartrate salt of (−) adrenaline.

quite different in that it is a neurotransmitter and is released from nerve terminals. Noradrenaline is most potent at α_1 and α_2 receptors but also has actions at β_1 and β_2. There are situations where both neurotransmitters act at the same β_1 receptors but via different routes. Thus noradrenaline increases heart rate by binding to receptors in the sinoatrial (SA) node upon release from sympathetic nerves adjacent to the SA node, while adrenaline binds to the same receptors when it is released into plasma from the adrenal medulla. The most potent adrenergic agonists have similar structural features to adrenaline. Thus one of the first agonists discovered was isoprenaline (Fig. 10.3) which has greater activity than adrenaline at the β receptors, indicating that an increase of the size of the alkyl group attached to the secondary amine group increases potency. This increase in the size of the alkyl group is carried to an extreme in the case of the selective β_2 receptor agonist salmeterol (Fig. 10.3). As might be expected, the activity of isoprenaline at α receptors, where noradrenaline is the natural ligand, is less than that of adrenaline, indicating the attachment of an alkyl group to the nitrogen represents a move away from the optimal pharmacophore at this receptor. However, in general, the structural requirements for action at α receptors are less precise than those required for activity at β-receptors. Thus clonidine (Fig 10.3), which bears little structural resemblance to noradrenaline, is an α receptor agonist albeit one which is much less potent than noradrenaline.

METABOLISM OF ADRENALINE AND NORADRENALINE

An important consideration in the development of drugs acting in the adrenergic system was to make them less suitable substrates for the enzymes which deactivate adrenaline

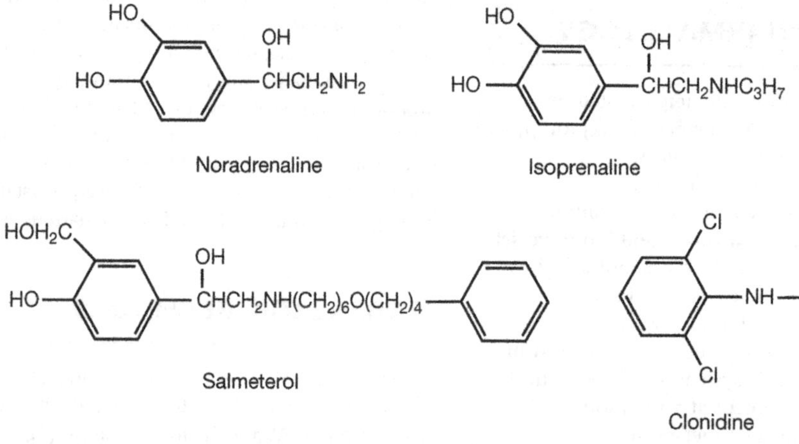

Figure 10.3 Some drugs which interact with the adrenergic system.

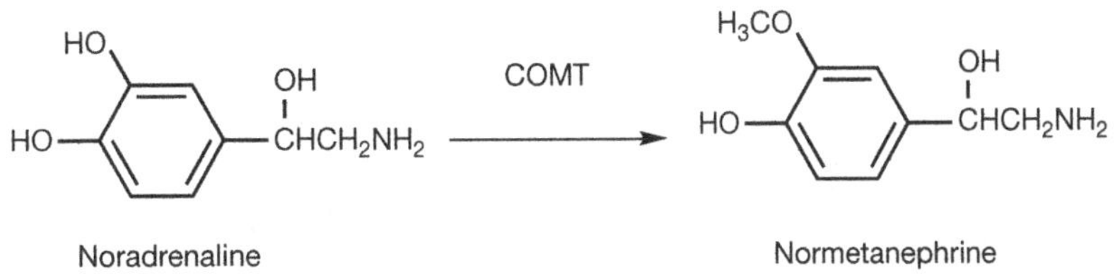

Figure 10.4 O-methylation of noradrenaline by COMT.

and noradrenaline by metabolism. Monoamine oxidase, discussed in Chapter 3, is an important route of metabolic deactivation for noradrenaline and adrenaline. In addition, catecholamines are deactivated via *O*-methylation by the action of the enzyme catechol *O*-methyl transferase (COMT). The action of this enzyme on noradrenaline is shown in Figure 10.4. The catecholamine group is essential for the biological activity of noradrenaline, and normetanephrine is inactive at adrenergic receptors.

COMMONLY USED DRUGS ACTING ON THE ADRENERGIC SYSTEM

Introduction

The adrenergic system is one of the most physiologically complex. The drugs discussed in this chapter will be described roughly in order of their frequency of usage. Thus we start with drugs acting at β_1 and β_2 receptors.

Drugs acting at β receptors

β_2 agonists

These drugs maintain structural similarities to adrenaline and follow on from isoprenaline which is a more potent agonist than adrenaline at β receptors. However, isoprenaline has potent effects on both β_1 and β_2 receptors and thus has undesirable effects on the heart. The agents that have replaced it are selective for the β_2 receptor and have reduced rates of metabolic deactivation. They are used in treating asthma and bronchospasm.

Terbutaline

Terbutaline (Fig. 10.5) was synthesised in 1968. As can be seen in Figure 10.5, it is an akanolamine like adrenaline. It is a selective agonist at β_2 receptors since the bulky t-butyl group abolishes activity at α receptors and reduces activity at β_1 receptors. Although it is a catecholamine the 3, 5 positions of the phenol groups prevent it being a substrate for COMT. The drug contains one chiral centre but it is administered as a racemate. Bambuterol is a prodrug of terbutaline where the phenolic groups in the molecule have been reacted to form carbamates. Carbamates are biologically very labile and hence bambuterol is readily converted to terbutaline in the body and offers a sustained delivery profile: a plasma half-life of 12 h as opposed to the 3–4 h obtained with terbutaline.

Description and preparations

Terbutaline sulphate is a crystalline solid soluble at 2% w/v in water and 0.12% in ethanol. Typical preparations include:

- Tablets 5 mg of terbutaline sulphate. Adult dose 2.5 mg to 5 mg 3× daily.
- Injection terbutaline sulphate 0.5 mg/mL. Adult dose 0.25–0.5 mg.
- Inhalation, nebuliser solution 2.5 mg/mL. Adult dose 0.25–0.5 mg metered dose.

Bambuterol hydrochloride preparations:

- Tablets 10 mg bambuterol hydrochloride. Adult dose 20 mg once daily.

Salbutamol

Salbutamol (Fig. 10.5) was synthesised in 1967. It is structurally very similar to terbutaline and its selectivity for β_2 receptors is similar to that of terbutaline. It is not a catecholamine and is thus not susceptible to deactivation by COMT. It has one chiral centre but is administered as a racemate.

Description and preparations

Salbutamol sulphate is a crystalline powder.

- Salbutamol sulphate tablets 2–4 mg. Adult dose 2–4 mg 3–4 times daily.
- Salbutamol sulphate injection 0.05–0.5 mg/mL. Adult dose subcutaneous injection 0.5 mg 4× daily.
- Sulbutamol sulphate aerosol inhalation. Adult dose: 0.1 mg metered dose.

Salmeterol

Salmeterol (Fig. 10.5) was introduced in 1988 and has 10 times the potency of salbutamol and is much longer acting. The large lipophilic chain attached to the amine in the side chain enhances activity at the β_2 receptor. Salmeterol can be used to control airways obstruction during sleep but is not used to control acute attacks. It is administered as a racemate.

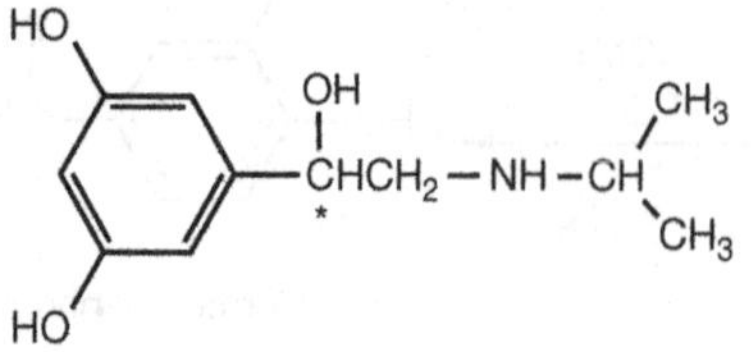

Orciprenaline

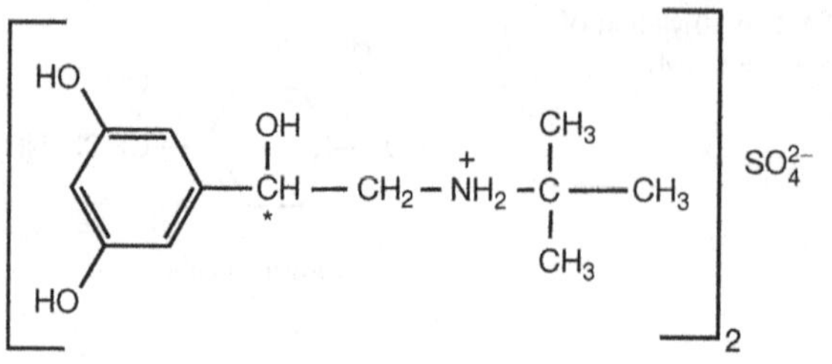

Terbutaline sulphate

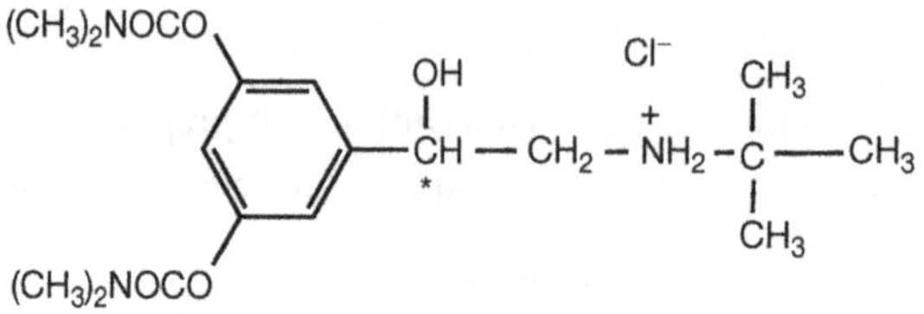

Bambuterol hydrochloride

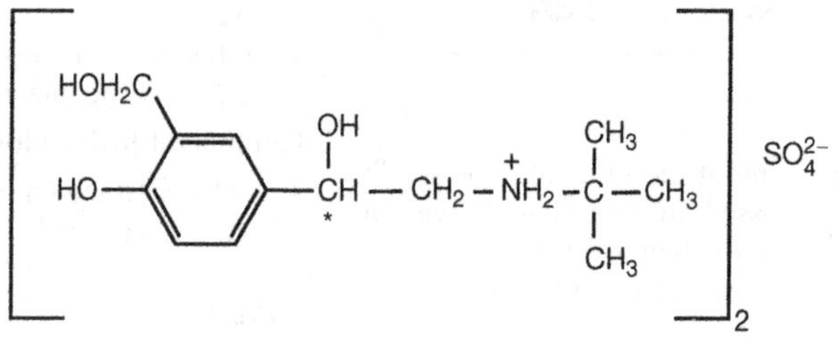

Salbutamol sulphate

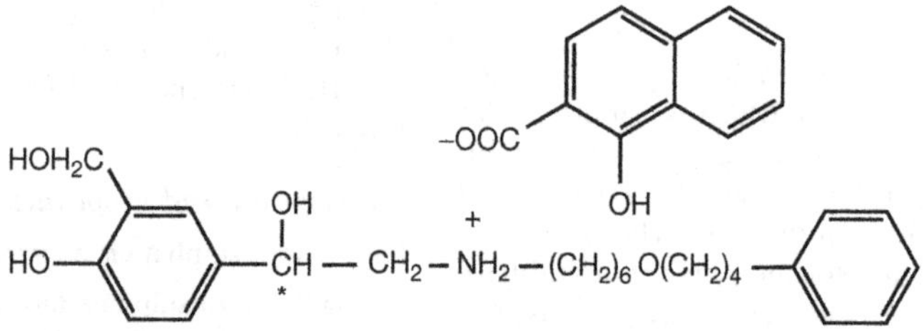

Salmeterol 1-hydroxy 2-naphthoate

Figure 10.5 Commonly used β_2-adrenergic agonists. * Denotes chiral centre.

Description and preparations

The drug is used as the 1-hydroxynaphthoate (Fig. 10.5) which is sparingly soluble in water and organic solvents apart from methanol in which it dissolves readily. Its poor water solubility, due to the use of a lipophilic counter-anion in the salt, makes it suitable for administration via dry powder inhaler.

- Salmeterol 1-hydroxynaphthoate formulated for dry powder inhalers. Adult dose 0.05 mg 2× daily from blister pack.

Formoterol

Formoterol (Fig. 10.6) is a variation on the structures discussed above in that it has lost a hydroxyl group from the

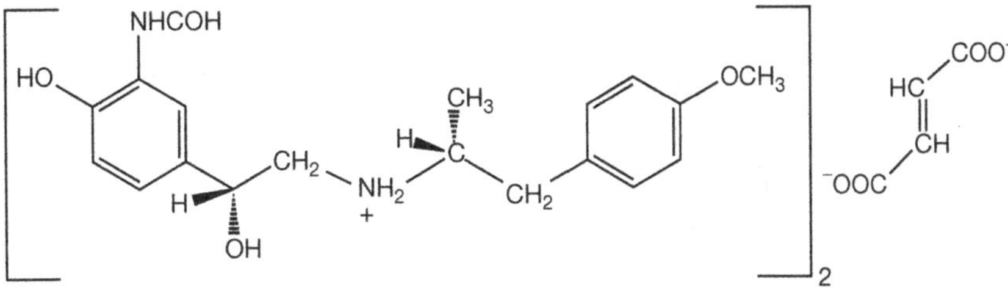

Formoterol fumarate RR isomer.
The drug is an enantiomeric mixture of RR and SS

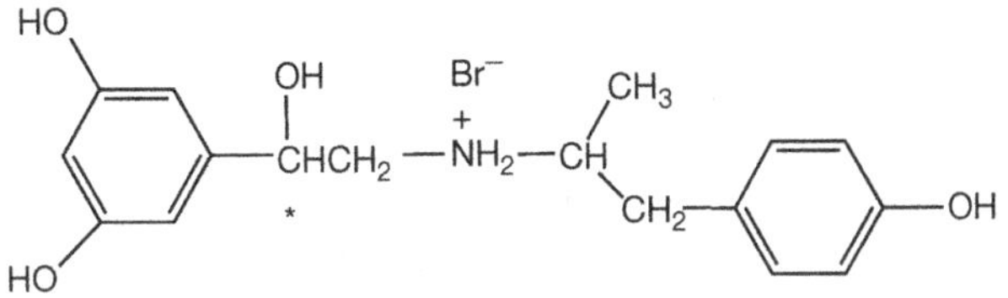

Fenoterol hydrobromide

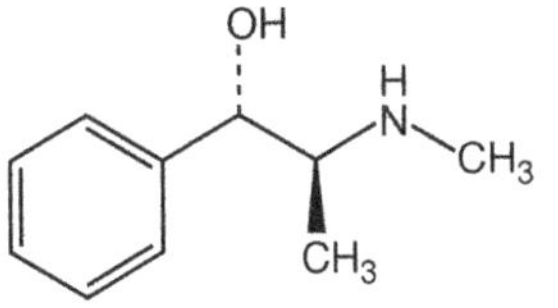

Pseudoephedrine

Figure 10.6

aromatic ring which has been replaced by a formamide. It contains two chiral centres and thus has four possible isomers composed of two pairs of enantiomers. The RR and SS pair of enantiomers (Fig. 10.6) is used therapeutically. Like salmeterol, fomoterol is a potent and long acting β_2 receptor agonist.

Description and preparations

Formoterol is used as its fumarate.

- Formoterol fumarate formulated for dry powder inhaler. Adult dose 0.012–0.024 mg twice a day from 0.012 mg dose unit.

Fenoterol hydrobromide

Fenoterol (Fig. 10.6) was patented in 1962 and was derived from orciprenaline (Fig. 10.4). It is a less selective β_2 agonist than, for instance, salbutamol.

Description and preparations

Fenoterol is used as its hydrobromide.

- Feneterol hydrobromide formulated for metered dose inhaler at either 0.1 or 0.2 mg per dose. Adult dose 0.1–0.2 mg 1–3 times daily.

Pseudoephedrine

Pseudoephedrine (Fig. 10.6) is a naturally occurring diastereoisomer of ephedrine and it is difficult to categorise because to some extent it resembles sympathomimetic amines (see Ch. 18). However, it has less vasoconstricting activity than these amines and it is widely used as a mild β_2 agonist being included in a wide range of proprietary cold cures.

Description and products

(+) R,R pseudoephedrine is used in the form of its hydrochloride.

- Pseudoephedrine hydrochloride tablets 60 mg. Adult dose 1 tablet 4 times daily as a nasal decongestant.

β_1 antagonists

The β_1 antagonists were developed over a similar timeframe as the β_2 agonists and in this case the goal was to achieve selectivity at the β_1 receptor so that therapeutic reduction of heart rate would not cause bronchoconstriction due to action at β_2 receptors or effects at α receptors. The structures were designed so that strong binding to the

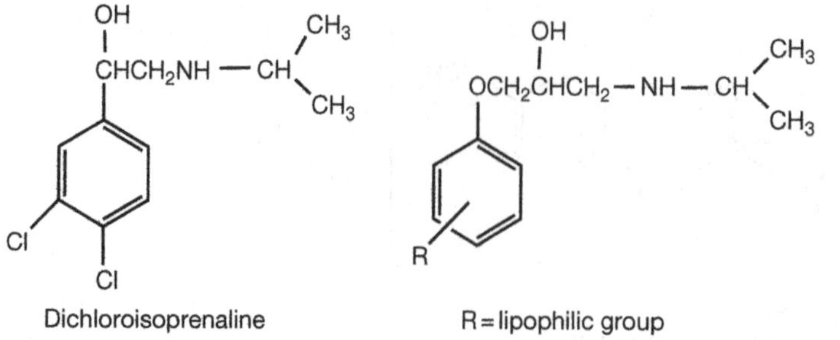

Figure 10.7 Dichloroisoprenaline, an early prototype of a β_1 antagonist and the general structure for later β_1 antagonists.

β_1 receptor would be achieved without triggering off the second messenger response linked to the receptor, i.e. the generation of cAMP. The generation of an agonist response at β receptors does require the structure of the agonist to resemble to quite a large extent the structure of adrenaline. The design strategy used was to omit the catecholamine group in the analogues initially synthesised. Thus one of the earliest agonists was dichloroisoprenaline which was discovered in 1957 (Fig. 10.7). Although this compound had antagonistic actions both at the β_1 and β_2 receptors it also had considerable agonist activity, i.e. essentially it behaved as a weaker agonist than adrenaline. Thus it was established that omitting the catechol group was a useful step towards pure antagonistic activity. The prototype for most β_1 antagonists was discovered in 1964 when the spacing between the aromatic ring and the side chain was changed by OCH_2 in comparison with adrenaline and propranolol (Fig. 10.8) was discovered. Propranolol remains in use as an antiarrythmic, antihypertensive and antianginal drug and most of the later drugs in this class are based on it. The majority of β_1 antagonists have the same side chain as propranolol but the substitution pattern of the aromatic ring varies a great deal. There are many β_1 antagonists now available and but it is often difficult to see clear advantages of one product over another. There have been no real advances in this therapeutic format in the last 25 years.

Propranolol

Propranolol is not completely selective as a β_1 antagonist and has antagonist activity at β_2 receptors causing bronchoconstriction; consequently, it is contraindicated in asthma. It does not have any agonist activity; thus it does not affect the heart rate at rest. It also, because of its high degree of lipophilicity, tends to enter the CNS and produce side effects such as bad dreams. Propranolol contains one chiral centre but it is used in the form of its racemate.

Description and products

Propranolol hydrochloride (Fig. 10.8) is freely soluble in water and ethanol but insoluble in organic solvents.

- Propranolol hydrochloride tablets 10–80 mg. Adult dose 80 mg twice daily for hypertension.
- Propranolol hydrochloride capsules 80 mg + 2.5 mg of the diuretic bendroflumethazide.
- Propranolol hydrochloride injection 1 mg/mL.

Atenolol

Atenolol (Fig. 10.8) was introduced in the 1970s and became the best selling β_1 antagonist during the 1980s. It is much less lipophilic than propranolol (Table 10.1) and thus it does not penetrate the blood–brain barrier as readily and cause bad dreams and other CNS effects. Unlike propranolol, it is β_1 selective and thus does not cause bronchoconstriction. This is also presumably due to its lower lipophilicity. It has one chiral centre but is administered as a racemate.

Description and products

Atenolol is used in the form of its free base which is freely soluble in methanol but only sparingly soluble in water and ethanol. N.B. The dosages on a weight basis may appear to be lower for this drug but that is because there is no counter-ion to account for part of the weight taken.

- Atenol free base in tablets 25 mg. Adult dose 50 mg daily for hypertension.
- Atenolol injection 0.5 mg/mL. Adult dose 2.5 mg.

Atenolol free base capsules 25 mg with 1.25 mg of bendroflumethiazide.

Oxprenolol

Oxprenolol was introduced in the 1960s. It acts as an antagonist both at β_1 and β_2 receptors but it does retain some agonist activity, i.e. it behaves as a weak analogue of adrenaline, blocking its action but exerting a small effect itself. The small amount of agonist activity is useful because it stimulates the heart when the patient is at rest and slows it down during exercise. The agonist stimulation is useful in heart failure where it is important not to block the resting heart rate. In addition, its agonist activities stimulate β_2 receptors in peripheral blood vessels thus reducing coldness in the extremities. Its β_2 agonist activity is not strong enough to reduce problems of β_2 antagonist activity in asthmatics. Clear

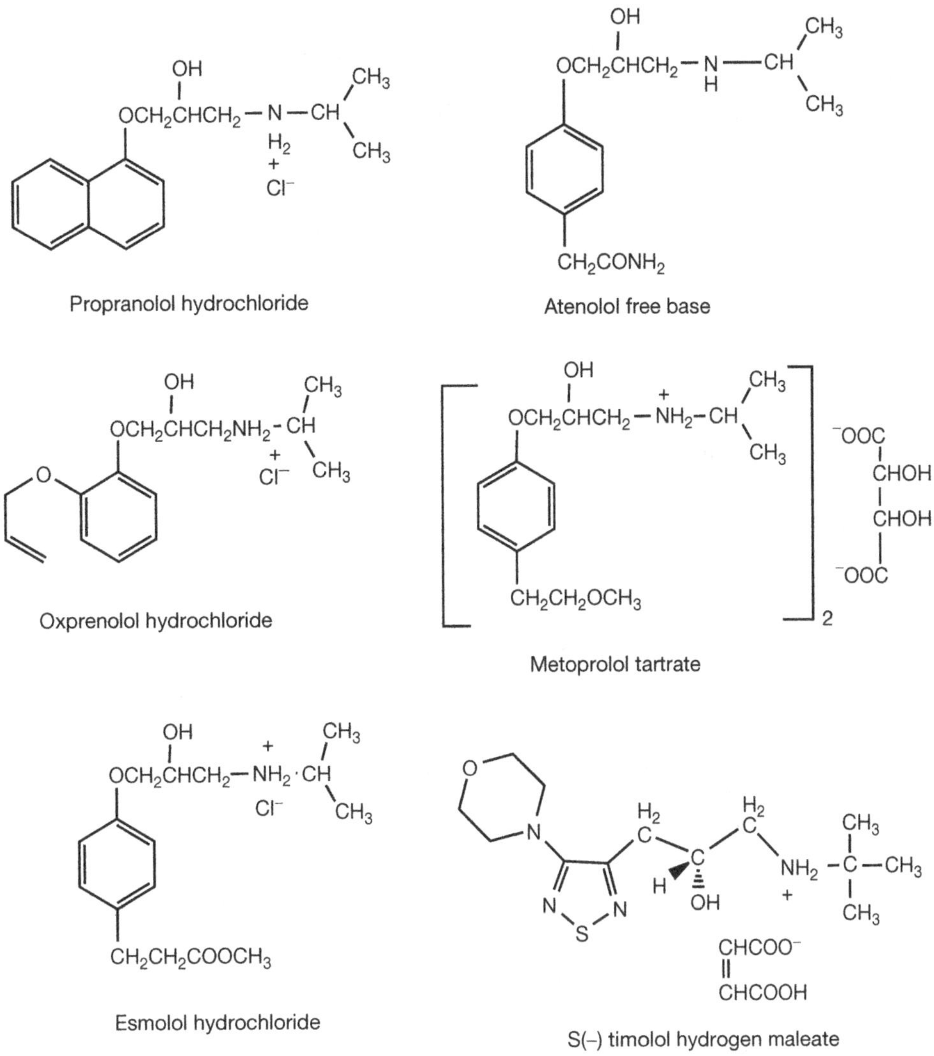

Figure 10.8 Commonly used β_1 antagonists.

Table 10.1 Log P values for some β_1 antagonists

Drug	Calculated log P	Literature log P
Propranolol	2.65	1.72
Atenolol	0.5	0.46
Oxprenolol	2.22	0.79
Metoprolol	1.72	1.59
Esmolol	1.83	
Timolol	2.34	1.08

clinical advantages for its additional properties have yet to be demonstrated. It is used in the form of the racemate.

Description and properties

- Oxprenolol hydrochloride tablets 20–160 mg. Adult dosage 80–160 mg daily in 2–3 doses for treatment of hypertension.

Metoprolol

Metoprolol is a selective β_1 antagonist. It is much more lipophilic than atenolol and thus has more potential to exert CNS effects. Like atenolol, its selectivity has made it one of the more frequently used β_1 antagonists. The drug is used in the form of its racemate.

Description and products

Metoprolol is used in the form of its tartrate which is soluble 1:1 in water and 1:2 in ethanol.

- Metoprolol tartrate tablets 50 or 100 mg. Adult dose 100–200 mg daily in 1–2 doses for hypertension.
- Metoprolol tartrate injection 1mg/mL. Adult dose 5 mg.

Esmolol

Esmolol (Fig. 10.8) has a different indication from the β_1 antagonists discussed above since it was designed to be short acting. It has a substituent on the aromatic ring which contains an ester grouping which is rapidly hydrolysed by plasma esterases to a free carboxylic acid, the hydrolysis product is inactive. The half-life of esmolol in plasma is *ca.* 9 minutes. Esmolol is valuable where prolonged depression of heart rate is not desirable such as before or after surgery or patients who are at risk from sustained β-blockade.

Description and products

The drug is used as its hydrochloride.

- Esmolol hydrochloride concentrated intravenous infusion 250 mg/mL. Adult dose: the infusion is diluted and administered at 0.05–0.2 mg/kg/min.

Timolol

Timolol (Fig. 10.8) departs in structure quite markedly from the majority of β_1 antagonists. The usual side chain is only altered slightly through having a t-butyl substituent on the nitrogen rather than an isopropyl substituent. However, the aromatic ring has been changed to a heterocyclic ring system. Timolol is the most widely prescribed β-blocker for the management of glaucoma, where the exact mode of action in terms of receptor binding remains unknown, although it is also used in the management of hypertension. It is one of the few β_1 antagonists which is administered as a single enantiomer, the S (−) enantiomer is used therapeutically. The increased potency resulting from 100% instead of 50% of active drug is evidenced by the lower dosages given in comparison with most other β_1 antagonists.

Description and products

Timolol is used as its hydrogen maleate salt which is freely soluble in water and ethanol.

- Timolol hydrogen maleate eye drops 0.25% or 0.5% w/v. Adult dose eyedrops twice daily.
- Timolol hydrogen maleate tablets 10 mg. Adult dosage: a maximum of 60 mg daily.

β_1 agonists

There are no drugs which are selective agonists at β_1 receptors but there are a few drugs with more wide-ranging activities which are used for their action at β_1 receptors in bringing about cardiac resuscitation. These include adrenaline itself and closely related agonists such as isoprenaline.

Adrenaline

R(−) adrenaline at a concentration of 0.01% w/v in the form of its acid tartrate is used in cardiac resuscitation. The dose used is 10 mL.

Isoprenaline

Isoprenaline has been described earlier in the chapter. Isoprenaline hydrochloride is used to stimulate the heart in heart block or severe bradycardia.

- It is given in an injection of 10 mL containing 0.002% w/v of the drug.

Dopamine

Dopamine (Fig. 10.9) is more associated with neurotransmission in the CNS but it can also act on β_1 receptors to stimulate the heart. Unlike adrenaline analogues, it can increase the force of contraction of the heart without increasing its rate, presumably because it is not an exact fit to the receptor since it lacks the side chain alcohol. It also promotes vasodilation and increased renal perfusion. It has a narrow therapeutic window which, when exceeded, can exacerbate heart failure by causing vasoconstriction.

- Intravenous infusion of dopamine hydrochloride at 1.6 mg/mL in 5% w/v glucose solution. Infusion: 2–5 μg/kg/min.

Dobutamine

Dobutamine (Fig. 10.9) derives from dopamine and has similar effects acting on β_1 receptors with minimal effect on heart rate.

- Dobutamine as hydrochloride 12.5 mg/mL concentrated solution for preparation of infusions. Infusion: 2.5–10 μg/kg/min.

Dopexamine

Dopexamine (Fig. 10.9) derives from dopamine but it is unusual in that it stimulates the heart via β_2 receptors which assume an increased importance in heart failure. It has a lesser tendency than dopamine to promote vasoconstriction but still promotes renal perfusion.

- Dopexamine as hydrochloride 10 mg/mL concentrated solution for preparation of infusions. Infusion: 0.5–6 μg/kg/min depending on response.

SUMMARY 10.1 DRUGS ACTING AT β RECEPTORS

- Selective β_2 agonists were desirable to treat bronchospasm and asthma.
- β_2 agonists derive from isoprenaline which is a potent agonist at both β_1 and β_2 receptors.

Figure 10.9 Drugs used to stimulate heart muscle.

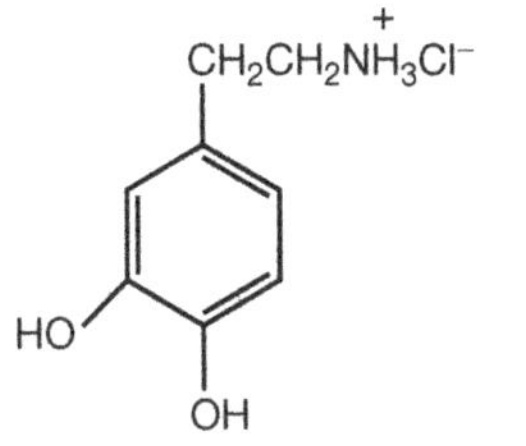

Dopamine hydrochloride

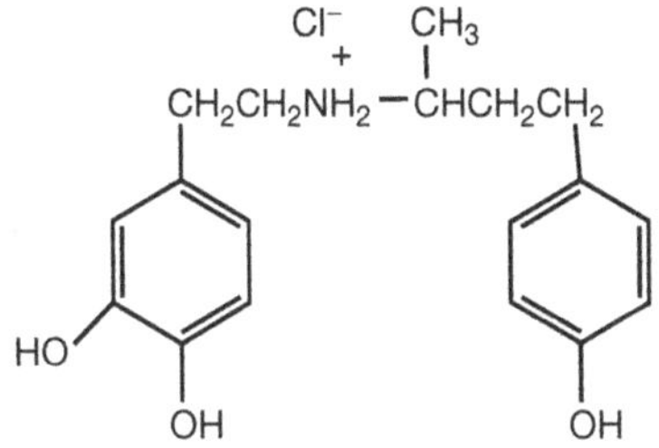

Dobutamine hydrochloride

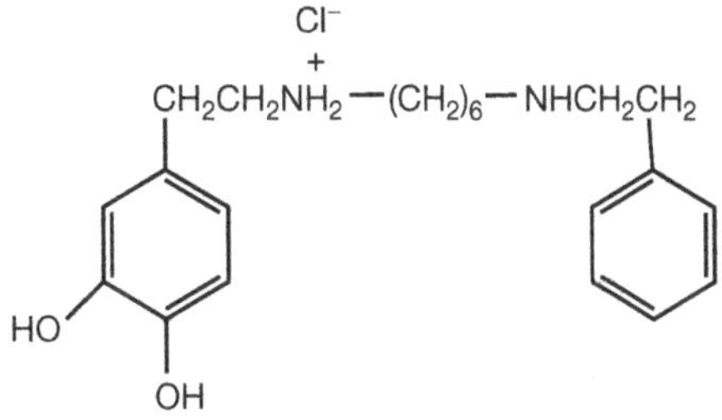

Dopexamine hydrochloride

- Slight modification of the ring substitution pattern and modfication of the substituent on the secondary amine group, most commonly to t-butyl, lead to selective agonists of the β_2 receptor.
- Selective β_1 antagonists were desirable to reduce cardiac output.
- β_1 antagonists derive from dichloroisoprenaline where agonist activity was reduced by elimination of the catechol group of isoprenaline.
- Addition of an extra OCH_2 to the side chain of isoprenaline and replacement of the catechol ring with napthyl led to propranolol the first selective β_1 blocker which still retained some action at β_2 receptors.
- Modifications to the ring, often leaving the side chain unchanged from that of propranolol, was carried out in order to achieve greater selectivity for β_1 receptors.
- There are a few β_1 agonists that are used to stimulate heart contraction following heart failure or heart block. Those derived from dopamine are particularly useful since they also promote renal perfusion.

Drugs acting at α-adrenergic receptors

Introduction

Drugs acting at α-adrenergic receptors are a smaller class than those that are active at β-adrenergic receptors. There is quite a number of agents that are known to act at α receptors but such compounds have often been found to be less useful as drugs. There is a fairly fine division between drugs that act directly on α receptors and those that either inhibit or promote noradrenaline release by other mechanisms. The picture is further confused by the fact that many α_2 receptors are presynaptic and thus mediate their effects by affecting noradrenaline release. Thus it is difficult to distinguish between drugs which act as α_2 receptors and those which modulate noradrenaline release via some other mechanism. This might explain why many of the drugs acting on α receptors do not have structures which have been clearly derived from the structure of noradrenaline.

α_1 agonists

Noradrenaline

Noradrenaline is, to some extent, a selective agonist for α receptors, whereas adrenaline shows little selectivity between α and β receptors. A goal of α_1 selectivity is to cause vasoconstriction without affecting the heart or lungs. Noradrenaline is used to selectively promote vasoconstriction in cases of acute hypotension. It is also sometimes incorporated in injections of local anaesthetics in order to prolong their action close to the site of injection.

Description and products

Noradrenaline is used therapeutically as its acid tartrate which is freely soluble in water.

- Noradrenaline acid tartrate 2 mg/mL for dilution to prepare infusions. Adult dose: 0.08 mg/mL i.v.; infusion: 0.16–0.33 mL/min.

Q Self Test 10.1

Indicate which of the following drugs are β_1, β_2 agonists or β_1 antagonists.

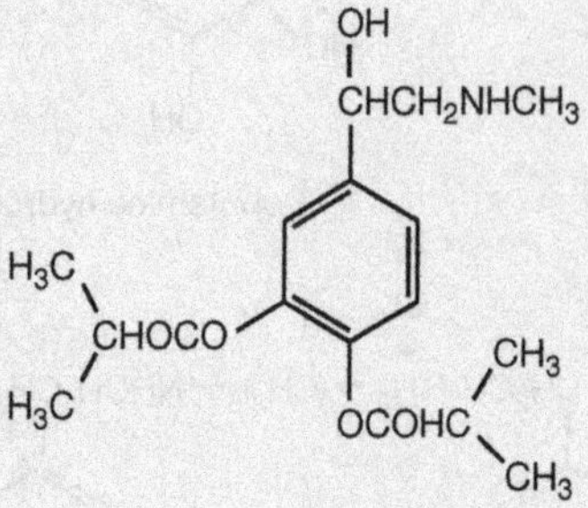

1. Ibopamine

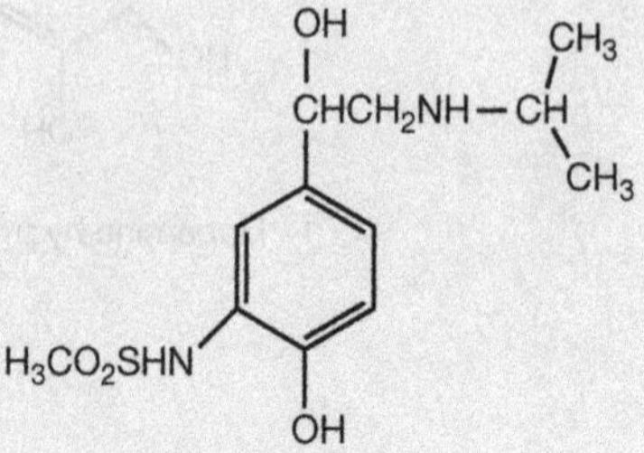

2. Soterenol

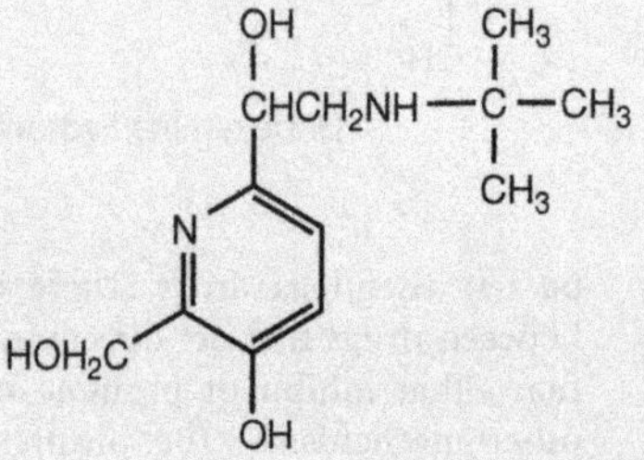

3. Pirbuterol

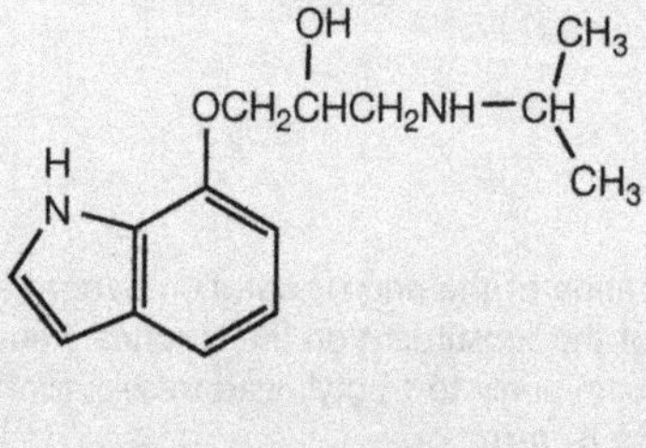

4. Pindolol

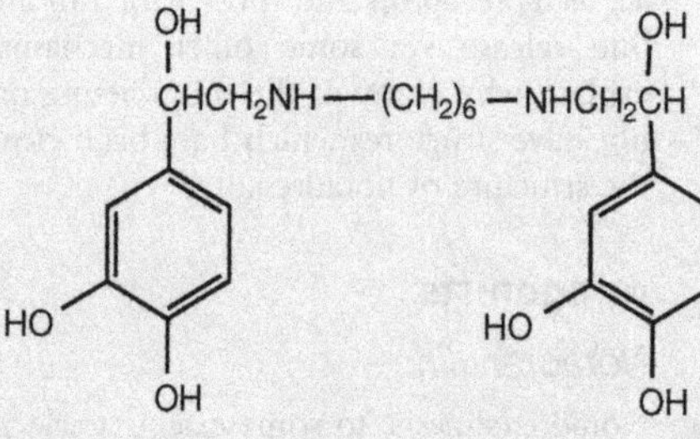

5. Hexoprenaline

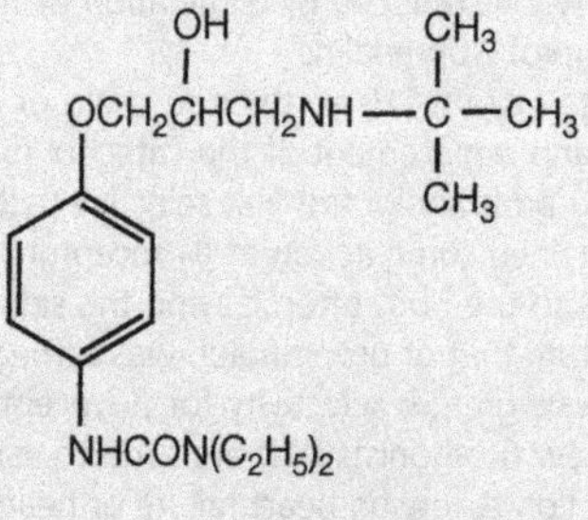

6. Celiprolol

Phenylephrine

The phenylephrine (Fig. 10.10) is derived from adrenaline via the removal of one phenolic hydroxyl group. It has limited action at β receptors and is an α_1 agonist although a weaker one than noradrenaline. It is also used to act on α_1 receptors in the ciliary muscle and cause dilation of the pupil of the eye (mydriatic). Another use is as a decongestant in a number of expectorant and demulcent cough preparations. In this case, it constricts the blood vessels close to the surface of mucous membranes thus inhibiting the secretion of mucus.

Description and products

Phenylephrine is used as the hydrochloride salt of its R (−) enantiomer. The drug consists of bitter crystals which are freely soluble in water and ethanol.

- Phenylephrine hydrochloride injection 10 mg/mL for dilution to prepare infusions. Adult dose: 1 mg/mL i.v.; infusion: 0.18–0.06 mg/min.
- Phenylephrine hydrochloride eyedrops 10% w/v.

Figure 10.10

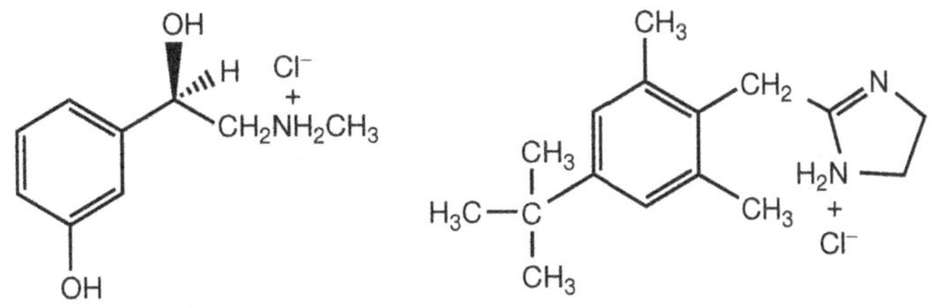

R(–) phenylephrine hydrochloride Xylometazoline hydrochloride

Xylometazoline

Xylometazoline (Fig. 10.10) is a representative of a class of α_1 agonists where a common feature is the imidazoline ring. These compounds are strongly basic and have p*Ka* values of around 10. The discovery of their selectivity for α_1 receptors was serendipitous. This class of compounds is used in nasal decongestants via local application acting through constricting the blood vessels in the mucous membranes.

Description and products

Xylometazoline is used as its hydrochloride salt which is soluble in water at up to 3% w/v.

- Xylometazoline hydrochloride nasal spray 0.1% w/v. Adult dose: spray into each nostril 2–3 times daily.

α_2 agonists

It was thought originally that α_2 receptors were largely presynaptic but they have been found to occur widely, e.g. in blood vessels and liver cells. There are few examples of direct agonists at α_2 receptors but there are examples of partial agonists, e.g. clonidine, but these really belong in the same category as antagonists since they are used to reduce the effects of noradrenaline rather than mimic it.

Metaraminol

Metaraminol (Fig. 10.11) derives directly from noradrenaline through removal of a phenolic hydroxyl group and addition of a methyl group to the side chain. It acts on α_2 receptors in blood vessels to promote vasoconstriction and is used in the same way as noradrenaline itself but produces a longer response. The drug has two chiral centres and is used in the form of the R, S diastereoisomer.

Description and products

Metaraminol is used in the form of its hydrogen tartrate salt which is freely soluble in water.

- Metaraminol tartrate injection 10 mg/mL.

Clonidine

Clonidine (Fig. 10.11) is another imidazoline compound but, unlike xylometazoline, it is not an agonist for vascular α_1 receptors. It is a weaker base (p*Ka* 8.25) than xylometazoline and it appears to be selective for presynaptic α_2 receptors which inhibit the release of noradrenaline. Presynaptic α_2 receptors essentially function as a feedback mechanism where the noradrenaline, released into the synaptic cleft, itself inhibits further release. Thus noradrenaline release is inhibited and the blood vessels are dilated. It is less often prescribed than many hypertensive agents because of its potential to produce a 'rebound effect' when it is withdrawn, resulting in a hypertensive crisis.

Description and products

Clonidine is used as its hydrochloride which is soluble 1:13 in water.

- Clonidine hydrochloride capsules 0.25 mg. Adult dose: 2–3 capsules daily as antihypertensive.

α antagonists

α antagonists are not a large class of drugs, the main use in this category being in antihypertensive therapy. There are a number of drugs in use which act as antagonists of both

Figure 10.11 Drugs acting at α-adrenergic receptors.

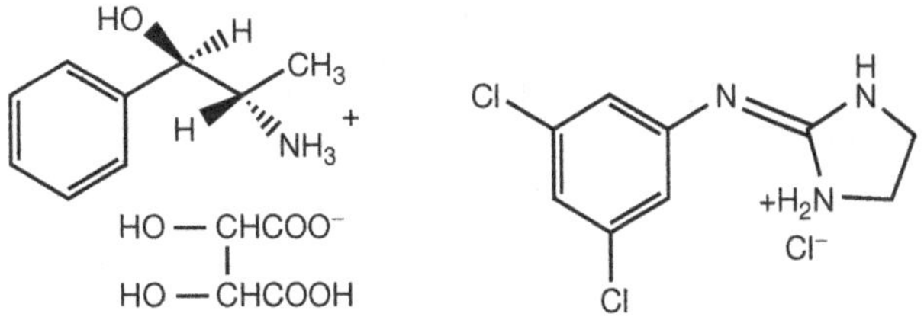

R,S metarominol hydrogen tartrate Clonidine hydrogen chloride

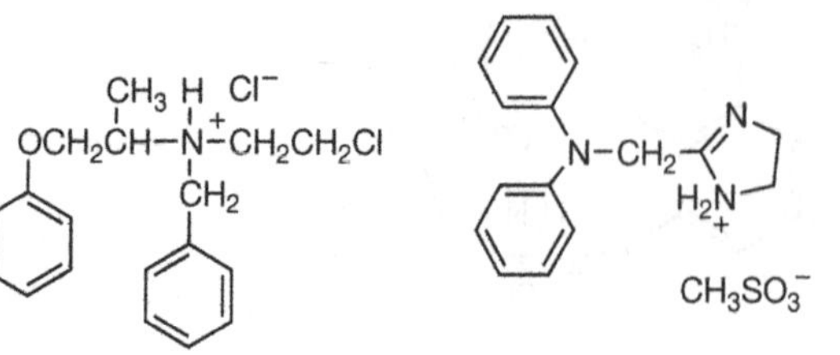

Figure 10.12

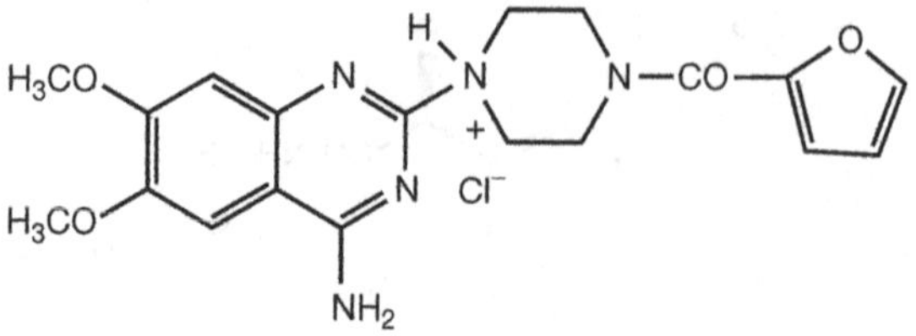

Figure 10.13

α_1 and α_2 receptors and some which are selective for α_1 receptors. There is none which is selective for α_2 receptors.

Phenoxybenzamine

Phenoxybenzamine (Fig. 10.12) is a powerful antagonist of α receptors. It is structurally well removed from noradrenaline and, as might be expected, does not act only on the adrenergic system. The drug contains a chlorine atom which is rendered more reactive than that of an ordinary alkyl halide by the proximity of the amine group. Thus the drug represents a rare example - aspirin being another one - outside of the area of chemotherapy, where a drug acts via covalent modification of a biological structure, in this case modification of α receptors. It is obvious that this type of action is not ideal since the effects of the drug can only be reversed with difficulty. However, there is one therapeutic area where it is important, which is in the management of phaeochromocytoma which is a tumour of the neural crest which excretes large amounts of catecholamines. Phenoxybenzamine is used in the short-term management of hypertensive episodes resulting from this condition.

Description and products

Phenoxybenzamine is used as its hydrochloride which is freely soluble in water. It is prone to hydrolysis under neutral or basic conditions.

- Phenoxybenzamine hydrochloride capsules 10 mg. Adult dose: 1–2 mg/kg daily for short-term management of phaeochromocytoma.

Phentolamine

The main indication of phentolamine is in the management of phaeochromocytoma but, unlike phenoxybenzamine, its action is reversible. It belongs to the imidazoline class of compounds like xylometazoline but functions as an α-receptor antagonist rather than an agonist. It is difficult to rationalise its antagonistic activity on the basis of its structure.

Description and products

Phentolamine (Fig. 10.12) is used as its mesilate salt which is freely soluble in water. The use of mesilate salt improves the stability of the imidazoline ring in aqueous solution. The ring is prone to base-catalysed hydrolysis.

- Phentolamine mesilate injection 10 mg/mL. Adult dose: 2–5 mg.

Prazosin, tetrazosin and doxazosin

Prazosin (Fig. 10.13) is a selective α_1-receptor blocker. Prazosin came out of research aimed at producing phosphodiesterase inhibitors which would cause vasodilation without acting directly on smooth muscle. However, it was eventually found to act through antagonism of α_1 receptors. Again, like many drugs in this category, its structure cannot easily be related back to that of noradrenaline. It is used in the treatment of hypertension, effecting a reduction in blood pressure without affecting the heart. It is also used for urinary retention by promoting urinary flow through relaxing the sphincter of the bladder which is mediated via α_1 receptors. Terazosin and doxazosin and very similar in structure to prazosin and have the same indications. Tetrazosin has a longer plasma half-life than prazosin, which permits once-a-day dosing.

Description and products

Prazosin and terazosin are used as hydrochlorides and dosazosin is used as its mesilate.

- Prazosin hydrochloride tablets 0.5 mg. Adult dose: 0.5 mg 2× daily to relieve urinary retention or in the treatment of hypertension.
- Terazosin hydrochloride tablets 1, 2, 10 mg. Adult dose: 2–10 mg once daily to relieve urinary retention or treat hypertension.
- Doxazosin mesilate tablets 1 mg. Adult dose: 1–2 mg once daily to relieve urinary retention or treat hypertension.

Tamsulosin

Tamsulosin (Fig. 10.14) represents a new departure in terms of therapeutic selectivity since it antagonises the α_{1A} subclass of receptors governing constriction of the bladder sphincter. Thus it can be used to relieve urinary retention without causing the same degree of hypotension

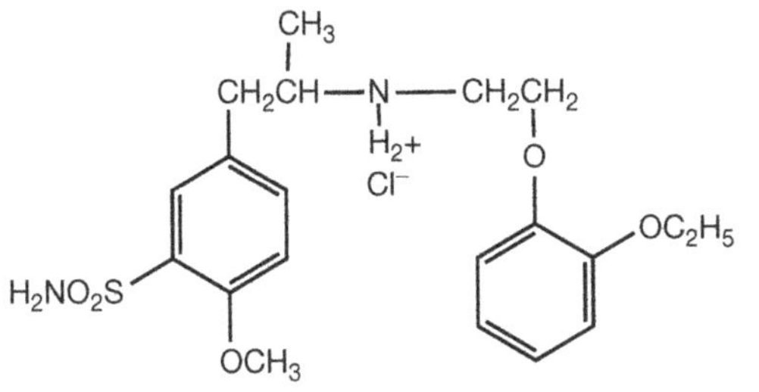

Tamsulosin hydrochloride

Figure 10.14

as other agents. Its specificity may owe something to the fact that is resembles noradrenaline more closely than other α antagonists.

Description and products

Tamsulosin is used in the form of its hydrochloride.

- Tamsulosin hydrochloride capsules 0.4 mg. Adult dose: 0.4 mg daily.

SUMMARY 10.2

- The structure–activity relationships of drugs acting at α receptors are not as clear as those of drugs acting at β receptors.
- The range of drugs developed with α receptors as their target is relatively small.
- Direct α agonists such as noradrenaline itself and phenylephrine are useful for treating hypotension.
- Drugs acting at α_1 receptors are used as nasal decongestants through their action in promoting vasoconstriction of the blood vessels in mucous membranes.
- Non-specific α antagonists are used in treating phaeochromocytoma.
- α_1 antagonists are used in the treatment of hypertension and urinary retention.

DRUGS INFLUENCING THE NORADRENALINE RELEASE PROCESS

Indirectly acting sympathomimetic amines

This class of drugs acts presynaptically. There are a number of compounds which fall into this category including the very ancient drug ephedrine through to more recent drugs such as amfetamine. However, ephedrine, its diastereoisomer pseudoephedrine and phenylpropanolamine are the only drugs in this category which are frequently used. The general structure for this type of agent has similarities with that of noradrenaline. The indirectly acting amines are taken up into the nerve terminal via reuptake 1, which has a high affinity for noradrenaline. Thus their first site of action is through competing with noradrenaline for reuptake, which has the effect of increasing the levels of noradrenaline in the synaptic cleft and hence the level of noradrenergic transmission. Once within the nerve terminal, these amines are stored within the noradrenaline-containing vesicles (see Fig. 10.1), and thus displace noradrenaline from these vesicles. The displaced noradrenaline is then either metabolised within the nerve terminal or released into the synaptic cleft by a mechanism which is independent of nerve depolarisation, thus increasing noradrenergic transmission. The increased release of noradrenaline means that the range of physiological effects mediated by adrenergic transmission is stimulated. A side effect of drugs with this action is that they deplete noradrenaline stores, thus creating a 'rebound effect' where noradrenergic activity is depressed. In this case, the 'false neurotransmitter', which is inactive at adrenergic receptors, that has accumulated in the noradrenaline containing vesicles, may be released instead of noradrenaline.

Examples of indirectly acting sympathomimetic amines

p-Tyramine

p-Tyramine (Fig. 10.15) was never used as a drug but it is common in food such as cheese and beer and is structurally related to noradrenaline. Under normal circumstances tyramine is metabolised by MAO in the gut wall but patients undergoing therapy with MAO inhibitors may suffer a hypertensive crisis provoked by dietary tyramine, which promotes noradrenaline release, the metabolic breakdown of noradrenaline also being inhibited by MAO inhibitors.

Amfetamine

Amfetamine (Fig. 10.15) has structural similarities to noradrenaline. In the form of the free base it is relatively volatile and was thus used as a nasal decongestant through promoting constriction of mucosal blood vessels. It also has appetite-suppressing effects which have been attributed to its ability to displace serotonin from synaptic vesicles, but since noradrenaline increases blood sugar levels this may also be part of its action. It is not frequently used because of it potential for being addictive since, because of its high lipophilicity, it can also enter the CNS. Its main indication in current practice is in the treatment of narcolepsy. Amfetamines are discussed in more detail in Chapter 18.

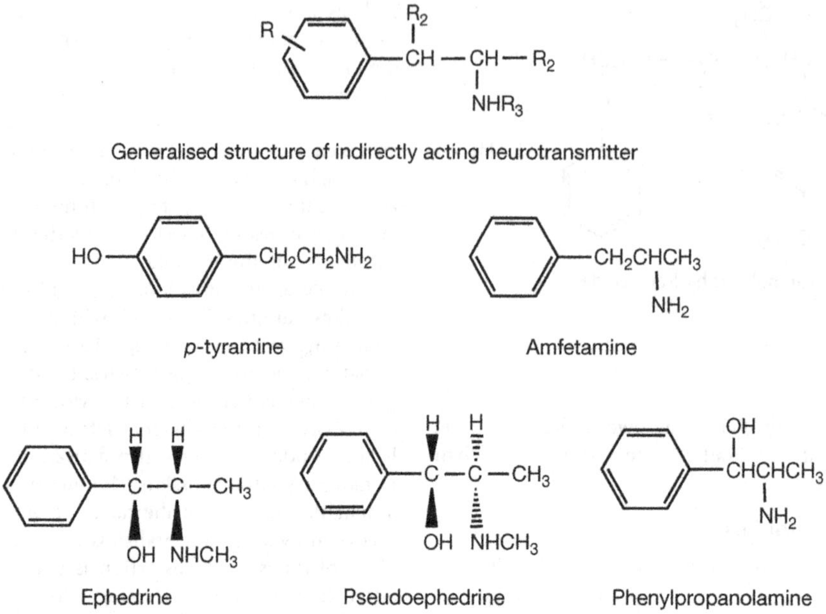

Figure 10.15 Sympathomimetic amines.

Description and products

The (+) isomer of amfetamine is used in the form of its sulphate, dexamfetamine sulphate.

- Dexamfetamine sulphate tablets 5 mg. Adult dose: 10 mg daily in divided doses for the treatment of narcolepsy.

Ephedrine

Ephedrine (Fig. 10.15) is found in the Chinese herb Ma Huang, which has been used in Chinese medicine for 3000 years. It was also used in Greek medicine. Its structural resemblance to adrenaline and noradrenaline is readily apparent. It was used in the treatment of asthma but has been superseded by selective β_2 agonists such as salbutamol. Its main application is as a nasal decongestant by promoting noradrenaline release, thus causing constriction of blood vessels in the nasal mucosa. It also has weak β-agonist activity. Its other actions are discussed in Chapter 18.

Description and products

Ephedrine is used as its hydrochloride salt which is freely soluble in water.

- Ephedrine hydrochloride nasal drops 0.5% w/v. Adult dose: 1–2 drops into each nostril 3 to 4 times daily.

Phenylpropanolamine

Phenylpropanolamine (Fig. 10.15) is the primary amine corresponding to ephedrine. This gives it a slightly closer resemblance to noradrenaline and it has stronger vasoconstricting activity than ephedrine. It is employed as a nasal decongestant and is included in cold preparations. It presumably exerts its action through constricting blood vessels in mucous membranes through promoting noradrenaline release.

Description and products

Phenylpropanolamine is used as its hydrochloride.

- A typical formulation containing phenylpropanolamine to reduce production of mucus is as follows: dextromethorphan (cough suppressant), paracetamol (anti-inflammatory) and phenylpropanolamine (decongestant).

Drugs affecting storage and release of noradrenaline

Noradrenaline is stored in phospholipid vesicles within nerve endings. The release of noradrenaline is mediated by calcium ions, which cause the vesicles to fuse with the membrane of the nerve terminal and thus release their contents into the synaptic cleft.

Guanethidine

Guanethidine (Fig. 10.16) reduces noradrenaline release, being taken up into the nerve terminal via uptake 1. As a large and stable cation it may act through binding to the noradrenaline-containing vesicles in the nerve terminal thus blocking the normal action of calcium ions. Guanethidine has the additional property of depleting

Figure 10.16 Drugs affecting noradrenaline release.

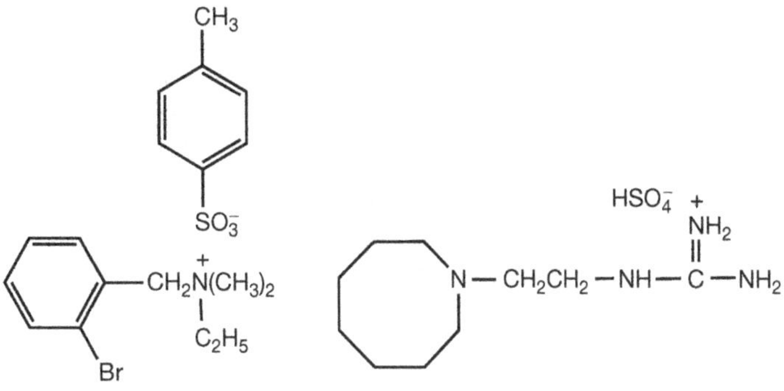

Bretylium tosylate

Guanethidine monosulphate

noradrenaline stores, possibly through disrupting vesicles prior to their fusion with the nerve terminal membrane. The drug is not widely used since it may cause severe hypotension. It is used for hypertension which will not respond to other treatments.

Description and products

Guanethidine is used in the form of its monosulphate.

- Guanethidine monosulphate injection 10 mg/mL. Adult dose: 10–20 mg by i.m. injection.

Bretylium tosylate

Bretylium (Fig. 10.16) works in a manner similar to guanethidine and is used in resuscitation.

Description

Bretylium is used in the form of its tosilate.

- Bretylium tosilate injection 50 mg/mL. Adult dosage: 5–10 mg/kg.

Drugs affecting the biosynthesis of noradrenaline

Methyldopa is used as an antihypertensive drug. It is useful since it is safe for treatment of hypertension in asthmatics, in cases of heart failure and in pregnancy. This is because it does not act directly on adrenergic receptors. The biosynthesis of noradrenaline is shown in Figure 10.17 with an indication where methyldopa acts

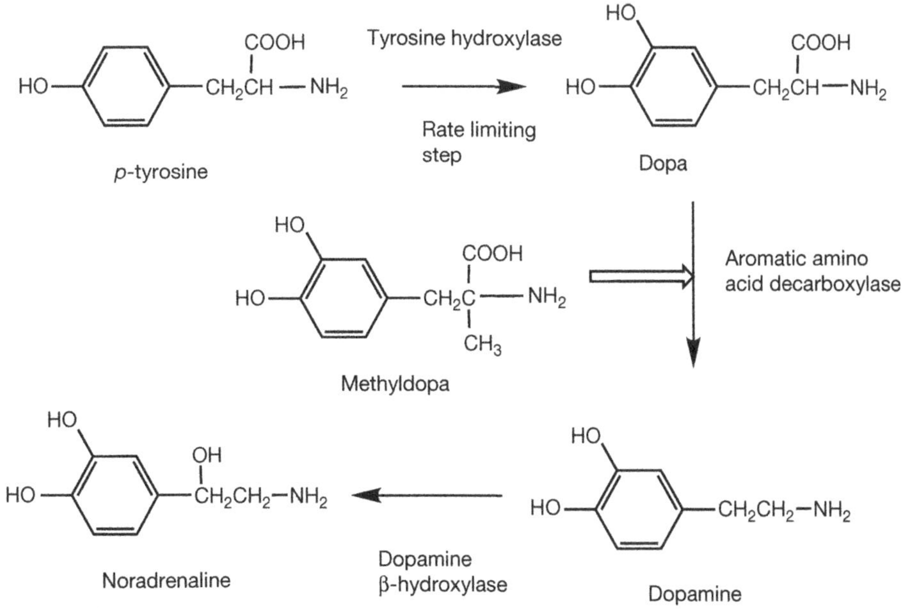

Figure 10.17 Biosynthesis of noradrenaline.

to inhibit decarboxylation of dopa to dopamine. It does this by competing with dopa for the decarboxylase enzyme. The decarboxylation of methyldopa is slower than that of dopa and since the enzyme only releases the substrate after decarboxylation the overall effect is a reduction in the rate of noradrenaline biosynthesis. Since methyldopamine is produced from methyldopa, the drug may also produce effects related to the action of the indirectly acting sympathomimetic amines.

Description and products

Colourless crystals or white to yellowish white fine powder. Soluble 1 in 100 of water, 1 in 400 of ethanol. Insoluble in many organic solvents.

- Methyldopa tablets containing 250 or 500 mg. Adult dose: 250 mg 2–3 times per day.

A Self Test 10.1

- β_1 agonist: 1; β_2 agonists: 2, 3, 5; β_1 antagonists: 4, 6.

Chapter 11

Drugs exerting non-adrenergic effects on cardiac output and vascular tone

Ahmed Saadi Ahmed

CHAPTER CONTENTS

INTRODUCTION

Physiological actions such as muscle contractions, hormone secretion, gene expression, protein synthesis, and the control of various intracellular actions, require a change in the cell potential from the polarised state (resting state) to the depolarised state. This change in cell potential is controlled by a number of ion channels such as the Ca^{2+} channel, Na^+ channel, and K^+ channel. Ca^{2+} plays a vital role in controlling different cellular activity through interaction with calcium-binding proteins (receptors), distributed all over the body, which in turn lead to enzyme activation or interaction with other proteins and promotion of the release of second messengers. Also it is believed that Ca^{2+} can affect neurotransmitter release through a specific cellular pathway.

Ca^{2+} influx through the cell membrane to the intracellular environment is controlled by different types of calcium channels: voltage-gated calcium channels (also refer to as voltage-operated calcium channels), receptor-activated calcium channels, and ligand-gated calcium channels. Some of these channels are endogenous and some are exogenous, and they are distributed all over the body and have different physiological effects and different mechanisms of action, activation and stimulation. In this chapter we will focus on drugs acting on voltage-gated calcium channels that have an important role in cardiac diseases. Also, we will talk about cardiac muscles, the mechanism of myocardial function, types of channels, nerve systems (type I fibre, type II A fibre, and type II B fibre), and cardiac disease.

DISEASES INVOLVING CALCIUM CHANNELS

A. Arrhythmia (ventricular and supraventricular)
B. Angina
C. Hypertension
D. Myocardial infarction

THE VOLTAGE-GATED CALCIUM CHANNEL (VGCC)

The voltage-gated calcium ion channel or voltage-dependent calcium ion channel family represents (according to the number of family members) the third largest family of signalling proteins, following the G protein-coupled receptors and the protein kinases. A change in the cell potential, from the polarised state to the depolarised state, is responsible for initiating an electrical signal required for contraction, secretion, neurotransmission, and various intracellular actions. This change in cell potential is controlled by voltage-gated calcium ion channels which control calcium ion influx during the depolarisation phase.

A significant change in cell membrane potential drives significant conformational changes in voltage-dependent calcium channels, and hence a change in the gating state of the channel for Ca^{2+} ion influx, with total opening or closing of the water-filled pores of the channel. The affinity of calcium channel blockers (CCBs) for Ca^{2+} channels is affected by the change in the conformation of the channel as it opens and closes. For example, the binding of CCBs to Ca^{2+} channels will increase as the channel is inactivated (i.e. in its depolarised or open state), while its affinity will decrease as the channel is activated (i.e. in its resting or closed state). Therefore, drugs acting as antagonists for Ca^{2+} channels seem to have high activity on the pathologically highly active cells with no antagonistic activity on normal or moderately active cells. According to assessment of electrophysiological and pharmacological properties, there are six types of voltage-gated Ca^{2+} channels; two of them are available in the heart and vascular smooth muscles: the transient channel (T-type) and the long-acting channel (T-type). Another four types of Ca^{2+} channels are available in the nervous system, namely N-channel, P/Q-channel, L-channel and R-channel. The T-channel and L-channel are triggered by a slight change in voltage of the cell from the polarised level to the depolarised level. In myocardium, both channels will be activated by the wave of depolarisation, while in vascular smooth muscles the initiator for the depolarisation process is still not recognised; some channels in smooth muscles seem to be self-activated.

The T-channel and L-channel are widely distributed in the conductive system of the heart, especially the sinoatrial (SA) node. The first phase of cell depolarisation in the SA node will be started via the activation of the T-channel (allowing fast influx of extracellular calcium ions), while the later phase of depolarisation will be controlled by the L-channel (slow influx). CCBs have no significant activity on the T-channel. Instead they shorten the L-channel opening time, which increases the penetration time required for Ca^{2+} ions to completely depolarise the cell and hence this reduces the heart rate (negative chronotropic effect).

Voltage-gated calcium channels are complex proteins which mainly consist of four subunits: α_1, α_2, β, and δ, while in skeletal muscles there is an additional γ-unit which explains why CCBs do not antagonise the calcium channel in skeletal muscles.

α_1 subunit of voltage-gated calcium channel

The calcium channel pore (α_1 subunit) represents the main action site for CCBs. When CCBs bind to this unit, they exhibit antagonistic effects by decreasing calcium ion influx though the cell membrane (Fig. 11.1), and this slows heart rate and decreases myocardium contractility. The α_1 subunit is a large transmembrane protein (165–260 kDa) and consists of four similar transmembrane domains, each of which consists of six helices, and one pore thought to be located between helices S5 and S6 of each domain. The four domains of the α_1 subunit are folded together, so that the four pores of the four domains will function as a single pore for a calcium ion per α_1 subunit, and Ca^{2+} selectivity seems to be controlled by amino acid sequence of the S5 and S6 linker region. The gating mechanism of the Ca^{2+} channel is thought to be controlled by S1 to S4 segments of these channels. According to extensive structure–function studies and recent X-ray crystallography, the positively charged amino acids of the S4 segments of the Ca^{2+} channel undergo outward and rotational movement leading to conformational changes in the protein structure of the channel and a change in the gating state of the channel.

Selectivity of Ca^{2+} channels for CCBs

The selectivity of the calcium channel is thought to be controlled by the peptide chains located between S5 and S6. This loop is called the H5 or P-loop (Fig. 11.2). The S3 and S3-S4 loops of domain I will determine whether the calcium channel is T-type or L-type, either fast activation

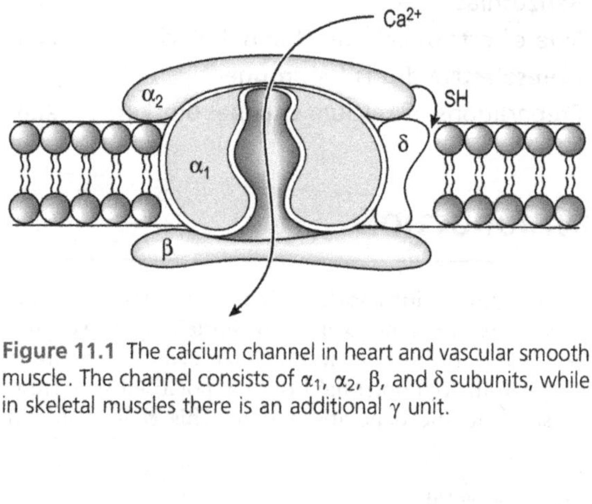

Figure 11.1 The calcium channel in heart and vascular smooth muscle. The channel consists of α_1, α_2, β, and δ subunits, while in skeletal muscles there is an additional γ unit.

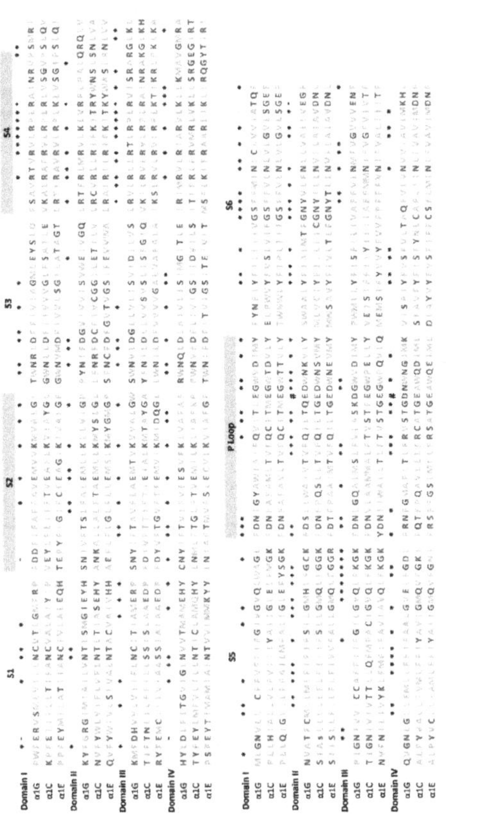

Figure 11.2 Amino acid sequences for the α_{1G}, α_{1C} and α_{1E} regions of the Ca^{2+} channel pore. Positively charged residues are marked with red, while negatively charged residues are marked with green. Neutral non-polar residues are marked with yellow, while neutral molecules with some polarity are marked with blue. Amino acids that are available in all mammalian α_1 subunits of voltage-activated Ca^{2+} channels are marked with an asterisk. Charge conservation is marked with a plus or minus sign. The hash symbol refers to glutamate residues in the pore loops that determine the Ca^{2+} channel selectivity.

like cardiac muscles, or slow activation like skeletal muscles. The selectivity and sensitivity of Ca^{2+} channels for CCBs is mainly controlled by the amino acid sequences in the transmembrane segments IIIS5, IIIS6, and IVS6 (Fig. 11.2). For dihydropyridines (DHPs), there are 13 amino acid sequences available in the L-type channel (nine amino acid sequences in non-L-type channels) which control the sensitivity of the channel: two amino acid sequences in IIIS5, seven amino acid sequences in IIIS6, and four amino acid sequences in IVS6. Sensitivity of L-type Ca^{2+} channels for phenylalkylamines (PAAs) is controlled by eight amino acid sequences in addition to the selectivity of the glutamate residues of each of the P-loops of repeats III and IV. The amino acid sequences are distributed as follows: four amino acid sequences in IIIS6 and four amino acid sequences in IVS6. For non-L-type Ca^{2+} channels, the four amino acid sequences in IVS6 and the selective glutamate residues are not available, and the selectivity of the non-L-type Ca^{2+} channels seems to be controlled only by the four amino acid sequences in IIIS6. The four amino acid sequences in IVS6, which control the selectivity of Ca^{2+} channels for PAAs, seem to play an additional role by controlling the selectivity of the channel for benzothiazepines (BTZs) in addition to two amino acid sequences in IIIS6 and some residues in the IVS5–IVS6 linker region. In vertebrates, there are about 10 α_1 subunits that have been identified and these have been categorised into three different isoforms: Ca_v1, Ca_v2 and Ca_v3 which possess different functions and distributions within vertebrates (Table 11.1). CCBs include phenylalkylamines, dihydropyridines, and benzothiazepines, which are a very significant treatment for cardiovascular diseases, bind selectively to $Ca_v1.2$ types of α_1 subunit of the L-type calcium channels. The $Ca_v\alpha_2$ and $Ca_v\delta$ subunits are incorporated in the gene responsible for production of extracellular α_2 subunit glycoproteins and transmembrane δ subunit glycoproteins, which have masses of 140 kDa and 27 kDa, respectively. Subunit $Ca_v\beta$ represents an intracellular protein with a significant role in cell surface expression and the control of the calcium channel. The $Ca_v\gamma$ subunits of the calcium channel may participate in the expression of membrane signalling proteins, and have the ability to bind to other calcium channels and more or less bind with other signalling proteins of the cell membrane. The calcium channel of the skeletal muscle ($Ca_v1.1$ channels) is characterised by the presence of the $Ca_v\gamma1$ subunit which is specific for such type of muscles. The toxicity of spider and cone snail venoms can be attributed for the ability of the neurotoxins secreted by these species to inhibit Ca_v2 subunits of calcium channels, which are widely available in the central and peripheral nervous systems.

L-type calcium channels, the main action site for calcium channel antagonists, need a significant change in cell potential in order to induce activation and opening of the channel, and because of the long depolarisation state in cardiac cells, they require a long time to be inactivated (slow inactivation).

Binding sites for CCBs

Binding site for nifedipine

Different DHPs interact specifically with a site in the calcium channel, which is believed to be located on the S6 helix of domains I, III, and IV of the α_1 subunit of calcium channel pore, while this receptor is not available on domain II.

Binding site for diltiazem

Benzothiazepines, such as diltiazem, have a specific interaction site on the α_1 subunit, which is supposed to be allosterically linked to the DHP receptor on the calcium

Table 11.1 Isoforms of α_1 subunits

α_1 isoforms	Subfamilies	Ca^{++} channel	Function	Auxiliary subunit
Ca_v1	$Ca_v1.1$ (α_{1S}) $Ca_v1.2$ (α_{1C}) $Ca_v1.3$ (α_{1D}) $Ca_v1.4$ (α_{1F})	L-type Channel	1. Muscle contraction 2. Endocrine secretion 3. Regulators for gene expression 4. Synaptic transmission in sensory input of the eye and ear 5. Other intracellular process	$Ca_v\alpha2$, $Ca_v\beta$, $Ca_v\gamma$, and $Ca_v\delta$
Ca_v2	$Ca_v2.1$ (α_{1A}) $Ca_v2.2$ (α_{1B}) $Ca_v2.3$ (α_{1E})	P/Q-type N-type R-type	Initiate fast synaptic transmission in the central and peripheral nervous systems	$Ca_v\alpha2$, $Ca_v\beta$, $Ca_v\gamma$, and $Ca_v\delta$
Ca_v3	$CA_v3.1$ (α_{1G}) $CA_v3.2$ (α_{1H}) $CA_v3.3$ (α_{1I})	T-type Channel	Play a significant role in the pacemaker cells of SA node in the heart	

channel. Once a benzothiazepine binds to its specific site on the calcium channel, it will enhance the interaction of a DHP with its receptors, so both drug types can be used together in order to have a synergistic effect.

Binding site for verapamil

Phenylalkylamine receptors are located somewhere near the S6 helix and around C-terminal chain of the four domains of the α_1 subunit in the calcium channel. In contrast to benzothiazepines, the binding of phenylalkylamines to their receptor will prevent binding of a DHP to its receptor. Table 11.2 summarises the characteristics of the three drug types.

Table 11.2 Summary of the characteristics of three types of calcium channel blockers

CCBs	Availability	Characteristics
DHPs	Vascular	High vascular selectivity, with minimal activity on myocardium and the conductive system of the heart
Benzothiazepine	Myocardium and conductive system of the heart (sinus node, and AV node)	??
Phenylalkylamine	Myocardium and conductive system of the heart (sinus node, and AV node)	??

Figure 11.3 summarises the different interaction sites for CCBs with L-type voltage-gated calcium channels. In addition, there may be another eight similar sites which are allosterically linked to calcium channels.

CALCIUM ANTAGONISTS

Calcium channel blockers are clinically used for the treatment of hypertension, angina pectoris, and arrhythmia (ventricular and supraventricular). Although all CCBs will slow down influx of extracellular Ca^{2+} through calcium channels it is quite clear that not all CCBs affect the same calcium channel. Different CCBs show different selectivity and activity toward different calcium channels in different tissues and organs, leading to specific bioactivity at that tissue or organ.

According to chemical structure, CCBs can be categorised into four groups: dihydropyridines, phenylalkylamines, benzothiazepines, and others.

Selectivity

Phenylalkylamines and benzothiazepines show a selective activity for Ca^{2+} channels in cardiac muscles while dihydropyridines show a maximum selectivity toward Ca^{2+} channels in the vascular smooth muscles with minimum activity on Ca^{2+} and Na^+ channels in the myocardium.

Stereospecificity of the receptors

The stereospecificity of Ca^{2+} channels has been demonstrated by the development of agonist activity for Ca^{2+} channels from CCBs through certain chemical modifications in their structures. It has been shown that the

Figure 11.3 Interaction sites for the three different types of CCBs.

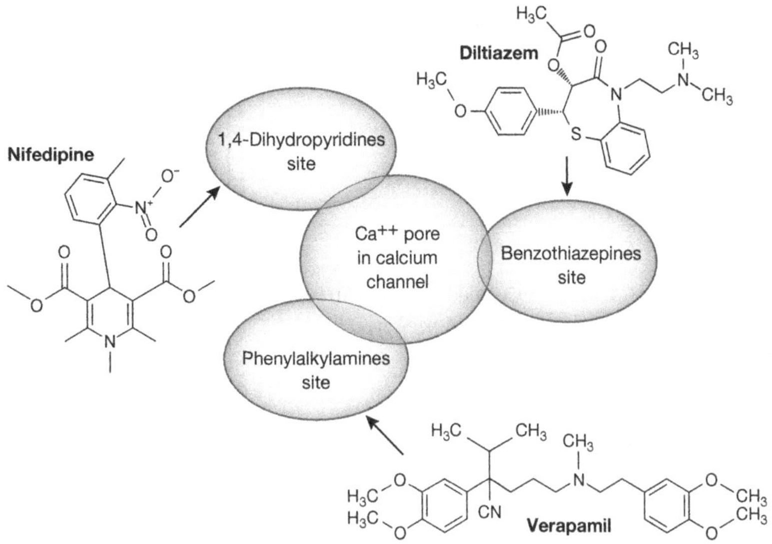

antagonist activity for nifedipine CCBs was increased if the methylester group was replaced with a NO_2 group at position 3 of nifedipine. This resulted in a new compound named Bay-K-8644. This new compound bound to the same binding site as CCBs but increased the Ca^{2+} influx through the channel leading to a positive inotropic effect and vasoconstriction which is the opposite to the normal action for CCBs.

The affinity of the Ca^{2+} channel for CCBs depends on the potential level of the cell. High affinity is correlated to the depolarised or inactivated state of the channel, whereas low affinity is correlated with the activated state or rest state where the cell is polarised. It is believed that the conformational changes in a channel which increase the affinity of the channel to CCBs is linked to the channel opening.

THE MECHANISM OF CHANNEL BLOCKING

Blockers for voltage-gated channels have an allosteric interaction with the gating mechanism of the channel. The affinity of the CCBs interaction with the channel is highly dependent on the conformation of the channel. Two mechanisms have been proposed which control the nature of drug binding with the channel: modulated receptor theory (MRT), and guarded receptor theory (GRT). MRT and GRT explain the mechanism of action for drugs acting on the Na^{+} channel such as local anaesthetics.

MRT states that there is a voltage-dependent conformation for each ion channel, and these conformations will be changed according to the change in the potential of the cell and the polarisation state. The different conformations of the channel will affect drug binding affinity and rate. The MRT model can explain the affinity of CCBs for the L-type Ca^{2+} channel and the voltage dependent block of the channel. Hence, the high-affinity conformation is associated with the inactivation state of the channel (depolarised state), while polarised state (resting state) provides a low-affinity conformation for drug molecule binding.

GRT proposes the presence of barrier in the channel that controls the access of the drug to its binding site in the channel, and this barrier will be opened and closed according to conformational changes in the ion channel. These conformational changes will not affect the binding affinity of the drug; rather, they affect the access of the drug to the binding site within the channel.

GRT is subdivided into two models: foot-in-the-door model, and the trapped-drug model. In the first model, the drug will have an access to its receptors in the channel through certain favourable conformations of the channel, and the drug molecule needs to be dissociated from its receptors before the channel will change to a non-favourable conformation. In the second model, the drug will interact with its binding sites in the channel through certain conformations but it does not need to be dissociated from its receptor in the channel before change to a non-favourable conformation occurs. Table 11.3 summarises the different models.

Dihydropyridines

The dihydropyridine (DHP) group of CCBs is characterised by the presence of the 1,4-dihydropyridine group within its structure (Fig. 11.4) which is believed to bind

Table 11.3 Models of binding to the Ca^{2+} channel

CCBs	Ca^{2+} channel	Mechanism of action	Subtype
Nifedipine	Ca_V1	MRT	
Verapamil	Ca_V1	MRT	
Diltiazem	Ca_V1	MRT	
	$Ca_V1.2$	Guarded Receptor Theory	Trapped molecule
Mibefradil	$CA_V2.1$	Guarded Receptor Theory	Foot-in-the-door
	$CA_V3.2$	MRT	
Isradipine	Ca_V1	Guarded Receptor Theory MRT	

to a specific site of the calcium-channel receptor identified in guinea pigs using ^{3}H-Nitrendipine (nifedipine analogue). The structures of the commonly used DHPs are shown in Figure 11.4.

Nifedipine

Nifedipine is a dihydropyridine L-type calcium channel blocker, widely used clinically as a coronary vasodilator. Pharmaceutical preparations are available as capsules, tablets and solutions, and the drug is usually administered orally or intravenously. The therapeutic range in plasma is 25–100 mg/L. The drug is practically insoluble in water, and is reported to be highly light sensitive, but there is controversy regarding its degradation products and the extent of degradation under different light conditions.

Nifedipine acts by antagonising L-type Ca^{2+} channels in myocardial and vascular tissues leading to inhibition of Ca^{2+} influx. An inhibition of extracellular Ca^{2+} influx will reduce the availability of the intracellular Ca^{2+} required for muscle contraction in the myocardium and smooth muscles of the vascular system leading to an improvement in the oxygen supply for myocardial tissue, dilation of the coronary and systemic arteries, and a decreased peripheral and systemic blood pressure.

Structure–activity relationship for dihydropyridines

Nifedipine was used as lead compound in order to carry out qualitative SAR studies for DHPs to determine the most significant structural components that affect the activity of DHPs. Such studies reveal:

1. DHP ring is an essential component for the activity of DHPs. Substitution of this ring with and oxidised pyridine ring or reduced piperidino ring will diminish the activity of the DHP analogue. Moreover, substitution at N1 will also reduce the activity of DHP analogues. Small alkyl groups such as: methyl (which is the preferable one), amino, cyano, and formyl group at carbon 2 and 6 can contribute to the activity of DHPs while hydrogen and a phenyl group at this position can decrease the activity.
2. Phenyl ring at C4 is also essential for optimum activity of DHPs. Substitution of the phenyl ring with cycloalkyl groups can reduce the activity while substitution with heteroaromatic rings can increase toxicity of the DHP analogues.
3. An ester group at the 3 position is also essential for vascular activity of DHPs, while an ester at the 5 position can add some lipophilicity to the drug molecules. The ester group at the 3 position will affect vascular activity and duration of action. Enantiomers may result from non-identical replacement at the carbon atoms 3 and 5, since this will generate a chiral centre at C4 atom. These two enantiomers will exhibit different in vitro and in vivo activity. The degree of hydrophilicity/lipophilicity is very important for the vascular activity of DHPs. The activity decreases as this ratio will increases.

DHPs are un-ionised normal physiological pH 7.4 since the neutral nitrogen atom of the DHP ring will not be protonated, in contrast to verapamil which will be completely protonated at pH 7.4. DHPs lose vascular activity as their degree of hydrophilicity increases. Amlodipine, a long acting drug (Norvasc®) (Fig. 11.5), has special features since replacement of NO_2 at R2 with a Cl atom reduces the photolability of the drug. Additionally, the aliphatic amine enhances the bioavailability of the drug and increases its duration of action to about 3 h as compared to 30 min for nifedipine. The strategy of introducing a basic group into a neutral molecule improves half-life. Amlodipine has a comparable hydrophobicity to nifedipine, which is neutral, but the introduction of a basic centre into amlodipine increases the volume of distribution for unbound form of the drug, increasing the half-life for the drug, and decreasing clearance of the drug. This increase in half-life (35 hours) and decrease in clearance allows a single daily dose of amlodipine compared to two or three doses for nifedipine. Amlodipine has a comparable antagonistic activity to nifedipine against L-type and N-type Ca^{2+} channels and also somewhat so against T-type channels. Amlodipine antagonistic activity is controlled by cell potential and extracellular pH, as the depolarisation state of the cell and high extracellular pH will enhance its antagonistic activity against the Ca^{2+} channel. Amlodipine activity requires less time (faster onset of action) as compared to the time required for the onset of action for nifedipine.

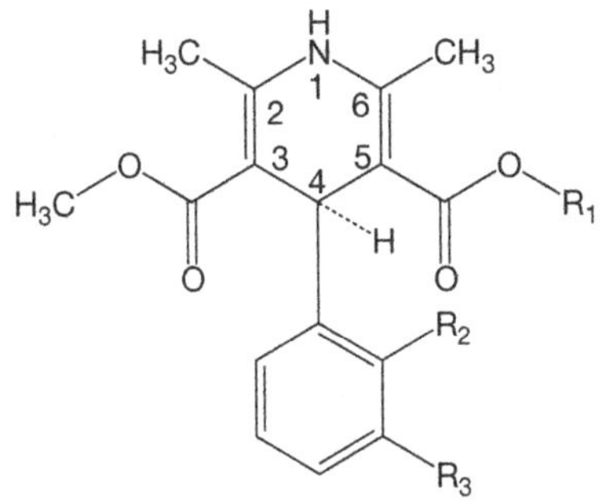

General dihydropyridines structure

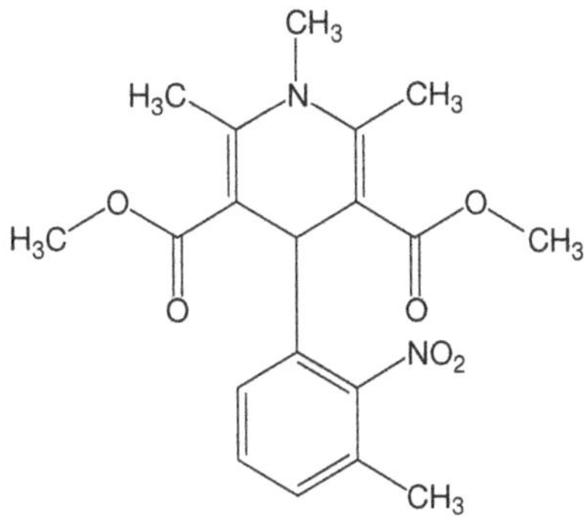

Nifedipine

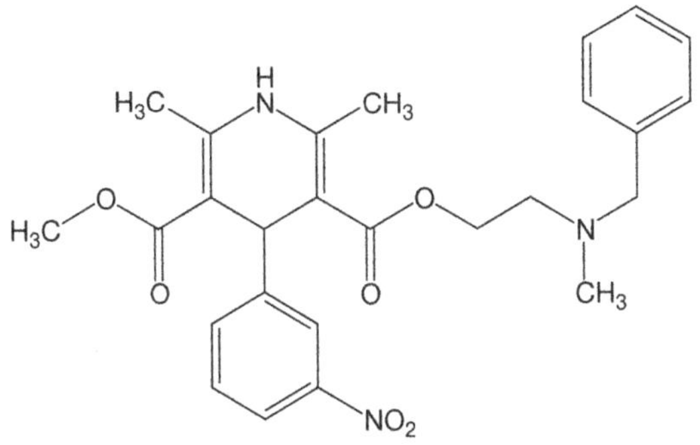

Nicardipine (Cardene®)

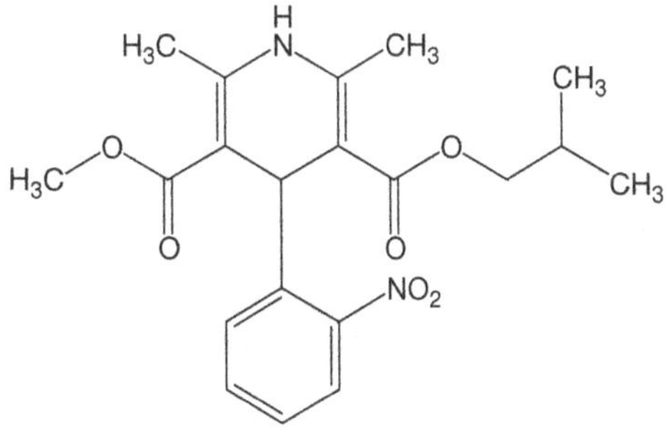

Nisoldipine

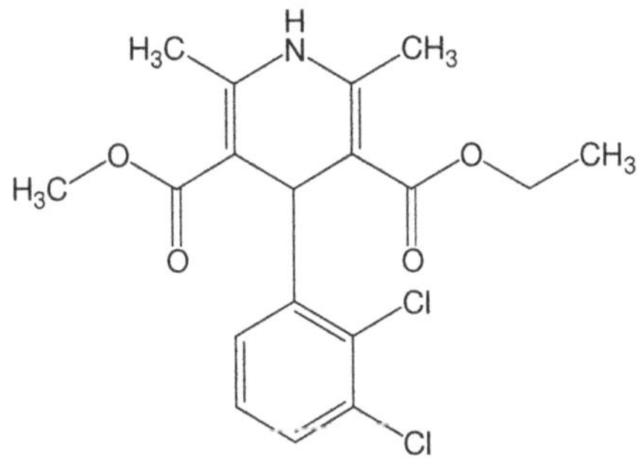

Felodipine (Plendil®)

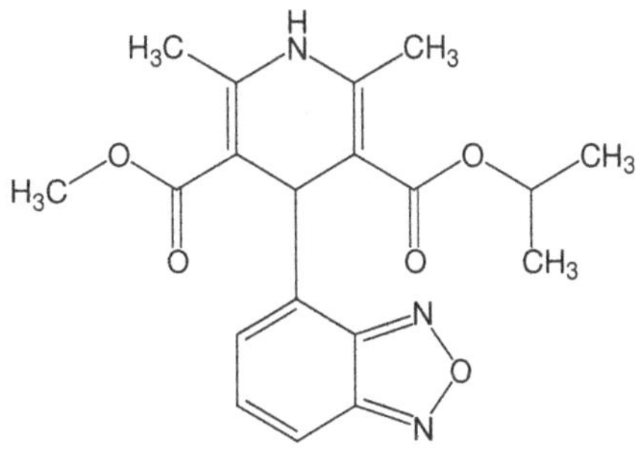

Isradipine (Dyna Circ®)

Figure 11.4 Chemical structures of the most commonly used dihydropyridines.

In comparison with amlodipine, nifedipine antagonises T-, L-, and N-type Ca^{2+} channels but its selectivity for L-type channels is much more than its selectivity for L- or N-type channels. (Nifedipine activity against L-type Ca^{2+} channels requires a concentration which is three- to fourfold less than that required for nifedipine activity against T-type channels.)

Formulation type plays a significant role in determining the pharmacological action of DHPs. A better pharmacological effect and fewer side effects can be obtained with long-acting DHPs (amlodipine, isradipine, and felodipine) or with extended-release formulations of nifedipine as compared to the short-acting ones. For example, in the case of the administration of nisoldipine, which is highly

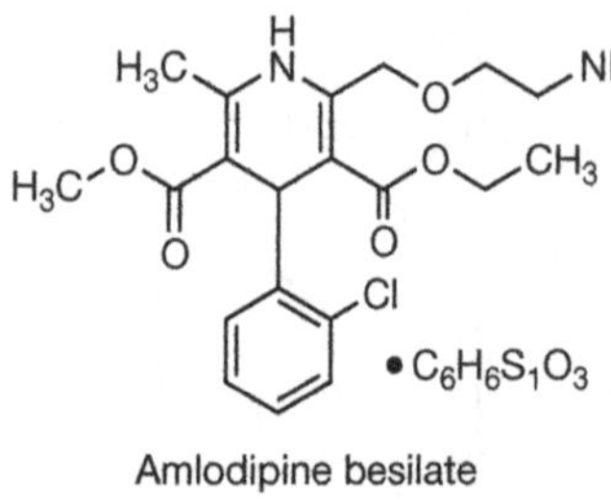

Figure 11.5 Amlodipine besilate.

selective for the calcium channels in the vascular system, the prolonged antianginal effect is obvious when this drug is taken as ultralong-acting core-coat preparation, while a moderate antianginal effect should be expected when this drug is taken as a twice-daily tablet.

The availability of single enantiomers of DHPs, where one enantiomer shows agonist activity and the other exerts antagonist activity, indicates the importance of stereoselectivity in DHP action. For example, a slight stereochemical modification of the 1,4-dihydropyridine analogue (Bay k8644) can result in a significant change in its pharmacological effect. This change in structure–activity relationship for Bay k8644 results from the availability of two enantiomeric forms for the same compound: The (S) form shows agonist activity for L-type voltage-gated Ca^{2+} channels, while the R form shows antagonistic activity (Fig. 11.6).

Metabolism of DHPs

Dihydropyridines are mainly metabolised by liver CYP3A4 which causes oxidation of the dihydropyridine group to the pyridine analogue (Fig. 11.7). This is then followed by hydrolysis of one of the ester groups at C3 or C5 via esterase activity. Sometimes, hydroxylation and ester hydrolysis (especially in nitrendipine) can result in the formation of γ-lactone groups.

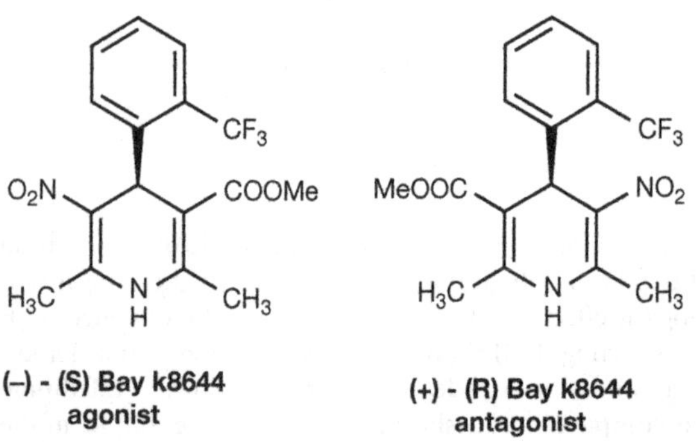

Figure 11.6 Enantiomers of Bay k8644.

Phenylalkylamines

Phenylalkylamines (PAAs) are characterised by the presence of the phenylalkylamine group (also called arylalkylamine) within its structure which is believed to bind to a specific site in the calcium-channel receptor identified by binding of ^{3}H-cinnarzine. Figure 11.8 shows the commonly used PAAs.

Structure–activity relationship for phenylalkylamines

Qualitative SAR studies for phenylalkylamines reveal the most essential components for their activity such as: (1) the levorotary form of the drug is the only active form; (2) two phenyl groups represent an important component of the activity; (3) meta substituents on the aromatic ring will increase the activity while ortho substituents exhibit steric hindrance for the interaction of the drug with receptors and this will decrease the activity. Such studies also confirm that the isopropyl group is not essential for the activity of verapamil-like drugs. Since only the levorotary form of the drug is active, any substituent near the chiral centre will affect the activity. Verapamil (p*Ka* 8.7) is mainly excreted by the kidney since at physiological pH 7.4, almost 95% of the drug will be protonated. The addition of two highly polar SO_2 groups in tiapamil increases the hydrophilicity to three times that of verapamil and the p*Ka* is slightly decreased (8.5) due to electron withdrawal from the nitrogen atom by the SO_2 groups.

Verapamil

Verapamil acts mainly by inhibiting extracellular Ca^{2+} ion influx through the transmembrane L- and T-type Ca^{2+} ion channels in the myocardial and vascular system. This blockade for the Ca^{2+} ion channel will result in negative inotropic effect (decrease in the contractility of cardiac and vascular system muscles), negative chronotropic effect (decrease in heart rate), and negative dromotropic effect (slowing down of the conductivity of the AV node). An improvement in the oxygen supply to the heart should be expected due to the dilation of the coronary arteries. Additionally, verapamil has the ability to inhibit the intracellular release of the Ca^{2+} ion from the endoplasmic reticulum.

The pharmaceutical dosage form is usually verapamil hydrochloride. Verapamil free base is practically insoluble in water, sparingly soluble in hexane, soluble in benzene, ether, freely soluble in the lower alcohols, acetone, ethyl acetate and chloroform. Verapamil hydrochloride is sparingly soluble in chloroform, soluble in ethanol, isopropanol, acetone, and ethyl acetate, and freely soluble in methanol. Verapamil is available as oral and i.v. dosage forms but the possibility of cardiotoxicity is much higher with the i.v. dosage form.

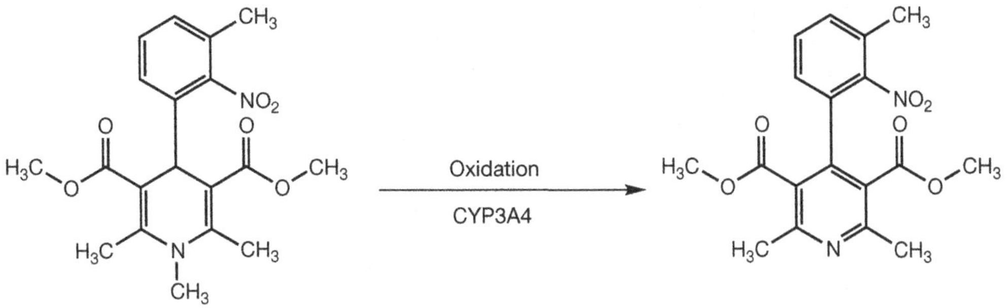

Nifedipine

Oxidised Nifedipine

Figure 11.7 Hepatic metabolism of nifedipine by CYP3A4.

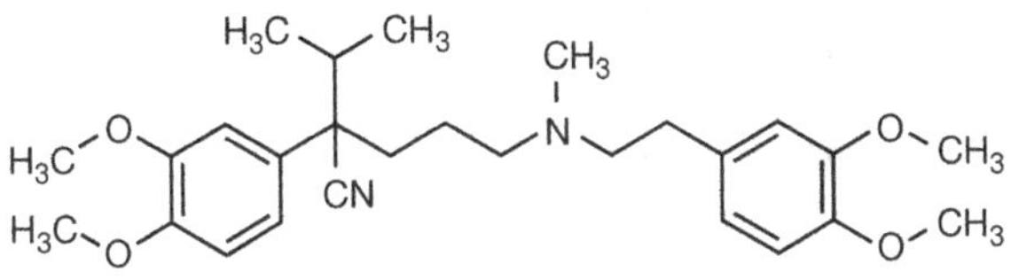

Verapamil

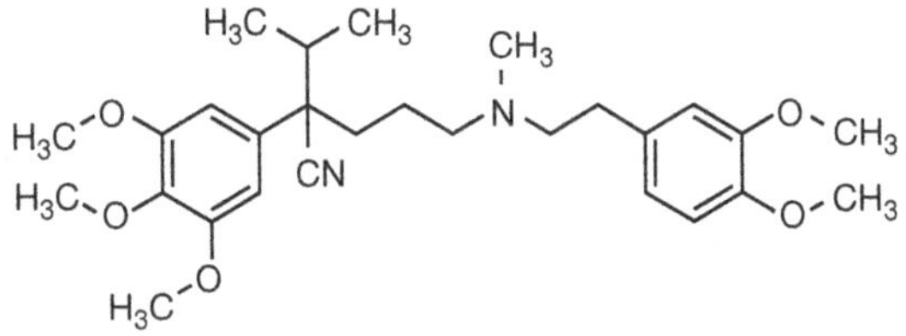

Gallopamil

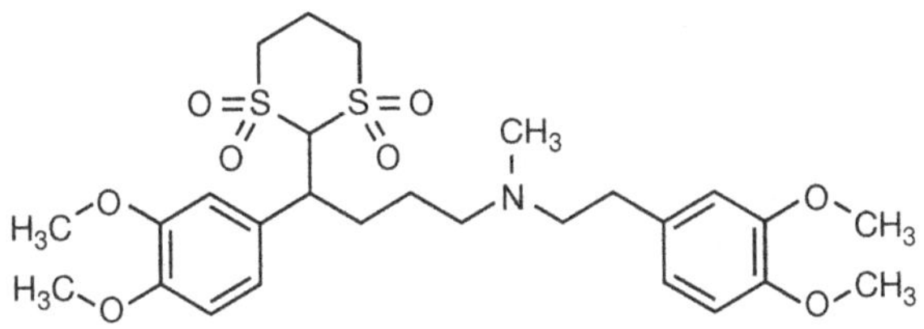

Tiapamil

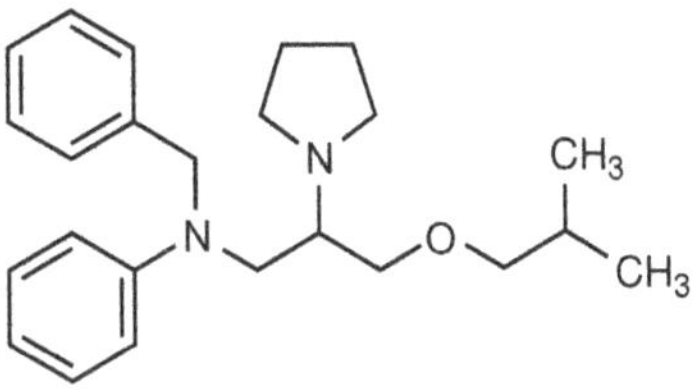

Bepridil

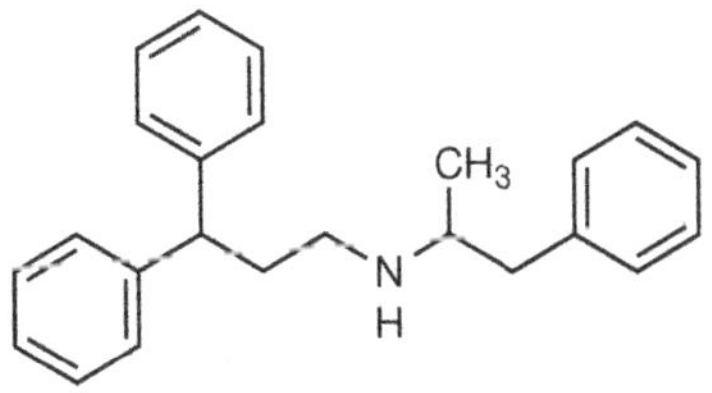

Prenylamine

Figure 11.8 The most commonly used phenylalkylamines.

The main indications for verapamil include:

1. Paroxysmal supraventricular tachycardia (PSVT): verapamil is the drug of choice due to its dromotropic effect.
2. Angina pectoris: due to its coronary vasodilatation effect and improved oxygen delivery to the myocardial tissue.
3. Hypertension: due to its arterial vasodilatation effect. Verapamil is considered as effective as nifedipine or nicardipine in the treatment of mild or moderate hypertension, without producing reflex tachycardia.

Verapamil can be used in patients with bronchospastic diseases, but there are several contraindications for using verapamil in patients with severe hypotension, left ventricular dysfunction, second- or third-degree atrioventricular block, heart failure, or a hypersensitivity to verapamil. The clinical signs for verapamil toxicity include: hypotension due to arterial vasodilatation; cardiogenic shock secondary to a negative inotropic effect; bradycardia and atrioventricular block.

Verapamil is characterised by a high level of absorption from the gastrointestinal tract (about 90%) when the drug is taken orally. The peak plasma level of verapamil will be attained over 30–120 min after oral administration. Bioavailability of verapamil is low (20–35%) in normal individuals, due to hepatic metabolism. Hepatic N-dealkylation of verapamil by the enzyme CYP3A4 will result in the formation of the main metabolite norverapamil (Fig. 11.9) which has the same elimination half-life as verapamil (4–8 hrs).

There is the possibility of another 12 metabolites which may result from the action of N- or O-dealkylating enzymes on the parent compound. About 70% of the dose is eliminated by the kidney as metabolites within 5 days of drug administration (3–4% is excreted as the parent compound). Moreover, 16% of the oral dose is eliminated by the gastrointestinal tract as metabolites within 5 days of administration. Additionally, there is a possibility of verapamil elimination via breast milk as the unchanged drug.

Verapamil provides an example of the importance of the stereoselectivity of a drug in a biological system, since verapamil is used as a racemic mixture of the pharmacologically active (−) enantiomer and the non-active (+) enantiomer. Verapamil undergoes stereoselective first pass metabolism after oral administration and the bioavailability of the active (−) form is 2–3 fold less than the non-active (+) form; thus the bioavailability of the active (−) is lower, and non-stereoselective chromatographic methods used to monitor the pharmacokinetics of the drug would miss this.

Gallopamil

Gallopamil (methoxyverapamil) is a CCB used for the treatment of coronary artery disease (angina pectoris). Gallopamil improves exercise tolerance in patients with chronic stable angina due to its protective effect on coronary arteries without negative effects on cardiac performance. The mechanism of action is similar to the mechanism of Na^+ channel blocking by tertiary amines. The drug, at normal physiological pH, is in equilibrium between neutral and cationic forms at the site of action on the Ca^{2+} channels, and the cationic form will block the channel from the intracellular side. Gallopamil undergoes extensive first-pass metabolism after oral administration, resulting in a low blood concentration of gallopamil and its metabolite norgallopamil. However, after chronic oral administration of gallopamil for 28 days, a higher blood concentration of gallopamil can be measured, which can be attributed to the saturation of gallopamil's metabolic pathways with repeated oral administration. A rapid decline in gallopamil's clearance after 28 days of oral administration can be considered as a strong evidence for the saturation of the metabolising enzymes in liver. Gallopamil has similar indications and mechanism of action to verapamil. It is a chiral compound and the oral dosage form is available as racemic mixture of R- and S-enantiomers. In contrast to verapamil, the metabolism of gallopamil is not stereoselective, and the rate of clearance

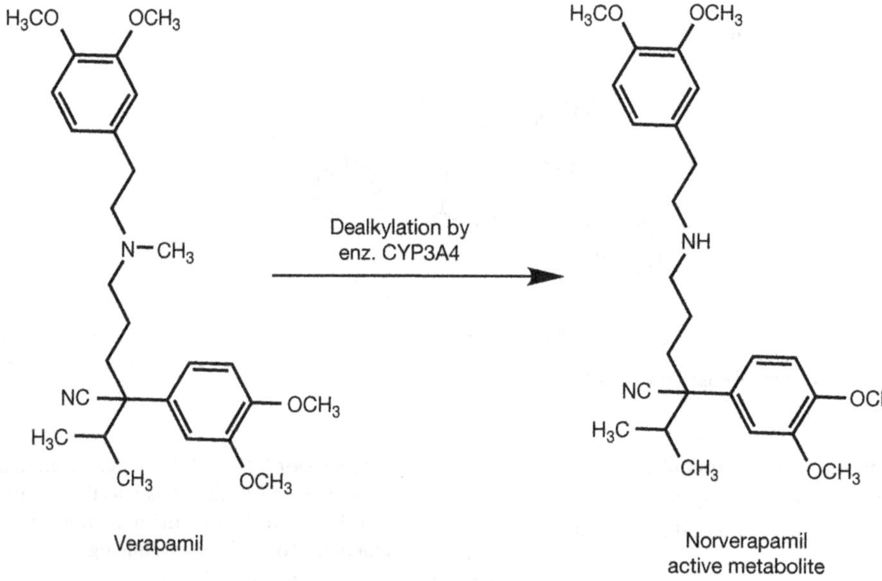

Figure 11.9 Hepatic metabolism of verapamil by CYP3A4.

of the R- and S-enantiomers is almost the same despite the similarity in structure to verapamil. Gallopamil is mainly metabolised by the hepatic enzyme CYP3A4 (an isoform of cytochrome P-450), which accounts for about 90% of the metabolic clearance through dealkylation of the tertiary amine in gallopamil structure (Fig. 11.10). Other metabolic pathways include O-demethylation of the methoxy groups at position 1–4 of the gallopamil which accounts for the remaining 10% of the metabolism of gallopamil.

Benzothiazepines

The benzothiazepine structure includes a benzene ring attached to 1,5-thiazepine (Fig. 11.11). Stereoisomerism is important in benzothiazepine (BTZs) due to the presence of two chiral centres at positions 2 and 3 of the 1,5-thiazepine ring, with significant vasodilatory activity being due to the cis form of the drug. Physiological action for BTZs may be also affected by presence of (−) or (+) enantiomers for the cis and trans forms of the drug molecule. The (+) cis-enantiomer for diltiazem (Fig. 11.12) exhibits a shorter duration of action (about 10-fold less) than the (−) trans-enantiomer. Introduction of an alkoxy or hydroxyl group in the phenyl group attached to C2 leads to a loss in activity. While introduction of a chlorine atom at C10 of the attached benzene ring increases the activity of the BTZ, other substitutions may decrease the activity. Substitution at C3 does not affect BTZ activity, as replacement of the acetoxy group at C3 with alkoxy, hydroxyl, aralkoxy, or aliphatic and aromatic acyloxy groups produces compounds with comparable activity to diltiazem. Alkylaminoalkyl substitution at N5 plays a significant role in the activity of the BTZs, while removing the substitutions from N5, by dealkylation, leads to inactivation of the compound.

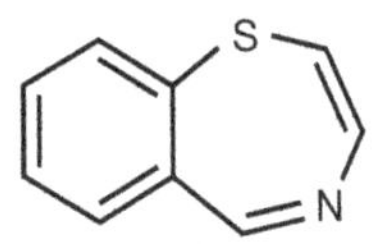

1,4-benzothiazepine

Figure 11.11

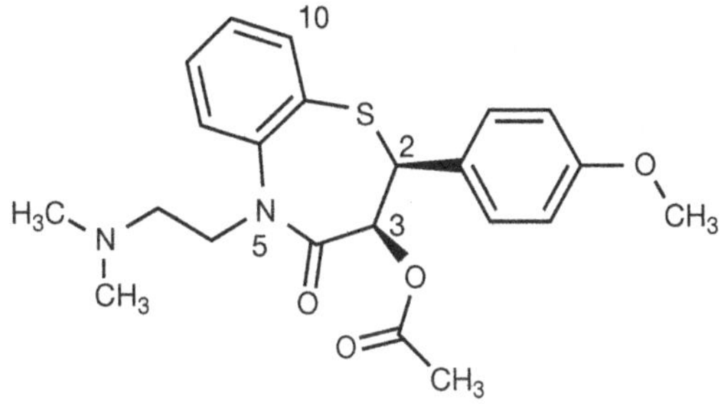

Diltiazem

Figure 11.12

Diltiazem has the same mechanism of action as verapamil, with the main indication as an antihypertensive agent, and an antianginal agent (for treatment of chronic stable angina and Prinzmetal's variant angina). Orally taken, diltiazem is subject to an extensive first-pass effect in liver by the action of the CYP3A4 enzyme. Sometimes, diltiazem may be prescribed as inhibitor of the CYP3A4

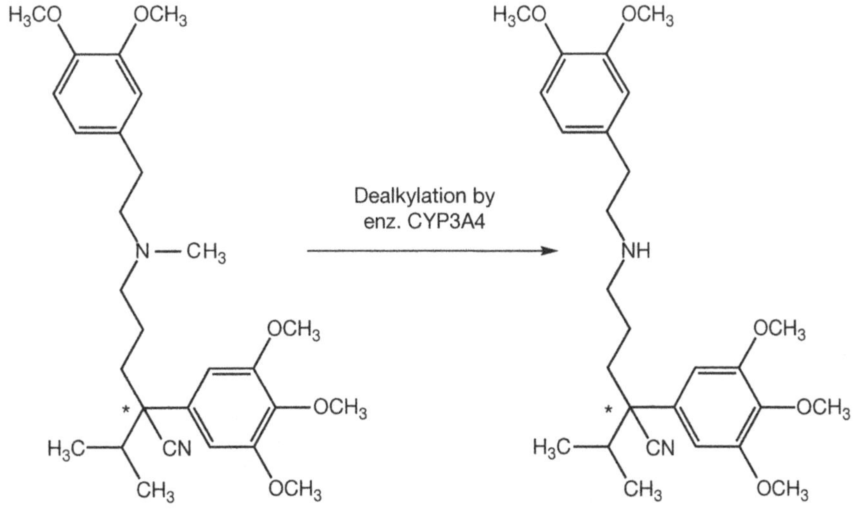

Gallopamil Norgallopamil

Figure 11.10 Hepatic metabolism of gallopamil by CYP3A4.

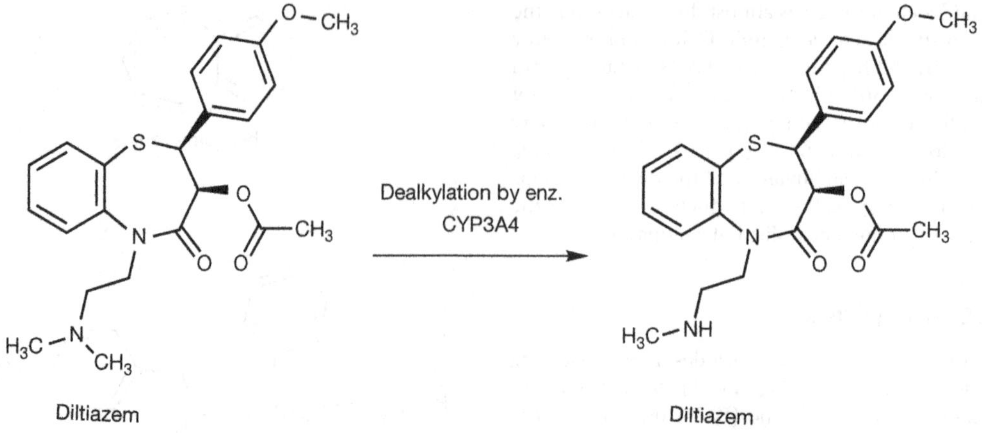

Figure 11.13 Hepatic metabolism of diltiazem by CYP3A4.

enzyme. Diltiazem is metabolised via a number of pathways: N-demethylation (hepatically by enzyme CYP3A4 (Fig. 11.13)), deacetylation, O-demethylation, ring hydroxylation and ester hydrolysis.

Side effects of calcium-channel blockers

Side effects for DHPs seem to be dependent on the type of formulation and type of drug release (fast acting, long acting), which controls the speed of drug bioavailability in blood. Slower-release formulations (long acting) will induce a slower elevation in DHPs level in blood, which may produce fewer side effects as compared with fast-acting ones. Headache, dizziness, acute vasodilatation, flushing and tachycardia are common side effects for fast-acting formulations. Second generation DHPs, such as isradipine, produce less ankle oedema as compared to felodipine, despite both of them being administered twice daily (both long acting), which suggest that ankle oedema is not directly related to the duration of drug action.

Headache, dizziness, acute vasodilatation, flushing and tachycardia are less common side effects for phenylalkylamines as compared to DHPs, while constipation is considered as the characteristic side effect for the phenylalkylamine group (with the exception of gallopamil), due to their ability to interact with calcium channels of the smooth muscles inside gut.

Side effects for benzothiazepines seem to be dose dependent (including oedema), since no side effects are expected at lower doses while headaches and oedema can be observed at higher doses. In contrast to the phenylalkylamines, constipation is a less common side effect for benzothiazepines, while depression of SA node function or AV nodal block would be expected for both benzothiazepines and phenylalkylamines.

Non-selective drugs (ungrouped)

The following drugs are also used for similar indications to the three main groups discussed above but in many cases their exact mechanism of action is not known: Amrinone, Anandamide, Anipamil, Azimilide, Bencyclane, Bepridil, Berbamine, Bevantolol, Canadine, Carboxyamido-Triazole, Cinnarizine, Conotoxins, Darodipine, Dauricine, Devapamil, Dimeditiapramine, Dotarizine, Emopamil, Enpiperate, Eperisone, Falipamil, Fantofarone, Fasudil, Fenamic acid, Fendiline, Flunarizine, Fosfedil, Gabapentin, Lamotrigine, Lidoflazine, Magnesium sulfate, Manoalide, Mepirodipine, Mibefradil, Monatepil, Naftopidil, Niguldipine, Niludipin, Norverapamil, Ochratoxin A, Octylonium, Osthol, Oxodipine, Perhexiline, Pinaverium, Piperidine, Prenylamine, Risedronic acid, Ryodipine, Sesamodil, Stepholidine, Terodiline, Tetrahydropalmatine, Tetrandrine, Tolfenamic acid, Tranilast. Table 11.4 summarises the mode of action of some of these drugs.

Preparations of calcium channel blockers

- Amlodipine: 5 mg and 10 mg tablets
- Felodipine: 2.5 mg, 5 mg, 10 mg tablets
- Isradipine: 2.5 mg, 5 mg tablets
- Lacidipine: 2 mg and 4 mg tablets
- Nicardipine: 20 mg, 30 mg and 45 mg capsules
- Nifedipine: 5 mg, 10 mg, 30 mg, 40 mg and 60 mg tablets, 10 mg and 20 mg controlled-release tablets, 10 mg, 20 mg and 30 mg capsules
- Nisoldipine: 10 mg tablets
- Verampamil: tablets 40 mg, 80 mg, 160 mg, tablets 120 mg and 240 mg modified release, injection 2 mg/mL
- Dilatiazem: tablets 60 mg, 90 mg and 120 gm, 120 mg controlled-release tablets, capsules 90mg, 120 mg, 180 mg and 300 mg, controlled-release capsules 120 mg, 180 mg, 240 mg and 300 mg.

Table 11.4 Non-selective calcium channel blocking drugs

Non-selective Ca^{2+} channel	Family	Compounds	Notes
1. Selectively binds to non L-type Ca^{2+} channel	Undefined binding site	Mibefradil Anandamide	
2. Non-selective Ca^{2+} channel modulator	a. Benzylisoquinoline	Tetrandrine Papaverine	
	b. Diphenylalkylamine	Bepridile	
		Cinnarzine	
		Flunarizine	Enhances dopamine release by nerve terminals
		Fendiline	
	c. Pyrazine	Amiloride	
	d. Diphenylbutylpiperidine	Pimozide Fluspirilene Penfluridol	

CALCIUM ANTAGONIST SUMMARY

DIHYDROPYRIDINE (DHPs)

Show negative inotropic effect by affecting vascular smooth muscles mainly.

- Amlodipine (Norvasc, Azor)
- Aranidipine (Sapresta)
- Azelnidipine (Calblock)
- Barnidipine (HypoCa)
- Benidipine (Coniel)
- Cilnidipine (Atelec, Cinalong, Siscard)
- Clevidipine (Cleviprex)
- Efonidipine (Landel)
- Felodipine (Plendil)
- Lacidipine (Motens, Lacipil)
- Lercanidipine (Zanidip)
- Manidipine (Calslot, Madipine)
- Nicardipine (Cardene, Carden SR)
- Nifedipine (Procardia, Adalat)
- Nilvadipine (Nivadil)
- Nimodipine (Nimotop)
- Nisoldipine (Baymycard, Sular, Syscor)
- Nitrendipine (Cardif, Nitrepin, Baylotensin)
- Pranidipine (Acalas)

PHENYLALKYLAMINE (PAAs)

Mainly act on heart by their negative chronotropic effect.

- Verapamil
- Bepridil
- Tiapamil
- Gallopamil

BENZOTHIAZEPINE (BTZs)

Have both negative inotropic and chronotropic effect.

- Diltiazem
- Clentiazem

OTHERS (UNGROUPED)

- Fendiline
- Flunarizine
- Mibefradil
- Norverapamil

RECOMMENDED READING

Smith DA, van de Waterbeemd H, Walker DK. *Pharmacokinetics and Metabolism in Drug Design.* 2nd revised ed. Weinheim: WILEY-VCH Verlag GmbH & Co. KGaA; 2006.

Opie LH. *Calcium antagonists and cardiovascular disease.* New York: Raven Press, c1984.

Godfraind T, with a contribution by Eric Ertel. *Calcium channel blockers.* Boston, MA: Birkhauser Verlag; 2004.

Gringauz A. *Introduction to Medicinal Chemistry: How Drugs Act and Why.* Weinheim: WILEY-VCH Verlag GmbH & Co. KGaA; 1996.

Triggle DJ, Copalakrishnan M, Rampe D, Zheng W. *Methods and principles in medicinal chemistry: Voltage-Gated Ion Channels as Drug Targets*. Vol 29. Weinheim: WILEY-VCH Verlag GmbH & Co. KGaA; 2006.

Katzung BG, Chatterjee K. Vasodilators and the treatment of angina pectoris. In: Katzung BG, ed. *Basic and clinical pharmacology*. New York, NY: McGraw-Hill; 2001: 181–199.

Rang HP, Dale MM, Ritter JM. *Pharmacology*. New York: Churchill Livingstone Inc; 1995.

Caira MR, Robbertse Y, Bergh JJ, Song M, De Villiers MM. Structural characterization, physicochemical properties, and thermal stability of three crystal forms of nifedipine. *J Pharm Sci*. 2003;92:2519–2533.

Perez-Reyes E, Cribbs LL, Daud A, et al. Molecular characterization of a neuronal low-voltage-activated T-type calcium channel. *Nature*. 1998;391:896–900.

Ertel EA, Campbell KP, Harpold MM, et al. Nomenclature of voltage-gated calcium channels. *Neuron*. 2000;25:533–535.

Lionel HO. Calcium channel antagonists in the treatment of coronary artery disease: Fundamental pharmacological properties relevant to clinical use. *Prog Cardiovasc Dis*. 1996;38:273–290.

Aso YYS, Otsuka T, Kojima S. The physical stability of amorphous nifedipine determined by isothermal microcalorimetry. *Chem Pharm Bull (Tokyo)*. 1995;43:300–303.

Mutlib AE, Nelson WL. Pathways of gallopamil metabolism. Regiochemistry and enantioselectivity of the O-demethylation processes. *Drug Metab Dispos*. 1990;18: 309–314.

Suzuki A, Iida I, Tanaka F, et al. Identification of Human Cytochrome P-450 Isoforms Involved in Metabolism of R(+)- and S(-)-Gallopamil: Utility of In Vitro Disappearance Rate. *Drug Metab Dispos*. 1999;27:1254–1259.

Chapter 12

Drugs interacting with mammalian enzymes

CHAPTER CONTENTS

SECTION A – LIPID-LOWERING DRUGS

Jeffrey Stuart Millership

INTRODUCTION

There are a number of systems within the body that are controlled by enzymatic systems and which function in the control of disease states. In certain cases these systems are involved in a relatively narrow area of activity, e.g. HMG-CoA reductase, whilst in other situations the enzyme systems are involved in a variety of functions, e.g. phosphodiesterases. The following sections detail aspects of lipid-lowering drugs including the action of statins with HMG-CoA reductase, the sulphonamide diuretics and carbonic anhydrase activity and their involvement with the Na/Cl/K symporter, ACE inhibitors, a number of different phosphodiesterase inhibitors involved in erectile dysfunction and chronic obstructive pulmonary disease and the proton pump inhibitors used in the treatment of gastric ulcers.

LIPID-LOWERING DRUGS

Cholesterol is an important steroid in various aspects of the function of human cells. It is a precursor of a number of important steroids, e.g. corticosteroids and the sex hormones. It is also important for the maintenance of cell wall integrity. Unfortunately, cholesterol can also cause problems when present in high levels in the body due to its involvement in atherosclerosis. Atherosclerosis results from a build-up of cholesterol in various forms in the arteries, thereby reducing the flow of blood. Blood clots can be produced and these can result in either heart attacks or strokes. Cholesterol is taken into the body either via the diet or is synthesised in the liver. Cholesterol is absorbed into the bloodstream; however, it is insoluble in its free form in the blood and is transported by means of lipoproteins. Lipoproteins are particles that have a hydrophilic outer shell comprising phospholipids, free cholesterol and apolipoproteins and an inner hydrophobic core containing the lipids such as cholesteryl esters and triglycerides. Although there are a number of lipoproteins associated with transport of cholesterol, two in particular are often discussed in relation to heart disease: low-density lipoproteins (LDLs) and high-density lipoproteins (HDLs). LDL cholesterol is often described as bad cholesterol whilst HDL cholesterol is good cholesterol. LDL cholesterol is bad cholesterol since it is associated with plaque formation, which is a fundamental cause of atherosclerosis. HDL, or good cholesterol, is associated with the removal of excess cholesterol in the body since it transports cholesterol to the liver for disposal. Since high levels of cholesterol in the blood (hypercholesterolaemia) is considered a major risk factor for atherosclerosis, its reduction is obviously of great importance given the level of this disease state in the population. High levels of triglycerides are also linked to heart disease, although the precise relationship is less clear than with cholesterol.

There are presently a number of drugs that may be applied to the lowering of lipids in the body and these include:

- anion exchange resins
- ezetimibe
- fibrates
- statins
- compounds of the nicotinic acid group.

These different classes of drugs work on a variety of different pathways in the body.

Anion exchange resins

Anion exchange resins such as Colestyramine and Colestipol (Fig. 12.1) have been used for some time as lipid-lowering agents. These two compounds act as bile acid sequestrating agents, binding to bile acids in the intestine via an electrostatic mechanism where the negatively charged acids bind to the positively charged resin. Through this process insoluble complexes are formed which are then excreted. As a result of this process plasma bile acid levels are reduced and subsequently cholesterol, which is the biosynthetic precursor of bile acids, is converted into bile acids and thus the levels of cholesterol in the body are reduced.

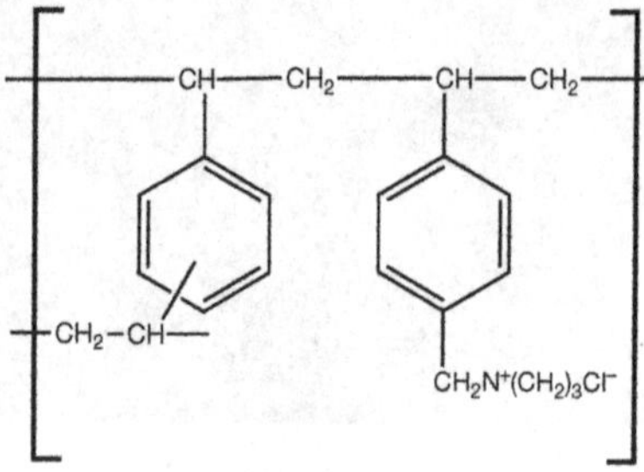

Cholestyramine

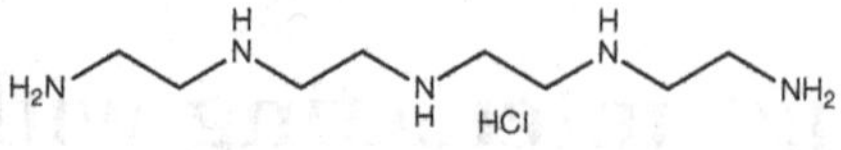

Colestipol

Figure 12.1 Bile acid sequestrating agents.

Fibrates

Fibrates are a class of lipid-lowering drugs that are all related to fibric acid (Fig. 12.2). It is reported that their

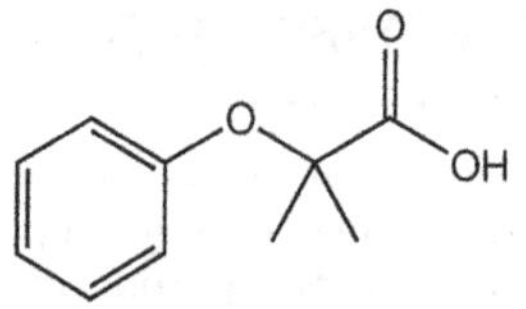

Fibric acid

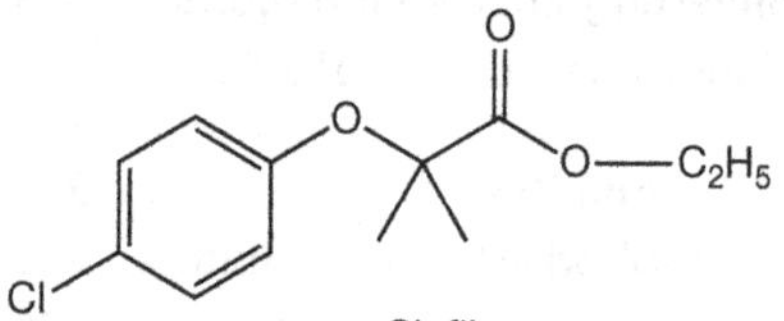

Clofibrate

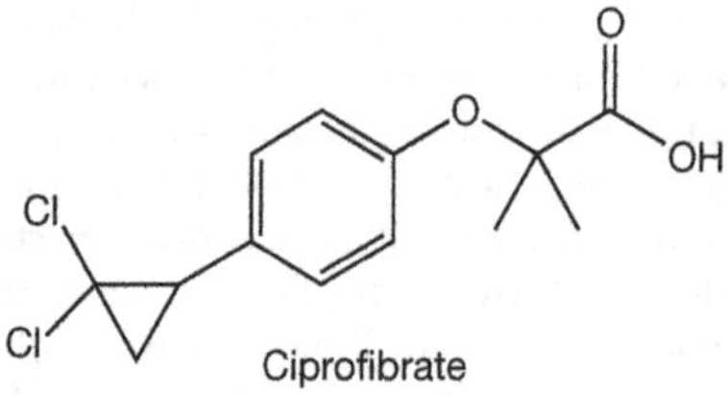

Ciprofibrate

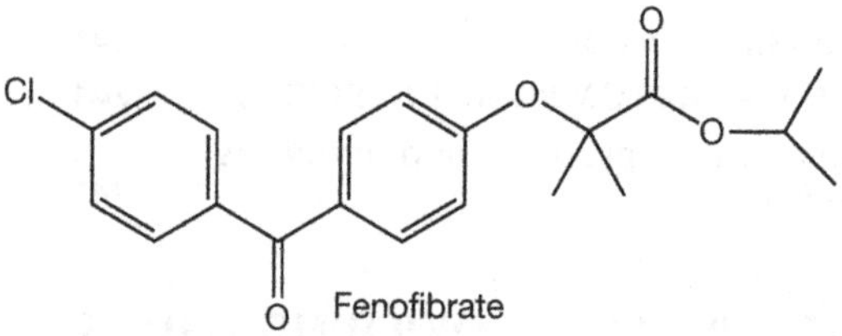

Fenofibrate

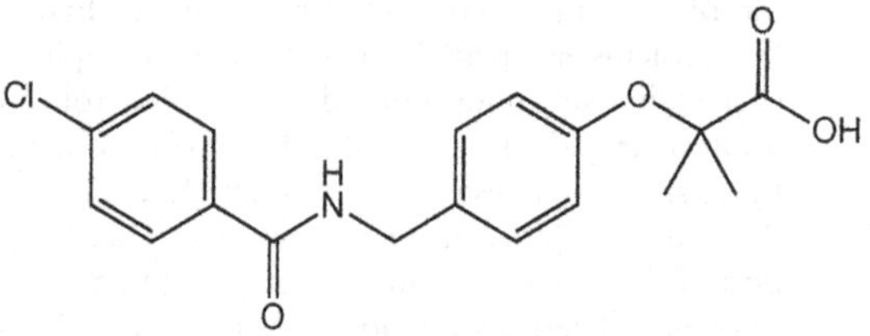

Bezafibrate

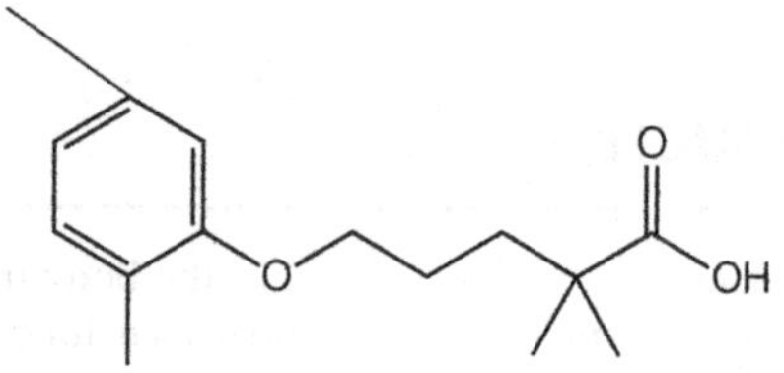

Gemfibrozil

Figure 12.2 Fibric acid and fibrates.

discovery was serendipitous. In the 1950s, available evidence suggested that androsterone was capable of reducing high levels of lipids in the blood. Formulation scientists trying to overcome the administration difficulties of androsterone used clofibrate as a solvent for the steroid. This product, subsequently known as Atromid, was shown to be effective as a lipid-lowering drug. Further studies eventually demonstrated that the lipid-lowering effect of this formulated product was due not to the androsterone but to the solvating agent clofibrate. Since the original discovery, a number of 'fibrates' have been introduced and several are still available clinically, however, the use of these drugs is less common nowadays due to the introduction of the newer lipid-lowering agents. Fibrates are, however, indicated as first-line therapy for patients with serum triglyceride levels greater than 10 mm/L. The fibrates that are clinically used at present include ciprofibrate, bezafibrate, fenofibrate and gemfibrozil (Fig.12.2).

Fibrates act as peroxisome proliferator activated receptors (PPAR) agonists and in particular PPARα agonists. PPARs, amongst other things, play an important role in the regulation of metabolism, including lipid metabolism. The action of the fibrates results in lowering of elevated cholesterol levels via increasing HDL levels and decreasing LDL (and very low-density lipoproteins VLDLs) levels as well as reducing triglyceride levels. The reduction in triglyceride levels is through reduced production in the liver and an increase in the rate at which they are removed from the blood stream.

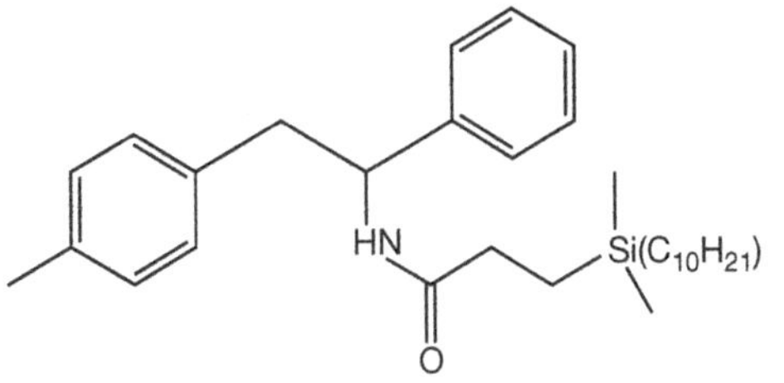

SA 58035

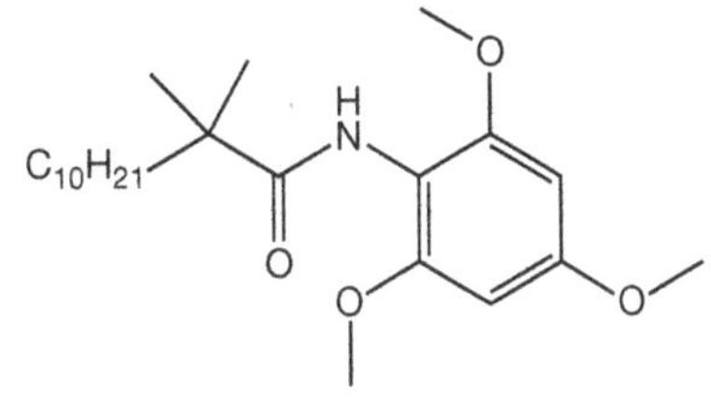

CI 976

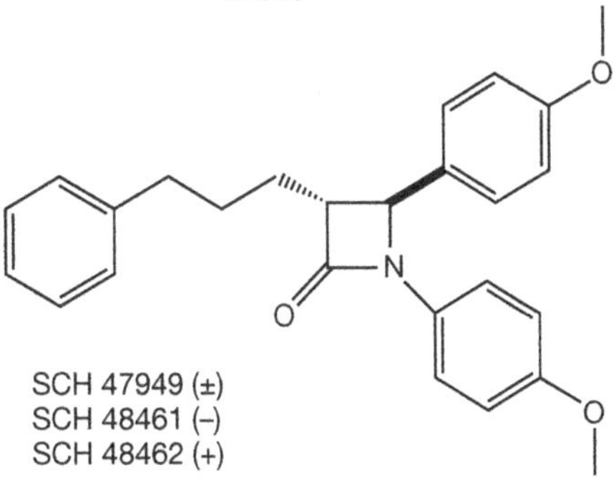

SCH 47949 (±)
SCH 48461 (–)
SCH 48462 (+)

Figure 12.4 Cholesterol absorption inhibitors.

Ezetimibe

Ezetimibe (Fig. 12.3) is a drug that works by reduction of blood cholesterol by inhibiting the absorption of cholesterol by the small intestine. As indicated above, cholesterol in the body is derived from dietary sources or is synthesised in the body. Acyl Coenzyme A: Cholesterol A Transferase (ACAT) is a membrane protein that catalyses the synthesis of cholesteryl esters from cholesterol. Inhibition of ACAT has therefore been investigated as a route to reducing blood cholesterol levels and thus a means of preventing atherosclerosis. Whilst investigating potential ACAT inhibitors, investigators at Schering-Plough discovered a group of azetidinon-2-ones (Fig. 12.4) that were inhibitors of cholesterol absorption.

This work involved a study of conformationally restricted forms of SA 58035 and CI 976, which are examples of two classes of compounds that act as ACAT inhibitors. During this work it was demonstrated that monocyclic β-lactams such as those shown in Figure 12.4 were inhibitors of cholesterol absorption. However, it was also discovered that they did not act as ACAT inhibitors, but via a different mechanism. From this work the now clinically used drug ezetimibe has been developed and it is now known that this drug acts by inhibiting cholesterol absorption in the intestines. It is believed that ezetimibe undergoes phase II metabolism to form the glucuronide of the phenolic hydroxy group. This metabolite appears to become localised in the brush border of the small intestine, thereby preventing cholesterol

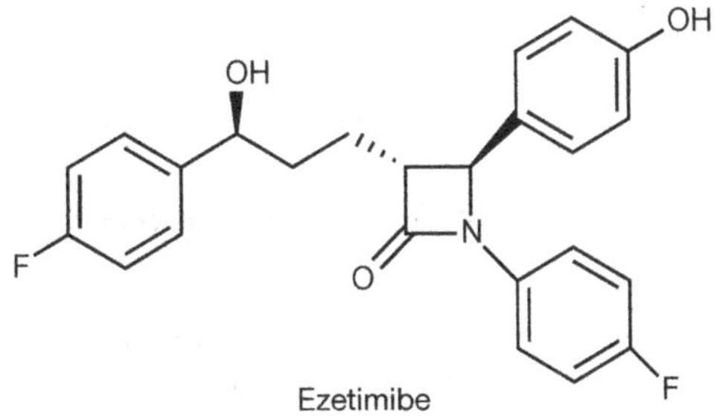

Ezetimibe

Figure 12.3 Structure of ezetimibe.

uptake. The precise mode of action of ezetimibe is still unclear. It has recently been reported that NPC1L1 (Niemann-Pick C1-Like 1) is the major target for ezetimibe; however, this has been contradicted.

Statins

The statins are a group of compounds that were discovered about forty years ago. During the 1960s, researchers had shown that cholesterol could be obtained from the diet or it could be synthesised in the body. It was observed that if humans consumed a diet rich in cholesterol then the body stopped synthesising it. This suggested that there was some form of feedback mechanism in the body that resulted in the inhibition of cholesterol synthesis. It was proposed that the enzyme system HMG CoA reductase was the enzyme system that was inhibited in this process.

The biosynthesis of cholesterol occurs in three main phases: stage one is the formation of mevalonic acid, stage two is conversion of mevalonate in farnesylpyrophosphate, and the final stage involves the head-to-tail condensation of two farnesylpyrophosphate units to yield squalene which subsequently yields cholesterol via lanosterol. The mevalonic acid (mevalonate) sequence is shown in Figure 12.5. In this sequence two molecules of acetyl coenzyme A condense to generate acetoacetyl CoA, which reacts with a further molecule of acetyl CoA to generate 3-hydroxy-3-methylglutaryl CoA (HMG CoA). HMG CoA is reduced by HMG CoA reductase to yield mevalonic acid. Note this last step is most important since it is inhibition of this enzyme system by statins which is pivotal in their lipid-lowering activity.

In the early 70s, in Japan, Drs Endo and Kuroda began studies to find chemical entities that would inhibit the activity of HMG CoA reductase and thus interfere with the synthesis of cholesterol in the human body. They investigated many microorganisms to find such inhibitors since they proposed that such organisms might produce inhibitors in order to combat attack on the mevalonic acid biosynthesis, which is prevalent in many organisms.

The action of the statins is related to their structural similarities to HMG CoA. In Figure 12.5, we can see the conversion of HMG CoA into mevalonic acid via the enzyme HMG CoA reductase. This process occurs via the intermediate mevalonyl CoA. The structure of both and the statin pharmacophore are shown in Figure 12.6. It is the dihydroxyheptanoic acid portion of the statins (circled in the diagram of the pharmacophore) that closely resembles the endogenous substrate for the HMG CoA reductase that allows the statins to act as inhibitors of the reductase. In some cases, such as with simvastatin (Fig. 12.7), the dihydroxyheptanoic acid portion exists as the lactone form and, as such, the statin is in fact a prodrug form of the parent molecule. Under physiological conditions the lactone form of the drug is in equilibrium with open chain form.

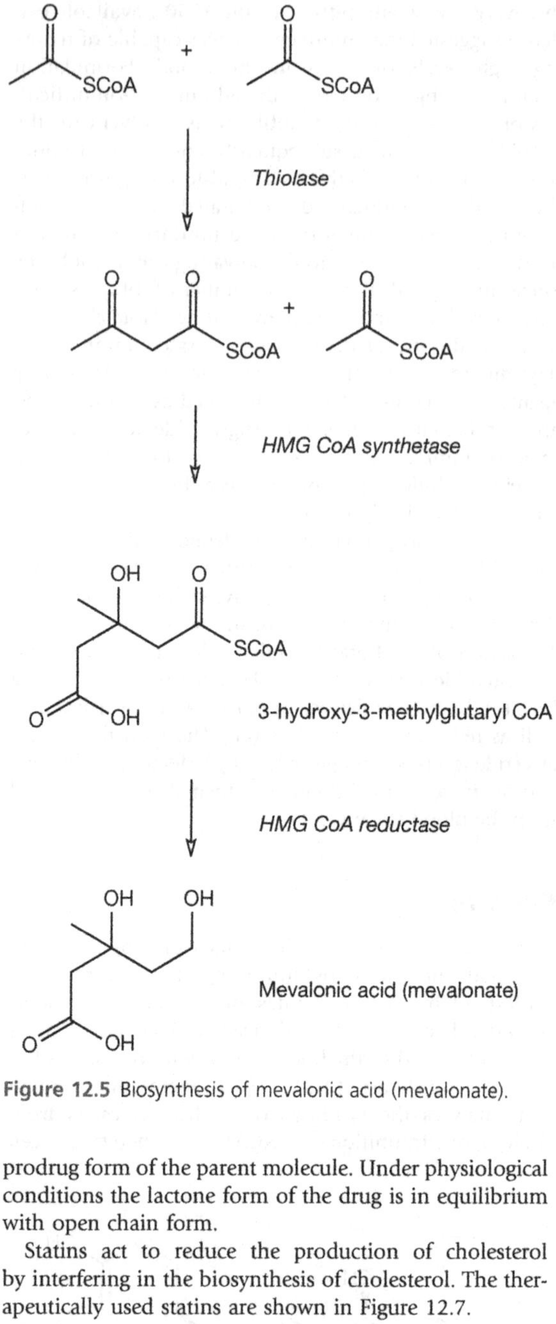

Figure 12.5 Biosynthesis of mevalonic acid (mevalonate).

Statins act to reduce the production of cholesterol by interfering in the biosynthesis of cholesterol. The therapeutically used statins are shown in Figure 12.7.

Compounds of the nicotinic acid group

Nicotinic acid and various analogues have been reported to produce lipid-modifying effects. At present, nicotinic acid (including modified release forms) and acipimox are available for clinical use (Fig. 12.8).

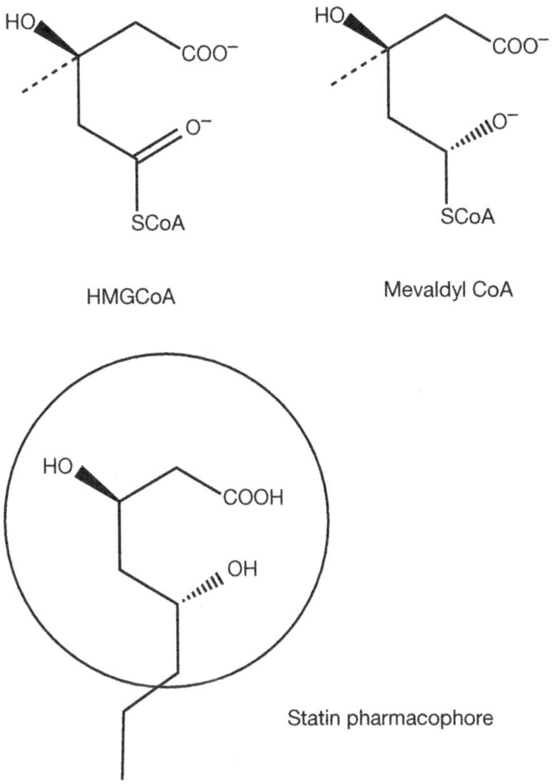

Figure 12.6 The statin pharmacophore.

These two compounds have been reported to act by lowering levels of LDLs and VLDLs whilst raising levels of HDLs. It is believed that this action arises from the blocking of the breakdown of adipose tissue fats, and that the recently reported nicotinic acid receptors may be involved.

ANGIOTENSIN-CONVERTING ENZYME INHIBITORS

Angiotensin-converting enzyme (ACE) inhibitors are indicated for the treatment of high blood pressure, heart failure and for the prevention of strokes. ACE inhibitors act on the renin-angiotensin-aldosterone system (Fig. 12.9). This system is involved in the regulation of various biological systems relating to hypotension, reduced blood volume, decreased sodium and sympathetic stimulation. In response to these factors renin, which is a proteolytic enzyme, is released into the circulation by the kidneys. Renin acts on circulating angiotensinogen and converts it to angiotensin I which is subsequently converted to angiotensin II by ACE.

Angiotensin II acts:

1. at the AT_1 receptor, resulting in constrictions of resistance vessels leading to increased arterial pressure,
2. on the adrenal gland with the release of aldosterone which subsequently acts on the kidney resulting in an increase in fluid and sodium retention,
3. on the kidneys, as in 1,
4. throughout the body it causes vasoconstriction,
5. results in the release of ADH from the pituitary gland.

The renin-angiotensin system is used clinically to treat high blood pressure by the use of ACE inhibitors. Thus we can see that in the system above angiotensin I is converted into angiotensin II via the action of ACE, which increases blood pressure. Therefore, if we can inhibit the action of this enzyme system there will be the opportunity to reduce high blood pressure in hypertensive patients.

The discovery and development of ACE inhibitors

Studies undertaken in the 1960s were based on the assumption that ACE was involved in hypertension. During this work, an extract from the venom of the Brazilian pit viper *Bothrops jararcara* was investigated and shown to be a potent inhibitor of ACE. From the one extract that demonstrated high activity, a number of peptides were isolated and the amino acid sequence was elucidated. One of these, the nonapeptide teprotide (Glu-Trp-Pro-Arg-Pro-Gln-Ile-Pro-Pro) was shown to be highly active but unfortunately it did not possess oral activity. The search then began for compounds with this ACE inhibitory activity that were also orally active. Following many investigations, captopril (Fig. 12.10) was introduced as the first potent orally active ACE inhibitor that was clinically effective.

When the drug was introduced into the clinic it was most efficacious, although a number of adverse side effects were observed including skin rash and loss of taste, and thus the search for better ACE inhibitors began. This has resulted in a large number of compounds presently available as ACE inhibitors. Some of these are: captopril, cilazapril, enalapril (maleate), fosinopril, imidapril, lisinapril, moexipril (hydrochloride), perindopril (erbumine, [t-butyl amine]), quinapril, ramipril and trandolapril (Figs 12.11, 12.12).

The side effects associated with captopril were thought to be associated with the sulphydryl moiety since similar observations had been made in the case of penicillamine. The search for improved ACE inhibitors led to the development of a number of compounds from an understanding of the nature of ACE and its substrates. Throughout the initial work on the development of ACE inhibitors it was known that:

1. If a peptide is a substrate, that substrate must be at least a tripeptide which contains a free carboxylic moiety.

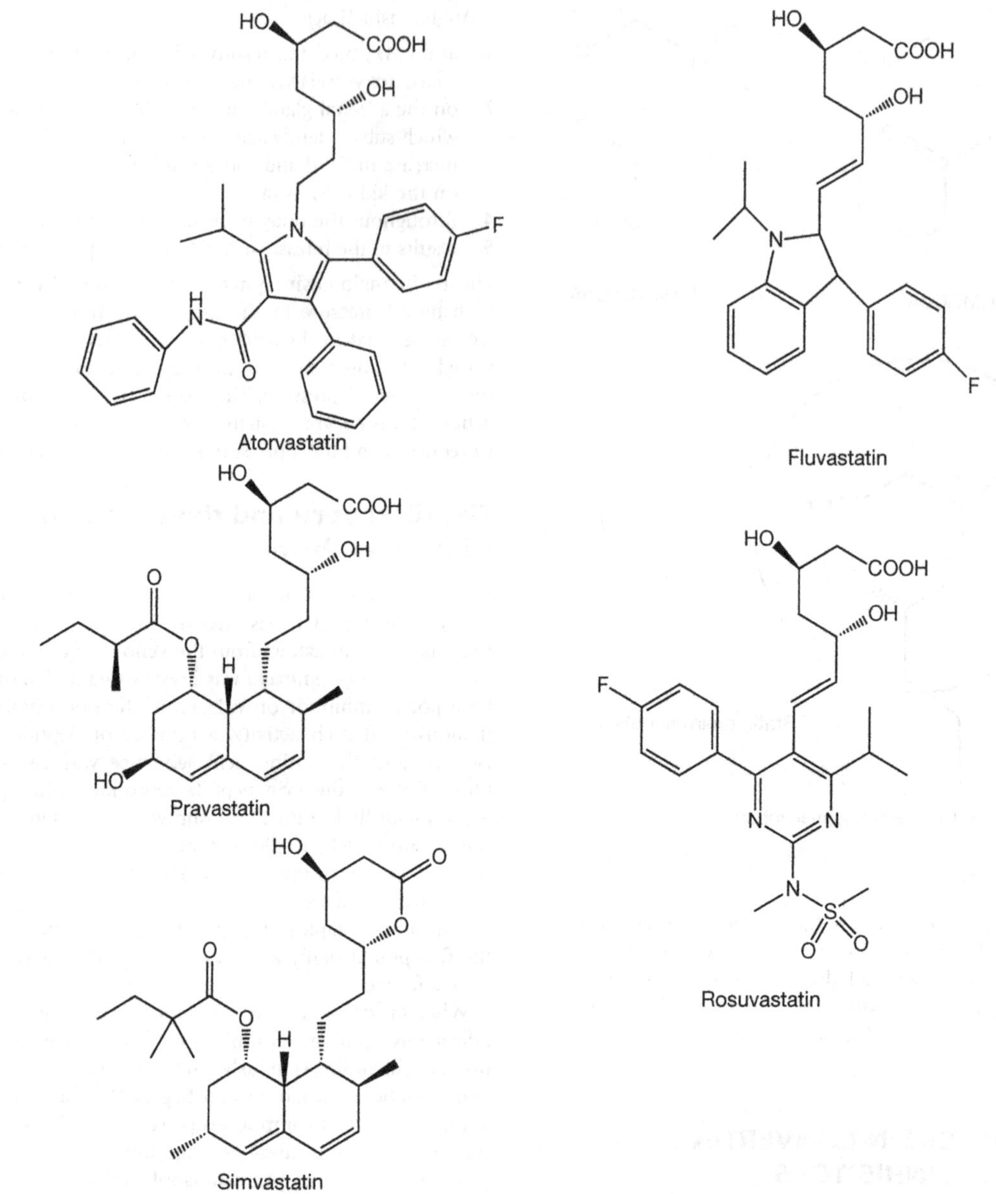

Figure 12.7 Structures of the statins.

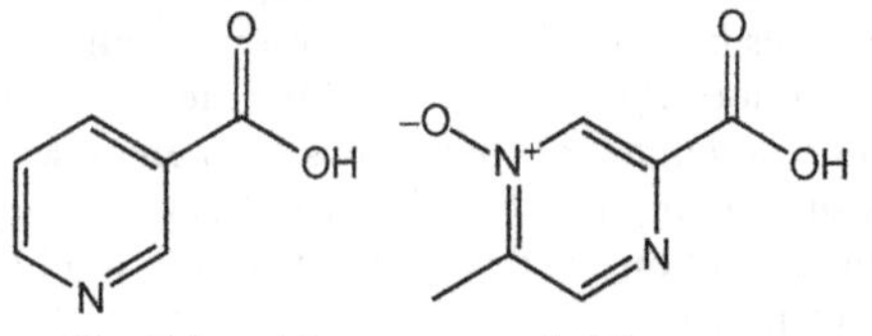

Nicotinic acid Acipimox

Figure 12.8 Structures of nicotinic acid and its synthetic analogue acipimox.

2. The binding site contains a Zn^{2+} site.
3. The enzyme will cleave a peptide linkage, removing a dipeptide group.
4. The enzyme will not cleave peptides with a proline residue close to the terminus.

Enalaprilat was the first member of the dicarboxylate class of ACE inhibitors introduced. In these compounds the sulphydryl group is replaced by a carboxylic acid. When this compound was developed it was found that, because of

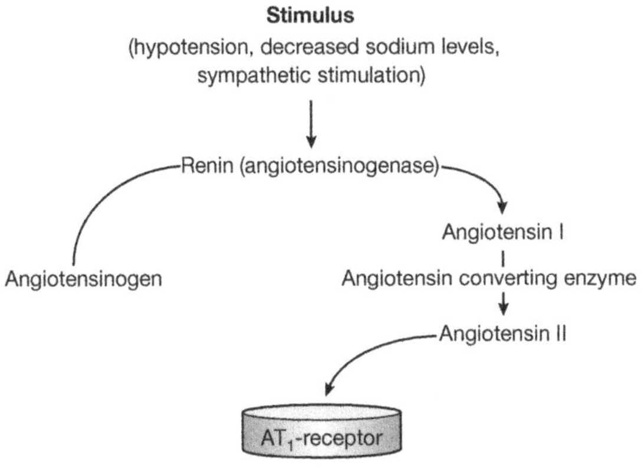

Figure 12.9 The renin-angiotensin-aldosterone system.

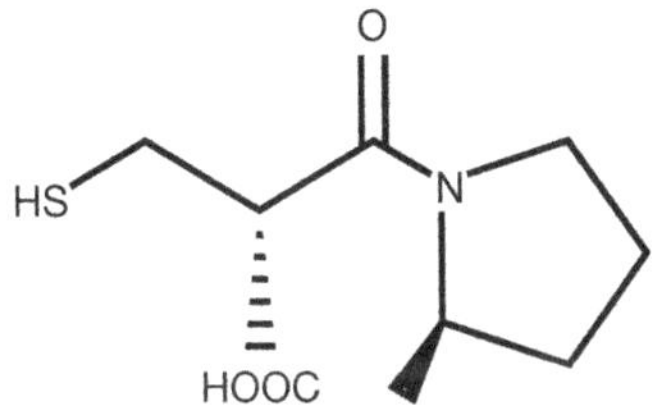

Figure 12.10 The structure of captopril.

the structural modifications introduced to deliver activity similar to captopril, the compound became orally inactive. In order to overcome these problems the ethyl ester prodrug enalapril was developed. This is rapidly metabolised in the body to release the active form. The quantitative structure–activity relationship (QSAR) studies that were undertaken around this time also indicated that there was a hydrophobic pocket present in ACE close to where the proline groups would sit and that by introducing a variety of modified ring systems, including bicyclic and spiro systems in place of the proline system, compounds with higher potency could be made (Figs 12.11, 12.12).

Another aspect that arose from these studies was the possibility that phosphinic acid groups could be incorporated into the inhibitors. Fosinopril (Fig. 12.11) is an example of such a product. However, once again note that this compound is a prodrug that is hydrolysed in vivo to the active form fosfinoprilat.

PHOSPHODIESTERASE INHIBITORS

Cyclic nucleotides such as cyclic adenosine 3′,5′-monophosphate (cAMP) and cyclic guanosine 3′,5′-monophosphate (cGMP) play an important role in cellular signalling as second messengers in response to, for instance, neurotransmitters or hormones. The initial action involves the (hormone) interacting with a G protein-coupled receptor that activates the enzyme systems adenyl cyclase or guanyl cyclase, which are able to convert adenosine triphosphate (ATP) or guanosine triphosphate (GTP) into their cyclic forms (Figs 12.13, 12.14). cAMP and cGMP, as second messengers, are then involved in binding to, and activation of, protein kinases that are themselves involved in a variety of actions via phosphorylation. These protein kinases are involved in wide ranging regulatory processes such as control of sugar, glycogen and lipid metabolism as well as the flow of Ca^{2+} through ion channels. Phosphodiesterases act by conversion of cGMP or cAMP into 5′-AMP or 5′-GMP which are inactive as shown in Figures 12.13 and 12.14. As such, these phosphodiesterases (PDEs) may be considered as regulators of the activity of these second messengers. Phosphodiesterase inhibitors are drugs that interfere with the action of the phosphodiesterases thereby modifying the inactivation of cGMP or cAMP.

There are at present 11 families of mammalian PDEs reported and within each family there are subgroups that have been classified. It is recognised that some PDEs are non-specific in that they can inactivate both cAMP and cGMP whilst others are selective for the inactivation of one or other of these cyclic nucleotides. In terms of PDE inhibitors, it has been discovered that some compounds may act as non-selective phosphodiesterase inhibitors whilst other compounds may act in a very specific fashion with useful clinical activity.

Non-selective phosphodiesterase inhibitors

A series of xanthine derivatives including theophylline, caffeine, theobromine and pentoxifylline (Fig. 12.15) that have bronchodilator properties have been shown to be non-selective phosphodiesterase inhibitors.

It has been proposed that these bronchodilator effects of xanthines result from a relaxant effect on bronchial smooth muscle and that the xanthines regulate the cAMP and cGMP in the smooth muscle via PDE inhibition.

Selective phosphodiesterase inhibitors

Within the last 10 years there have been a number of important developments in terms of selective PDE inhibitors with the licensing of phosphodiesterase 5 (PDE5) inhibitors in the late 1990s paving the way for a range of new clinical applications.

Phosphodiesterase 5 selective inhibitors

Researchers at Pfizer who were investigating compounds that possessed antianginal and antihypertensive properties discovered this group of compounds. The researchers were interested in atrial natriuretic factor (ANF), because

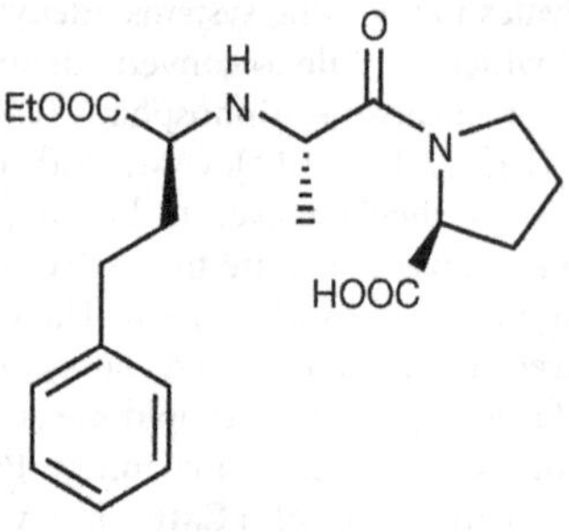

Enalapril

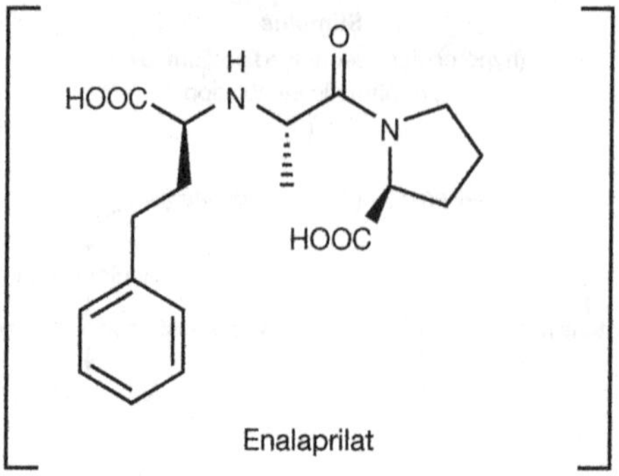

Enalaprilat

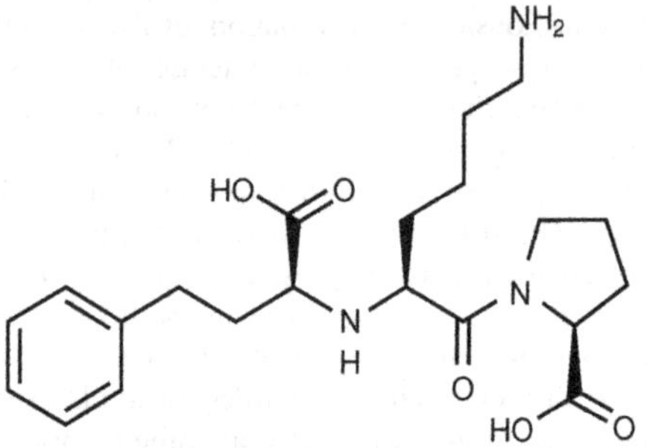

Lisinopril

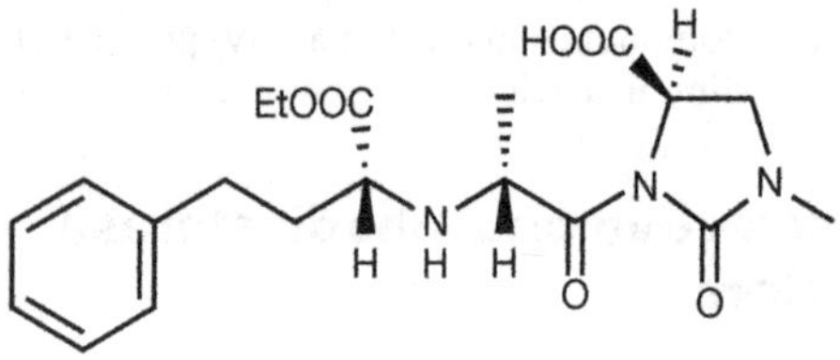

Imidapril

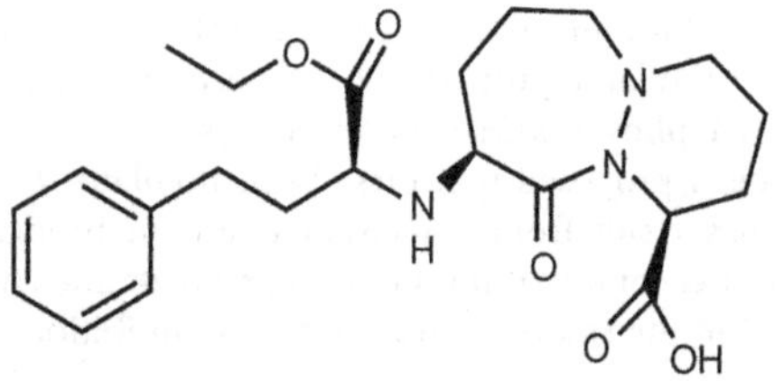

Cilazapril

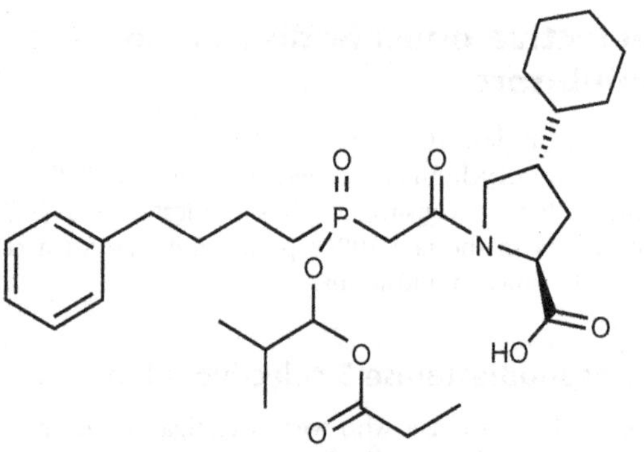

Fosinopril

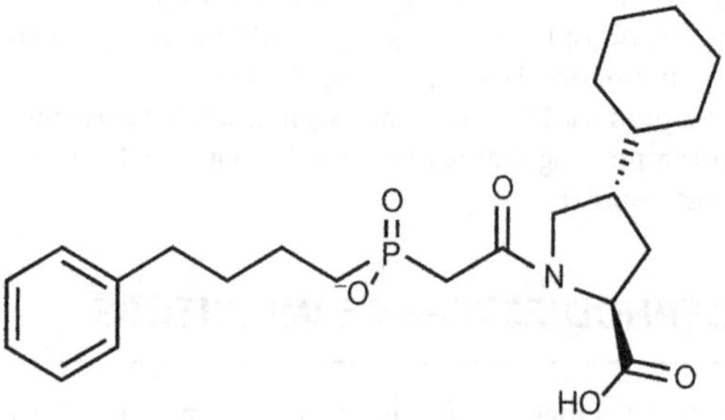

Fosinoprilat

Figure 12.11 ACE inhibitors.

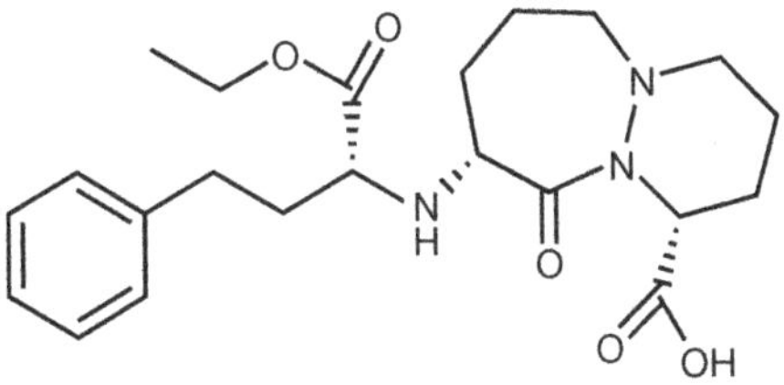

Cilazapril

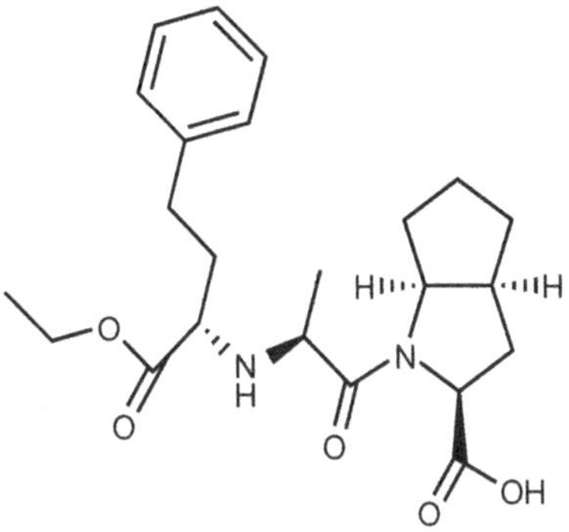

Ramapril

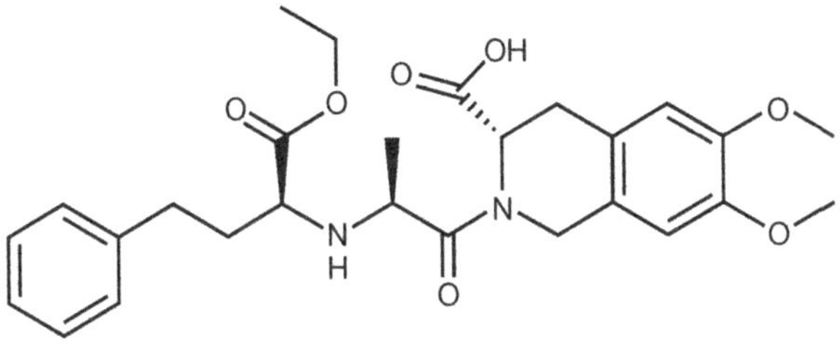

Moexipril

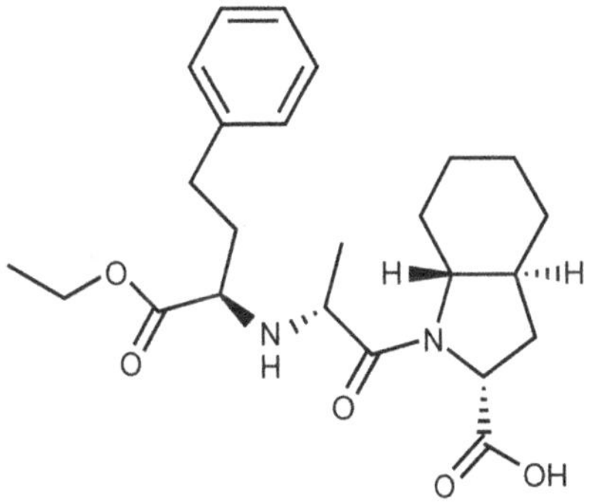

Trandolapril

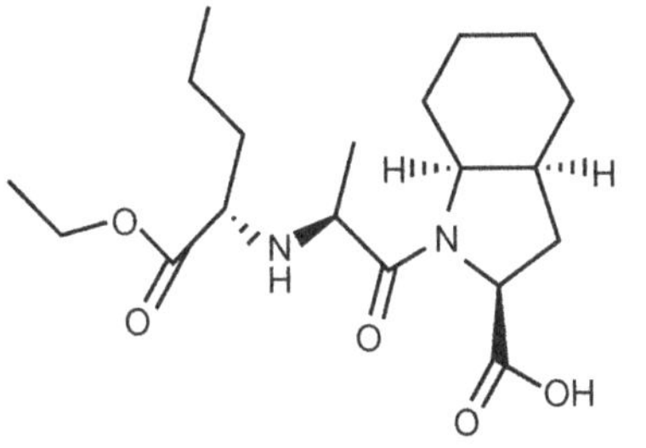

Perindopril

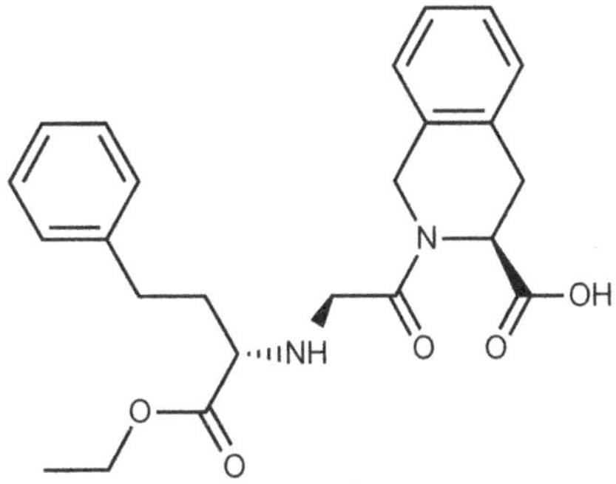

Quinapril

Figure 12.12 ACE inhibitors.

of its vasodilator and natriuretic properties, in cGMP and PDEs. They were working on the hypothesis that because ANF produced its effects via the stimulation of guanyl cyclase, which resulted in an increase in cGMP, and that this was degraded by PDEs. They proposed that compounds that inhibited the action of the PDEs would reduce the degradation of cGMP and hence potentiate the vasodilator and natriuretic properties of ANF. This group began by studying zaprinast (Fig. 12.16). This drug had been shown to have antiallergy drug properties but also had vasodilator properties resulting in smooth muscle relaxation allowing increased flow of blood. Zaprinast was found to be a poorly selective PDE inhibitor but from this basic work information was obtained that led to investigations concerned with improving the selectivity towards PDE5 and also the potency. Investigations of dipole moments of zaprinast and cGMP showed similarities. Computational studies were able to

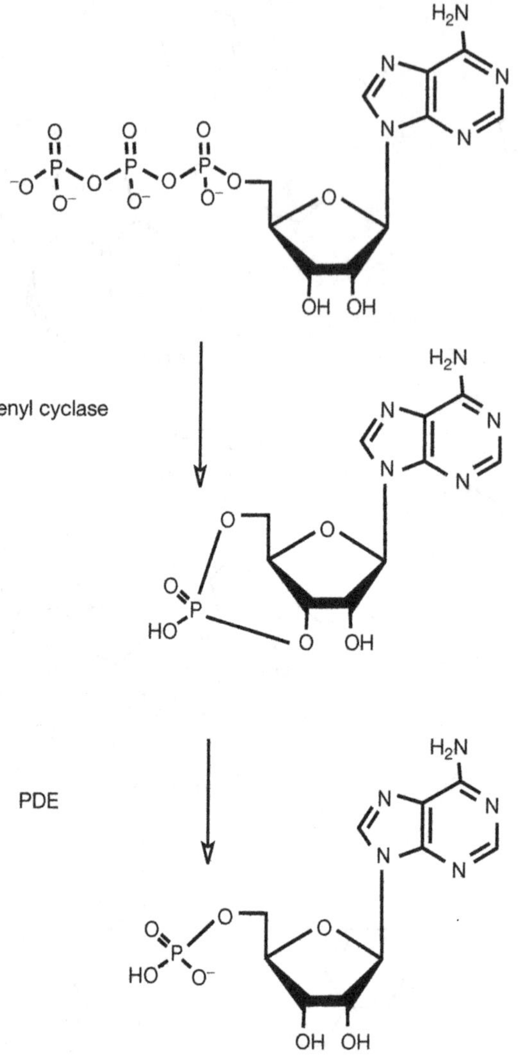

Figure 12.13 Structures of ATP, cyclic AMP and 5′-AMP.

show that cGMP could adopt a *syn* conformation and that modification of the skeleton of zaprinast would enable the inclusion of isosteric moieties for the cyclic phosphate portion of the cGMP. X-ray studies indicated co-planarity via intramolecular hydrogen bonding within the molecule; therefore, this portion of the molecule was left intact. Following several investigations the pyrazolopyrimidinone lead compound shown in Figure 12.16 was synthesised and shown to have significant activity and selectivity towards PDE5. Further studies led to the discovery of sildenafil, which had a 100-fold increase in PDE5 inhibitory activity compared to zaprinast, and exceptional selectivity for PDE5 versus other PDEs. When the drug was taken forward into clinical trials in a study of patients with coronary heart disease, the results were somewhat less promising than had been hoped for. A number of side effects were noted during the trial, one of which was an increase in erectile function, and thus the research then focused on the possibility of using the drug for patients suffering from erectile dysfunction.

The mechanism by which sildenafil produced this change in erectile function was investigated. It was found that through sexual stimulation nitric oxide (NO) is released in the penis, which causes guanyl cyclase to increase the levels of cGMP in the corpus cavernosum. The cGMP causes relaxation of the smooth muscle, increased blood flow and this results in an erection; then, through the action of PDE5, the cGMP is converted to GMP and the erection stops. Sildenafil was shown to

Figure 12.14 Structures of GTP, cyclic GMP and 5′-GMP.

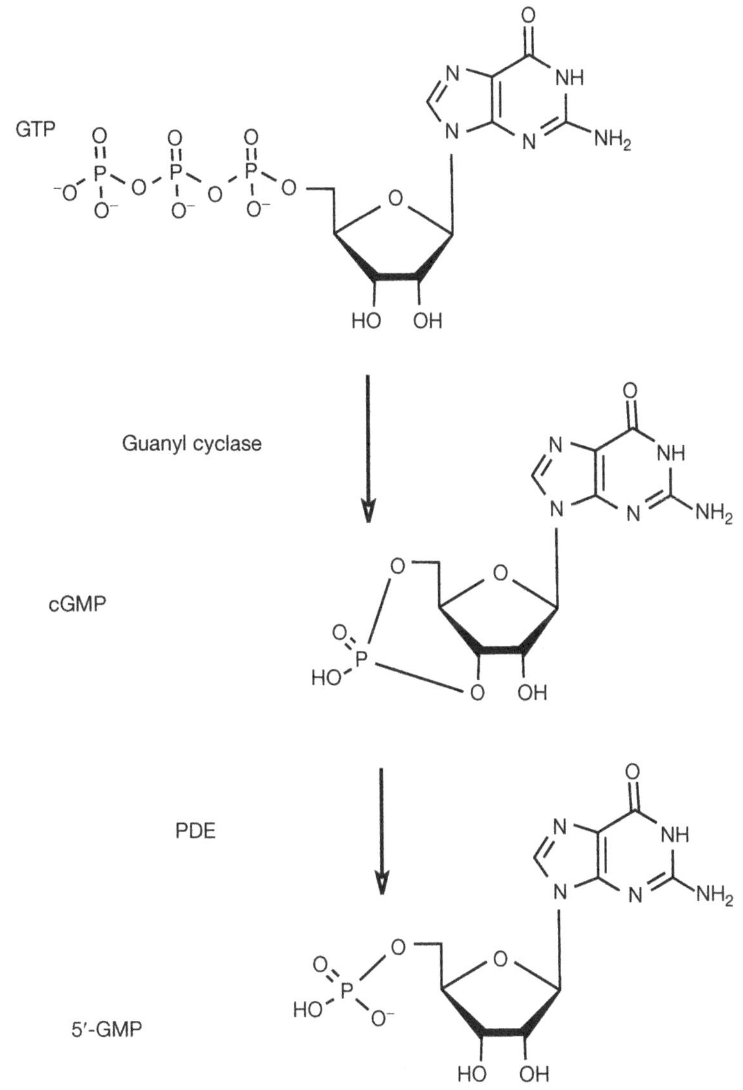

inhibit the breakdown of cGMP by interaction with the active site of the PDE5 system thus reducing the hydrolysis and thereby improving erectile function. Since the introduction of sildenafil, other agents that are also capable of treating erectile dysfunction have been reported, e.g. vardenafil and tadalafil (Fig. 12.17).

Other selective phosphodiesterase inhibitors

Following on from the introduction of sildenafil, a number of other selective PDE inhibitors have been introduced, including PDE3 and PDE4 inhibitors. The PDE3 selective inhibitors milrinone and enoximone (Fig. 12.18) are indicated for congestive heart failure, whilst cilostazol, also a selective PDE3 inhibitor, is used in the treatment of intermittent claudication.

The PDE4 selective inhibitors being studied at present are roflumilast and cilomilast (Fig. 12.19); these compounds are being investigated for use in chronic obstructive pulmonary disease because of their possible effects on inflammatory mediators.

SULPHONAMIDE DIURETICS

Diuretics are drugs that promote the formation/secretion of urine in the kidney. There are a number of different classes of drugs that are used to achieve this promotion

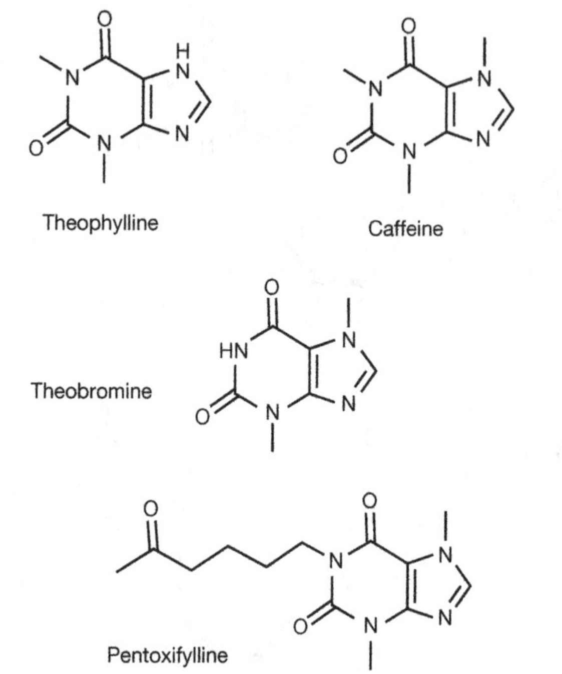

Figure 12.15 Non-selective phosphodiesterase inhibitors.

of urine formation, and a variety of mechanisms by which this may occur including mercurial diuretics, which are no longer used, osmotic diuretics, carbonic anhydrase inhibitors, thiazide and thiazide-like diuretics, loop diuretics and potassium-sparing diuretics. Diuretic drugs are used to aid medical situations where there is a build-up of fluid in the body that occurs, for instance in high blood pressure, congestive heart failure, liver and kidney disease. Additionally some diuretics are also used in the treatment of glaucoma. In this section we will concentrate on those compounds that contain a sulphonamide functional group, i.e. thiazide/thiazide-like and loop diuretics, and we shall consider the mechanisms of action of these compounds, including consideration of their carbonic anhydrase inhibitory activity and their involvement with the Na/Cl/K symporter.

There are a relatively large number of compounds that might be grouped together under the heading of sulphonamide diuretics. Within the group of compounds containing this functionality, we have a variety of different classes of diuretics based on their mechanism of action. These compounds are considered active as carbonic anhydrase inhibitors (acetazolamide), inhibitors of the reabsorption of Na^+ Cl^- (thiazide and thiazide-like diuretics [benzthiazide, hydrochlorothiazide]) and inhibitors of the Na K Cl symporter (furosemide).

The development of sulphonamide diuretics arose from early observations concerning the use of sulfanilamide as an antibacterial agent. Sulfanilamide was shown to be the active metabolite of prontosil (Fig. 12.20) when used in vivo.

It was observed that this compound produced a diuretic effect although the diuresis was somewhat limited. Attempts were made to synthesise a range of compounds related to sulfanilamide to improve the diuretic effect. The basic premise in this work appears to have been based on synthesising compounds, which contained the -SO_2NH_2 moiety, attached to an aromatic or a heterocyclic ring system. From this early work based on the investigation of heterocyclic ring usage, acetazolamide (Fig. 12.21) was developed.

Sulfanilamide and acetazolamide were shown to be carbonic anhydrase inhibitors.

In addition to the development of acetazolamide, work was also undertaken on the substitution of the benzene ring of sulfanilamide. Many compounds were prepared including a number with sulphonamide groups present.

One of the compounds that resulted from these studies was 4-amino-6-chloro-3-benzenedisulfonamide (Fig. 12.22). This compound displayed some diuretic properties; however, it was never used as a routine clinical diuretic. Further modifications of this compound were attempted, involving the derivatisation of the 4-amino functionality. Treatment of this compound with, for

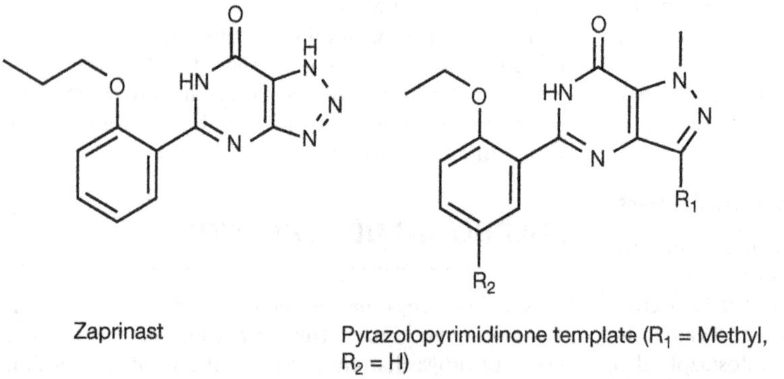

Figure 12.16 Structure of zaprinast and pyrazolopyrimidinone template.

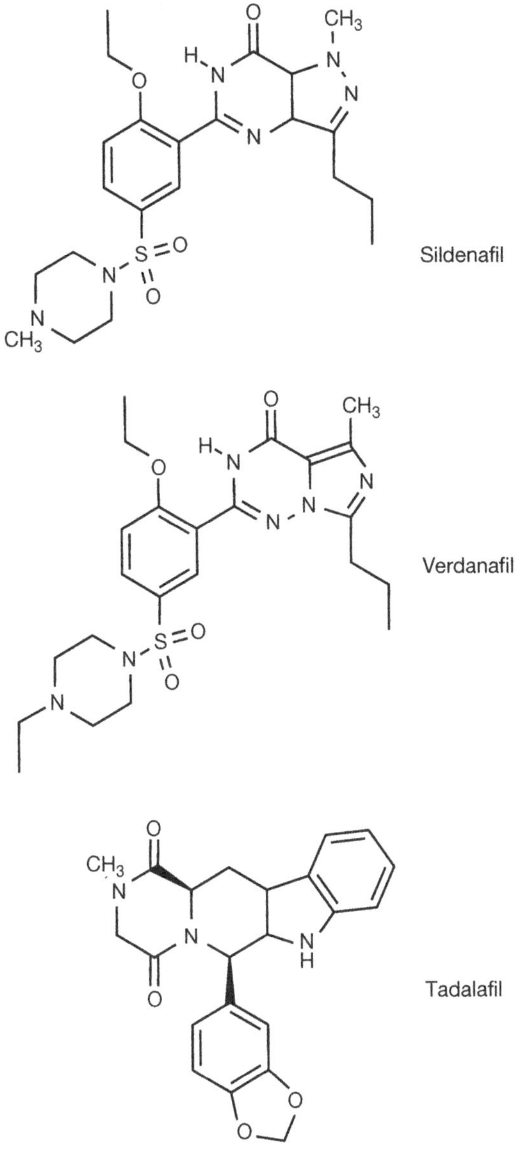

Figure 12.17 Structures of sildenafil, vardenafil and tadalafil.

instance, formamide, resulted in cyclisation with the formation of thiazides, whilst reaction with aldehydes and ketones resulted in the preparation of hydrothiazides (Fig. 12.23).

Further investigations in this area led to the preparation of a range of compounds classified as thiazide-like diuretics, e.g. indapamide, metolazone and chlortalidone, and other compounds such as furosemide (Fig. 12.24).

The BNF lists a number of other compounds that can be classified as sulphonamide diuretics and these compounds are detailed in Figures 12.25 and 12.26.

Mechanism of action

The functioning unit of the kidney is the nephron, and blood is brought into the nephron via the afferent arteriole where it enters the renal corpuscle, which consists of the glomerulus and Bowman's capsule. About one-fifth of the blood (plasma) passing through the nephron in any given time is filtered by this system. The filtrate that passes into Bowman's capsule contains water, nutrients, minerals (salts) and waste material, but red and white blood cells, platelets and large molecules such as proteins will not pass into Bowman's capsule. On leaving the renal corpuscle, the blood enters a set of capillaries known as the peritubular capillaries, whilst the filtrate enters the proximal convoluted tubule and then to the proximal straight tubule, the loop of Henle, the distal convoluted tubule and thence to collecting tubule. During this process there is the possibility for a series of exchanges of both liquid and solutes between capillaries and the tubules. Throughout the passage through the nephron there are changes in the osmolarity of the plasma via exchanges that can occur through concentration gradients within the various sections; these are controlled by different mechanisms. Through these processes liquid, electrolytes and nutrients (salts, amino acids, glucose) are reabsorbed whilst the waste material (e.g. urea) is taken on to the collecting duct and thence to the bladder. In those disease states where diuretics are employed, the diuretics act by reducing the reabsorption of water and salts, thereby increasing urine production. As explained in the earlier section, the majority of the sulphonamide diuretics were developed from the initial idea that sulfanilamide and acetazolamide were carbonic anhydrase inhibitors. It is now well known that the thiazide and thiazide-like diuretics act by different mechanisms. Thiazides act in the distal tubule by interfering with the reabsorption of sodium and chloride ions; this action results from binding with the Na/Cl/K symporter.

The loop diuretics such as furosemide, torasemide and bumetanide act in the thick ascending loop of Henle, inhibiting the reabsorption of sodium, potassium and chloride ions.

SECTION B – PROTON PUMP INHIBITORS

David G Watson

Observations on the effect of the potential antviral drug pyridylthioacetamide (Fig. 12.27) in reducing gastric acid secretion (GAS) led to the lead compound H124/26 which was highly effective in reducing GAS. It was found that this compound was metabolically converted to timoprazole (Fig. 12.27) which was the active form of the drug. The sulphoxide group was thus found to be an important element in the drug action and picoprazole was developed and found to be free from the antithyroid effects exhibited by timoprazole.

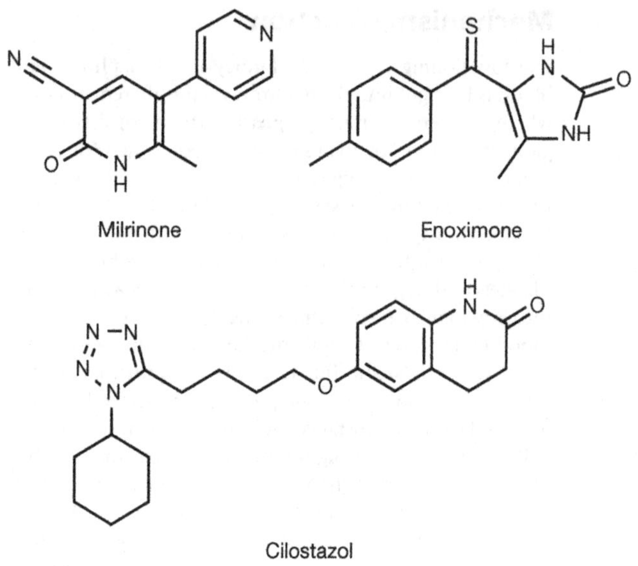

Figure 12.18 Selective PDE3 inhibitors.

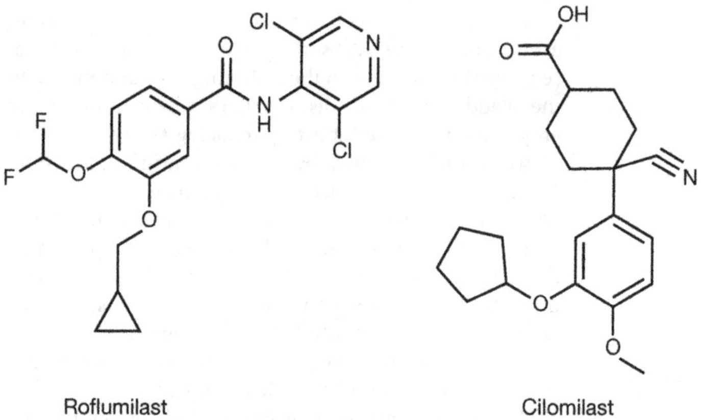

Figure 12.19 Selective PDE4 inhibitors.

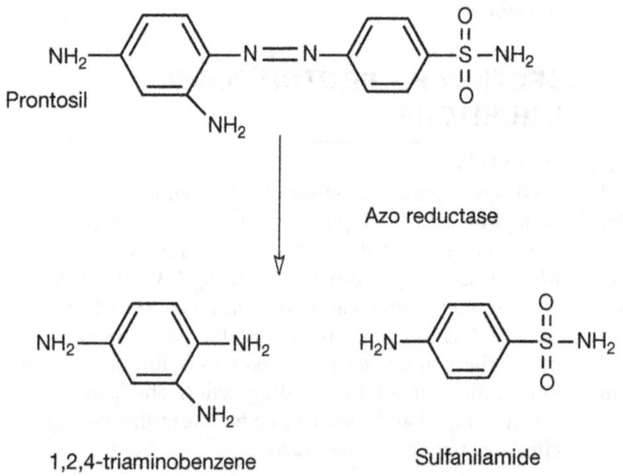

Figure 12.20 The conversion of prontosil into sulfanilamide via azo reductase.

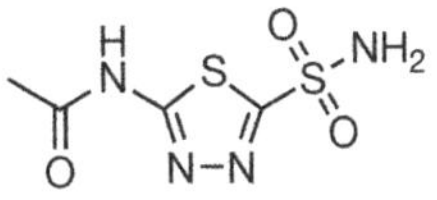

Acetazolamide

Figure 12.21 Structure of acetazolamide.

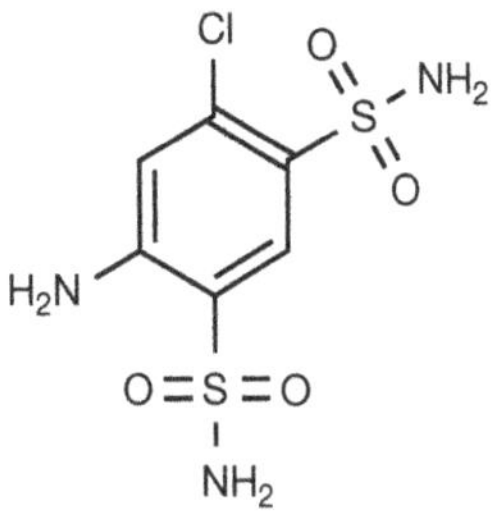

Figure 12.22 4-amino-6-chloro-3-benzenedisulfonamide.

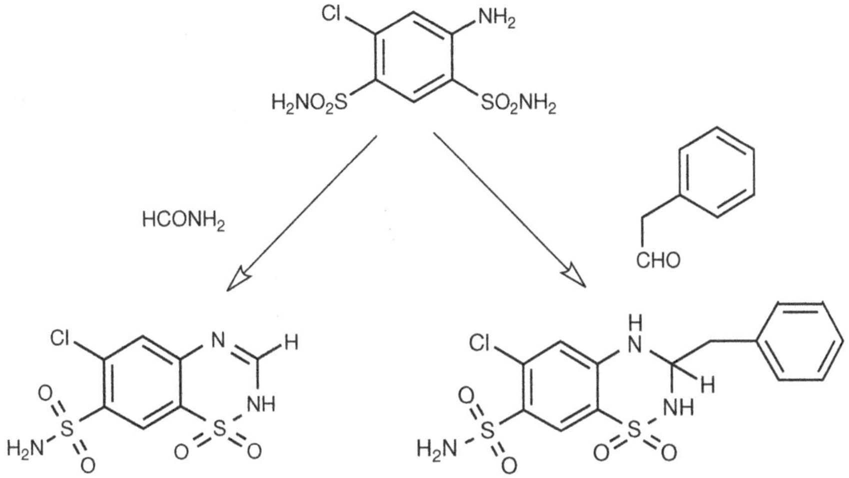

Figure 12.23 Synthesis of thiazide and hydrothiazide diuretics.

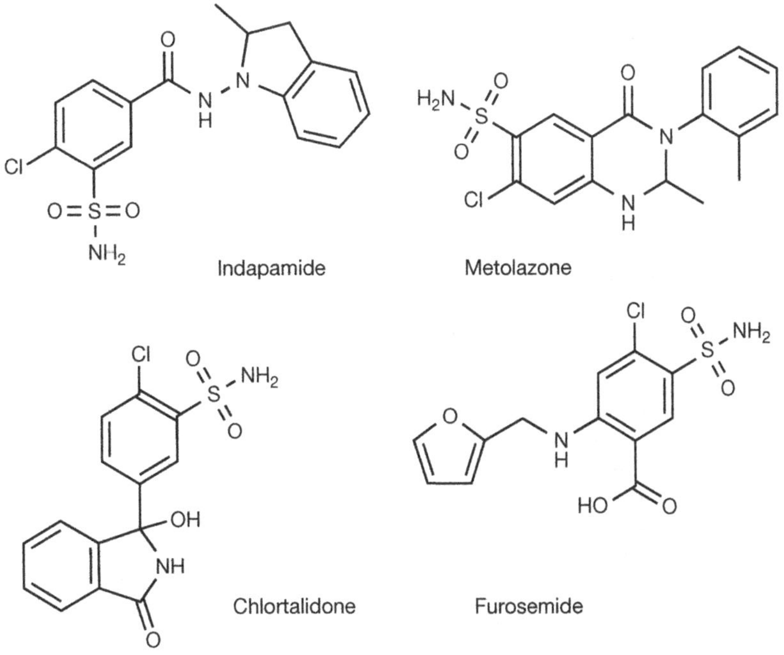

Figure 12.24 Thiazide-like diuretics.

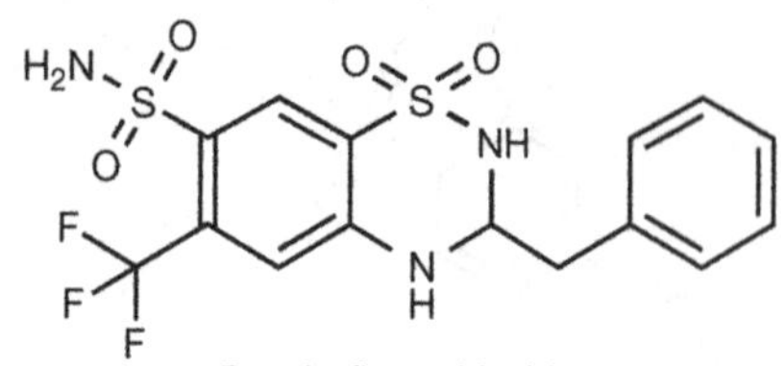

Bendroflumethiazide

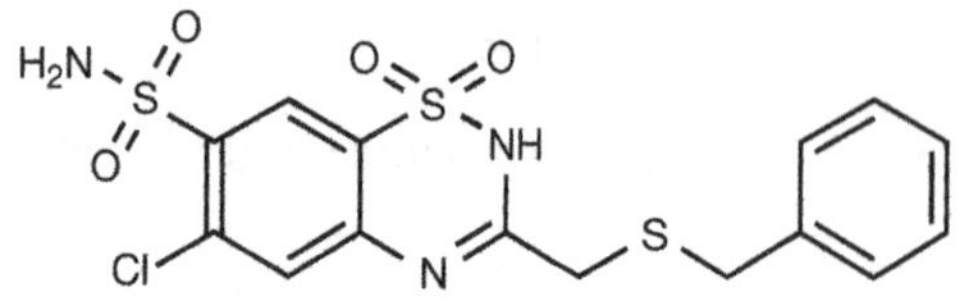

Benzthiazide

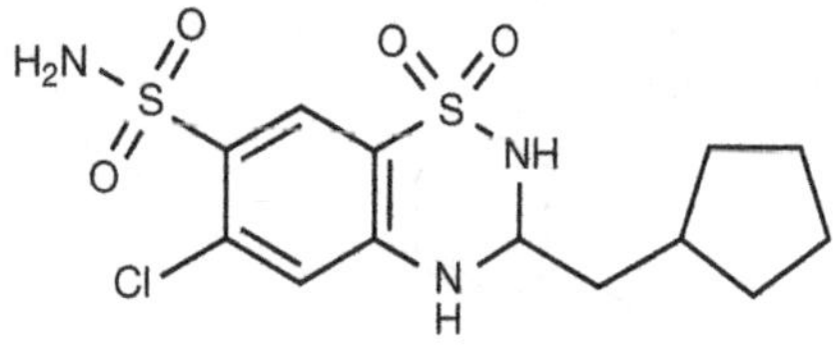

Cyclopenthiazide

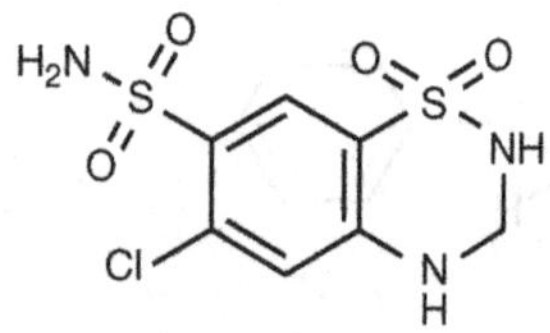

Hydrochlorothiazide

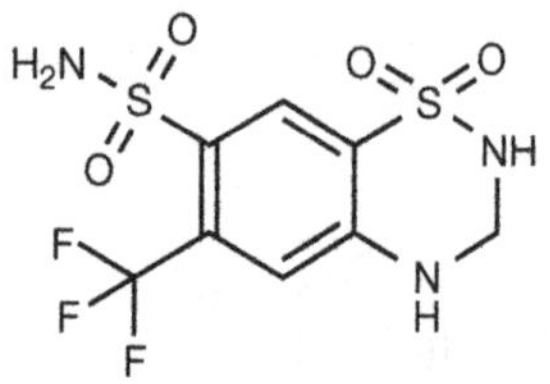

Hydroflumethiazide

Figure 12.25 Clinically used thiazide diuretics.

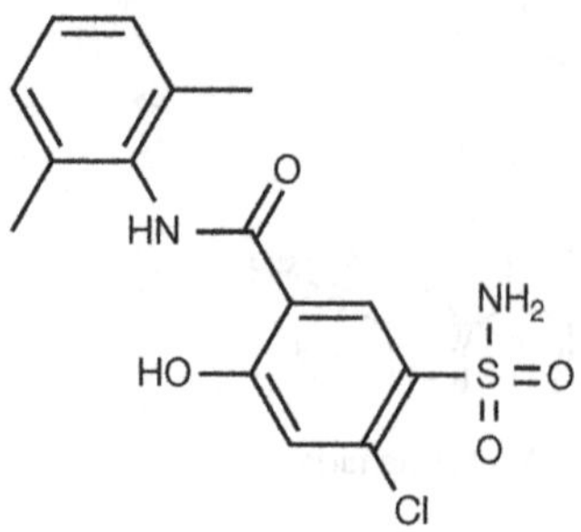

Xipamide

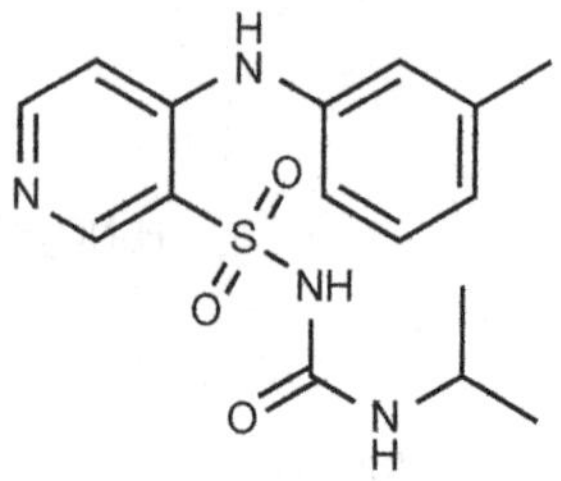

Torasemide

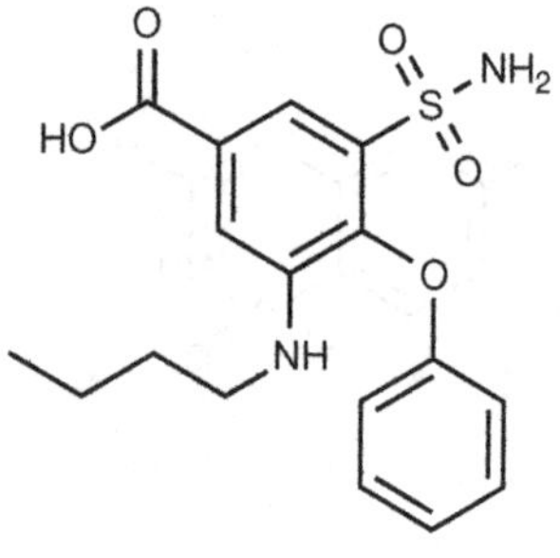

Bumetanide

Figure 12.26 Clinically used loop diuretics.

More potent analogues were achieved by increasing the basicity of the pyridine, eventually resulting in omeprazole (Fig. 12.27). The addition of a 4-methoxy group to a pyridine ring raises its p*Ka* from 5.2 to 7.1 due to the electron-rich substituent increasing the electron density in the ring;[1] the methyl groups also increase the electron density in the ring. Thus it would seem that the measured p*Ka* value of 8.7 for omeprazole[2] refers to the nitrogen in the pyridine ring which is thus a strong nucleophile. Radiolabelled ^{3}H omeprazole was given i.v. and found to accumulate in parietal cells in the gastric mucosa. Parietal cells contain the membrane channel protein H^+K^+ATPase which is involved in exporting H^+ (and Cl^-) out of the cell in exchange for K^+ (and HCO_3^-) into the cell. Figure 12.28 shows a proposed mechanism for the export of H^+ out of the parietal cells via phosphorylation of the membrane channel protein.

Omeprazole becomes completely ionised and thus trapped in secretory channels of the parietal cells due to an acid-catalysed rearrangement which converts it into a quaternary amine. The mechanism of the structural rearrangement is not known exactly. It seems likely that it is the sulphenic acid (Fig. 12.29) intermediate that reacts with the H^+K^+ATPase and rather than the sulphenamide (Fig. 12.29), which is a more stable end product of the rearrangement.[2]

The sulphenic acid intermediate reacts with a cysteine residue in the H^+K^+ATPase (Fig. 12.30) preventing it from functioning properly and thus preventing acid secretion by the parietal cell. Regeneration of the enzyme takes 3–5 days. There is a cysteine residue one amino acid removed from the phosphorylation site of the protein which may be the target of the drug. Since the drug undergoes rearrangement when exposed to acidic

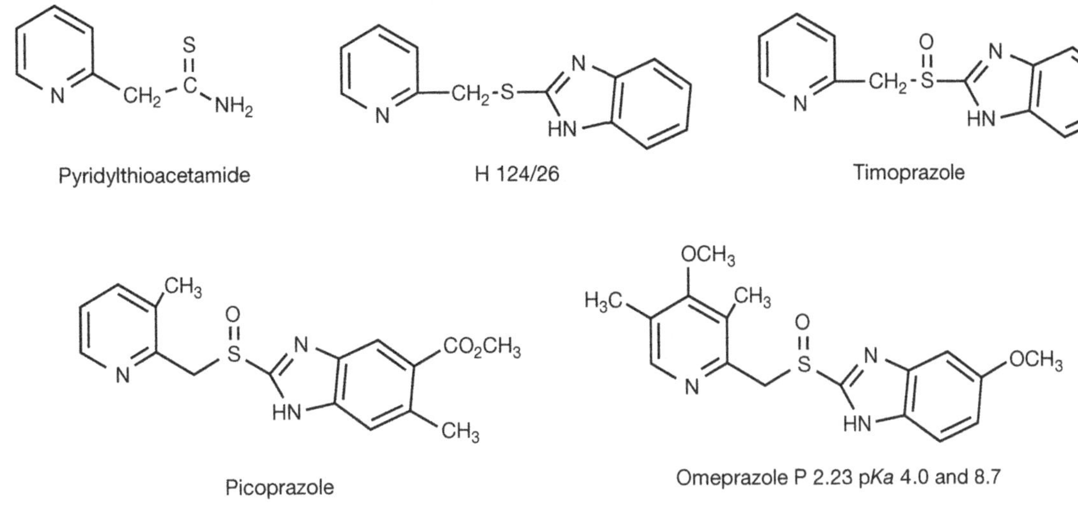

Figure 12.27 Omeprazole and its lead compounds.

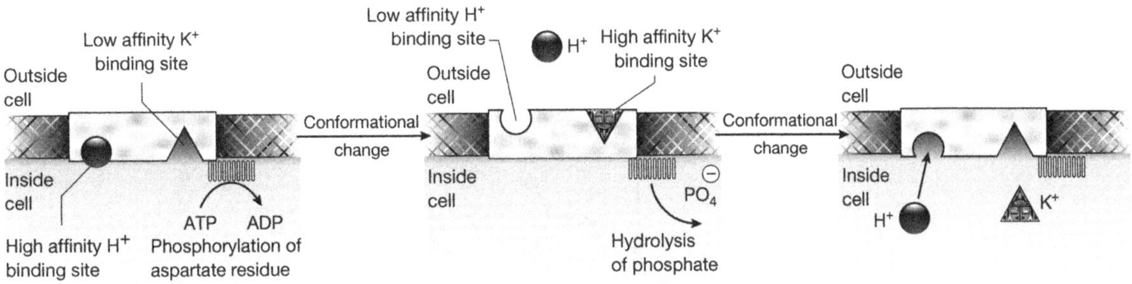

Figure 12.28 Proposed mechanism for the export of protons out of the parietal cells.

conditions it has to be administered in the form of capsules or enterically coated tablets which are resistant to the stomach acid and pass through the stomach, releasing the drug in the small intestine. The drug can also be given intravenously.

Sulphoxides have a tertrahedral geometry and, like carbon atoms, can exhibit chirality, with the lone pair on the sulphur atom taking lowest priority in the same manner as a proton attached to a carbon atom has lowest priority. Omeprazole can exist as R and S enantiomers (Fig. 12.31). The S isomer contibutes 90% inhibition of gastric acid production compared with 20% for R-isomer, and greater efficacy has been claimed for it. The S enantiomer is marketed as esomeprazole.

Since omeprazole reached the market, a number of compounds with similar actions have been marketed (Fig. 12.32). They all act via the same mechanism, as can be seen from the essential pharmacophore which is present in all the structures, and there is no particularly strong argument for using one over another.

Formulations of proton pump inhibitors in the BNF

- Esomeprazole: tablets 20 mg and 40 mg; intravenous injection 20 mg.
- Lansoprazole: capsules 15 mg; orodispersible tablet (disperses to give enterically coated microgranules); suspension 30 mg per sachet (composed of enterically coated microgranules).
- Omeprazole: capsules 10 mg; dispersible tablets 10 mg, 20 mg, 40 mg (composed of enterically coated pellets); capsules 10 mg, 20 mg, 40 mg; injection 40 mg.
- Pantoprazole: tablets 20 mg, 40 mg; injection 40 mg.
- Rabeprazole: tablets 10 mg, 20 mg.

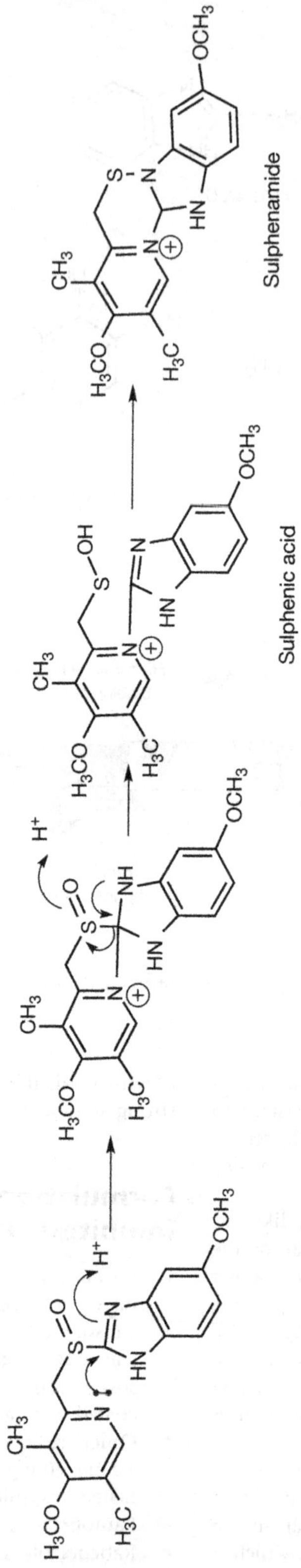

Figure 12.29 Acid catalysed re-arrangement of omeprazole in the parietal cells.

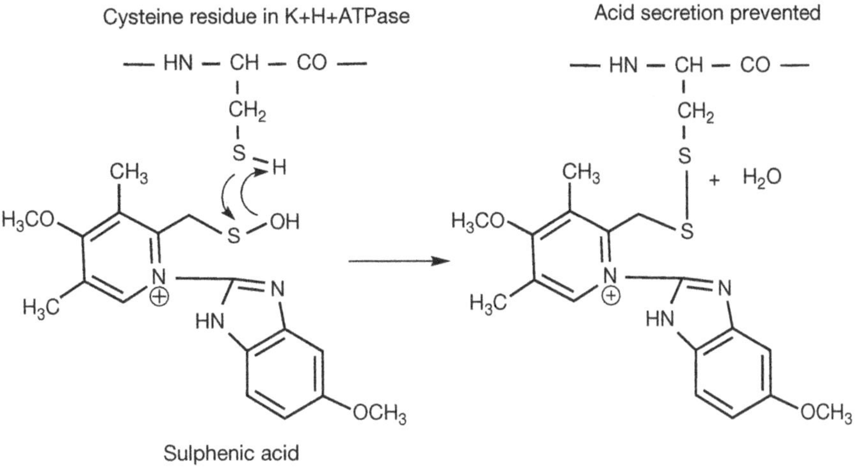

Figure 12.30 Reaction of the sulphenic acid intermediate with a cysteine residue in $H^+K^+ATPase$.

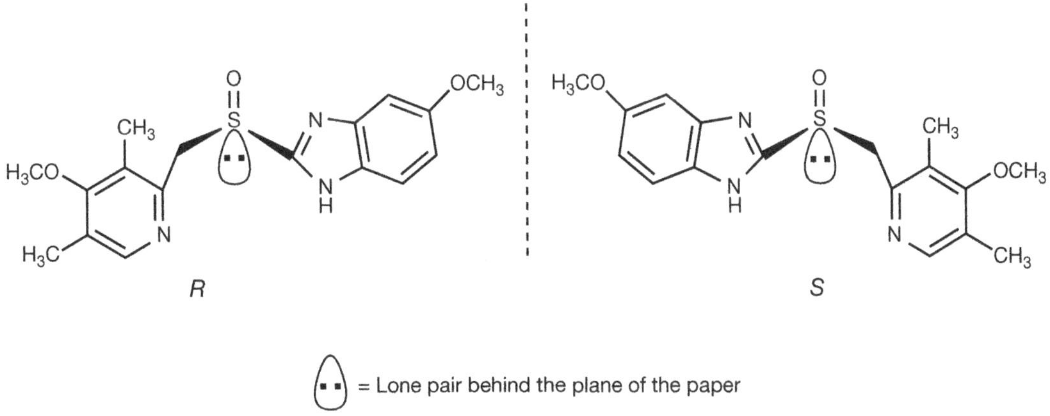

Figure 12.31 Enantiomers of omeprazole.

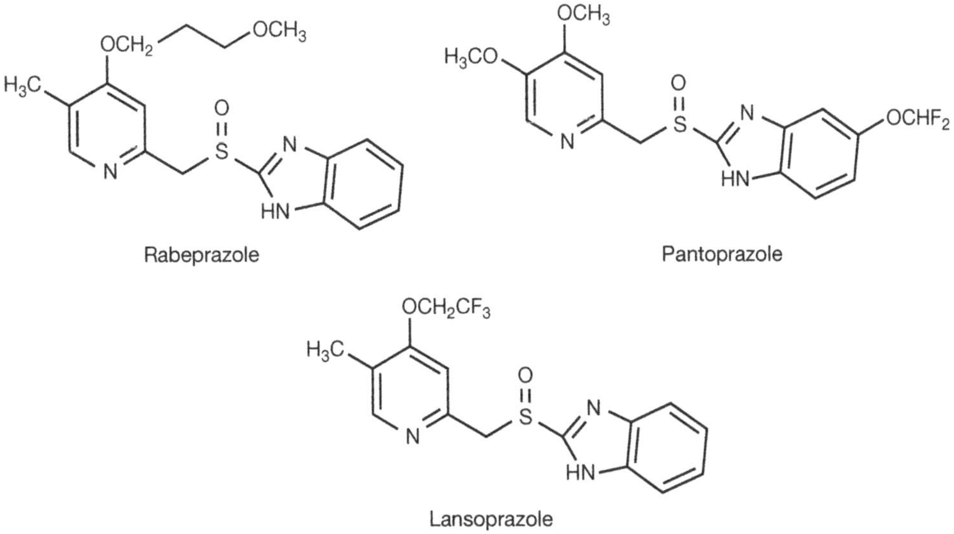

Figure 12.32 Additional proton pump inhibitors.

REFERENCES

1. Grandberg I, Faizova GK, Kost AN. Comparative basicities of substituted pyridines and electronegativity series for substituents in the pyridine series. *Khimiya Geterotsiklicheskikh Soedinenii.* 1966;2:561–566.
2. Qaisi AM, Tutunji MF, Tutunji LF. Acid Decomposition of omeprazole in the absence of thiol: A differential pulse polarographic study at the static mercury drop electrode (SMDE). *J Pharm Sci.* 2006;95:385–391.

Chapter | 13 |

Central nervous system depressants

Jeffrey Stuart Millership

CHAPTER CONTENTS

INTRODUCTION

Within the group of compounds that may be classified as central nervous system (CNS) depressants there are many different drugs and a range of effects that can result from the use of the said drugs. The use of these drugs may result in anaesthesia, sleep, relief from anxiety, sedation and relief from schizophrenia. The compounds within these classes act within the brain at a series of sites such as receptors, ion channels, etc. The compounds active within this general heading have a wide variety of structures from simple molecules such as chloral hydrate to multisubstituted, multiring structures such as midazolam. Within each section of this chapter the application of each drug class will be considered and, where possible, an indication of the structure–activity relationships within and between each section will be detailed.

GENERAL ANAESTHETICS

General anaesthetics are used to allow surgical procedures to be undertaken without the patient suffering the pain and discomfort that would be felt in the absence of these drugs. It is accepted that the general anaesthetics lead to unconsciousness during these surgical procedures and they also provide analgesia and hopefully lead to loss of skeletal muscle activity. Nowadays, general anaesthetics are subdivided into inhalation and intravenous anaesthetics. The structures of the presently used agents in these categories are presented in Figures 13.1 and 13.2, respectively.

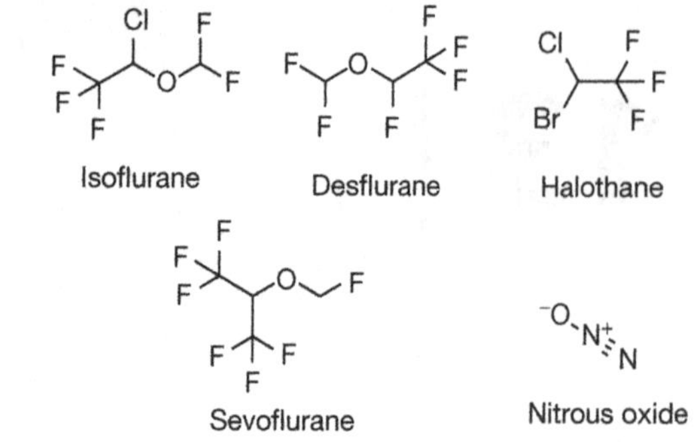

Figure 13.1 Inhalation anaesthetics.

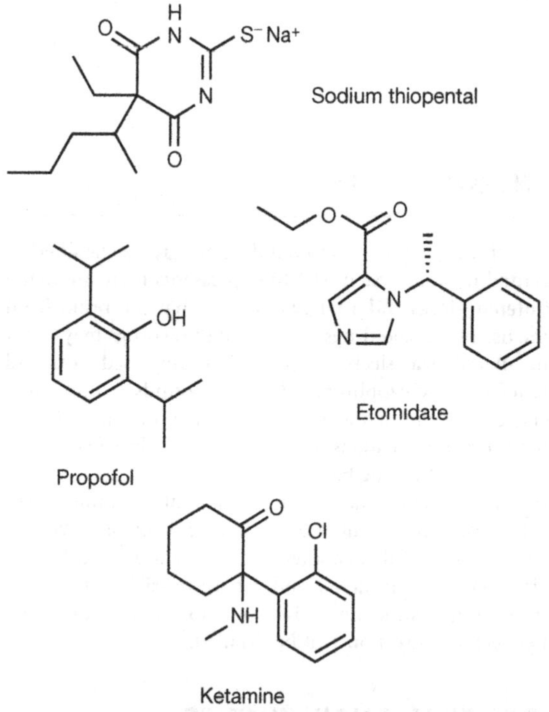

Figure 13.2 Intravenous anaesthetics.

The history of anaesthesia reportedly stretches back to ancient times and through the medieval period. It is documented that as far back as 1500 BC opium-based preparations were in use for anaesthetic purposes. In the Middle Ages the use of the *Spongia somnifera* was reported. This was a sponge, soaked with a mixture of 'herbal' agents (poppy, henbane, mandrake), and was allowed to dry and then, when the operation was due to commence, the sponge was placed over the nose of the patient and treated with hot water. The infusion produced the anaesthesia. Alcohol was also commonly used to produce a state of anaesthesia in historical times.

The modern basis of anaesthesia began in the middle of the nineteenth century with the discovery of ether (1846) and chloroform (1847) as inhalation anaesthetic agents. Nitrous oxide had first been isolated in the eighteenth century, and although its anaesthetic action was known, it was not seriously considered for surgical procedures until 1846. Over the next hundred years a number of other agents were investigated, including saturated and unsaturated hydrocarbons, diverse halogenated hydrocarbons and a variety of ethers. Subsequently, halothane was introduced in 1956 and then a series of halogenated ethers containing multiple fluorine substituents were developed, a number of these compounds (isoflurane, sevoflurane and desflurane) now form the bulk of inhalation anaesthetics used in modern practice. The era of intravenous anaesthetics is thought to have commenced in the 1930s with the use of barbiturates. Since that time a number of compounds with a variety of functional moieties have been developed and the commonly used agents are presented in Figure 13.2.

MECHANISM OF ACTION OF ANAESTHETICS

Inhalation anaesthetics

There have been many attempts to produce a unified theory detailing the mechanism of action of inhalation anaesthetics but no single theory has been accepted. Early theories on the mechanism of action of inhalation anaesthetics can by summarised by means of the Meyer-Overton theory, which indicated that the potency of anaesthetic action was related to the lipophilicity of an anaesthetic compound. The Meyer-Overton theory suggested that lipids within the brain could be dissolved by anaesthetic agents, thereby interfering with brain cell activity, leading to anaesthesia.

Correlations of the oil (olive oil)/gas partition coefficient of the anaesthetic agent against potency (expressed as the minimum alveolar concentration [MAC]) showed a linear relationship. Over time, evidence was presented which led to the conclusion that this theory did not adequately describe the action of anaesthetic agents. In a number of cases, where homologous series of anaesthetics agents have been studied, a sudden loss of anaesthetic activity is observed even though the lipophilicity is increased. A second aspect that challenges the theory is that enantiomers of anaesthetic compounds can display different anaesthetic potency yet the lipophilicity will be identical. This has resulted in a number of newer theories regarding the mechanism(s) of anaesthetic action.

There appears to be no clear, unified indication of a single explanation emerging in this area; rather there are ideas being postulated that indicate a number of possible mechanisms. It has been suggested that the inhaled anaesthetics cause a modification to the activity of ion channels, for example those relating to the action of acetylcholine, γ-aminobutyric acid-A (GABA-A), glutamate and nicotinic receptors. It may be that such anaesthetics are able to interact in a way that causes enhancement of the activity of the inhibitory GABA-A receptors whilst inhibiting the activity of the excitatory acetylcholine, glutamate and nicotinic receptors. It is postulated on the basis of considerable experimental evidence that the inhaled anaesthetics do not act specifically via a lock-and-key mechanism but rather act via a modification of the speed with which the receptors operate.

Intravenous anaesthetics

In terms of the intravenous anaesthetics, it is believed that the anaesthetic activity of propofol, sodium thiopental and etomidate arises from enhancement of the activity of the inhibitory GABA-A receptors. It is worth noting that etomidate is formulated as a single enantiomer, the R (+) isomer, which is approximately 20-fold more active as an anaesthetic than the S (−) enantiomer. Despite the fact that many anaesthetic agents contain elements of chirality, etomidate is the only member of this class that is formulated as a single enantiomer. Ketamine, however, acts in a different way by inhibition at the N-methyl-D aspartate (NMDA) receptor. Ketamine is a chiral compound with the S (+) ketamine being two to three times more potent than its enantiomer in terms of anaesthetic properties. The drug is administered as a racemic mixture despite the fact that R (−) isomer has been shown to possess a number of undesirable emergence side effects including aggression, combativeness, and hallucinations.

HYPNOTICS, ANXIOLYTICS AND BARBITURATES

Benzodiazepines

Hypnotics and anxiolytics are used as antianxiety agents, with hypnotics being prescribed to promote sleep whilst anxiolytics are used for the relief of daytime anxiety. There is a variety of drugs used in these areas, with the benzodiazepines being used both as hypnotics and anxiolytics. The benzodiazepine drugs were discovered serendipitously in the mid 1950s at the Hoffmann-La Roche laboratories. The first compound of the class, chlordiazepoxide, was synthesised by Leo Sternbach and, when tested, was shown to be an effective hypnotic and anxiolytic. Since this initial finding a large number of benzodiazepines have been synthesised and tested. The basic structure of this class of compounds is the 1,4-benzodiazepine ring structure shown in Figure 13.3.

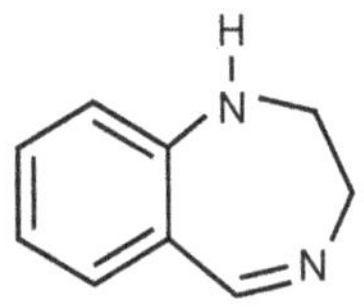

Figure 13.3 The benzodiazepine ring structure.

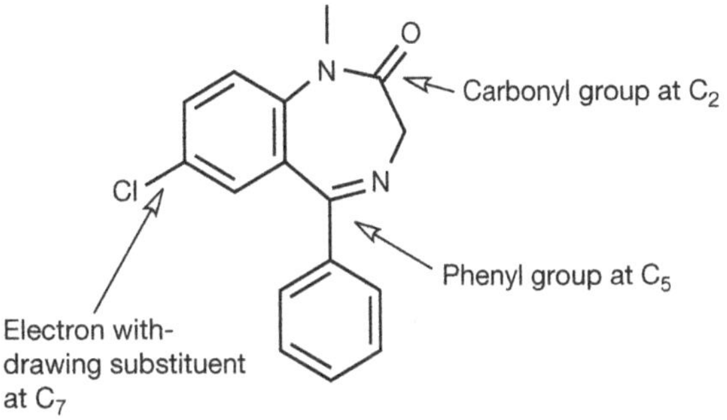

Figure 13.4 Structural characteristics of active benzodiazepines.

Many of the benzodiazepine compounds that are active as hypnotics and anxiolytics have other structural features as indicated in Figure 13.4.

Benzodiazepines are widely used as hypnotics and anxiolytics and the currently available drugs that are clinically available under the heading of hypnotics include nitrazepam, flurazepam, loprazolam, lormetazepam and temazepam (Fig. 13.5). The anxiolytic benzodiazepines are detailed in Figure 13.6.

Mode of action

The benzodiazepines act by interaction with the benzodiazepine site at the GABA-A receptor. GABA, γ-aminobutyric acid (Fig. 13.7), is the major inhibitory neurotransmitter in the CNS of vertebrates.

Within the brain we have the amygdala, which are two almond-shaped organs present in the temporal lobe. The amygdala play an important role in anxiety because when stress is felt the excitatory neurons of the amygdala fire rapidly, causing a sensation of fear and panic. To overcome this situation the inhibitory neurotransmitter GABA is released so as to modulate these sensations. The released GABA acts at the postsynaptic GABA-A receptor site, thereby modulating these feelings of anxiety by inhibition of excitatory signal transmission. The benzodiazepines act at the GABA-A receptor site, not at the active site for GABA but at an allosteric site. In doing so, they increase the affinity of the receptor site for GABA.

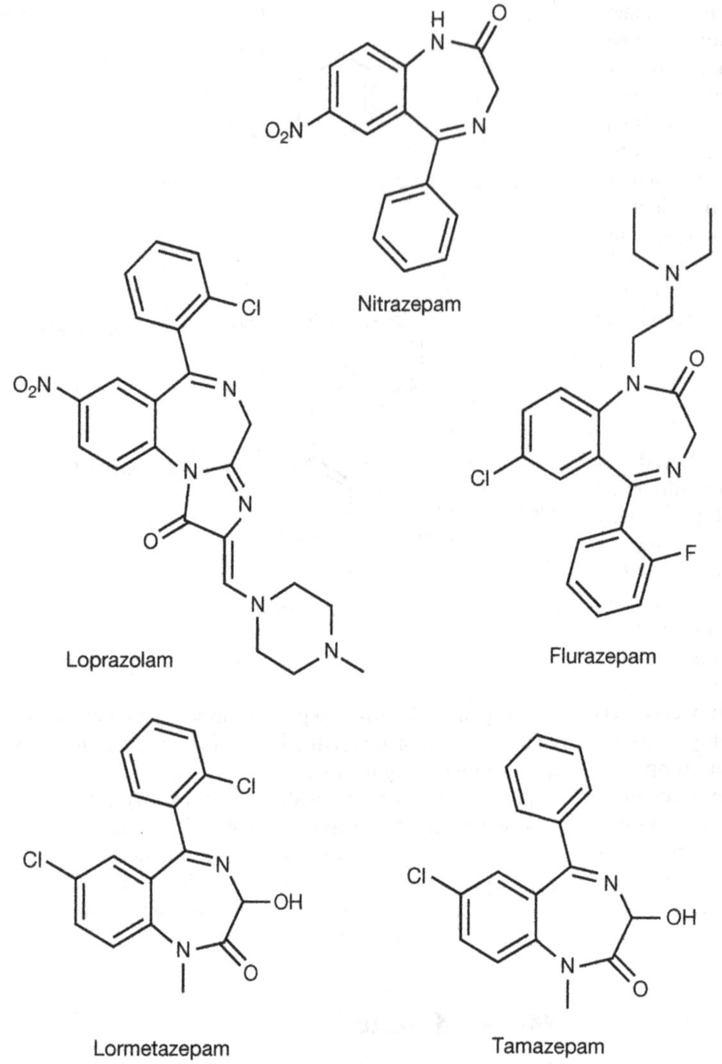

Figure 13.5 Structures of benzodiazepines employed as hypnotics.

The 'Z drugs'

The so-called 'Z-drugs' zopiclone, zolpidem and zaleplon (Fig. 13.8) were discovered through systematic screening of molecules that possessed binding characteristics and in vivo activity similar to that of the benzodiazepines. These three drugs are non-benzodiazepine drugs, as can be seen from their structural characteristics. However, they bind at the same site on the GABA-A receptor as do the benzodiazepines themselves.

It is worth noting that more recently the S (+)-enantiomer of zopiclone, eszopiclone (Fig. 13.9) has been licensed. The S(+)-enantiomer is reported to have greater activity than the R(−)-enantiomer with a 50-fold higher affinity for the GABA-A receptor and it is also suggested that it is superior in terms of the side effects profile.

Miscellaneous hypnotics and anxiolytics

For many years the mainstay of the clinician's armamentarium in the area of hypnotics and anxiolytics were the barbiturates. These compounds are essentially derivatives of barbituric acid, with the clinically used compounds often possessing dual substitution at the 5 position of the ring. Barbituric acid (Fig. 13.10) has no biological activity itself and it was only with the synthesis of barbital (Fig. 13.10) that the hypnotic/anxiolytic activity was observed.

Several thousand barbiturates have been synthesised and shown to possess hypnotic/anxiolytic activity and were for many years used for this purpose. However, they are seldom used in a routine fashion for this indication

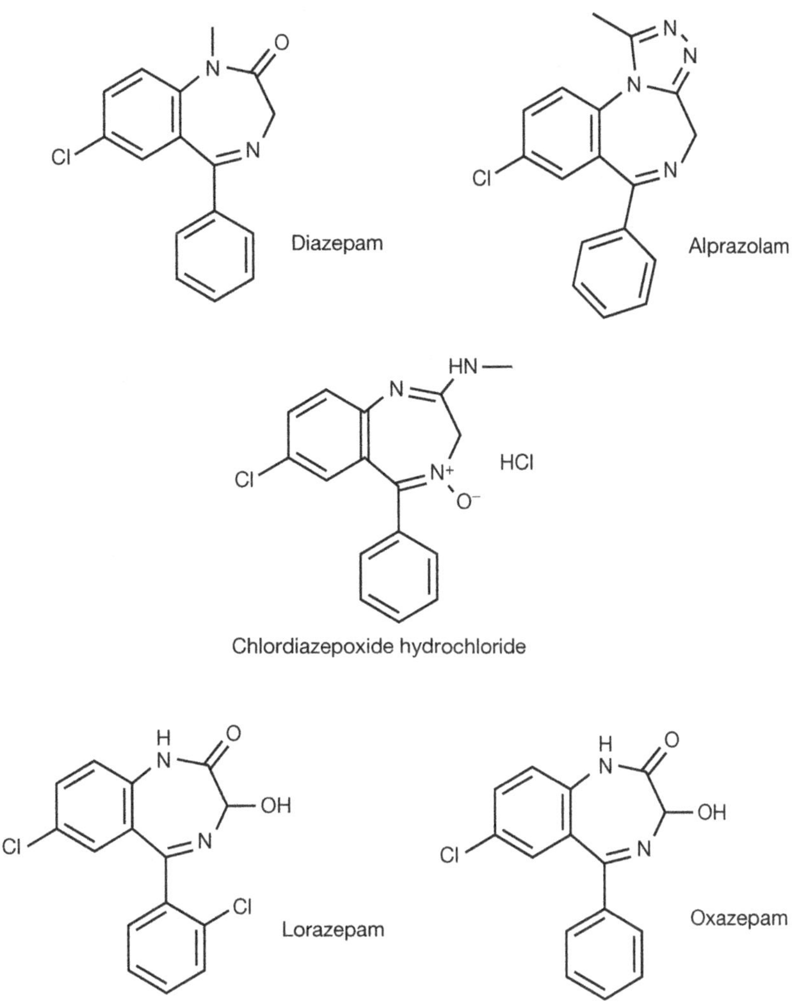

Figure 13.6 Anxiolytic benzodiazepines.

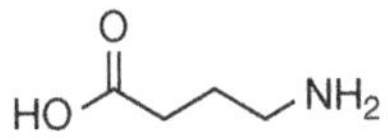

Figure 13.7 γ-aminobutyric acid.

these days because of the addictive problems associated with their use and also because of greater likelihood of death in overdose situations. The benzodiazepines and the Z-drugs have largely replaced the barbiturates in the routine treatment in this area, as indicated above. Some barbiturates are still used; for example, phenobarbital is still employed as an anticonvulsant and sodium thiopental as an intravenous anaesthetic. Additionally, three barbiturates, amobarbital, butobarbital and secobarbital (Fig. 13.11), are still indicated in the treatment of severe intractable insomnia.

The barbiturates act in a similar fashion to the benzodiazepines in that they bind to a site on the GABA-A receptor, although this site is distinct from the benzodiazepine site.

A range of other drugs is still indicated as hypnotics and anxiolytics although their use is somewhat restricted nowadays. Chloral hydrate and trichlofos (Fig. 13.12) are prodrugs that are converted into trichloroethanol in the body. The actual mechanism of action of trichloroethanol is uncertain. However, it is suggested that it may act as a CNS depressant in a similar manner to ethanol or that it exerts its activity via binding to the GABA receptor. Historically, chloral hydrate was a constituent of a Mickey Finn when mixed with ethanol.

Clomethiazole (Fig. 13.12) is a hypnotic agent, which has limited indications at present; it is indicated only for use in elderly patients. It acts at the barbiturate site of the

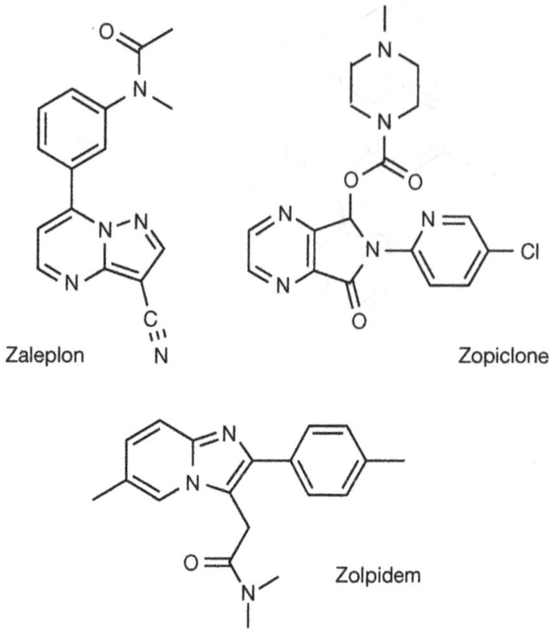

Figure 13.8 The Z-drugs.

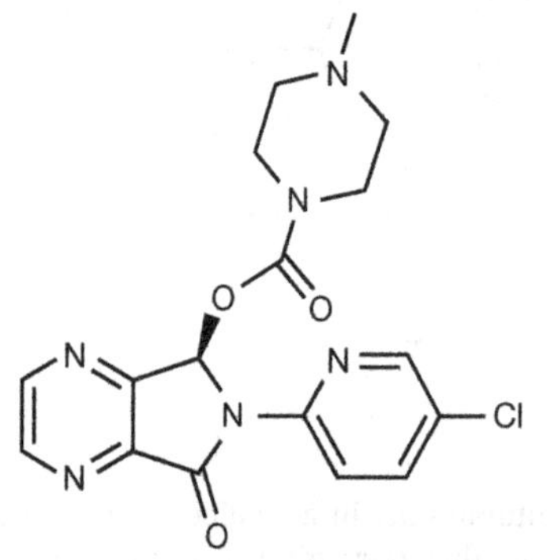

Figure 13.9 The structure of eszopiclone.

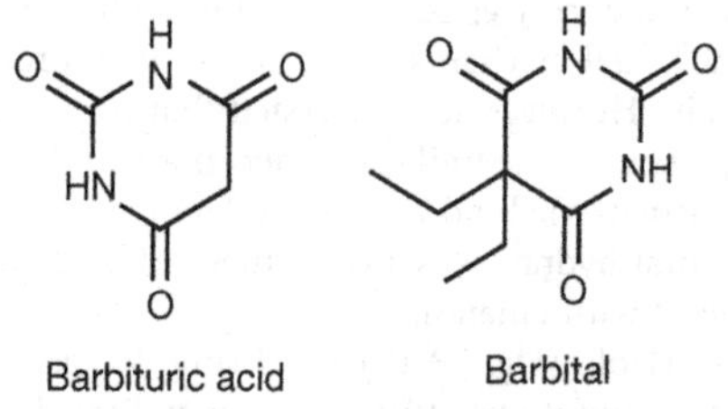

Figure 13.10 Structures of barbituric acid and barbital.

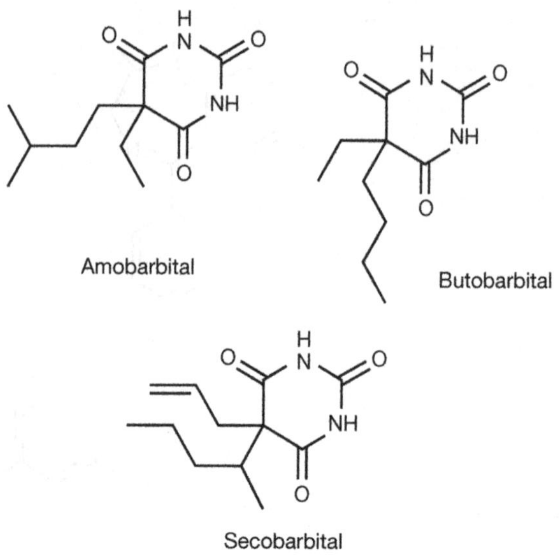

Figure 13.11 Barbiturates used in the treatment of severe intractable insomnia.

GABA-A receptor thereby enhancing the action of GABA. Sodium oxybate is the sodium salt of γ-hydroxybutyrate, commonly referred to as GHB. This drug has a very specific indication which is the treatment of cataplexy in narcolepsy. Narcolepsy is a chronic sleep disorder and the narcoleptic patient will often present as having severe insomnia. Cataplexy is a sudden loss of muscle tone and strength, usually caused by an extreme emotional stimulus. This occurs regularly (approximately 75% of cases) in patients with narcolepsy. Treatment with sodium oxybate is reported to improve the symptoms of narcolepsy and also to reduce the number of occurrences of cataplexy.

A number of antihistamines are also available for the treatment of insomnia, promethazine and diphenhydramine (Fig. 13.12) being examples of such drugs. It has been proposed that antihistamines cause sedation by the blockade of central histamine H_1-receptors.

Two further drugs have been described that have applications in this area, namely buspirone and melatonin (Fig. 13.13).

Buspirone is a member of a class of compounds that are designated azapirones, based on the functionality circled in Figure 13.13. This drug was first synthesised in the late 1960s whilst searching for neuroleptic compounds. The compound showed no antipsychotic properties although it was later identified as an anxiolytic. It is active as an agonist at both pre- and postsynaptic 5-HT_{1A} receptors and it is generally acknowledged not to display its anxiolytic activity immediately, but after a lead-in period of several weeks.

Melatonin is a hormone that is involved in the regulation of circadian rhythms in the body and its production is greater during darkness than during daylight hours.

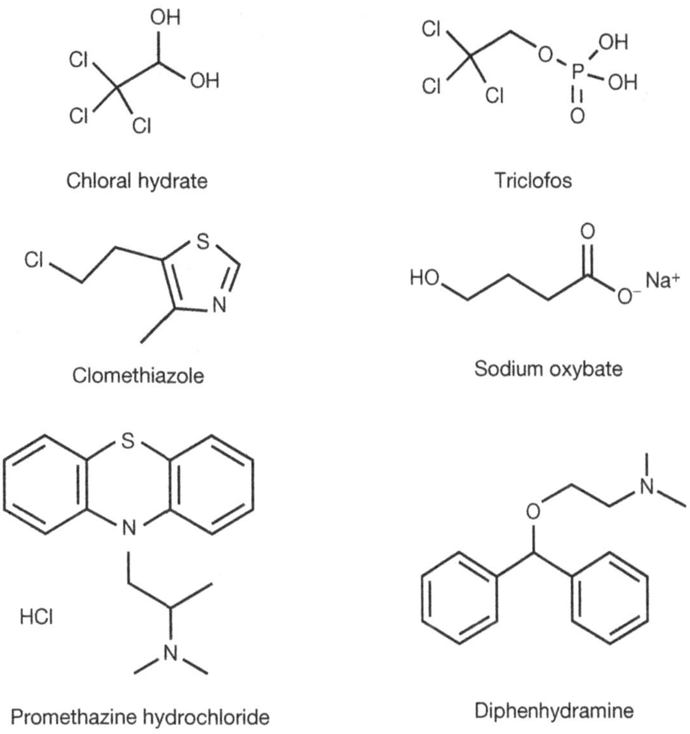

Figure 13.12 Miscellaneous hypnotics and anxiolytics.

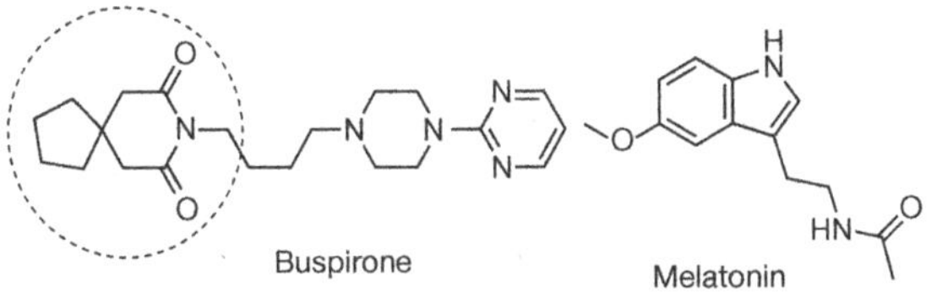

Figure 13.13 The structures of buspirone and melatonin.

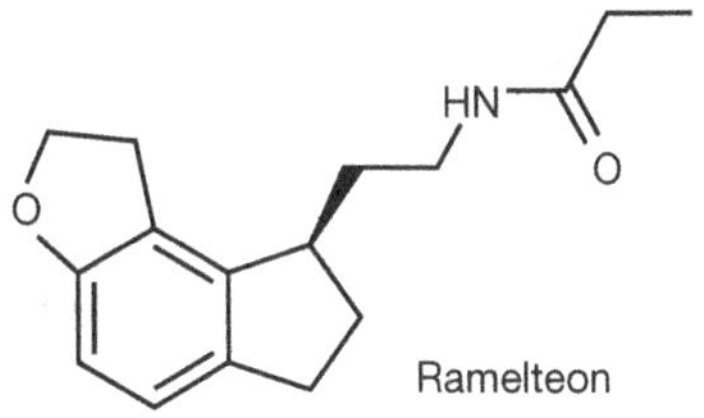

Figure 13.14 Structure of remelteon, a specific MT_1 and MT_2 receptor agonist.

The increased production of melatonin later in the day is thought to aid sleep via the binding of melatonin to MT_1 and MT_2 receptors in the brain, and in doing so reduces alertness. It has been suggested (though there are dissenting viewpoints as well) that melatonin may be useful in the treatment of age-related insomnia. There is evidence that as people age they have poorer sleep patterns with an increase in both the frequency and extent of waking. It has also been shown that during aging people show a decreased melatonin production and that this may have an influence on insomnia. As a result, studies have investigated the ability of melatonin to assist in improving insomnia in patients over 50. These studies indicated that a dose of about 0.3 mg is appropriate and that doses achievable using 'health food store' melatonin tablets may provide doses that are too high to assist insomniac patients. Recently, a new class of drugs has been reported, and this class of drugs is known as specific MT_1 and MT_2 receptor agonists. Ramelteon (Fig. 13.14), the first drug in this class, has recently been licensed in the USA and it is proposed that because of the specificity for these receptors (and the lack of GABA-A receptor affinity) the common side effects of anxiolytics are not observed.

EPILEPSY AND ANTIEPILEPTIC (ANTICONVULSANT) DRUGS

Epilepsy is a chronic neurological disorder that has been known since ancient times, with reports that Hippocrates (460–377 BC) was aware of this condition; in fact, it has been reported that his writing on this topic was the first ever medical monograph. The word epilepsy is derived from the Greek word 'epilamabanie/epilamabanien' which means to seize. Historically, it was known as the 'sacred disease' since it was thought that the seizures and the visions reported by epileptics were sent by the gods. Epilepsy is a disorder in which the normal low-frequency discharge of cortical neurons is replaced by an abnormal burst of high-frequency discharges. When groups of neurons discharge together in this way, a seizure may result. These seizures may or may not be accompanied by loss of consciousness and convulsions. Neurons in the brain allow information to be received and transmitted between one another in the form of electrical signals. These processes occur through the action of brain chemicals known as neurotransmitters. During an epileptic seizure the electrical signals produced by the neurons are produced more quickly than normal, are stronger than normal, and less organised than under normal neuronal activity.

The prevalence of epilepsy is reportedly 5 to 8 per 1000 population although there are indications that in Latin America and Africa this number may be double. The occurrence of a single seizure is not in itself an indication of epilepsy; only when a person has two or more can he or she be diagnosed as having epilepsy. There are many different types of epilepsy and these were detailed in the 1981 International League Against Epilepsy (ILAE) common seizure list, which has recently (2006) been updated, although work is still ongoing. A simplified version of the 1981 common seizure list is presented in Table 13.1. Note that partial seizures are seizures that involve only one region of the brain, whereas generalised seizures spread throughout the brain.

Table 13.1 The ILAE 1981 – Common seizure list

Partial or focal onset
Simple partial seizures (consciousness not impaired) Complex partial seizures Partial seizures evolving to secondary generalised seizures
Generalised onset
Absence seizures Myoclonic seizures Clonic seizures Tonic seizures Tonic clonic seizures Atonic seizures
Unclassified epileptic seizures
Neonatal seizures Rhythmic eye movements Chewing Swimming movements

Although there are many instances where the factors contributing to the development of epilepsy are unknown, there are also a variety of known factors such as head injuries, cerebral tumours, brain infections and strokes which can be associated with the development of the condition. It has long been thought that heredity played a role in the development of epilepsy but only recently has a genetic link been found. However, the precise nature of this genetic aspect is still under investigation.

Anticonvulsant drugs used in the treatment of epilepsy

The BNF details a range of drugs that are available for the treatment of epilepsy; these drugs are commonly referred to as antiepileptic drugs or AEDs. Figure 13.15 details the structures of these AEDs. As can be seen, the compounds have a wide range of diverse structures. This group of drugs may be classified in various different ways. One of the simplest is to classify the drugs in terms of established and newer AEDs as is shown in Table 13.2.

In the left-hand column of Table 13.2 we have what are classified as established AEDs. In terms of treatment of epilepsy in the modern era, this really began in the 1850s with the introduction of potassium bromide. In the early years of the twentieth century, potassium bromide was superseded by phenobarbital. Over the next 50 years, several other compounds such as phenytoin, ethosuximide, carbamazepine and valproic acid came into routine usage. It is only in the last 20 years that the newer AEDs have begun to appear. These drugs are reportedly as effective as the older drugs and are said to have fewer side effects although some surveys still indicate widespread usage of some of the older drugs and some problems with the newer ones.

A series of drugs is also available for the treatment of status epilepticus, which will be dealt with separately.

The mechanism of action of antiepileptic drugs

There are three proposed major mechanisms of action of AEDs: (1) sodium channel inactivation, (2) calcium channel blockade, and (3) interaction with GABA-A receptors/channels. With sodium channel inactivation antiepileptic drugs have the ability to extend the inactivation of sodium channels which reduces the frequency of the firing of the neurons, which is a feature of the seizures. Drugs that are associated with this inactivation include phenytoin, carbamazepine and valproate. Calcium channel blockade (T-type) is related to the modulation of neuronal firing associated with absence of seizures and is associated with ethosuximide and zonisamide activity. L-type calcium channel blockade is reportedly associated

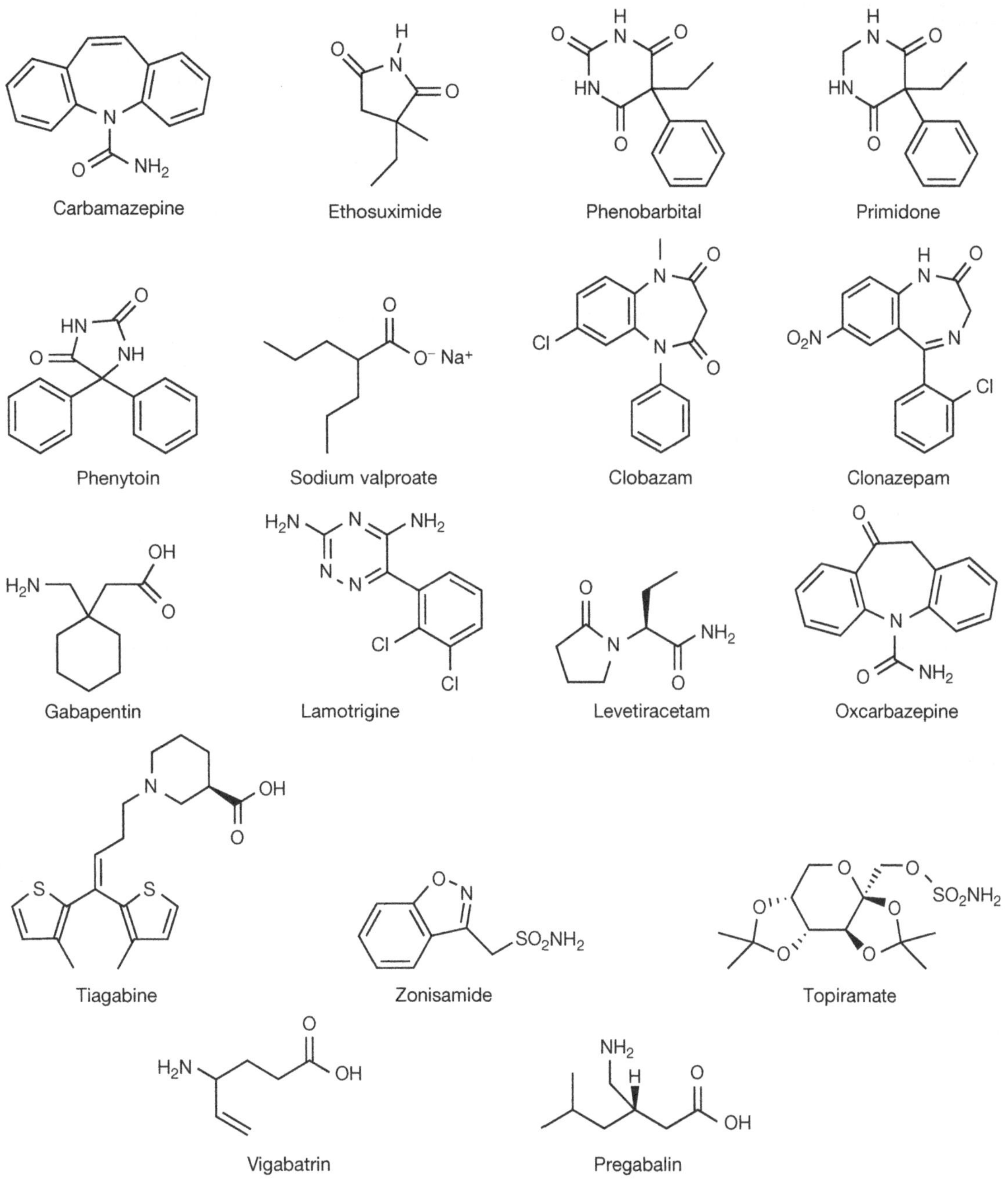

Figure 13.15 Structures of commonly used AEDs.

with modulation of neurotransmitters at presynaptic nerve terminals, and such activity is indicated for gabapentin. The third major mechanism is associated with interaction at the GABA-A receptor. The rapid firing of neurons associated with an epileptic seizure is modulated via the action of certain AEDs. In certain instances the action is via direct action with the GABA-A receptors whilst with others the action is related to the synthesis and turnover of GABA itself. Finally, it has been reported that in some instances interaction with glutamate receptors is proposed for the action of certain AEDs. It is also worth noting that in some instances an AED might be

Table 13.2 AEDs classified based on age

Established AEDs	Newer AEDs
Carbamazepine	Gabapentin
Ethosuximide	Lamotrigine
Phenobarbital [Primidone]	Levitracetam
Phenytoin	Oxcarbazepine
Valproate	Tiagabine
Clobazam	Zonisamide
Clonazepam	Topiramate
	Vigabatrin
	Pregabalin

indicated as acting via a single mechanism of action. For example, the activity of ethosuximide in the treatment of absence seizures is designated as being via the (T-type) calcium channel blockade whilst in other cases a drug may be indicated as acting through a number of different processes. Details of the proposed mechanisms of action of a number drugs are detailed in Table 13.3.

When considering treatment for epilepsy, there are several points that must be noted. The details presented above indicate a wide range of seizure types, as listed in Table 13.1, and a large number of AEDs to treat epilepsy and an indication of a number of different mechanisms by which these drugs work. Despite this, the treatment of patients who suffer from epilepsy is difficult. In some instances a patient may be stabilised with good seizure control with only one AED (approximately 70%) whilst in other cases polytherapy is necessary, and in some instances even this is unsuccessful and surgery may be necessary. The details presented in Table 13.2 listing the newer antiepileptic drugs indicate that many of these drugs are as effective as the established drugs but would have superior side effect profiles. However, a reduction in side effects has not been overwhelmingly proven and indeed there are other 'newer' drugs that have been introduced and not stood the test of time. In recent years there has been considerable research into genetic aspects of epilepsy, and with these developments a more fundamental understanding of epilepsy is developing. Thus, more realistic, evidence-based treatment may follow from this work.

Table 13.3 Mechanisms of action of various AEDs

AED	Enhancement of GABA-mediated excitation	Blockade of sodium channels	Blockade of calcium channels	Inhibition of glutamate	Other
Benzodiazepines	+	+*			
Carbamazepine		+			
Ethosuximide			+ (T-type)		
Phenobarbital	+	+		+	
Phenytoin		+			
Valproate	+	+			+
Gabapentin			+ (L-type)		
Lamotrigine		+	+ (L-type)		
Levitracetam					+
Oxcarbamazepine		+	+ (L-type)		
Tiagabine	+				
Topiramate	+	+	+ (L-type)	+	+
Vigabatrin	+				
Zonisamide		+	+ (T-type)	+	+

*Based on data in Mechanisms of Action of Antiepileptic Drugs, P. Czapriski et al. Current Topics in Medicinal Chemistry, 2005, 5, p3–14.

Status epilepticus

Status epilepticus is traditionally defined as a situation where there is continuous seizure activity for a period of 30 minutes or where there are a continuous series of seizures during which the sufferer does not regain consciousness. More recently, it has been suggested that any continuous seizure period of longer than 5 minutes should be classified as status epilepticus. In these situations the treatment employed may well consist of one of the previously indicated antiepileptic drugs such as clonazepam (Fig. 13.15), phenobarbital and phenytoin (Fig. 13.15) or alternatively diazepam, fosphenytoin (a prodrug of phenytoin), lorazepam, midazolam and paraldehyde (Fig. 13.16) may be employed. For the drugs used in the treatment of status epilepticus, the formulation and dose differ from conventional doses due to the situation and thus many of these will be administered by intravenous injection, intravenous infusion, buccal or rectal administration.

ANTIPSYCHOTIC DRUGS

There are many drugs that are used to treat psychoses such as schizophrenia or manic behaviour. The antipsychotic drugs, sometimes referred to as neuroleptics, are nowadays generally classified under the headings of typical and atypical. The typical antipsychotics are essentially the older, well-established drugs that work mainly by blocking dopamine D_2 receptors, whilst the atypical antipsychotics are the newer members of the class, which often work via a similar mechanism of action, although within the atypical group other actions are sometimes involved.

It is believed that the production of excessive amounts of the neurotransmitter dopamine in the mesolimbic region of the midbrain is associated with psychotic behaviour. Dopamine is generated in the presynaptic side of the synapse from tyrosine via DOPA (Fig. 13.17).

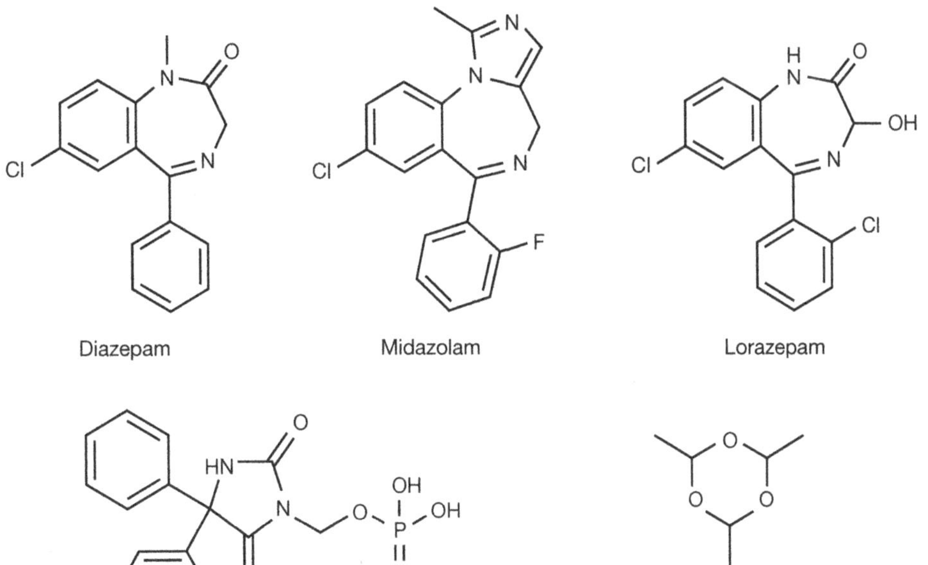

Figure 13.16 Additional drugs used in the treatment of status epilepticus.

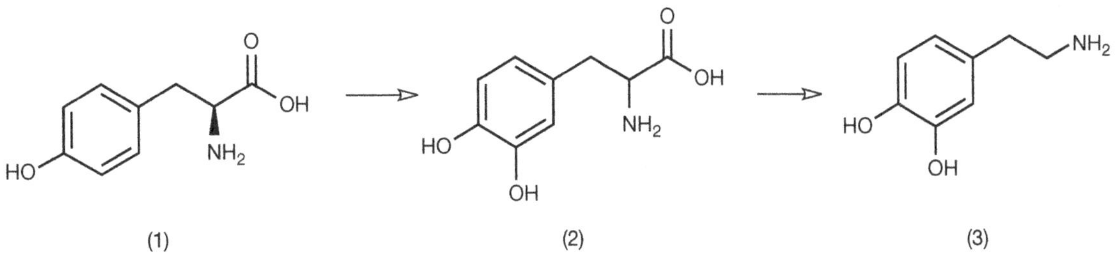

Figure 13.17 Metabolic conversion of tyrosine into dopamine.

Table 13.4 Typical and atypical antipsychotic drugs

Typical	Atypical
Chlorpromazine	Amisulpride
Levomepromazine	Aripiprazole
Pericyazine	Clozapine
Perphenazine	Olanzapine
Prochlorperazine	Paliperidone
Trifluoperazine	Quetiapine
Benperidol	Risperidone
Haloperidol	Sertindole
Pimozide	Zotepine
Flupentixol	
Zuclopenthixol	
Zuclopenthixol acetate	

Tyrosine is hydroxylated to DOPA via tyrosine hydroxylase and the final production of dopamine involves DOPA decarboxylase. The generated dopamine can then bind to the dopamine receptors on the postsynaptic side of the synapse. Dopamine is an inhibitory neurotransmitter which, when it interacts with the receptor, prevents the neuron from firing. It has been observed that psychotic-like behaviour can result from excessive use of drugs such as cocaine and amfetamines. It is known that these drugs result in an increase in dopamine levels in the brain; thus the proposal that in schizophrenic and manic patients excessive dopamine production in the brain is a cause. From this we have the idea that many of the antipsychotic drugs act by blocking the dopamine receptors in the mesolimbic region, thus alleviating the psychotic behaviour. The nature of this action and other modes of action will be discussed in more detail in the following sections.

As indicated above, the antipsychotic agents are generally classified as typical or atypical. Table 13.4 details these agents.

Phenothiazine antipsychotic drugs

The first class of antipsychotic agents discovered was the phenothiazines and the first clinically used member of this group was chlorpromazine. The compounds are all based on the phenothiazine ring structure shown in Figure 13.18.

The parent compound phenothiazine was first prepared in 1883 and derivatives of this compound have been used in a variety of non-pharmaceutical applications, for example

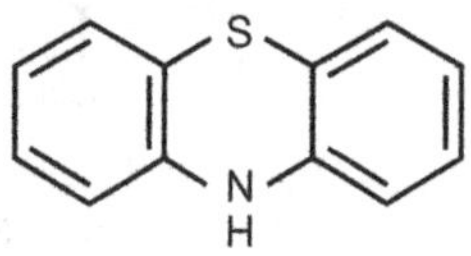

Figure 13.18 The basic structure of phenothiazine.

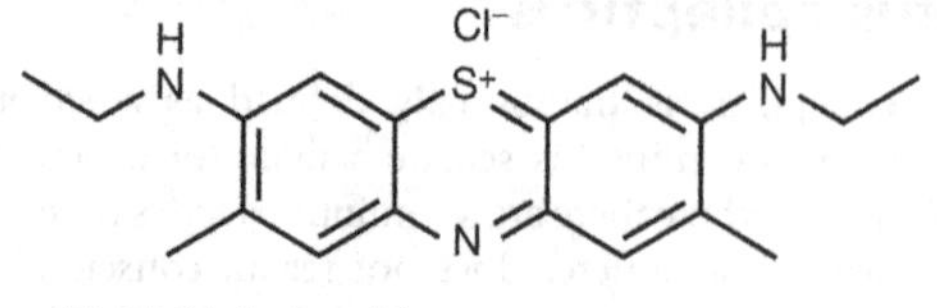

Figure 13.19 Methylene blue.

methylene blue (Fig. 13.19), which is used as an indicator and as a biological stain. There has been a revival of interest in methylene blue as a drug and it has recently been tested in the treatment of Alzheimer's and Parkinson's diseases.

In the early 1950s, the antipsychotic activity of substituted phenothiazines was discovered and chlorpromazine (Fig. 13.20) was introduced as the first clinically used member of this class.

The drugs that belong to the class of active antipsychotic drugs have functionalities substituted on the nitrogen of the central ring system and on the aromatic rings within the phenothiazine molecule. The active compounds are often designated with the type of basic substitution pattern shown in Figure 13.21.

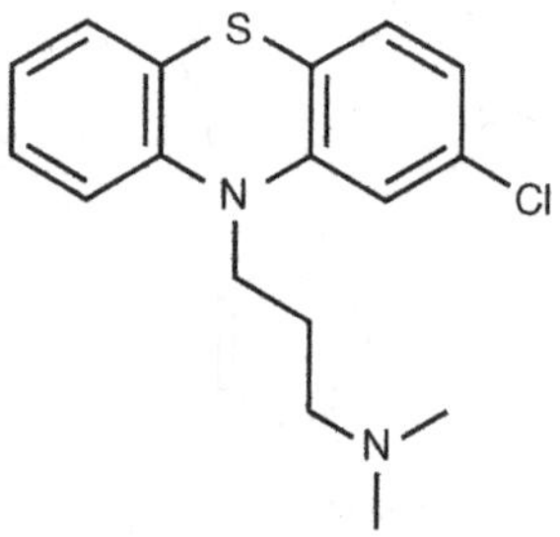

Figure 13.20 Chlorpromazine.

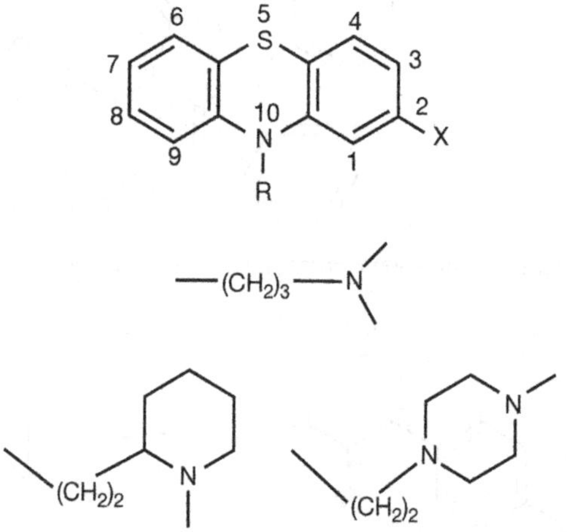

Figure 13.21 General structure of antipsychotic phenothiazines and three common N_{10} substituents of active phenothiazines: (1) a propyl dialkyl amino side chain, (2) an alkyl piperidyl side chain or (3) a propyl piparazine side chain.

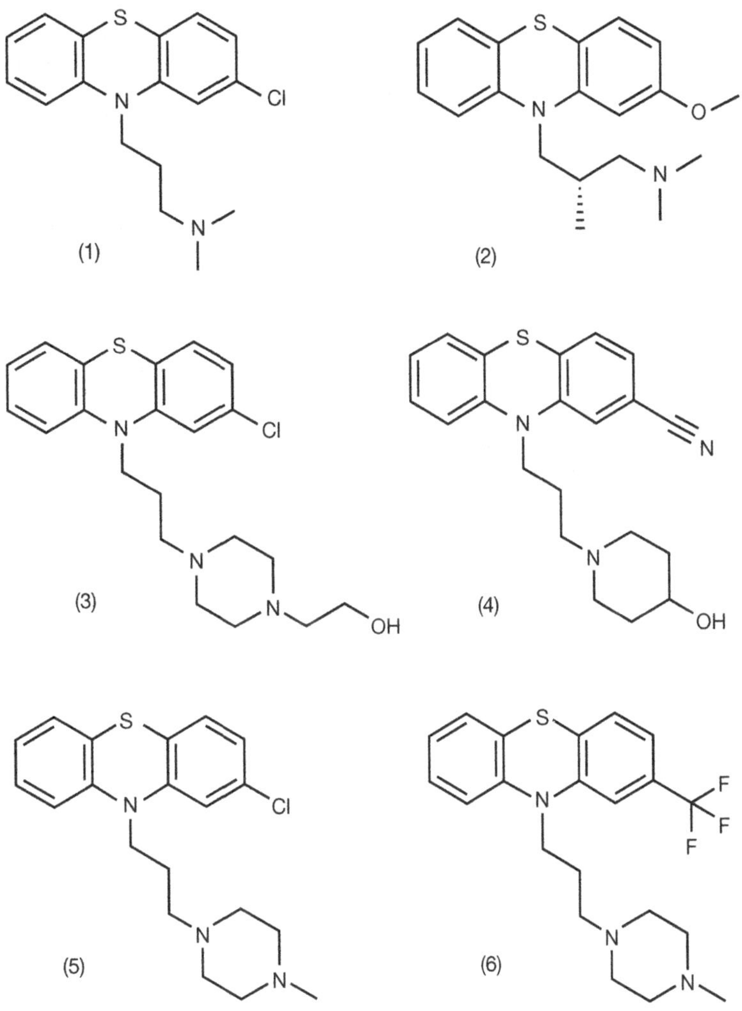

Figure 13.22 Some of the clinically used phenothiazines. (1) Chlorpromazine, (2) Levomepromazine, (3) Perphenazine, (4) Pericyazine, (5) Prochlorperazine, (6) Trifluoperazine.

Within this group of compounds we find that the compounds that are clinically active may have a range of moieties at the C_2 position, for example H, Cl, SMe, O=SMe, CF_3, whilst the side chain attached to the ring nitrogen is one of three chain systems a propyl dialkyl amino side chain, an alkyl piperidyl side chain or a propyl piparazine side chain (Fig. 13.21). Some of the presently clinically used phenothiazines are shown in Figure 13.22. As stated above, it is believed that the mode of action of this class of drugs related to the blocking of the dopamine receptors in the mesolimbic region of the mid brain. The structural similarity between these phenothiazines and dopamine is proposed as the reason for the activity. In Figure 13.23, the structural characteristics of dopamine and chlorpromazine are presented, both as the separate entities and also superimposed on one another.

From this two-dimensional representation we can observe that the central portion of these clinically active phenothiazines has a number of structural similarities to dopamine. There have been detailed studies into the activity of these compounds that have also focused on the three-dimensional aspects. It has been suggested that within the whole class of tricyclic antidepressants there are some 3-D aspects that are important in relation to whether the compounds possess antipsychotic properties or not. Thus, for instance, the structural characteristics of the phenothiazines and the thioxanthenes (see below) are such that they display neuroleptic properties, whilst closely related compounds such as amitryptyline (Fig. 13.24) do not possess this activity but do possess antidepressant (thymoleptic) properties.

The difference in properties is believed to be due to the shape of the molecules and Figure 13.25 shows how certain geometric features of this group of compounds may be classified. The angle of flexure α is the angle between the planes of the two aromatic rings when projected

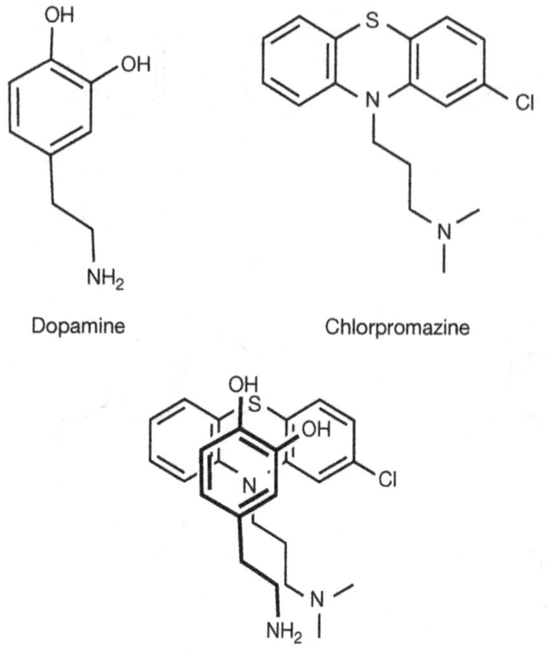

Figure 13.23 Separate and overlaid structures of dopamine and chlorpromazine.

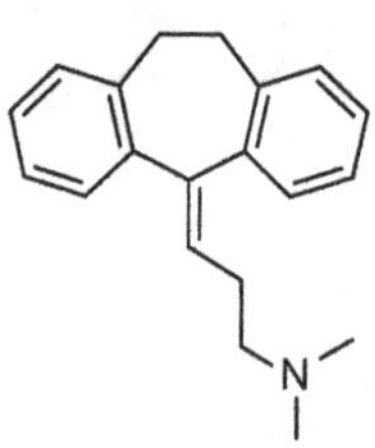

Figure 13.24 Amitryptyline.

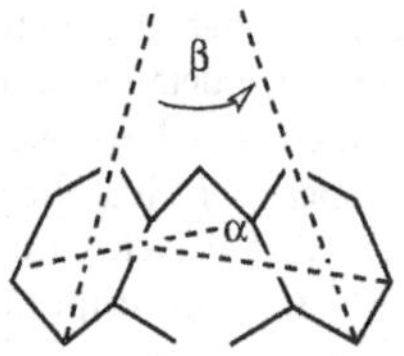

Figure 13.25 Geometric features associated with the neuroleptic or thymoleptic properties of the tricyclics.

towards the molecule's centre. The angle of annelation β is a measurement of how much the two sides of the aromatic rings are from being parallel. The lower the values of α and β are, the more likely it is that the compounds will possess neuroleptic properties. Additionally it is understood that the nature of the 3-D shape adopted by the side chain in phenothiazines and thioxanthenes is important in relation to their antipsychotic activity.

Thioxanthenes

The clinically active thioxanthenes are structurally similar to the corresponding phenothiazines (Fig. 13.26). The difference in structure is due to the replacement of the linkage from the nitrogen to the side chain in phenothiazines via a single bond with a carbon double bond as shown below. Despite this change, the activity of the thioxanthenes is similarly based on the interaction with the dopamine receptors and it has been shown that the cis-isomer of the thioxanthenes is generally more active than the trans-isomer, as can be observed in the clinically used examples described in Figure 13.27. The clinically used thioxanthenes are substituted both in the ring and in the side chain with similar moieties as the phenothiazine analogues. Some of the presently used thioxanthenes are shown in Figure 13.27.

Fluorobutyrophenones and diphenylbutylpiperidines

The final group of typical antipsychotics are the fluorobutyrophenones and diphenylbutylpiperidines that were discovered in the late 1950s by the pharmaceutical company Janssen. The fluorobutyrophenones were discovered during investigations aimed at improving the activity of pethidine. In their studies in this area, the Janssen group synthesised a derivative of pethidine in which the N-methyl group was replaced with a propiophenone moiety. This compound was shown to possess significantly greater (more than 100-fold) analgesic activity than pethidine (Fig. 13.28). A range of other derivatives was then prepared, one of which was the butyrophenone analogue which showed potent but short-lived analgesic activity but additionally cataleptic activity similar to that of chlorpromazine. This led the Janssen workers to search for analogues that might be useful as antipsychotics but without the analgesic properties of pethidine and over four hundred derivatives were synthesised. The outcome of this work was discovery of haloperidol (see below), which was the first of the fluorobutyrophenones introduced clinically and which was approximately 50 times more potent than chlorpromazine. Figure 13.29 details the structures of the present clinically used fluorobutyrophenones.

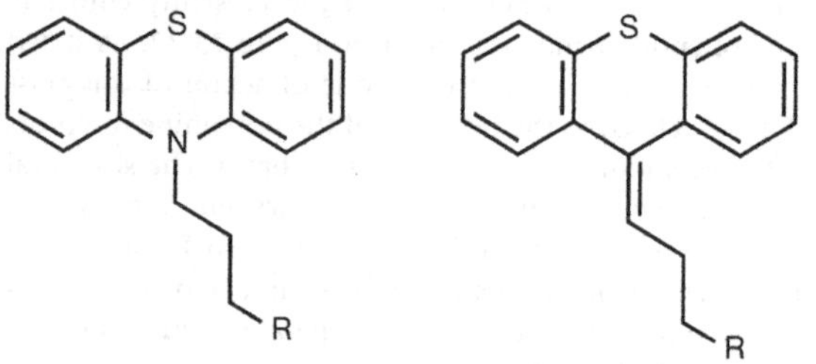

Figure 13.26 Structures of a phenothiazine compared with a thioxanthene.

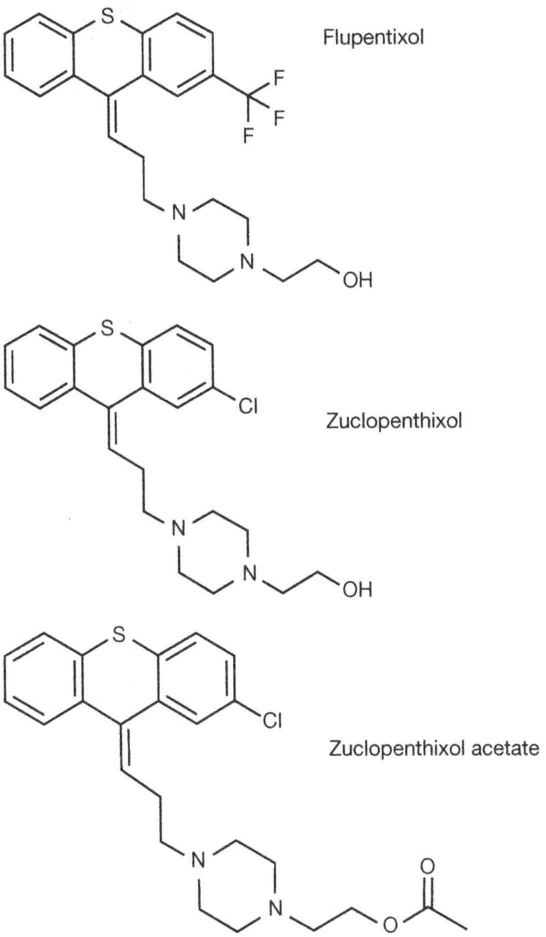

Figure 13.27 Clinically used thioxanthenes.

Further studies into modifications of the butyrophenones in which the fluoroketone functionality was replaced by a difluorophenyl moiety resulted in the discovery of a group of neuroleptic agents, the diphenylbutylpiperidines. These compounds have similar levels of activity to the butyrophenones but have a longer duration of activity.

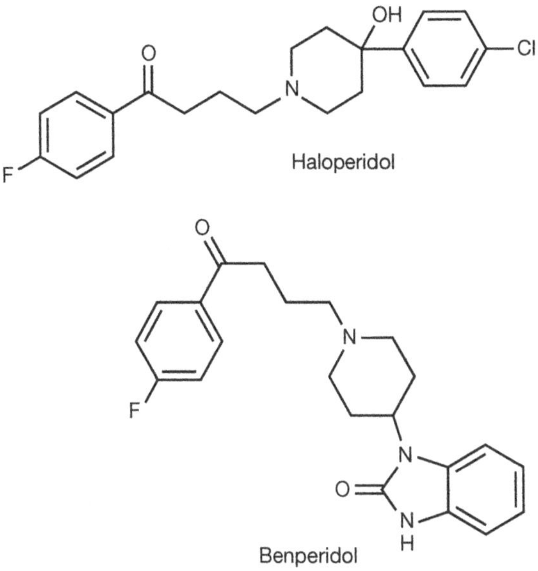

Figure 13.29 Structures of haloperidol and benperidol.

Pimozide (Fig. 13.30) is essentially the diphenylbutylpiperidine derivative of benperidol and is a useful antipsychotic. It is also indicated for Tourette's syndrome.

Atypical antipsychotic drugs

The group of compounds that is detailed under the heading of atypical antipsychotic drugs is often thought of as the second generation of this class of drugs because they are some of the more recently introduced compounds. They are also generally thought of as antipsychotics that have a reduced propensity to cause the extrapyramidal side effects (EPS) associated with the typical antipsychotic. The EPS associated with the typical antipsychotics include slurred speech, tremor, akathesia and dystonia, and drug treatment to control these problems is sometimes required. The atypical antipsychotics are reportedly less likely to cause these problems although this idea has been challenged. The atypical antipsychotics presently indicated for the treatment of

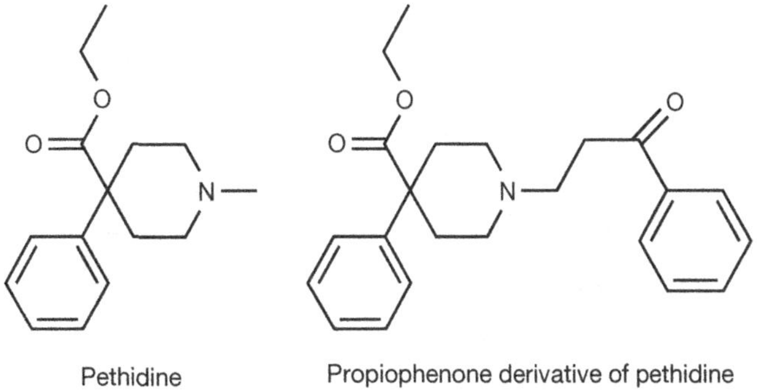

Figure 13.28 Structure of pethidine and its propiophenone analogue.

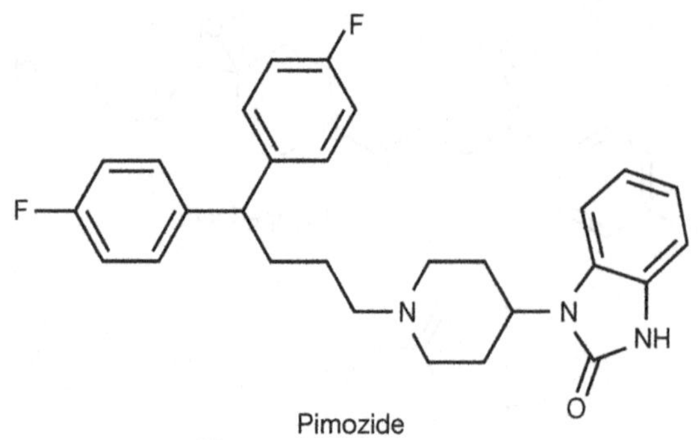

Figure 13.30 The diphenylbutylpiperidine pimozide.

schizophrenia and manic disorders include amisulpride, aripiprazole, clozapine, olanzapine, paliperidone, quetiapine, risperidone, sertindole and zotepine. Their structures are shown below in Figures 13.31 and 13.32.

As can be seen from these two figures, this class of drugs contains many drugs with diverse structures. There is much discussion of the mode of action of the atypical antipsychotics and some diversion of opinions of the exact details. It is believed that the atypical antipsychotics exhibit their activity, at least to a certain extent, in a manner similar to the typical agents in that interaction with dopamine receptors is partially involved. It has been suggested that with some atypical antipsychotics the binding to the D_2 receptors is looser than that of the typical compounds and that they can rapidly dissociate from these receptors, thereby allowing a more normal dopamine activity in terms of neurotransmission, which reduces the EPS. There is some evidence that 5-HT receptors also play an important role in the activity of these atypical agents. It is also proposed that the ratio of the blockage of 5-HT to D_2 is important in distinguishing typical from atypical agents. It is reported that different affinities for different dopamine receptors (e.g. D_2/D_3 with amisulpride) is important in its activity.

Antipsychotic depot injections

With some patients who require antipsychotic medication there is a problem with adherence (compliance); i.e. they do not remember to take their drugs as prescribed. In such

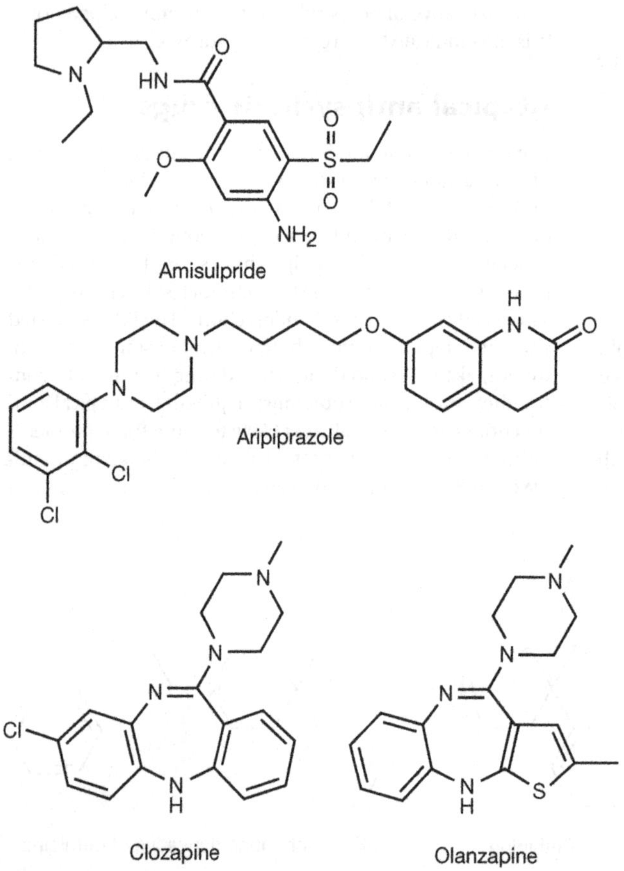

Figure 13.31 Atypical antipsychotic drugs (1).

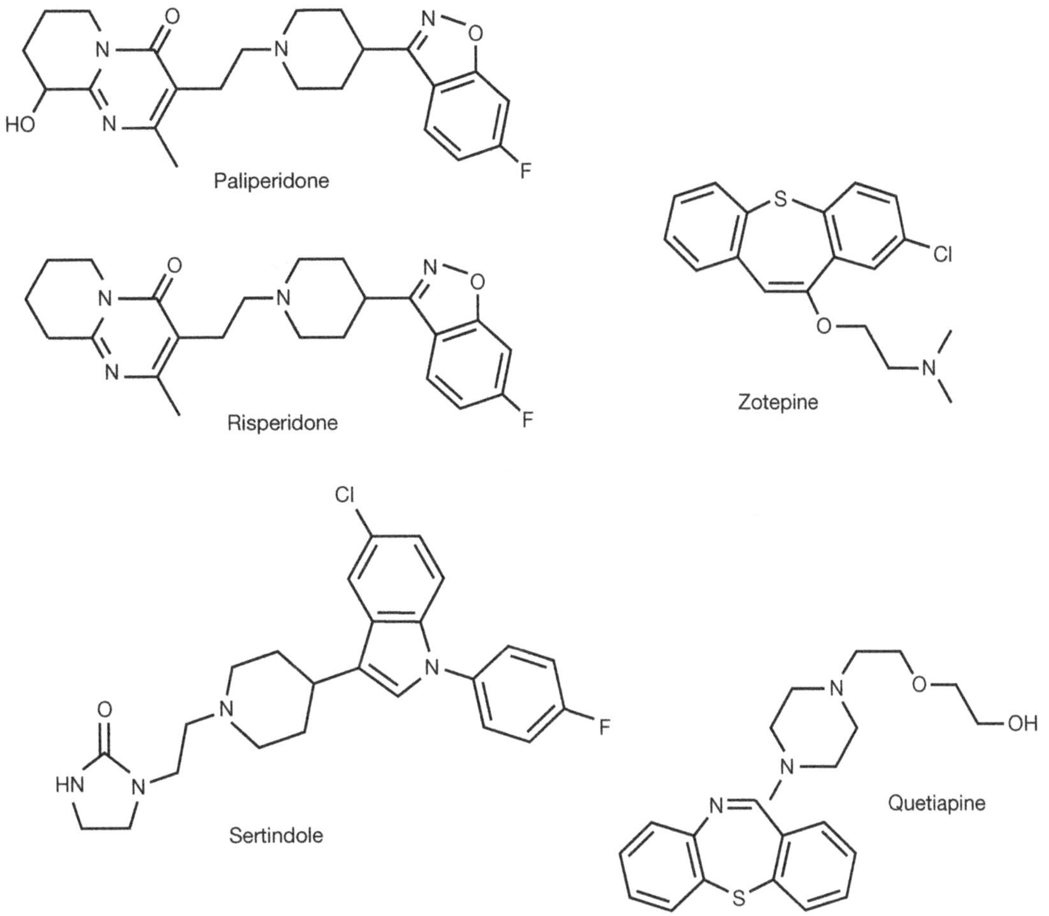

Figure 13.32 Atypical antipsychotic drugs (2).

cases the schizophrenia/mania will not be controlled and this will lead to behavioural problems. To overcome this difficulty there are a number of depot injections available. The antipsychotics available for such purposes include haloperidol decanoate, flupentixol decanoate, flufenazine decanoate, pitoatiazine palmitate, zuclopenthixol decanoate and risperidone (Fig. 13.33). The first five of these are available as oily injections that are administered by deep intramuscular injection. They are all prodrugs of their parent drug and are all essentially highly lipophilic ester derivatives. Following the deep injection into the gluteal muscle, these compounds are slowly released into the bloodstream where they are rapidly converted into the parent drug by non-specific esterases. Thus the patients receiving these injections have a continuous release of the antipsychotic over the period between injections, which is between 2 and 4 weeks. With risperidone, the parent drug is administered and it is the drug delivery system itself that provides the sustained release of the drug. Risperdal CONSTA contains risperidone encapsulated in biodegradable microspheres made of poly(lactide-co-glycolide). The drug is provided as these microspheres for reconstitution in a diluent solution provided by the manufacturers. Following its preparation, the drug is administered by injection into the gluteal muscle. The slow release is brought about by degradation of the microspheres through hydrolysis, which allows the diffusion of the drug out of the polymer system and thus into general circulation.

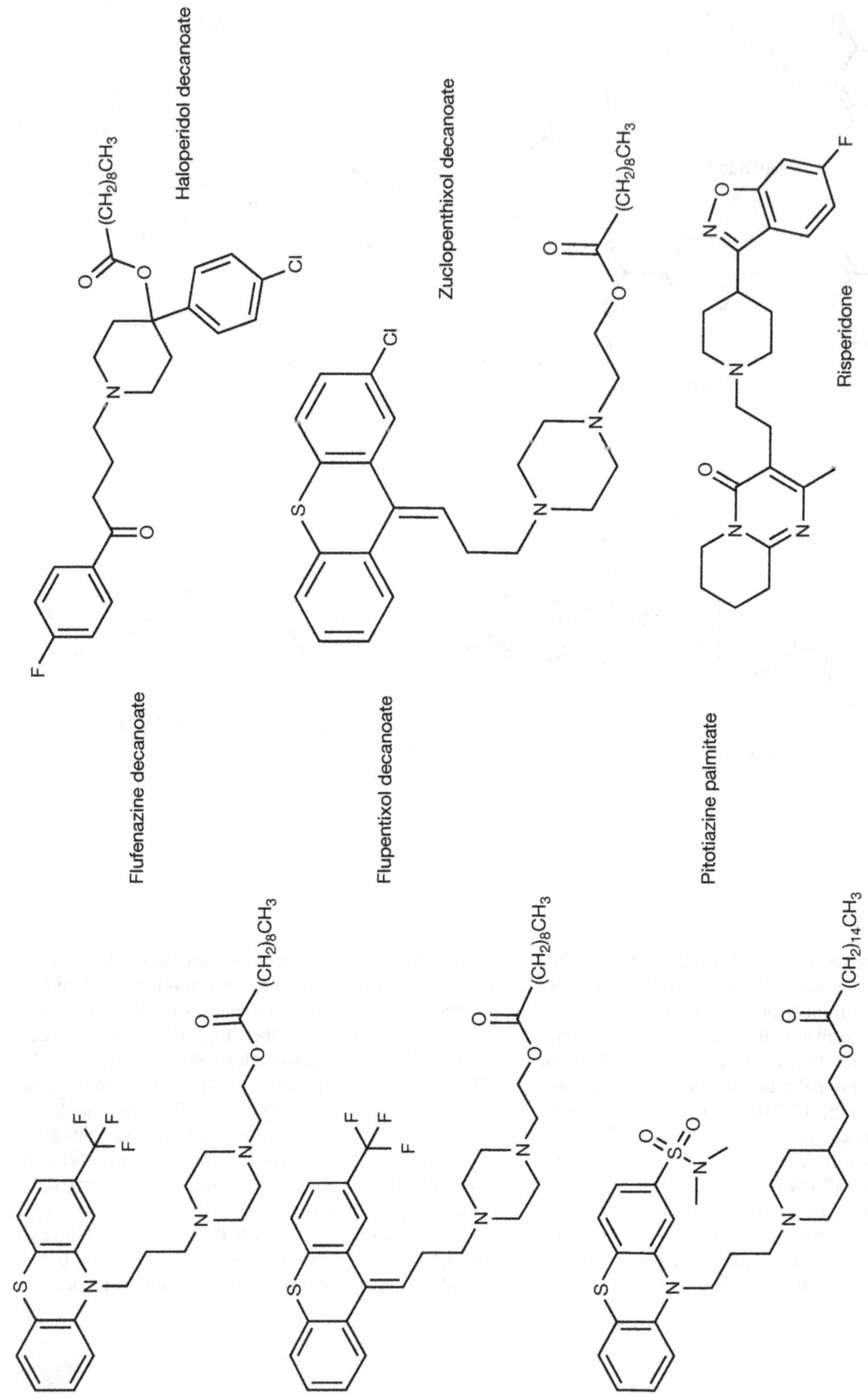

Figure 13.33 Depot antipsychotics.

Q Self Test 13.1

Classify the drugs shown below as: phenothiazine, haloperidol type, thioxanthine, atypical tranquilliser, not a tranquilliser.

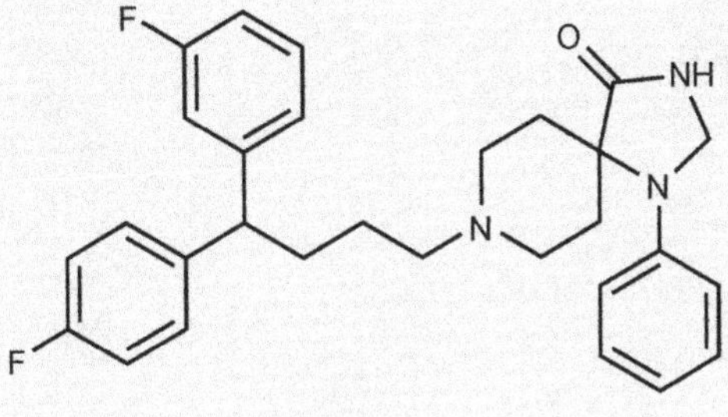

Fluspirilene

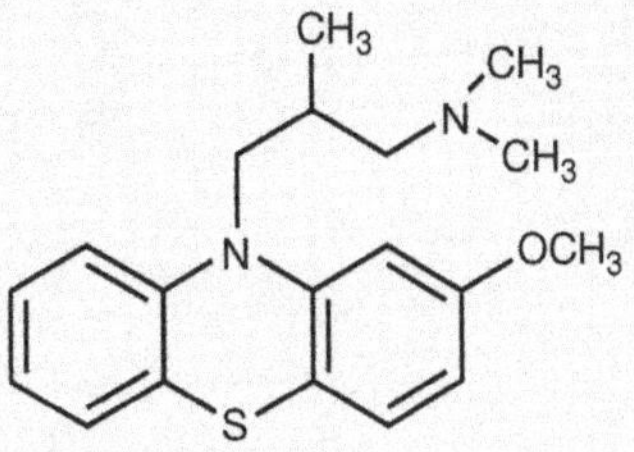

Levomepromazine

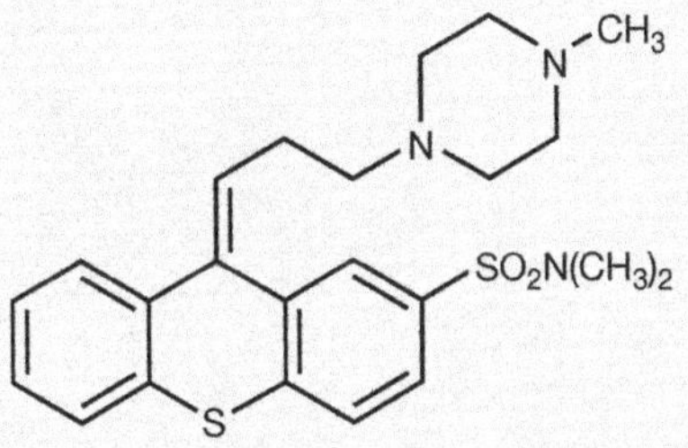

Tiotixine

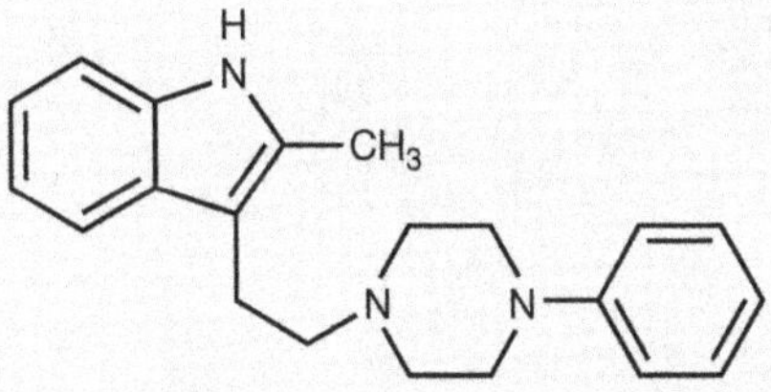

Oxypertine

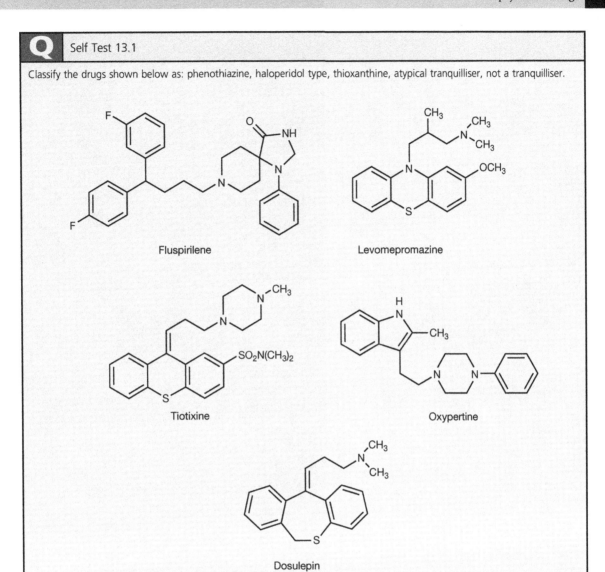

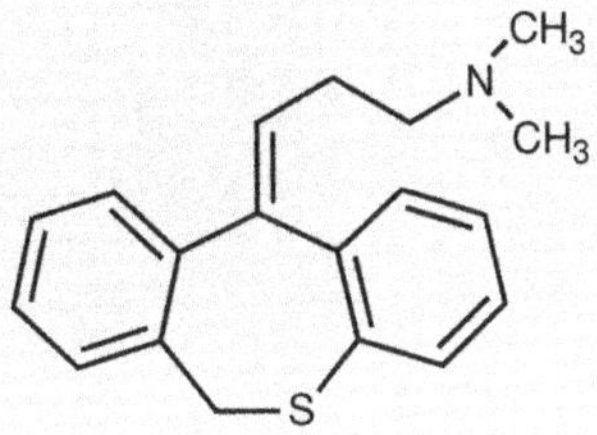

Dosulepin

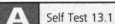

A Self Test 13.1

Fluspirilene (haloperidol type), levomepromazine (phenothiazine), tiotixine (thioxanthine), oxpertine (atypical), dosulepin (not a tranquilliser).

Chapter | 14 |

Analgesics

RuAngelie Edrada-Ebel

CHAPTER CONTENTS

A BRIEF HISTORICAL BACKGROUND

Pain management can be traced back as early as the Fifth Dynasty (2450 BC) in Egypt.[1] The Egyptians utilised various pain-relieving strategies, especially in the long hours of ancient surgery. The technique known today as cryo-analgesia was used in circumcision, one of the earliest forms of surgery carried out, during this period. In this procedure a mixture of calcium carbonate and acetic acid was used to produce carbon dioxide, causing local cooling and analgesia.[2] Opium obtained from the poppy seed capsules of *Papaver somniferum* was widely yet controversially administered. The bark extract of the willow tree, *Salix alba*, was a less-debated joint pain adjuvant (Box 14.1).[3]

Greek medicine was based on Egyptian scientific knowledge. The word 'pain' originates from the Latin *poena* and the Greek *poine*, which means penalty or punishment. On the other hand, the word *analgesic* was derived from Greek *an-* (without) and *algos* (pain). In classical Greek civilisation, Hippocrates (460–370 BC) unwittingly used the chemical precursor of acetylsalicylic acid (aspirin) from willow tree bark extract, which is presently known to contain salicylic acid, to treat pain. In the 1900s, aspirin became an established treatment for pain and migraine.

By the Middle Ages, the knowledge of analgesic remedies containing poppy, mandrake (*Mandragora officinarum*), and henbane (*Hyoscyamus niger*) is well recorded in prescriptions in medical literature. This was complimented by the remarkable variety of applications which included drug-soaked sponges, compresses and plasters, oils, ointments, smoke and smelling salts, drinks and waters, pills and troches, powders, electuaries, and confections.[4] One example is a combination of mandrake root and almond oil for analgesia and general anaesthesia which was commonly used by the Anatolian Seljuck dynasties.[5–7] Mandrake has the general properties of belladonna, is also a member of the Solanaceous family of plants, and was formerly used as a narcotic and sedative. It contains the alkaloids mandragorine, hyoscyamine, and scopolamine. *Mandragora officinarum* was used like opium for anaesthesia and as a pain killer.[7] The use of analgesics in ancient civilisation has been well documented in the Egyptian Ebers Papyrus and medical books written by Dioscorides, Galen, and Avicenna.

With the discovery of the New World, The Badianus Manuscript (Codex Barberini, Latin 241), an Aztec Herbal of 1552, described the native Aztec Indian remedies, and among the most of interest are the narcotics and analgesics. Pain-relieving remedies were applied externally or combined in potions to be taken internally. The Aztecs referred to various species by specific native names, tlapatl (*Datura stramonium*); toloatzin (*Datura innoxia*) and nexehuac (*Datura ceratocaula*). The juice of cocoxihuitl (*Baccconia arborea*) was applied externally as an analgesic to relieve pain locally.[8] A number of these remedies were taken to Europe and incorporated into the pharmacopoeias of the sixteenth to the early eighteenth centuries.

Box 14.1 **Timeline in the development of analgesia**

2450 BC	Egyptian Fifth Dynasty, Egyptian Ebers papyrus Cryo-Analgesia in long hours of ancient surgery Opium was obtained from poppy seeds and used to relieve pain
460–370 BC	Hippocrates used salicylic acid from the willow tree extract
AD 100	Dioscorides noted in his medical books the use of willow leaves to relieve pain
AD 130–200	Galen developed the first pain classification system of the sensory nerves
AD 400–476	Mandrake and henbane were recorded as analgesic remedies
1552	The Badianus manuscript recorded the use of *Datura* by the Aztecs as a pain remedy
1672	Rev. Edward Stone begun the research on salicylates as a analgesics and antipyretics
1806	Sertürner isolated morphine from the poppy plant
1828	Büchner isolated salicin from willow bark
ca. 1831	Samuel James confirmed the results of Stone
1897	Large-scale production of aspirin by Hoffman and Eichengrun of Bayer
1953	Acetaminophen was released to the market by Sterling-Winthrop

PAIN MECHANISM

SUMMARY OF PHARMACOLOGY

- The ascending pain pathway commences at the afferent nociceptive fibres which send information to the brain via the spinal cord where they form synapses with its dorsal horn where pain is comprehended.
- In the descending pain pathway, the endogenous central analgesia system is mediated by the periaqueductal grey matter, the nucleus raphe magnus and the nociception-inhibitory neurons within the dorsal horns of the spinal cord, which act to inhibit nociception-transmitting neurons located in the spinal dorsal horn thus modulating pain.

Galen (AD 130–200), the greatest physician of the Roman Empire, made important contributions in understanding the mechanism of pain through his discovery of the sensory nerves; his description of vision, hearing and taste; and his development of the first pain classification system.[9] In the twentieth century, several pain theories were prevalent, including Weddell and Sinclair's pattern or summation theory in 1955 and Livingston's central stimulation theory in 1943. In 1965, Melzak and Wall conceptualised the gate control theory which stated that a mechanism in the dorsal horn cells of the spinal cord controlled the course of impulses from the periphery.[10] Hitherto, pain is defined by the International Association for the Study of Pain (IASP) as 'an unpleasant sensory and emotional experience associated with actual or potential tissue damage, or described in terms of such damage'. Pain is a major symptom in many medical conditions and is a sensation that could be described from unpleasant to intolerable and could be categorised into two types: nociceptive and neuropathic.

1. Nociceptive pain is stimulation of a nociceptor (pain receptor) due to a chemical, thermal, or mechanical event that has the potential to damage body tissue.
2. Neuropathic pain is damage to the nervous system itself due to disease or trauma which could either be referred to as peripheral, which is caused by damage to nerves, or central, which is caused by damage to the brain, brainstem, or spinal cord.

Afferent nociceptive fibres send information to the brain through the spinal cord where they form synapses with its dorsal horn (Fig. 14.1). This nociceptive fibre located in the periphery is a first-order neuron. The cells in the dorsal horn are divided into physiologically distinct layers called laminae. Different types of fibre form synapses in different lamina. Aδ fibres form synapses in laminae I and V, C fibres connect with neurons in lamina II, Aβ fibres connect with lamina I, III, and V. After reaching the specific lamina within the spinal cord, the first-order nociceptive fibre proceeds to second-order neurons and cross the midline. The second-order neurons send information through the anterolateral system to the thalamus where the information is processed in the ventral posterior nucleus and sent to the cerebral cortex in the brain. This is known as the ascending pathway to the brain, instigating the conscious recognition of pain. The descending pain pathway modulates pain sensing where the brain can request the release of specific hormones or endogenous chemicals from the hypothalamus to reduce or inhibit pain sensation (Fig. 14.2). This effect of descending inhibition can be exhibited by electrically stimulating the periaqueductal grey area of the midbrain to propel other areas involved in pain regulation, such as the raphe magnus, which also receives similar afferents from reticularis paragigantocellularis. The raphe magnus sends off signals to the substantia gelatinosa region of the dorsal horn and mediates the sensation of spinothalamic inputs.

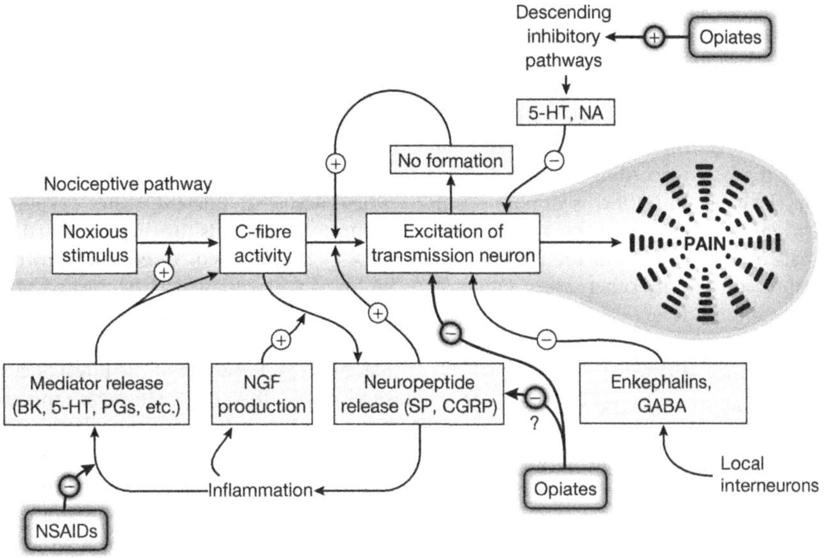

Figure 14.1 Summary of modulatory mechanisms in the nociceptive pathway. 5-HT, 5-hydroxytryptamine; BK, bradykinin; CGRP, calcitonin gene-related peptide; NA, noradrenaline; NGF, nerve growth factor; NO, nitric oxide; NSAID, non-steroidal anti-inflammatory drug; PG, prostaglandin; SP, substance P (from Rang HP, Dale MM, Ritter JM, Flower RJ, 2007. Pharmacology 6th edn., St Louis, Elsevier, with permission).

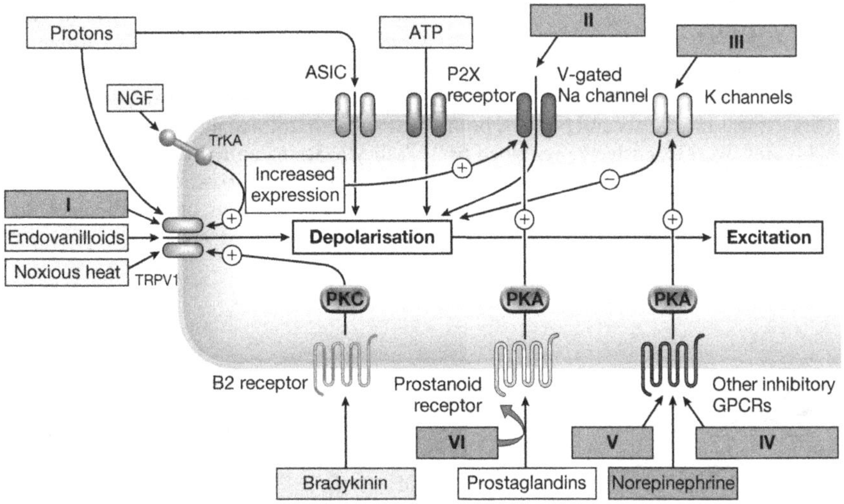

Figure 14.2 Channels, receptors and transduction mechanisms of nociceptive afferent terminals. Only the main channels and receptors are shown. Ligand-gated channels include acid-sensitive ion channels (ASICs), ATP-sensitive channels (P2X receptors) and the capsaicin-sensitive channel (TRPV1), which is also sensitive to protons and to temperature. Various facilitatory and inhibitory G-protein-coupled receptors (GPCRs) are shown, which regulate channel function through various second messenger systems. Growth factors such as nerve growth factor (NGF) act via kinase-linked receptors (TrkA) to control ion channel function and gene expression. B2 receptor, bradykinin type 2 receptor; PKA, protein kinase A; PKC, protein kinase C (from Rang HP, Dale MM, Ritter JM, Flower RJ, 2007. Pharmacology 6th edn., St Louis, Elsevier, with permission).

Analgesia alters the sense of pain without loss of consciousness. The body has an endogenous analgesia system, which can be supplemented with painkillers or analgesic drugs to regulate nociception and pain. Analgesia may occur in the central nervous system or in peripheral nerves and nociceptors. The perception of pain can also be modified by the body according to the gate control theory of pain. The gate control theory of pain postulates that nociception is 'gated' either by non-noxious stimuli or by signals that descend from the brain to the spinal cord to suppress, and in other cases enhance, incoming nociceptive information.

Pain sensation can be treated as follows:

- elimination of the cause of pain
- lowering the sensitivity of nociceptors (antipyretic analgesics, local anaesthetics)
- interrupting nociceptive induction in sensory nerves (local anaesthetics).

Based on the increasing epidemiology of various painful conditions, the worldwide analgesic market is expected to nearly double to US$75 billion by the year 2010. Unfulfilled needs for analgesics are currently being identified and strategies are outlined to develop novel analgesic drugs.

MAJOR CLASSES OF ANALGESICS

Cyclooxgenase inhibitors

Discovery of aspirin and other non-steroidal anti-inflammatory drugs

Analgesics from the family of the non-steroidal anti-inflammatory drugs (NSAIDs) have been used for more than 2000 years. Bark extracts of willows and poplars, both from the Salicaceae family, were extensively prescribed by Hippocrates to reduce pain and lower fever. The use of willow leaves was noted in the medical books written by Dioscorides in AD 100, while 100 years later willow was again described as a drug by Pliny the Elder and Galen. In the twelfth century, Hildegard von Bingen widely recommended willow bark extract for joint pains. Folk medicine during the Middle Ages employed willow together with meadowsweet for their pain-relieving effects.[11] Research on salicylates as analgesic, antipyretics as well as antiphlogistic cyclooxygenase inhibitors began when Reverend Edward Stone (1702–68) of Chipping Norton in Oxfordshire experimented with the willow bark.[12] He gathered, dried, and powdered a pound of willow bark with which he treated about fifty persons suffering with agues and intermitting disorders. On 25 April 1763 he sent a letter announcing his success to Lord Macclesfield, President of the Royal Society, and this letter survives to this day. However, this received a weak response. It was 30 years later when the physician Samuel James (*ca.* 1763–1831) of Hoddesdon confirmed the results of Stone which eventually influenced later chemists in their search for specific compounds.[12]

In the nineteenth century, natural science was at its renaissance and natural products chemistry was at its beginning. Pharmacists and chemists were isolating active compounds from their plant sources. In 1806, the German pharmacist Sertüner isolated morphine from the poppy plant.[13] In 1820, the French chemists Caventou and Pelletier isolated quinine from cinchona bark. And in 1828, the pharmacist Büchner in Munich isolated salicin from willow bark. Salicin is the alcoholic β-glucoside of hydroxymethyl phenol (Fig. 14.3). In 1838, Piria in Paris hydrolysed salicin to glucose and the free phenol.

A French chemist, Charles Frederic Gerhardt, was the first to prepare acetylsalicylic acid in 1853. In the course of his work on the synthesis and properties of various acid anhydrides, he mixed acetyl chloride with sodium salicylate (Fig. 14.4). Since no structural theory existed at that time, Gerhardt assigned the compound he synthesised as 'salicylic-acetic anhydride'. Six years later, in 1859, in Marburg, Kolbe successfully performed the structure elucidation and synthesis of salicylic acid. In the same year, von Gilm obtained analytically pure acetylsalicylic acid

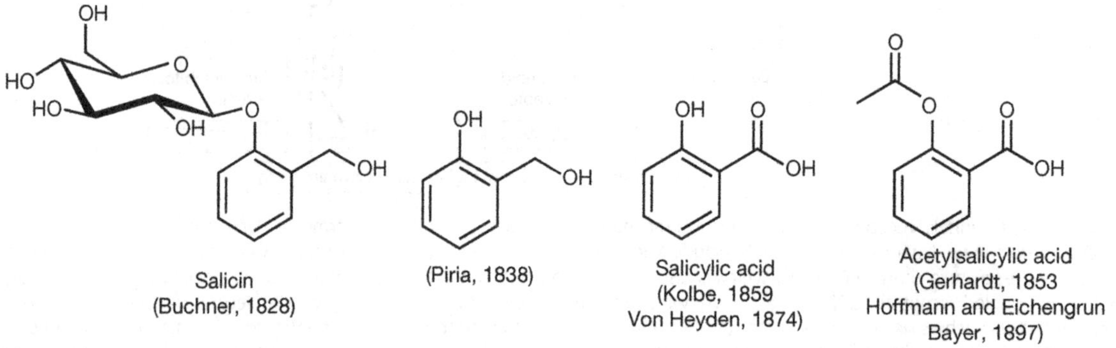

Figure 14.3 Aspirin and related compounds.

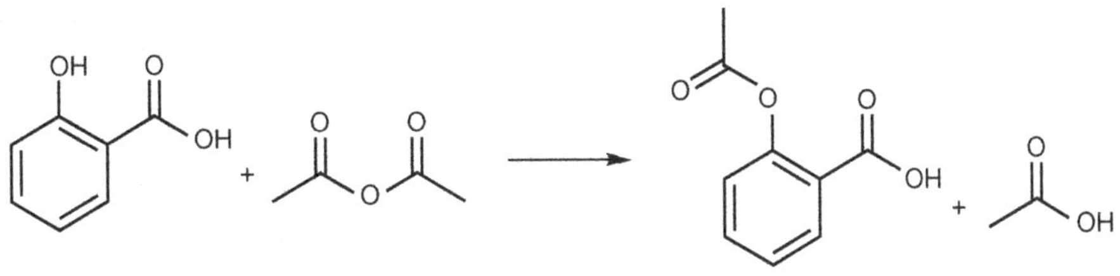

Figure 14.4 Acetylation of salicylic acid to produce aspirin. The synthesis of aspirin is classified as an esterification reaction. Salicylic acid is treated with acetic anhydride, an acid derivative, causing a chemical reaction that turns salicylic acid's phenol group into an acetyl group, (R-OH®R-OCOCH3). This process yields aspirin and acetic acid, which is considered a byproduct of this reaction. Small amounts of sulphuric acid (and occasionally phosphoric acid) are almost always used as a catalyst.

(which he called 'acetylierte Salicylsäure', acetylated salicylic acid) by a reaction of salicylic acid and acetyl chloride. In 1869, Schröder, Prinzhorn and Kraut repeated both Gerhardt's (from sodium salicylate) and von Gilm's (from salicylic acid) syntheses, concluding that both reactions synthesised identical compounds - acetylsalicylic acid (Fig. 14.4). They were the first to assign to it the correct structure with the acetyl group connected to the phenolic oxygen.

Von Heyden, Kolbe's student as well as apprentice, developed the large-scale synthesis and later started pharmaceutical production of salicylic acid in Dresden, Chemiewerke von Heyden, in 1874. In 1876, Traube and Stricker in Berlin and McLagan in Dundee were already investigating the antiphlogistic effect of salicylic acid on patients suffering with rheumatism. In 1897, the chemists Felix Hoffmann and Arthur Eichengrun, of the drug and dye firm Bayer, were doing large-scale derivatisation of salicylic acid by reacting sodium salicylate with acetyl chloride to form the less corrosive compound, and a less irritating drug, acetylsalicylic acid (ASA). ASA became a registered trademark under the name Aspirin™ from 23 November 1899. The name Aspirin is derived from A = Acetyl and 'Spirsäure' = an old (German) name for salicylic acid.[12]

The release of ASA into the market played an important role in the discovery of new anti-inflammatory drugs. At the University of Erlangen, the chemist Knorr successfully synthesised phenazones, and their antipyretic and analgesic activities were proven by the pharmacologist Filehne. The phenazone, Antipyrine™ (Fig. 14.5) was patented in 1884 and was produced by a small chemical firm (Farbwerke, vorm. Meister, Lucius und Bruning) near Frankfurt. Later Höchst bought the increasing production of Antipyrine™, which later made the company a world renowned pharmaceutical firm.

In 1886, acetanilide was prescribed as an antipyretic but was then substituted with phenacetin and paracetamol (Fig. 14.5), which were less toxic and easier to synthesise from the waste products of aniline dye production. Bayer was marketing phenacetin as the third antipyretic analgesic available during that time. The English company, Sterling-Winthrop, substituted phenacetin with its metabolite paracetamol, also known as acetaminophen, and registered it under the trademark Panadol™. Within one century, Central Europe was able to produce three prototypes of antipyretic, antiphlogistic analgesics: aspirin, antipyrine, and phenacetin. It was the beginning of the growth of the pharmaceutical industry.

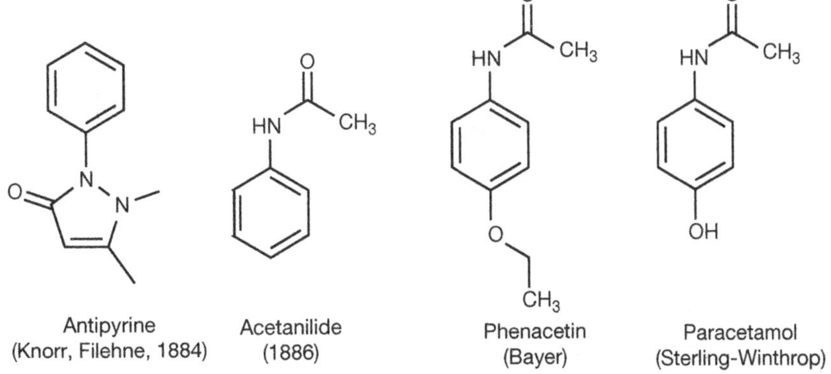

Figure 14.5 The first NSAIDs.

Aspirin's popularity grew over the first half of the twentieth century, spurred on by its effectiveness in the wake of the Spanish flu pandemic of 1918, and aspirin's profitability led to fierce competition and the proliferation of aspirin brands and products, especially after the American patent held by Bayer expired in 1917.

For decades, the pharmaceutical companies were restricted to the idea of either synthetically modifying or introducing new adjuvants to these three drug prototypes available from the nineteenth century:

- Other companies combined ASA with antipyrine or phenacetin.
- Höchst combined antipyrine with caffeine and came up with a series of new phenazone derivatives (Fig. 14.6) to improve potency, absorption and elimination. Filehne suggested that increasing the number of nitrogen units in the structure would increase efficacy.
- On the other hand, Roche synthesised a propylphenazone derivative which to date is still being employed as an analgesic.
- Bayer also tried to acetylate other analgesics in order to increase their potency, including the acetylation of morphine thereby synthesising heroin.

Aspirin's popularity in the market dropped after release of paracetamol (acetaminophen) in 1953 and ibuprofen in 1969. In the 1960s and 1970s, John Vane and others discovered the basic mechanism of aspirin's effects, while clinical trials and other studies from the 1960s to the 1980s established the efficacy of aspirin as an anti-clotting agent that reduces the risk of thrombosis. Aspirin sales revived considerably in the last decades of the twentieth century, due to widespread use as a preventive treatment for heart attacks and strokes.

The mechanism of action of non-steroidal anti-inflammatory analgesics

The first plausible theory on the mechanism of action of salicylate on inflammation and pain was published in 1967. In addition to its analgesic and antipyretic activities, aspirin exerts an anti-inflammatory effect. This can be attributed to inhibition of cyclooxygenase (COX), which hampers the conversion of arachidonic acid to prostaglandin. Arachidonic acid is an eicosatetraenoic acid, a C_{20} fatty acid containing four double bonds, which is a component of the cell membrane phospholipids and is released by phospholipase A2. Synthesis of prostaglandins proceeds through intermediary cyclic endoperoxides by forming a cyclopentane ring in the acyl chain (Fig. 14.7). Prostaglandins are primarily inactivated by the enzyme 15-hydroxyprostaglandin-dehydrogenase.

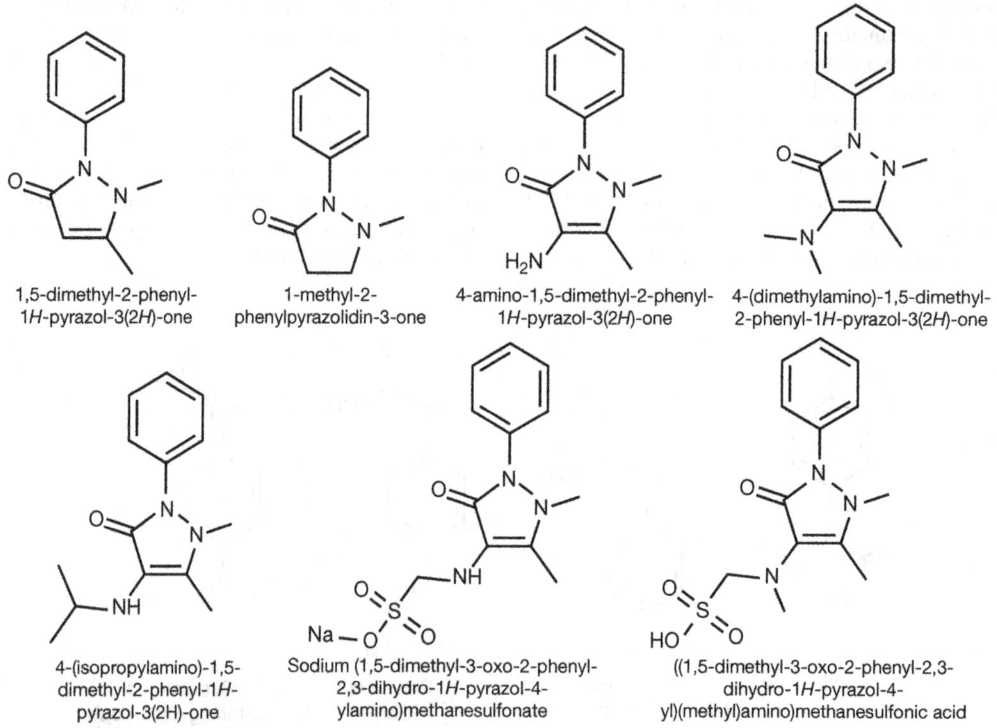

Figure 14.6 Phenazone analgesics.

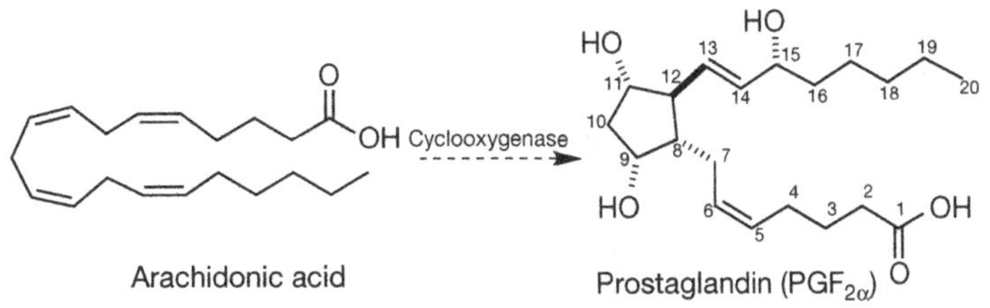

Figure 14.7 Cyclooxygenase action. *Prostaglandin nomenclature*: Prostaglandins are abbreviated PG followed by a letter indicating the type of functionality present at positions 8–12 and 15; the number subscript refers to the number of double bonds; and the Greek letter designates the orientation of the extra hydroxyl group on the ring. Numbering always starts at the carboxylic acid (1 position) and continues around the molecule for the entire 20-carbon atoms.

Prostaglandins are local mediators attaining their biologically effective concentration only at their site of formation. The individual prostaglandins possess different biological effects that include the following:

- *Nociceptors*: Prostaglandins increase the sensitivity of the sensory nerve fibres where the rate of evoked potentials is dependent on the given stimulus strength.
- *Thermoregulation*: Prostaglandins augment the set point of the preoptic thermoregulatory neurons, thereby increasing the body temperature which results in fever.
- *Vascular smooth muscle*: Prostaglandins (PGE_2 and PGI_2) produce arteriolar vasodilation and ($PGF_{2\alpha}$) venoconstriction.
- *Gastric secretion*: Prostaglandins promote the production of gastric mucus and reduce the formation of gastric acid.
- *Endometrium and uterine muscle*: Prostaglandins ($PGF_{2\alpha}$) are responsible for the ischaemic necrosis of the endometrium and the relative proportions of individual PGs are said to be altered in dysmenorrhoea and excessive menstrual bleeding. Prostaglandins stimulate labour contractions.
- *Bronchial muscle*: PGE_2 and PGI_2 induce bronchodilation and $PGF_{2\alpha}$ induces constriction.
- *Kidney function*: Vasodilating prostaglandins are released when the renal blood flow is lowered.

COX exists in two forms: COX-1 and COX-2. COX-1 is present in most tissues and through PG synthesis promotes the functions listed above. COX-2 is expressed in inflammatory cells and mainly produces PG mediators of inflammation. Many of the side effects of NSAIDs are due to non-selective inhibition of COX-1 as well as the desired target, COX-2.

Pharmacokinetics of non-steroidal anti-inflammatory analgesics

Acetylsalicylic acid (ASA)

Acetylsalicylic acid (ASA) can be administered in tablet form, as effervescent powder, or injected systemically as its lysinate. Following a single dose of 0.5–1 g, ASA undergoes ester hydrolysis in the gut and subsequently in the blood. Salicylic acid is a weak acid and very little of it is ionised in the stomach after oral administration. ASA is poorly soluble in the acidic conditions and therefore poorly absorbed in the stomach. ASA irritates the gastric mucosa due to a direct acid effect and also inhibits the synthesis of cytoprotective prostaglandins (i.e. PGE_2) which can lead to bronchoconstriction ('aspirin asthma').

In the small intestine, more of the salicylate is dissolved at elevated pH and is rapidly absorbed due to the increased surface area in that region of the gut. The effects of ASA outlast its presence in plasma where $t_{1/2}$ is approximately 20 min since cyclooxygenases are irreversibly inhibited due to covalent binding of the acetyl residue to serine-530 in the enzyme. Then the duration of the effect depends on the rate of re-synthesis of the enzyme (Fig. 14.8). Aspirin is more selective for COX-1 in its inhibitory action. Furthermore, the concentration of free salicylate in the plasma may contribute to the affect. About 50–80% of salicylate in the blood is protein bound. Saturation of binding sites leads to more free salicylate and increased toxicity. The volume of distribution is 0.1–0.2 L/kg. ASA inhibits platelet aggregation and thus prolongs bleeding time; thus it should not be used in patients with impaired blood coagulation.

As much as 80% of the therapeutic dose of salicylic acid is metabolised in the liver. Salicylate conjugates with glycine to produce salicyluric acid, while with glucuronic acid, salicyl acyl and phenolic glucuronide are generated. Small amounts of salicylic acid are also hydroxylated to gentisic acid. With large salicylate doses, the kinetics switch from first order to zero order, as metabolic pathways become saturated and renal excretion becomes increasingly important.[14] Salicylate is excreted by the kidneys as:

- salicyluric acid (75%)
- free salicylic acid (10%)
- salicylic phenol (10%)
- acyl (5%) glucuronides
- gentisic acid (< 1%).

At small doses (less than 250 mg in an adult), all pathways proceed by first-order kinetics, with an elimination

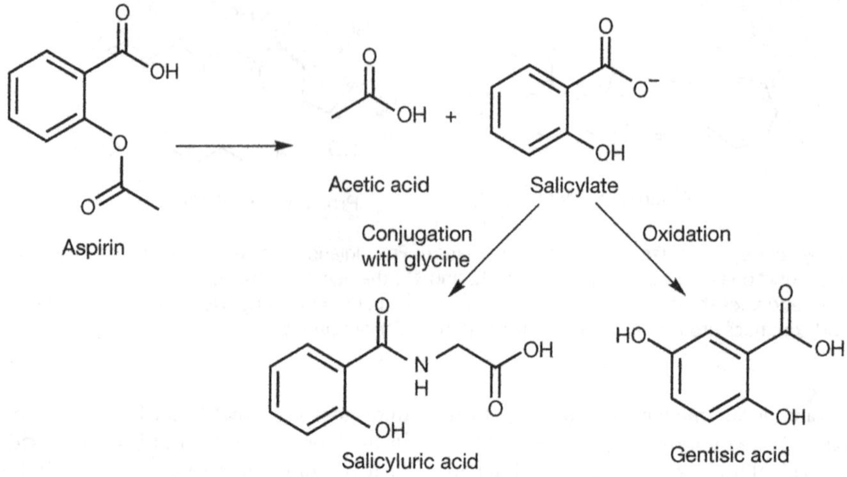

Figure 14.8 ASA metabolism.

half-life of about 2–4.5 hours, while at higher doses of salicylate (more than 4 g) the half-life is at about 15–30 hours as the biotransformation pathways to salicyluric acid and salicyl phenolic glucuronide become saturated.[15] Renal excretion of salicylic acid becomes increasingly important as the metabolic pathways become saturated resulting in a 10- to 20-fold increase in renal clearance.

Metamizole (antipyrine)

Dipyrone, also known as metamizole sodium, Analgin, Novalgin or Melubrin, displays the highest efficacy among antipyretic analgesics and is effective in visceral pain associated with smooth muscle spasm. It is rapidly absorbed when administered orally or via the rectal route. It is water soluble and is also available for intravenous administration. Dipyrone is a prodrug which, after oral administration, is rapidly hydrolysed in the gastric environment to its major metabolite 4-methyl-amino-antipyrine (MAA) and absorbed in this form (Fig. 14.9). MAA is then converted to 4-formyl-amino-antipyrine and 4-amino-antipyrine, which is further acetylated to 4-acetyl-amino-antipyrine by the polymorphic enzyme N-acetyl-transferase.[16] The drug metabolites are eliminated from the plasma with a $t_{1/2}$ of 4–6 h. Despite being an old drug, it has recently been shown that the main metabolite, MAA, exhibited suppression of COX-2 at the peripheral site.[17] Dipyrone has been associated with a low incidence of fatal agranulocytosis, which has led to it being banned in many countries although it is still available in some. In sensitised patients, cardiovascular collapse can occur, especially after intravenous injection.

Acetaminophen (paracetamol)

Paracetamol is chemically classified under the 'aniline analgesics' along with acetanilide and phenacetin. Acetaminophen is a widely used analgesic and antipyretic

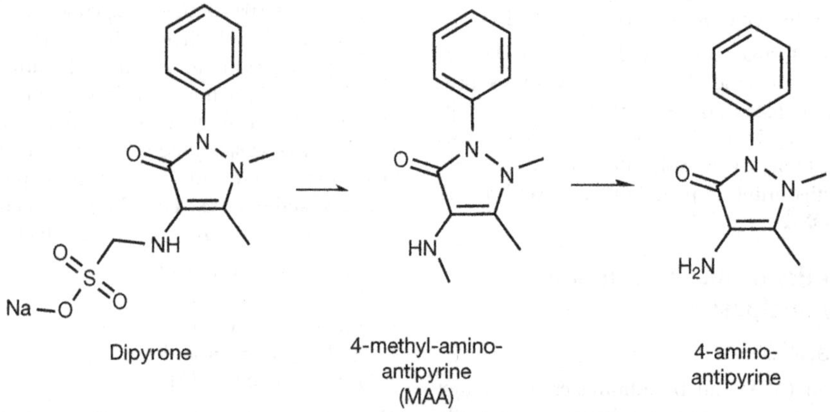

Figure 14.9 Metabolic activation of metamizole.

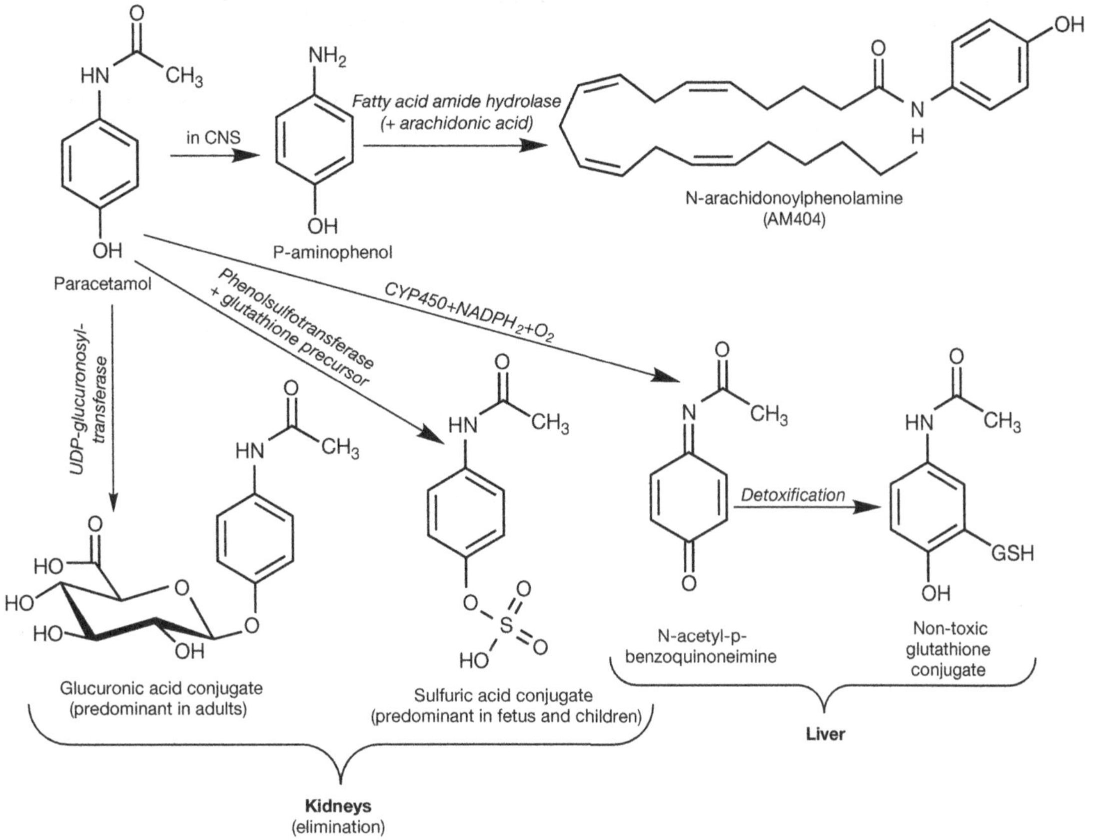

Figure 14.10 The molecular basis of paracetamol action and its metabolism.

which is not associated with gastric side effects. It can be administered orally or rectal in the form of suppositories at a single dose of 0.5–1.0 g. It is efficacious against toothaches and headaches. However, unlike the antipyrines, paracetamol is not effective for visceral pain. Unlike the other NSAIDs, it possesses no anti-inflammatory activity. On the other hand, it has been shown that the antipyretic effect is due to the inhibition of COX in the brain.[18] It has been confirmed that, provided the ambient concentration of peroxides is kept low, paracetamol can inhibit COX. This consequently explains why paracetamol is not active at the site of inflammation where the peroxide level is high while the peroxide concentration in the brain is low. The in vivo effect of paracetamol is comparable to those of the selective COX-2 inhibitors. In 2006, the groups of Bertolini and Zygmunt demonstrated that the analgesic effect of paracetamol is due to the indirect activation of cannabinoid CB_1 receptors[19] in human. Like dipyrone, acetaminophen is a prodrug. The active metabolite N-arachidonoylphenolamine (AM404) is formed in the brain by conjugation of the primary amine (p-aminophenol) of paracetamol with arachidonic acid in the presence of a fatty acid amide hydrolase (FAAH).[20] AM404 is an already known compound, previously described as an endogenous cannabinoid (Fig. 14.10). It is a TRPV1 (transient receptor potential vanilloid) ion channel receptor agonist which indirectly activates the CB_1 receptors by further increasing the levels of endogenous cannabinoids; moreover, it inhibits cyclooxygenases in the brain at concentrations not attainable with analgesic doses of paracetamol.

Prior to renal elimination, the drug undergoes conjugation at its phenolic hydroxyl moiety with glucuronic or sulphuric acid. A small fraction is oxidised to N-acetyl-p-benzoquinone which is detoxified by coupling with gluthathione. At high doses (*ca.* 10 g), the hepatic glutathione reserve is depleted and the quinone-imine metabolite reacts with the liver cells, resulting in necrosis. As an antidote, N-acetylcysteine is given intravenously within 6–8 h. Table 14.1 shows the large number of formulations which contain paracetamol or aspirin or both.

Table 14.1 Brand names of paracetamol/aspirin in combination with other ingredients

Brand name	Other ingredients present
Anadin Extra	paracetamol 200 mg, aspirin 300 mg, caffeine 45 mg
Alka-Seltzer XS	aspirin 267 mg, paracetamol 133 mg, caffeine 40 mg, sodium bicarbonate 1606 mg, citric acid 954 mg
Dispirin	aspirin 300 mg, paracetamol 200 mg
Boots Cold & Flu Relief Tablets	paracetamol 400 mg, ascorbic acid 50 mg, caffeine 30 mg, phenylephrine HCl 5 mg
Day Nurse	paracetamol 500 mg, pseudoephedrine HCl 30 mg, pholcodine 5 mg
Feminax	paracetamol 500 mg, codeine phosphate 8 mg
Hedex Extra	paracetamol 500 mg, caffeine 65 mg
Lemsip Max	paracetamol 1000 mg, phenylephrine HCl 12.2 mg, guaifenesin 200 mg
Migraleve	paracetamol 500 mg, codeine phosphate 8 mg, buclizine HCl 6.25 mg
Night Nurse	paracetamol 500 mg, promethazine HCl 10 mg, dextromethorphan HBr 7.5 mg
Paracodol	paracetamol 500 mg, codeine phosphate 8 mg
Paramol	paracetamol 500 mg, dihydrocodeine tartrate 7.46 mg
Propain Plus	paracetamol 50 mg, doxylamine succinate 5 mg, caffeine 30 mg, codeine phosphate 10 mg
Resolve	paracetamol 1000 g, sodium bicarbonate 1408 mg, caffeine 60 mg
Sinutab	paracetamol 500 mg, pseudoephedrine HCl 30 mg
Solpadeine	paracetamol 500 mg, codeine phosphate hemihydrate 8 mg, caffeine 30 mg
Veganin	paracetamol 500 mg, codeine phosphate 8 mg, caffeine 30 mg
Vicks Medinite	paracetamol 600 mg dextromethorphan HBr 15 mg, pseudoephedrine hydrochloride 60 mg, doxylamine succaine 7.5 mg

More recently developed non-steroidal anti-inflammatory analgesics

Since platelets have no DNA, they are unable to synthesise new COX once aspirin has irreversibly inhibited the enzyme. Other NSAIDs cyclooxygenase inhibitors such as ibuprofen, diclofenac, and indomethacin act similarly to aspirin in that they bind to COX but they do not covalently modify the enzyme and thus do not irreversibly inhibit the platelet function (Fig. 14.11). NSAID analgesics can be chemically classified as shown in Table 14.2. Ibuprofen was the first of these compounds to be marketed and it was followed by a number of other compounds such as naproxen and ketoprofen, which are more potent than ibuprofen.

Chronic use of NSAIDs, as in rheumatoid arthritis, is likely to cause adverse effects which include: gastric and duodenum ulceration, impaired renal function with sodium and water retention, bone marrow depression, allergic skin rash and bronchial asthma, and the search has continued for more selective agents.

Newer NSAIDs, called COX-2 selective inhibitors, have been developed that inhibit only COX-2, with the intent to reduce the incidence of gastrointestinal side effects in comparison with non-selective drugs. However, several of the new COX-2 selective inhibitors have been withdrawn recently after evidence emerged that COX-2 inhibitors increase the risk of heart attack. It is proposed that endothelial cells lining the microvasculature in the body express COX-2, and, by selectively inhibiting COX-2, prostaglandins, specifically PGI_2 prostacyclins, are down-regulated with respect to thromboxane levels, as COX-1 in platelets is unaffected. Thus, the protective anticoagulative effect of PGI_2 is decreased, increasing the risk of

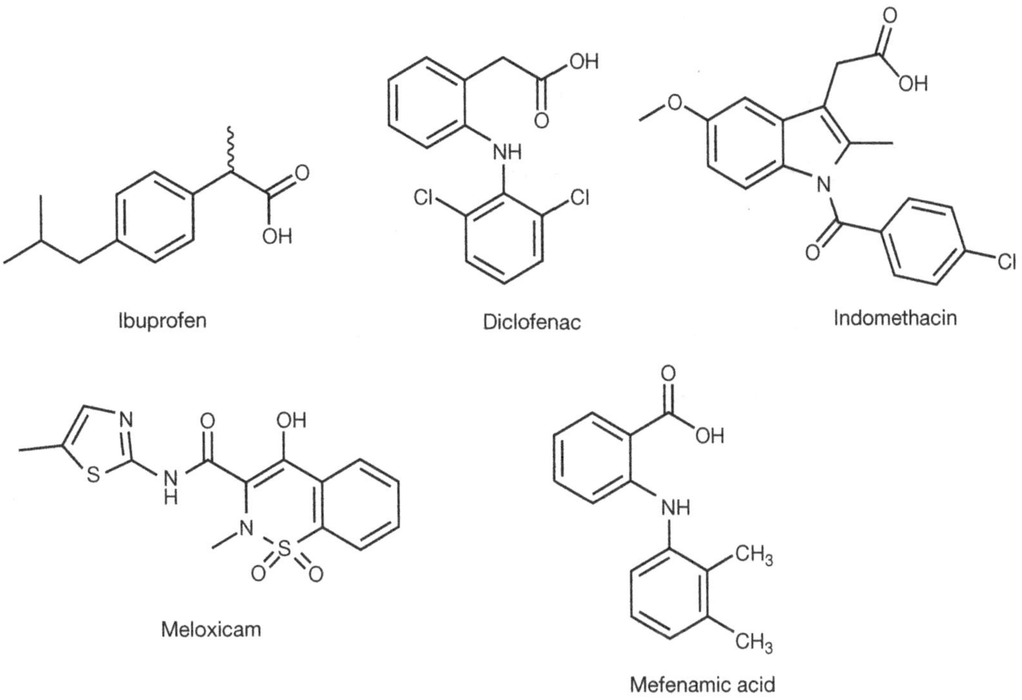

Figure 14.11 Some NSAIDs.

Table 14.2 Chemical classes of NSAID

Phenylpropionic acid class	Fenoprofen · flurbiprofen · ibuprofen · ketoprofen · naproxen · oxaprozin
Oxicam class	Meloxicam · piroxicam
Acetic acid class	Diclofenac · indometacin · ketorolac · nabumetone · sulindac · tolmetin
Anthranilic acid (fenamate) class	Meclofenamate · mefenamic acid

Table 14.3 The current status (2009) of COX-2 inhibitors

COX-2 inhibitors	
Celecoxib	Under FDA alert
Etoricoxib	Withdrawn by FDA
Lumiracoxib	Registration cancelled
Parecoxib	Withdrawn by FDA
Rofecoxib	Withdrawn from market
Valdecoxib	Withdrawn from market

thrombus and associated heart attacks and other circulatory problems. Due to these foreseen risks, COX-2 inhibitors are being withdrawn from the market. The current status of these agents is shown in Table 14.3.

Opioids and opiates

Opioids are analgesics that work by binding to the opioid receptors found on neurons in various areas of the brain and spinal cord as well as intramural plexuses that regulate the motility of the gastrointestinal and urogenital tracts. Opiates are by definition limited to natural opium alkaloids and their semi-synthetic derivatives. Morphine, a benzylisoquinoline alkaloid, is a stronger analgesic than any of the antipyretic analgesics mentioned previously in this chapter. Other than morphine, the opium poppy also yields other related alkaloids generally called opiates (Fig. 14.12) and these include codeine which is used primarily as an antitussive, thebaine which is more a stimulant rather than a depressant, papaverine which is an antispasmolytic and noscapine which is a cough suppressant rather than an analgesic. Thebaine is not used therapeutically due to its toxicity which causes strychnine-like

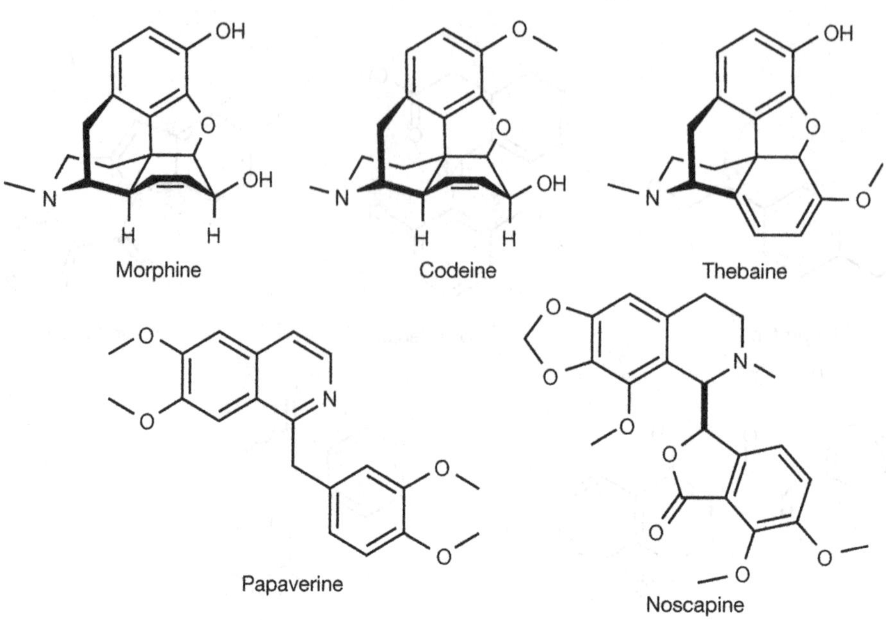

Figure 14.12 Morphine and some of its congeners.

convulsions at higher doses. However, thebaine is utilised as a raw material to industrially produce oxycodone, oxymorphone, nalbuphine, naloxone, naltrexone, buprenorphine and etorphine. Of more than 120 poppy species, only two produce morphine, while there are many species that yield abundant amounts of thebaine. Closely related to morphine are morphine-N-oxide (genomorphine) and pseudomorphine, an alkaloid which exists in opium as a degradation product of morphine.

Although morphine is a precursor for illicit drugs such as heroin (diacetylmorphine, Fig. 14.13) and hydromorphone, along with other opiates, it has been used to semi-synthesise new derivatives to optimise the drug's efficacy as well as reduce and reverse its side effects. The modification of morphine has also augmented the development of non-narcotic drugs with other therapeutic uses such as emetics, stimulants, antitussives, anticholinergics, muscle relaxants, local anaesthetics, general

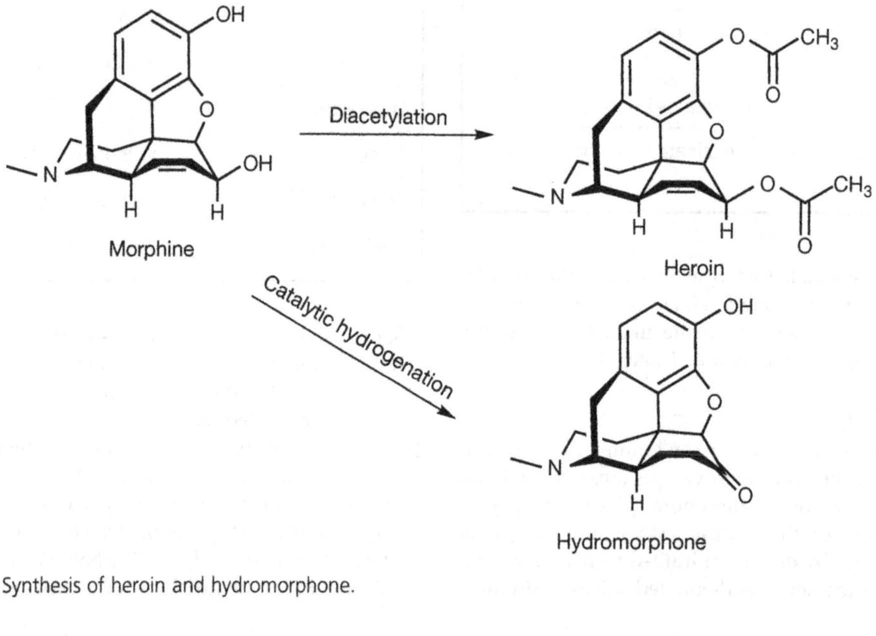

Figure 14.13 Synthesis of heroin and hydromorphone.

anaesthetics and others. One of the most common examples is that morphine is used to produce the antitussive drugs codeine and pholcodine. Morphine-derived agonist-antagonist drugs have also been developed. Powerful opioid antagonists include naloxone (Narcan™), naltrexone (Trexan™), and nalorphine (Nalline™) for human use and also the strongest antagonists known, such as diprenorphine (M5050), the reversing agent in the Immobilon™ large animal tranquilliser dart kit which contains etorphine (M99) as an agonist.

To date, there are more than 200 morphine derivatives that have been developed since the last quarter of the nineteenth century. These drugs range from codeine which has 25% the strength of morphine to drugs which have several hundred times the potency of morphine. Most semi-synthetic opioids, both of the morphine and codeine subgroups, are created by modifying one or more of the following (numbers of the positions are given in Figure 14.14):

- Functional group at positions 1 and/or 2 on the morphine carbon skeleton can be substituted.
- The 3 position is methylated in morphine producing codeine, producing a prodrug which yields morphine by demethylation. Methylation is used to produce prodrugs of other morphine analogues as in: hydrocodone and hydromorphone, oxycodone and oxymorphone, nicocodeine and nicomorphine, dihydrocodeine and dihydromorphine (Fig. 14.14).
- The bond between positions 7 and 8 can be saturated and functional groups can be added to these positions. For example, oxidation of the hydroxyl group to a carbonyl and saturation of the 7–8 double bond along with oxidation of the 3-hydroxyl group changes codeine into hydromorphone, and attaching a functional group at position 14 yields oxymorphone.
- Catalytic reduction, hydrogenation, or oxidation of positions 2, 4, 5 or 17 on the morphine skeleton produces stronger derivatives (agonists) of morphine and codeine.
- The substitution of an allyl moiety for the methyl group on the nitrogen atom of morphine produced the opioid receptor antagonists, nalorphine and naloxone (Fig. 14.15).

In order to reduce the narcotic qualities of opiates which elicit habituation, physical dependence, or addiction, new opioid analogues have been developed with the objective of diminishing or reversing these side effects and on the other hand improving potency or optimising other therapeutic activity. Such compounds are fully synthetic drugs that are structurally different from morphine and include anilidopiperidines, phenylpiperidines, diphenylpropylamines, benzomorphans, and morphinans (Fig. 14.16).

Opioid receptors and mode of action of opioids

There are several subtypes of opioid receptors, designated as μ, δ, and κ, that mediate the various opioid effects. All opioid receptors are G-protein coupled to inhibition of adenylate cyclase. They facilitate the opening of the potassium ion channels causing hyperpolarisation while they inhibit opening of the calcium ion channels, thus inhibiting neurotransmitter release. Opioid receptors have many other and more important roles in the brain and periphery, however, modulating pain, cardiac, gastric and vascular functions as well as possibly panic and satiation, and receptors are often found at postsynaptic locations as well as presynaptically. Opioids can differ in their affinities and, correspondingly, in the pattern of their therapeutic actions.

- *μ-Receptors* are responsible for the majority of the analgesic effects of opioids and their side effects. Such opioids are classed as μ-receptor agonists. μ-Receptors are the main receptor through which morphine acts. Classically, μ-receptors are presynaptic, and inhibit neurotransmitter release. They thereby inhibit the release of the inhibitory neurotransmitter GABA, and thus trigger the dopaminergic pathways, causing more dopamine to be released. By hijacking this process, exogenous opioids cause inappropriate dopamine release, and lead to aberrant synaptic plasticity, which causes addiction.
- *δ-Receptors* significantly contribute to analgesia in the periphery.
- *κ-Receptors* have two subtypes identified as κ1- and κ2-receptors. They contribute to analgesia at the spinal level, eliciting sedation and dysphoria as side effects, but they induce relatively few unwanted effects and do not spawn dependence. Some analgesics are κ-receptor selective. Nalorphine, which counters the effect of morphine, also produces limited analgesia by mediating through κ-receptors.

Neurons react to opioids through hyperpolarisation due to increase in K^+ conductance as mediated either by the μ- or δ-receptors. κ-Mediated decrease in Ca^{2+} influx into the nerve terminals during excitation leads to a decrease in the release of excitatory transmitters and a decrease of synaptic activity. Depending on the population of the affected cells, synaptic inhibition may translate into either a depressant or excitant effect.

The analgesic effect occurs at the spinal cord level and results in an attenuation of the impulses spread to the brain which produce pain perception. However, the ability to concentrate is impaired while tranquillisation and hypnotic effects become prominent.

Endogenous opioids

The high analgesic efficacy of opioids is due to their affinity for receptors normally acted upon by ligands known as

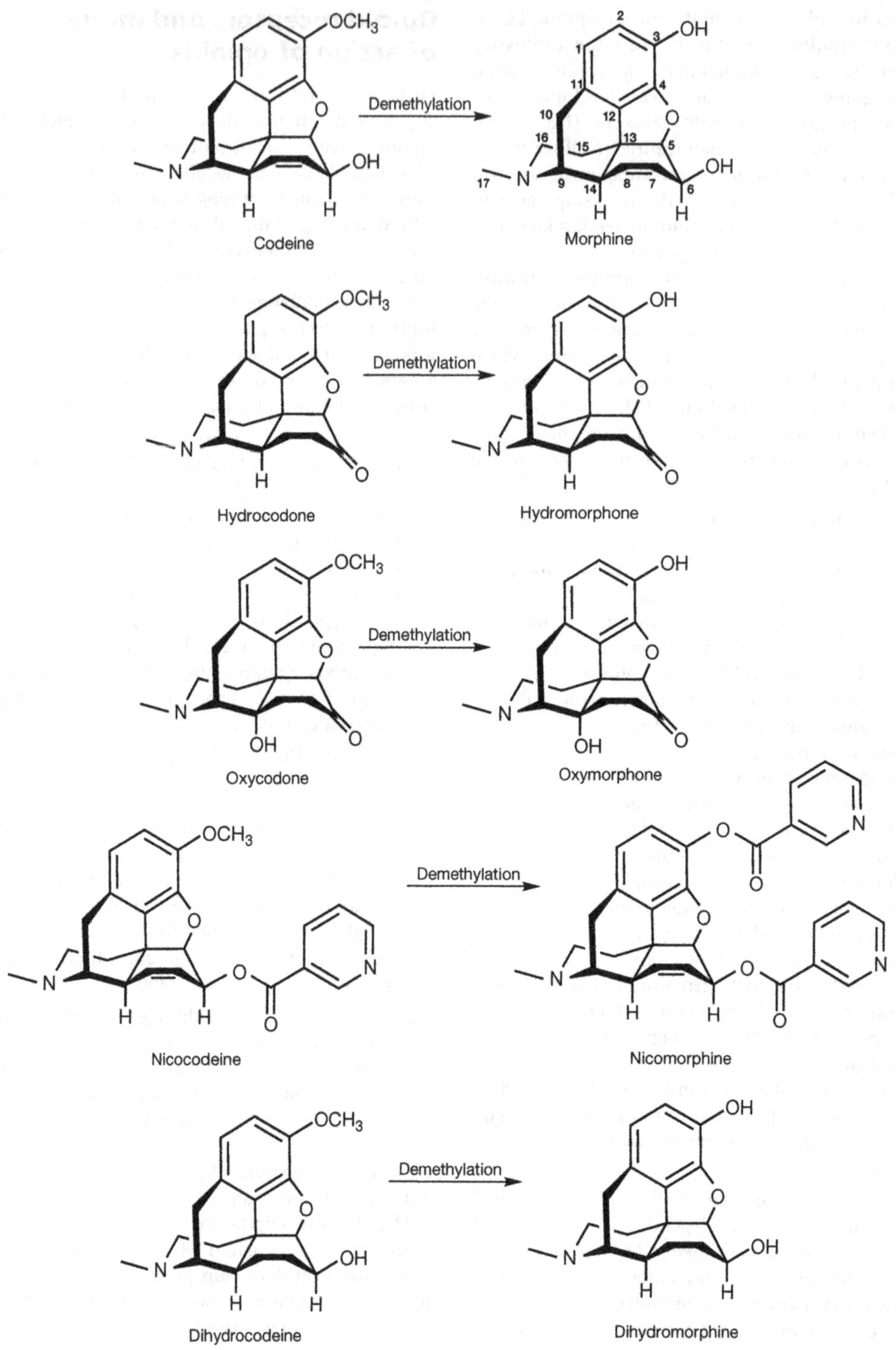

Figure 14.14 3-methyl pro-drugs of morphine derivatives.

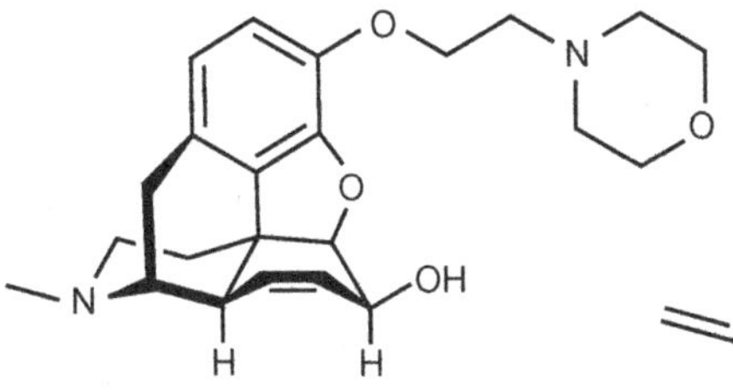

Pholcodine

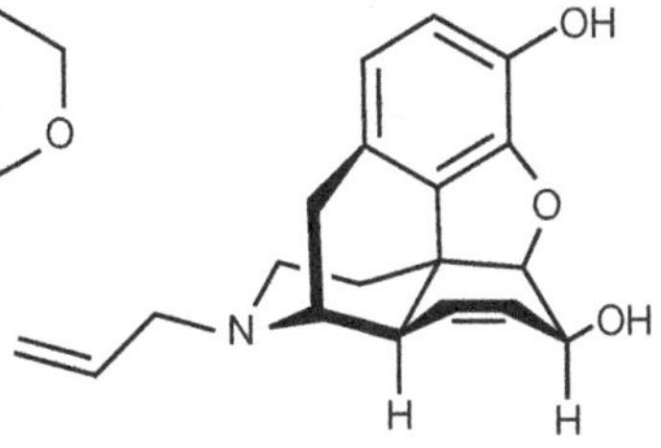

Nalorphine

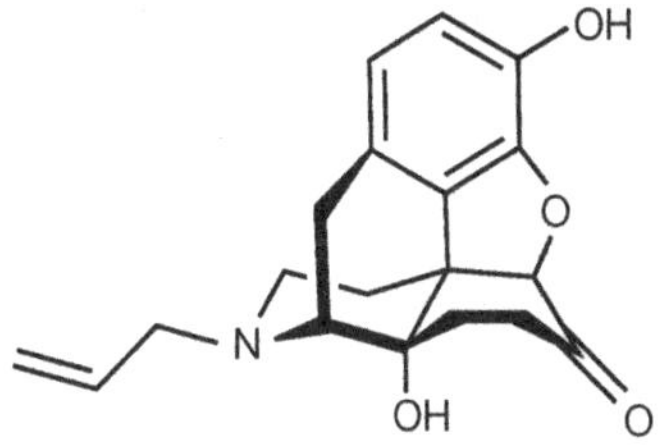

Naloxone

Figure 14.15 Opiod receptor antagonists.

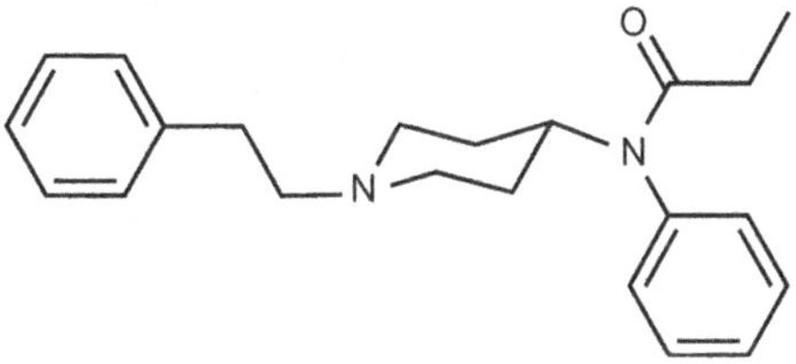

Fentanyl

Also:
Alphamethylfentanyl
Alfentanil
Sufentanil
Remifentanil
Carfentanyl
Ohmefentanyl

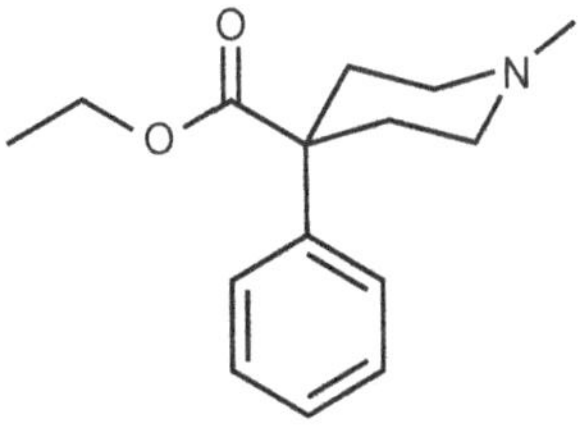

Pethidine

Also:
Ketobemidone
MPPP
Allylprodine
Prodine
PEPAP

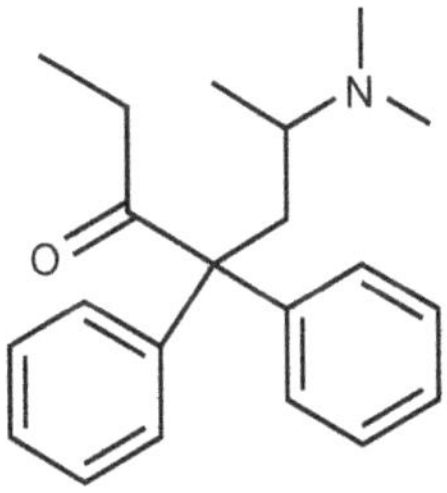

Methadone

Also:
Propoxyphene
Dextropropoxyphene
Dextromoramide
Bezitramide
Piritramide
Dipipanone
Levomethadyl acetate
Loperamide diphenoxylate

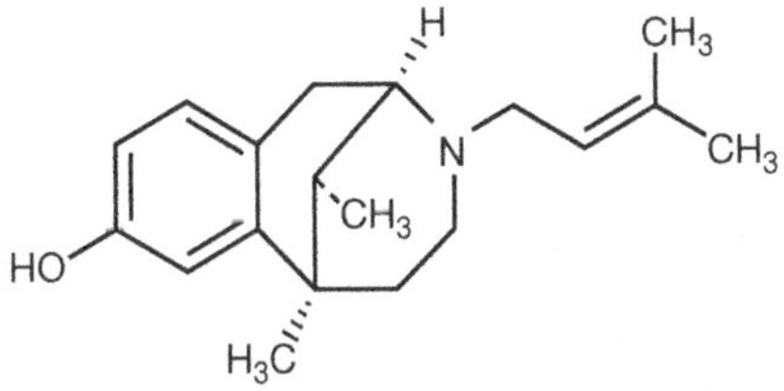

Pentazocine

Also:
Dezocine
Phenazocine

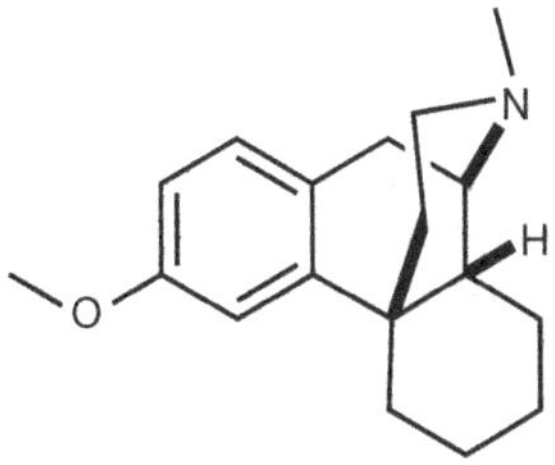

Levomethorphan

Also:
Butorphanol
Nalbuphine
Levorphanol

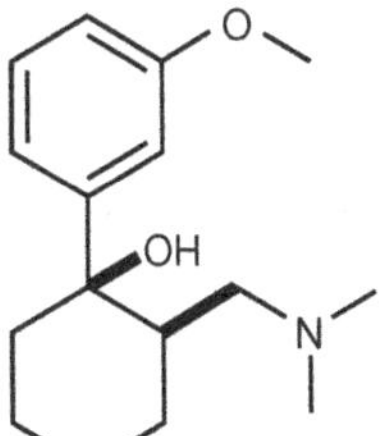

Tramadol

Also:
Lefetamine
Meptazinol
Tilidine
Tapentadol

Figure 14.16 Wholly synthetic opioid agonists and other drugs in their classes.

endogenous opioids. These physiological ligands are opiopeptides that mimic opioid activity and activate the opioid receptors. The four classes of opiopeptides produced by the body are:

- *Enkephalins* have two isoforms: Met-enkephalin (Tyr-Gly-Gly-Phe-Met) and Leu-enkephalin (Tyr-Gly-Gly-Phe-Leu). The met-enkephalin peptide is coded by the pro-enkephalin gene and endorphin gene (also known as the POMC gene) while the leu-enkephalin peptide is coded by the pro-enkephalin gene and dynorphin gene. Met-enkephalin is widely distributed in the CNS and acts on μ- and δ-opioid receptors. Leu-enkephalin acts only on the δ-opioid receptors.
- *Endorphins*, also known as β-endorphin, are released into the blood (from the pituitary gland) and into the spinal cord and the brain through the hypothalamic neurons. β-endorphin is a cleavage product of pro-opiomelanocortin which is also the precursor hormone for adrenocorticotrophic hormone (ACTH). In situations where the level of ACTH is increased, the level of endorphins also increases slightly. β-endorphin has the highest affinity for the μ1-opioid receptor, slightly lower affinity for the μ2- and δ-opioid receptors and low affinity for the κ1-opioid receptors. β-Endorphins are more hormone-like in nature.
- *Dynorphins* arise from the precursor protein prodynorphin. When prodynorphin is cleaved, dynorphin A, dynorphin B, and α/β-neo-endorphin are released. Depolarisation of a neuron containing prodynorphin stimulates proprotein convertase 2, which occurs within synaptic vesicles in the presynaptic terminal. Occasionally, prodynorphin is not fully processed, leading to the release of 'big dynorphin'. Structurally, this 32-amino acid molecule consists of both dynorphin A and dynorphin B. Dynorphin A and dynorphin B contain a high proportion of basic amino acid residues, particularly lysine and arginine. Although dynorphins are found widely distributed in the CNS, they have their highest concentrations in the hypothalamus, medulla, pons, midbrain, and spinal cord. Dynorphins are stored in large (80–120 nm diameter) dense-core vesicles that are considerably bigger than vesicles storing neurotransmitters. These dense-core vesicles differ from small synaptic vesicles in that a more intense and prolonged stimulus is needed to cause the large vesicles to release their contents into the synaptic gap. Dynorphins mainly wield their effects through the κ-opioid receptor. Although κ-opioid receptor is the primary receptor for all dynorphins, the peptides also have some affinity for the μ-opioid receptor, δ-opioid receptor, N-methyl-D-aspartic-type glutamate receptor,[21] and bradykinin B2 receptor.[22] Different dynorphins show different receptor selectivities and potencies at receptors. Big dynorphin and dynorphin A have the same selectivity for human κ-opioid receptor, but dynorphin A is more selective for κ-opioid receptor over μ-opioid and δ-opioid receptor than is big dynorphin. Big dynorphin is more potent at κ-opioid receptors than is dynorphin A. Both big dynorphin and dynorphin A are more potent and more selective than dynorphin B.[23]
- *Endomorphins* include two endogenous opioid peptides. Endomorphin-1 (Tyr-Pro-Trp-Phe-NH_2) and endomorphin-2 (Tyr-Pro-Phe-Phe-NH_2) are tetrapeptides with the highest known affinity and specificity for the μ-opioid receptor. Endomorphin-1 is located in the nucleus of the solitary tract, the periventricular hypothalamus, and the dorsomedial hypothalamus, where it is found within histaminergic neurons and may regulate sedative and arousal behaviours. It is assumed that endomorphins are the cleavage products of a larger precursor, but this polypeptide or protein has not yet been identified.

Pharmacokinetics of opioids

Both morphine free base and its hydrated form are sparingly soluble in water, where only 1 gram of the hydrate will dissolve in 5 litres of water. For this reason, pharmaceutical companies produce sulphate and hydrochloride salts of the drug, both of which are over 300 times more water-soluble than the parent molecule. Since they are derived from a strong acid and weak base, in solution they are at about pH 5; as a consequence, morphine salts are mixed with small amounts of NaOH to make them suitable for injection.

A number of morphine salts are currently in clinical use, the most frequently used ones being hydrochloride, sulphate, tartrate, acetate and citrate salts. Less commonly used salts include methobromide, hydrobromide, hydroiodide, lactate, chloride, and bitartrate salts. Natural alkaloidal salts occurring in poppy plants are morphine meconate, pectinate, and nitrate. Like codeine, dihydrocodeine and other, especially older opiates, morphine has been used as the salicylate salt by some suppliers, thus imparting the therapeutic advantage of both the opioid and the NSAID. Several barbiturate salts of morphine were also used in the past as well as morphine valerate, the salt of the acid found in the perennial flowering plant valerian (*Valeriana officinalis*). Calcium morphenate is an intermediate in various latex and poppy-straw methods of morphine production. Morphine ascorbate and other salts such as the tannate, citrate, and acetate, phosphate, valerate and others may be present in poppy tea, depending on the method of preparation. Morphine valerate produced industrially was one ingredient of a medication available for both oral and parenteral administration, popular many years ago in Europe and elsewhere, called

Trivalin (not to be confused with the current, unrelated herbal preparation of the same name) which also included the valerates of caffeine and cocaine, with a version containing codeine valerate as a fourth ingredient being distributed under the name Tetravalin.

Morphine salts can be given orally or parenterally, as well as epidurally or intrathecally in the spinal cord. However, morphine is less bioavailable when given orally because it is subject to presystemic elimination. Morphine has a duration of action of 4 hours and is metabolised to morphine-6-glucoronide which, surprisingly, has greater analgesic efficacy than morphine. However, morphine-6-glucoronide is a highly polar metabolite and is unlikely to easily re-enter the CNS but produces analgesia via the peripheral opioid receptors.[24] In treating patients with severe chronic pain, it is necessary to maintain a steady plasma level within the effective range, which requires larger doses at increased dose intervals when break-through pain occurs. Since this entails a temporary increase in plasma level beyond the needed therapeutic concentration, the risk of unwanted side effects is enhanced. Sustained-released morphine preparations or long-acting opioids such as L-methadone offer better alternatives to frequent dosing.

In opiate abuse, administration by intravenous injection known as 'mainlining' avoids the first-pass effect and achieves a faster increase of the drug's concentration in the brain, resulting in psychological effects. The effect of opioids can be obliterated by the antagonist naloxone. This antagonist is used as an antidote in morphine poisoning. In normal individuals, naloxone has little or no effect. However, in opioid-dependent individuals, it causes acute withdrawal symptoms. Oral dosing with methadone stabilises the patient by stopping the opioid withdrawal syndrome. At present, methadone is used in the treatment of opioid dependence. It has cross-tolerance with other opioids including heroin and morphine and a long duration of effect. Methadone also blocks the euphoric effects of heroin, morphine, and similar drugs in higher doses (60–80 mg). As a result, properly dosed methadone patients can reduce or stop altogether their use of morphine and heroin. Methadone is only approved for the treatment of opioid dependence and it is not intended for use in the reduction of the use of non-narcotic drugs such as cocaine, methamfetamine, or alcohol.

Cannabinoid receptors

The cannabinoid receptors are classified under the G-protein-coupled receptor superfamily. There are two known subtypes, CB1[25,26] found predominantly in the brain, but also in the lungs, liver and kidneys, while CB2 is principally found in T cells of the immune system, on macrophages and B cells, and in haematopoietic cells. The protein sequences of CB1 and CB2 receptors are about 44% similar. In addition, minor variations in each receptor have been identified. Cannabinoids bind reversibly and stereoselectively to their receptors.

Activation of the CB1 receptors in the brain is due to an endocannabinoid-mediated depolarisation-induced suppression by retrograde signalling, which means that endocannabinoids control a negative feedback of synaptic activity against the usual synaptic transmitter flow. They are released from the depolarised neuron, then bind to the CB1 receptor in the presynaptic neuron, and cause a reduction in GABA release. Activation of presynaptic CB1 receptors inhibits sympathetic innervations of blood vessels and contributes to the suppression of the neurogenic vasopressor response in septic shock.[27] CB1 receptors are responsible for the euphoric and anticonvulsive effects of cannabis. CB1 agonists provide neuroprotection after brain injury. On the other hand, CB2 receptors play a role in nociception and the anti-inflammatory effects of cannabis. In the brain, they can also be expressed by so-called microglial cells in the cerebellum. After the receptor is engaged, multiple intracellular signal transduction pathways are activated. However, separation of the therapeutically undesirable psychotropic and the clinically desirable effects of agonists that bind to cannabinoid receptors has not been reported.

By definition, cannabinoids comprise a variety of distinct chemical classes which bind to the cannabinoid receptor. These include the classical cannabinoids structurally related to tetrahydrocannabinol, the non-classical cannabinoids, the aminoalkylindoles, the eicosanoids related to the endocannabinoids, 1,5-diarylpyrazoles, quinolines and arylsulphonamides and additional compounds that do not fall into these standard classes. According to their production and origin, there are three types of cannabinoids: phytocannabinoids, endogenous cannabinoids, and synthetic cannabinoids.

Phytocannabinoids

Cannabinoids are a group of more than 60 terpenophenolic compounds found in cannabis (*Cannabis sativa* L). All classes are derived from cannabigerol-type and vary in the manner in which the precursor is cyclised. Tetrahydrocannabinol (THC, Fig. 14.17) is the primary psychoactive constituent in the plant. However, unlike THC, the congeners, cannabinol (CBN, Fig. 14.17) and cannabidiol (CBD, Fig. 14.17) have negligible psychoactive properties. In other analogues, the pentyl side chain is replaced with a propyl chain which is named using the suffix 'varin' and is designated as THCV, CBDV, or CBNV. The latter congeners are presumably biosynthesised from butyryl-CoA as the starting unit rather than hexanoyl-CoA. It appears that shorter chains increase the intensity but decrease the duration of the bioactivity of the compounds. Sativex is a whole-plant cannabinoid extract oral spray used for neuropathic pain and spasticity in Canada and Spain.

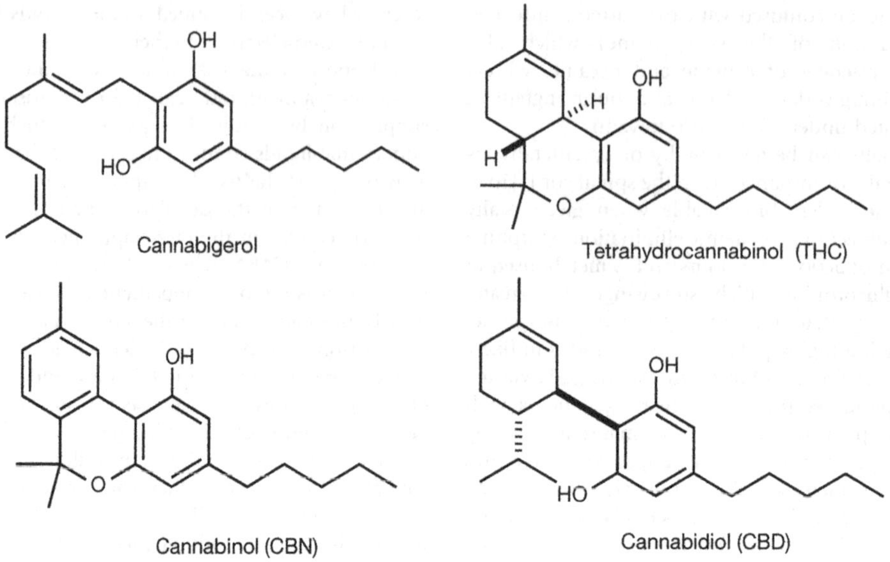

Figure 14.17 Some naturally occurring cannabinoids.

Endogenous cannabinoids

Endogenous cannabinoids have been identified to be polyunsaturated fatty acid derivatives. Endocannabinoids are lipophilic molecules that are not very soluble in water. Two major endogenous compounds are anandamide and 2-arachidonylglycerol that produce their effects by binding to both the CB1 and CB2 cannabinoid receptors. Anandamide is the natural ligand of CB1 which mimics many of the pharmacological properties of tetrahydrocannabinol. By interaction with CB1 or CB1-like receptors, located on peripheral endings of sensory neurons involved in pain transmission, anandamide (Fig. 14.18) pacifies both the early and late phase of the pain pathway produced by formalin-induced chemical damage. The natural ligand of CB2 is 2-arachidonoylglycerol (Fig. 14.18) and its levels in the brain are 800 times greater than anandamide. However, they are not stored in vesicles and do not exist as essential constituents of the membrane bilayers that make up cells but are synthesised on demand. Due to their hydrophobicity, they cannot move independently for any great distance in the aqueous phase surrounding the cells from which they are diffused; therefore, they act locally on target cells. In comparison to hormones, that can affect cells all through the body, endocannabinoids have a restricted sphere of influence.

Synthetic cannabinoids

Synthetic THC is prescribed today under the generic name Dronabinol (Marinol™) to treat vomiting and for enhancement of appetite, mainly in AIDS patients. Synthetic cannabinoids are particularly valuable for determining structure–activity relationships by making systematic, incremental modifications of cannabinoid molecules. Levonantradol (Fig. 14.19) is a synthetic cannabinoid analogue of THC developed by Pfizer in the 1980s. It is 30 times more potent than THC, exhibiting antiemetic and analgesic effects via activation of both the CB1 and CB2 receptors. However, levonantradol is not currently used in medicine but is widely utilised in research of potential therapeutic applications of cannabinoids. Nabilone (Fig. 14.19), marketed as Cesamet™, is a synthetic cannabinoid indicated as an antiemetic and as an adjunct analgesic for neuropathic pain. Dimethylheptylpyran (DMHP, Fig. 14.19), is a synthetic analogue of THC which is similar in structure to THC, but differs in the position of the alicyclic double bond, and the 3-pentyl chain was

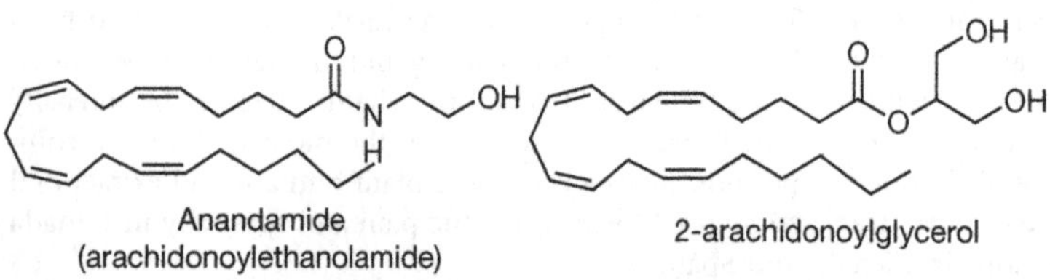

Figure 14.18 Endogenous cannabinoids.

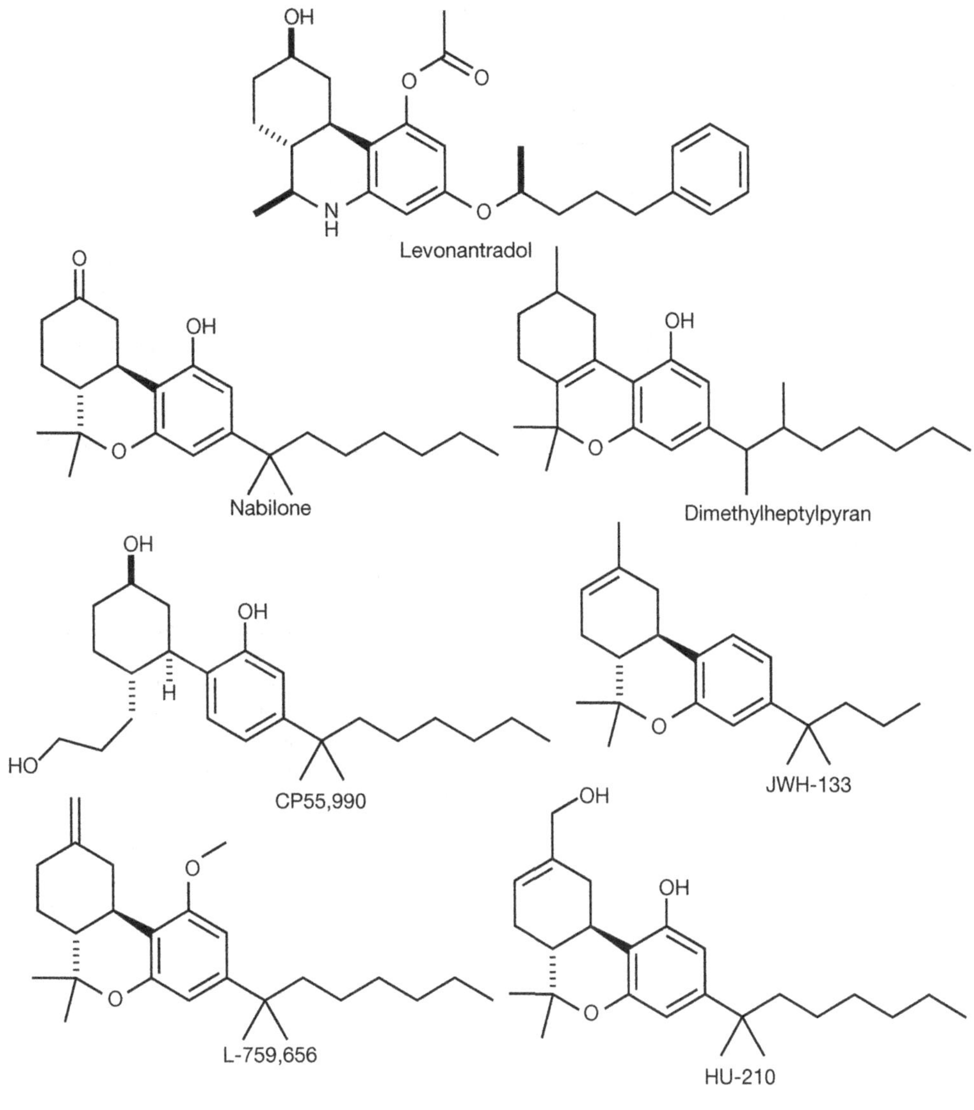

Figure 14.19 Synthetic cannabinoids.

replaced with a 3-(1,2-dimethylheptyl) chain. DMHP exhibits comparable activity to THC, such as sedative effects, but is considerably more potent and has stronger analgesic and anticonvulsant effects than THC with relatively weaker psychological effects. CP 55,990 (Fig. 14.19), produced in 1974, is a cannabinoid receptor agonist which is many times more potent than THC.

Several synthetic cannabinoids have been shown to have higher affinity for the CB2 than for the CB1 receptor,[28] and most of these compounds exhibit modest selectivity. CB2 selective agonists are effective in the treatment of pain, various inflammatory diseases. L-759,656 (Fig. 14.19) is a classical THC-type cannabinoid congener, in which the phenolic hydroxyl group is methylated and has a CB2/CB1 binding ratio of greater than 1000. Other synthetic CB2 selective agonists which are currently in clinical trials are JWH-133 and HU-210 (Fig. 14.19). The anti-inflammatory action of HU-210 is induced by hindering microglial activation that elicits inflammation. HU-210 is implicated in preventing inflammation caused by the amyloid β proteins involved in Alzheimer's disease, in addition to preventing cognitive impairment and loss of neuronal markers.

Cannabinoid agonists and antagonists that are not structurally related to THC have been synthesised for diverse therapeutic indications. One of them is Rimonabant™

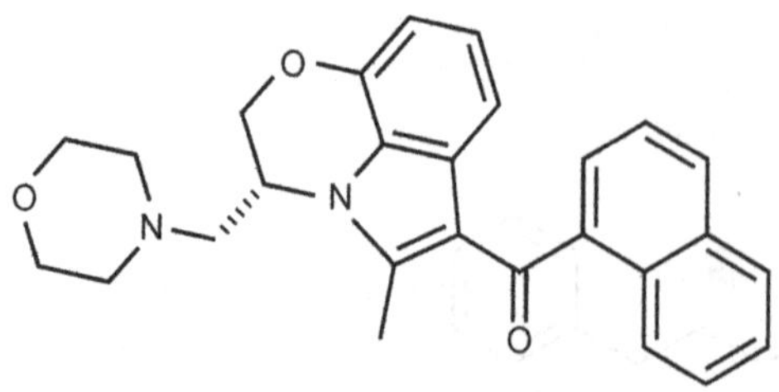

WIN 55,212-2

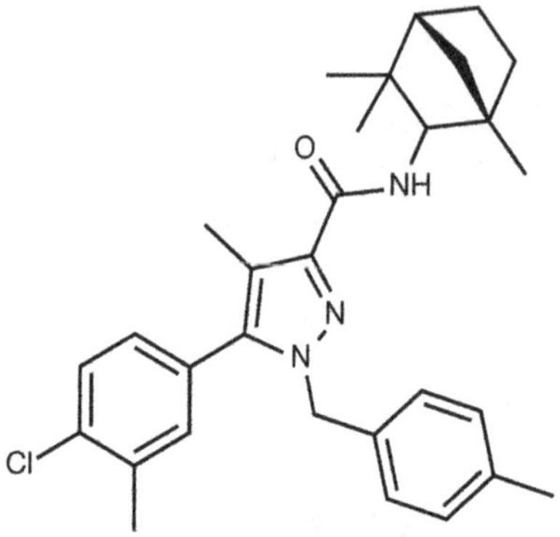

SR144528

Figure 14.20 Non-structurally related cannabinoid agonist and antagonist.

(Fig. 14.20), a CB1 selective antagonist used for weight reduction and smoking cessation, while a non-selective cannabinoid agonist, WIN-55,212-2, an aminoalkylindole derivative (Fig. 14.20), induces the regression or eradication of malignant brain tumours in rats and mice.

Pharmacokinetics of cannabinoids

Cannabinoids can be administered by vaporisation, oral ingestion, transdermal patch, intravenous injection, sublingual absorption, or rectal suppository. They are metabolised in the liver by cytochrome P450 mixed-function oxidases, particularly by CYP2C9 (abbreviated for Cytochrome P450, family 2, subfamily C, polypeptide 9). Thus, supplementing with CYP2C9 inhibitors control extended toxicity. Δ^9-THC is metabolised to 11-hydroxy-Δ^9-THC, which is consequently further metabolised to 11-*nor*-Δ^9-carboxy-THC (Fig. 14.21). Unlike 11-hydroxy-Δ^9-THC and the precursor itself, 11-*nor*-Δ^9-carboxy-THC is not psychoactive, but has a long half-life in the body of up to several days or even weeks in very heavy users, making it the major metabolite tested in blood or urine for cannabis use. The metabolites could also be stored in fat. Thus, cannabis metabolites can be detected in the body even after several weeks.

Ion channel blockers and mediators

Voltage-gated ion channels are permeable to specific ions and are found in excitable cells in muscle, glial cells, neurons, etc. At physiologic or resting membrane potential, the channels are normally closed. They are activated and opened at depolarised membrane potentials and this is the source of the 'voltage-dependent' epithet. Activation of particular channels allows ions to enter the cell, which, depending on the cell type, results in muscular contraction, excitation of neurons, up-regulation of gene expression, or release of hormones or neurotransmitters.

Electrical potential differences of excitable membranes are dependent on ion channels that open in response to depolarisation allowing current to enter the cell. The major inward current that steers the depolarising phase of the action potential is driven through the voltage-gated ion channels. Voltage-gated ion channels are a class of transmembrane ion channel that are activated by changes in the electrical potential difference of their environment and directionally propagate electrical signals. These ion channels consist of several subunits (one large α of *ca.* 180 kDa and one or two β-subunits) of pore-forming proteins arranged

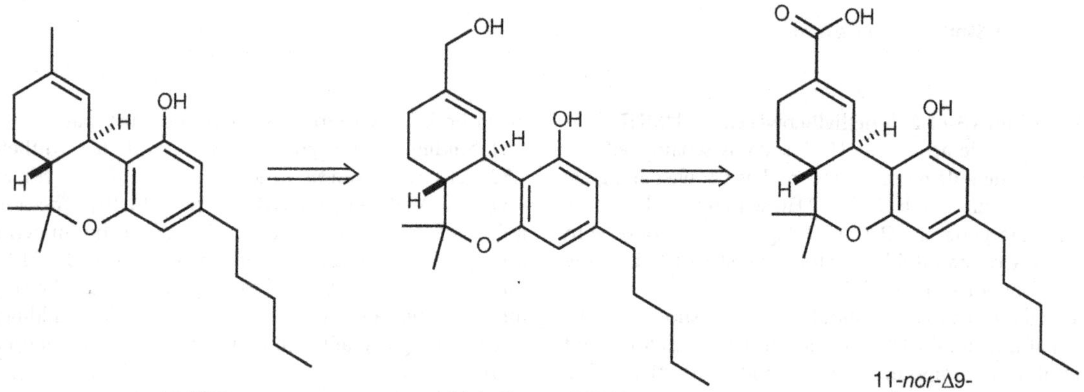

Δ9-THC   11-hydroxy-Δ9-THC   11-*nor*-Δ9-carboxy-THC

Figure 14.21 THC metabolism.

in such a way that there is a central pore that helps to establish and control the small voltage gradient across the plasma membrane of all living cells by allowing the flow of ions down their electrochemical gradient.[29] The central pore is located on the α-subunit while its combination with the β-subunits influences the overall gating pattern. Ion channels are found along the axon and at the synapse and play a crucial role in neuronal and muscle tissues, allowing a rapid and coordinated depolarisation in response to triggering voltage change. The channels are ion-specific, although similarly sized and charged ions may sometimes travel through them. The sodium and potassium voltage-gated channels are found in nerve and muscle tissues, while voltage-gated calcium channels play a role in neurotransmitter release in presynaptic nerve endings.

An electrical potential difference occurs when a cell membrane is adequately stimulated and sufficiently depolarised to open a voltage-gated ion channel, producing an inward current to overcome the outward current. These impulse-generating stimuli occur at the distal sensory endings or postsynaptic receptors of the CNS. Application of analgesics to the peripheral nerve results in the inhibition of propagating electrical potentials through voltage-gated ion channels. The drug binds at a site in the inner pore of the channel which is accessible from the cytoplasmic portal and blocks the voltage-gated ion channel. The ability of the drug to bind to these channels is dependent on their conformation and their affinity for the open inactivated channel states induced by membrane depolarisation. The potency of the drug for blocking pain-related impulses increases during a high frequency of repetitive firing and depolarisation of an injured nerve. On the other hand, blockade of voltage-gated ion channels by local anaesthetics suppresses neurogenic inflammation and the release of neurotransmitters at distal and central terminals. In general, blockade of the action potential relies on the inhibition of the voltage-gated ion channels. Drugs targeting these channels have been found to have analgesic activity both in human and animal models.

Sodium channel blockers

In neuropathic and inflammatory pain, nine isoforms ($Na_v1.1$ to $Na_v1.9$) of the voltage-gated sodium channel α-subunit are expressed by somatosensory primary afferent neurons but not by skeletal or cardiovascular muscle.[30] Voltage-gated sodium channels provide the inward current that generates the upswing of an action potential in response to the depolarisation threshold of the membrane potential. Sodium channel blockers, which act as anaesthetics at high concentrations, are acknowledged for their analgesic activity at lower dosage. Local anaesthetics bind to sodium channels in a state-dependent manner. Activation of the channels increases the accessibility for the drug through the cytoplasmic opening to selectively block the channels that are firing at higher frequency. They either decrease or do not change the action potential duration in partially depolarised cells. At low doses of local anaesthetics, nociceptors are therefore activated and selectively targeted. These drugs also tend to be much more specific for voltage-gated sodium channels. Lidocaine (Fig. 14.22) in particular selectively blocks sodium channels in their open and inactive states, while it has little binding capability in the resting state. This introduces the possibility that some local anaesthetics are isoform-specific drugs as analgesics, which make them non-cardiotoxic and non-neurotoxic. Cardiotoxicity and/or neurotoxicity limit the use of sodium channel blockers such as bupivacaine (Fig. 14.22), which is markedly cardiotoxic. Other sodium channel blockers include mexiletine (Fig. 14.22), tocainide, and phenytoin.

Tetrodotoxin (TTX) and saxitoxin (Fig. 14.23) are alkaloid-based toxins from the puffer fish that block sodium channels by binding to and occluding the extracellular pore opening of the channel. TTX has been utilised as a biochemical probe in order to elucidate voltage-gated sodium channel isoforms. These channel isoforms were functionally classified in conjunction with their degree of sensitivity to TTX. Channel isoforms have diverse electrophysiological properties. They vary in the length of time that they remain open and the time that they spend in their inactivated state as well as in the effect of the membrane potential on this kinetic parameter. Touch receptors, which are low-threshold mechano-receptive dorsal root ganglion neurons, appear to express isoforms $Na_v1.1$, 1.2, 1.3, 1.4, 1.6, and 1.7 that are TTX-sensitive and have fast kinetics. TTX-resistant sodium current in dorsal root ganglion neurons is believed to be carried

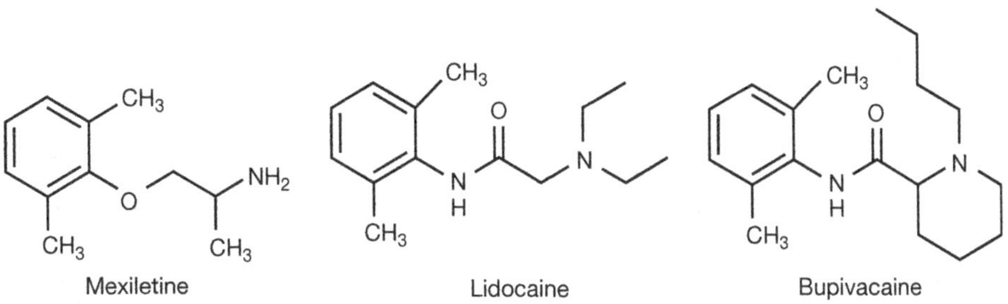

Figure 14.22 Sodium channel blockers.

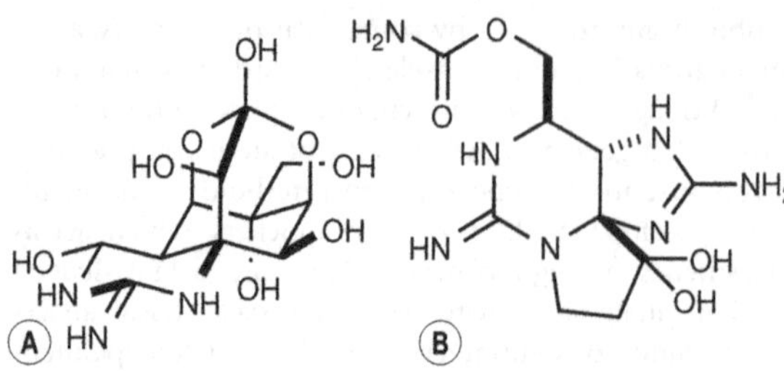

Figure 14.23 Alkaloid toxins which block sodium channels. **A** Tetrodotoxin. **B** Saxitoxin.

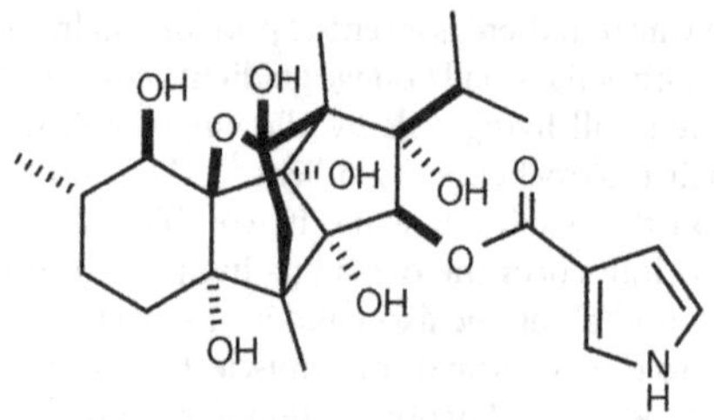

Figure 14.24 Calcium channel blocker ryanodine.

primarily via the isoforms $Na_v1.5$, 1.8, and 1.9, preferentially expressed in nociceptive afferents, where it appears to be localised in the peripheral receptor and central terminals within the spinal cord dorsal horn.[31,32] Most nociceptive neurons in the dorsal root ganglion have a mixture of channel isoforms with both TTX-sensitive fast kinetics and TTX-resistant slow kinetics. On the other hand, inflammatory mediators (e.g. prostaglandin [PGE_2]), algogenic substances (e.g. endothelin-1), and neurotransmitters (e.g. serotonin) can also alter the TTX-resistant channel gating through promoting enzymatic phosphorylation of the intracellular portions of the α- and β-subunits. However, there is little evidence that TTX-sensitive channels are subject to such receptor-driven phosphorylation in primary nociceptors. Isoform-selective drugs that modify the function in primary afferent neurons can avoid cardiac side effects and exclude toxicity from the CNS.

Calcium channel blockers

Opening of the voltage-gated or L-type calcium channels is caused by smooth muscle cell depolarisation brought about by cell stretching, agonist-binding to a G protein-coupled receptor, or autonomic nervous system stimulation. Opening of the L-type calcium channel causes an influx of extracellular Ca^{2+}, which then binds to a CALcium MODULated protein (calmodulin). The activated calmodulin molecule activates myosin light-chain kinase, which phosphorylates the myosin in thick filaments. Phosphorylated myosin forms cross-bridges with actin, thin filaments assisting the smooth muscle fibre to contract. L-type calcium channels are found in cardiac and skeletal myofibres. In the cardiac muscle, opening of the L-type calcium channel permits influx of calcium into the cell. In the skeletal muscle, the calcium-release channel in the sarcoplasmic reticulum open when calcium binds to them, which is a calcium-induced calcium release mediated by ryanodine receptors. The receptors are named after the plant alkaloid ryanodine (Fig. 14.24) to which they show high affinity, and ryanodine was utilised as a biochemical probe to study pain pathways in voltage-gated calcium channels. Ryanodine is a toxic alkaloid found in the South American plant *Ryania speciosa* (Flacourtiaceae) which was originally used as a natural insecticide. At nanomolar concentrations, ryanodine blocks the voltage-gated calcium channel in a half-open state, whereas it fully closes the channel at micromolar concentration. Ryanodine binds at nanomolar levels which cause release of calcium from calcium reservoirs into the sarcoplasmic reticulum, leading to massive muscular contractions.[33]

Voltage-gated calcium channels are formed as a complex of several different protein subunits: α1 (170 kDa), α2δ (150 kDa), β1-4 (52 kDa), δ (17-25 kDa) and γ (32 kDa). The α1-subunit forms the ion-conducting pore while the associated subunits have several other functions including modulation of gating. There are several different kinds of high-voltage-gated as well as low-voltage-gated calcium channels. They are structurally homologous but not structurally identical. In the laboratory, it is possible to tell them apart by studying their physiological roles and their inhibition by specific toxins. High-voltage-gated calcium channels include: the neural N-type channel ($Ca_V2.2$) which can be blocked by ω-conotoxin GVIA as well as by endogenous opioid peptides; the R-type channel ($Ca_V2.3$) which is involved in poorly defined processes in the brain; the closely related P/Q-type channel ($Ca_V2.1$) which is blocked by the ω-agatoxins (e.g. Fig. 14.25) of the funnel web spider venom; and the dihydropyridine-sensitive L-type channels ($Ca_V1.1$, $Ca_V1.2$, and $Ca_V1.3$) which are responsible for excitation-contraction coupling of skeletal, smooth, and cardiac muscle and for hormone secretion in endocrine cells. On the other hand, the T-type channels ($Ca_V3.1$, $Ca_V3.2$, and $Ca_V3.3$) are low-voltage-gated calcium channels. $Ca_V2.2$, $Ca_V2.3$, and $Ca_V3.2$ play a crucial role in pain sensation and are interesting analgesic drug targets.

Peptides derived from the venom of the marine cone snails (genus *Conus*) have been powerful tools in identifying and characterising the function of $Ca_v2.2$ and $Ca_v2.1$ in neurons.[34] Derived from the cone snail *Conus magus*, ziconotide (Fig. 14.26), which is known under the drug name Prialt™, is the synthetic form of the cone snail peptide ω-conotoxin MVIIA, an N-type calcium channel blocker.[35] Ziconotide blocks the N-type calcium channels on the primary nociceptive nerves in the spinal cord. Moreover, the peptide is the first therapeutic agent to

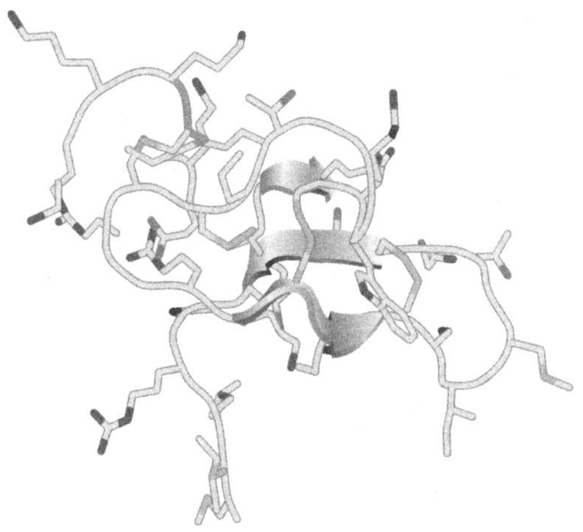

ω-Agatoxin IVA (MW 5210 kDa)

Figure 14.25 ω-agatoxin – calcium channel blocker (MW 5210 kDa).

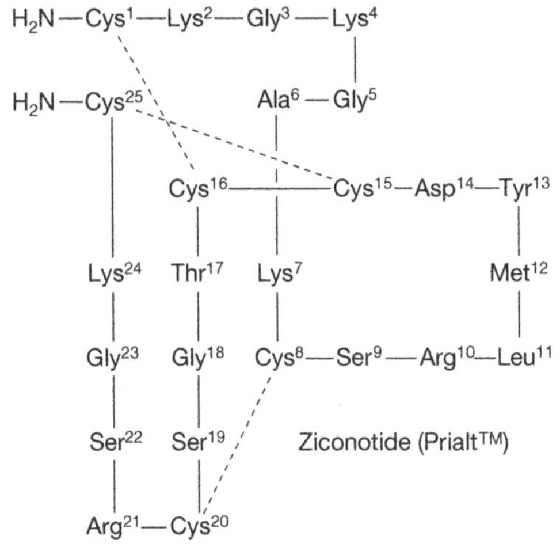

Figure 14.26 Ziconotide N-type calcium channel blocker (Prialt™).

specifically target and block the $Ca_v2.2$ channel. Ziconotide was approved by the United States Food and Drug Administration in December 2004 to be administered as an infusion into the cerebrospinal fluid via an intrathecal pump system for the treatment of intractable, chronic pain. Due to the profound side effects or lack of efficacy when delivered orally or intravenously, ziconotide must be administered directly into the spine. As this is an expensive and invasive procedure of drug delivery, ziconotide therapy is generally considered appropriate only for management of severe chronic pain in patients who are intolerant of or

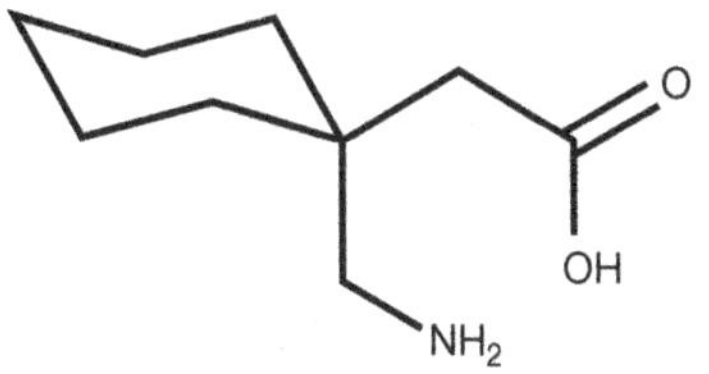

Gabapentin (Neurontin™)

Figure 14.27 Gabapentin.

noncompliant to other treatment, such as systemic analgesics, adjunctive therapies or intrathecal morphine. Intrathecal ziconotide was found to be more potent, longer acting, and more specific than intrathecal morphine. However, this must be weighed against the high level of pain management, both in terms of degree and length, as well as the apparent lack of tolerance[36] and indication of dependence[37] even after extended treatment, along with the need for alternatives to other therapies that have not worked for the patient. Ziconotide is contraindicated for patients with pre-existing mental disorders due to evidence that they are more susceptible to certain severe side effects.

Gabapentin is another effective analgesic used in neuropathic pain therapy that selectively targets calcium channel subunits α2δ-1 in the CNS[38] and binds to high affinity sites in the brain (Fig. 14.27). Gabapentin is a GABA analogue and is known under the brand name Neurontin™. It was originally developed for the treatment of epilepsy but is currently widely used to relieve neuropathic pain. It has been found to be effective in prevention of frequent migraine headaches.[39] Gabapentin is administered to patients with postoperative chronic pain and nerve pain associated with spinal cord injury. It was also reported to be effective in reducing pain and spasticity in multiple sclerosis.[40]

Transient receptor potential (TRP) channel mediators

Transient receptor potential or TRP channels (Table 14.4) are loosely linked ion channels that are non-selectively permeable to cations which include sodium, calcium,

Table 14.4 TRPV temperature sensing receptors

TRPV1	43°C
TRPV2	52°C
TRPV3	31°C (also known as the camphor receptor)
TRPV4	27°C
TRPM8	<15°C

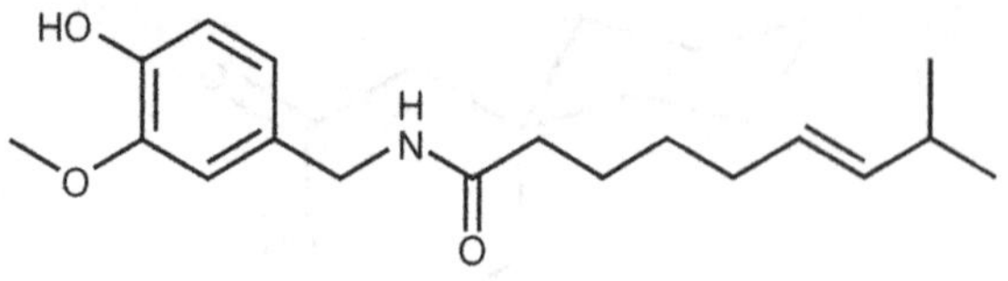

Figure 14.28 Capsaicin.

and magnesium. They are also described as ligand-gated ion channels. TRP channels were first identified in the *trp* mutant strain of a fruit fly, *Drosophila*, where they are involved in visual signalling. Later, TRP channels were found in vertebrates where they are ubiquitously found in many cell types and tissues. Mammalian TRP includes at least 20 related cation channels. They are activated and regulated by a broad range of chemical and physical stimuli. Their functions in sensory neurons include responding to painfully hot temperatures (TRP vanilloid receptors) as well as to noxious cold (TRP menthol receptors). The receptors exist in two conformations, OPEN for heat-activated and CLOSED for cold-activated.

Capsaicin and dihydrocapsaicin are the major capsaicinoids in chilli peppers. Minor capsaicinoids found in chilli are nordihydrocapsaicin, homodihydrocapsaicin, and homocapsaicin. Capsaicin (Fig. 14.28) is biosynthesised in the interlocular septa of chilli peppers by addition of the branched-chain fatty acid, n-nonanoic acid, to vanillylamine. In the genus *Capsicum* (family Solanaceae), capsaicin is present in large quantities in the placental tissue and to a lesser extent in the fleshy part of the fruit. Opposing the popular belief, the seeds do not produce any capsaicin, although the highest concentration of capsaicin can be found in the white pith around the seeds. The seeds of *Capsicum* plants are predominantly dispersed by birds. Birds do not have the receptor to which capsaicin binds, so it does not function as an irritant for them. Thus, natural selection may have led to increasing capsaicin production because it makes the plant less likely to be eaten by animals.

It is common for people to experience gratifying and even ecstatic effects from eating capsaicin-flavoured foods. This attributes to pain-stimulated release of the endogenous opioid, endorphins, which have a different mechanism of action from that of the local receptor overload that makes capsaicin effective as a topical analgesic. The effect can be blocked by compounds that compete for receptor sites with endorphins and opiates.[41]

The burning and painful sensations associated with capsaicin result from its chemical interaction with sensory neurons. Pain can only be eased by cooling and mechanical stimulation, and if no actions are carried out, the burning impression just gradually disappears. Capsaicin binds to the protein of the transient receptor potential channel called vanilloid receptor subtype 1 (TRPV1) which is most densely expressed in C-fibre neurons.[42] The research team led by David Julius of UCSF showed in 1997 that capsaicin selectively binds to TRPV1 on the membranes of pain- and heat-sensing neurons.[43] The identification of the capsaicin receptor as a vanilloid receptor within the TRP family led to the classification of the TPRV class of receptors. TRPV1 is a heat-activated calcium channel, which opens between 37°C and 45°C, while the human heat threshold is at 43°C. When capsaicin stimulates TRPV1, it causes the channel to open below 37°C at the normal body temperature. TRPV1 is stimulated by heat and physical abrasion, permitting cations to pass through the cell membrane and into the cell when activated. The resulting depolarisation of the neuron stimulates it to send the signal to the brain. Capsaicin does not cause actual chemical burn or any physical tissue damage. By binding to TRPV1, the same sensation as that generated by excessive heat or abrasive damage is generated, which explains the burning sensation produced by capsaicin. There are a number of other TRP ion channels that have been described to be sensitive and are responsive to different ranges of temperature sensation (see Table 14.4). Prolonged activation of these neurons by capsaicin depletes presynaptic substance P, a neurotransmitter for pain and heat, causing extended numbness. Neurons that do not contain TRPV1 are unaffected.

Capsaicin is currently used in topical ointments to relieve the pain of peripheral neuropathy such as post-herpetic neuralgia caused by shingles. It is used as a cream for the temporary relief of minor aches and pains of muscles and joints associated with arthritis, simple backache, strains and sprains at concentrations of between 0.025% and 0.075%. Capsaicin is also available as bandages that can be topically applied. As a topical anaesthetic, capsaicin is applied to the aching area until numbness occurs. Capsaicin remains on the skin until the patient begins to feel the heat, at which point it is promptly removed. Capsaicin seems to mimic the burning sensation while the nerves are overwhelmed by the influx of calcium ions; no sense of pain is conveyed for an extended period of time. With chronic exposure to capsaicin, neurons are depleted of neurotransmitters and it leads to reduction in sensation of pain and blockade of neurogenic inflammation. Capsaicin is the key ingredient in the experimental drug Adlea™, which has just completed phase-three trials as a long-acting analgesic to treat post-surgical and osteoarthritis pain for weeks to months after a single injection at the site of pain.[44]

Self Test 14.1

Indicate which of the classes in Table 14.2 the NSAIDs shown below belong to.

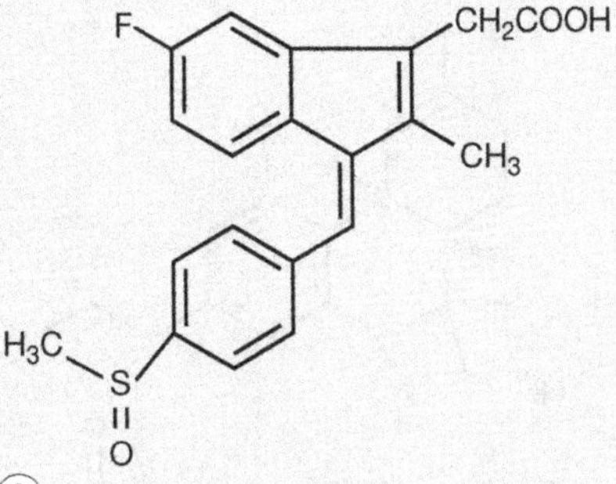

A

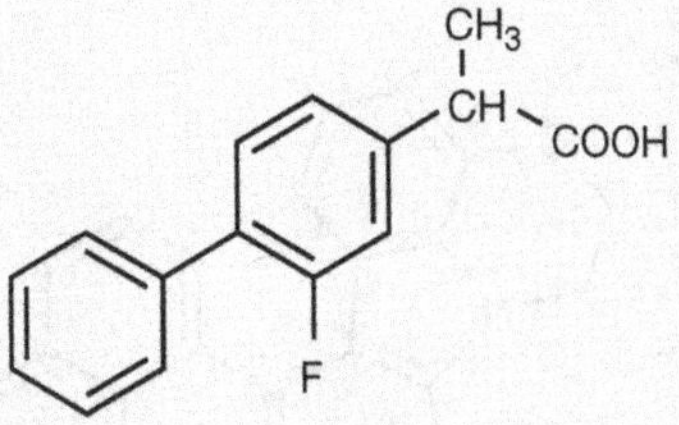

B

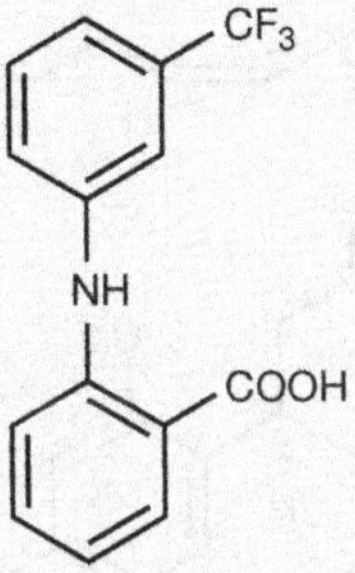

C

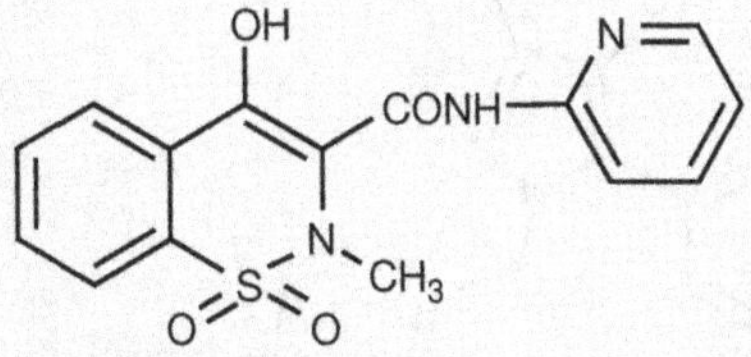

D

Self Test 14.2

Identify which target sites will be blocked or mediated by the following drugs or chemicals:

a. Ryanodine
b. Aspirin
c. Paracetamol
d. Sativex™
e. Prialt™
f. L-methadone
g. Lidocaine
h. Adlea™
i. Dynorphin A

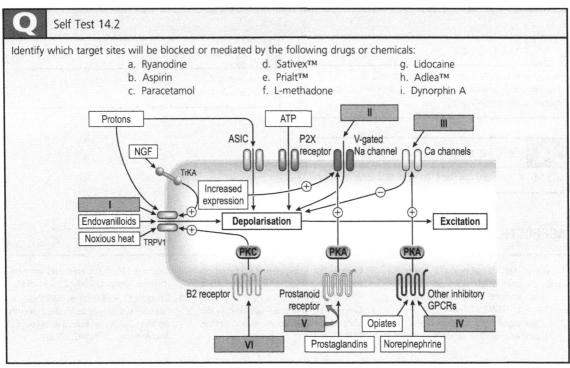

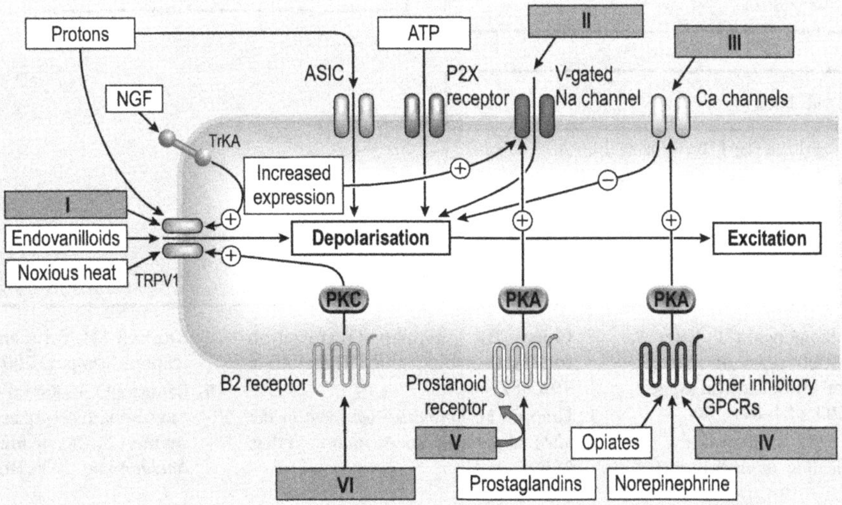

Q Self Test 14.3

Identify the antagonist and the agonist.

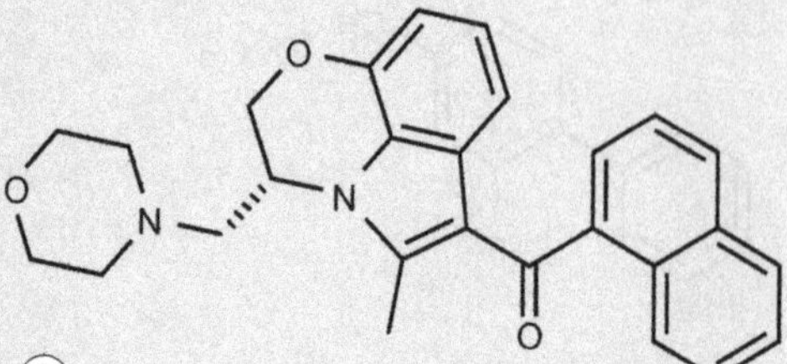

(A)

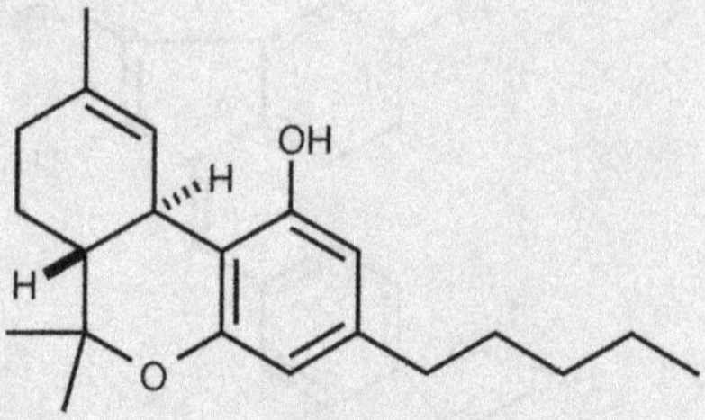

(B)

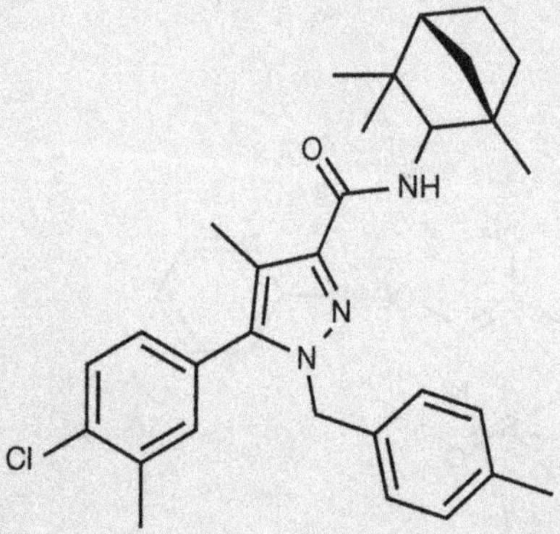

(C)

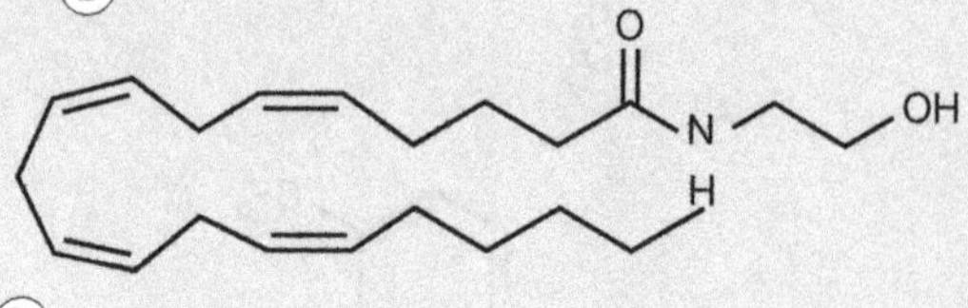

(D)

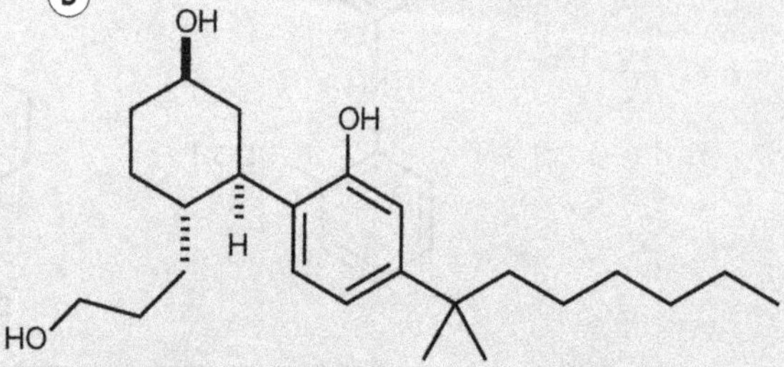

(E)

A Self Test 14.1

Acetic acid class (sulindac), phenylpropionic class (flurbiprofen), anthranilic acid class (flufenamic acid), oxicam class (piroxicam).

A Self Test 14.3

Antagonists: C, D.
Agonists: A, B, E

A Self Test 14.2

a. III; b. V; c. V; d. IV; e. III; f. IV; g. II; h. I; i. VI.

REFERENCES

1. Ansary ME, Steigerwald I, Esser S. Egypt: over 5000 years of management – cultural and historical aspects. *Pain Pract.* 2003;3:84–87.
2. Ghalioungui P, El-Dawakhly Z. *Health and healing in ancient Egypt.* Cairo: The Egyptian Organization for Authorship and Translation; 1965:87.
3. Grapow H. *Grundriss der Medizin der alten Aegypter.* Berlin: Akademie-Verlag; 1959.
4. Brunsch SH. Schmerzmittel im Mittelalter. *Schmerz.* 2007;21:331–338.
5. Basagaoglu I, Karaca S, Salihoglu Z. Anesthesia techniques in the fifteenth century by Serafeddin Sabuncuoglu. *Anesth Analg.* 2006;102:1289.

6. Buyukunal SN, Sari N. Serafeddin Sabuncuoglu, the author of the earliest pediatric surgical atlas: Cerrahiye-i Ilhaniye. *J Pediatr Surg*. 1991; 26:1148–1151.
7. Demirhan EA, Sifali B. *Dogal ilaçlarla geleneksel tedaviler (Medicinal Plants: Traditional Treatments with Natural Drugs)*. 1st ed Istanbul: Alfa; 2001: 100–101.
8. *The Badianus Manuscript (Codex Barberini, Latin 241) translated by Emily Walcott Emmart*. Johns Hopkins Press; 1940.
9. El-Ansary M. The concept of pain by Galen versus avicenna pain. *The J ESMP*. 1987;5:1–10.
10. Melzak H, Wall PD. Pain mechanism: new theory. *Science*. 1965;971–979.
11. Brune K. The early history of non-opioid analgesics. *Acute Pain*. 1997; 1:33–40.
12. Pierpoint WS. Samuel James (c1763–1831) of Hoddesdon and the medicinal use of willow bark. *J Med Biogr*. 2007;15:23–30.
13. Sertürner FW. Darstellung der reinen Mohnsäure (Opiumsäure) nebst einer chemischen Untersuchung des Opiums mit vorzüglicher Hinsicht auf einen darin neu entdekten Stoff und die dahin gehörigen Bemerkungen. *J der Pharmacie f Ärzte, Apotheker u Chemisten*. 1806;14.
14. Chyka PA, Erdman AR, Christianson G, et al. Salicylate poisoning: an evidence-based consensus guideline for out-of-hospital management. *Clin Toxicol (Phila)*. 2007; 45:95–131.
15. Prescott LF, Balali-Mood M, Critchley JA, Johnstone AF, Proudfoot AT. Diuresis or urinary alkalinisation for salicylate poisoning? *Br Med J (Clin Res Ed)*. 1982;285: 1383–1386.
16. (a) Noda A, Goromaru T, Tsubone N, Matsuyama K, Iguchi S. In vivo formation of 4-formylaminoantipyrine as a new metabolite of aminopyrine. *Chem Pharm Bull*. 1976;24:1502–1505. (b) Volz M, Kellner HM. Kinetics and metabolism of pyrazolones (propyphenazone, aminopyrine and dipyrone). *Br J Clin Pharmacol*. 1980;10 (suppl 2): 299S–308S.
17. Hinz B, Cheremina O, Bachmakov J, et al. Dipyrone elicits substantial inhibition of peripheral cyclooxygenases in humans: new insights into the pharmacology of an old analgesic. *FASEB J*. 2007;21:2343–2351.
18. Flower RJ, Vane JR. Inhibition of prostaglandin synthetase in brain explains the anti-pyretic activity of paracetamol (4-acetamidophenol). *Nature*. 1972;240:410–411.
19. Bertolini A, Ferrari A, Ottani A, Guerzoni S, Tacchi R, Leone S. Paracetamol: new vistas of an old drug. *CNS Drug Rev*. 2006;12:250–275.
20. Hogestatt ED, Jonsson BAG, Ermund A. Conversion of acetaminophen to the bioactive N-acylphenolamine AM404 via fatty acid amide hydrolase-dependent arachidonic acid conjugation in the nervous system. *J Biol Chem*. 2005;280: 31405–31412.
21. Bodnar RJ. Endogenous opiates and behaviour. 2006. *Peptides*. 2007;28 (12):2435–2513.
22. Lai J, Luo MC, Chen QM, et al. Dynorphin A activates bradykinin receptors to maintain neuropathic pain. *Nat Neurosci*. 2006;9:1534.
23. Merg F, Filliol D, Usynin I, Bazov I, Bark N, Hurd YL. Big dynorphin as a putative endogenous ligand for κ-opioid receptor. *J Neurochem*. 2006; 97: 292–301.
24. Tegeder I, Meier S, Burian M, Schmidt H, Geisslinger G, Lotsch J. Peripheral opioid analgesis in experimental human pain models. *Brain*. 2003;126:1092–1102.
25. Lambert DM, Fowler CJ. The endocannabinoid system: drug targets, lead compounds, and potential therapeutic applications. *J Med Chem*. 2005;48:5059–5087.
26. Begg M, Pacher P, Bátkai S, et al. Evidence for novel cannabinoid receptors. *Pharmacol Ther*. 2005;106: 133–145.
27. Morgan CJ, Curran HV. Effects of cannabidiol on schizophrenia-like symptoms in people who use cannabis. *Br J Psych J Mental Sci*. 2008;192: 306–307.
28. Bisogno T, Ligresti A, Di Marzo V. The endocannabinoid signalling system: biochemical aspects. *Pharmacol Biochem Behav*. 2005;81:224–238.
29. Hille B. *Ion channels of excitable membranes*. 3rd ed Sunderland, Mass: Sinauer Associates; 2001.
30. Amir R, Argoff CE, Bennett GJ, et al. The role of sodium channels in chronic inflammatory and neuropathic pain. *J Pain*. 2006;7(5 suppl 3): S1–S29.
31. Hong S, Morrow TJ, Paulson PE, Isom LL, Wiley JW. Early painful diabetic neuropathy is associated with differential changes in tetrodotoxin-sensitive and tetrodotoxin-resistant sodium channels in dorsal root ganglion neurons in the rat. *J Biol Chem*. 2004;279:29341–29350.
32. Jeftinija S. The role of tetrodotoxin-resistant sodium channels of small primary afferent fibers. *Brain Res*. 1994;639:125–134.
33. Bertil H. *Ionic Channels of Excitable Membranes*. 2nd ed. Sunderland, MA: Sinauer Associates; 01375.
34. Olivera BM, Miljanich GP, Ramachandran J, Adams ME. Calcium channel diversity and neurotransmitter release: the ω-conotoxins and ω-agatoxins. *Annu Rev Biochem*. 1994; 63:823–867.
35. Skov MJ, Beck JC, de Kater AW, Shopp GM. Nonclinical safety of ziconotide: an intrathecal analgesic of a new pharmaceutical class. *Int J Toxicol*. 2007;26:411–421.
36. Prommer E. Ziconotide: a new option for refractory pain. *Drugs Today*. 2006;42:369–378.
37. Klotz U. Ziconotide – a novel neuron-specific calcium channel blocker for the intrathecal treatment of severe chronic pain – a short review. *Int J Clin Pharmacol Ther*. 2006;44: 478–483.
38. Davies A, Hendrich J, Van Minh AT, Wratten J, Douglas L, Dolphin AC. Functional biology of the alpha(2) delta subunits of voltage-gated calcium channels. *Trends Pharmacol Sci*. 2007;28:220–228.
39. Mathew NT, Rapoport A, Saper J, et al. Efficacy of gabapentin in migraine prophylaxis. *Headache*. 2001;41: 119–128.
40. Mack A. Examination of the evidence for off-label use of gabapentin. *J Manag Care Pharm*. 2003;9:559–568.
41. Francesco C, Giuseppe G, Leonardo R, Giampiero G. *J Altern Complement Med*. 2002;8:341–349.
42. Story GM, Crus-Orengo L. Feel the burn. *Amer Sci*. 2007;95:326–333.
43. Caterina MJ, Schumacher MA, Tominaga M, Rosen TA, Levine JD, Julius D. The capsaicin receptor: a heat-activated ion channel in the pain pathway. *Nature*. 1997;389: 816–824.
44. http://www.anesiva.com/wt/page/adlea.

Chapter | 15 |

Local anaesthetics

David G Watson

CHAPTER CONTENTS

SUMMARY OF PHARMACOLOGY

- Nerve cells contain Na^+ at a concentration of *ca.* 12 mM and K^+ at a concentration of *ca.* 140 mM. Outside the cell Na^+ is at a concentration of *ca.* 150 mM and K^+ at a concentration of *ca.* 4 mM.
- The unexcited nerve is permeable to K^+ but much less permeable to Na^+. Thus, since the inside of the nerve contains greater levels of K^+, it has a negative potential of *ca.* −70 mV and an outward K^+ ion current.
- When a nerve fires, sodium channels open and the membrane becomes more permeable to Na^+ ions and the inward current of Na^+ ions becomes much greater than the outward flow of K^+ ions. The membrane potential thus rises to + 40 mV before the inward flow of Na^+ ions ceases and the negative membrane potential is restored.
- Local anaesthetics (LAs) work by blocking sodium channels in nerve cells. Nerve depolarisation (firing) depends upon sodium channels opening to allow Na^+ ions to enter the cell. Blocking Na^+ channels prevents nerve depolarisation.
- Side effects include: cardiotoxicity which is due to the anaesthetic entering the systemic circulation and blocking Na^+ channels in the heart and effects on the central nervous system (CNS) due to the anaesthetic crossing the blood–brain barrier.

INTRODUCTION

Local anaesthetics (LAs) were developed starting from observations on the naturally occurring alkaloid cocaine which occurs in shrub *Erythoxylon coca* which is found in both South America and South-east Asia. South American

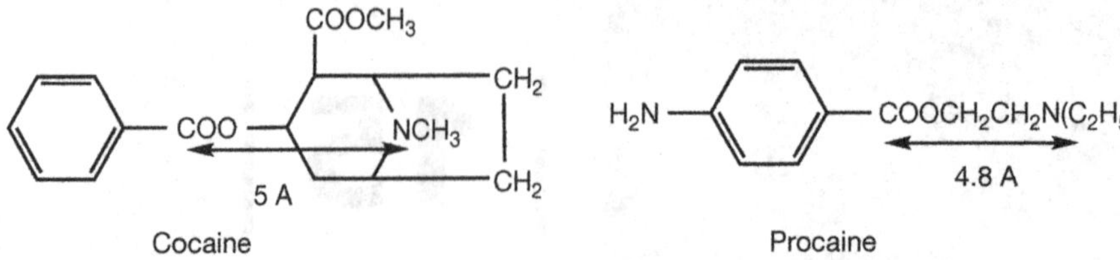

Figure 15.1 Comparison of the structures of cocaine and procaine.

Indians chew the leaves, mixed with lime or alkaline fire ash to ensure that the cocaine is largely in the form of the readily absorbable/lipophilic free base, in order to ward off hunger and fatigue during hunting expeditions and also in the high Andes to overcome the effects of altitude through its effects on respiration. Cocaine was first isolated from coca leaves in 1860 and shortly thereafter infusions of the leaves formed the basis of popular beverages, including, allegedly, the original Coca-Cola®, where it was considered to be a stimulant similar to caffeine. In 1884, the results of experiments with cocaine in producing local anaesthesia in the human eye were reported and subsequently cocaine anaesthesia had a great impact on surgical practice. Unfortunately, cocaine proved to be both toxic and addictive and was deemed to be more appropriate for topical anaesthesia of, for instance, the eye, nose and throat. Following the elucidation of the structure of cocaine in the late nineteenth century many synthetic analogues were produced and tested. Procaine was one of the first effective synthetic LAs and its resemblance to cocaine can be seen in Figure 15.1. Despite the apparent structural differences the distance between the benzoyl carbonyl carbon and the tertiary amine group is very similar to the equivalent distance in cocaine. At physiological pH procaine is less lipophilic than cocaine; thus it is less likely to penetrate into the CNS and is therefore not addictive. The structural elements required for local anaesthetic activity and the drugs with this activity are discussed in more detail below.

SODIUM AND POTASSIUM CHANNELS

There are many similarities between the membrane pores for Na^+, K^+ and Ca^{2+} ions. The pores for Na^+ ions are formed from single polypeptide with four identical domains, each domain having six membrane-spanning helices. However, the pores are not identical for all three ions, and although Na^+ ions have a smaller ionic radius than K^+ ions, they require a larger pore size because they are more extensively bound to water molecules and the pore has to accommodate the solvating water as well as the Na^+ ion. Thus the pore dimensions are quite specific for each ion and probably the structures of the LAs are too large to enter the K^+ channels. The Na^+ channel is known to be less selective than the K^+ channel and will allow a wider range of ions to enter it. As might be expected the pores are somewhat negatively charged in order to have a degree of attraction for positively charged ions. The sections of peptide chain that line pores contain some glutamic acid residues. However, the predominant type of amino acid found in these pores is of the hydrophobic type, e.g. tryptophan and valine, and this ensures that the amino acid side chains are pushed away from the channel by the water present in it. The LAs which block the Na^+ channel will bind to negatively charged glutamate residues within the channel and their hydrophobic portion will interact strongly with the hydrophobic walls of the channel. It is known that the action of the specific K^+ channel blocker tetraethylammonium (TEA) ion is reduced by deletion of a glutamate residue from the mouth of the K^+ channel (Fig. 15.2). TEA is not active in blocking the larger Na^+ channel, presumably because its hydrophobic portion is not sufficiently large.

LAs enter the sodium channel by diffusion of the un-ionised molecule through the lipophilic membrane of the nerve cell. Thus they must be sufficiently un-ionised at physiological pH for them to have a favourable partition coefficient into the membrane. Thus most LAs are fairly weak bases and have p*Ka* values in the range 7.5–9. It has been proposed that LAs act by binding to the pore from the intracellular side of the membrane and that they are not able to pass directly into the pore. However, a number of mechanisms can be envisaged. The pH partition mechanism is illustrated in Figure 15.3. The LA may enter the pore either by partitioning right into the cell and then entering via the open gate or through partitioning laterally into the pore from the membrane. Most of the anaesthetics are sufficiently lipophilic for their partition coefficients to be appreciable even if they are quite highly ionised, as illustrated below for bupivacaine.

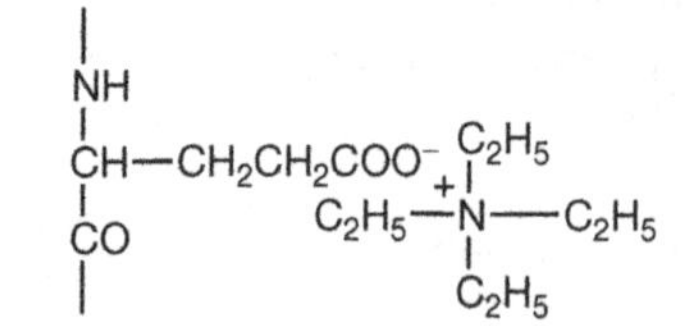

Figure 15.2 Interaction between glutamate and tetraethylammonium.

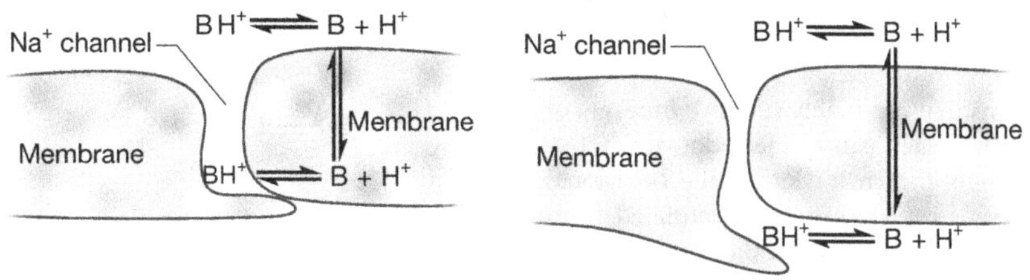

Figure 15.3 Partitioning of a local anaesthetic into a cell membrane.

CALCULATION EXAMPLE 1

Bupivacaine has a literature p*Ka* value of 8.1 and a calculated octanol/water partition coefficient of 7244. Calculate its partition coefficient at pH 7.4.

Substituting into the equation given on page 36 for the variation in the partition coefficient of a base with pH:

$$\text{Papp} = \frac{7244}{1 + 10^{8.1-7.4}} = \frac{7244}{6} = 1207$$

Q Self Test 15.1

Ropivacaine has a p*Ka* value of 8.2 and a calculated partition coefficient of 2754. Calculate the partition coefficient for ropivacaine at pH 7.4. Which is the more potent local anaesthetic?

SUMMARY 1

- LAs interact with acidic and lipophilic structures within the Na^+ channels in the membranes of nerves, blocking the normal influx of Na^+ ions into response to stimulus.
- The LAs can at least partially enter the relatively large Na^+ channels but are too large to enter K^+ channels.
- LAs are weak bases with p*Ka* values between 7.5 and 9 with a high degree of lipophilicity. This ensures that the LAs are sufficiently lipophilic at physiological pH to diffuse through the nerve cell membrane and block the intracellular end of the Na^+ channel.

LOCAL ANAESTHETICS STRUCTURE-ACTIVITY RELATIONSHIPS

Thousands of compounds have been tested which exhibit some kind of nerve conduction blocking activity. Indeed, many compounds which are known for other types of pharmacological activity such as antihistamines, compounds with activity at adrenergic receptors and tranquillisers block nerves to some extent. The wide range of compounds which have been used over the years has been narrowed down to a few effective agents. The earlier used esters such as procaine have been largely superseded by amides. The utility of these agents has been refined by development of advanced procedures for their administration, such as the use of epidural and spinal injection.

Drugs with non-specific action on the nerve membrane

There are a number of LAs which do not stem directly from cocaine and these include eugenol (Fig. 15.4), which is present in clove oil used in dentistry, benzyl alcohol and chlorobutanol. Benzocaine (Fig. 15.4) also falls into this category although it would seem as if it belongs to the cocaine-related compounds because it is present as a structural element in some of the drugs in this series. Benzocaine produces mild local anaesthesia and is used in throat lozenges and for mild topical anaesthesia of the skin. The drugs in this class probably act through a non-specific association with the nerve cell membrane causing disordering of the lipid structure that results in blocking of the Na^+ channel.

Figure 15.4 Non-specific local anaesthetics.

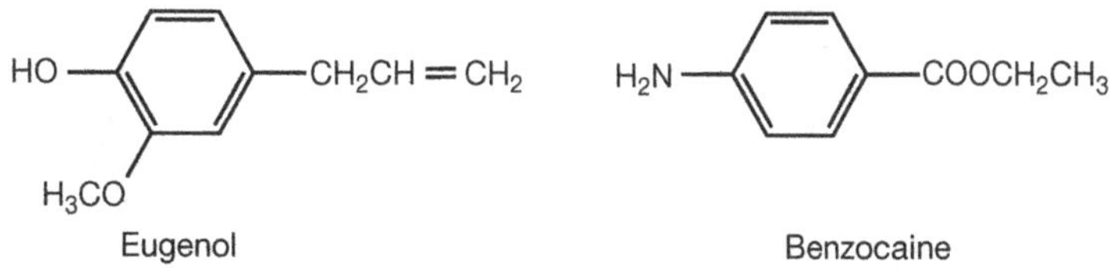

Compounds acting at the mouth of the Na^+ channel

There are some toxins that are highly selective blockers of the Na^+ channel such as saxitoxin and tetrodotoxin. Tetrodotoxin is perhaps best known for killing the occasional adventurous Japanese diner since it is accumulated from toxic algae by the puffer fish which, if not prepared properly, can produce more than indigestion. The toxin is so selective that it has been used to purify the sodium channel protein by affinity chromatography. Tetrodotoxin (Fig. 15.5) bears a highly basic guanidinium group which binds to the Na^+ channel at its mouth, probably to a glutamate group, while the rest of the molecule blocks the channel. The Na^+ channel is known to allow the guanidinium ion itself to pass through it quite rapidly, while the K^+ channel excludes this base almost completely. Toxins like tetrodotoxin and the related saxitoxin are limited in their applications due to their toxicity and the fact that they are complex natural products that are difficult to synthesise chemically.

Local anaesthetics following from the cocaine structure

A generalised structure can be drawn for this type of drug as shown in Figure 15.6. The main structural elements are:

- A lipophilic ring
- A moderately hydrophilic portion
- A lipophilic chain
- A secondary or tertiary amine that may have a variety of lipophilic groups attached to it.

ESTER-TYPE LOCAL ANAESTHETICS IN CURRENT USE

Procaine

As indicated above, procaine was the first potent analogue of cocaine to be produced. In recent years it has become less popular because, in comparison with more recent agents, it has greater effects on the CNS. However, from 1906 it dominated local anaesthesia for nearly 50 years, being marketed

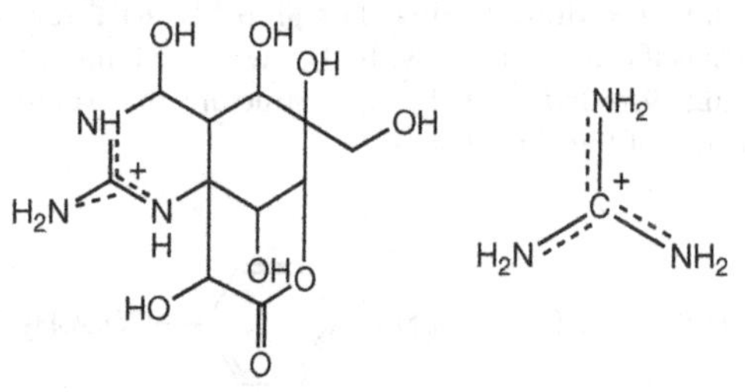

Figure 15.5 Tetrodotoxin.

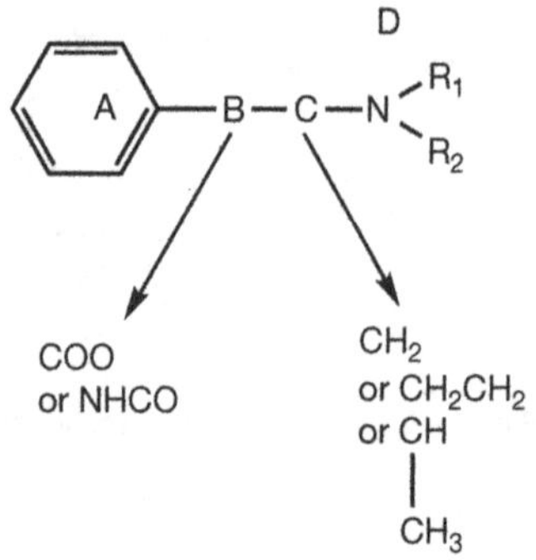

Figure 15.6 Generalised structure for a local anaesthetic.

as Novocaine®. It is used most commonly as a hydrochloride salt, and injections of procaine also include 0.0005% w/v adrenaline as a vasoconstrictor in order to decrease the rate at which the anaesthetic is dispersed into the blood stream from the site of injection. Procaine has a similar potency to lidocaine (see below) but a shorter duration of action. This is because it is rapidly hydrolysed by esterases in the plasma which break it down into *p*-aminobenzoic acid and an amino alcohol (Fig. 15.7). Hydrolysis of procaine in plasma is extremely rapid and it has a half-life of less than a minute. Sterilisation of procaine injections by heating them to a high temperature can also result in ester hydrolysis, which is another disadvantage of this class of anaesthetic.

Description and preparations

The hydrochloride of procaine is the most commonly used form. It is soluble in water in a 1:1 ratio and in alcohol 1:30. The hydrochloride is insufficiently lipophilic to be used in preparations for topical application to the skin. It is currently used occasionally being administered by infiltration injection.

- Typically, a 1-g dose may be administered during surgery being infused in 100 mL of solution. Adrenaline at a concentration of 0.0005 % w/v is also included in the infusion.

Tetracaine

Tetracaine (Fig. 15.8) was synthesised in 1932. It is close in structure to procaine but has the advantage that it is less prone to hydrolysis than procaine in aqueous solution. In addition, it is hydrolysed by plasma esterases (mainly pseudocholinesterase) four times more slowly than procaine. The latter effect may be due to its bulky butyl group that prevents it from fitting into the active site of the esterase as readily as procaine. The butyl group also makes the free base form of the drug lipophilic so that it may be incorporated readily into creams or gels for topical application. The salt form also partitions readily into membranes, which renders it suitable for topical application to the eye.

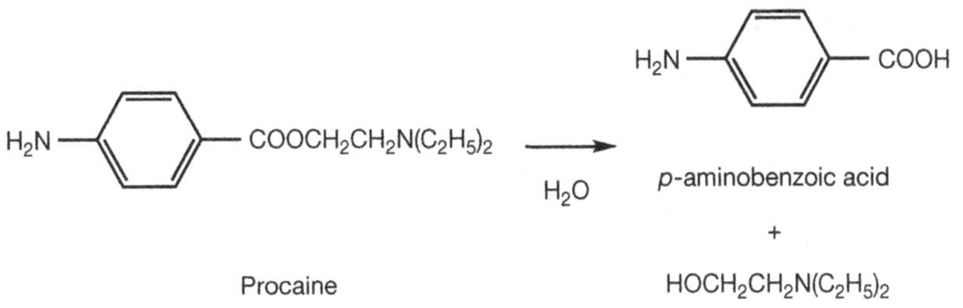

Figure 15.7 Hydrolysis of procaine.

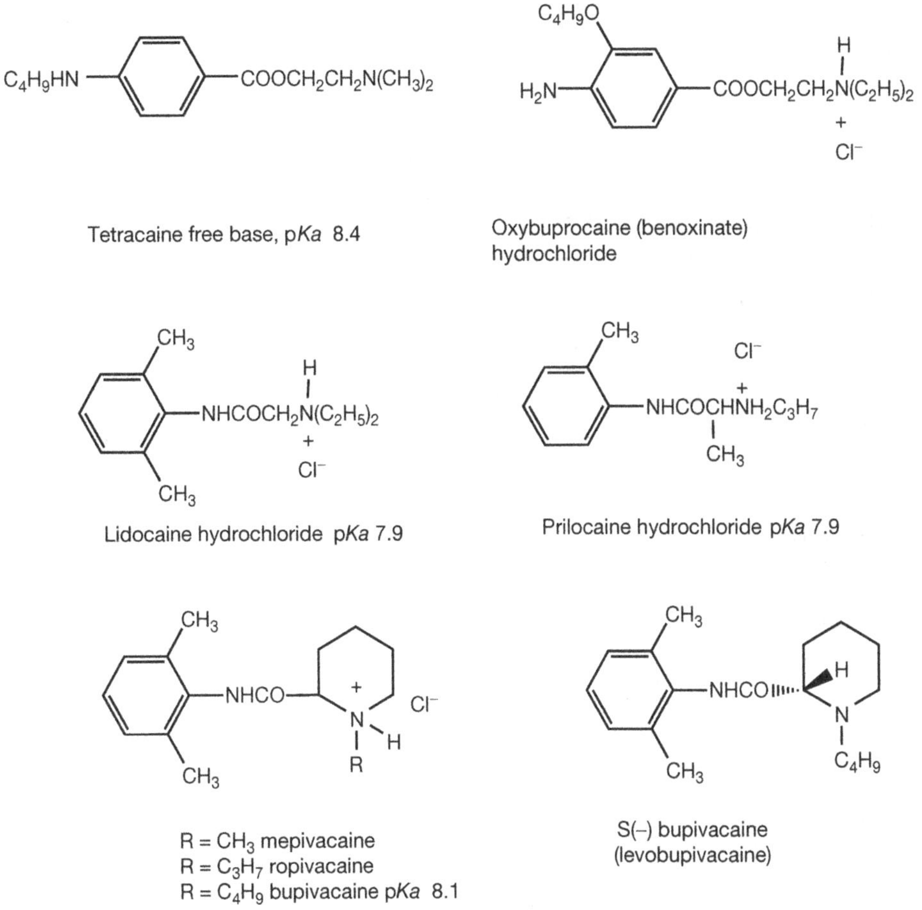

Figure 15.8 Commonly used ester and amide LAs.

Description and preparations

The free base of tetracaine is freely soluble in organic solvents but insoluble in water. The hydrochloride salt is soluble 1:7.5 in water and 1:30 in ethanol.

- The free base is used in anaesthetic gels. Typically, it is available as a gel 4% w/w. The gel should not be applied to mucous membranes or inflamed tissues because the free base is rapidly absorbed and can produce effects upon the CNS due to its lipophilicity.
- The hydrochloride is used in eye surgery for minor surgical procedures such as suture removal. It is available as either 0.5% w/v or 1% w/v eye drops.

Oxybuprocaine (benoxinate)

Oxybuprocaine (Fig. 15.8) is another example of an anaesthetic with an ester-linked side chain. Like tetracaine, it is more stable to hydrolysis in aqueous solution than procaine. The presence of the butylether group makes it more lipophilic than procaine and thus readily absorbed following topical application.

Description and preparations

The hydrochloride salt is soluble in water, ethanol and chloroform. Its main use is in anaesthesia during minor surgical procedures carried out on the eye, such as tonometry (determination of intraocular pressure).

- Oxybuprocaine hydrochloride is formulated in a 0.4% w/v eyedrop.

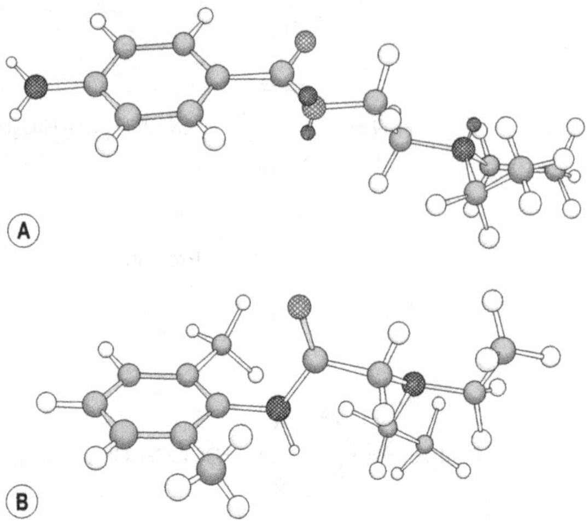

Figure 15.9 3-D models. (**A**) Procaine, displaying flexible side chain. (**B**) Lidocaine, showing conformational rigidity introduced by the presence of two methyl groups in the aromatic ring adjacent to the amide bond so that the side chain is not able to rotate into the same plane as the aromatic ring.

AMIDE-TYPE LOCAL ANAESTHETICS

Lidocaine (Lignocaine)

Lidocaine was synthesised in the early 1940s and was first marketed by Astra in 1948. It would have appeared to have no marked therapeutic advantages over ester-type LAs if it were not for its resistance to hydrolysis. Two per cent w/v solutions of lidocaine buffered at pH 7.3 were found to degrade only by 0.05% after autoclaving. Treatment of procaine under these conditions would cause more or less complete hydrolysis of the ester. The distance between the carbonyl group and the basic centre in lidocaine and the related amide-containing LAs is much less than the corresponding distances in the ester-type LAs. However, in most of the esters there is quite a degree of flexibility in the side chain that may assist in binding. In contrast side chains of the amide anaesthetics are less flexible due to restricted rotation about the CO–N bond due to it being involved in resonance stabilisation (see Ch. 4). In addition, in many cases the benzene ring is 2,6-substituted with two methyl groups that force the amide bond away from being in the same plane as the aromatic ring. This is shown for procaine in comparison with lidocaine in Figure 15.9. The lack of flexibility in binding reduces the potency of the amide anaesthetics with respect to binding. However, the proximity of the carbonyl group to the basic centre in the amide LAs has a base-weakening effect and the p*Ka* values of all these drugs are around 8.0, which increases their partition coefficients into membranes at physiological pH in comparison with esters such as procaine, which has a p*Ka* of 8.8. Thus the amide LAs are in general more potent than the ester LAs.

The amide anaesthetics are not hydrolysed by plasma enzymes and their metabolic inactivation takes place in the liver. This also increases their duration of action in comparison with the esters since they have to be removed from their site of action before they are inactivated.

Description and preparations

Lidocaine free base is virtually insoluble in water but is soluble in organic solvents. Lidocaine hydrochloride is freely soluble in water and ethanol but insoluble in organic solvents.

- Injections of lidocaine hydrochloride are available as 0.5%, 1% and 2% w/v. The injections may or may not contain 0.00005% w/v adrenaline. The dose for infiltration anaesthesia is determined by the patient's weight but a typical maximum is 200 mg or 500 mg if the injection includes adrenaline.
- Creams typically contain lidocaine and prilocaine free bases both at 2.5% w/w. Prilocaine does not affect the CNS as much as lidocaine but it does have toxicity problems of its own (see below).
- Lidocaine hydrochloride is formulated into a spray at 4% w/v for use in anaesthesia of the larynx and trachea. Use of this product requires particular caution.
- Lidocaine free base at 10% w/v is formulated into a pump spray for use in dentistry and obstetrics.

Q Self Test 15.2

An infant weighing 6.4 kg requires an injection of bupivacaine at a dosage of 0.5 mg per kg. How many millilitres of 0.25% w/v injection are required?

Prilocaine

Prilocaine was synthesised in 1960 and was found to be very similar to lidocaine. It has a wider safety margin which is probably because it has a lower partition coefficient (Table 15.1) than lidocaine and also the amide bond is more readily enzymatically hydrolysed than that in lidocaine. It does have an additional problem in that the 2-methyl aniline hydrolysis product of metabolism (Fig. 15.10) can cause methaemoglobinaemia, a condition where the oxygen-carrying capacity of blood cells is reduced due to oxidation of iron (II) in haemoglobin to iron (III). Prilocaine has a chiral centre but it is administered as racemate. However, it is only one of the enantiomers which are rapidly hydrolysed in the liver causing toxicity; this provides an example of how chirality can influence therapeutic activity.

Description and preparations

Prilocaine hydrochloride is freely soluble in water and alcohol and slightly soluble in chloroform.

- Injections of prilocaine hydrochloride are available at 1% w/v. The dose is according to the weight of the patient to a maximum of 400 mg or to 300 mg if a vasoconstrictor is used.
- Injections of prilocaine hydrochloride are available for dental use at 4% w/v or 3% w/v with the vasoconstrictor felypressin.

Table 15.1 Calculated log P values for some amide type LAs

Drug	Log P	P
Lidocaine	2.41	257
Prilocaine	2.18	151
Bupivacaine	3.86	7244
Ropivacaine	3.44	2754
Mepivacaine	2.62	417

Bupivacaine

Bupivacaine (Fig. 15.8) was synthesised in 1957. The duration of action of bupivacaine is considerably longer than those of lidocaine and prilocaine although it has a slow onset of action. (This may be due to less flexibility in the structure when it comes to binding to its site of action.) As can be seen from Table 15.1, its partition coefficient is *ca.* 30 times greater than that of lidocaine which, given that the p*Ka* values are similar, accounts for its long duration of action since it resides in the lipophilic membrane of a nerve cell for longer. Thus its properties indicate that it is obviously not appropriate for dentistry. It is the most frequently used drug for spinal anaesthesia during surgical procedures and childbirth. Bupivacaine is most frequently administered as a mixture of two enantiomers but recently the pure S (−) enantiomer (levobupivacaine) has become available. Levobupivacaine has a similar degree of potency to that of R (+) bupivacaine but it is more selective for sensory neurons and there is less risk of motor neuron block and associated cardiotoxicity. In addition, it has been reported that levobupivacaine on its own acts as its own vasoconstrictor, eliminating the need for inclusion of adrenaline in injections.

Properties and products

Bupivacaine hydrochloride is soluble 1:40 in water and 1:125 in ethanol. It is insoluble in most other organic solvents.

- Bupivacaine hydrochloride injection at 0.25% w/v for infiltration injection. Dosage depends on the patient but the maximum recommended dose is 60 mL.
- Bupivacaine hydrochloride injection 0.5% w/v with 8% w/v glucose (reduces loss of anaesthetic by diffusion). For spinal anaesthesia. Dose 2–4 mL.
- Bupivacaine hydrochloride injection 0.25 of 0.5% w/v with 0.0005% w/v adrenaline.
- Levobupivacaine hydrochloride 0.25% w/v.

Ropivacaine

Ropivacaine (Fig. 15.8) was synthesised in 1985 as a single S (-) enantiomer. It has similar properties and potency to bupivacaine but has somewhat shorter duration of action as a result of its lower partition coefficient.

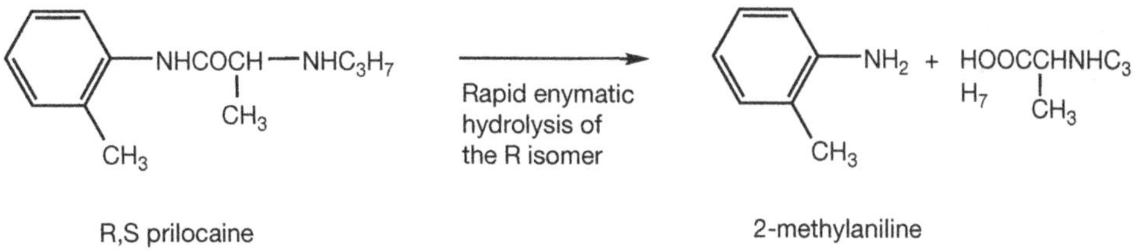

Figure 15.10 Enzymatic hydrolysis of prilocaine.

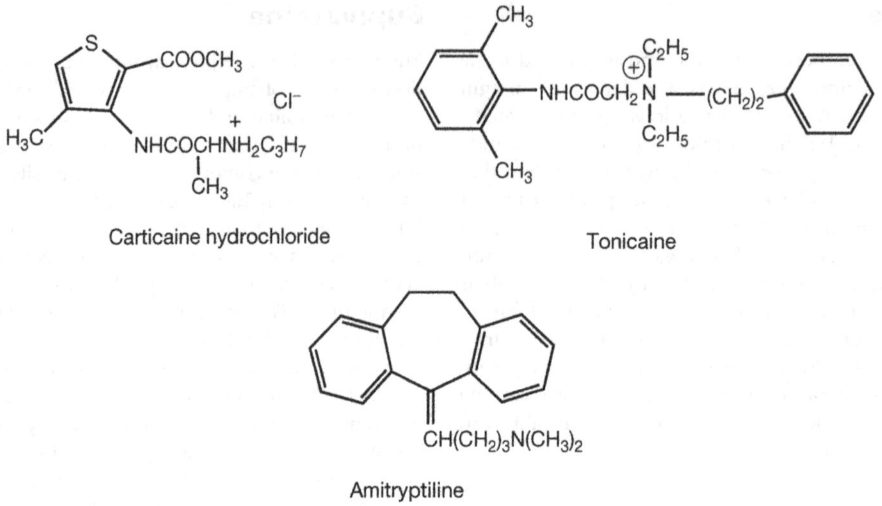

Figure 15.11 New and experimental LAs.

Properties and preparations

Ropivacaine hydrochloride is quite soluble in water and ethanol.

- Ropivacaine hydrochloride injection 0.2% w/v and infusion 0.2% w/v for epidural pain relief.

Additional agents

Mepivacaine (Fig. 15.8) is a less potent analogue of bupivacaine which is used in dentistry. Carticaine (Fig. 15.11) has recently been introduced for dental use. It retains the amide side chain but the aromatic ring has been replaced by a substituted thiophene ring. This ring contains an ester that may be useful in reducing the duration of action of the drug since hydrolysis of the ester reduces the partition coefficient of the drug. Tonicaine (Fig. 15.11) is an experimental anaesthetic that is highly selective in blocking sensory neurons in comparison with motor neurons. It is highly lipophilic and has a long duration of action. However, it has a narrow therapeutic index and displays neurotoxicity, and these factors have delayed its development. Amitryptiline (Fig. 15.11) is a tricyclic antidepressant but it is also a potent LA, having a longer duration of action than bupivacaine. Its use may be limited by its cardiotoxicity but it may become a useful topical LA.

ADDITIONAL PHARMACEUTICAL CONSIDERATIONS

Formulation

The problems of the stability of the ester LAs have been discussed above. The amide LAs are very stable under aqueous conditions. Another problem, particularly with highly lipophilic anaesthetics, is that many LAs have limited water solubility as the free base. The p*Ka* values of these compounds are in many cases close to 8.0 and thus at a physiological pH of 7.4 there may be *ca.* 20% of un-ionised drug. Even if the injection formulation is buffered at a low pH to ensure solubility, the buffering action of physiological fluids will cause particularly lipophilic compounds to precipitate, producing risk of tissue irritation. Buffering very low pH values may also be irritating. Attempts were made to formulate in non-aqueous vehicles but these proved to be an irritant. Thus the problem has not been entirely solved and there remains some scope for innovative formulation in this area. Liposomal formulations show some promise as a system for delivering prolonged and selective sensory blockade by LAs.

The influence of salts

It has been proposed that some salts may give better anaesthetic performance than the hydrochlorides. For instance the use of carbonate salts of LAs may potentiate their activity.

SUMMARY 2

- Mild anaesthesia may be achieved with non-amine agents that act on nerve membranes in a non-specific manner.
- The LAs in use originate from the ester/amine cocaine. The ester LAs are unstable in solution and readily hydrolysed and have been largely replaced by amide LAs which are stable to both chemical and biological hydrolysis.
- The potency of a LA depends on a combination of its lipophilicity and p*Ka* value. Lower doses of highly lipophilic/low p*Ka* value LAs such as bupivacaine are required.
- Precipitation of highly lipophilic LAs at physiological pH causing tissue irritation is a potential problem.

Q Self Test 15.3

Examine the structures of the following less used LAs and order them in terms of increasing potency and duration of action.

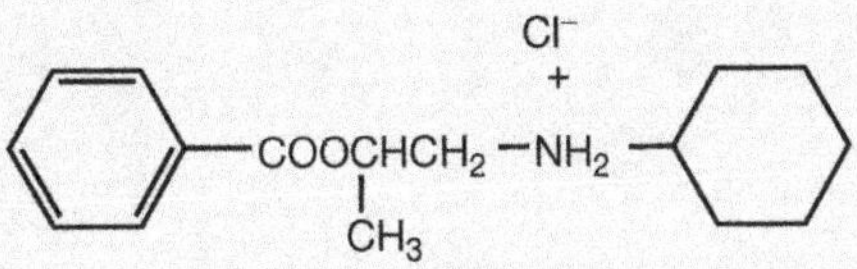

1. Hexycaine hydrochloride

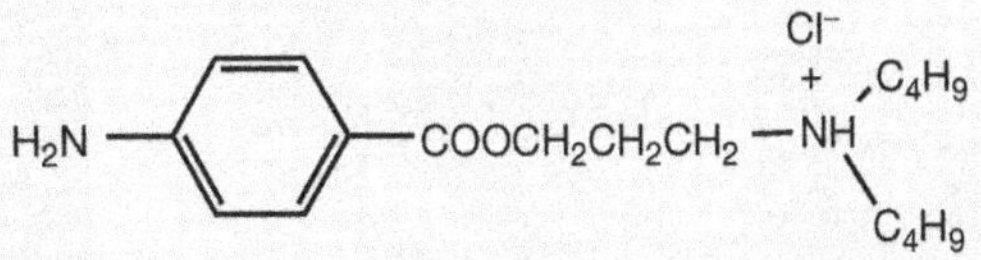

2. Butacaine hydrochloride

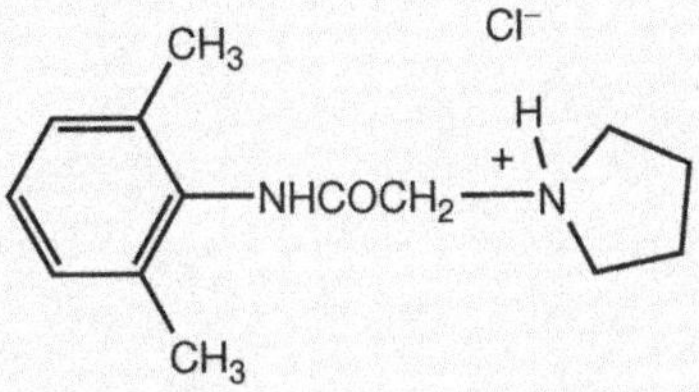

3. Pyrrocaine hydrochloride

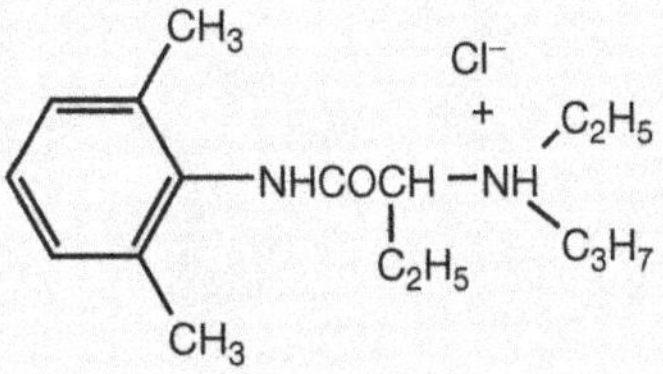

4. Etidocaine hydrochloride

A Self Test 15.1

437.

A Self Test 15.2

1.28 mL.

A Self Test 15.3

Potency: 3, 1, 2, 4. Duration of action: 1, 2, 3, 4.

Chapter 16

Anticholinergic agents

Muhammad Anas Kamleh

CHAPTER CONTENTS

INTRODUCTION

In this chapter, we will discuss drugs acting on the cholinergic system. The cholinergic receptors are part of the autonomic nervous system. They are well distributed in all tissues of the body, and play major roles in the homeostasis of physiological functions. The intervention at cholinergic activity level can help in many disease states. Some of them have been extensively studied (e.g. glaucoma, myasthenia gravis and peptic ulcer) and some of them have only recently been discovered to have a cholinergic dimension (e.g. Parkinson's disease, Alzheimer's syndrome, psychosis, obesity and cancer).[1,2,3,4] Moreover, the control of cholinergic activity is highly desirable during surgical operation, and this has had a great impact on the facilitation of surgical procedures.

Naturally occurring anticholinergic compounds have long been used in history for very different reasons. *Atropa belladonna* (the beautiful lady), the natural source of atropine, was used by Italian women to dilate the eye pupils in order to give a charming look. Calabar beans, the natural source of physostigmine, were used to test alleged criminals for innocence, death indicating a 'guilty suspect'. The dry extract of curare was rubbed against the arrows used by American Indians during their fights and for hunting. Moreover, the psychological/neurological effects of these drugs have made them a good material for detective novel writers.

The botanical origin of the first receptor ligands is a common feature among all drug categories related to the cholinergic activity. Muscarine from the amanite mushroom and nicotine from tobacco leaves were the two alkaloids which exhibited agonistic activity on the muscarinic and nicotinic cholinergic receptors, respectively. Atropine from *A. belladonna* was the first antimuscarinic agent to be discovered. Tubocurarine (or calabash curare) was the first compound to be discovered to have nicotinic receptor antagonist activity and physostigmine was the first known anticholinesterase substance.

Drugs acting on the cholinergic systems may be divided into two main categories, each being subdivided into subgroups which will have different therapeutic indications:

I. drugs enhancing cholinergic activity
    a. cholinergic receptor agonists
        i. acetylcholine-like agonists

b. antiacetylcholine esterase agents
   i. competitive antagonists
   ii. short-acting inhibitors (carbamates)
   iii. long-acting inhibitors (organophosphorus)

II. drugs suppressing the cholinergic activity
   a. muscarinic antagonists
   b. nicotinic antagonists.

The potency of these drugs makes them dangerous poisons, and it is very common throughout the chapter to mention the use of one agonist in treating the toxicity of an antagonist, and the same antagonist for treating the toxicity of that very same agonist.

PHYSIOLOGY OF THE AUTONOMIC SYSTEM

The cholinergic receptors are well spread throughout the whole human body with varying abundance of one subtype of the receptors over the others in a specific tissue.

The early observation of the different responses elicited by application of muscarine and nicotine suggested two different receptors. Both receptors share the neurotransmitter acetylcholine (ACh), thus both were named cholinergic receptors, but a further nomenclature was followed to distinguish between those preferably affected by muscarine (muscarinic receptors) and those affected by nicotine (nicotinic receptors).

Nicotinic receptors (AChNR) are found in synapses between sympathetic and parasympathetic nerves, synapses between a nerve and a skeletal muscle, at the end plates of the somatic motor nerves and the adrenal medulla. Muscarinic receptors (AChMR) are distributed in the synapses between a parasympathetic nerve and a smooth muscle and cardiac muscles (Fig. 16.1).

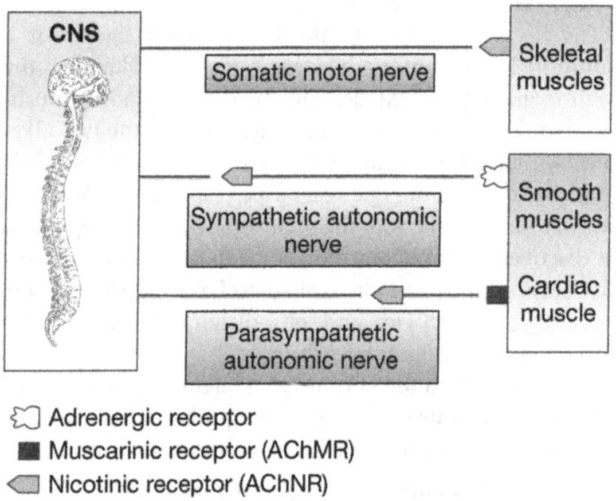

Figure 16.1 Distribution of the cholinergic receptors in the nervous system.

The two sets of receptors vary a great deal, but all share the neurotransmitter acetylcholine and the general structure required to accommodate it, and these differences are not detected by the natural activator ACh. However, they are sufficient for the selective acceptance/rejection of the binding of other molecules. Both types of cholinergic receptor have been isolated.

The muscarinic receptor is a seven-helix membrane-spanning G-protein-type receptor and the associated second messenger is either activation of inositol-3-phosphate (IP3) or inhibition of cyclic adenosine monophosphate (cAMP). There are five subtypes of the muscarinic receptors (M1–M5). All share the same general structure and the active site, but they differ in their tissue distribution, their second messenger mechanism and the associated physiological response.[5,6]

The nicotinic receptor is a channel-type receptor composed of four non-identical subunits which open an ion gate upon activation, allowing the build-up of a membrane potential which in turn transmits the signal further down the nerve or muscle. The structure of the receptors will be discussed in more detail later. The effects resulting from the activation of the muscarinic and nicotinic receptors in different tissues are summarised in Table 16.1.

We should bear in mind that some of the above actions, especially those in the cardiovascular system, are controlled by a complex system. For example, the direct slowing effect on sinoatrial rate will result in hypotension which in turn leads to a sympathetic reflex discharge. Additionally, the muscarinic agonist can act indirectly via EDRF (endothelium-derived release factor which is nitrous oxide [NO]) or directly in high doses which will elicit opposing effects, i.e. dilation, contraction, respectively. That is why the net effect of acetylcholine agonist is dependent on its relative availability in the blood and vessels and the sympathetic reflex responsiveness.

THE RECEPTOR ACTIVATION PROCESS

The activation of the cholinergic receptor starts with the synthesis of ACh from choline by the enzymatic action of choline acetyl transferase. ACh is then stored in vesicles pending the arrival of nerve signals interacting with the cell membrane which result in releasing ACh to the synaptic cleft. ACh then binds to its receptor and produces a physiological response and leaves the receptor. The neighbouring acetylcholinesterase captures any dissociated ACh and hydrolyses it to acetate and choline, thus inactivating it. The latter is recycled into the nerve cell by a choline carrier protein (Fig.16.2).

On the basis of the information shown in Figure 16.2, the targets for cholinergic drug action could be:

- choline acetyltranseferase: synthesis of ACh (nerve ends)
- ACh carrier protein (nerve ends)

Table 16.1 Summary of physiological responses of muscarinic and nicotinic receptors

Receptor type	Organ/tissue	Response	Treatment/treatment modulation
Muscarinic	Eye-sphincter muscle of the iris	Contraction (miosis) – promotes the flow of aqueous humour into the canal of Schlemm	Closed angle glaucoma Ophthalmic examination
	Eye – ciliary muscle	Accommodation (contraction for near vision) – response as above	
	Cardiovascular system – sinoatrial node	Decrease in heart rate and the strength of heart contractions	Treatment of tachycardia Treatment of excessive vagal discharge
	Cardiovascular system – atria	Decrease in contractile strength and refractory period	
	Cardiovascular system – atrioventricular node	Decrease in conduction velocity Increase in refractory period	
	Cardiovascular system – ventricles	Small decrease in contractile strength	
	Cardiovascular system – arteries	Dilation (via EDRF) Contraction (direct action in high doses)	Severe hypertension
	Cardiovascular system – veins	Dilation (via EDRF) Contraction (direct action in high doses)	
	Lung – bronchial muscle	Contraction	Treatment of COPD
	Lung – bronchial glands	Stimulation (increase in secretion)	
	GI tract – gastrointestinal smooth muscles	Contraction/peristaltic activity increased	Treatment of ulcer
	Salivary and gastric glands	Stimulation of secretion	Treatment of Parkinson's syndrome symptoms
	GU tract – Detrusor	Stimulation – promote voiding	Nocturnal urination
	Sphincter	Relaxation	
	CNS – brain	Tremor, hypothermia and antinociception – M2 receptors	Alzheimer's syndrome symptoms
	CNS – brain	Seizure – M1 receptors	
Nicotinic	CNS – brain	Mild alerting action (low doses) Tremor, emesis and stimulation of respiratory centre (large doses) Coma (very large doses)	
	Postganglionic neurons – cardiovascular tissues	Hypertension and tachycardia	
	GI/GU tract tissues	Nausea, vomiting, diarrhoea and voiding of urine	
	Skeletal muscles – neuromuscular junction	Contraction, when the effect is prolonged it leads to a depolarisation blockade resulting in a flaccid paralysis	Muscle relaxation in surgery

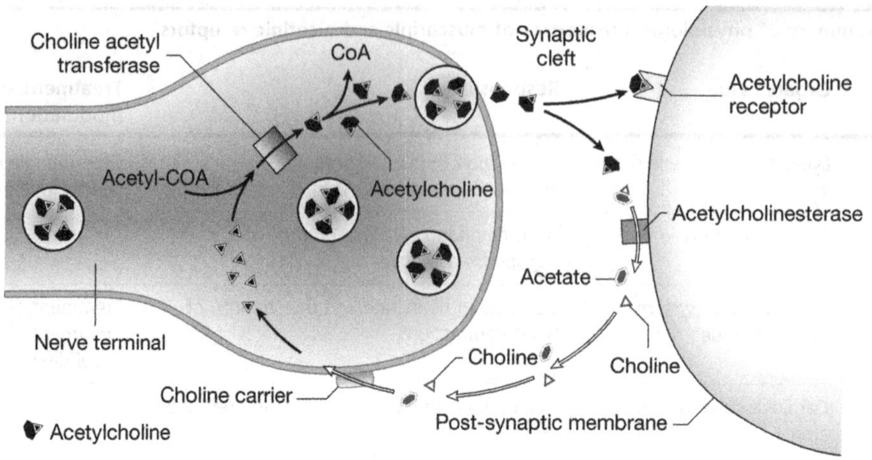

Figure 16.2 The acetylcholine (ACh) receptor activation cycle (from Rang HP, Dale MM, Ritter JM, Flower RJ 2007 *Pharmacology*, 6th edn. St Louis, Elsevier, with permission).

- cholinergic receptor (muscarinic – nicotinic) receiver cell (nerve or muscle)
- acetylcholinesterase receiver cell (nerve or muscle)
- choline receptor (presynaptic nerve)
- choline carrier protein. Synaptic cleft.

Acetylcholine (ACh) was the first neurotransmitter to be characterised. It binds efficiently to both AChNR and AChMR despite the differences in the active sites of the receptors. The dissimilarity of the active site is good news with regards to the different responses elicited by the activation of the two receptors, as it makes possible the rational design of highly selective receptor agonists or antagonists.

ACh itself is a small molecule freely rotating on its backbone (choline). This gives rise to numerous potential freely interconvertible conformations, and ACh can switch on all cholinergic receptors, but it probably does so at each receptor with a different conformation. This is supported by the selectivity of muscarine and low-dose nicotine on one group of receptors rather than the other. ACh adopts a specific conformation at different receptors where the 'active' part of the molecule is locked into a limited number of conformations by incorporating a part of it into a cyclic moiety (Fig. 16.3).

ACh contains an ionic quaternary ammonium entity and dipolar ester with accompanying electrostatic fields.[7] Experiments of varying groups indicated maximum activity to be associated with the cationic nitrogen. In explorations of the role of the cationic head, the primary amine analogue, aminoethyl acetate, is inactive. However, tertiary amine counterparts, such as dimethylaminoethyl acetate, are strong enough bases to be almost totally ionised at pH 7.4, thus retaining cationic character along with lipophilic character. The importance of charge is shown by inactivity of the neutral, quaternary substance resulting from replacement of N by C. Other necessary features are the polarised carbonyl oxygen and probably the non-carbonyl oxygen.The ester group has to be in the optimum position, and extending the carbon bridge between the nitrogen and the carbonyl to more than two methylene units diminishes the activity significantly. Alkane chains with no ester group show essentially no activity. Structure–activity relationship (SAR) studies revealed that the presence of hydrogen-bond acceptor groups close to the quaternary nitrogen is detrimental for AChNR binding. (SAR results for ACh are valid for both receptors.) Box 16.1 shows the important factors in SAR at cholinergic receptors.

The active site of the receptor is thought to be an asparagine motif which interacts with the dipole of the carbonyl group in the ester side of the transmitter, while the interaction on the other quaternary ammonium side is thought to be either an ion-pair interaction with an aspartic acid residue or an interaction between the delocalised positive charge on the quaternary nitrogen+ three methyl groups and an electron-rich pocket formed by three tyrosine motifs in the receptor (cation-π-donor interaction).

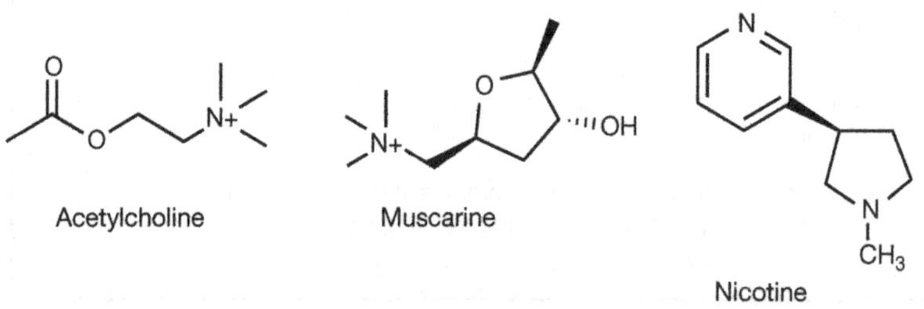

Figure 16.3 Acetylcholine (ACh) and the ligands which bind to the subclasses of ACh receptors.

Box 16.1 **When studying structure–activity relationship, these rules apply:**

- The charged amine is important.
- The ester bond is important.
- The bridge of two carbons between the two ends can not be expanded or shrunk.
- The size of the ester function can not be greatly increased as it seems to fit into a very small hydrophobic pocket.

CHOLINERGIC AGONISTS

The SAR of ACh indicates a very tight fit interaction at the receptor, resulting in a very limited space for the medicinal chemist for a rational drug design. ACh itself is rapidly hydrolysed by acetylcholinesterase (AChE). The effect of a large-bolus i.v. injection wears out in 5–20 seconds (there is large variation between individuals). ACh is very labile to hydrolysis of its ester function via either chemical or enzymatic activity. Chemical hydrolysis makes it orally inactive. This instability arises from the proximity of a quaternary ammonium function to an ester group, as it attracts the electron pairs on the oxygen to move towards its positive charge, thus withdrawing the electrons from the carbon–oxygen bond on the ester function towards the oxygen. This will make the dipole C–O greater, hence more prone to attack by a nucleophile (even weak nucleophile such as water, Fig. 16.4).

Hydrolysis by esterases (pseudocholinesterase, butyrylcholinesterase) in the circulation gives ACh a very short plasma half-life, in addition to its specific hydrolysis by AChE at the active site. Exogenous ACh has been employed therapeutically for restoring the gastrointestinal or urological

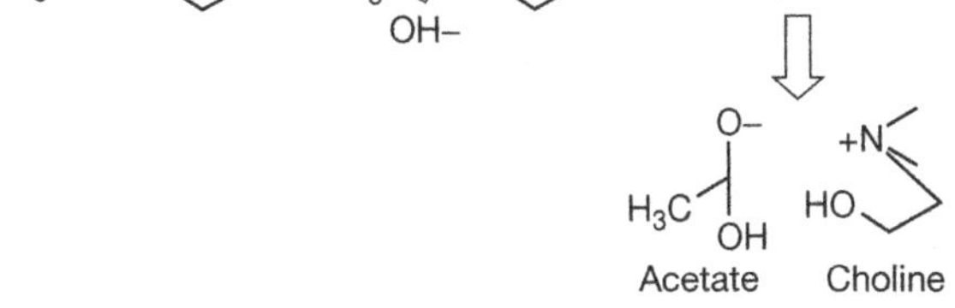

Figure 16.4 Effect of the proximity of quaternary ammonium group on the hydrolysis of ACh.

movement post surgery. The minimum effective dose of ACh is 20–50 μg/min and it has no selectivity at all.

ACh as a therapeutic agent is not convenient, and modifications are needed to ensure:

- stability against acid hydrolysis (oral drugs)
- stability against chemical hydrolysis in the blood (longer lasting)
- stability against enzymatic hydrolysis (longer lasting)
- organ selectivity (pharmacokinetic)
- receptor type (e.g. cholinergic over adrenergic receptor, e.g. of nicotine and muscarine) and subtype (e.g. M1 over M4) selectivity (pharmacodynamic).

Modifications of the acetylcholine structure

When designing a drug to be a cholinergic agonist, selectivity is highly desirable but not a simple term, as therapeutic candidates should be selective for the cholinergic receptor among other neurological receptors, selective for nicotinic or muscarinic, or selective for specific subtypes or tissue types. Selectivity could be achieved on the pharmacodynamic level, where the structure of the drug molecule makes it more active at one receptor than another, or on the pharmacokinetic level where the molecular structure of the drug makes it more available to specific tissues. Equally important, the new structure should retain ACh's activity (see Box 16.1).

Adding an alkyl group on the beta position relative to the quaternary ammonium group will provide a shield which will inhibit nucleophilic attacks and also provide an electroinductive group which will decrease the dipole activity of the ester function. The tight fit at the receptor mentioned previously dictates this alkyl group should be only a small one; in fact, anything larger than a methyl group yields better stability but a poorer activity. Methacholine (Fig. 16.5) is mainly used via inhalation for the diagnosis of asthma (challenge test). It is a water-soluble drug and it is not active via oral absorption and does not cross the blood–brain barrier (BBB). The addition of an extra methyl group creates a chiral centre.

The extra methyl group led to enhanced selectivity at the muscarinic receptor and diminished activity at the nicotine receptor. Methacholine was designed to ensure stability against chemical hydrolysis, but the additional group appeared to provide hindrance to access of cholinesterase as well, and methacholine is three times more resistant to esterase hydrolysis than ACh.

Another approach to reduce the attacks of nucleophiles is to decrease the dipole activity by countering the positive dipole charge on the carbonyl carbon. This could be achieved by replacing the alkyl function with an amine group to create a carbamate (carbachol, Fig. 16.5). The lone pair of electrons on the nitrogen delocalises, countering the partial positive charge formed on the carbonyl carbon, hence making it less vulnerable to nucleophilic attack.

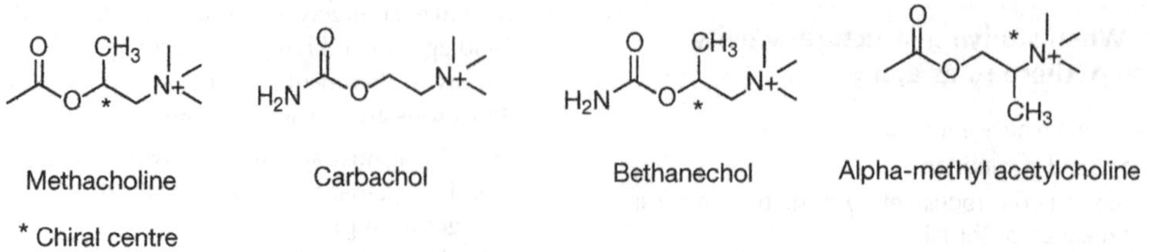

Figure 16.5 Modifications of the acetylcholine structure.

Carbachol (carbamylcholine) is mainly used in eyedrops for the treatment of glaucoma, an ophthalmic disease resulting a high pressure inside the oculus which can be relieved by cholinergic agonist action. Carbachol induces miosis and increases the drainage of aqueous humour. Carbachol has a very slight increased preference for the nicotinic receptor, but is still considered a non-selective cholinergic agent just like ACh. It is introduced in 0.01% w/v sterile eyedrops (carbachol chloride) for the treatment of open-angle glaucoma.[8]

Bethanechol combines the two modifications described above. It is resistant to both chemical and enzymatic hydrolysis and consequently has a relatively long half-life of 60–90 minutes. Bethanechol is a chiral drug due to the methyl addition at the β-position relative to the quaternary ammonium. The muscarinic receptor is strongly stereoselective and (S)-bethanechol is 1000 times more potent than (R)-bethanechol.[9] But these agents are still produced as racemates.

Q Self Test 16.1

Which is R and which is S bethanecol?

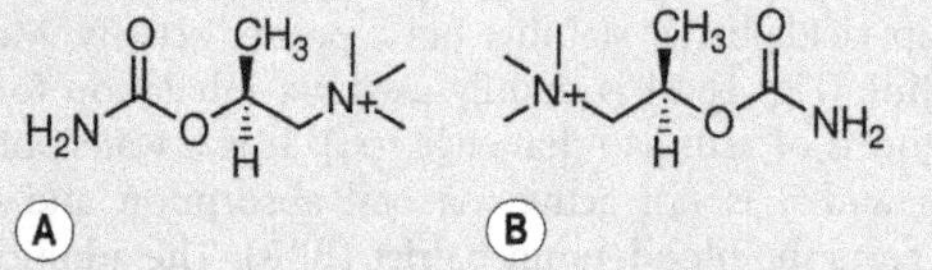

Bethanechol is, like methacholine, highly selective for the muscarinic receptor and shows no appreciable nicotinic action. It is reported to be selective for M3 muscarinic subtype as well. Cholinergic drugs are used to restore bowel movement following surgical manipulations or congenital megacolon, and to counteract urinary retention, for instance resulting from trauma. Bethanechol is the drug of choice for treating these conditions. It is used orally (10–25 mg three to four times per day). It shows systemic activity when administered subcutaneously and it is used in doses of 5 mg. Notice the low oral bioavailability. There is a very strict rule regarding the use of cholinergic drugs in these conditions. The depressed smooth muscles should be obstruction free; otherwise application of the drug will increase the pressure and could lead to perforation.[10]

ADDITIONAL INFORMATION

- It is noteworthy that adding a methyl group to the δ-position relative to quaternary ammonium in ACh has led to significant selectivity at the nicotinic receptor (δ-methylacetylcholine; Fig. 16.5). All these agents are cleared mainly via the kidneys, and acidification of urine (e.g. by ingestion of ascorbic acid) enhances excretion.
- Cholinergic agonists are used for the treatment of glaucoma. Glaucoma is characterised by increased intraocular pressure.
- Cholinergic activity leads to reducing the secretion, as well as relaxing the ciliary body, allowing for outflow of aqueous humour which decreases intraocular pressure.
- Angle-closure glaucoma is an emergency state which can be controlled by muscarinic agonist drug treatment until the patient is stable and ready for an inevitable surgery.
- Open-angle glaucoma is a chronic disease which should be corrected to avoid vision loss. Recently introduced laser techniques have superseded drug treatment of glaucoma.
- Cholinergic receptor agonists are used in correcting accommodative esotropia, an ocular disease in young children.

Other cholinergic agonists

Demecarium (Fig.16.6) is used in veterinary medicine for the treatment of glaucoma in animals.

Pilocarpine (Fig. 16.6) is another botanical alkaloid structurally related to muscarine acting on the cholinergic system. It was first extracted from the leaves of plants from the genus *Pilocarpus*. Pilocarpine shows a muscarinic agonist activity, with selectivity to M3 which is found in the eye. The selectivity made it a first-line choice for the treatment of both types of glaucoma (open and closed angle). It is given as eyedrops (concentration of 4% w/v), as long-acting plastic implants in the conjunctival sac, or as eyedrops in combination with physostigmine in the case of treatment of closed-angle glaucoma. Pilocarpine is also used as an antidote for toxicity caused by scopolamine or atropine.

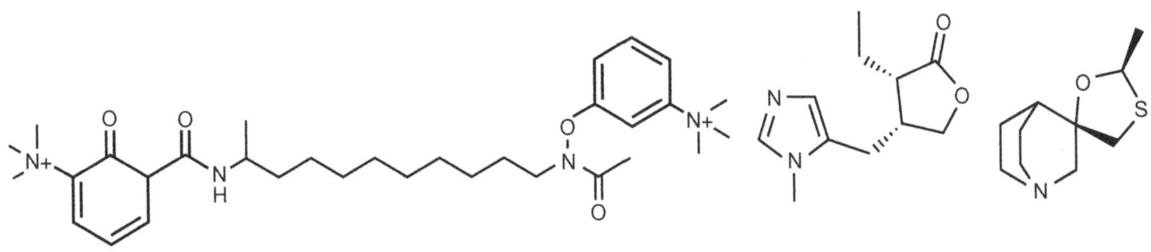

Figure 16.6 Additional miscellaneous cholinergic agonists.

Cevimeline (Fig. 16.6) is a new direct-acting muscarinic agonist highly selective for the M3 receptor. It is used for the treatment of dry mouth associated with Sjögren's syndrome, an autoimmune disease where atypical antibodies destroy the glands which produce tears and saliva.

ANTIACETYLCHOLINESTERASE DRUGS

Acetylcholinesterase (AChE) is situated next to any cholinergic receptor. It catches the molecule once it has departed its active site and renders it inactive by breaking the ester bond to give choline, which is taken by the presynaptic terminus, and acetate. Hydrolysis of acetylcholine and restoration of the active site of the enzyme completes in about 150 microseconds. AChE is a treelike enzyme, with the stem implemented in the cell membrane and the branches (three) protruding out of the cell membrane. Each branch holds four active sites composing an army of twelve active sites ready to capture any unbound ACh. This makes AChE activity one of the most efficient hydrolysis processes in biology. The active site was thought to include an aspartic acid residue which was supposed to hold ACh by ionic bonding, and a tyrosine residue which interacts with an oxygen ester group via a H-bond. However, recent studies have shown the active site to be buried deep in the enzyme, with no negatively charged residues. Instead, the positive charge of the quaternary ammonium interacts with a series of aromatic residues, possibly via a charge transfer interaction (see Ch. 1). AChE holds the ACh molecule in place by a peripheral site composed of a tryptophan at position 279 and tyrosine at position 121. This peripheral site fixes the ACh in the right orientation in preparation for the action of the catalytic site which consists of the catalytic triad (serine–histidine–aspartate) and two additional aromatic amino acids tryptophan 84 and phenylalanine 330 which may play a further role in orientation of the ACh. The whole arrangement holds the ester region in an orientation where it is in a proximity to a serine residue situated next to a histidine residue. This arrangement is essential for the hydrolysis efficiency, where histidine plays a vital rule in fortifying the nucleophilic activity of serine which, in the absence of the acid/base catalysis of histidine, is just an aliphatic alcohol and thus too weak a nucleophile to hydrolyse an ester by itself. Drugs which inhibit the hydrolysis action of cholinesterase will preserve endogenous ACh in the synaptic cleft, thus eliciting a drug action exactly like the injection of ACh, with a duration of action which can be modified (see below). The mechanism of the hydrolysis by AChE is shown in Figure 16.7.

The work on anticholinesterase drugs is a good example for the impact of chemical knowledge on the outcome in medicinal chemistry. In this case, a best fit in the enzyme active site may not be the most active compound, as chemistry of hydrolysis rather than enzyme binding seems to be the determinant factor of activity. Cholinesterase inhibitors have less effect on smooth muscles, thus on blood pressure, than direct acting cholinergic agonists.

The antiacetylcholinesterase drugs

According to their mechanism of action, the anti-AChE agents can be divided into three groups.

Competitive antagonists

Quaternary alcohols such as edrophonium (Fig. 16.8) act as competitive antagonists with ACh to AChE. Edrophonium works without the involvement of any covalent bonds, which form in the case of other antagonists. It is used for diagnosis and dose titration purposes before and within the therapeutic regimen used for the treatment of myasthenia gravis, an autoimmune disease where the body destroys the nicotinic receptors (AChNR) (see Box 16.3). It is of vital importance to choose the right dose used for anticholinesterase treatment as low doses will keep the patient in agony, and higher doses will elicit muscarinic hyperactivity (abdominal cramps, bronchial constriction and increased secretions, among other symptoms) and an

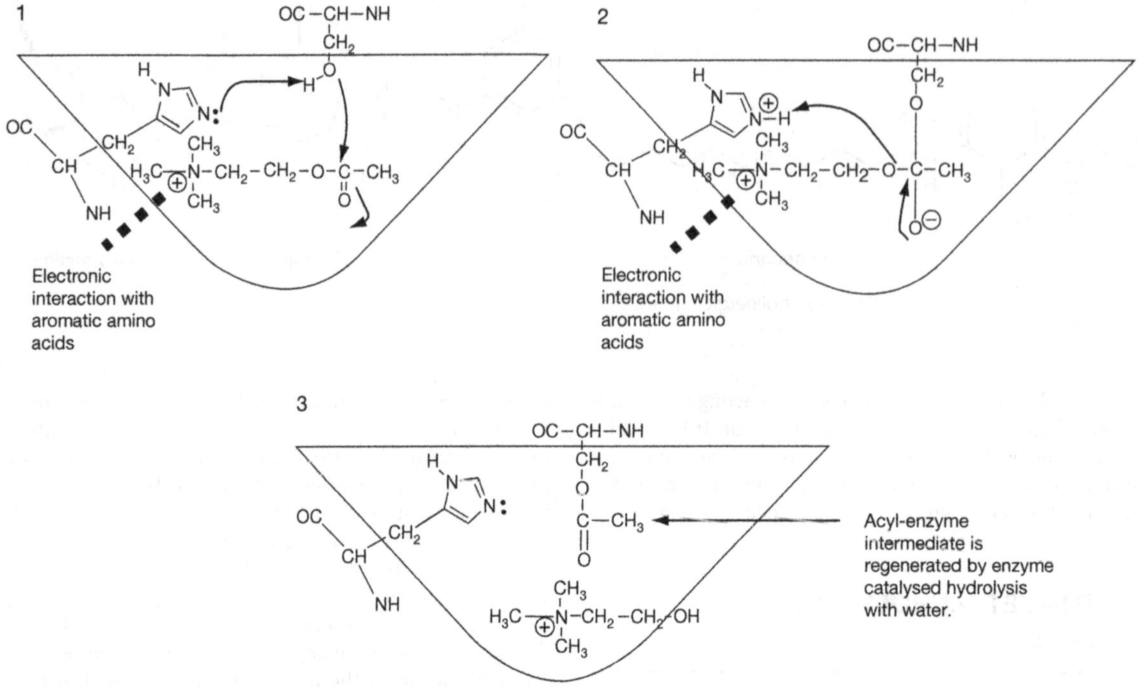

Figure 16.7 The mechanism of hydrolysis of ACh by AChE.

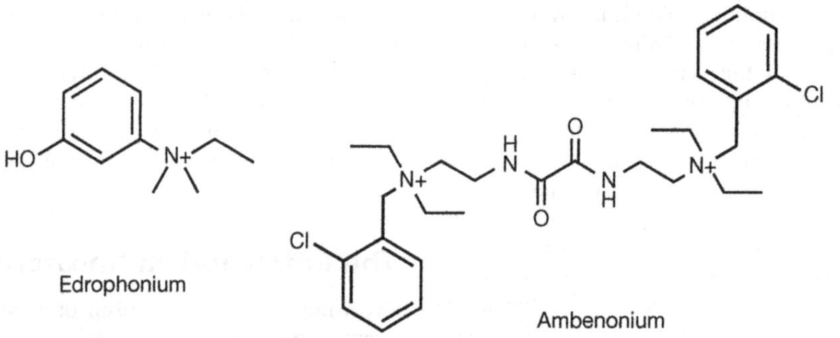

Figure 16.8 Competitive antagonists of AChE.

excessive dose may worsen the situation by evoking a nicotinic depolarising blockade (a clinical situation termed as cholinergic crisis). The edrophonium (Tensilon) test uses an injection of edrophonium chloride (10 mg). The activity starts 30–60 seconds after the injection and lasts for 10 minutes. Edrophonium was used to treat supraventricular arrhythmias, but has been superseded by newer agents of different pharmacological classes.

Ambenonium is another competitive inhibitor of AChE. It is composed of two moieties structurally related to edrophonium connected by an oxaldiamide bridge. This is thought to provide a competitive shield of the two active sites in the AChE. It is used as its bromide salt for treating myasthenia gravis in dose intervals of 3–6 hours.

Short-acting carbamate anticholinesterase agents

The remaining groups of anti-AChE drugs all cause formation of a covalent bond with the serine residue in AChE, which is more resistant to nucleophilic attack by water than the normal acetyl group and thus slows down recycling of the enzyme. A good anticholinesterase drug should:

1. contain a leaving group which is equal in efficiency of dissociation to the acetyl group in ACh.

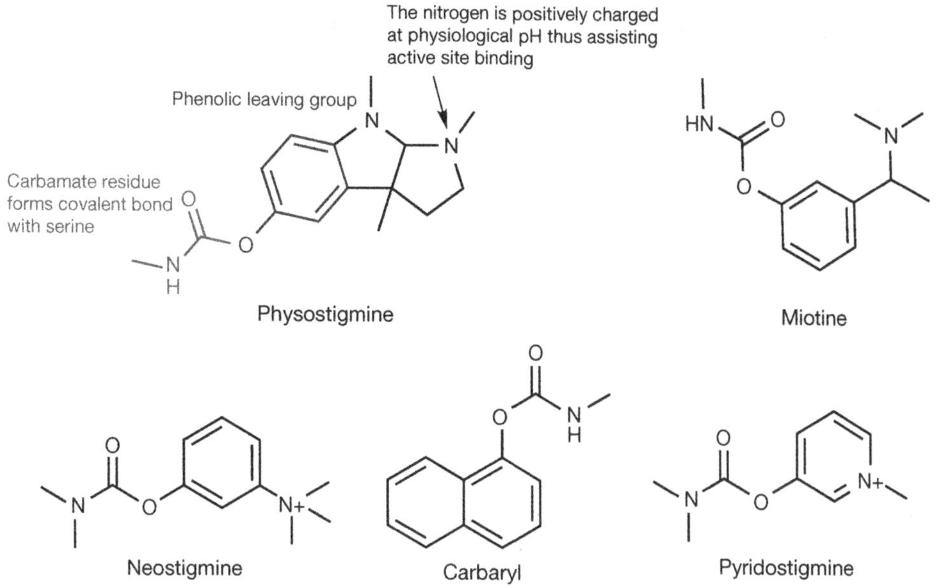

Figure 16.9 Anti-AChE agents which transfer a carbamate group.

2. the leaving group should produce a residual group bound to serine, which is less susceptible to hydrolysis than acetate.
3. contain a positively charged motif to fix the molecule in the right position/orientation in the enzyme's active site.

Physostigmine (Fig. 16.9) was discovered in 1864 and its structure was established in 1925. It is extracted from the plant *Physostigma venenosum* (calabar bean) and it was the first compound found to show anti-AChE activity. Physostigmine has serious side effects which limit its use, but it provided a prototype which medicinal chemists could use as a lead compound and improve it. The important structural elements within the molecule are shown in Figure 16.9.

The three structural elements mentioned above with regard of the structure of physostigmine are as follows:

1. A phenol carbamate is required since it is easily hydrolysed (*cf.* aspirin) thus it readily transfers its carbamate group to serine. The hydrophobic interaction produced by the benzene is thought to be important as well.
2. The carbamate group works exactly as the nitrogen in carbachol which stabilises the linkage by providing its lone pair to the positive carbonyl carbon, making it less attractive to weak nucleophiles (water in this case). Thus carbamate agents such as physostigmine undergo the hydrolysis via the action of AChE, but form a carbamoyl serine (or methyl carbamoyl serine), which is more stable than acetate against hydrolysis required for the restoration of the active site. Regeneration takes 30–60 minutes compared with 150 microseconds in the case of the acetylated enzyme. This is forty million times slower than the hydrolysis of serine acetate.
3. In physostigmine the methyl pyrrolidine is not a quaternary ammonium, yet it is protonated at physiological pH, hence satisfying the third rule which requires a positively charged group for binding to the active site.

Physostigmine is used as a drug either locally in the treatment of glaucoma, or in the treatment of atropine poisoning. It exhibits serious side effects including psychoneurological effects, being originally used to extract the truth from criminals who were made to swallow an extract of calabar beans (ordeal beans). The drug is susceptible to chemical hydrolysis. It is available as physostigmine salicylate injection (1 mg). It is not permanently charged, and can cross the BBB (Box 16.2), causing central side effects. Antimuscarinic and tricyclic antidepressant toxicity cause severe muscarinic blockade. Physostigmine has been employed in treating toxicity due to muscarinic receptor blockers and tricyclic antidepressants via promoting an increase in ACh levels. The ability of this agent to cross the BBB makes it the chosen drug for this condition. However, it produces its own toxic effects, which restrict its use to severe cases uncontrollable with symptomatic therapy.

The task for medicinal chemists was to produce analogues of physostigmine with similar activity and fewer side effects (especially on CNS) and with better chemical stability. Miotine (Fig. 16.9) followed physostigmine as a first synthetic AChE inhibitor. It is still prone to chemical hydrolysis and its non-permanently charged tertiary

> Box 16.2 **Blood–brain barrier (BBB)**
>
> Only un-ionised drugs cross the BBB. One could ask, if the tertiary amines are all protonated, when they access their receptor, i.e. at physiological pH, how come they still can cross the BBB? This is because most, but not all, the molecules are protonated. For instance, at pH = 7.4, physostigmine (p*Ka* = 8.2) will be only 86% protonated and 14% unprotonated. This ratio is always constant. The unprotonated lipophilic form will cross the BBB and disrupt the balanced status, leading to production of new unprotonated molecules which will, in turn, cross BBB and so on.

amine group grants it access to the CNS, leading to undesired side effects there.

Neostigmine (Fig. 16.9) is a further modification on miotine where the methylcarbamate group is replaced with dimethylcarbamate, making the compound more resistant to chemical hydrolysis due to the added inductive effect of the second methyl group. This permanently charged quaternary nitrogen in neostigmine prevents it from crossing the BBB, making it a safe drug from a CNS perspective, and encourages binding to the enzyme active site. The quaternary ammonium is directly attached to the benzene ring, which forces nitrogen into the same plane as the ring, making a stable/fixed conformation for the whole molecule. This is thought to contribute to the enhanced activity of neostigmine. It was historically used as a pregnancy test as it induces menstrual bleeding in the absence of pregnancy, but was superseded by hormonal tests. Neostigmine has additional direct effect at nicotinic receptors, which makes it a better treatment for myasthenia gravis syndrome. The dose is titrated according to the edrophonium test, but its short duration of action requires an inconvenient frequency of dosing (every 2–3 hours). Sustained-release products are available for night usage. Neostigmine is used for treating postoperative depression of smooth muscles (paralysis of stomach or bowel, or urinary retention). It is used orally (15 mg) or subcutaneously (0.5–1 mg). Note the high oral dose which indicates its very low oral bioavailability. It is used as well in congenital megacolon and other clinical situations involving depression of smooth muscles. Neostigmine is used to promptly reverse anaesthesia-produced paralysis. The prompt effect necessitates the use of intravenous or intramuscular dosage forms. A final indication for neostigmine is its use as an antidote for atropine poisoning.

Carbaryl is another carbamate anti-AChE agent which has a high fat solubility. It was designed for rapid distribution into the CNS of insects and it was used until 2004 as a lotion for the treatment of head lice.

Pyridostigmine (Fig. 16.9) is close in structure to both neostigmine and miotine. The aromatic ring (leaving group) is preserved but attached to a methylpyridine ring rather than a benzene ring. A permanent charge is provided by the aromatic ring as well. It is used for myasthenia gravis and it leads to better patient compliance than neostigmine as the dose frequency is less (every 3–6 hours). The dose is determined by the edrophonium test.

> Box 16.3 **Myasthenia gravis**
>
> Myasthenia gravis is an autoimmune disease where antibodie to the nicotinic receptors are produced which decrease the number of functional nicotinic receptors. The syndrome is associated with general weakness in all muscles, especially the small ones such as those in the head, neck and extremities. Providing strong agonists of the nicotinic receptor or keeping a high concentration of the acetylcholine at the postsynaptic junction will improve the patient's condition and help improve daily activities. The drug class of choice for treating the symptoms of myasthenia gravis is the short-acting anticholinesterase agents. The dose requirement in this disease changes too rapidly to allow for the use of longer-acting anticholinesterases. Any observed muscarinic activity may be treated with antimuscarinic drugs such as atropine.

Pyridostigmine is used to reverse anaesthesia-produced paralysis in the same fashion as neostigmine.

Long-acting organophosphate agents

Irreversible inhibitors of AChE act in a similar way as the carbamates, but the phosphate bond is stable for hundreds of hours. It is further strengthened by the ageing phenomenon, where the phosphorylated serine on the active site loses one of its oxygens, leading to a phosphine–serine bond, which is even more resistant to hydrolysis.

These compounds were first intended to be (but fortunately never used) as chemical warfare agents. The prototype compounds were dyflos and sarin (nerve gases). These compounds irreversibly phosphorylate the serine hydroxyl motif in AChE. The reaction product is very stable and can not be hydrolysed by weak nucleophiles, even with histidine catalysis. This increases the availability of endogenous ACh in the synaptic gap, leading to a constant signalling at the smooth and skeletal muscles, paralysis and death.

Dyflos and sarin (Fig. 16.10) are extremely active and have serious side effects, thus limiting their use to local ophthalmic administration for the treatment of glaucoma. The binding of these agents is irreversible and a new enzyme is needed in order for the cells to restore ACh hydrolysing capacity.

The number of organophosphates synthesised as insecticides is estimated to be 50 000. Organophosphates are generally very lipid soluble (ecothiopate is an exception, and is soluble and stable in aqueous solutions), and many of them are chemically unstable. Among the organophosphates, ecothiopate, malathion and parathion have

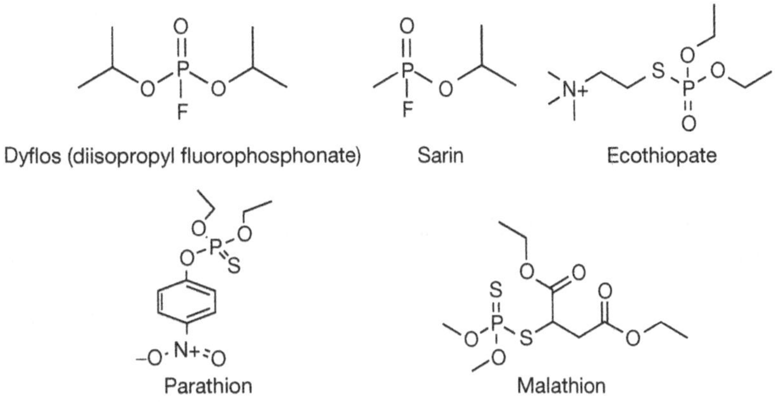

Figure 16.10 Organophosphate AChE inhibitors.

satisfactory stability. This led to the widespread use of these agents since environmental stability determines the frequency of application. Ecothipate was developed to selectively bind to AChE. This was achieved by introducing a quaternary ammonium group at a suitable distance (the two carbon bridge rule) from the phosphorylating head group. Ecothiopate is more potent than dyflos, and its stability in aqueous solutions (up to several weeks) enables its use as eyedrops for the treatment of glaucoma. It dissociates from AChE over a few days. It is manufactured as ophthalmic drops of ecothiopate iodide (1.5–12.5 mg/5 mL) for the treatment of glaucoma and accommodative esotropia, an ocular disease in young children. Despite its toxicity, ecothiopate is considered the second line for the treatment of open-angle glaucoma uncontrollable by short-acting cholinergic agonists.

Parathion and malathion (Fig. 16.10) are examples of insecticides which function by irreversibly inhibiting AChE. These compounds have a phosphorylating head group similar to dyflos and sarin, but with one oxygen substituted by a sulphur. Surprisingly, these compounds, despite their potent insecticidal activity, are relatively safe for humans. The design of these compounds stemmed from a knowledge of the differences in biosynthetic pathways between vertebrates and insects. The compounds are inactive in both insects and humans, but they are converted to their active forms where the sulphur is changed to an oxygen by metabolism in the body. This metabolic process happens in both insects and vertebrates, but in the latter it happens in parallel with metabolic detoxification, which makes these agents rather safe.[11] Parathion is prone to detoxifying metabolism with a slower rate than malathion, which makes the latter safer. Fish are not able to detoxify these agents, and fish deaths have been reported when using parathion and malathion insecticides in areas of proximity to water. In spite of the proposed safety, these compounds, owing to their high lipid solubility, can be absorbed via the skin and accumulate in fatty tissues. Thus they should be treated with extra care.

Antidote for irreversible antiacetylcholinesterases

Phosphorylated AChE, but not the phosphinylated (post aging) enzyme, is susceptible to hydrolysis when treated with a strong nucleophile such as hydroxylamine. Again, the design here is heavily based on the chemical knowledge of the designer. The serine phosphate ester created by agents such as dyflos is extremely stable, and requires a strong nucleophile to break it. Hydroxylamine seems to be the most suitable candidate for the job, but it is also very toxic. The antidote was designed as a prodrug which would release hydroxylamine, or provide a hydroxylamine moiety only at the site of action. Specific binding to the AChE enzyme is strongly needed to increase potency and reduce side effects. This could be achieved by providing an ACh-like tail separated judiciously from a hydroxylamine head. Pralidoxime (Fig. 16.11) was the outcome of this combined knowledge, with a quaternary ammonium tail which interacts with the hydrophobic pocket in AChE securing better approachability for the hydroxylamine head to attack the phosphorylated serine.

Pralidoxime is permanently charged, hence, it can not counteract the organophosphorylation in the CNS (remember, irreversible anti-AChEs are lipid soluble, thus expected to easily pass to the CNS). ProPAM (Fig. 16.11) is a prodrug of pralidoxime, and was designed as a

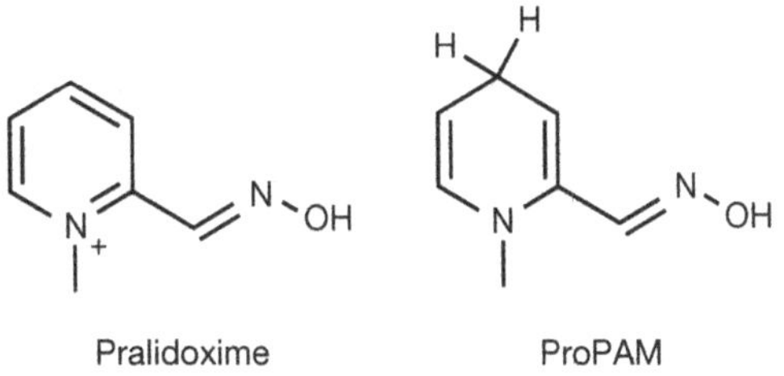

Figure 16.11 Antidotes to irreversible AChE inhibitors.

reduced form of pralidoxime. The permanent charge (necessary for drug activity) is lost by reduction, allowing Pro-PAM to cross the BBB where the charge (thus the activity) can be regained by enzymatic oxidation. The permanently charged molecule cannot leave the CNS, which improves the availability of the antidote in the desired site.

CENTRALLY ACTING CHOLINERGIC DRUGS

Acetylcholine neurotransmission was found to play an essential role in memory function, Alzheimer's disease and parkinsonism. This has added a new (CNS) dimension to the therapeutic portfolio of cholinergic drugs, specifically muscarinic agents, as muscarinic subtype receptors are predominant in the CNS.[12]

Tacrine (Fig. 16.12) is an AChE inhibitor which exerts its action in the CNS as an anticholinesterase and a cholinergic agonist as well. However, it causes hepatotoxicity. It has poor absorption from the gut which necessitates an inconvenient four-times-daily dosage regimen.[13] Donepezil (Fig. 16.12) is a more selective, less hepatotoxic member of this family. It has an excellent oral absorption, passes across the BBB and has a long half-life (70 hours) allowing for a once-daily (5–10 mg) treatment. Both drugs are approved to be used to ameliorate the cognitive deterioration associated with Alzheimer's disease, and donepezil has been tested for the treatment of other types of secondary dementia. The two drugs do not seem to be structurally related, or related to other cholinesterase inhibitors.

Huperzine A (Fig. 16.12) from the plant *Huperzia serrata*, which has a long history of use in the Chinese herb library, was found to have AChE activity. It is safer than tacrine and donepezil and has been used in clinical trials for treating Alzheimer's disease and epilepsy.

Galanthamine (Fig. 16.12, galantamine) is another example of a drug of botanical origin. It is now chemically synthesised for large-scale production purposes, but was first isolated in 1959 from *Galanthus woronowii* (Voronov's snowdrop). It is a competitive and reversible cholinesterase inhibitor with a very good oral bioavailability (80–100%) and a half-life of 7 hours. The side effects of galantamine may not be tolerable, and dose titration is necessary to improve tolerability. It is available as a tablet, extended-release capsule or oral solution in doses of 4–12 mg.

ANTICHOLINERGIC DRUGS

Countering the action of ACh leads to several physiological responses which have been therapeutically exploited for treatment of diseases or for synergising with the action of other medications. It is of great importance for this antagonism to be selective for a specific receptor subtype or even a specific tissue. As the muscarinic (AChMR) and nicotinic (AChNR) cholinergic receptors are not structurally similar, and they do not function in the same manner, we can classify the cholinergic antagonists into two categories: muscarinic antagonists and nicotinic antagonists.

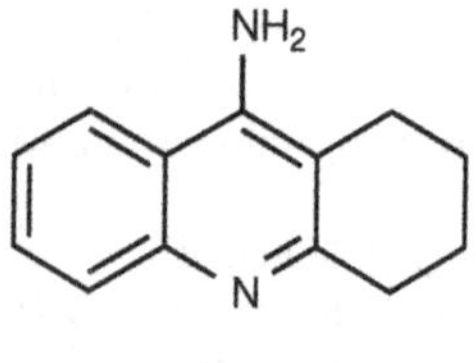

Tacrine

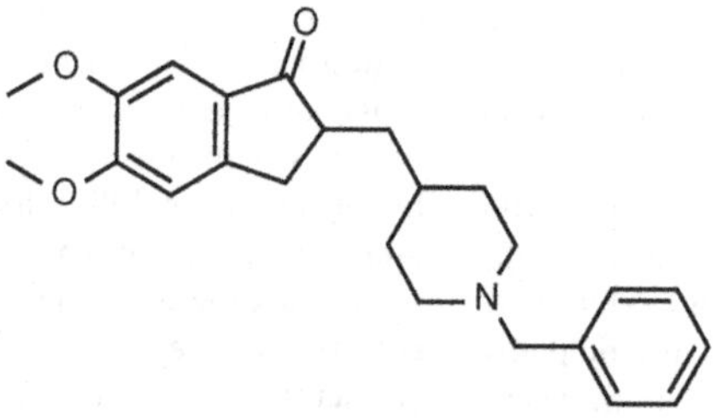

Donepezil

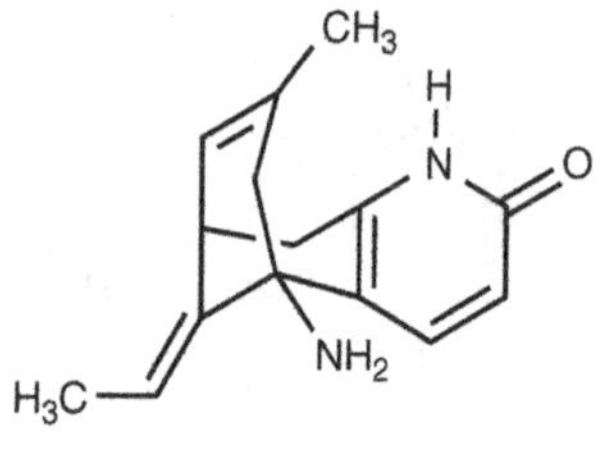

Huperzine A

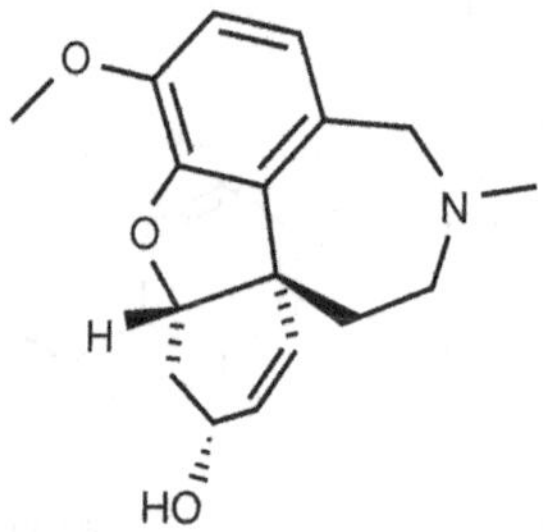

Galantamine

Figure 16.12 Centrally acting cholinergic drugs.

Muscarinic antagonists

The muscarinic receptors are of the G-protein family. They are all composed of seven transmembrane segments arranged in a serpentine fashion where the third cytoplasmic loop is coupled to a G-protein. Five different subtypes of muscarinic receptors have been identified by DNA cloning. Three of these subtypes M1, M2 and M3, have been assigned definite functions, where as M4 and M5 are suspected to be related to a CNS cholinergic activity.[5] The activation of these subtypes results in different post-receptor second messenger signals, with M1, M3 and M5 activating the inositol-3-phosphate and diacylglycerol cascade and M2 and M4 leading to inhibition of cAMP production.[14] The tissue distribution of muscarinic receptors varies as well. M1 is found in nerves, cortex, hippocampus and secretory glands. M2 is dominant in the heart and smooth muscles; hence M2 is called the cardiac M2 receptor.[15] M3 is found in glands (exocrine glands), smooth muscles and endothelium.[16] M4 is found in the neostriatum, and M5 in substantia nigra. It is necessary that the antimuscarinic agent has a considerable selectivity for cholinergic receptors rather than any other types of receptor and for muscarinic receptors rather than nicotinic receptors. Ideally, activity should be at a specific subtype of the muscarinic receptor in harmony with the desired action. The effect of a specific drug varies across tissues and this can be attributed to the pharmacokinetic (distribution) and pharmacodynamic (selectivity) properties of the drug.

Antimuscarinic agents

The first-discovered muscarinic antagonist was atropine which occurs as a secondary metabolite in the roots of the plant *Atropa belladonna* and other plants of the species *Solanaceae*. Atropine is an ester of tropine with hydroxymethylphenylacetic acid. The cosmetic use of extracts of belladonna for dilating the pupils to render women more attractive eventually led to its use (mydriatic) in the examination of the cornea in ophthalmology. Atropine is biosynthesised as a single enantiomer (called L-hyoscyamine), but once in solution, it easily racemises due to the carbonyl group situated in the alpha position to the chiral centre (Fig. 16.13).

Pure atropine was isolated in 1831 and is still in use as a drug today. It is highly selective for cholinergic receptors and specifically for the muscarinic receptor. Its action at the nicotinic receptor is undetectable at subtoxic doses. It is more selective for muscarinic receptors than any of the synthetic antimuscarinic agents which may show ganglionic blocking effects or histamine blocking effects. However, it is non-selective for the subtypes of muscarinic receptors. Atropine has a half-life of 2 hours and the effect of the drug declines after this time in all organs but the eye. Certain species, e.g. rabbits, have an atropine esterase which will deactivate the drug more rapidly. It is most effective in salivary, bronchial and sweat glands, and least effective in the parietal cells in the stomach.

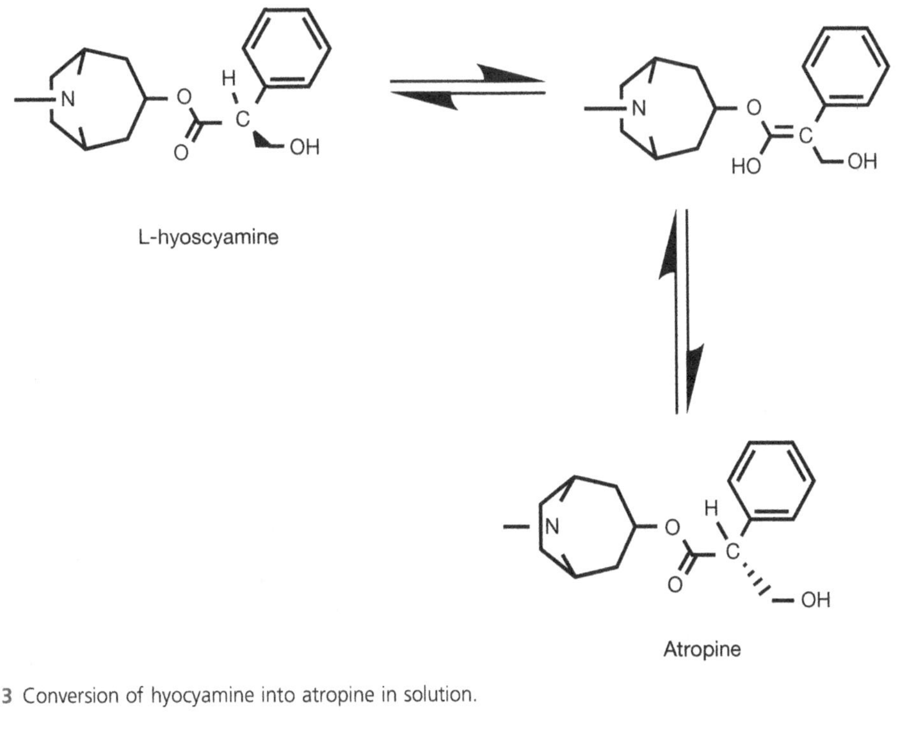

Figure 16.13 Conversion of hyocyamine into atropine in solution.

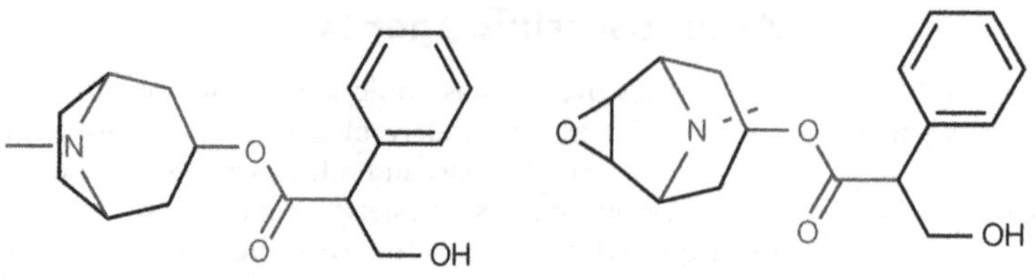

Figure 16.14 The active moiety in the structure of atropine and scopolamine.

Atropine is used to inhibit the secretion induced by the irritant effect of inhaled anaesthetic agents at the bronchi. It is given in i.v. injection prior to anaesthesia with doses of 0.5–1 mg. Parenteral atropine has an emergency site use in countering the vagal depression of the sinoatrial node function resulting from myocardial infarction. It is used as well in myasthenia gravis for controlling the muscarinic side effects associated with prolonged anti-AChE therapy.

Atropine, owing to its long duration of action on the eye, is suitable for preventing adhesion formation in uveitis. Other ocular uses include the preparation for ophthalmic examination of non-compliant patients (e.g. children) as eyedrops (1% of atropine sulphate).

Atropine has shown a great efficacy against diarrhoea, especially when combined with a morphine receptor agonist. The commercial combination Lomotil (atropine sulphate 0.025 mg/dephenoxylate. HCl 2.5 mg) is one of the best treatments for diarrhoea. However, atropine in this case is used to produce some side effects which will discourage the abuse of diphenoxylate.

Atropine suppresses sweating, which is tolerable in adults, but can cause atropine fever in children, even at ordinary doses. Urinary retention and gastric hypomotility, usually expected post surgery, are exacerbated with antimuscarinic use.

Hyoscine (scopolamine, Fig. 16.14) is another natural antimuscarinic agent. It was isolated in 1879 from *Datura stramonium* (thorn apple). The structure has the addition of an oxygen bridge to the complex tropine ring system in atropine. This seems to increase the activity, especially in the CNS. This is probably because it is a much weaker base p*Ka* 7.6 compared with atropine (p*Ka* 9.9), this being due to the electron withdrawing effect of the oxygen reducing the availability of the lone pair on the nitrogen. Scopolamine has been used for many years as a prophylaxis and for the treatment for motion sickness. It is as effective as any other recently introduced treatment. It is given by mouth (0.3 mg three times daily), injection or transdermal batches (1.5 mg). It induces a dry mouth and sedation via all routes of administration.

Scopolamine is interchangeable with atropine in preventing laryngospasm (by reducing bronchial secretion) in surgery. Its central effect, especially induced amnesia, is considered desirable in such traumatic events. The precautions in the use of atropine still apply to scopolamine.

Both compounds have in their skeleton an acetylcholine like section, i.e. a nitrogen, protonated at physiological pH, and an ester separated by three carbons (coloured with red in Fig. 16.14). Both compounds are tertiary amines which cross the BBB and produce CNS side effects, scopolamine being more likely to do this in view of its lower p*Ka* value.

The two compounds occur naturally as the S (−) isomers but they are used therapeutically as racemic mixtures although with decreased activity compared to the natural form since The S (−) form is at least 100 times more potent than the R (+) form which reflects the enantioselective nature of the muscarinic receptor.

Q Self Test 16.2

Which enantiomer of scopolamine is shown below? Why is centre 2 not chiral?

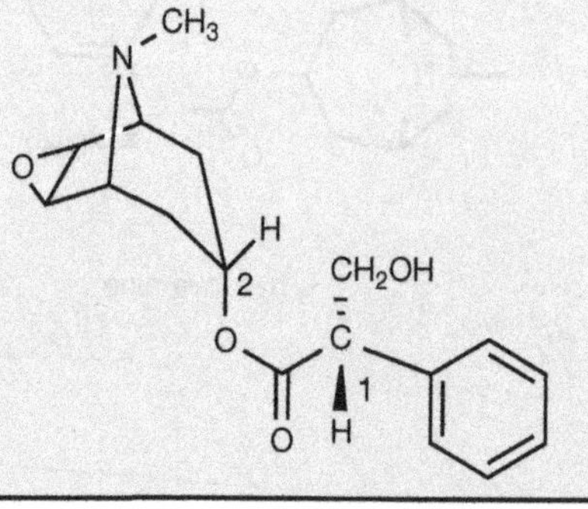

Starting from these two compounds, synthetic compounds were produced taking into consideration the need to diminish the disadvantages of the natural compounds. Note here that there is more flexibility with the length of the carbon bridge between the ester and the nitrogen, and there is no restriction with regard to alkyl substitution on the nitrogen or with regard to the acetyl motif on the ester side, as was discussed earlier in cholinergic agonists. This is because we do not need an exact fit on the receptor here to switch it on, but rather we are a seeking a mechanism to

Figure 16.15 Quaternary ammonium agents related to atropine.

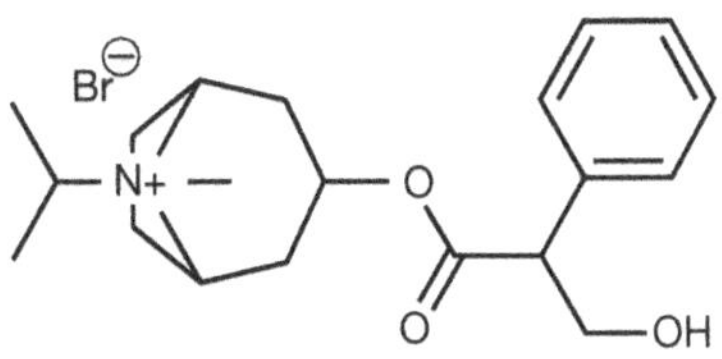

Ipratropium bromide

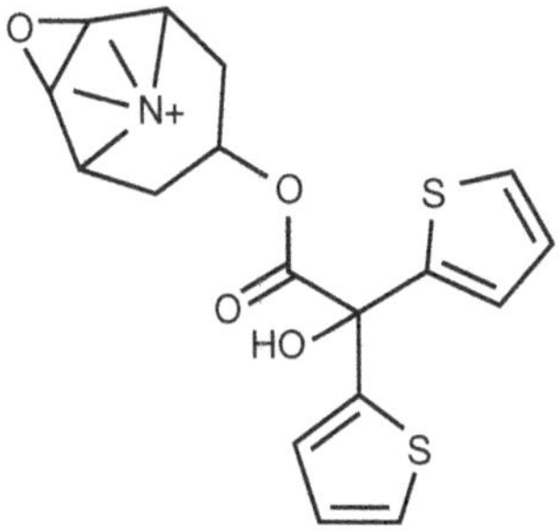

Tiotropium

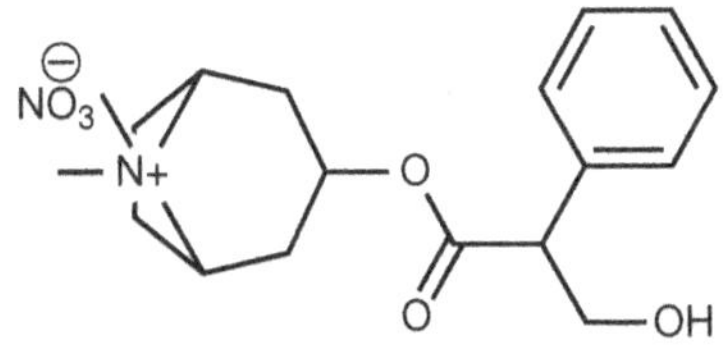

Atropine methonitrate

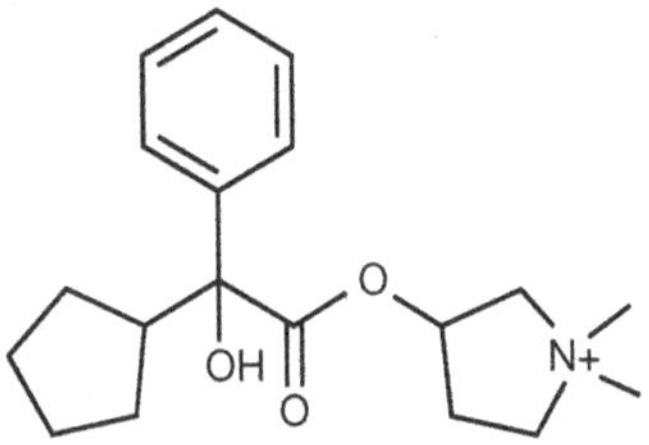

Glycopyrronium bromide

prevent endogenous ACh from accessing the active site on the receptor.

Ipratropium bromide (Fig. 16.15) is a synthetic quaternary ammonium compound made by adding an isopropyl alkyl group to the tertiary nitrogen in atropine (think of the name as three syllables ipr-atrop-ium (ipr from isopropyl, atrop from atropine, and ium) because it is a quaternary ammonIUM). Antimuscarinic activity at the muscarinic receptor M3 leads to bronchodilation and reduction of bronchial secretion. This effect is more significant in patients with chronic obstructive pulmonary diseases (COPD). The selectivity of M3/M2 for the chosen antimuscarinic agent is crucial for these effects, as blocking M2 will remove the autoinhibitory effect of ACh and trigger a stronger cholinergic discharge in postganglionic nerves, releasing more ACh to compete more with the muscarinic M3 antagonist. Ipratropium seems to be highly selective for M3, and is employed in metered-dose aerosols for the treatment of COPD (such as asthma) with a concentration of 40 μg/actuation. The dosage form provides maximum drug distribution at the desired tissue of action, and minimum systemic side effects. Ipratropium does not cross BBB due to its permanent charge; hence it shows very few CSN side effects. The dose varies widely according to the severity of the condition (2–6 actuations per dose) and the short half-life of ipratropium requires a frequent dosing (2–4 times per day).

Tiotropium (Fig. 16.15) is a long-acting antimuscarinic agent with a similar selectivity profile to ipratropium. It is structurally related to scopolamine with substitution of the phenyl ring with two aromatic thiazol rings, and replacement of the hydroxymethyl group alpha to carbonyl group with a hydroxyl group. Tiotropium combines the ACh-like skeleton with the branched hydrophobic rings (discussed below). In clinical trials, tiotropium was superior to ipratropium in improving asthmatic patients, and allowed a reduction of the concomitant use of salbutamol. The long half-life of tiotropium (dissociation half-life of M3=35 hours) allows for a once-daily (18 μg) use. The dosage form is a dry powder inhalation, provided as capsules applied via an inhalation device. The capsules are ineffective when taken orally and may cause intolerable side effects.[17,18,19]

Atropine methonitrate (Fig. 16.15) is a methylated quaternary ammonium atropine. It was found to increase the activity of the myenteric plexus (a plexus of sympathetic and parasympathetic nerves supplying the two layers of muscles in the small intestine). Its permanent charge prevents its absorption by the gastrointestinal tract where it works locally for treating intestinal cramps.

The complex ring system is not really crucial for the antimuscarinic activity. This is illustrated by the potency of glycopyrronium bromide. The ester group seems to be important but not vital. Some compounds such as benzhexol (trihexyphenidyl (Fig. 16.16) have shown antimuscarinic activity even with no ester group at all. Glycopyrronium bromide (Fig. 16.15) is an example of an antimuscarinic compound which does not have the tropine ring system. The tropinium in atropine methonitrate was replaced by a simple pyrrolydinium ring, while the phenyl in the bulky blocking unit found in atropine was preserved,

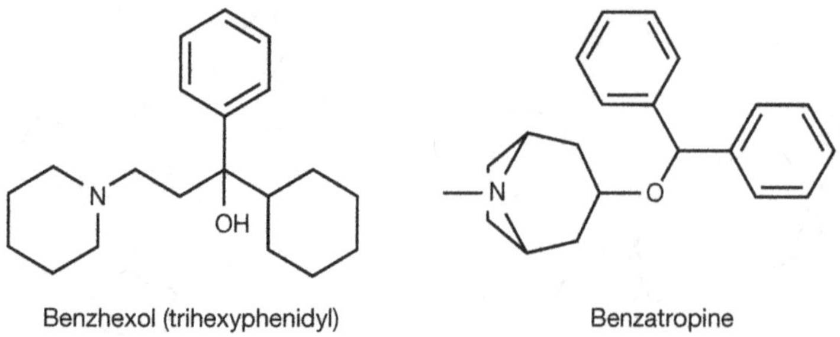

Figure 16.16 Non-ester cholinergic antagonists.

with the addition of a branched cyclopentanoyl group to the position alpha of the carbonyl. Glycopyrronium bromide is used interchangeably with atropine and scopolamine for reducing bronchial excretion and preventing laryngospasm. It is used as well to reduce or prevent the muscarinic effects of neostigmine. Glycopyrronium bromide is also used orally as an adjunctive therapy for peptic ulcer (2 mg) and topically as an antiperspirant (1% w/w and 3% w/w creams).

Recent experiments in animals have shown that glycopyrronium bromide, a quaternary amine, has conjunctival penetration and onset of action and duration of action as good as atropine when applied in ophthalmic solutions. This is contrary to the general belief which had previously prevailed that quaternary ammonium agents were not well absorbed by the eye.

Antimuscarinic compounds with no ester groups in the skeleton have a branched hydrophobic ring system, the rings are six-member or more or less, but there should be two rings which are *NOT* aliphatically attached to each other. These hydrophobic rings are thought to fill a hydrophobic cavity with a 'T' or 'Y' shape inside the active site, thus fixing the tail of the molecule in an orientation where the ACh-like head group blocks the access of the endogenous neurotransmitter, thus preventing the necessary conformational changes in the receptor which lead to the cholinergic activity.

The potency of molecules which lack the ester groups suggests that there are two mechanisms of binding to the receptor, one involves hydrogen bond interaction with the electron pairs on the ester oxygens and the other involves a van der Waals hydrophobic interaction with the hydrophobic rings (look at the structure of tiotropium, Fig. 16.15, which may combine the two mechanisms).

Parkinson's disease is associated with tremor and rigidity in muscles. These symptoms seem to result from the imbalance of acetylcholine–dopamine ratio at the ganglia-stratum in favour of the first. Blocking ACh activity was the first drug treatment strategy for this disease. Latterly, dopamine treatment was deemed more important. Nevertheless, combination of both treatments yields significant synergism and is desirable when the anticholinergic treatment is tolerated by the patient. Benzhexol is used centrally to treat the symptoms of Parkinson's disease and is added as well to the antischizophrenic therapy regimens to alleviate the extrapyramidal (Parkinson's-like) side effects of antipsychotic drugs (see Box 16.5). It is available in tablets of 2 or 5 mg, injection (10 mg) and elixir (2 mg/5 mL). It is used in doses up to 15 mg per day. Benzhexol causes, as do other tertiary amine antimuscarinic agents, hallucinogenic effects, which puts it on the list of 'drugs of abuse'.

Benztropine has similar uses and administration to benzhexol. It shares the tropine ring with atropine but the ester is replaced with an ether and branched benzyl groups. It has some antihistamine and local anaesthetic activity but is not indicated for such uses. Benzatropine (used as the mesilate salt) has a longer half-life than benzhexol and is used as a single daily dose (1–6 mg). It is available in oral (tablet) or injectable (i.m.) dosage forms.

Antimuscarinic agents have a remarkable effect on the gastrointestinal tract, and reduced saliva, gastric section, amount of stomach acid, pepsin and mucine are all observed. Motility is affected as well, with the walls of the viscera being relaxed and both the tone and propulsive movements being diminished upon antimuscarinic therapy. These effects make antimuscarinic drugs potential agents for the treatment of peptic ulcers, diarrhoea and intestinal cramps. Specific agents have been optimised for each of these three indications.

Pirenzepine (Fig. 16.17) makes a special antimuscarinic case. It is selective for the M1 receptor compared to its activity against M2 or M3. It is 20 and 4 times less potent at the M3 receptor than at M1 and M2, respectively. As discussed before, M1 is found in secretory glands and M2 is found in the heart. This selectivity gives pirenzepine a good activity against gastric acid secretion with no cardiac side effects. However, pirenzepine was superseded by H_2-receptor antagonist and proton pump inhibitors (which are discussed in Ch. 17 and Ch. 12, respectively).

The antispasmodic agents make use of the muscle relaxation effect of the antimuscarinic agents, but seem to depend on other additional mechanisms for success in obtaining the desired action, which is directly proportionate to the ability to relax the gut muscles in the absence, as well as the presence, of cholinergic stimulation. Examples of these types of drugs are propantheline, hyoscine-*N*-butyl bromide and dicycloverine (Fig. 16.17).

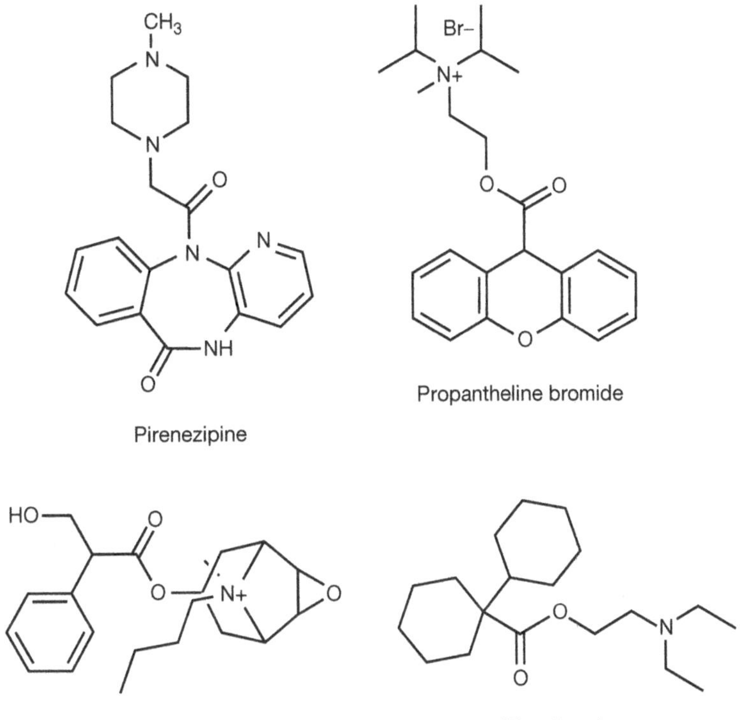

Pirenezipine

Propantheline bromide

Hyoscine N-butylbromide

Dicycloverine

Figure 16.17 Additional atypical cholinergic antagonists.

Propantheline provides another example of the branched ring system. It is a quaternary ammonium with the bromide salt used to relieve spasms of the intestine or to treat involuntary urination in doses of 15–30 mg.

Hyoscine-*N*-butyl bromide is a quaternary ammonium variant of hyoscine (scopolamine) formed by adding a butyl group to the tertiary amine group. It is mainly used to relieve temporal spasms of the intestine or menstrual cramps. It produces very moderate side effects, especially in the CNS. The long-term use of hyoscine-*N*-butyl bromide for the treatment of irritable bowel syndrome (IBS) has been reported as well (three daily doses of 10 mg). The drug is available in oral dosage forms with doses of 10–35 mg.

Injectable hyoscine-*N*-butyl bromide has been successfully used as an antisecretory drug in combination with haloperidol in palliative care.[20]

Dicycloverine is another example of an antimuscarinic agent which binds by both hydrogen bonding and hydrophobic van der Waals forces to the receptor. It is used as a gastrointestinal spasmolytic agent for the treatment of abdominal cramps and symptoms of IBS. It is available as oral capsules (10–20 mg), syrup (20 mg/5 mL) and an injection (20 mg/2 mL) of the hydrochloride salt.

Otilonium bromide is a new generation antispasmodic. It has an ACh-like moiety (red colour) attached to an aromatic system which ends with an octyl ether. The oral bioavailability of otilonium bromide is very low, and it was found to accumulate in the lower intestine, making it a locally active agent. Otilonium bromide is highly tolerable with very few side effects due to poor absorption of the drug. Even the effect on gastric secretion, which occurs with other antimuscarinic agents, was not reported at therapeutic doses. The antimuscarinic (M3) spasmolytic activity of otilonium bromide is fortified by other mechanisms including blockade of calcium channels and binding to tachykinin neurokinin-2 receptors. Its specific indication lies in treating the symptoms of IBS, especially with associated diarrhoea, in doses of 40 mg three times daily.[21]

The prolongation of gastric emptying time subsequent to the diminished gastric motility makes antimuscarinic agents, even the selective agent pirenzepine which is used for peptic ulcer, contraindicated in gastric ulcer as they increase the acid–ulcer contact time. Another observation about the same effect is the interaction with drug absorption, which is affected by the emptying time, and this should be taken into consideration when adding any antimuscarinic agents to a current ongoing therapeutic regimen.

The effect of antimuscarinic agents on the eye is mydriasis, cycloplegia and reduction of lacrimal secretions. These effects are desirable in ophthalmic examination of noncompliant patients (e.g. children) but considered to be side effects (blurred vision, dry [sandy] eye) in the systemic use of these agents. Cyclopentolate and tropicamide

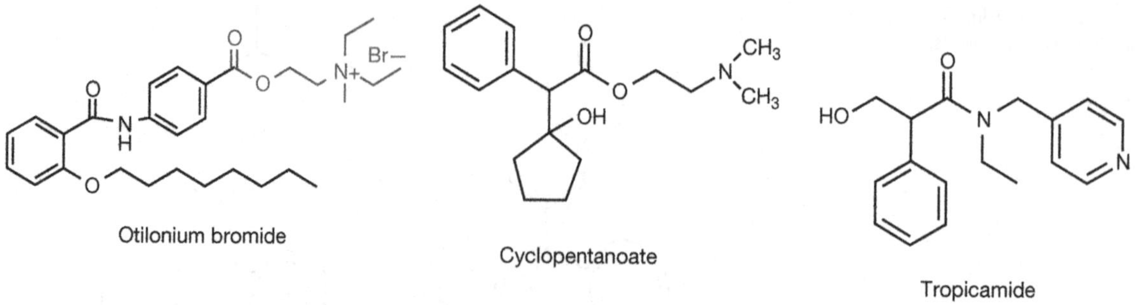

Figure 16.18 Antimuscarinic agents with no structural relationship to atropine.

(Fig. 16.18) are antimuscarinic agents used in ophthalmic examinations. They have shorter duration of action, 1 and 0.25 days respectively, in comparison to atropine (7–10 days). They are not structurally related, or related to any other antimuscarinic agent. However, in cyclopentolate it can be seen that there is an ester group separated by two methylene units from an amine group, as in ACh. They may also be used before or after eye surgery, such as lens replacement surgery. Both cyclopentolate and tropicamide are available in eyedrops at concentrations 0.5% and 1% w/v.

Upon antimuscarinic treatment, smooth muscles of the ureters and bladder wall are relaxed. This leads to urinary retention which is desired for patients with urinary incontinence but is contraindicated in males with prostate hyperplasia where filling the bladder increases pressure on the prostatic walls. Oxybutynin (Fig. 16.19) has shown some pharmacokinetic/pharmacodynamic selectivity towards the urinary tract. It is used orally (5–15 mg/day) in patients with overactive bladder and has been proven valuable as well in relieving bladder spasm after urological surgery. Tolterodine (Fig. 16.19) is an M3 selective antimuscarinic agent. It is used for urinary incontinence in adults.

Many antihistamines, antipsychotics and antidepressants have structural similarities with muscarinic receptor antagonists and, predictably, show antimuscarinic effects which are considered in many cases the major side effects of these drug categories. Imipramine (Fig. 16.19) is a

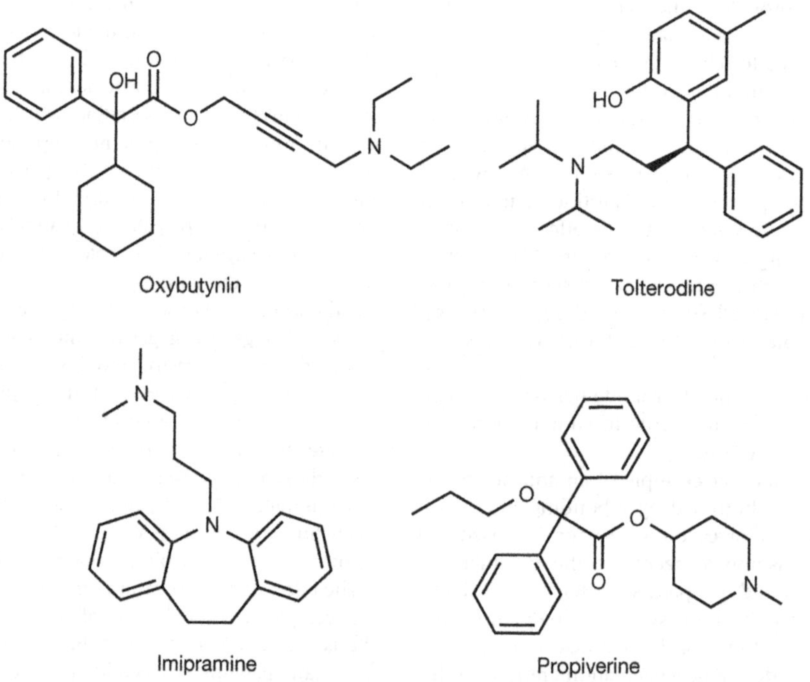

Figure 16.19 Antimuscarinic agents which belong to other drug classes.

tricyclic antidepressant with a chemical structure which fits that of a muscarinic blocker. The muscarinic blockade is considered a side effect (Box 16.4) when used for treating depression, but imipramine is also employed for treating urinary incontinence in the elderly.

Propiverine (Fig. 16.19) is a newer antimuscarinic approved for the specific use of urinary incontinence in doses of 5–75 mg. The rules for the use of antimuscarinic agents are summarised in Box 16.5.

Box 16.4 Effects of antimuscarinic agents on the cardiovascular system

The antimuscarinic agents elicit these effects on the cardiovascular system:

1. Blockade of vagual discharge (tachycardia)
2. Ventricles are under a lesser degree of control than the sinoatrial node and atria and are therefore less affected by antimuscarinic agents.
3. Blockade of the muscarinic provokes the release of EDRF (endothelium-derived release factor which is nitrous oxide [NO]).

The most notable net effect is tachycardia. The effect on blood pressure is compensated by other control mechanisms.

Box 16.5 Rules for the use of quaternary and tertiary amines as antimuscarinic agents

Quaternary amines are poorly absorbed by the gut and poorly distributed to the CNS owing to their hydrophilicity and are used when a peripheral effect devoid of central effects is desirable.

Tertiary amines are well absorbed from the intestine and conjunctival membrane. They easily cross the BBB, with scopolamine showing the highest preference for central residency among all antimuscarinic agents.

All antimuscarinic agents work in a surmountable competitive fashion; reversal of their actions can be concluded easily by infusing acetylcholine or any other cholinergic agonists, but the reversing agents should be selected carefully according to a peripheral (quaternary amine) or peripheral/central (tertiary amine) toxicity that needs to be surmounted.

Q Self Test 16.3

Categorise the following agents according to whether or not they are centrally or peripherally acting antimuscarinic agents: benzhexol, otilonium, atropine methonitrate, scopolamine. Indicate in each case an appropriate agent for reversing the antimuscarinic effects.

ANTINICOTINIC DRUGS

The nicotinic receptor AChNR is quite different from the muscarinic receptor. It is a ligand-gated ion channel and does not operate with a second messenger system. Activation of the nicotinic receptor leads to a flow of Na^+ and K^+ across the cell membrane and a depolarising effect on the effector cell (nerve cell or neuromuscular end plate).

AChNRs are subdivided into two subtypes, which vary in structure and distribution. The muscular nicotinic receptors are distributed in the neuromuscular junctions of the skeletal muscles and the postganglionic nicotinic receptors in the ganglia of the autonomic nervous system. Both nicotinic subtypes are pentamer proteins, but the subunits are not the same.

The nicotinic receptors in muscle and neural tissues have a large N-terminal domain, consisting of four hydrophobic transmembrane domains, called TM1–TM4 regions, a large cytoplasmic loop, and a short extracellular C-terminus. The transmembrane loop is thought to form the ion pore for the nicotinic ACh receptor. Binding of ACh and AChNR agonists to the muscular AChNR takes place at the amino-terminal regions of the α/γ and γ/β interfaces, whereas binding to the neuronal AChNR takes place at the two α/β interfaces of the heteromers and to the five subunit interfaces in the homomers.[22]

The nicotinic receptor is found in the CNS as well. It plays a central role in nicotine (smoking) addiction. Nicotine binds strongly to the brain cholinergic receptor due to a strong cation–π donor interaction to a specific aromatic amino acid of the receptor, TrpB (tryptophan 149). The interaction is enhanced by a hydrogen bond to the carbonyl at the backbone of TrpB. This interaction is absent in the muscular AChNRs, explaining why absorption of nicotine via smoking does not cause muscle contractions. Although the amino acid sequence in the active site is similar in muscular and neurological AChNRs, a neighbouring disparity in amino acid residues (a lysine in neurologic and a glycine in muscular receptors at position153) which affects the active site shape explains the differences in nicotine-binding strength between the two receptor types. The lysine is thought to form a backbone hydrogen bond between loop B and loop C (remember, AChNRs have four transmembrane loops) whereas glycine discourages this bond.[23]

All AChNR have two alpha subunits, each carries one active site. To give the greatest probability of channel opening, both active sites should be occupied by agonists. Activation of only one site still can lead to channel opening but only with a moderate probability. Large amounts of ACh released by nerve impulses cause the muscle action potential. There are two types of muscle relaxation produced by manipulation of AChNR. Depolarising muscle relaxation happens when agonists occupy the active site for a prolonged period, resulting in the constant depolarisation of the effector cells (postganglionic neurons and muscular end-plate cells), which will then not fire any new signals, and this leads to muscle relaxation. This action is irreversible and is constant as long as the agonist is occupying the active site on the receptor. The non-depolarising muscle relaxants act by competitively antagonising the active site, and this is reversible by cholinergic agents.[24]

Non-depolarising neuromuscular blockers

Non-depolarising neuromuscular blockers (NMBs) in normal doses act by competitive inhibition of the interaction between acetylcholine and nicotinic receptors. In higher doses, they are thought to block the ion channel as well, which explains the decreased effectiveness of AChE inhibitors in treating non-depolarising neuromuscular blocker toxicity.

The non-depolarising agents vary according to their duration of action and cardiac effects. The paralysis is desirable only during surgery, and a speedy recovery is in favour of the patient. This has been an incentive to medicinal chemists to design short-acting agents.

The duration of action of non-depolarising neuromuscular blockers is basically dependent on their metabolism, with agents excreted by the kidney being the longer acting. Here, we should take into consideration that patients under surgery have different liver and kidney functions from aware patients, as do elderly and young patients.

Tubocurarine-like drugs

As with all the drug categories in this chapter, the first compound with antinicotinic activity came from a natural source. Curare was used by the American Indians as a dry extract of the plant *Chondrodendron tomentosum* (the curare vine) rubbed onto the tip of their arrows. The actual name, curare, is a corruption of two Tupi Indian terms meaning 'bird' and 'to kill'. The name indicates the potency of this plant as a weapon. Curare extracts contain several alkaloids, the most potent of which is tubocurarine, which was isolated in 1935, but it took 35 years to determine its structure. Tubocurarine has a complex structure with two amine functions, one being quaternary and the other tertiary, and both are thought to be involved in the mechanism of action of tubocurarine (Fig. 16.20). Tubocurarine is the natural prototype of the non-depolarising neuromuscular relaxants. Its first medical use goes back to 1912 and it was introduced into anaesthesia in 1942. Tubocurarine causes a hypotension due to a moderate release of histamine and blocks the autonomic ganglionic nicotine receptors,

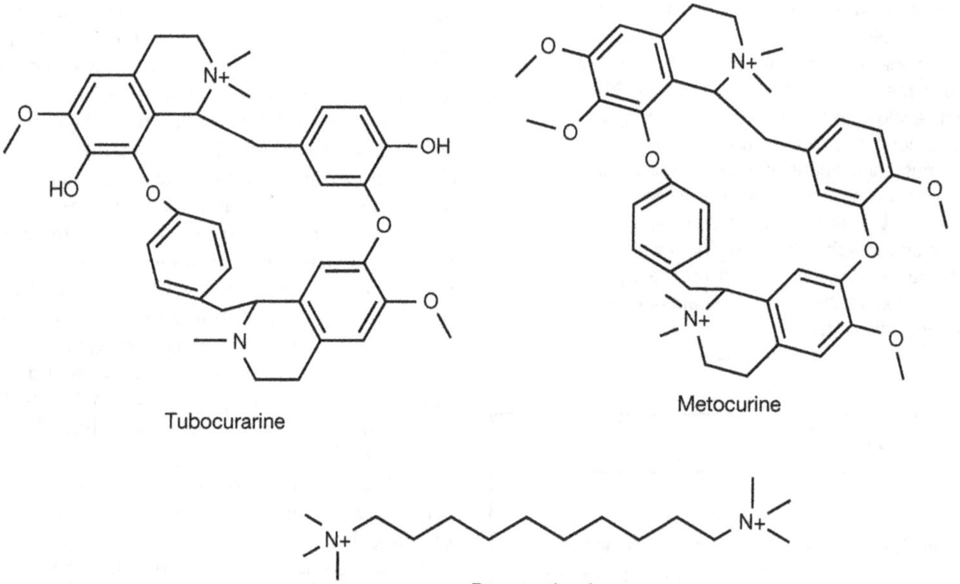

Figure 16.20 The early compounds to be used as NMBs.

producing a vagolytic effect (tachycardia). It is still employed in doses of 0.12–0.4 mg/kg and its action lasts for 60–90 minutes. However, its side effects make it less favoured than newer agents. Metocurine (Fig. 16.20) was introduced as an attempt to reduce the side effects of tubocurarine. It is a slight modification of the tubocurarine structure where both free hydroxyl groups were methylated, with the tertiary nitrogen being rendered quaternary by addition of a methyl group as well. The modification succeeded in decreasing histamine release, but had no impact on the vagolytic effect. Both tubocurarine and metocurine are highly selective towards the nicotinic receptor compared to the muscarinic receptors.

Several hypotheses have been suggested for the mechanism of binding of tubocurarine and later analogues to the nicotinic receptor, which seems puzzling considering the total absence of the ester function in these compounds. The most plausible hypothesis suggests an interaction between one of the charged nitrogens with the active site, with the other nitrogen interacting with a cysteine residue 0.9–1.2 Å away from the active site. This is supported by the distance between the two nitrogens in tubocurarine, and the fact that decamethonium (Fig. 16.20), a very simple molecule where two quaternary nitrogens are separated by an aliphatic chain of ten carbons, has shown potency comparable to tubocurarine.

Thus the active site of the receptor is blocked competitively, preventing the access of the endogenous ACh. The proposed mechanism indicates the importance of the distance between the two charged nitrogens in any antinicotinic compound to be designed, also bearing in mind that these distances change with the conformation that the molecule takes, in the case of a highly flexible molecule such as decamethonium.

Decamethonium was used as a replacement for tubocurarine but it had multiple disadvantages of its own. Decamethonium is a partial agonist giving a brief contraction of muscles which delays its onset of action, it is non-selective for the neuromuscular junction and gives cardiac side effects including tachycardia and hypotension which may persist for a considerable time given the strong interaction between the drug and the receptor. The lack of selectivity in decamethonium can be understood in terms of the flexibility of the molecule, which can take so many conformations, some of which are suitable to switch off the muscarinic receptor as well.

The design of effective analogues of tubocurarine and decamethonium took into consideration the introduction of conformationally restricted groups, as well as the mechanism governing the rate of elimination of the drug from the body while at the same time preserving the crucial distance between the two charged amines. The later non-depolarising agents have a relatively rigid structure and can be divided, from a chemical perspective, into steroid and isoquinoline derivatives.

Q Self Test 16.4

Based on the hypothesis given for NMB activity, do you think the compound below will give improved antinicotinic properties compared to decamethonium? Why?

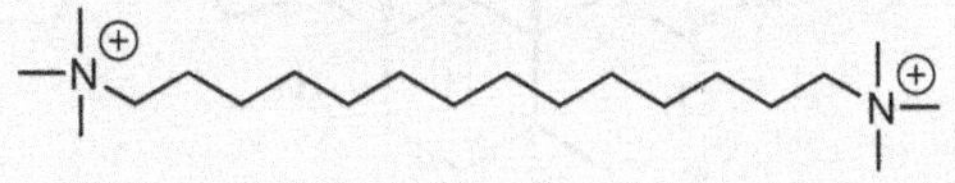

Steroid-like neuromuscular blocking agents

Pancuronium (Fig. 16.21) was the first steroid-like neuromuscular blocking (NMB) agent employed in clinical use. It is composed of two acetylcholine motifs separated by a rigid steroid-like structure. The acetylcholine motifs use parts of the steroid as the two-carbon separator bridge, and the quaternary ammonium groups are incorporated into a piperidenium ring (outlined in red). This structure ensures a good occupancy of the active sites on both alpha subunits in the nicotinic receptor to prevent its switching on by acetylcholine. It is a potent muscle relaxant (six times more potent than tubocurarine) and has a prolonged duration of action (120–180 minutes). However, the onset of action is relatively slow (2–4 minutes) and its renal excretion (80%) makes it better avoided for patients with kidney diseases. It is inactive via the oral route and is given by i.v. injection as a bromide salt with a concentration of 1 mg/mL or 2 mg/mL. Pancuronium has been cited many times in forensic investigations of suicides and murders, and as a part of the euthanasia procedure.

Vecuronium is an N-desmethylpancuronium, the minor change resulting in a substantial impact on the rate of elimination of the drug. Removing the methyl from one of the quaternary ammonium groups will convert it into a tertiary amine with a loss of the permanent charge. This reduces the hydrophilicity and, since the general structure is steroid-like, this facilitates elimination of the drug into the bile. Vecuronium has a shorter duration of action of 20–35 minutes (compared to 120 minutes for pancuronium), fewer cardiac side effects with comparable potency (very slightly more than pancuronium).[25] The salt used is the bromide and is available in multiple-injection vials of 20 mg/20 mL concentration. The paralysing action is noticed in approximately 1 minute for a 0.08–1 mg/kg initial dose.

Pancuronium and vecuronium both have faster onset of action than tubocurarine, and they do not have significant cardiovascular side effects. Their intermediate duration of action makes them suitable for medium-sized surgical procedures (e.g. caesarean section). However, faster onset of action, fewer side effects and a shorter duration of action are still desirable features demanded by anaesthetists.

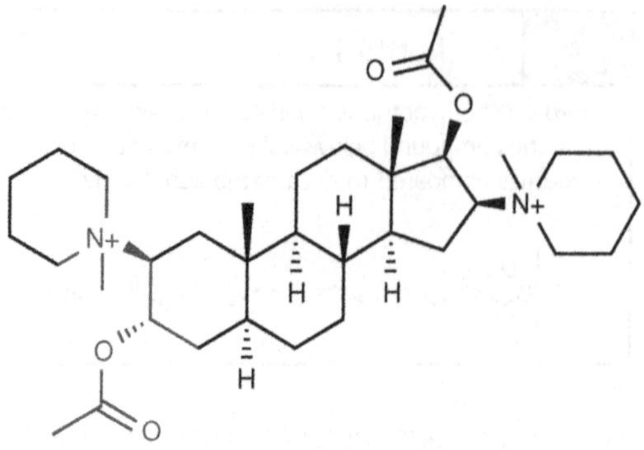

Pancuronium

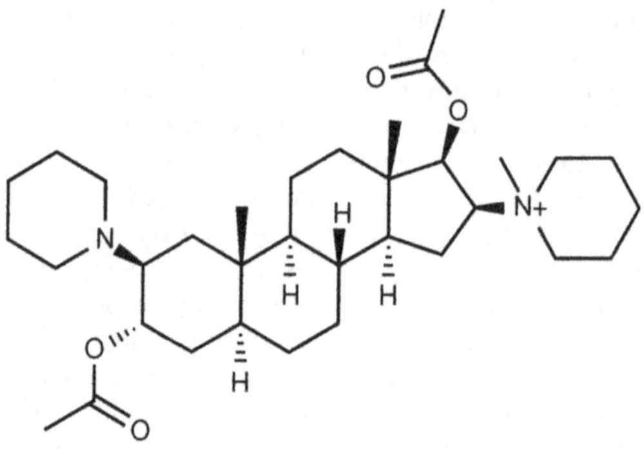

Vecuronium

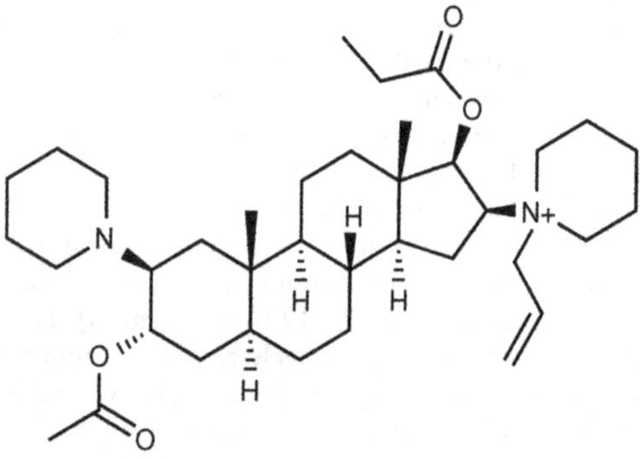

Rapacuronium

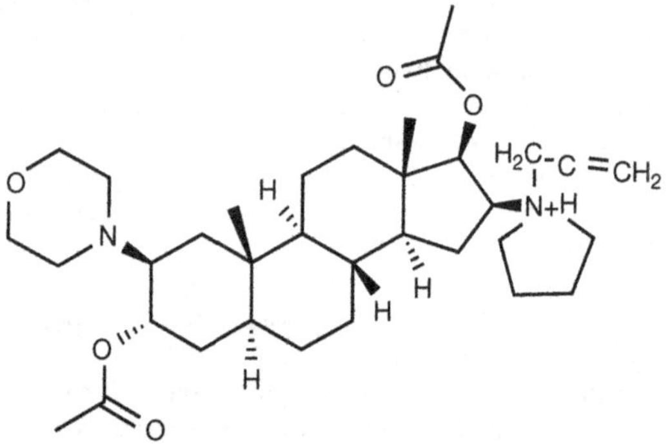

Recuronium

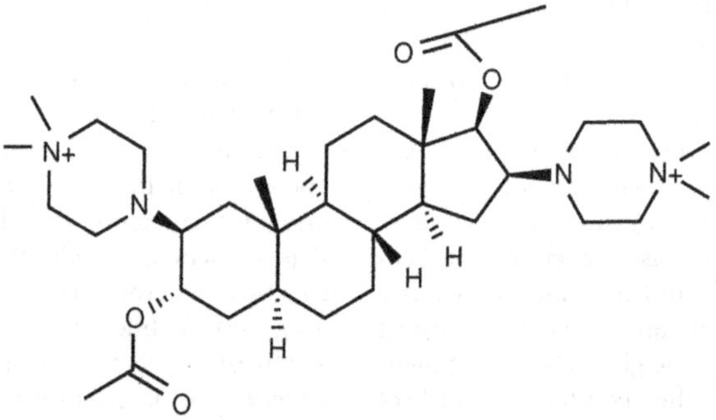

Pipecuronium

Figure 16.21 Steroid based neuromuscular blocking agents.

N-desmethylation on one quaternary nitrogen, and replacing the methyl with an allyl group on the other, resulted in rapacuronium (Fig. 16.21), the most rapid onset of action of non-depolarising muscle relaxants. Rapacuronium has a short duration of action as well (10–20 minutes), it is eliminated mainly by liver, and its potency is 15 times less than pancuronium. However, it was voluntarily withdrawn in 2001 by its manufacturing company because of reports of severe bronchospasm.[26]

Rocuronium (Fig. 16.21) preserves the vecuronium trend of tertiary versus quaternary nitrogens, but with further modifications on the nitrogen substitutes. The drug has a similar pharmacokinetic, duration of action, and toxicity profile to vecuronium but six times less potent.[27] It has a fast onset of action (about 2 minutes). Recuronium is supplied as its bromide salt in multiple-dose vials containing volumes of 50 or 100 mL at a concentration of 10 mg/mL.

Pipecuronium is a modification of pancuronium where both quaternary ammonium groups were desmethylated, but quaternary nitrogens were introduced into what was a piperidine ring in pancuronium. Pipecuronium is similar to pancuronium in efficacy. It shows some elimination by liver but this is not as predominant as in recuronium or vecuronium. Pipecuronium has a half-life of 1.7 hours in normal renal function and 4 hours in renal function impairment. The onset of action is reported to be 2.5–3 minutes and the duration of action about 45 minutes. Pipecuronium is supplied in a sterile injection containing 10 mg of the bromide salt.[28]

The early steroid-like neuromuscular blockers show very little histamine release or ganglionic effects, but still cause cardiac side effects due to non-selective binding to the cardiac muscarinic receptor, with pancuronium showing a moderate block on that receptor. The problem was partially resolved in rocuronium and rapacuronium and diminished further in vecuronium and pipecuronium but with some loss of potency. The steroid-like agents are prone to metabolism. Of the different metabolites, the 3-hydroxy shows 40–80% activity compared to the parent compound which may cause problems upon long term accumulation of the metabolite. This should be taken into consideration in patients with liver and kidney diseases. However, this is a concern only in intensive care units (ICUs), as accumulation of the metabolite is negligible during surgery. Box 16.6 summarises the importance of muscle relaxation in anaesthesia.

Box 16.6 **Importance of muscle relaxation in anaesthesia**

Complications of surgeries, especially those on the abdomen or throat, necessitate skeletal muscle relaxation prior to surgery. Before the introduction of muscle relaxation, this was achieved by deep anaesthesia which itself is a hazard for patients (cardiac complications, respiratory suppression). Deep anaesthesia is no longer required by virtue of neuromuscular blocking agents providing adequate muscle relaxation for all surgical requirements.

Muscle relaxation is desirable in surgical operations and also in ICUs where paralysis is of benefit to the patient.

Isoquinoline derivative neuromuscular blocking agents

The design of these agents was based on the properties of both tubocurarine and decamethonium. The bulky ring system, which gave tubocurarine conformational restriction and thus selectivity and linear space between the two quaternary ammonium groups present in decamothenium, were combined. Isoquinoline derivatives were intended to be similar in structure to the bulky groups in tubocurarine (the natural compound) and still conserve a linear chain with a 1.1–1.2 Å distance separating two nitrogen atoms. In the atracurium structure, two exactly similar isoquinoline derivatives were connected by a 13-atom bridge. The linear (non-branched) bridge provides the necessary distance between the two quaternary ammonia. Additionally, it contains two beta-carbonyl groups which facilitate the degradation of atracurium via the Hofmann elimination. Atracurium (Fig. 16.22) was first synthesised in the Department of Pharmacy at the Strathclyde University in 1974, which was part of a remarkable double since the pharmacological screening which led to vecuronium was carried out in the Department of Pharmacology at Strathclyde at about the same time. The commercial drug is a mixture of ten stereoisomers.

Atracurium has a duration of action similar to that of vecuronium and is eliminated by a rationally designed, purely chemical degradation mechanism via the Hofmann elimination (see Box 16.7) which occurs in an aqueous environment with the rate increasing with higher pH (Fig. 16.23). Atracurium is supplied as a sterile injection of 10 mg/mL.

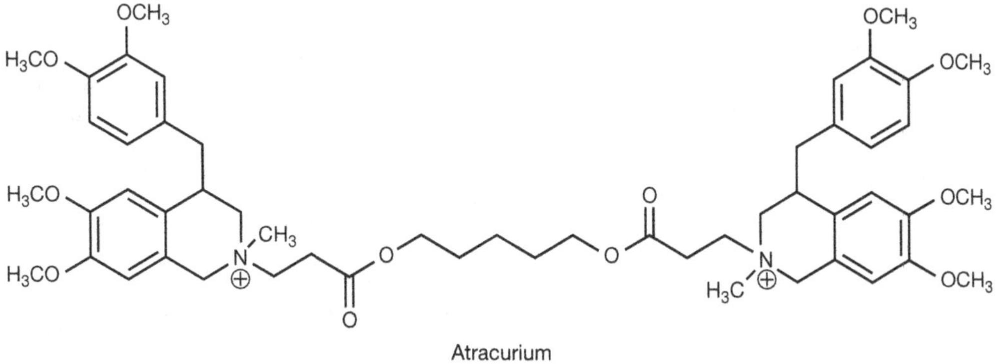

Figure 16.22 The chemical structure of the most ubiquitous component of atracurium.

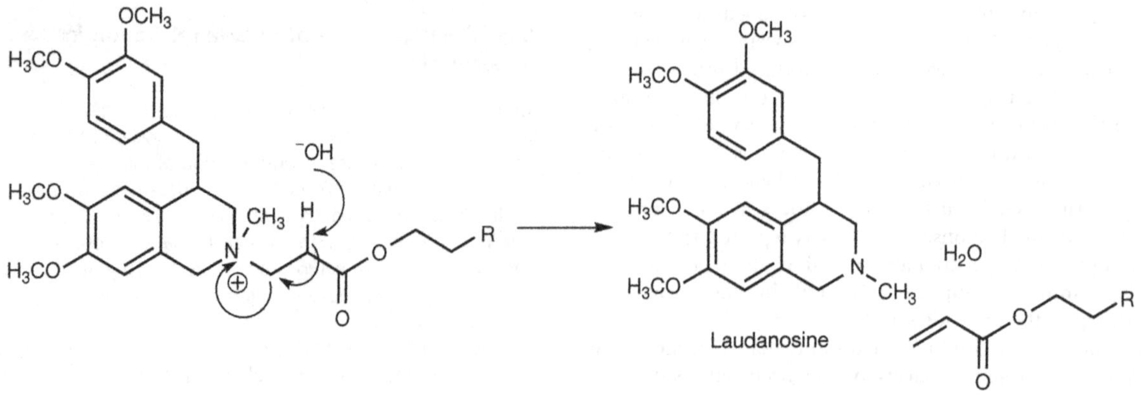

Figure 16.23 Hofmann elimination leading to the degradation of atracurium.

The main product of the Hofmann elimination of atracurium is laudanosine, an alpha-adrenoreceptor blocking agent which causes hypotension.[29] Moreover, laudanosine crosses the blood–brain barrier (in contrast to the parent compound) and may cause excitement and seizure activity which leads to an increase in anaesthetic requirement by 30%. Accumulation and corresponding problems with laudanosine arise only in infants and with prolonged application in ICUs.[30] Laudanosine-caused hypotension is enhanced by histamine released from tissue stores as a side effect of atracurium.[31]

To counter the problems produced by laudanosine, the stereoisomers of atracurium were isolated in order to allow a dose reduction. Cisatracurium (Fig. 16.24) is an R-cis R-cis isomer of atracurium. It is degraded by Hofmann elimination just like atracurium. However, plasma concentrations of laudanosine do not reach such high levels as in the case of atracurium, leading to fewer cardiac side effects. Cisatracurium also releases less histamine from tissue stores. The potency and duration of action are similar in both drugs. Cisatracurium besilate is provided in sterile injections with a concentration equivalent to 2 mg/mL of cisatracurium in 5- or 10-mL vials, or 10 mg/mL of cisatracurium in 20-mL vials intended for use in ICUs only.

The spontaneous chemical elimination makes these agents a better option for patients with renal or hepatic diseases and allows less patient-to-patient variability. The Hofmann elimination does not occur in acidic pH, and these drugs are stable when stored at a pH = 3–4. This pH level is achieved by the addition of benzenesulphonic acid which provides some buffering capacity compared to, say, hydrochloric acid. However, even at this pH, an observed loss of potency by a rate of 6% per annum has been reported to both agents at 4°C. This rate increases to 5% per month at 25°C and thus refrigerator storage is necessary for these agents.

Mivacurium (Fig. 16.25) is another bisbenzylisoquinolinium neuromuscular blocking agent. One structural difference from atracurium is the additional methoxy group on each of the benzyl rings in the benzylisoquinoline, but the greatest change is the addition of a third carbon to separate the carbonyl group from the quaternary ammonium. This has made the elimination of the drug less dependent on chemical degradation mechanisms and more reliant on plasma cholinesterase (pseudocholinesterase). Additionally, the introduction of a double bond in the centre of the unbranched chain separating the two quaternary ammonium centres allowed multiple geometric isomers to emerge. The commercial drug is a mixture of trans-trans [52–62%], cis-trans [34–40%] and cis-cis [4–8%]. These forms, especially the first two, are easy targets for plasma cholinesterase, and the result is a

Box 16.7 Hofmann elimination as a chemical degradation mechanism of isoquinoline NMBs

Hofmann elimination occurs in quaternary amines where one of the attached alkyl groups leaves the nitrogen in the form of an alkene. The reaction happens in an alkaline medium, usually with the aid of heating and vacuum. With unsymmetrical amines, the major alkene product is derived from the least substituted and generally the least stable alkyl group, an observation known as the Hofmann rule. This is in direct contrast to normal elimination reactions where the more substituted, stable product is dominant.

The conditions required for Hofmann elimination can never be achieved in vivo, but the introduction of a nearby electron withdrawing group, a carbonyl in this specific case, supported by the slightly alkaline (pH = 7.4) medium will facilitate the process. The reaction products are inactive and can no longer block the active site of the nicotinic receptor, and in the best case, the elimination products can occupy one of the two active sites on the nicotinic receptor, which, as discussed, is not sufficient for a complete blockage of ACh action.

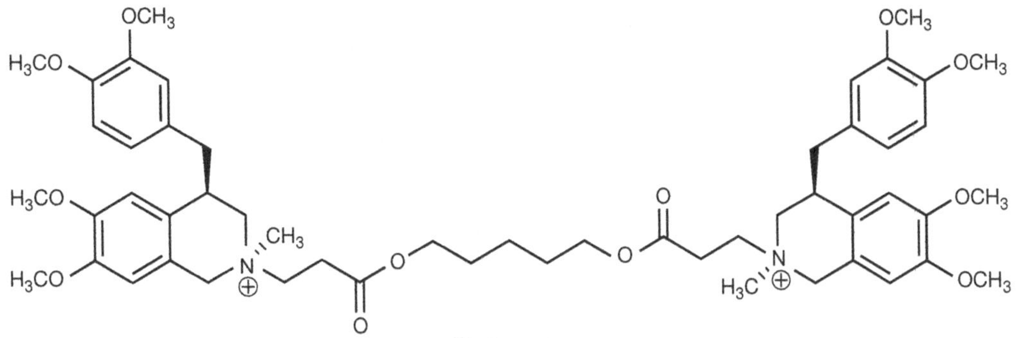

Cisatracurium

Figure 16.24 The chemical structure of cisatracurium indicating the geometric positions.

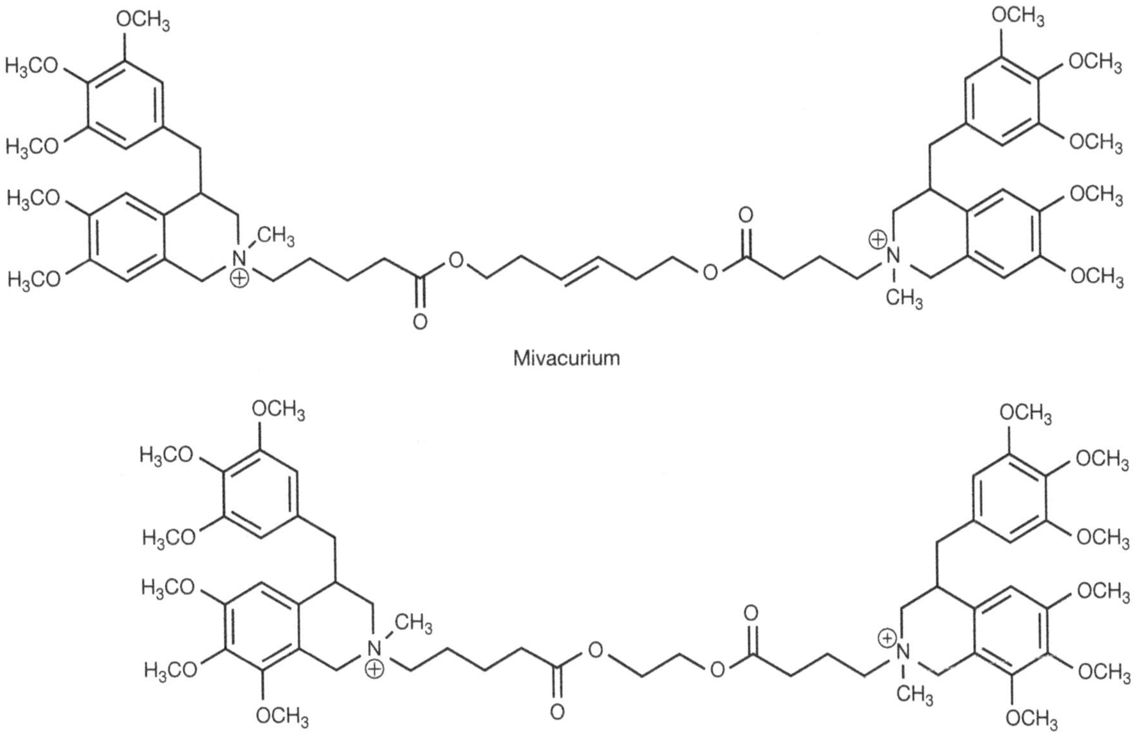

Mivacurium

Doxacurium

Figure 16.25 Second generation isoquinolinium NMBs.

very short-acting neuromuscular blocking agent (10–20 minutes). Nevertheless, the duration of action is prolonged in kidney disease patients as they have decreased pseudocholinesterase levels and in individuals with genetically variable levels of pseudocholinesterase. The separating bridge in mivacurium consists of 16 atoms (compared to 13 in atracurium) but surprisingly it is three times more potent than atracurium. Mivacurium causes histamine release comparable to that caused by atracurium. It is provided as mivacurium dichloride and the pharmaceutical dosage form is a sterile injection with a concentration of 2 mg/mL.

Doxacurium is a middle case between atracurium and mivacurium. The non-branched bridge was modified from atracurium by shifting the carbonyl group to the gamma position relative to the quaternary ammonium,

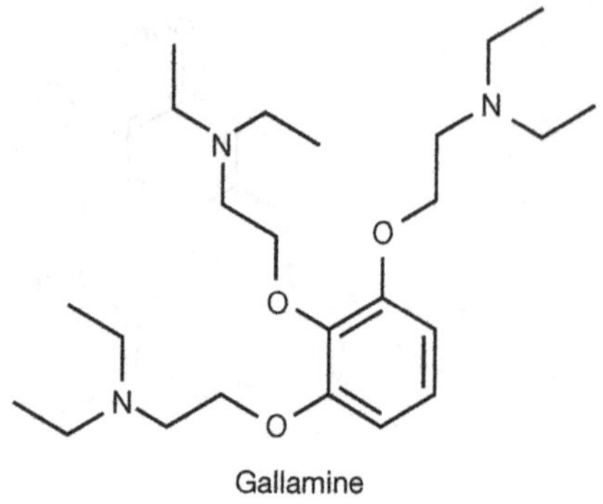

Figure 16.26 The chemical structure of gallamine, a unique NMB non-related to any NMB chemical class.

and by eliminating three of the methylene units from the centre of the bridge. This modification (as in mivacurium) limits the Hofmann elimination and disposes doxacurium to renal elimination. Other modifications include one extra methoxy group on each of the four aromatic rings in the structure. Its duration of action is prolonged (40 minutes) and its potency is enhanced compared to atracurium (four times). The renal elimination of doxacurium makes it less optimal in patients with kidney diseases. It is supplied in sterile injections of doxacurium dichloride with a concentration equivalent to 1 mg/mL of the active compound.[32]

Gallamine (Fig. 16.26) was developed in 1947 as a non-depolarising neuromuscular blocker. It does not chemically belong to any of the groups above. The effect of gallamine lasts for 40–60 minutes and its potency is 20% that of tubocurarine. It is used as its tri-iodide salt and the presence of the iodide salt means that it is unsuitable for patients with thyroid problems. Gallamine blocks the cardiac muscarinic receptor very strongly, resulting in a remarkable increase in heart rate and cardiac output with occasional hypertension.

Depolarising neuromuscular blocking agents

Suxamethonium (Fig. 16.27) is the only depolarising NMB agent in clinical use. Suxamethonium (succinylcholine) was designed by introducing two ester groups in symmetric positions in the middle of the decamethonium molecule. The ester has labile functions which degrade in the circulation both chemically and enzymatically via the action of pseudocholinesterase (PAChE). The hydrolysis product, succinylmonocholine, binds only to one alpha unit of the active site of the nicotinic receptor. This produces only a mild depolarisation, not enough to cause a continuous depolarising and a subsequent neuromuscular blockade. Succinylmonocholine shows no toxicity. Plasma cholinesterase has a very large capacity, and can metabolise suxamethonium very rapidly, explaining the short duration of action (5–10 minutes). Suxamethonium is not metabolised by end-plate cholinesterase, and is removed by diffusion (Fig. 16.27). The elimination in the plasma makes the diffusion equilibrium directed towards extracellular fluid (then plasma) and prevents accumulation. This allows for pseudocholinesterase to play a great role in the potency and duration of action of suxamethonium, and makes it, as in the case of mivacurium use, highly variable in patients with kidney disease and among individuals deficient of this enzyme for genetic reasons (0.05% of humans lack PAChE).

The blockade process passes through two phases. It starts with a depolarisation just like that induced by ACh, the natural ligand for the nicotinic receptor, causing random, very brief muscle contractions. Suxamethonium is not metabolised by synaptic AChE. Thus it produces a prolonged depolarisation compared to ACh. The longer depolarisation state of the membrane makes it refractory to new excitements and results in a flaccid paralysis. This phase can be augmented by AChE inhibitors (e.g. neostigmine), as they usually inhibit PAChE as well, and increase synaptic exposure to suxamethonium.[33] The unsynchronised

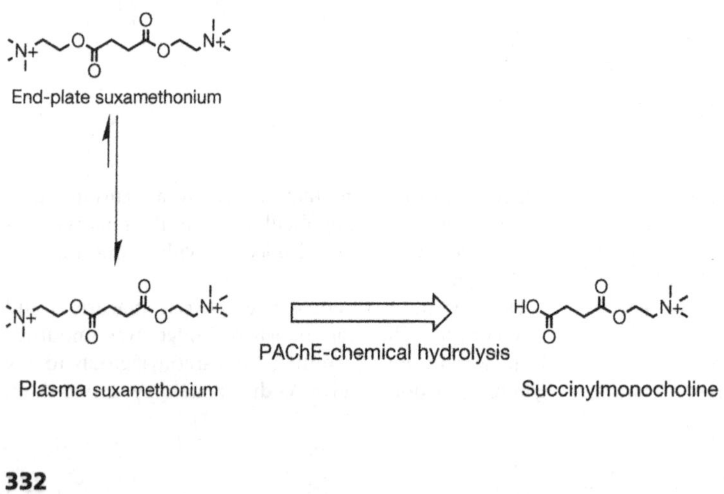

Figure 16.27 Hydrolysis of and removal of suxamethonium from the AChNR.

nature of the muscle contractions in this phase causes damage in the neighbouring muscle fibres, explaining the complaints of muscle pain post surgery where suxamethonium was used. In the second phase, repolarisation is achieved but the end plates are still not responsive to new depolarisation. This is described as desensitisation of the motor end-plate cells. Evidence suggests that suxamethonium acts by occupying the receptor and blocking the ion channel itself, to which the desensitisation phenomena can be attributed. Suxamethonium has the fastest onset of action (<1 minute) among all neuromuscular blocking agents. The onset of action determines how soon the patient's trachea can be intubated, which is necessary in life-threatening emergencies. It is given in doses of 1–2 mg/kg intravenously or 3 mg/kg intramuscularly, reconstituted from a clear solution of a concentration of 50 mg/mL. Suxamethonium activates cholinergic receptors in a non-selective manner. All nicotinic (neuromuscular and ganglionic) and muscarinic receptors are affected by this drug and it causes various cardiac arrhythmias. The contradictory effect of activating cholinergic receptors in different sites (e.g. ganglionic receptors versus muscarinic receptors in the sinus node) means its effect on the cardiovascular system varies according to dose and individuals. Other side effects of suxamethonium include increased intraocular pressure and intragastric pressure. Suxamethonium occasionally causes an exaggerated release of potassium into the blood. This may lead to cardiac arrest in children. In 1993, the FDA prevented the use of suxamethonium in children, and then modified the risk level to a warning. Additionally, since suxamethonium's basic elimination mechanism is by enzymatic hydrolysis with PAChE which varies significantly between individuals, this leads to difficulties in dose determination and recovery time prediction.

NMB agents, whether depolarising or non-depolarising, are polar compounds owing to the positive charge carried on the quaternary ammonia. This makes them biologically unavailable when given by the oral route, and less able to distribute to the central nervous system. The polarity makes their volume of distribution close to that of the blood.

> **Box 16.8 Drug combinations in anaesthesia**
>
> The addition of neuromuscular blockers to the anaesthetic regimen has proven significantly valuable. However, additional therapeutic measures are necessary to combat the adverse effects of the different agents. Hence, the histamine release caused by tubocurarine, metocurine, atracurium and mivacurium are eliminated by a pre-surgery dose of an antihistamine. The muscarinic activity of suxamethonium is reversed by a dose of atropine and the post-surgery muscle pain resulting from the fasciculation caused by suxamethonium is relieved by a small dose of a non-depolarising muscle relaxant. These measures, albeit complicating the anaesthetic regimen, are in favour of the patient when measured by a risk/benefit assessment.

Box 16.8 summarises some of the drug combinations that are used in anaesthesia.

Ganglionic blockers

Ganglion blocking drugs are anticholinergic agents which block the nicotinic receptor at the ganglionic level. Nicotinic ion gate blockers, which work on the nicotinic receptor but at a site of interaction different from the ACh active site, are classified with this category of drugs. The lack of selectivity in the action elicited by these drugs allows for high interpersonal variability in response and limits their clinical use. These agents block the postganglionic acetylcholine signal for both sympathetic and parasympathetic nerves. For tissues innervated by both types, the net effect of this blockade is dependent on the predominant tone in the tissue.

Hexamethonium (Fig. 16.28) is a quaternary ammonium agent. It was the first successful antihypertensive treatment. However, its side effects led to discontinuation of its use. It is thought to exert its action by blocking the ion channel rather than the acetylcholine active site. Blocking the ganglionic nicotinic receptor will stop the

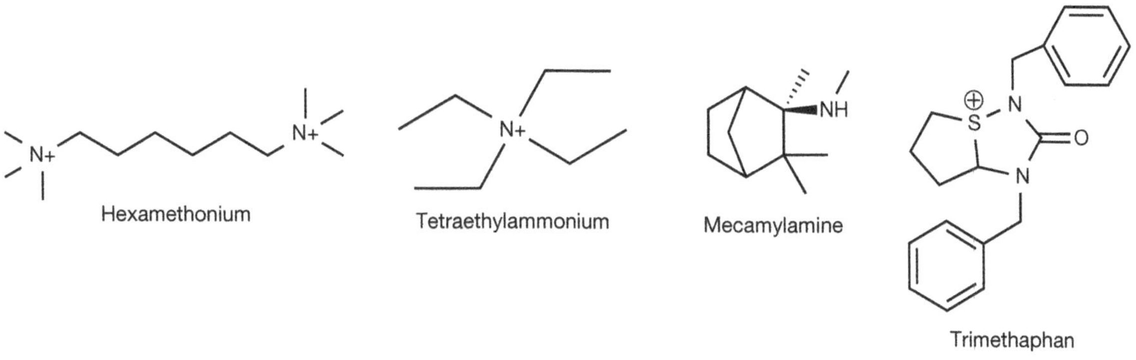

Figure 16.28 Ganglionic blocking drugs.

sympathetic discharge to the veins and arteries, resulting in a vasodilation.

Tetraethylammonium (Fig. 16.28) is a quaternary ammonium agent with a very short duration of action. Mecamylamine is a secondary amine designed to improve the oral bioavailability of ganglionic blockers. Central side effects are not unexpected. It was used for the emergency treatment of malignant hypertension but has been superseded by safer agents such as sodium nitroprusside. Trimethaphan (Fig. 16.28) is a short-acting anticholinergic agent working at the ganglionic site. It has a complex structure compared to other agents in this class. It bears two adjacent tertiary amides, but still can not be absorbed by the gut or cross the BBB owing to the positive charge of its sulphonium ion. The structure does not seem to be related to acetylcholine. It is given i.v. for the emergency treatment of malignant hypertension.

A Self Test 16.1

A = S. C – O > C – C – N > C – H. B = R. Hydrogen is behind the plane of the paper.

A Self Test 16.2

Isomer S. C – C = O > C – C – O > C – C = C. Hydrogen is in front of everything thus reverse the assignment.

Centre 2 is not chiral because the carbon 2 is attached to two identical carbon atoms due to symmetry in the tropine ring.

A Self Test 16.3

Centrally acting: Benzhexol and scopolamine. Both are reversed with physostigmine.

Peripherally acting: Otilonium, atropine methonitrate. Neostigmine can be used to reverse the effects of these agents.

A Self Test 16.4

No. The aliphatic chain is too long to fit in the space necessary for the interaction with the active site on the receptor from one side and the cysteine residue on the other side.

REFERENCES

1. Dean ESaB. Role of the cholinergic system in the pathology and treatment of schizophrenia. *Expert Rev Neurother.* 2009;9:73–86.
2. Koch HJHS, Jürgens T. On the physiological relevance of muscarinic acetylcholine receptors in Alzheimer's disease. *Curr Med Chem.* 2005;12:2915–2921.
3. Laura Paleari AG, Cesario A, Russo P. The cholinergic system and cancer. *Semin Cancer Biol.* 2008;18:211–217.
4. Maresca ASC. Muscarinic acetylcholine receptors as therapeutic targets for obesity. *Expert Opin Ther Targets.* 2008;12:1167–1175.
5. Jtirgen Wess NB, Mutschler E, Bluml K. Muscarinic acetylcholine receptors: structural basis of ligand binding and G protein coupling. *Life Sci.* 1995;56:915–922.
6. Zlotos DP, Buller S, Tränkle C, et al. Bisquaternary caracurine V derivatives as allosteric modulators of ligand binding to M2 acetylcholine receptors. *Bioorg Med Chem Lett.* 2000;10:2529–2532.
7. Kovacic P, Pozos RS, Draskovich CD. Unifying electrostatic mechanism for receptor-ligand activity. *J Recept Signal Transduct Res.* 2007;27:411–431.
8. Jensen AA, Mikkelsen I, Frolund B, et al. Carbamoylcholine homologs: novel and potent agonists at neuronal nicotinic acetylcholine receptors. *Mol Pharmacol.* 2003;64: 865–875.
9. Frank Dorje JW, Lambrecht G, Tacke R, Mutschler E, Brann MR. Antagonist binding profiles of five cloned human muscarinic receptor subtypes. *J Pharmacol Exp Ther.* 1991; 256:727–733.
10. Bikádi ZSM. Muscarinic and nicotinic cholinergic agonists: structural analogies and discrepancies. *Curr Med Chem.* 2003;10:2611–2620.
11. Patrick GL, ed. *An introduction to medicinal chemistry.* Oxford; New York: Oxford University Press; 2005.
12. Hanna Kaduszkiewicz TZ, Beck-Bornholdt H-P, van den Bussche H. Cholinesterase inhibitors for patients with Alzheimer's disease: systematic review of randomised clinical trials. *Br Med J.* 2005;331:321–327.
13. Maltby N, Broe GA, Creasey H, Jorm AF, Christensen H, Brooks WS. Efficacy of tacrine and lecithin in mild to moderate Alzheimer's disease: double blind trial. *Br Med J.* 1994;308: 879–883.
14. van Koppen CJ, Kaiser B. Regulation of muscarinic acetylcholine receptor signaling. *Pharmacol Ther.* 2003;98: 197–220.
15. May LT, Avlani VA, Langmead CJ, et al. Structure-function studies of allosteric agonism at M2 muscarinic acetylcholine receptors. *Mol Pharmacol.* 2007;72:463–476.
16. Zhiguo Wang HSaHW. Functional M3 muscarinic acetylcholine receptors in mammalian hearts. *Br J Pharmacol.* 2004;142:395–408.

17. Keam SJKG. Tiotropium bromide. A review of its use as maintenance therapy in patients with COPD. *Treat Respir Med.* 2004;3:247–268.
18. Mundy C, Kirkpatrick P. Tiotropium bromide. *Nat Rev Drug Discov.* 2004;3:643–644.
19. van Noord JA, Bantje TA, Eland ME, et al. A randomised controlled comparison of tiotropium and ipratropium in the treatment of chronic obstructive pulmonary disease. *Thorax.* 2000;55:289–294.
20. Barcia E, Reyes R, Luz Azuara M, et al. Compatibility of haloperidol and hyoscine-N-butyl bromide in mixtures for subcutaneous infusion to cancer patients in palliative care. *Support Care Cancer.* 2003;11: 107–113.
21. Susanne Lindqvist JH, Sharp P, Johns N, et al. The colon-selective spasmolytic otilonium bromide inhibits muscarinic M3 receptor-coupled calcium signals in isolated human colonic crypts. *Br J Pharmacol.* 2002;137:1134–1142.
22. Villeneuve G, Cécyre D, Lejeune H, et al. Rigidified acetylcholine mimics: conformational requirements for binding to neuronal nicotinic receptors. *Bioorg Med Chem Lett.* 2003;13: 3847–3851.
23. Xiu X, Puskar NL, Shanata JAP, et al. Nicotine binding to brain receptors requires a strong cation-[π-π] interaction. *Nature.* 2009;458:534–537.
24. Lee C. Conformation, action, and mechanism of action of neuromuscular blocking muscle relaxants. *Pharmacol Ther.* 2003;98:143–169.
25. Vizi ES, Lendvai B. Side effects of nondepolarizing muscle relaxants: Relationship to their antinicotinic and antimuscarinic actions. *Pharmacol Ther.* 1997;73:75–89.
26. Gyermek L. Development of ultra short-acting muscle relaxant agents: history, research strategies, and challenges. *Med Res Rev.* 2005;25: 610–654.
27. Sluga M, Ummenhofer W, Studer W, et al. Rocuronium versus succinylcholine for rapid sequence induction of anesthesia and endotracheal intubation: a prospective, randomized trial in emergent cases. *Anesth Analg.* 2005;101: 1356–1361.
28. Katzung BG, ed. *Basic and clinical pharmacology.* New York, London: McGraw-Hill; 2001.
29. Chuliá S, Ivorra MD, Lugnier C, Vila E, Noguera MA, D'Ocon P. Mechanism of the cardiovascular activity of laudanosine: comparison with papaverine and other benzylisoquinolines. *Br J Pharmacol.* 1994;113:1377–1385.
30. Fodale V, Santamaria LB. Laudanosine, an atracurium and cisatracurium metabolite. *Eur J Anaesthesiol.* 2002;19:466–473.
31. Chiodini F, Charpantier E, Muller D, et al. Blockade and activation of the human neuronal nicotinic acetylcholine receptors by atracurium and laudanosine. *Anesthesiology.* 2001; 94:643–651.
32. Harald J. Sparr TMBaTF-B. Newer neuromuscular blocking agents 1–1 how do they compare with established agents. *Drugs.* 2001;61:919–942.
33. Views E. Succinylcholine: new insights into mechanisms of action of an old drug. *Anesthesiology.* 2006; 104:633–634.

Chapter 17

Antihistamine drugs

David G Watson

CHAPTER CONTENTS

INTRODUCTION

Histamine (Fig. 17.1) was isolated in *ca.* 1908 from an extract of the ergot fungus which had been found to stimulate the uterine muscle of the cat to contract. It was already a known compound but its pharmacological action had not been previously assessed. It was found that histamine was present in the human body and was widely distributed in connective tissues and in the capsular membranes of organs. Histamine is a very polar molecule with two amine functionalities. The primary amine in the side chain has a p*Ka* value of around 9.7 and thus is completely protonated at physiological pH, while the nitrogen in the imidazole ring is a weaker base having a p*Ka* value of around 6, which means that at physiological pH the lone pair on the nitrogen is readily available to interact with electophilic groups. Histamine is stored in mast cells in the form of granules in association with the polysulphate molecule heparin and it seems that electrostatic interaction with the heparin is an important factor in granule formation. Histamine also occurs in basophils in association with another polysulphated polysaccharide chondroitin sulphate. Release of histamine occurs as part of the inflammatory response and is provoked by mediators such as the chemotaxins (small peptides) or by IgE. Histamine acts via four different receptor subtypes: H_1–H_4. The effects of its interaction with the different receptors are summarised in Table 17.1.

The development of drugs affecting the histaminergic response has focused on interactions with H_1 and H_2 receptors, leading to two main categories of drugs: the antihistamines which are antagonists of the H_1 receptor and reduce allergic reactions, and the H_2 antagonists which reduce the secretion of stomach acid. The structural requirements for histamine are quite specific and thus its closely related metabolite 1-methylhistamine (Fig. 17.1) is inactive, while substitution with a single methyl group on the side chain producing 2′-methylhistamine reduces activity to about 20%. Other metabolic inactivation products include imidazole acetic acid and 2′-N-acetylhistamine (Fig. 17.1).

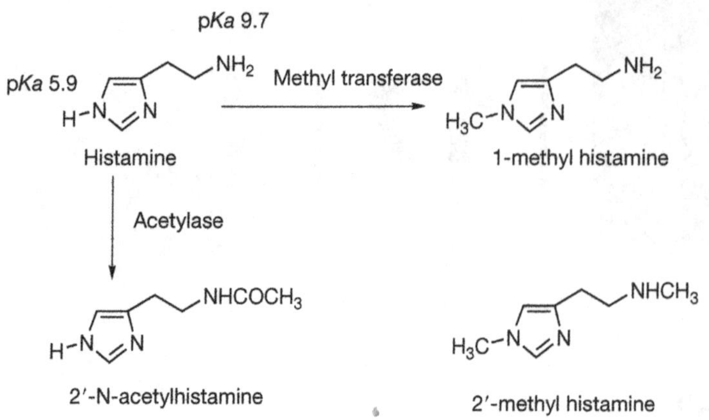

Figure 17.1 Histamine metabolism.

pKa 9.7

pKa 5.9

Histamine

Methyl transferase

1-methyl histamine

Acetylase

2'-N-acetylhistamine

2'-methyl histamine

Table 17.1 Histamine receptors

Receptor	Tissue/cell	Physiological effects
H_1	Smooth muscle, endothelium, neurological tissue	Dilates blood vessels and increases their permeability, contracts lung and other smooth muscle tissues
H_2	Parietal cells Heart tissue	Increased stomach acid secretion, stimulates heart
H_3	Located in neural tissue in the CNS	Reduces release of: adrenaline, serotonin and acetyl choline and histamine
H_4	Found in immune cells	Modulates the immune response

ANTAGONISTS OF HISTAMINE H_1 RECEPTORS

Figure 17.2 shows the amino acid sequence of the histamine H_1 receptor. It is a typical transmembrane G-protein with seven membrane-spanning helices (five of the putative hydrophobic/transmembrane regions are shown in blue). Three important amino acid residues have been found to play a role in the binding of histamine: the aspartic acid residue at 116, the lysine residue at 200, and the asparagine residue at 207.[1,2] These residues occur in the middle of the hydrophobic transmembrane regions which group together quite closely in space, and the force exerted by the binding of histamine changes the conformation of the G-protein. In the case of the H_1 receptor, the G-protein is coupled to a Gq protein which results

MSLPNSSCLLEDKMCEGNKTTMASPQLMPLVVVLSTIDLVTVGLNLLVL YAVRSERKLHT
2nd 116
VGNLYIVSLSVADLIVGAVVMPMNILYLLMSKWSLGT PLCLFWLSMDYVASTASIFSVFIL
4th 161 167
CIDRYRSVQQPLRYLKYRTKTRASATILGAWFLSFLWVIPILGWNHFMQQTSVRREDKCE
5th 200 207
TDFYDVTWFKVMTAIINFYLPTLLMLWFYAKIYKAVRQHCQHRELINRSLPSFSEIKLRPE

NPKGDAKKPGKESPWEVLKRKPKDAGGGSVLKSPSQTPKEMKSPVVFSQEDDREVDKL

YCFPLDIVHMQAAAEGSSRDYVAVNRSHGQLKTDEQGLNTHGASEISEDQMLGDSQSFS

RTDSDTTTETAPGKGKLRSGSNTGLDYIKFTWKRLRSHSRQYVSGLHMNRERKAAKQLG
6th 433 436
FIMAAFILCWIPYFIFFMVIAFCKNCCNEHLHMFTIWLGYINSTLNPLIYPLCNENFKKTFK

RILHIRS

Figure 17.2 Primary amino acid sequence of H_1 receptor showing transmembrane regions in blue and important binding residues for histamine and its antagonists in red.

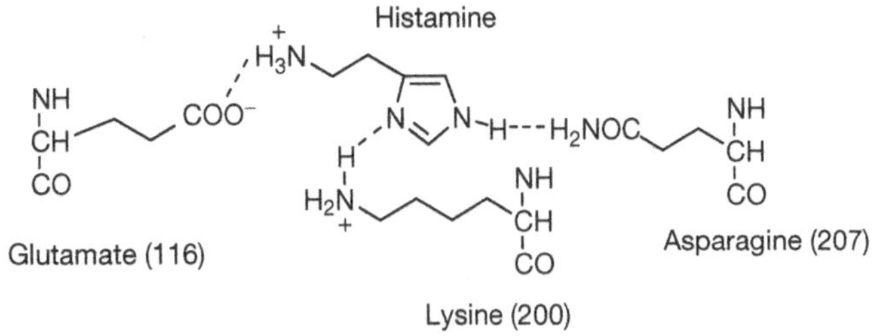

Figure 17.3 Binding of histamine to the H_1 receptor.

in the activation of phospholipase C which cleaves phosphatidyl inositol. Figure 17.3 shows the hypothetical interaction of histamine with its receptor.

After the identification of the effects of histamine in the early twentieth century, screening for potential histamine antagonists was carried out. The first effective antihistamine compound to be found was cyclizine, which was discovered in the 1940s (Fig. 17.4). It was effective both in treating allergy and as an antiemetic. Investigations of the phenothiazine class of compounds led to the discovery of promethazine (Fig. 17.4) which is a very effective long-acting antihistamine. Diphenhydramine (Fig. 17.4) was also synthesised in the 1940s. These compounds defined a distinct pharmacophore shown in Figure 17.4 where the important interaction with the aspartate residue at 116 is present but the interactions promoting binding with the lysine and asparagine residues have been replaced by π–π/lipophilic interactions between the aromatic rings in the antagonist and aromatic rings in the fourth and sixth membrane-spanning helices (Fig. 17.5). Thus the agonist binds but does not cause the conformational change required for receptor activation.

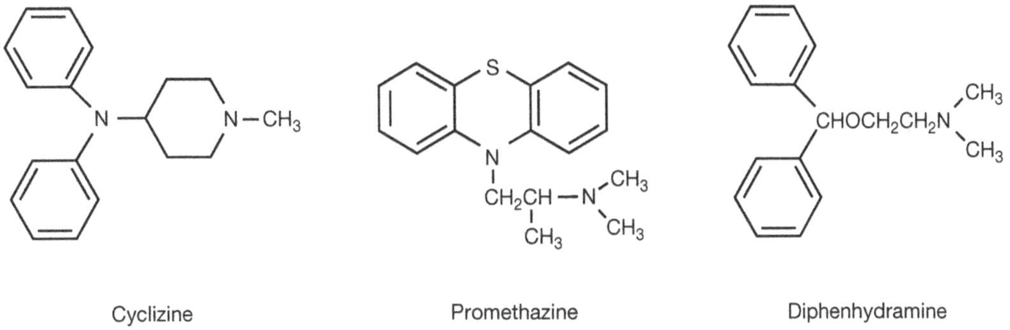

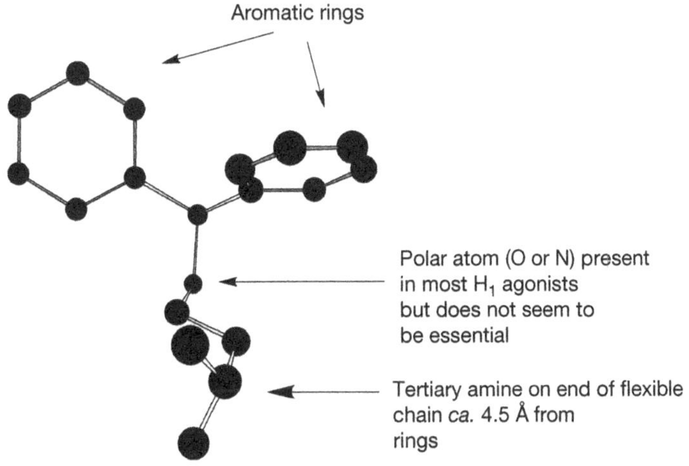

Figure 17.4 Early antihistamines and the H_1-antagonist pharmacophore.

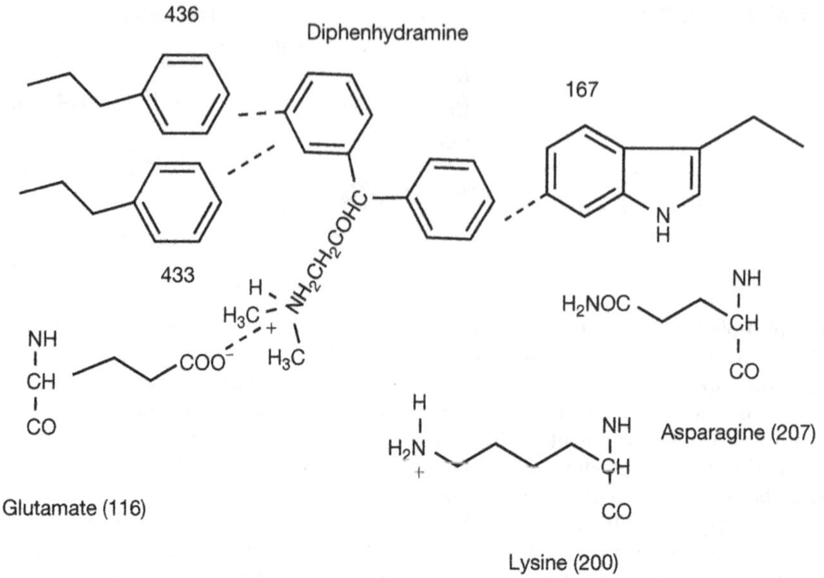

Figure 17.5 Putative interaction of diphenhydramine with glutamate 116 and tryptophan and phenylalanine residues in the fourth and sixth helices.

The pharmacophore present in the first generation of antihistamines was more or less carried forward into the next generation with the development of pheniramine, bromopheniramine and chlorphenamine (Fig. 17.6) except that in these compounds there is a nitrogen atom in one of the aromatic rings, which may enhance the interaction of one of the aromatic rings with asparagine 207. Chlorphenamine is the only compound still used. It is a more potent antagonist than the first generation of antihistamines and its high partition coefficient ensures that, like the first-generation antihistamines, it penetrates into the CNS and causes sedation in addition to having antihistamine activity. The sedating activity may be useful in some cases but if the patient needs to be alert, then obviously this is a disadvantage. A series of stereochemically rigid antihistamines which included cyproheptadine and ketotifen (Fig. 17.6) was produced. The rigid stereochemistry of these analogues favours stronger interaction with the phenylalanine and tryptophan residues in the fourth and sixth helices and these are more potent analogues. However, they are lipophilic and retain the sedating activity of the first-generation antihistamines.

Thus, the next generation of antihistamines were designed to have a lower partition coefficient whilst retaining their activity at the H_1 receptor. The initial discovery of non-sedating antihistamines was accidental. Terfenadine (Fig. 17.7) was designed to be a sedative but was found to be a non-sedating antihistamine. Its structure

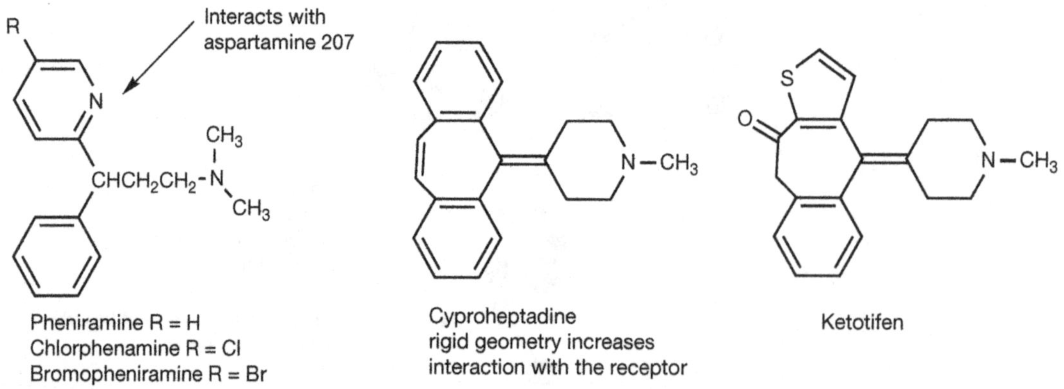

Figure 17.6 Second-generation antihistamines.

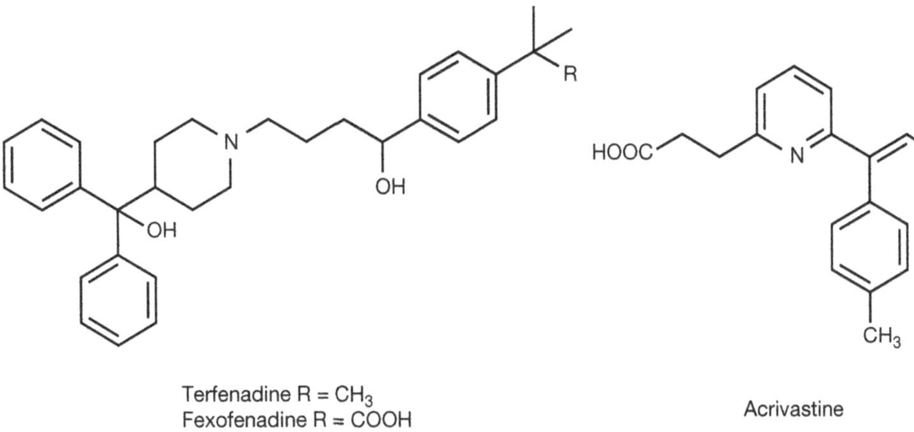

Figure 17.7 Non-sedating antihistamines.

looks similar to that of diphenhydramine and it might be expected to penetrate into the CNS but that it does not is in part due to the fact that it is metabolised via CyP450 activity to fexofenadine (Fig. 17.7) which has a much reduced partitioning into the CNS due to the presence of a carboxylate group in its structure.

Fexofenadine has replaced terfenadine as a drug and is one of the most popular antihistamines. Acrivastine (Fig. 17.7) is another antihistamine which obviously derived from the observation that terfenadine was converted to its carboxy metabolite. It has been proposed that the presence of the carboxy group in some of the non-sedating antihistamines increases binding to the H_1 receptor via interaction with lysine 200 (see Fig. 17.2). Loratadine and its metabolite desloratadine (Fig. 17.8), sold separately as a drug, are also non-sedating antihistamines but it is difficult to explain the lack of CNS penetration from their structures, which are more like those of sedating antihistamines. Mizolastine is a relatively new non-sedating antihistamine, and its lack of CNS penetration might be attributed to its rapid and extensive metabolism.

Figure 17.8 Recently developed non-sedating H_1 antagonists.

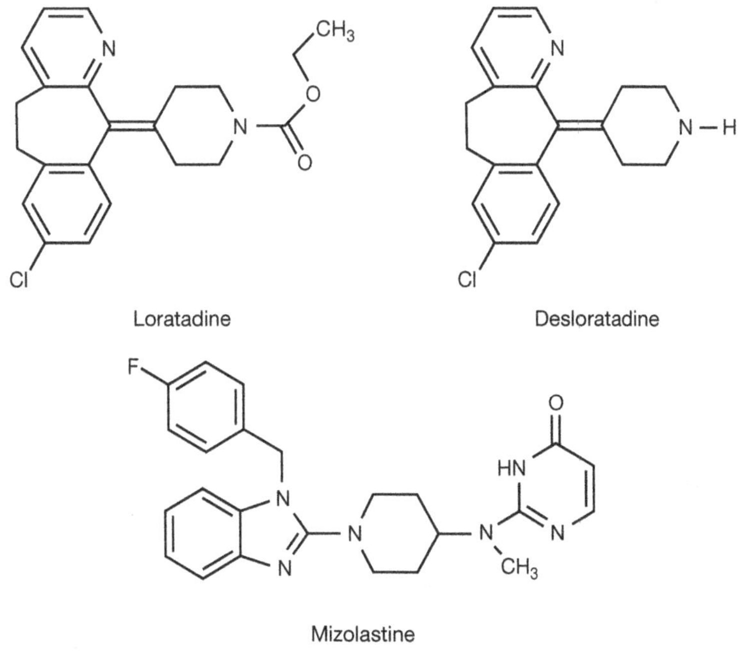

Self Test 17.1

Indicate which category the following antihistamines belong to: a. sedating low potency. b. sedating high potency. c. non-sedating.

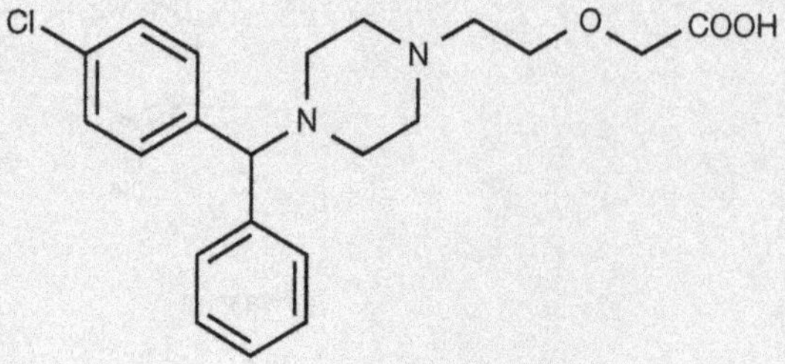

Cetirizine

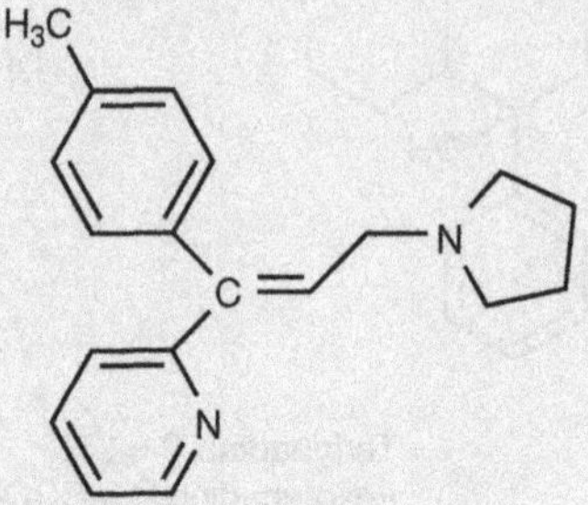

Triprolidine

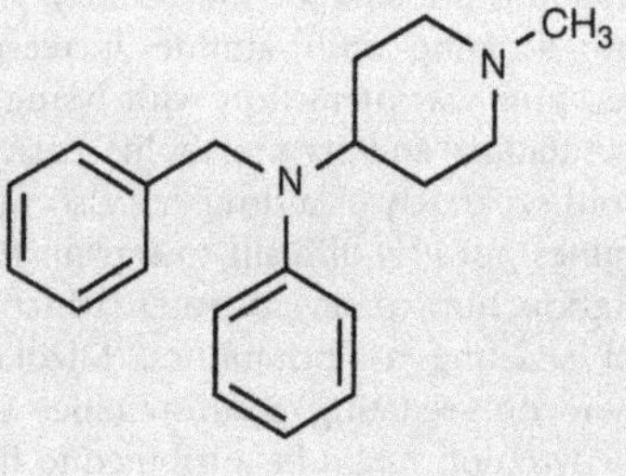

Bamipine

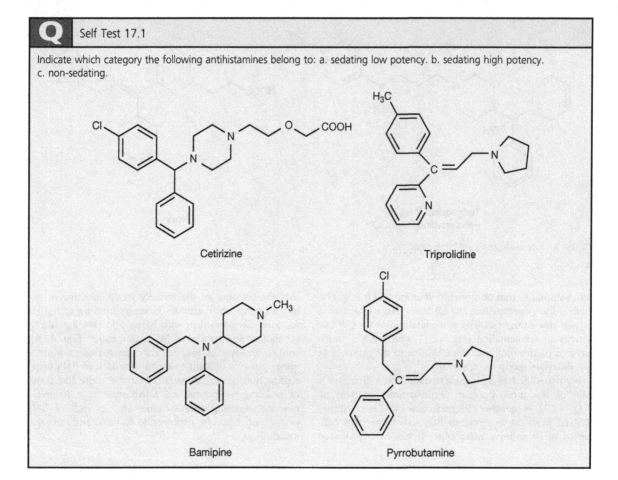

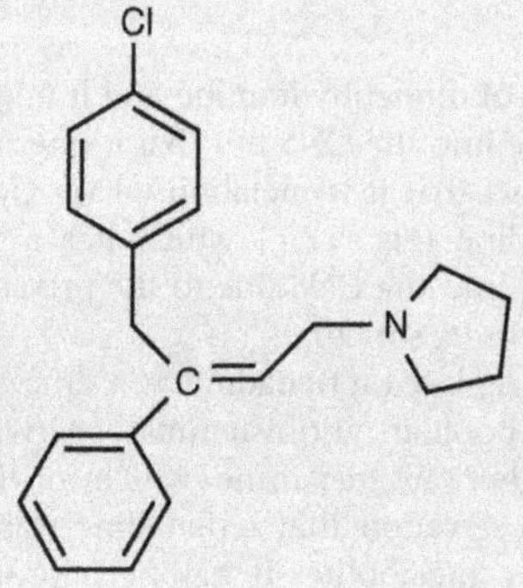

Pyrrobutamine

PREPARATIONS OF ANTIHISTAMINES

Systemic treatments

Non-sedating

- Cetrizine hydrochloride: tablets 10 mg, oral solution 5 mg/5 mL
- Desloratadine: tablets 5 mg, syrup 2.5 mg/5 mL
- Fexofenadine hydrochloride: tablets 30 mg
- Levocetirizine hydrochloride: tablets 5 mg
- Loratadine: tablets 10 mg.
- Mizolastine: tablets 10 mg.

Sedating

- Alimemazine tartrate: tablets 10 mg, syrup 7.5 mg/5 mL and 30 mg/5 mL
- Chlorphenamine maleate: tablets 4 mg, oral solution 2 mg/5 mL, injection 10 mg/mL
- Clemastine hydrogen fumarate: tablets 1 mg
- Cyproheptadine hydrochloride: tablets 4 mg
- Hydroxyzine hydrochloride: tablets 10 mg and 25 mg, syrup 10 mg/5 mL
- Ketotifen hydrogen fumarate: tablets 1 mg, elixir 1 mg/5 mL.

Cough and decongestant preparations

Many cough and decongestant preparations contain sedating antihistamines and sometimes non-sedating antihistamines.

Self Test 17.2

Find out which antihistamines are used in the following commercial cough or decongestant preparations: a. Benylin Chesty Coughs; b. Night Nurse; c. Actifed Chesty Coughs; d. Benadryl Plus Capsules.

Eyedrops

- Antazoline sulphate 0.5% w/v eyedrops
- Emedastine difumarate 0.05% w/v
- Epinastine hydrochloride 0.05% w/v
- Ketotifen fumarate 0.025% w/v.

Topical antihistamines

Antihistamines used in creams for topical application include mepyramine, diphenhydramine, and antazoline.

Allergic rhinitis

- Azelastine hydrochloride 0.1% w/v metered nasal spray
- Levocabastine hydrochloride 0.05% w/v aqueous nasal spray.

HISTAMINE H_2 ANTAGONISTS

Classical antihistamines were found to have no effect on the secretion of gastric acid and this led Sir James Black to speculate that there might be a separate histamine receptor controlling gastric acid secretion which could be exploited in order to treat peptic ulcers and reflux oesophagitis. Classical antihistamine receptors were subsequently termed H_1 receptors and the receptors controlling gastric acid secretion were termed H_2 receptors. Like the H_1 receptor, the H_2 receptor has seven transmembrane-spanning helices. However, it only has 33% amino acid similarity within its primary structure to the H_1 receptor. The primary amino acid sequence is shown in Figure 17.9 with the transmembrane helices and binding sites for histamine highlighted in red and the binding sites for the coupled G-protein on the third intracellular loop highlighted in blue. The proposed mode of binding[3] is shown in Figure 17.10 where the primary interaction with charged side chain on histamine is with the aspartic acid residue at position 98 in the third helix. The two nitrogen atoms in the imidazole ring interact with the aspartic acid and threonine residues at 186 and 190, respectively. The interaction with the aspartic acid residue might be either hydrogen bonding or electrostatic since at physiological pH the imidazole nitrogen (p*Ka* 5.9) is barely charged. As with all G-coupled receptors, binding of the histamine agonist causes a change in the conformation of the receptor which then activates the G-protein and the chain of events resulting from this activation. Site-directed mutagenesis studies[4] indicated that the aspartic acid residue at position 98 was essential for histamine activity but that mutation of the aspartic acid and threonine residues at 186 and 190 did not cause complete loss of histamine agonist activity but did reduce the binding affinity of H_2-receptor antagonists. Later studies[5] have suggested that the tyrosine residue at position 182 (Fig. 17.9) might also be important in the binding of histamine to the receptor.

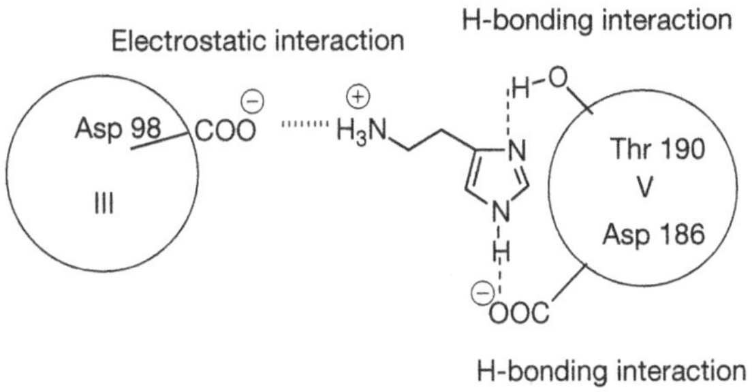

Figure 17.10 Original three-point attachment model for histamine action at the H_2 receptor.

1st

MAPNGTASSFCLDSTACKITI**TVVLAVLILITVAGNVVVCLAVG**LNRRLR NLTNCFI

2nd 3rd 98

VSLAITDLLLGLLVLPFSAIYQLSCKWSFGKVFCN**IYTSLDVMLCTASILNLFMISL**DRYCA

4th

VMDPLRYPVLVTPVR**VAISLVLIWVISITLSFLSIHLGWN**SRNETSKGNHTTSKCKVQVNE

5th 182 186 190 6th

VYGLVDGLVTFYLPLLIMCITYYRIFKVARDQAKRINHISSWKAATIREHKATVT**LAAVMGA**

7th

FIICWFPYFTAFVYRGLRGDDAINE**VLEAIVLWLGYANSALNPILYA**ALNRDFRTGYQQ

LFCCRLANRNSHKTSLRSNASQLSRTQSREPRQQEEKPLKLQVWSGTEVTAPQGATDR

Figure 17.9 Primary structure of the histamine H_2 receptor with the binding sites for histamine and the coupled G-protein highlighted in red and blue, respectively.

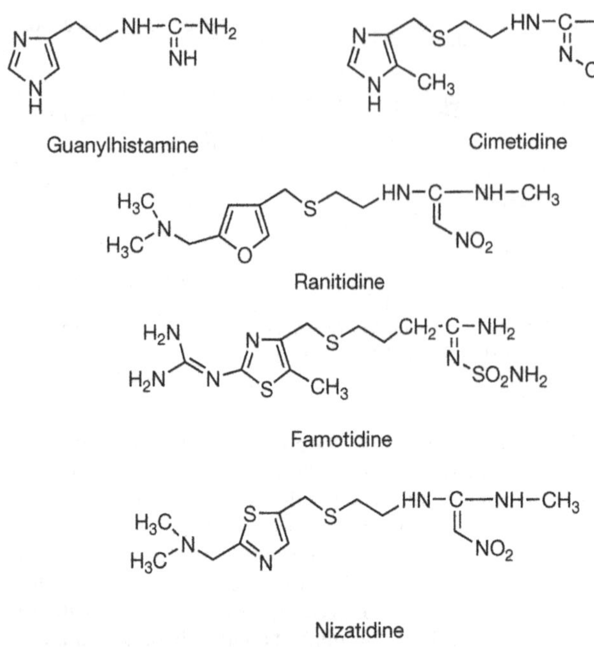

Figure 17.11 H_2-receptor antagonists.

The two major H_2-receptor blocking drugs cimetidine and ranitidine (Fig. 17.11) were discovered before anything was known about the structure of the binding site of the H_2 receptor. The lead compound produced by Sir James Black and his team was guanylhistamine (Fig. 17.11), where the primary amine group in histamine has been replaced by the more strongly basic guanine group. This compound functions as a partial agonist, binding to the receptor and blocking histamine binding but at the same time producing a lower level of acid secretion. Presumably, the presence of the guanine group reduces the binding to the two other points of attachment in helix V since it would be likely to bind strongly to asp 98. It was assumed that by reducing the interaction of the basic side chain with the aspartic acid residue at 98 it would be possible to get the same antagonism without the partial agonist activity. The first commercially successful H_2 receptor antagonist was cimetidine and in this structure imidazole ring is retained but the side chain is lengthened and the basic guanidine group is substituted with a cyano group which more or less abolishes its basicity due to the electron withdrawing effect of the CN group. Despite the substituted guanine group no longer being basic, cimetidine binds strongly to the receptor without exhibiting any agonist activity. Cimetidine exhibited side effects due to absorption into the CNS and also interferes with CyP450 oxidation of other drugs, and thus ranitidine (Fig. 17.11) was developed. The ranitidine structure is quite remote from the structure of histamine but is an effective antagonist. It retains the modified guanidine group of cimetidine which in the case of ranitidine is rendered non-basic via substitution of a strongly electron withdrawing nitro group, but the histidine ring has been replaced by a side chain containing a tertiary amine group. The tertiary amine group has a higher p*Ka* value than the imidazole ring thus ensuring the molecule is completely ionised at physiological pH and reducing penetration into the CNS and also increasing the binding to the H_2 receptor. Ranitidine is about three times more potent than cimetidine in vivo. Following on from ranitidine, two more H_2-receptor antagonists were launched on to the market: famotidine (Fig. 17.11), which is about 20 times more potent than cimetidine, and nizatidine (Fig. 17.11) which has similar potency to ranitidine. There are no clinical advantages of famotidine and nizatidine over ranitidine.

OTHER AGENTS USED IN TREATMENT OF PEPTIC ULCERS

The use of proton pump inhibitors in the treatment of ulcers is covered in Chapter 12. However, there is a disparate collection of compounds used in therapy of ulcers which do not fall into a particular class. These are described below.

Bismuth salts

Bismuth salts were used in the eighteenth and nineteenth centuries as antimicrobial compounds and also as antacids. With the discovery that *Helicobacter pylori* was the causative agent of ulcer formation, there was revival of interest in their use in the 1990s. The most commonly used water-soluble form of bismuth is tripotassium dicitratobismuthate

($[Bi_2(C_6H_4O_7)]^{2-}2K^+$) which has a complex structure.[6] This salt is unstable in the stomach acid and precipitates out to form complex cationic species which form complexes with proteins in the stomach wall protecting ulcers from gastric acid and pepsin, and these complexes are also toxic to *H. pylori*. The basis of the toxicity of bismuth salts to the bacteria may be due to formation of complexes with the urease (which produces ammonia from urea) that the bacteria produce in large amounts in order to maintain the pH of their environment at around 6 so that they can survive under the acidic conditions in the stomach.[7] Bismuth salts are usually used in combination with an H_2-receptor antagonist and a tetracycline (see Ch. 22) which is also used to kill the bacteria.

Sucralfate

Sucralfate is a basic salt of aluminium with sucrose octasulphate. Its mechanism of action is not fully understood but it appears to strengthen the mucosal layer in the stomach by binding to proteins on the stomach wall. In addition, there is some evidence that it stimulates PGE_2 formation which in turn strengthens the mucosal layer.[8]

Misoprostol

Misoprostol is a synthetic prostaglandin which is used to treat gastric and duodenal ulcers. It is the methyl ester of PGE_2, which has various activities including promotion of the secretion of mucus. The ester is rapidly converted into the biologically active free acid in the body. It is used particularly to mitigate the side effects of non-steroidal anti-inflammatory drugs.

Preparations of H_2-receptor antagonists and other drugs promoting ulcer healing

- Cimetidine: tablets 200 mg, suspension 200 mg/5 mL, oral solution 200 mg/5 mL, syrup 200 mg/5 mL, injection 100 mg/mL
- Ranitidine: tablets 150 mg and 300 mg, effervescent tablets 150 mg and 300 mg, oral solution 75 mg/5 mL, syrup 75 mg/5 mL and ranitidine 25 mg/mL
- Famotidine: tablets 20 mg and 40 mg, tablets chewable 10 mg
- Nizatidine: capsules 150 mg and 300 mg, injection 25 mg/mL
- Ranitidine bismuth citrate: tablets 400 mg
- Sucralfate: tablets 1 g and suspension 1 g/5 mL
- Misoprostol: Tablets 200 μg.

A Self Test 17.1

c. Cetirizine; b. Triprolidine; a. Bamipine; b. Pyrrobutamine.

A Self Test 17.2

a. Diphenhydramine; b. Promethazine; c. Triprolidine; d. Acrivastine.

REFERENCES

1. Leurs R, Smit MJ, Meeder R, Ter Laak AM, Timmerman H. Lysine 200 located in the fifth transmembrane domain of the histamine H_1 receptor interacts with histamine but not with all H_1 agonists. *Biophysical Res Comm.* 1995;214:110–117.
2. Wieland K, Ter Laak AM, Smit MJ, Kuhne R, Timmerman H, Leurs R. Mutational analysis of the agonist-binding site of the histamine H_1 receptor. *J Biol Chem.* 1999;274:29994–30000.
3. Gantz I, Del Valle J, Wang L, et al. Molecular basis for the interaction of histamine with the histamine H_2 receptor. *J Biol Chem.* 1992;267:20840–20843.
4. Nederkoorn PHJ, van Gelder EM, Donné-Op den Kelder GM, Timmerman H. The agonistic binding site at the H_2 receptor II. Theoretical investigations of histamine binding to the seven α-helical transmembrane domain. *J Comp Aided Mol Des.* 1996;10:479–489.
5. Del Valle J, Gantz I. Novel insights into histamine H_2 receptor biology. *Am J Physiol Gastrointest Liver Physiol.* 1997;273:987–996.
6. Sandler PJ, Guo Z. Metal complexes in medicine: Design and mechanism of action. *Pure Appl Chem.* 1998;70:863–871.
7. Zhang L, Mulrooney SB, Leung AFK, et al. Inhibition of urease by bismuth(III): Implications for the mechanism of action of bismuth drugs. *Biometals.* 2006;19:503–511.
8. Slomiany BL, Murty VLN, Piotrowski E, Morita M, Piotrowsky J, Slomiany A. Activation of arachidonoyl phospholipase A, in prostaglandin-mediated action of sucralfate. *Gem Pharmar.* 1994;25:261–266.

Chapter | 18 |

CNS stimulants and CNS-active drugs affecting the serotonergic system

Simon D Brandt

CHAPTER CONTENTS

INTRODUCTION

Noradrenaline, adrenaline, dopamine and serotonin (5-HT, 5-hydroxytryptamine) (Fig. 18.1) are monoamines of fundamental importance in the central nervous system (CNS) because of their function as neurotransmitters. It is therefore not surprising that these compounds serve as structural templates for medicinal products in the attempt to influence brain signalling mechanisms. Health may often be defined as the absence of illness and, correspondingly, most currently available drugs have been developed to compensate for a reduced capability of the brain to maintain functioning. An additional perspective refers to the fact that health and well-being may be viewed as a potential for enhancement beyond what would otherwise be considered as normal physiological and psychological performance.

This chapter aims to provide a basic introduction to the idea that even the smallest structural modifications of a particular neurotransmitter template can result in fascinating alterations of their activity on brain chemistry and behaviour. It is quite likely that most treatments for CNS-related disorders involve the application of derivatives which were derived from these templates. Equally so, a large number of structurally related compounds have been found to be powerful drugs of abuse, including hallucinogens and psychostimulants.

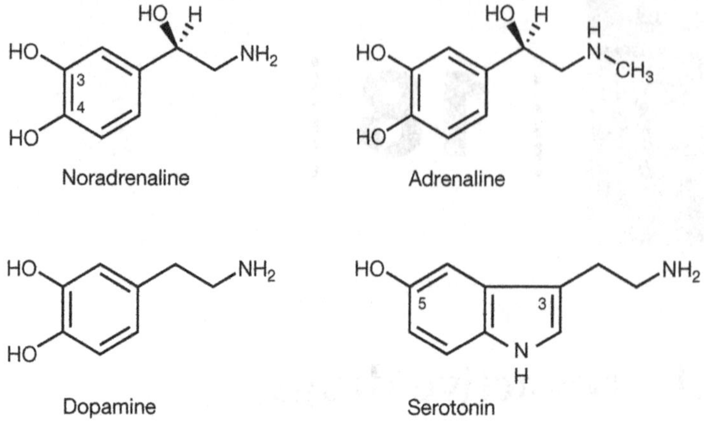

Figure 18.1 Template neurotransmitters.

As far as structure–activity relationships (SAR) and mechanisms of action are concerned, it is important to remember that only a few basic principles with regard to primary targets can be mentioned here. This is in part based on the fact that a rational approach is not always possible but, more importantly, the understanding of these complex phenomena also depends on the perspective. For example, observation of a behavioural response towards drug exposure may be used to evaluate SAR of potential drug candidates. The overall response or output of this test system may appear to be identical but the corresponding neurochemical correlates (e.g. human brain or animal) may actually be quite different. Advances in molecular biology and neurochemistry allow us to gain increased insights into these mechanisms but also make us realise the complexities involved. This parallels the experience we have when we revise for exams where it sometimes seems that the more we look into the details of a particular subject, the less we understand. Drug intake can have a tremendous effect on gene expression patterns of protein products which effect signalling processes. Also, several different compounds may interact with the same receptor subtype but trigger substrate-specific, i.e. independent, signal transduction pathways. This is sometimes called functional selectivity and may indicate that the traditional view of a key–lock model of the fit between ligand and receptor may need modification. Drug interactions with primary targets may help to predict or understand a particular mechanism. Cocaine (Fig. 18.2), for example, is known for its psychostimulant and reinforcing properties. One primary target is the dopamine reuptake transporter where blockage leads to increased availability of dopamine. However, not every molecule that interacts with the same target will result in an identical pharmacological and behavioural response. Compounds such as mazindol, GBR 12935 and nomifensine (Fig. 18.2) are known to be effective inhibitors of dopamine transport but do not seem to show any of the reinforcing properties of cocaine, which means that these derivatives are not addictive. The primary target is the same but obviously something else is going on here. Nevertheless, the identification of certain primary targets can help to direct research and development in the right direction.

CENTRAL NERVOUS SYSTEM STIMULANTS

In the context of this chapter, the term CNS stimulant refers to a behavioural definition and includes a variety of compounds with psychostimulatory properties based on their interaction with catecholamine, i.e. monoamine, systems. This means that these derivatives are able to induce a number of dose-dependent behaviour-activating responses such as increased levels of alertness, vigilance and self-confidence, elevation of mood, anorexia and reduced fatigue. Physiologically, the body activates several parameters typically involved in a fight-or-flight reaction, particularly when these derivatives are administered at high dosages. Increased blood glucose levels, heart rate and blood pressure are characteristic manifestations and muscle tissues are supplied with increased blood flow and oxygen levels. In other words, psychostimulants lead to the innervation of the sympathetic system. As discussed in Chapter 10, stimulation of peripheral α- and β-adrenergic receptors have powerful effects on vasoconstriction, bronchodilation and the cardiovascular system. An inherent characteristic of certain psychostimulants is their ability to reinforce consumption which is part of the human condition to repeat exposure to an experience that is perceived as pleasurable. This brings the dopaminergic system into the equation, which is involved in the mediation of natural and drug-induced reward, habituation and dependence. Tolerance can develop relatively rapidly and increased dosages have to be ingested in order to maintain elevated mood and euphoria, which can precipitate in a variety of very detrimental conditions, as described later.

Figure 18.2 Inhibitors of dopamine transport.

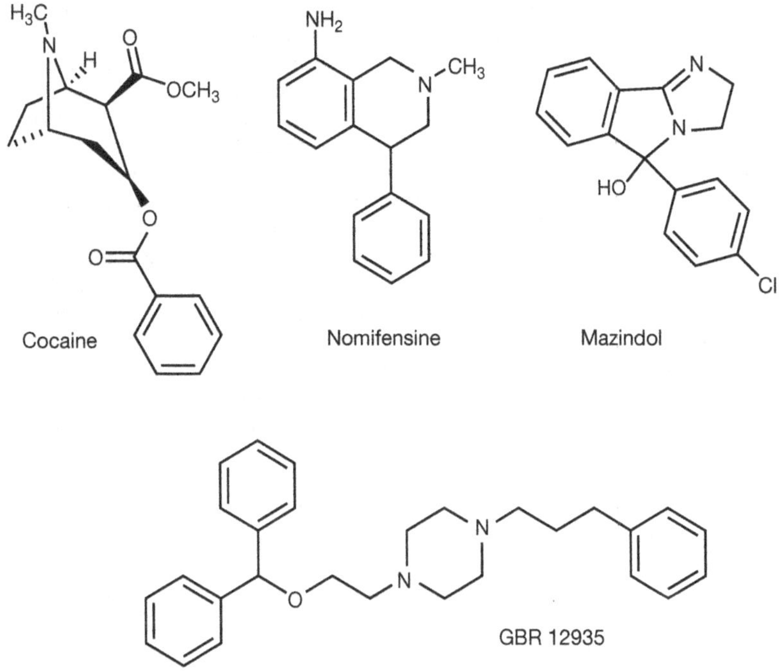

A number of indications for the clinical use of CNS stimulants have been identified over the years and included depression in terminal illness, chronic shift work sleep disorder, Parkinson's disease and, paradoxically, narcolepsy and attention deficit hyperactivity disorder (ADHD). A large number of psychostimulants are used for the short-term treatment of obesity due to their anorectic effects but are usually not recommended for this application any more due to the development of tolerance. The abuse potential of several medically relevant psychostimulants has led to a more stringent control, and global research activities keep focused on the development of alternative medicines with reduced potential for misuse.

Several psychostimulant anorectics have been withdrawn from the market or are less often prescribed due to increased numbers of reported adverse reactions such as hepatotoxicity (e.g. pemoline, Fig. 18.3) and cardiovascular problems (e.g. fenfluramine, Fig. 18.3, and phentermine, Fig. 18.4). It seems worthwhile to point out that despite these concerns many products remain to be used, either legally or illegally, in different countries. A large number of performance-enhancing and anorectic stimulants can be purchased over the Internet, which places the consumer at additional risk because of the potential presence of counterfeit or mislabelled products. Another reason for concern is the adulteration of plant materials and extracts. One example includes the availability of traditional Chinese slimming medicines which were found to contain unknown plant matter spiked with a variety of psychostimulants.

Basic mechanisms

Psychostimulant pharmacology involves an augmented release of noradrenaline and dopamine into the synaptic cleft. The presence of monoamine neurotransmitters in the synaptic cleft is regulated in a variety of ways in response to an action potential. Around 70–80% of all transmitter molecules return into the presynaptic neuron by uptake using an energy-dependent reuptake transport protein that is embedded in the neuronal membrane. A smaller fraction

Figure 18.3 Less commonly used psychostimulant anorectics.

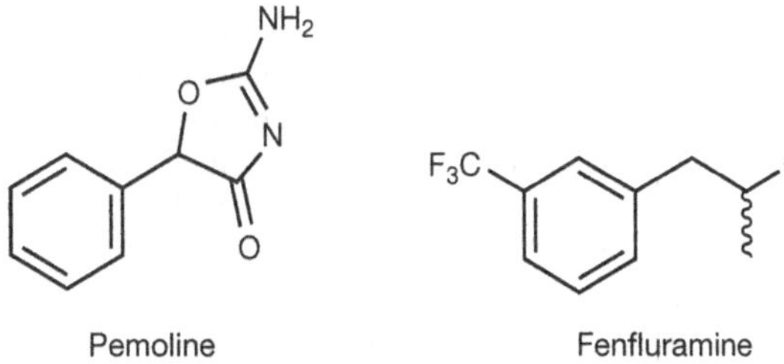

can also be inactivated by catechol-O-methyltransferase (COMT) and via oxidative deamination by monoamine oxidase (MAO). Increased neurotransmitter availability is thought to be caused either directly or indirectly. A direct mechanism of action prohibits neurotransmitter reuptake by blockage where drug binding induces conformational changes within a binding site that prevents the transporter from removing and recycling the neurotransmitter, which thus increases availability in the synaptic cleft. A typical example of this mechanism is found in the interaction of cocaine with the dopamine transporter.

The indirect principle is currently believed to involve two synergistic mechanisms. Certain drugs are substrates at the transport protein based on structural similarity with the particular neurotransmitter. Transporter blockage would not be observed but drug binding still occurs. This leads to transport reversal where the drug is transported into the cytoplasm in exchange for the monoamine transmitter which then gets released into the synapse. In addition, a particular drug may be able to interact with what is called a vesicular monoamine transporter (VMAT-2) which facilitates the transport of monoamines from the cytoplasm back to the synaptic vesicles where they are stored and protected from degradation. In other words, VMAT-2 accumulates both newly synthesised and freshly returned neurotransmitter molecules from the synapse. A psychostimulant is able to enter the storage vesicles and cause the monoamine to be released into the cytoplasm and also prevents reuptake back into the vesicles.

In order to provide a rough indicator for the mechanism of action, a psychostimulant can either be classified as a monoamine 'blocker' or 'releaser'. For example, certain amfetamines may be called dopamine releasers, rather than being classified as dopamine reuptake blockers. It is important to consider, however, that these derivatives often possess both qualities, although one mechanism normally dominates. As mentioned previously, it is important to note that additional neurotransmitter systems, such as serotonin and glutamate, may be involved in the regulation of these effects. Cocaine is also able to block the serotonin and noradrenalin plasma membrane transporter in addition to blockage of dopamine reuptake. The dopamine system can also be regulated by cortical glutamatergic and inhibitory amino acid γ-aminobutyric acid (GABA) systems.

Dopamine

It has been estimated that dopamine contributes at least 50% to the total CNS catecholamine content. A number of neurological diseases are based on the activity of dopamine and examples include drug addiction, Tourette's syndrome, Parkinson's and Huntington's disease and schizophrenia. Four major dopamine systems have been identified in the brain.

1. The nigrostriatal pathway resides in the substantia nigra and provides the connection to the dorsal striatum, i.e. putamen and caudate nuclei. This pathway is implicated in the control of fine motor function and is fundamentally involved in Parkinson's disease where dopamine transmission is severely impaired. In other words, this is part of the extrapyramidal system. On the other hand, hyperactivity of this pathway has been correlated with involuntary movements (dyskinesias) and tics.
2. The short tuberoinfundibular pathway connects the hypothalamic arcuate nucleus with the pituitary gland via the median eminence. In this case, dopamine functions include suppression of prolactin release.
3. The mesocortical pathway connects the ventral tegmental area of the midbrain with the prefrontal cortex which involves the regulation of several cognitive processes such as selective attention and working memory.
4. The mesolimbic pathway also originates in the ventral tegmentum but leads to several centres of the limbic system, including the amygdala and the nucleus acumbens. This is thought to involve the perception of pleasure, i.e. natural or drug-induced reward, which plays a fundamental role in the determination whether a drug has addictive potential. Mesolimbic overactivity has been suggested to be involved in positive symptomatology of psychosis. There are indications that several dopamine receptor agonists may also serve as positive reinforcers, while antagonist action may decrease the perception of reward. Currently, five metabotropic G-protein coupled receptors are known. The D_1-like family comprises D_1 and D_5 subtypes whereas the so-called D_2-like family consists of D_2, D_3 and D_4 subtypes.

Any neurotransmitter system is interrelated with a number of modulating networks that influence signalling, which adds complexity to the challenge of gaining an understanding when talking about structure–activity relationships. For example, increased serotonergic activity, either stress- or drug-induced, is known to attenuate dopamine release in the mesolimbic system, depending on the involved serotonin receptor subtypes.

Amfetamines

Amfetamine (Fig. 18.4) is often named as a representative example for an indirect dopamine-releasing psychostimulant. The presence of the β-phenylethylamine nucleus is a common theme in a variety of psychoactive derivatives. CNS activity and adverse reactions typically found with amfetamines are shared by most psychostimulants, albeit to a different degree and intensity. Amfetamine itself can be used safely, provided that dose and route of administration are followed as prescribed for a particular condition. The two most common areas of application include narcolepsy and ADHD.

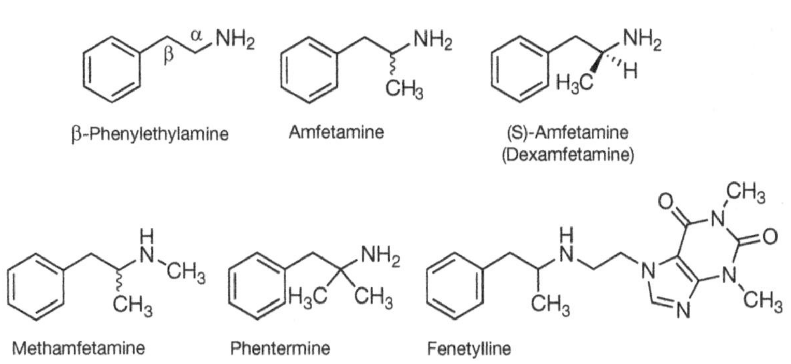

Figure 18.4 Amfetamine derivatives.

Description and preparations

Amfetamine is obtainable as a variety of salts including sulphate, phosphate, aspartate and saccharate. Dexamfetamine is available as the phosphate and sulphate salts and is formulated using the (*S*)-isomer. It is a white crystalline powder and soluble in water.

- Dexamfetamine sulphate 5 mg tablets. Adult dose 10–60 mg daily (narcolepsy). Children max. 20–40 mg (ADHD), age-dependent.

Its adrenergic component induces characteristic cardiovascular responses described in Chapter 10. Low to moderate doses increase blood pressure, slow heart rate, relax bronchial muscle and produce a variety of other responses that follow from the body's alerting response. In the CNS, amfetamine is a potent psychomotor stimulant, producing increased alertness, euphoria, excitement, wakefulness, a reduced sense of fatigue, loss of appetite, mood elevation, increased motor and speech activity, and a feeling of power. At chronic and high doses, a number of severe side effects may occur such as tachycardia, anxiety, restlessness, insomnia, tremor and severe arrhythmias. Stereotypical behaviours may also be observed and include purposeless, repetitive acts, paranoia, outbursts of aggression and manifestation of a so-called amfetamine psychosis.

In the amfetamine group of compounds it has generally been found that the (*S*)-enantiomer is significantly more potent when compared with either racemic or (*R*)-amfetamine. Ring substitution generally seems to reduce amfetamine-like activity. *N*-Methylation leads to the much more potent methamfetamine. It was formerly used for the treatment of ADHD but has gained negative publicity as a widely abused drug, particularly after the widespread inhalation of the free base vapour. One of the differences between smoking free base cocaine (crack) and methamfetamine is the long half-life of the latter of around 12 hours.

Both *N*-ethylamfetamine and the (*S*)-enantiomer of *N*-benzyl-*N*-methylamfetamine (adult dose 25 to 150 mg of the hydrochloride salt daily) have been marketed in the past as anorectics and they have shown weaker amfetamine-like properties. Removal of the α-methyl group of amfetamine gives β-phenylethylamine which is not a stimulant. Extension of the α-methyl group appears to diminish amfetamine-like characteristics.

Phentermine, possessing two methyl groups on the α position, retains the indirect-acting sympathomimetic properties and is also used for the short-term treatment of obesity. The association of primary pulmonary hypertension with certain anorectics, including phentermine, has led to reduced prescription and removal from the market in several countries. The usual adult dose of phentermine hydrochloride is 15 to 30 mg once daily before breakfast and 8 mg three times daily has also been recommended.

Fenetylline is an interesting example where the molecule consists of a combination of sympathomimetic-like entities. In this compound the caffeine derivative theophylline is fused to amfetamine and it has been used for the treatment of ADHD and narcolepsy. It has been claimed that fenetylline showed fewer amfetamine-type side effects such as elevated blood pressure, tremor and fine motor activity, but became illegal due to increased numbers of abusers. A typical adult dose of fenetylline hydrochloride is 25–50 mg once or twice a day. Fenetylline abuse has been reported to be particularly prominent in the Middle East and a large number of counterfeit products are circulating.

Ephedrine derivatives

A comparison with Chapter 10 confirms that the β-phenylethylamine feature is also present in a variety of drugs that affect the adrenergic system. Noradrenaline (NA) and its derivatives were shown to possess two hydroxyl groups on the 3 and 4 position of the benzene ring, these contributing to their ability to interact directly with α- and β-receptor subtypes, leading to the expected peripheral effects. A closer look at the molecules in Figure 18.5 allows us to realise that a few structural modifications have taken place when compared with the NA derivatives and, as one might expect, this introduces some changes in their pharmacological properties.

Ephedrine and its derivatives are present in *Ephedra sinica* Stapf, used for millennia as a stimulant. The absence

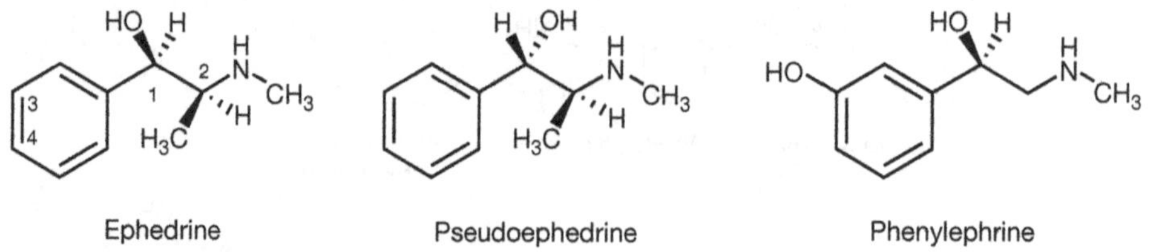

Figure 18.5 Ephedrine derivatives.

of hydroxyl groups on the aromatic ring increases lipophilicity which results in improved membrane permeability at the intestinal mucosa–blood and the blood–brain barriers. Another important difference is the presence of an additional methyl group on the ethylamine side chain. This position is also referred to as the α-position, which, strictly speaking, gives a β-phenylisopropylamine derivative. The presence of the α-methyl group also protects the molecule from metabolism by MAO. This means that both reduced polarity and increased metabolic stability result in prolonged bioavailability and the induction of pronounced stimulating effects on the CNS. Ephedrine is a mild stimulant and can be found, either alone or in combination preparations (e.g. with caffeine), in a variety of products, particularly cold cures.

Description and preparations

Ephedrine is available as the anhydrous free base, the hemihydrate (· ½ H_2O), hydrochloride or sulphate salts and appears as white crystalline powder or crystals. It is soluble in water and ethanol and exposure to light and air should be avoided.

- Ephedrine hydrochloride nasal drops 0.5% (w/v), nasal decongestion. Adult dose 1–2 drops into each nostril up to 3 or 4 times daily when required.
- Ephedrine hydrochloride 3 mg/mL solution, reversal of hypotension from spinal or epidural anaesthesia by slow intravenous injection; adult dose 3–6 mg repeated every 3–4 minutes according to response to max. 30 mg.
- Ephedrine hydrochloride tablets 15 mg, bronchodilation; adult dose 15–60 mg, 3 times daily.

In addition to pharmacopoeial preparations, a number of diverse preparations are available for purchase, often via the Internet. These include *Ephedra* spp. herbal extracts and teas (e.g. *Cao Ma Huang*, used in traditional Chinese medicine) and are marketed in context with sports supplement weight loss products. Dosages can vary greatly and several additives, sometimes unknown, are often encountered.

Stereochemistry

Ephedrine contains two chiral centres giving rise to four possible stereoisomers, with ephedrine and pseudoephedrine being dominant in the *Ephedra* plant. Ephedrine itself, (Fig. 18.5) is identifiable as the (1*R*,2*S*)-stereoisomer and also named (−)-ephedrine. Correspondingly, (+)-ephedrine is represented by the (1*S*,2*R*)-derivative. In pseudoephedrine, the configuration of the hydroxyl group changes, which makes it the (1*S*, 2*S*)-derivative of ephedrine. Accordingly, (−)-pseudoephedrine would typically be defined as (1*R*,2*R*)-ephedrine. (+)-Pseudoephedrine is more commonly used in decongestion products than ephedrine. Removal of the α-methyl group from ephedrine and addition of a hydroxyl group on the *meta*-position of the benzene ring leads to phenylephrine that can be classified as a (1*R*)-derivative of ephedrine, which lacks significant stimulatory effects.

Cathinones

Fresh leaves of the khat bush (*Catha edulis* Forssk.), found for example in several African countries and the Arabian Peninsula, are chewed for their psychostimulant properties and evidence suggests that khat use may predate coffee drinking. The consumption of fresh leaves is based on the fact that potency diminishes drastically within two days. Correspondingly, khat use has remained endemic, but modern transportation allows for daily shipments to a variety of European countries and the United States. A large number of β-phenylethylamine derivatives have been detected but the main constituents are (*S*)-cathinone, (1*S*,2*S*)-cathine and (1*R*,2*S*)-norephedrine. Psychoactivity is, however, predominantly determined by cathinone and cathine (Fig. 18.6). The plant material is legally available in some countries, whereas both cathinone and cathine are controlled. (*R*)-cathinone has yet to be detected in leaves.

Cathinone was found to be significantly more potent than cathine and the reason for fresh consumption reflects the fact that cathinone is converted rapidly into the less active, mild stimulatory cathine. Note that cathine is a common name for (1*S*,2*S*)-pseudonorephedrine (Fig. 18.6). Inspection of the cathinone structure shows that it may also be described as β-keto amfetamine and it is not surprising that its effects are very similar to amfetamine. *N*-Methylation of cathinone leads to methcathinone which is only synthetically available on the streets and may not be a plant constituent (Fig. 18.7). Increased lipophilicity leads to increased potency which mirrors the relationship found between amfetamine and methamfetamine. Studies with rats indicated that (S)-methcathinone appeared to be more potent than (S)-cathinone, (S)-methamfetamine and (S)-amfetamine and around ten times more potent than

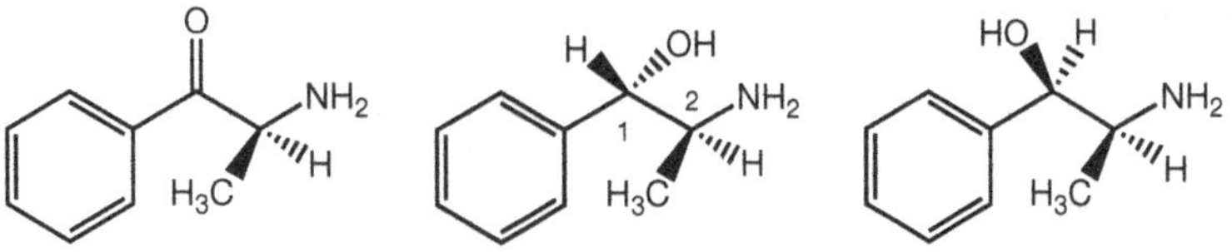

Figure 18.6 Cathinone alkaloids.

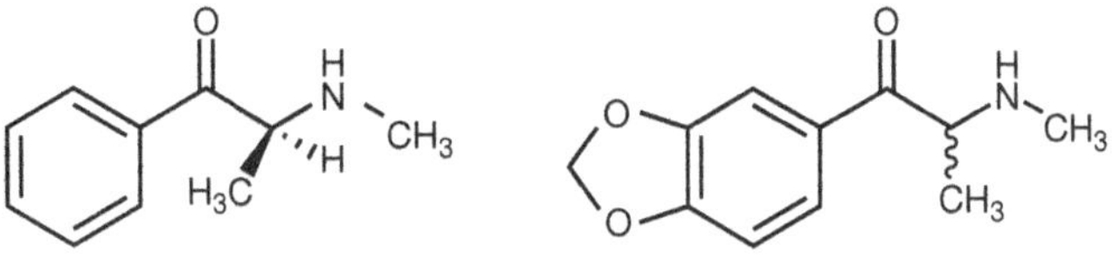

Figure 18.7 Synthetic analogues of cathinone.

cocaine. (S)-Methcathinone is more commonly found on the street than the (R)-isomer or the racemic mixture which reflects the fact that the (S)-isomer can be easily prepared by the oxidation of ephedrine which, as we have seen, is the (1R,2S)-diastereoisomer. Correspondingly, cathinone is the oxidised analogue of norephedrine. Recent reports indicated that commonly available ephedrine or pseudoephedrine containing over-the-counter decongestion products have been used for the illegal production of methcathinone. A distinctive extrapyramidal, i.e. Parkinsonian, syndrome has been observed in users of these products, which was correlated with very high manganese blood levels, reflecting the use of potassium permanganate as the oxidising agent required for their production.

Methylone (3,4-methylenedioxymethcathinone) was originally developed as an analeptic in the 1950s but appeared in the recreational context in recent years and is classified as an illegal drug. It would appear that both methcathinone and methylone share psychopharmacological similarities with methamfetamine and 3,4-methylenedioxy-*N*-methamfetamine (MDMA, *Ecstasy*) (see Fig. 18.39), based on the ability to both block and release catecholamines. Recent research has indicated that methylone may also inhibit serotonin and dopamine reuptake.

A tert.-butyl β-keto derivative of the basic pharmacophore carrying a chlorine atom on position 3 of the benzene ring results in bupropion (Fig. 18.8). The psychostimulant properties are not pronounced in this case and it has been suggested that it exerts its effects via non-selective inhibition of both the dopamine and noradrenaline transporter. This feature is found in a variety of antidepressants and the two most commonly involved indications are depression and smoking cessation. Bupropion has also been reported to act as an antagonist at neuronal nicotinic acetylcholine receptors and does not seem to have significant sympathomimetic properties. A more detailed understanding of the mechanism involved in its antidepressant activity is needed.

Description and preparations

Bupropion is available as the hydrochloride salt and is obtainable in several bioequivalent oral formulations including immediate, sustained and extended release. Film-coated tablets (f/c) are also available.

- Bupropion hydrochloride f/c tablets 150 mg. Adult dose: 150–300 mg for 7–9 weeks (smoking cessation). In severe cases of depression, up to 450 mg of the hydrochloride salt have been recommended.

Diethylpropion (diethylcathinone) is the *N,N*-diethyl derivative without the presence of the chlorine atom and displays amfetamine-like effects in humans. When

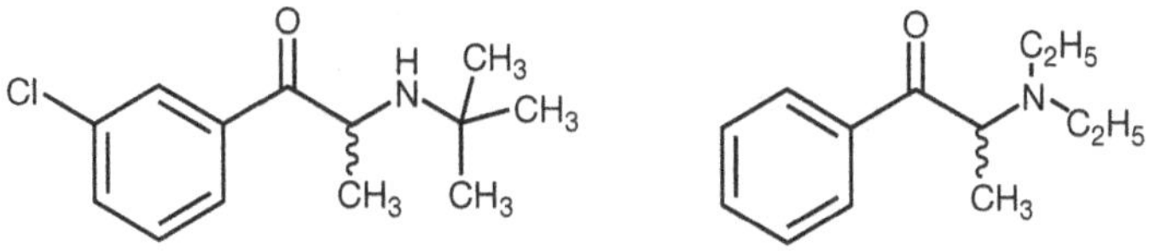

Figure 18.8 Synthetic cathinones used within a medicinal context.

compared with bupropion, it was found to exhibit significantly stronger ability to release noradrenaline. The fact that this results in stronger sympathomimetic effects led to its use as an anorectic for the short-term treatment of obesity. Interestingly, there has been some indication that diethylpropion metabolites may be responsible for noradrenaline release, and not the parent compound.

Diethylpropion hydrochloride is manufactured in 25 mg and 75 mg controlled-release tablets.

- Diethylpropion hydrochloride tablets 25 mg. Adult dose: 25 mg three times daily.

Caffeine

Caffeine and some of its derivatives have been of great interest since ancient times for their diuretic, analgesic, decongestant, anorectic, respiratory and central stimulant properties. Caffeine derivatives are methylated xanthines which are naturally present in several natural products including coffee beans (*Coffea arabica* Linnaeus), tea leaves (*Camellia sinensis* (Linnaeus) O. Kuntze), and chocolate derived from cacao beans (*Theobroma cacao* Linnaeus), maté (*Ilex paraguariensis* Saint-Hilaire) and guaraná (*Paullinia cupana* Kunth ex H.B.K.). A number of soft and energy drinks, and over-the-counter pain and weight loss products contain significant amounts as well.

Caffeine is represented by 1,3,7-trimethylxanthine (Fig. 18.9) and its naturally occurring catabolic products are characterised by demethylation, leading to 1,3-(theophylline), 3,7-(theobromine) and 1,7-dimethylxanthine (paraxanthine). The latter is less commonly reported to be a major plant constituent but appears to be the major caffeine metabolite in humans due to *N*-demethylation catalysed by CYP1A2. However, more than 25 metabolites have been identified and many are pharmacologically active. Theophylline exhibits psychostimulant activities to some extent but is also involved in bronchodilation and anti-inflammatory activity in the airway.

A detailed mechanistic understanding of the pharmacology of caffeine currently remains elusive but a key concept is based on the antagonism at adenosine receptors when considering normal doses of caffeine consumption (50 to 300 mg, one to three cups of coffee). Four adenosine receptors have been cloned and are classified as A_1, A_{2A}, A_{2B}, and A_3. The two main reasons for the belief that only A_1 and A_{2A} subtypes appear to be primarily involved in caffeine pharmacology are based on the fact that these subtypes have sufficiently high affinity to be activated by physiological concentrations of extracellular adenosine and recreational dosages of caffeine, and in addition, both receptor subtypes are predominantly expressed in the brain. The arousal-enhancing activity of caffeine is based on the antagonism of sleep-promoting effects of adenosine. The extent of this seems to depend on subregional differences in brain areas and complex interactions involve the presence of A_{2A}-D_2, A_1-D_1, A_1-A_{2A} receptor heteromer formation and A_1 receptor-mediated control of glutamate and possible other neurotransmitters as well. In other words, a number of pre- and postsynaptic mechanisms regulate and modulate dopamine release and transmission, which is a feature shared with other CNS stimulants such as cocaine and amfetamine. However, at normal recreational dosages, caffeine does not activate the brain circuit of addiction and reward, although it appears to act as a positive reinforcer.

The xanthine backbone forms the basis of a large number of derivatives acting as adenosine receptor antagonists, and higher potencies than caffeine have been observed (Fig. 18.10). One common approach is based on 1,3-dialkyl and 8-aryl or 8-cycloalkyl substitution patterns. For example, the A_1-receptor antagonist KW-3902 (1,3-dipropyl-8-(3-noradamantyl)xanthine) has been shown to be potentially useful for the treatment of heart failure. A carboxylic acid functionality of BG-9928 shows increased water solubility over KW-3902, which would be generally more desirable for intravenous applications. KW-6002 (istradefylline) was found to be a potent A_{2A}-receptor antagonist with potential antiparkinsonian effects. A theophylline derivative carrying a dioxolane group in position 7 (doxofylline) has also displayed some promising bronchodilating properties via A_1-receptor antagonism.

Methylphenidate

An example of a non-amfetamine behavioural stimulant is methylphenidate (Ritalin) (Fig. 18.11) and, correspondingly, it is used for the treatment of ADHD and narcolepsy. It shows both a direct cocaine-like action via dopamine

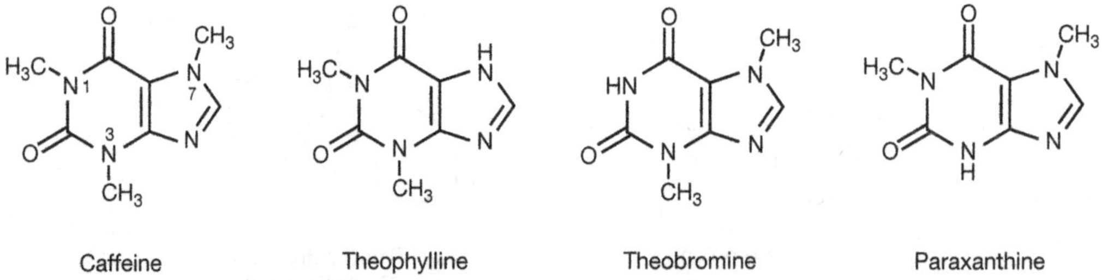

Figure 18.9 Caffeine and its catabolites.

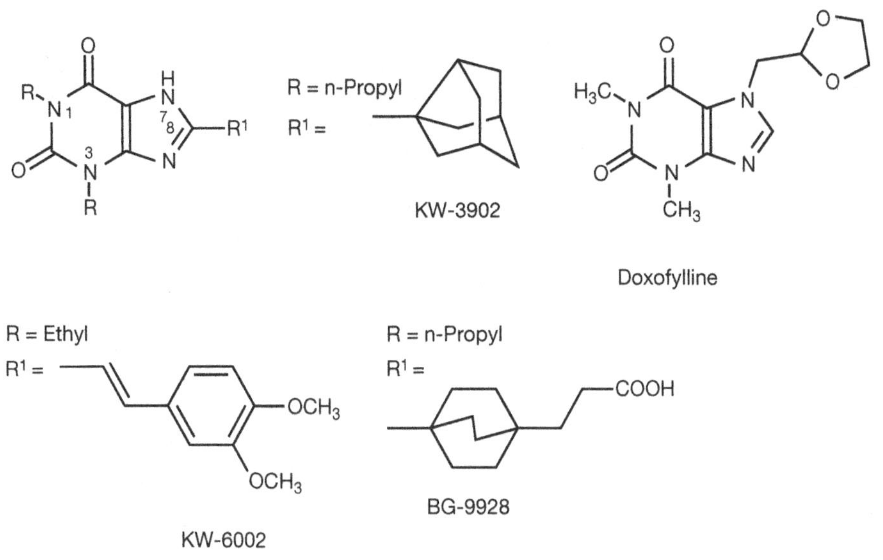

Figure 18.10 Adenosine receptor antagonists.

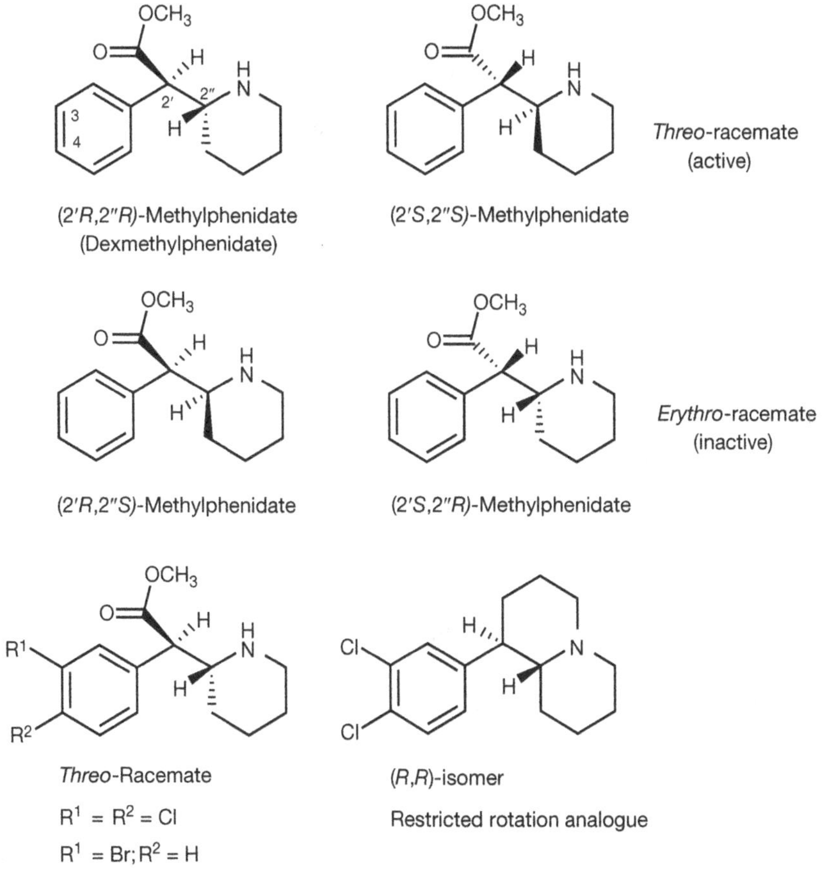

Figure 18.11 Methylphenidate and its analogues.

transporter blockage and an indirect amfetamine- or ephedrine-like action via dopamine release. As is the case with most psychostimulants, an increase in noradrenergic transmission is also thought to be involved. However, when compared with the reinforcing properties of cocaine and several stimulatory amfetamines, methylphenidate does not seem to display such a self-rewarding property, which may result in a reduced potential for abuse. Overall, it has been reported that methylphenidate may offer a safe alternative to amfetamine-type stimulants with a significantly reduced side-effect profile. One possible reason for a reduced rate of positive reinforcement after oral administration has been suggested to involve a slow uptake into the brain. Figure 18.11 shows that methylphenidate has two chiral centres, which results in the presence of four stereoisomers. We have seen a similar example with ephedrine mentioned above. The *erythro*-racemate refers to the 50:50 ratio of (2′*R*,2″*S*)- and (2′*S*,2″*R*)-methylphenidate which shows negligible stimulant activity and hence is not used. The racemic *threo*-racemate was shown to exert the desired effects and it also became clear that the (2′*R*,2″*R*)-enantiomer (dexmethylphenidate) displayed a more powerful inhibition of catecholamine uptake. One of the factors that stimulated the development of several modified and extended-release formulations was based on the observed variability in dose-response and clearance, which resulted in unpredictable absolute bioavailability and the need for individual titration during treatment. Racemic *threo*-methylphenidate displays enantioselective metabolism where a variety of pharmacokinetic parameters differ significantly between dexmethylphenidate and its (2′*S*,2″*S*)-enantiomer after oral administration.

Interestingly, several structural modifications of *threo*-mixtures led to increased potencies with regards to dopamine reuptake blockage. Examples include halogenated substituents in the *meta*- and/or *para* position of the benzene ring. A more recent study revealed that a number of restricted-rotation analogues (Fig. 18.11) also showed significant potencies. The absence of the ester group in these derivatives may produce improved metabolic stability since it would prevent esterase-mediated formation of ritalinic acid. The evaluation of these restricted-rotation analogues demonstrates a common theme within the context of drug development. The methylphenidate molecule contains a flexible side chain that is able to rotate freely and this means that the molecule can adopt a variety of rotational conformers. Intramolecular interactions are often responsible for these phenomena. In this case, formation of hydrogen bonds between the ester group and the N–H may induce the preference for a potential bioactive conformation. Preparation of a particular rigid, i.e. cyclised, analogue can therefore help the medicinal chemist to get an insight into the bioactive candidate that most effectively binds to the receptor.

Description and preparations

Methylphenidate is both available as the racemic mixture and its (*R*,*R*)-stereoisomer. It is used as the hydrochloride salt and preparations include immediate (i/r)- and modified-release (m/r) formulations and transdermal patches.

- Methylphenidate hydrochloride 5–20 mg i/r tablets. Paediatric dose age-dependent, ranges from up to 1.4 mg/kg daily (4–6 years) to max. 60 mg daily in divided dose (>6 years) (ADHD). Treatment of narcolepsy requires 20–30 mg, twice daily.
- Methylphenidate hydrochloride 18–36 mg m/r tablets, and 10–40 mg m/r capsules.
- Transdermal patches for once-daily applications (ADHD) in children (6–12 years). Delivery can range from 1.1 to 3.3 mg/hour.

Modafinil

Modafinil (Fig. 18.12) is also a non-amfetamine with psychostimulant properties, used for the treatment of narcolepsy, ADHD, obstructive sleep apnea/hypopnea syndrome and may show potential for the treatment of cocaine withdrawal symptoms. Inspection of the structural representation indicates that modafinil contains a diphenylmethyl moiety and hence is dissimilar from an

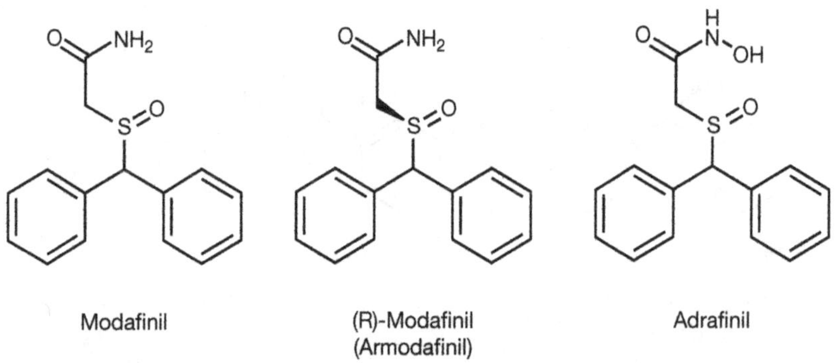

Figure 18.12 Non-amfetamines with psychostimulant properties based on modafinil.

amfetamine structure. The exact mechanism is not yet fully elucidated but enhanced glutamate function, synthesis and striatal glutamate brain levels have been observed. Inhibition of dopaminergic neurons via agonism at presynaptic dopamine D_2 receptors has also been correlated with the induction of stimulant-like effects. Modafinil and its derivatives have also been termed 'wakefulness-promoting agents', possibly in the attempt to differentiate these molecules from the classical sympathomimetic stimulants.

The (*R*)-enantiomer of modafinil is called armodafinil, which sustained higher plasma levels than racemic modafinil and hence resulted in longer wakefulness. It may not be immediately obvious but the sulphur atom of the involved sulphoxide group is a chiral centre because the free electron pair on the sulphur atom provides a tetrahedral molecular geometry similar to an sp^3 carbon. The *N*-hydroxylated derivative of modafinil is called adrafinil and has similar uses. One major metabolite is modafinil and this conversion may be the reason why the elimination half-life of adrafinil is longer than modafinil after oral administration. Increased alertness without stimulation has been claimed and it has been suggested to potentially classify these derivatives as potential nootropics. Adrafinil, for example, shows promising performance and cognitive-enhancing properties.

Description and preparations

- Modafinil 100 mg tablets; adult dose 200–400 mg daily (narcolepsy, obstructive sleep apnoea syndrome and chronic shift work sleep disorder).
- Armodafinil 50–250 mg tablets; adult dose 150–250 mg daily (same indication as above).
- Adrafinil 300 mg tablets; adult dose up to 900 mg daily (same indication as above).

Cocaine

The leaves of the South American coca bush (*Erythroxylum coca* Lamarck and *Erythroxylum novogranatense* (Morris) Hieronymus) have been used and cultivated for millennia. Among the most important alkaloids is cocaine, which is characterised by the simultaneous occurrence of three effects. As described in Chapter 16, cocaine is a potent local anaesthetic that also constricts blood vessels. Vasoconstriction is quite helpful as it delays diffusion into tissue. Cocaine is normally known for its powerful psychostimulant traits with very strong reinforcing, i.e. addictive, properties. This appears to be particularly the case for the pure compound that is obtained by extraction from leaves. Adverse systemic reactions, such as cardiac complications, and abuse potential restrict the medical use to surgical procedures on eyes, ear and throat. The most common forms of the drug are the hydrochloride and sulphate salts. The free base form (crack cocaine) is often smoked in the attempt to intensify the experience, followed by severe forms of toxicological reactions and dependency. Removing the electrostatic interaction between the charged base on its anion counterion increases the volatility of the drug. Cocaine is a tropane-type derivative with several chiral centres (Fig. 18.13) and only the (1*R*,2*R*,3*S*,5*S*)-stereoisomer, also called (−)-cocaine, appears to have appreciable psychostimulant properties, and the remaining stereoisomers have been shown to display significantly decreased affinities for the transport protein. One of the primary targets is the dopamine transporter and, as mentioned previously, blockage of reuptake is defined as a directly mediated mechanism. As a consequence, increased dopaminergic innervation is observed in the caudate, putamen and nucleus acumbens.

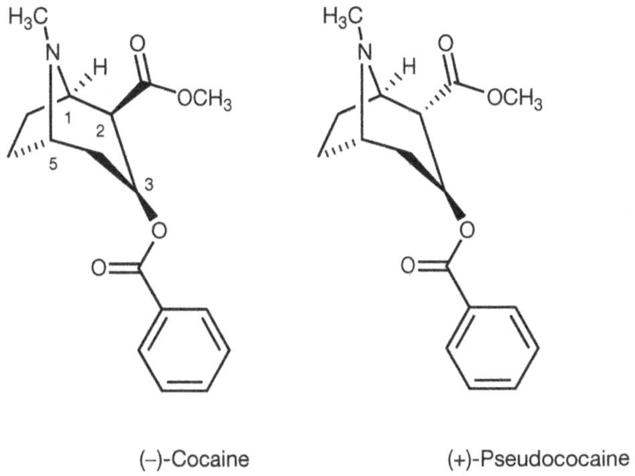

Figure 18.13 (−)-Cocaine and its (2*S*)-stereoisomer called (+)-pseudococaine.

A large number of cocaine analogues have been evaluated for their ability to block the dopamine transporter. One of the reasons for this is to attempt better to understand the binding characteristics of this protein because it was observed that not every transporter inhibitor with high affinity displays psychostimulant effects, a phenomenon that is generally possible with all ligand–receptor interactions. The reasons for this are not yet fully elucidated but one proposal involves the presence of potentially distinct binding sites for both dopamine and cocaine. A corollary of this possibility is the attempt to develop derivatives for the treatment of cocaine abuse and addiction. In this scenario, a potential cocaine antagonist or partial agonist may be able to displace cocaine from its binding site without interfering with dopamine reuptake.

The dopamine transporter appears to tolerate several structural modifications of the cocaine molecule while retaining the ability to block reuptake. Of particular interest was the manipulation of the 2 and 3 position, provided that both substituents remained in the 2β- and 3β-configuration, i.e. (2*R*,3*S*). Several 2β-alkyl and -aryl ester derivatives retained affinity, one of which was the phenyl ester RTI-15 (Fig. 18.14). Removal of the 3β-ester linkage at position 3 led to a number of phenyltropane analogues such as WIN-35,065-2. Placement of substituents at the *para* position of the phenyl ring gave valuable

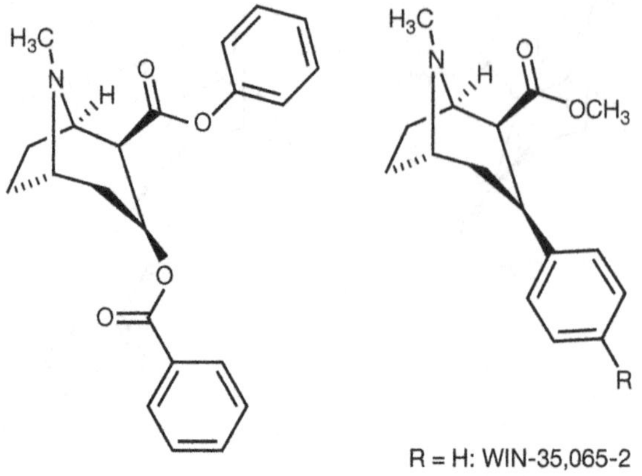

Figure 18.14 RTI and WIN derivatives based on the cocaine template.

compounds used for in vivo studies. Examples include the *para*-halides RTI-55 and WIN-35,428 which have been used as radiotracers in order to determine dopamine transporter occupancy within the brain. *N*-Alkylation of a number of RTI-55 derivatives did not show any significant reduction in dopamine transporter affinity. When mentioning the reuptake transporter as a primary target of cocaine, it is important to note, however, that additional receptor interactions are also involved including inhibition of the noradrenaline and serotonin transporters. Thus, a large number of 2β,3β-analogues are well tolerated by the dopamine transporter but not necessarily by the noradrenaline or serotonin counterparts. Such effects are, however, beneficial in the determination of drug selectivity.

Description and preparations

- Cocaine hydrochloride aqueous solutions. Adult dose up to 4% (ophthalmology). Solutions up to 10% are applied to the nasal mucosa (otolaryngological procedures). Maximum total adult dose recommended for use on the nasal mucosa is 1.5 mg/kg in order to avoid risk of arrhythmias.

Psychostimulants summary

Psychostimulants are able to induce a number of dose-dependent behaviour-activating features including the activation of fight-or-flight-type responses. A fine line can exist between therapy and potential for misuse or abuse and sometimes the differentiation appears to be somewhat arbitrary. Psychomotor stimulant pharmacology involves an augmented release of noradrenaline, dopamine, and to a lesser extent serotonin, into the synaptic cleft. Increased availability of monoamines is predominantly caused by inhibition of the corresponding monoamine reuptake transporter. Two dominating modes of action are particularly important for this increased availability. In case of substrate-type releasers a synergistic procedure includes reversed transporter-mediated neurotransmitter exchange and cytoplasmic accumulation involving vesicular monoamine transporters (VMAT-2). The second mode is based on reuptake inhibition.

The β-phenylethylamine structure serves as the basis for many biologically active drugs. A large number of psychostimulants are based on this principle as well, and what differentiates them structurally from, for example, the adrenergic drugs described in Chapter 10, is the absence of hydroxyl groups on the benzene ring and the ethylamine side chain. Amfetamine and methamfetamine are such examples where the lack of hydroxylated substituents facilitates transport through the blood–brain barrier. The presence of the α-methyl group increases metabolic stability towards monoamine oxidase. This also renders the α-carbon optically active where the (*S*)-enantiomer displays higher potencies. Amfetamines are classified as dopamine releasers.

Ephedrine derivatives may be viewed as hybrids between amfetamines and adrenergic drugs. They lack the 3,4-dihydroxylated component but retain the presence of the β-hydroxyl group on the side chain, thus attenuating stimulatory pharmacology. Ephedrines have two chiral centres which give rise to four stereoisomers. The naturally occurring ephedrine is identifiable as the (1*R*,2*S*)-stereoisomer. The (1*S*,2*S*)-stereoisomer is known as (1*S*,2*S*)-cathine or (1*S*,2*S*)-pseudonorephedrine.

Oxidation of the β-hydroxyl in ephedrine group gives rise to cathinone or methcathinone derivatives with psychostimulatory properties. Bupropion, used for the support of smoking cessation, is a tert.-butyl derivative and appears to act as a non-selective dopamine and serotonin reuptake inhibitor. *N*,*N*-diethylcathinone, also called diethylpropion, has been used as an appetite suppressant but showed potentially neurotoxic side effects.

The xanthine family give rise to a number of natural products such as caffeine (1,3,7-trimethylxanthine). Caffeine pharmacology involves adenosine receptor antagonism but details remain elusive. The xanthine backbone forms the basis of a large number of derivatives acting as adenosine receptor antagonists.

Methylphenidate (Ritalin) is a behavioural stimulant used for the treatment of narcolepsy and attention deficit hyperactivity disorder (ADHD). It is commonly classified as a non-amfetamine but its nucleus is still present in that structure. The *erythro*-racemate, i.e. (2′*R*,2″*S*)- and (2′*S*,2″*R*)-methylphenidate, shows negligible stimulant activity and is not used. The racemic *threo*-racemate is responsible for activity but the (2′*R*,2″*R*)-enantiomer (dexmethylphenidate) displayed a more powerful inhibition of catecholamine uptake.

Modafinil contains a diphenylmethyl moiety and hence is truly dissimilar from the amfetamine structure. The (*R*)-enantiomer of modafinil appears to sustain higher plasma levels than racemic modafinil, resulting in longer wakefulness. The presence of a sulphur atom of the involved sulphoxide group is a chiral centre based on the tetrahedral molecular geometry similar to a sp^3 carbon.

Cocaine is a tropane-type derivative with several chiral centres and only the (1*R*,2*R*,3*S*,5*S*)-stereoisomer, also called (−)-cocaine, appears to have appreciable psychostimulant properties. Its primary mode of action is based on blockage of the dopamine transporter which is defined as a directly mediated mechanism. Cocaine is therefore classified as a dopamine blocker rather than dopamine releaser, as is the case with some amfetamines. A large number of 2β,3β-cocaine analogues are well tolerated by the dopamine transporter but not necessarily by the noradrenaline or serotonin counterparts. This means that dopamine reuptake blockage alone is not necessarily sufficient to reinforce consumption, and appropriate structural modifications could lead to the development of treatment options for cocaine abuse.

Self Test 18.1

Select the shape of the rings labelled A and B in dexmethylphenidate:

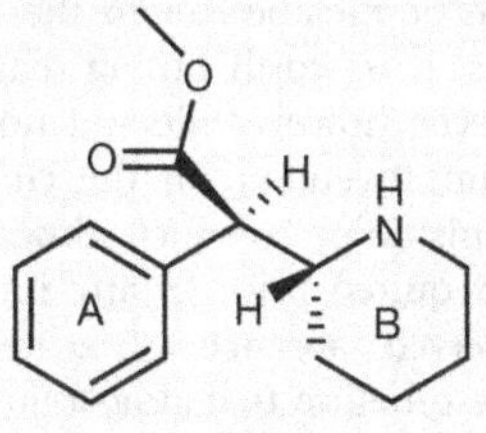

Dexmethylphenidate

	Ring A	Ring B
A	Planar	Chair
B	Chair	Planar
C	Planar	Planar
D	Chair	Chair
E	Linear	Planar

Self Test 18.2

Select the hybridisation of the nitrogen atom and the carbonyl group:

	N	C=O
A	sp^2	both atoms sp^2
B	sp^2	both atoms sp^2
C	sp^2	both atoms sp^2
D	sp^2	both atoms sp^2
E	sp^2	C is sp^2, O is sp^3

Self Test 18.3

Dexmethylphenidate can be described in pharmaceutical terms as:

A. A strong acid
B. A weak acid
C. A neutral compound
D. A weak base
E. A strong base

CNS-ACTIVE DRUGS AFFECTING THE SEROTONERGIC SYSTEM

Serotonin (5-HT, 5-hydroxytryptamine) (see Fig. 18.1) is involved in the regulation of a large number of physiological processes. Over 90% of the total 5-HT present in the body is produced by enterochromaffin cells which are located in the gastrointestinal mucosa. Release of enteric 5-HT may be influenced by mechanical or vagal stimulation, which impacts on motility of intestinal gastric and smooth muscle. Regulation of smooth muscle in the cardiovascular system can also be influenced by 5-HT. Platelet aggregation is enhanced by 5-HT, for example, in response to a damaged endothelium. 5-HT release, stored in secretory granules, may also lead to vasoconstriction. 5-HT storage is carried out by active transport by the circulation because synthesis is not possible. Around 10% of the total amount of 5-HT is found in the CNS and fundamental processes are driven and modulated by this neurotransmitter. These processes include appetite, sex, sleep, cognition and memory, sensory perception, mood, nociception, endocrine function, temperature regulation, motor activity and behaviour.

5-HT neurons originate in the raphe nuclei in the midline region of the pons and upper brain stem. There are several serotonergic pathways in the CNS that innervate a variety of lower (e.g. medulla and spinal cord) and higher CNS centres such as cerebellum, thalamus, neocortex and the limbic system. Serotonergic nerve terminals are able to synthesise their own 5-HT from L-tryptophan, an ability they share with enterochromaffin cells. Neuronal reuptake and vesicular storage protects 5-HT from deamination by MAO.

Based on one current classification system, fourteen serotonin receptor subtypes have been described for the peripheral and central actions of 5-HT. A brief summary is provided in Table 18.1 but the reader is referred to the appropriate pharmacological literature for details. Only the 5-HT_3 receptor is a ligand-gated ion channel; the remaining subfamilies are G-protein coupled receptors. It is also worth noting that the situation is more complicated based on the presence of additional receptors which

Table 18.1 Basic serotonin receptor classification

Human 5-HT families	Coupling	Representative signalling pathway
$5\text{-}HT_{1:\ 1A,1B^*,1D,1E,1F^\dagger}$	$G_{i/o}$ type	Inhibition of adenylyl cyclase; decreased production of cAMP; membrane hyperpolarisation; inhibition of neuronal firing.
$5\text{-}HT_{2:\ 2A,2B,2C}$	$G_{q/11}$ type	Formation of diacyl glycerol and inositol phosphates via phospholipase C: protein kinase C activation.
$5\text{-}HT_3$	Ion channel	Gating of Na^+ and K^+. Activation leads to desensitising depolarization.
$5\text{-}HT_4$	G_s type	Stimulation of adenylyl cyclase; increased production of cAMP: protein kinase A activation. Also, phosphorylation of cAMP-responsive transcription factors.
$5\text{-}HT_5$	$G_{i/o}$ type	See $5\text{-}HT_1$
$5\text{-}HT_6$	G_s type	See $5\text{-}HT_4$
$5\text{-}HT_7$	G_s type	See $5\text{-}HT_4$

*The $5\text{-}HT_{1B}$ subtype is also referred to as $5\text{-}HT_{1D\beta}$; †also referred to as $5\text{-}HT_{1E\beta}$.

derive from alternative splicing of genes or mRNA editing. An impressive example is found in the human $5\text{-}HT_{2C}$ receptor where at least 32 different mRNAs and 24 different proteins are known. Furthermore, signalling may also be influenced by receptor dimerisation and functional selectivity. In the latter case, different agonists may be able to trigger differential downstream responses after induction of distinguishable ligand–receptor conformations within the same protein. Intense research activities will hopefully shed more light on these issues, which ultimately may also results in the development of more subtype-selective agonists and antagonists.

In this section the emphasis is placed on the serotonergic system in the context of the CNS. The chemical manipulation of the serotonergic system within the CNS can be achieved either directly, for example by the use of 5-HT receptor agonists (e.g. migraine, depression) or antagonists (e.g. emesis), or indirectly by the manipulation of serotonin synthesis and turnover. The latter principle is of particular importance when treating a variety of depressive disorders.

Antidepressants

Antidepressants cover a wide range of indications and include depression, obsessive-compulsive disorders, anxiety, pain, panic, eating disorders or social phobia. The 'monoamine hypothesis' of depression is an often-used term that describes a concept that arose over 50 years ago when a direct link was observed between major depression and imbalance/deficiency of available monoamines such as serotonin and catecholamines. Consequently, most of the currently available drugs aim to increase availability of monoamines either by inhibition of reuptake or metabolism in the attempt to alter our mood states. It is worth noting that the immediate biochemical effects, however, do not normally result in an immediate improvement on the clinical level since continual administration of such drugs for at least 3 weeks is often required prior to any improvement. The commonly observed absence of acute antidepressant effects, and the estimation that almost 50% of all patients treated with antidepressants fail to show a full response, led to the idea that monoamines may function as modulators, rather than simply being 'happiness' molecules. An advanced understanding in the areas of gene expression, neuroplasticity and brain circuitry will hopefully shed more light on the causal factors involved in the precipitation of these conditions. Nevertheless, the progress of antidepressant therapy and drug discovery within the last 50 years would have been inconceivable without the skilful research in the area of monoamine neurochemistry and behaviour.

Tricyclic antidepressants

Tricyclic antidepressants (TCAs) were the first monoamine reuptake inhibitors available and it is believed that one important mechanism of action for antidepressant activity includes the inhibition at the serotonin (SERT) and noradrenaline (NAT) reuptake transport protein. An inspection of the tricyclic structures below indicates high lipophilicity that results in good absorption after oral administration. Around 80–99% of the TCA concentration present in the circulation is bound to plasma proteins and their elimination half-life commonly lies between 10 and 40 hours, although longer-lasting exceptions are known. A mean adult maintenance dose often ranges between 75 and 150 mg per day. High selectivity for only one binding site is not observed with TCA derivatives and interactions with additional receptor sites contribute to a number of unwanted, and sometimes toxic and potentially dangerous, side effects. These are comprehensively covered in pharmacology textbooks. Briefly, the most characteristic side effects involve antagonism at H_1, M_1 and α_1-adrenergic receptor sites and effects may include sedation (sometimes desired), dry mouth, blurred vision, urinary retention, orthostatic hypotension, cardiac effects (arrhythmia and arrest), restlessness/activation and others. A more serious disadvantage is based on the relatively narrow therapeutic window of certain derivatives which means that serious toxicity may arise from overdose that ultimately may be fatal. This particular side effect profile often requires that the dose of a particular TCA is gradually tailored to the patient's needs according to tolerance and clinical response. It is recommended that the elderly receive lower dosages.

Basic structure–activity relationships

The tricyclic structure of TCA derivatives consist of a central, seven-membered, non-aromatic ring that is flanked by two benzene rings (Fig. 18.15). A commonly found structural feature is the presence of a tertiary or secondary amine attached to the central ring which is, in most cases, a three-carbon chain. The amine can also be part of an alicylic, i.e. non-aromatic, ring. The ring topology of tricyclic derivatives, i.e. the three-dimensional structure of this pharmacophore, appears to play an important role in psychoactivity. For example, it has been suggested that the dihedral angle (α) between the two benzene rings can impact on the extent of antidepressant activity (Fig. 18.15). The structurally related phenothiazine ring systems appear to be nearly flat with the side chain nitrogen projecting away from the nucleus. The imipramine-type structure allows for the formation of a larger dihedral angle ('butterfly shape') which also positions the side chain nitrogen directly above the ring system. The replacement of -S- by -CH_2-CH_2- is an example of classical bioisosterism, a key principle in medicinal chemistry and lead modification. The results of such modifications are not always predictable.

The tricyclic skeletal structure of TCA derivatives can generally accommodate several isosteric modifications. Replacement of carbon atoms by nitrogen, oxygen and sulphur heteroatoms give active derivatives such as imipramine, doxepin and dosulepin, respectively. Also, antidepressant activity does not appear to require the presence of an sp2 hybridised carbon atom. Aromatisation of the central ring gives a planar molecule with complete loss of antidepressant activity. The presence of heteroatoms in the ring is not necessarily required for antidepressant activity.

The tertiary amine groups are often metabolised by demethylation, which leads to the formation of secondary amines which often possess antidepressant properties. As a rule of thumb, secondary amines appear to show higher selectivity for NAT whereas their parent, tertiary counterparts tend to be either less selective (mixed SERT/NAT) or display a somewhat higher selectivity for SERT. The other major transformations are based on hydroxylation followed by glucuronidation and, in some cases, formation of *N*-oxides.

Iminodibenzyl derivatives

Imipramine is the prototype TCA and was the first clinically potent antidepressant drug. Imipramine and its derivatives are iminodibenzyl derivatives (Fig. 18.16). Both desipramine and lofepramine appear to be more selective towards noradrenaline reuptake (NA) whereas the remaining derivatives are considered to be more non-selective towards SERT and NAT (5-HT/NA), respectively.

Description and preparations

Imipramine is most commonly available as the hydrochloride salt.

- Imipramine hydrochloride tablets 10 and 25 mg. Adult dose 75–300 mg daily in divided doses (depression).
- Children >7 years 25–75 mg at bedtime (nocturnal enuresis, i.e. bed-wetting).

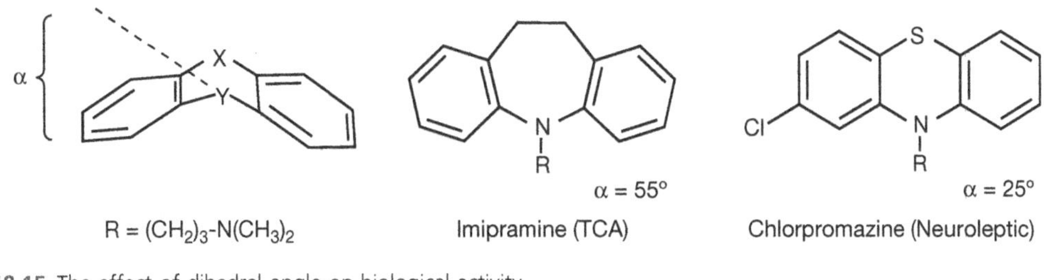

Figure 18.15 The effect of dihedral angle on biological activity.

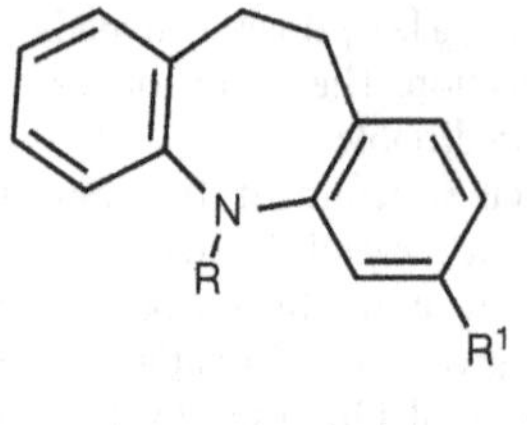

R = $(CH_2)_3$-$N(CH_3)_2$; R^1= H: Imipramine [SERT/NAT]
R = $(CH_2)_3$-$N(CH_3)_2$; R^1= Cl: Clomipramine [SERT/NAT]
R = $(CH_2)_3$-$NHCH_3$; R^1= H: Desipramine [NAT]
R = CH_2-$CH(CH_3)$-CH_2-$N(CH_3)_2$; R^1= H: Trimipramine [SERT/NAT]
R = $(CH_2)_3$-$N(CH_3)CH_2$-CO-(C_6H_4)-4′-Cl; R1= H: Lofepramine [NAT]

Figure 18.16 Iminodibenzyl derivatives.

Clomipramine is used as the hydrochloride salt and is prepared in capsules, modified-release (m/r) or film-coated (f/c) tablets. It appears to be more 5-HT-selective. Note that clomipramine is the chloro derivative of imipramine.

- Clomipramine hydrochloride tablets 10–50 mg. Adult dose 30–150 mg daily in divided doses or up to 250 mg as single dose at bedtime (depression, phobic states). Not recommended for children and adolescents under 18 years.

Desipramine is the principle metabolite of imipramine after demethylation and shows comparatively high selectivity for NAT. It is available as hydrochloride salt tablets and 100–200 mg are usually given in the treatment of depression.

Trimipramine maleate is available in capsules (50 mg) and tablets (10 and 25 mg). The presence of a methyl group on the tertiary amine side chain renders this carbon chiral but trimipramine is currently used as the racemate.

- Trimipramine maleate. Adult dose 50 to 75 mg initially and increased as necessary to 150 to 300 mg.

Lofepramine, a NA-selective TCA, is available as hydrochloride salt tablets and oral suspension at 70 mL/5 mL. It is considered to be less toxic in overdose and one of the metabolites is desipramine. Lofepramine shows high plasma protein binding around 99%.

- Lofepramine hydrochloride tablets 70 mg. Adult dose 140–210 mg daily in divided doses.

Iminostilbene derivatives

Description and preparations

Protriptyline (Fig. 18.17), available as hydrochloride salt tablets (5 and 10 mg), shows slow absorption with peak plasma concentration being reached between 8 and 12 hours. Elimination half-life has been found to vary between 55 and 198 hours.

- Protriptyline hydrochloride. Adults 15 to 60 mg in divided doses.

Opipramol is available as 50, 100 and 150 mg film-coated tablets as the dihydrochloride salt (· 2 HCl). Opipramol shows the typical TCA structure but does not appear to display the expected mixed reuptake inhibition profile. Currently, it would appear that it is more prominently prescribed on the German market where it is used for its dominating anxiolytic properties. The exact mechanisms for the benzodiazepine-like activities are not yet fully understood but there are indications that opipramol may interact with sigma-1 and sigma-2 receptors.

- Opipramol dihydrochloride. Adults 150 to 300 mg daily.

Dibenzocyloheptadiene derivatives

Amitriptyline is considered a classic TCA and was launched soon after imipramine in 1961. It is widely prescribed and most commonly described side effects in the pharmacological literature are applicable to most of the remaining TCAs. Amitriptyline overdose is considered to be particularly dangerous. Nortriptyline is the demethylated metabolite and also individually available (Fig. 18.18).

Description and preparations

Amitriptyline is available as hydrochloride salt tablets (10, 25 and 50 mg) but the embonate (i.e. the pamoic acid salt) has also been described. Oral solutions (25 mg/5 mL) are also used. A multi-ingredient preparation (sugar-coated tablets) containing 25 mg amitriptyline and 2 mg

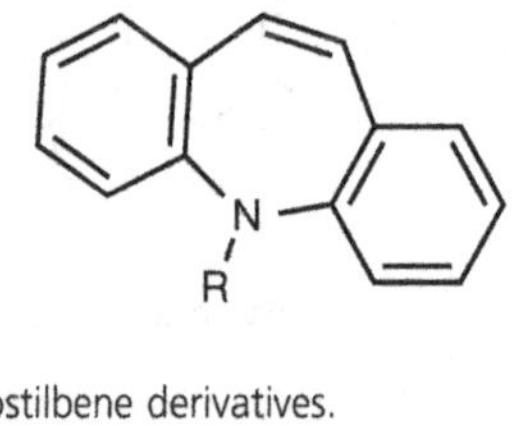

R = $(CH_2)_3$-$NHCH_3$: Protriptyline [NAT]
R = $(CH_2)_3$—N N—$(CH_2)_2$OH Opipramol

Figure 18.17 Iminostilbene derivatives.

Figure 18.18 Dibenzocyloheptadienes.

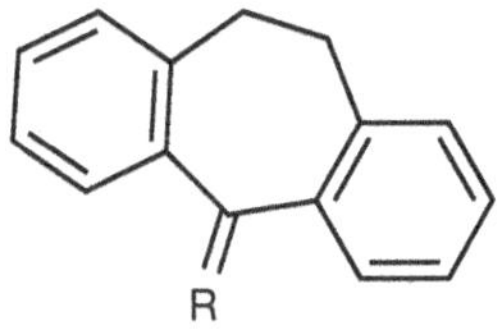

R = CH-$(CH_2)_2$-$N(CH_3)_2$ Amitriptyline [SERT/NAT]
R = CH-$(CH_2)_2$-$NHCH_3$ Nortriptyline [NAT]

perphenazine (phenothiazine antipsychotic with anxiolytic properties).

- Amitriptyline hydrochloride. Adult dose up to 150–200 mg in divided doses (depression).
- Children >7 years 25–75 mg at bedtime (nocturnal enuresis, i.e. bed-wetting). Maximal period of treatment 3 months.
- Neuropathic pain (unlicensed indication), initially 10–25 mg, up to 75 mg daily at night.
- Migraine prophylaxis (unlicensed indication), initially 10 mg, up to 50–75 mg daily at night.

Nortriptyline hydrochloride (10 and 25 mg tablets) is used for similar clinical purposes including unlicensed indications. It appears to show fewer sedation and anticholinergic effects than amitriptyline and also displays longer plasma half-life.

Dibenzoxepine and dibenzothiepine derivatives

The only structural difference between these two examples (Fig. 18.19) is represented by the heteroatom which makes them classical bioisosteres since both oxygen and sulphur have the same valence. Both may be classified as mixed 5-HT/NA reuptake inhibitors but replacement of the oxygen atom with sulphur appears to shift the selectivity from NAT to SERT.

Description and preparations

Doxepin hydrochloride capsules (most commonly 25 and 50 mg) are used but oral solutions exist as well as concentrates at 10 mg/mL. It consists of a mixture of *E*- and *Z*-isomers (85:15). Strong interactions with histamine H_1 and H_2 receptors are the basis for its use in the topical treatment of severe pruritus.

- Doxepin hydrochloride. Adult maintenance dose 30–300 mg daily in divided doses (depression).

Dosulepin hydrochloride capsules (25 mg) or tablets (25 or 75 mg) are quite commonly prescribed. As with amitriptyline, a dangerous overdose potential has been reported. Dosulepin, also known as dothiepin, exists mainly as the *E*-isomer although pharmcopoeial monographs allow up to 5% of the Z-isomer. Oxidative transformation of dosulepin during phase-I metabolism leads to the formation of sulphoxide metabolites, i.e. they carry an R-(S=O)-R′ functionality. The free electron pair that belongs to the sulphur atom contributes to a tetrahedral molecular geometry and, as a consequence, (*R*)- and (*S*)-configurations are possible within the metabolites.

- Dosulepin hydrochloride. Adult dose 75–150 mg daily in divided doses (depression).

Monoamine oxidase inhibitors

Monoamine oxidase (MAO) uses flavin adenine dinucleotide (FAD) as the enzyme-bound cofactor and catalyses the oxidative transformation of biogenic amines that results in the formation of a corresponding aldehyde and a free amine. A second step is required to reoxidise the reduced $FADH_2$ with the help of oxygen which in turn generates hydrogen peroxide as a by-product. Figure 18.20 shows a representative example using serotonin. The aldehyde is relatively short-lived because it gets oxidised further to the corresponding acid for excretion. A similar principle applies to other amines as well such as adrenaline, dopamine, etc.

Most mammalian tissues display the presence of MAO-A and MAO-B isoforms with different substrate specificities. For example, MAO-A catalyses the oxidative deamination of serotonin, whereas MAO-B displays higher specificity for benzylamine and β-phenylethylamine. Noradrenaline, adrenaline, tyramine, tryptamine and dopamine are deaminated by both isozymes. In the human brain the hypothalamus and basal ganglia (striatum) show high MAO activity and it has been observed that

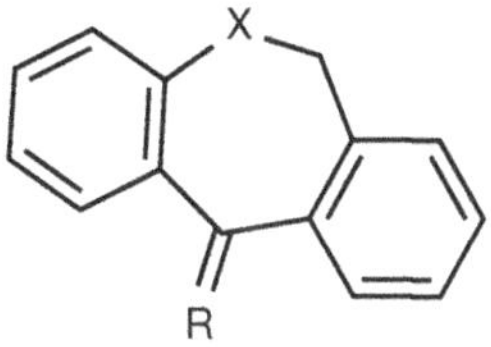

Dibenzoxepine derivative

R = CH-$(CH_2)_2$-$N(CH_3)_2$; X = O: Doxepin [SERT/NAT]

Dibenzothiepine derivative

R = CH-$(CH_2)_2$-$N(CH_3)_2$; X = S: Dosulepin [SERT/NAT]

Figure 18.19 Dibenzoxepines and dibenzothiepines.

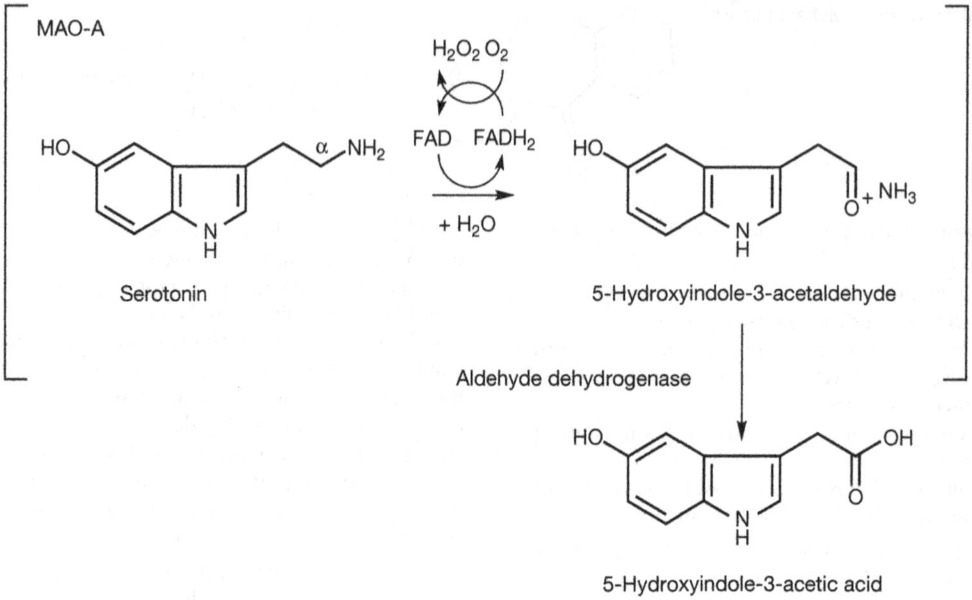

Figure 18.20 Oxidation of serotonin by MAO.

neocortex and cerebellum, for example, display relatively low activity. Another interesting observation is the fact that MAO-A does not appear to tolerate the presence of a substituent at the α-carbon (Fig. 18.20) since it would have to break a C–C bond in order to produce the acidic product. For example, the presence of alkyl groups can prevent oxidative transformation by MAO which increases metabolic stability. This is the case for amfetamine derivatives which carry an α-methyl group.

Originally, the 'monoamine hypothesis' of depression has gained support from the fact that increased serotonergic neurotransmission led to symptom alleviation in humans after exposure to MAO inhibitors (MAOIs). Over the years the use of MAOIs has declined due to the development of new drugs such as the selective monoamine reuptake inhibitors and because of potentially severe interactions with other drugs and the toxicity of MAOIs. Nevertheless, MAOIs are still considered to be important for individuals who do not respond to other drug classes. They are also relevant for a number of specific applications in the areas of anxiety and phobias.

The first MAOIs that appeared on the market during the 1950s had non-selective and irreversible properties. Apart from tranylcypromine (phenylcyclopropanamine), a number of developed MAOIs were hydrazine derivatives (Fig. 18.21).

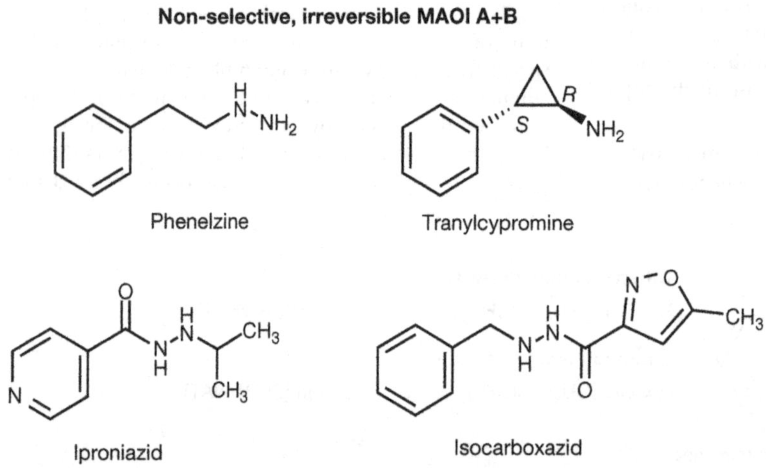

Figure 18.21 MAOIs.

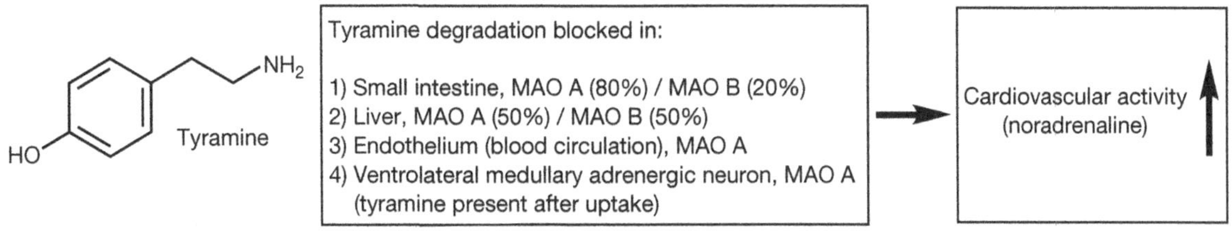

Figure 18.22 The 'cheese effect'.

There are two issues of concern which are associated with irreversible MAOIs involving the display of liver toxicity, particularly with hydrazines, and the permanent inactivation of both MAO-A and -B isoforms. The replacement of MAOs requires protein synthesis which may take up to 14 days. From the antidepressant viewpoint, only a selective blockage of serotonin metabolism may be of interest in order to increase serotonin availability. However, this long-term effect significantly reduces metabolism of a variety of other biogenic amines, which leads to their accumulation, which is not necessarily desired. This leads to an excessive availability of tyramine and others, which ultimately leads to increased release of noradrenaline that may result in the stimulation of cardiovascular sympathetic nervous system activity. As a consequence, potentially fatal hypertensive crises and cerebral haemorrhage can occur (Fig. 18.22). This phenomenon has often been termed the 'cheese effect', in order to reflect the fact that tyramine is present in a variety of foods such as wine, cheese and other fermented food and drink products. It would appear, however, that under carefully controlled and restricted dietary conditions such a risk can be minimised.

Current knowledge suggests that irreversible inhibition of MAO is based on a process called mechanism-based enzyme inactivation. Studies with derivatives such as phenelzine and tranylcypromine indicated that the inhibitor is turned from an inactive into a reactive species as a consequence of the interaction with the binding site. Hydrazines or amine groups are able to undergo single electron transfers from the non-bonding electron pair to the flavin which leads to the presence of a radical cation ($^{\bullet+}$). A sequence of steps converts the biogenic amine into an aldehyde that gets released as part of oxidative deamination, but the inactivator has been suggested to react with a cysteine residue in MAO rather than undergoing conversion into an aldehyde. Worthy of note, this mechanism differs from irreversible inhibition of prostaglandin synthase (cyclooxygenase) by acetylsalicylic acid (aspirin). In this scenario, aspirin is already a reactive species and the acetyl group is transferred (acetylation) to the serine-530 residue, hence leading to inactivation.

Description and preparations

Iproniazid phosphate is not in use any more due to the occurrence of severe liver toxicity. Phenelzine is available as its sulphate as film-coated tablets (15 mg). Irreversible MAOIs are generally not recommended for children.

- Phenelzine sulphate. Adult dose initially 15 mg 3 times daily. After two weeks, increased if necessary to 4 times daily, then reduced gradually to lowest possible maintenance dose.
- Isocarboxazid 10 mg tablets. Adult dose 10–60 mg daily.
- Tranylcypromine sulfate 10 mg tablets. Adult dose 10–30 mg daily.

MAO-A and -B are pharmacologically distinguishable by their differential sensitivities towards clorgyline and selegiline (Fig. 18.23). Clorgyline hydrochloride is an irreversible MAO-A inhibitor that is not used for treatment any more, but it serves as a valuable pharmacological tool. Selegiline (*L*-deprenyl) irreversibly inhibits MAO-B, which does not appear to display antidepressant properties. Instead, it is used within the context of anti-Parkinson's treatment. MAO-B inhibitors do not carry the risk of provoking the 'cheese effect' because the intestine does

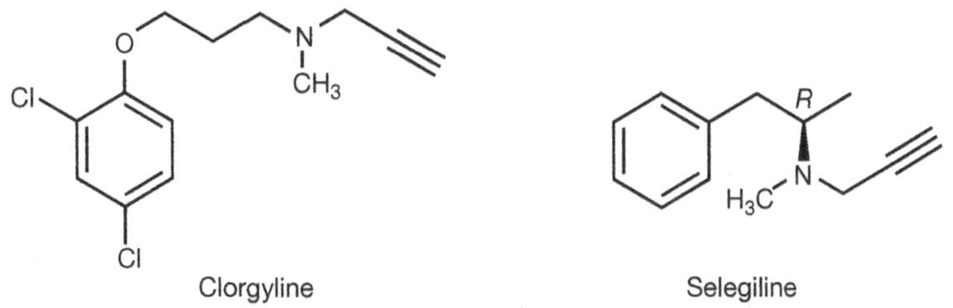

Figure 18.23 Selective, irreversible MAO-A and MAO-B inhibitors.

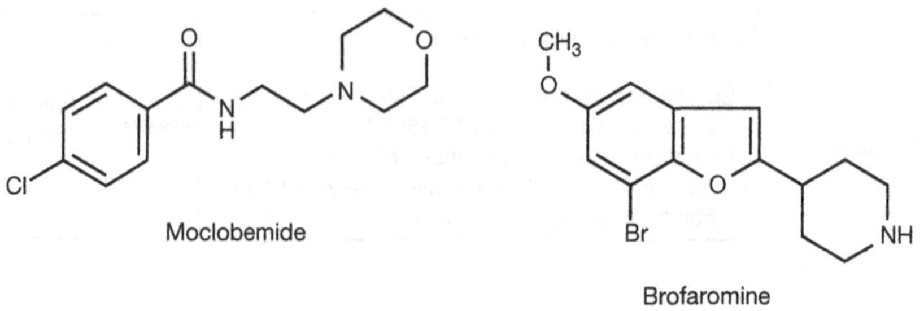

Figure 18.24 Selective, reversible MAO-A inhibitors.

not express large amounts of MAO-B and tyramine can be effectively metabolised by MAO-A.

Introduction of reversible MAO-A inhibitors resulted in significantly improved safety during antidepressant therapy. The potential for hypertensive problems is virtually absent because tyramine is able to displace the drug from the binding site. Furthermore, selectivity for only MAO-A allows for metabolism with MAO-B. The benzamide derivative moclobemide (Fig. 18.24) was launched in 1990 and represents the most commonly used drug for this particular purpose. Brofaromine, a benzofuran derivative, has been found to show very similar properties when compared with moclobemide. It also displayed some promising potential as a weak selective serotonin reuptake inhibitor but clinically studies have been abandoned due to lack of corporate interest.

Moclobemide preparations include tablets and film-coated tablets (150 and 300 mg).

- Moclobemide. Adult dose 150–600 mg daily (depression) and 300–600 mg (social anxiety disorder).

Selective serotonin reuptake inhibitors

In 1987, the United States Food and Drug Administration (FDA) approved the use of fluoxetine for the treatment of depression and this derivative is now considered to be the prototype of a drug class called selective serotonin reuptake inhibitors (SSRIs). As the name suggests, this term refers to the reuptake blockage of serotonin into the presynaptic membrane in order to indirectly increase neurotransmitter availability. A number of these derivatives showed beneficial effects for the treatment of a variety of additional conditions such as obsessive-compulsive disorders (OCD), bulimia nervosa, anxiety disorders, obesity, anorexia, post-traumatic stress disorders (PTSD) and others. SSRIs have become the first-line therapy for depression, which is based on improved side effect profiles when compared with TCA derivatives or MAOIs. A number of adverse effects are described in the pharmacological literature and include sexual dysfunction, gastrointestinal bleeding, impaired platelet function, agitation and many others. The popularity of SSRIs (possibly in part stimulated by the economic success and the overall euphoria) has also led some to consider using these derivatives as lifestyle drugs! The focus, however, has been expanded and now includes the consideration of noradrenaline (NA) reuptake inhibition as well, which has led to the development of mixed 5-HT/NA and selective NA inhibitors (NARIs).

Fluoxetine and some of its derivatives contain a phenoxyphenylpropylamine nucleus and a mono- or dimethylated aminoethyl- or aminopropyl side chain. Figure 18.25 provides a summary of the current five most commonly used SSRIs. A structural comparison indicates that their similarity is not as obvious as one might expect. It appears that only slight modifications of the fluoxetine structure change the affinity towards other binding sites such as NAT, as we will see a bit later. This means that the structure–affinity relationships of SSRIs are not necessarily straightforward. A commonly used approach in medicinal chemistry is based on what is sometimes called 'scaffold-hopping'. This procedure involves the use of computational 2-D or 3-D modelling tools which aim to identify similar bioactive compounds (biomimetics) when compared with a given reference ligand. Although these may be based on non-related structures, a number of similar factors may be shared such as pharmacophores, topological motifs and shapes.

Description and preparations

Fluoxetine hydrochloride is available in a variety of preparations which include capsules (20 mg) and oral solutions at 4 mg/mL. Elimination half-life appears to be around 2–3 days but the main demethylated and pharmacologically active metabolite norfluoxetine displays an even longer half-life of 7–9 days. Fluoxetine is prepared as the racemic hydrochloride salt but a number of stereoselective preparative methods are now available. (*R*)-Fluoxetine, however, may not be suitable due to the occurrence of cardiac side effects such as increased QT intervals. Its metabolite, (*R*)-norfluoxetine, is virtually inactive. Also, the (*S*)-norfluoxetine enantiomer (seproxetine) is significantly more potent than its (*R*)-counterpart.

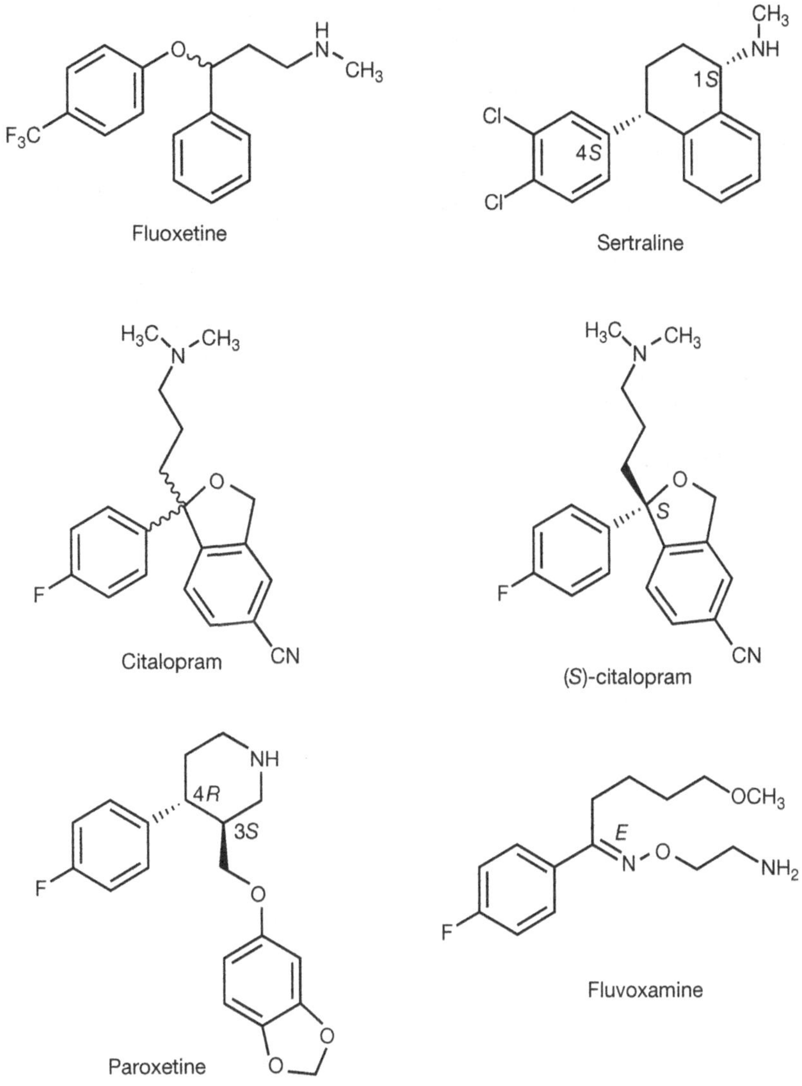

Figure 18.25 SSRIs.

- Fluoxetine hydrochloride. Adult dose 20–60 mg (major depression), 60 mg once daily (bulimia nervosa), 20–60 mg (OCD). Not recommended <18 years.

Sertraline is used as the hydrochloride salt as tablets or film-coated tablets (50 mg). The (1*S*,4*S*)-diastereoisomer appeared to be the most potent and selective SSRI when compared with the remaining three candidates. The main metabolite *N*-desmethylsertraline did not appear to have any significant SSRI properties. Sertraline was shown to be around fivefold more potent than fluoxetine.

- Sertraline hydrochloride. Adult dose 50–200 mg daily (depression, OCD, PTSD).

Paroxetine is available as the hydrochloride salt (10–30 mg) but the anhydrous and hemihydrate forms exist as well. An oral suspension of the hydrochloride salt is also used at 2 mg/mL. Note also the presence of two chiral centres and that the preparation consists of the (3*S*,4*R*)-isomer. Metabolism leads to inactive products.

- Paroxetine hydrochloride. Adult dose 10–40 mg, sometimes 60 mg daily (major depression, social anxiety and panic disorder, PTSD and OCD).

Fluvoxamine is available as the maleate salt in tablets (50 and 100 mg).

- Fluvoxamine maleate. Adult dose 50–300 mg (depression, OCD).

Citalopram can be obtained as both the hydrochloride and hydrobromide salts. The hydrochloride salt is available as oral drops at 40 mg/mL. Tablets (10, 20 and 40 mg) contain the hydrobromide salt. Citalopram is prepared as the racemic mixture. Metabolism appears to lead to the formation of inactive species. The (*S*)-enantiomer of citalopram, called escitalopram, showed more than two orders of magnitude higher potency than the (*R*)-derivative which led to a follow-up approval of the oxalate salt (Note that although oxalic acid is toxic the doses given in this case are well below the toxicity threshold). In other words, the major part of antidepressant activity resides with this enantiomer. It also showed improved potential to be used for the treatment of social anxiety disorders.

- Citalopram hydrobromide. Adult dose 10–60 mg (depressive illness and panic disorder).
- Escitalopram oxalate. Adult dose 10–20 mg (depressive illness), 5–20 mg (panic disorder) or 10–20 mg (social anxiety disorder).

Shifting reuptake selectivities

Minor structural modifications to the fluoxetine structure may have an impact on selectivity. For example, removal of the trifluoromethyl group on the *para* position of the phenoxy ring and attachment of a methoxy group to the *ortho* position resulted in the discovery of nisoxetine, an effective blocker of the noradrenaline reuptake transport protein NAT (Fig. 18.26). Replacement of the methoxy with a methyl group appears to be tolerated by NAT, which leads to atomoxetine, a selective NAT inhibitor. This derivative has non-stimulant properties and is used in the treatment of ADHD in adults and children. It is available as the hydrochloride salt and dosages can range between 40 and 100 mg. The formulated product only contains the (*R*)-enantiomer.

Reboxetine can also be viewed as a rigid fluoxetine derivative. The methylated aminopropyl side chain that

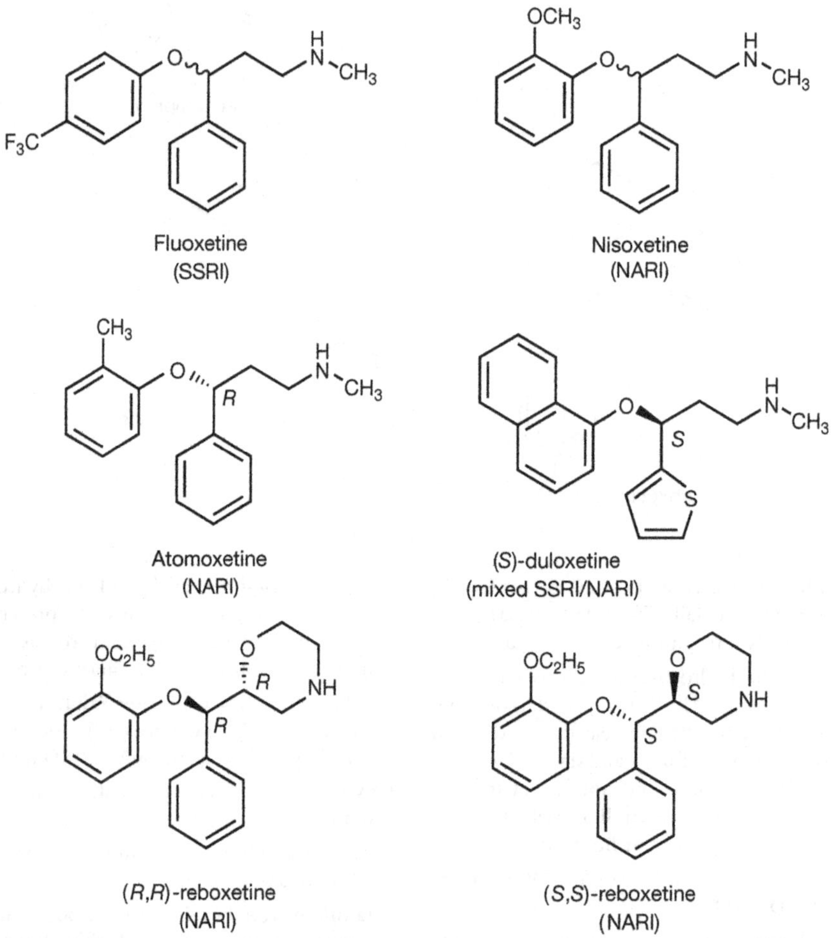

Figure 18.26 Shifting monoamine reuptake selectivities using the fluoxetine template.

was present in the previously mentioned drugs has undergone a chain-ring transformation which potentially impacts on conformation, and pharmacodynamic properties of the molecule. Its structural modifications led to selective NAT inhibition. Ring formation introduced an additional chiral centre and the commercially available preparation contains a racemic mixture of the (*R*,*R*)- and (*S*,*S*)-isomer. There are indications that the (*S*,*S*)-isomer may show significantly higher affinity and selectivity towards NAT. Reboxetine mesilate (methanesulphonate salt) is currently available as tablets (4 mg) and is prescribed for major depression at 4–12 mg daily. Reboxetine and atomoxetine may also be effective for the treatment of chronic pain disorders such as low back pain.

In the case of duloxetine, a benzene ring has been replaced by a thiophene nucleus which is a commonly used approach during the process of lead modification. The number of atoms is not the same; hence it may be described as a non-classical isostere. The phenoxy group has also been transformed, which provides an example of a ring fusion, resulting in the presence of a naphthalenyloxy group. This drug is non-selective, which makes it a mixed SERT/NAT inhibitor. It is indicated for the treatment of major depression, diabetic neuropathy and urinary incontinence. Duloxetine is used as the (*S*)-enantiomer hydrochloride salt and is available as capsules (30 mg). A typical adult daily dose for the treatment of major depression and diabetic neuropathy is 60 mg. In case of urinary incontinence, 40 mg twice daily have been recommended.

Another example of a dual SSRI/NARI is venlafaxine (Fig. 18.27), which one can view as a *N*,*N*-dimethylated and *para*-methoxy-phenylethylamine derivative, substituted with cyclohexanol at the β-position. It only weakly inhibits dopamine transport and is commonly prescribed for depression but also for general and social anxiety disorder.

Sibutramine is also a mixed inhibitor of SERT and NAT but does not display any antidepressant properties. Instead, it is used in the management of obesity, following an observed reduction of food intake. Structurally, one can observe the substituent at the α-carbon, in this case an isobutyl group, which gives an amfetamine-type derivative.

Description and preparations

Venlafaxine hydrochloride is currently available as the racemic mixture. It would appear that the (*R*)-enantiomer is able to inhibit both SERT and NAT while the (*S*)-enantiomer selectively acts as the SSRI.

- Venlafaxine hydrochloride tablets (37.5 and 75 mg). Adult dose 75–150 mg in two divided doses (depression).
- Venlafaxine hydrochloride modified-release capsules (75 and 150 mg). Adult dose 75 mg as single dose (depression, general and social anxiety disorder).

Sibutramine is available as the hydrochloride salt and is prepared as the racemate. The (*R*)-enantiomer of the mono- and didemethylated metabolite appear to show an increased affinity towards the dopamine reuptake transporter, which led to the question as to whether they may be useful for the treatment of ADHD.

- Sibutramine hydrochloride tablets (10 mg). Adult dose 10–15 mg daily (obesity), maximum period of treatment 1 year.

It was mentioned above that both citalopram, and its (*S*)-enantiomer have SSRI properties. Inspection of Figure 18.28 shows that slight modifications give talopram, which is a potent NARI, despite the structural similarity to citalopram. Both share the phenyl substituted phthalane (1,3-dihydroisobenzofuran) and propylamine moiety. Talopram may therefore be viewed as a secondary amine derivative of citalopram after removal of the two aromatic substituents and attachment of a 1,1-dimethyl group to the 3 position. The NARI property, however, remains when the oxygen is replaced with an isosteric sulphur atom. This provides talsupram, the thiophthalane (1,3-dihydrobenzo[*c*]thiophene) derivative of talopram, which is a bioisostere.

Hallucinogens

A large number of derivatives are known to induce altered states of consciousness which means that they are characterised by their powerful impact on perception, mood and

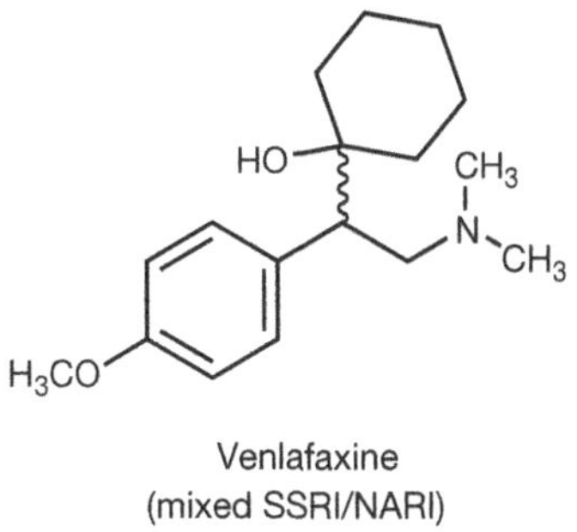

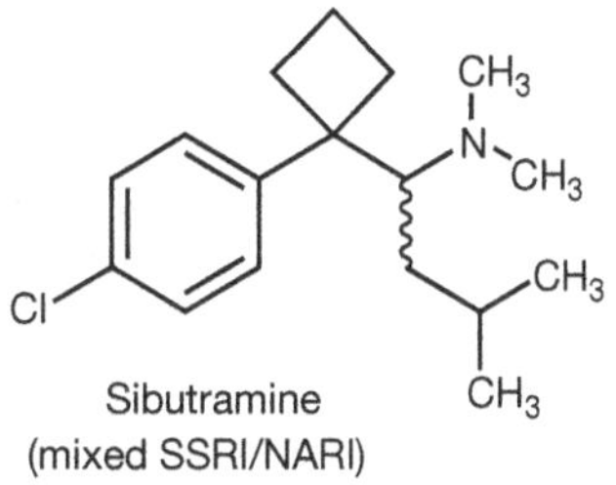

Figure 18.27 Examples of dual SSRI/NARI derivatives.

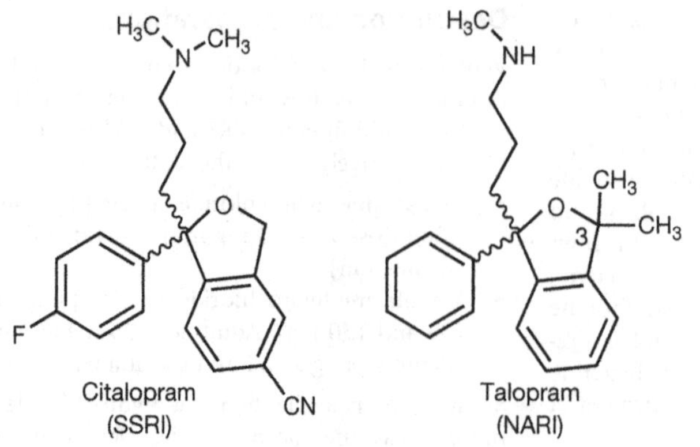

Figure 18.28 Citalopram and some of its derivatives.

cognition. Some of the naturally occurring compounds are found in plants and fungi and have been used since ancient times for recreational and religious purposes within an indigenous context. This section places the attention on the so-called classical hallucinogens, which refers to their ability to interact with the serotonergic system and the fact that they share structural similarities with neurotransmitters such as dopamine, adrenaline and serotonin. Another commonly used term is 'psychedelic', which is normally translated to 'mind-manifesting'. Research into the details of molecular and human psychopharmacological principles is still ongoing but current knowledge suggests that classical hallucinogens exert their effects, at least in part, by agonist or partial agonist action at the 5-HT_{2A} receptor. It has to be noted, however, that this is a massive oversimplification and that the dopamine and cortical glutamate systems are also believed to potentially play a key role.

The so-called 'classical' hallucinogens, represented by mescaline, *N,N*-dimethyltryptamine (DMT), psilocybin or lysergic acid diethylamide (LSD) (Fig. 18.29), do not appear to show significant toxicological or addictive properties but produce profound dose-dependent alterations of consciousness in humans. An individual's mindset and the immediate surroundings (setting) have been reported to dramatically influence the nature of the experience, which often leads to irreproducible psychodynamic effects. Research so far suggests that classical hallucinogens such as psilocybin may be well tolerated in psychologically healthy subjects under carefully controlled conditions and supervision. Unsupervised and recreational high-dose consumption of these derivatives has been observed to increase the possibility to experience psychotic ego dissolution, anxiety, psychosomatic symptoms and paranoid ideation ('horror trip'). Classical hallucinogens are controlled substances and therefore are illegal to possess, but a number of these compounds have a long (but interrupted) history to be investigated within the context of alcoholism, model psychosis research and schizophrenia. Since the early 1990s, however, human clinical research activities have dramatically increased which, in combination with the availability of advanced medical and diagnostic technology, has led to significant contributions to the understanding about the functioning of the human mind.

Structural modifications of the classical hallucinogen-like templates have led to a number of important

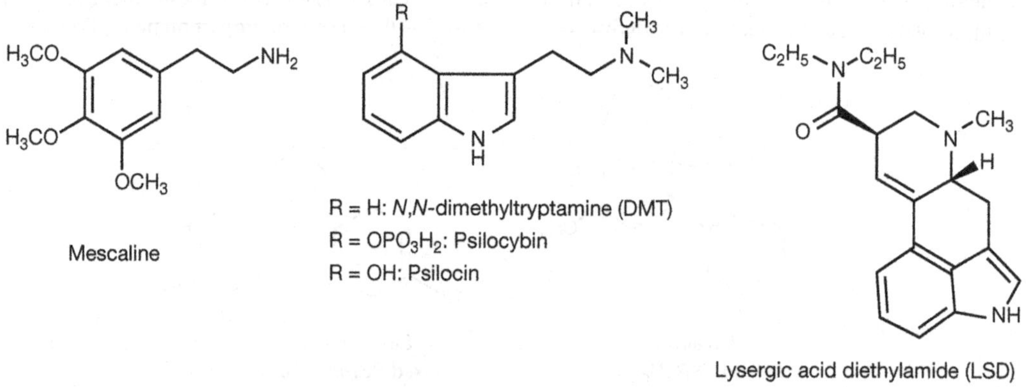

Figure 18.29 Examples of the 'classical' hallucinogens.

neurobiochemical probes with sometimes high selectivities at serotonin receptor subtypes. This has allowed researchers to shed some light on some neurochemical correlates of altered states of consciousness and possible underlying factors of mental disorders. Moreover, based on recent research activities, it has been suggested that some of these derivatives may show interesting potential within the area of psychotherapy. On the other end of the spectrum lies the recreational consumption of these derivatives, and the term 'designer drugs' is often quoted in order to describe drugs which are based on the structural template of classical hallucinogens. The pharmacology and toxicology is very often unknown.

One commonly used classification system of hallucinogenic drug-induced phenomena in humans is based on A. Dittrich's description of the following basic dimensions: (1) 'oceanic boundlessness', which includes positively experienced loss of ego boundaries, positive changes in mood ranging from heightened feelings to sublime happiness and mystical states or mania-like grandiosity; (2) 'visionary restructuralisation' involving visual illusions, hallucinations, synaesthesias and changes in the meaning of various precepts; (3) 'anxious ego dissolution', manifested as thought disorder, ego disintegration, loss of autonomy and self-control variously associated with arousal, anxiety, and paranoid feelings of being endangered; (4) 'acoustic alterations', i.e. hypersensitivity to sound or noise and auditory hallucinations; and (5) 'altered vigilance'.

A very large number of structurally modified phenylethylamines, tryptamines and lysergamides have been evaluated based on human self-experimentation by A.T. and Ann Shulgin and published in the scientific and popular literature including the Internet. As one might imagine, this has led to controversial discussions. One position is based on the argument that this approach may lead to popularisation of drug misuse, and an often used counter-argument centres around the opinion that these data will be of use to the public, helping to inform potential consumers about the nature, pharmacology and potential toxicology of psychoactive drugs that may circulate on the streets.

Phenylethylamines

Mescaline (Fig. 18.30) is a natural product found, for example, in the peyote cactus *Lophophora williamsii*. Mescaline contains the 3,4,5-trimethoxyphenylethylamine unit that structurally resembles some of the previously described adrenaline and dopamine derivatives. Masking of the hydroxyl functionality with methyl groups gives compounds with increased lipophilicity and thus increased ability to cross the blood–brain barrier. Methoxylation of the benzene ring in a number of phenylethylamines and amfetamines at specific positions plays a key role in hallucinogenic activity. Mescaline and other phenylalkylamines are most commonly found as the hydrochloride or sulphate salt. Mescaline is of relatively low potency when compared with other hallucinogens. The active oral adult dose is reported to be around 200–400 mg of the salt with a threshold of around 100 mg. Effects are known to last up to 10–12 hours.

Structural modifications of the mescaline-type 3,4,5-substitution pattern revealed a particular influence of the *para* (position 4) on human psychoactivity. Potency appears to increase with an increase in alkyl chain length attached to the oxygen at this position but then drops beyond a chain length of three atoms. A tenfold increase in potency over mescaline has been observed with 4-allyloxy-3,5-trimethoxyphenylethylamine (AL). Thiomescaline represents an example of isosterism where oxygen has been replaced by sulphur that has the same valency. This modification also displayed a tenfold increase in potency when compared with mescaline. An extended duration of action of 10–15 hours has been reported for thiomescaline.

Another arrangement follows the 2,4,5-trisubstitution pattern which gives rise to the so-called 2C-X and 2C-T-X series where X refers to a large variety of alkyl and halogen substituents (Fig. 18.31). Within this group a similar trend has been observed for the impact of structural modification of the 4 position on biological activity. An increase in alkyl chain length from CH_3 (2C-D) to C_3H_7 (2C-P) within the 2C-X series led to increased potency from around 8-fold to 40-fold when compared with mescaline. The 2C-T-X group, which can be viewed as the 2,4,5-counterpart of the thiomescalines, appeared to follow a similar trend and attachment of a fluorine atom in 2C-T-21 showed 30-fold increase in potency relative to mescaline.

Amfetamines

The previous section on CNS stimulants described the fact that amfetamine and its *N*-methylated derivative show stimulatory properties. This was attributed to the lack of

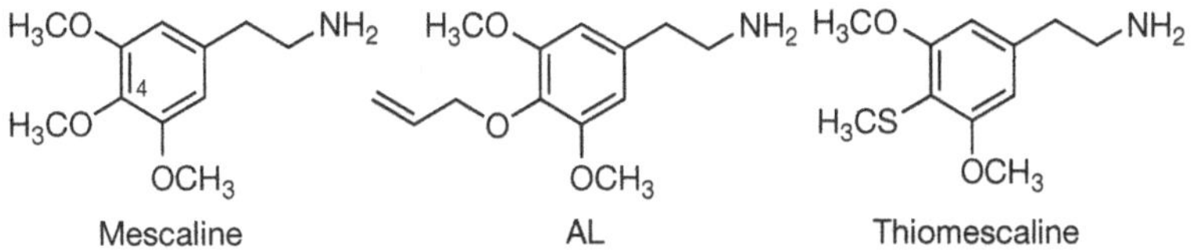

Figure 18.30 Mescaline and some of its psychoactive derivatives leading to increased potency.

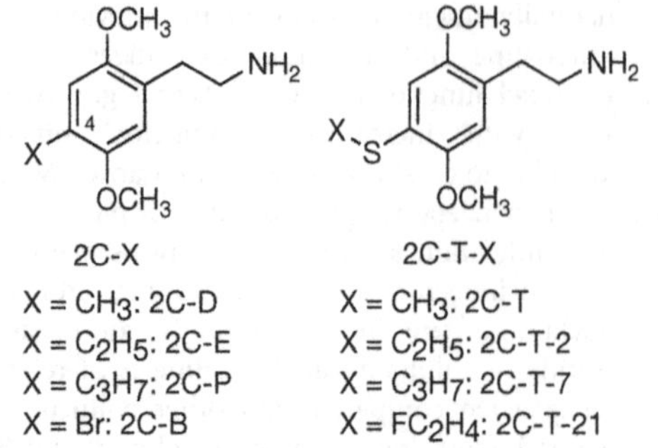

Figure 18.31 Highly potent phenylethylamine derivatives called the 2-C-X and 2C-T-X series, respectively. They share the presence of two methoxy groups at positions 2 and 5.

polar hydroxyl groups on the benzene ring and the presence of a CH_3 group at the α-position which contributes to protection from deamination by monoamine oxidase. In phenylethylamine, absence of the α-methyl results in a structure that lacks these properties. Within the group of hallucinogenic phenylethylamines mentioned above, addition of an α-methyl group is known to give hallucinogenic amfetamines with unusually high potencies (Fig. 18.32). Consequently, addition of an α-methyl group to 2,5-dimethoxy-4-methylphenylethylamine (2C-D) gives 2,5-dimethoxy-4-methylamfetamine (DOM) which increases potency from 8-fold to about 50-fold relative to mescaline. DOM became known on the streets in the 1960s and has also been termed STP. As mentioned before, increased alkyl chain length potentiates biological activity and prolonged duration up to 30 hours. Halogen replacement at this position was found to increase potencies around 150-fold. The commercially available 2,5-dimethoxy-4-iodoamfetamine (DOI) and DOB are valuable neurochemical tools for both in vivo (e.g. drug discrimination studies with rats) and in vitro studies. Attachment of the α-methyl group to compounds of the 2C-T-X series results in the formation of the corresponding amfetamines of the ALEPH-X series with up to 50-fold increased potencies. There is some indication in the literature that ALEPH-2 may show anxiolytic properties which may be partly rationalised by its ability to act as a monoamine oxidase inhibitor. In the section on the stimulatory amfetamines, we have seen that introduction of a substituent at the α-position produces a chiral carbon and the (*S*)-enantiomer was said to show higher potencies. In the world of the hallucinogenic amfetamines, such as DOM, DOB and DOI, it would appear that the (*R*)-enantiomers are more potent than their (*S*)-counterparts.

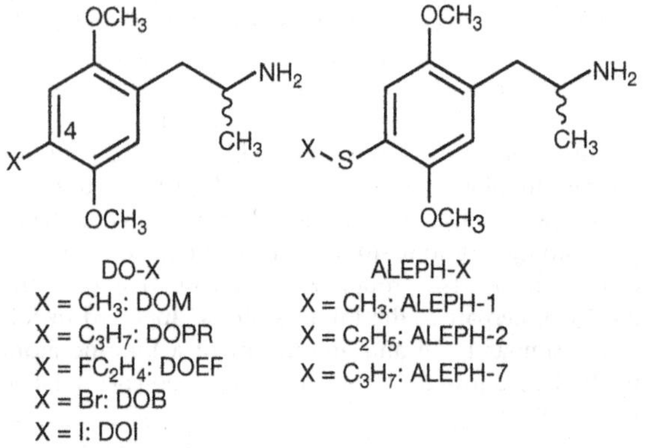

Figure 18.32 Amfetamine counterparts (additional presence of the α-carbon) of 2-C-X and 2C-T-X compounds give rise to the DO-X and ALEPH-X series.

Tryptamines

N,N-Dimethyltryptamine (DMT) is a representative of the tryptamine, i.e. indole-3-alkylamine, family. Note the structural similarity to serotonin which is 5-hydroxytryptamine (Fig. 18.33). DMT is parenterally, but not orally, active at around 60–100 mg of the free base since rapid deamination by monoamine oxidase occurs following oral administration. Pharmacological effects are therefore induced by inhalation of the free base vapour or by injection of a water-soluble salt. The fumarate salt has been used in a number of human clinical studies and it was reported that the psychoactive effects are relatively short-lived, with durations less than 1 hour. Smoking of the free base leads to very intense but short-lived effects for around 5–15 minutes. A number of *N*-mono and dimethylated tryptamines are also present in several human tissues. Their exact function has been debated for several decades but so far no definite conclusion has been reached.

Inhibition of monoamine oxidase, on the other hand, renders DMT orally active. A fascinating example of the

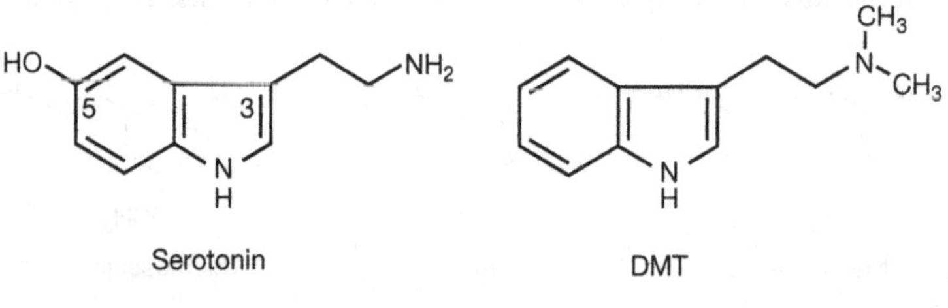

Figure 18.33 Serotonin (5-hydroxytryptamine) and the naturally occurring hallucinogen *N,N*-dimethyltryptamine (DMT).

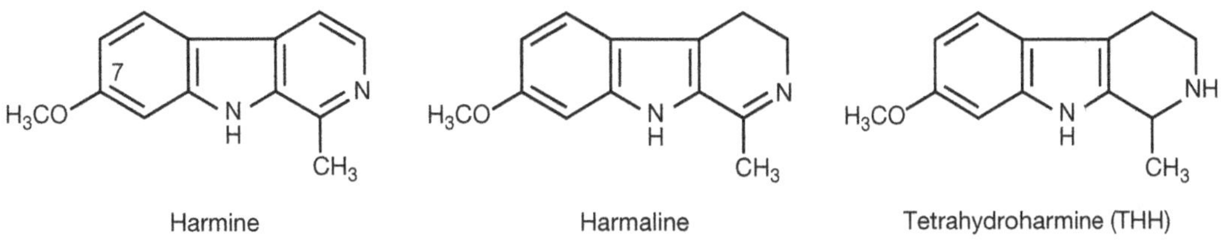

Figure 18.34 Harmala alkaloids and their different degree of ring saturation.

application of this principle is found in *ayahuasca*, a psychoactive beverage that has been used in South America for millennia by a large number of indigenous cultures for religious and medicinal purposes. This beverage is often prepared by the combination of DMT-containing plants, e.g. *Psychotria viridis*, a member of the coffee plant family, with *Banisteriopsis caapi*. This wooden liana is known to contain a number of reversible MAO inhibitors such as harmine, harmaline and tetrahydroharmine (Fig. 18.34) which also appear to possess some form of serotonin reuptake inhibiting properties. Inspection of these so-called β-carboline-type structures reveals some resemblance to the tryptamine nucleus. Indeed, tetrahydroharmine (THH), for example, may be synthetically accessible by the Pictet-Spengler reaction where the 7-methoxytryptamine precursor undergoes cyclisation with a suitable carbonyl source such as acetaldehyde. The presence of double bonds in harmaline and harmine indicates that oxidation of THH must have occurred. The use of *ayahuasca* is not restricted to indigenous populations and a variety of urban syncretic churches employ the brew as sacraments for healing purposes. Within the recreational underground community the combination of DMT-containing plants with pharmaceutical MAO inhibitors has been reported and termed *pharmahuasca*. Hyperserotonergic activity can potentially be lethal (serotonin syndrome), particularly when MAO inhibitors are consumed in combination with compounds that increase serotonergic activities such as serotonin reuptake inhibitors.

3-(2-Dimethylaminoethyl)-1H-indol-4-yl dihydrogen phosphate (psilocybin), the *O*-phosphoryl-4-hydroxy derivative of DMT (Fig. 18.35), is a major constituent of 'magic mushrooms' of the *Psilocybe* genus that is found in most areas of the world. The presence of the phosphate ester renders the molecule relatively stable but the active principle is now believed to be the 4-HO-DMT derivative psilocin. Psilocybin is orally active at around 5–20 mg and effects do not normally exceed 4–6 hours. Administration of psilocybin at subpsychoactive dosages has been found to show impressive potential for the treatment of cluster headaches, presumably involving 5-HT$_1$-receptor agonism.

Due to the polarity of the hydroxyl group in the 5 position and rapid deamination by monoamine oxidase, oral administration of serotonin will not lead to passage through the blood–brain barrier. Tryptamine itself, although present in the brain as a so-called trace amine, is also not psychoactive. Protection from metabolic attack is facilitated by the introduction of the α-methyl group which renders α-methyltryptamine (AMT) orally active at the 15–30-mg level (Fig. 18.36). The duration of effects have also been reported to be dramatically extended up to 16 hours. A 20-fold increase in potency has been observed for the 5-methoxy counterpart of AMT when compared to DMT (3–5 mg) where lipophilicity has been increased by *O*-methylation. Several α-alkylated derivatives also show strong monoamine oxidase inhibiting properties which have generated interest in the field of antidepressant therapy. In contrast to the hallucinogenic amfetamines, in the case of both AMT and 5-MeO-AMT higher potency resides with the (*S*)-enantiomers.

Generally, psychoactivity is greatly affected by substitution on the indole ring, the side chain carbons and by

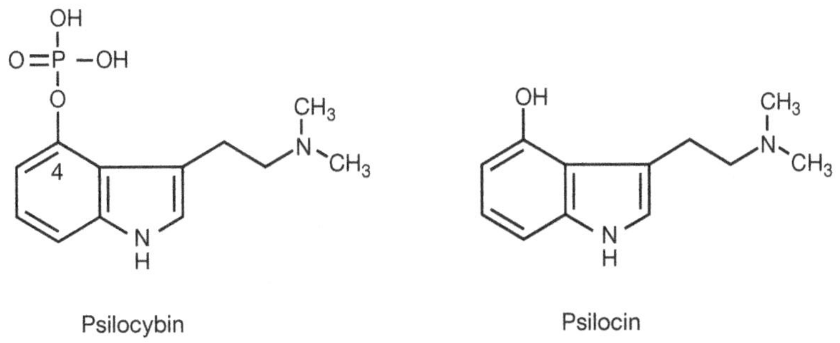

Figure 18.35 Psychoactive key constituents of 'magic' mushrooms.

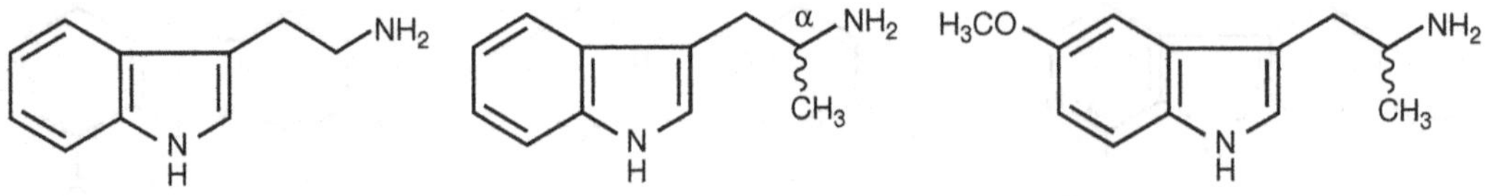

Tryptamine AMT 5-MeO-AMT

Figure 18.36 α-Methylation of the inactive tryptamine gives psychoactive derivatives.

alkylation of the side chain nitrogen. Most of the psychoactive *N,N*-disubstituted derivatives known may show oral activity, presumably due to their lack of sufficient substrate specificity to the metabolising enzyme monoamine oxidase. Homologation of the *N,N*-dialkyl substituents retains psychoactivity but this appears to diminish with alkyl groups larger than four carbons. In other words, the most commonly found side chain alkylation pattern is represented by either symmetrically substituted *N,N*-dimethyl-, diethyl-, dipropyl-, diallyl and diisopropyltryptamines or by asymmetrically substituted derivatives including *N*-methyl-*N*-ethyl or *N*-methyl-*N*-isopropyl derivatives. Figure 18.37 shows a few selected examples of typically found derivatives. In comparison with *N,N*-dialkylated tryptamines unsubstituted on the benzene ring, the presence of hydroxyl groups on the 4 position and methoxy groups on the 5 position have been observed to show increased potencies. The presence of substituents on the remaining position of the benzene ring leads to attenuation or inactivity. In contrast with a large number of hallucinogenic phenylalkylamines, which show significant affinities towards the 5-HT_{2A} and 5-HT_{2C} receptor, several so far explored hallucinogenic tryptamines show significant affinities towards the 5-HT_{2A} and 5-HT_{1A} receptors. Another difference between tryptamines and phenylalkylamines is the fact that *N*-alkylation of the side chain nitrogen of the latter leads to significant loss in activity which is not observed in tryptamines.

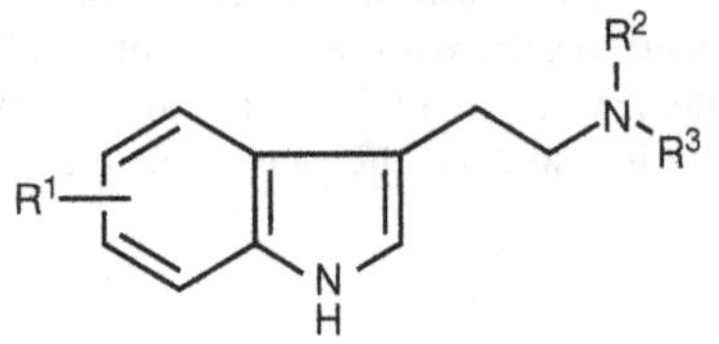

R^1 = H; R^2 = R^3 = C_2H_5: DET

R^1 = H; R^2 = R^3 = C_3H_7: DPT

R^1 = 4-OH; R^2 = CH_3; R^3 = $CH(CH_3)_2$: 4-OH-MIPT

R^1 = 5-MeO; R^2 = R^3 = $CH(CH_3)_2$: 5-MeO-DIPT

Figure 18.37 Representative examples of neuroactive *N,N*-dialkylated tryptamines. Structural key features also include the presence of H, OH or CH_3O at the 4 and 5 position of the benzene ring.

Lysergamides

Lysergic acid diethylamide (LSD, Fig. 18.38) is one of the most potent hallucinogens currently known and the psychoactive properties of this derivative were discovered by A. Hofmann in 1943. It is orally active in the 50–200 μg range with effects lasting up to 12 hours. Its stereochemistry plays a fundamental role in its high activity. The active isomer carries the (5*R*,8*R*)-configuration and is called *d*-LSD. Epimerisation to the (5*R*,8*S*)-derivative, easily triggered, for example, by exposure to light, gives the inactive iso-LSD. LSD has mostly been prepared as the tartrate salt. Most structural modifications of the LSD template led to reduced psychoactivity but an exemption was observed for several compounds alkylated at N(6) where replacement of the methyl group of LSD with ethyl, propyl and allyl groups appeared to slightly increase potencies (Fig. 18.38).

Lisuride is a dopamine DA D_2-receptor agonist (it has been considered for the management of Parkinson's disease), a feature that is also shared with LSD. Lisuride has been observed to be inactive in humans despite high affinity towards the $5HT_{2A}$ and other serotonin receptor subtypes. Recent research has provided support for the concept of functional selectivity where LSD may be able to stabilise a distinct G-protein coupled receptor conformation which leads to differential activation of signalling pathways and neurobehavioural responses.

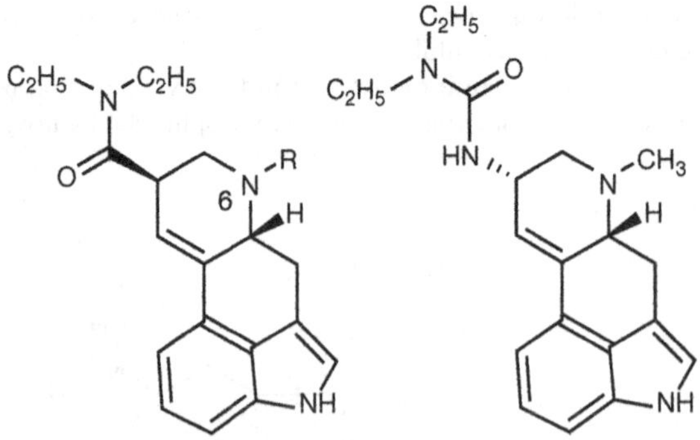

Lisuride

R = CH_3: MethLAD = LSD
R = C_2H_5: EthLAD
R = C_3H_7: ProLAD
R = allyl: AllyLAD

Figure 18.38 LSD and some of its derivatives.

Entactogens (3,4-methylenedioxyamfetamines)

Substituted amfetamine derivatives containing a 3,4-methylenedioxy component attached to the phenyl ring form the structural basis of the so-called entactogens. The most commonly encountered representative is 3,4-methylenedioxy-*N*-methamfetamine (MDMA), also known as *ecstasy* (Fig. 18.39). This illicit derivative has been observed to have been consumed recreationally by an increasing proportion of young adult populations since the early 1980s. The main reason for its popularity is based on a number of distinctive subjective effects, normally not commonly observed with stimulants and hallucinogens. These include emotional closeness, fearlessness, empathy and the ability for peaceful self-reflection. This particular feature contributed to the renewed interest within the context of clinical studies evaluating the potential of MDMA-assisted psychotherapy for the treatment of anxiety related to advanced-stage cancer and post-traumatic stress disorder.

A large body of evidence has provided support for the notion that repetitive and particularly high-dose consumption of MDMA may cause a number of psychopathological and neuropsychological deficits in humans, such as depression, mood disturbances and cognitive impairments. A number of contributing factors, such as polydrug use, consumption of contaminated drug tablets, physical distress (dancing, high temperature, lack of fluids) and the presence of premorbid conditions, have been reported to increase the risk of suffering from a number of acute complications. In severe cases these may include cardiac arrhythmias, seizures, coma and in rare cases death.

One primary neurochemical mode of action of MDMA involves an indirectly mediated release of monoamines via reversed plasma membrane monoamine transport function and disruption of vesicular storage. Increased 5-HT release appears to be the dominating feature and DA, NA and acetylcholine release are also observed to be involved, although to a lesser degree. Additional mechanisms include inhibition of tryptophan hydroxylase and MAO-A, as well as involvement of 5-HT_{2A} receptors.

MDMA is orally active in the 80–150 mg range with psychoactive effects usually lasting 4–6 hours. This derivative is most commonly found as the hydrochloride salt but the phosphate and sulphate salts have also been described. The (*S*)-enantiomer is significantly more potent

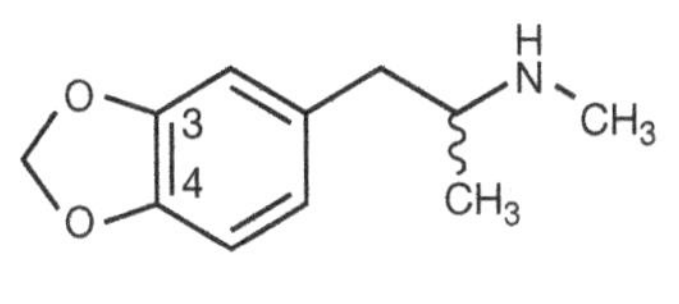

Figure 18.39 MDMA (*ecstasy*), the entactogen prototype.

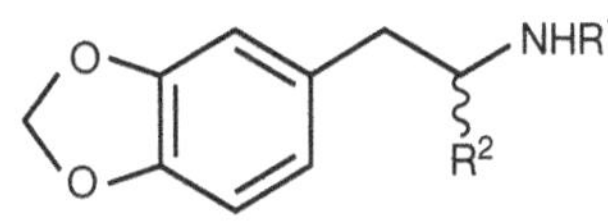

Figure 18.40 MDMA derivatives based on modification of the α-carbon and/or the alkyl group on the side chain nitrogen.

than its (*R*)-counterpart, a feature that appears to apply to other entactogen derivatives as well.

Figure 18.40 shows the product of *N*-ethylation that gives rise to 3,4-methylenedioxy-*N*-ethylamfetamine (MDEA or MDE). A slight drop in duration (3–5 hours) and potency has been observed, resulting in an oral dosage range of 100–200 mg but MDMA-like activity appears to be retained. Current knowledge suggests that the (*S*)-enantiomer may be responsible for the induction of elevated mood and entactogenic effects whereas the (*R*)-isomer may contribute more significantly to the observation of neurotoxic conditions. The α-ethyl derivative of MDMA also retains MDMA-like activity and stereoselectivity. MBDB, i.e. 1-(1,3-benzodioxol-5-yl)-*N*-methylbutan-2-amine (Fig. 18.40), has also been observed to display a slight drop in potency, as indicated by an active range of 180–210 mg. Duration of effects appear to be similar to MDMA.

The triptans

The triptan series refers to a class of drugs which act as selective 5-$HT_{1D/1B}$-receptor agonists. These derivatives, used for the acute treatment of migraine attacks (constriction of intracranial blood vessels), are based on the structural template of the prototype called sumatriptan (Fig. 18.41). The most important structural requirements are based on the presence of a hydrogen bond acceptor at the 5 position of an indole nucleus and a flexible *N*,*N*-dialkylated ethylamine-type side chain. In other words, most of these compounds can be viewed as 5-substituted derivatives of the hallucinogenic DMT described above (Fig. 18.41). Also note the structural similarity to the magic mushroom-derived psilocybin which is a 4-substituted DMT derivative. Introduction of the substituent at the 5 position abolishes hallucinogenic activities and gives way to selective 5-$HT_{1D/1B}$-receptor agonism. As mentioned above, administration of subhallucinogenic doses of psilocybin have been reported to abolish acute cluster headache episodes and it might not be too surprising if similar triptan-type interactions may be involved. This mixed selectivity can result in undesired cardiovascular side effects (vasoconstriction) that appear to include agonist activity at the 5-HT_{1B}-receptor subtype. Sumatriptan showed relatively low bioavailability after oral or nasal administration (14–17%) which

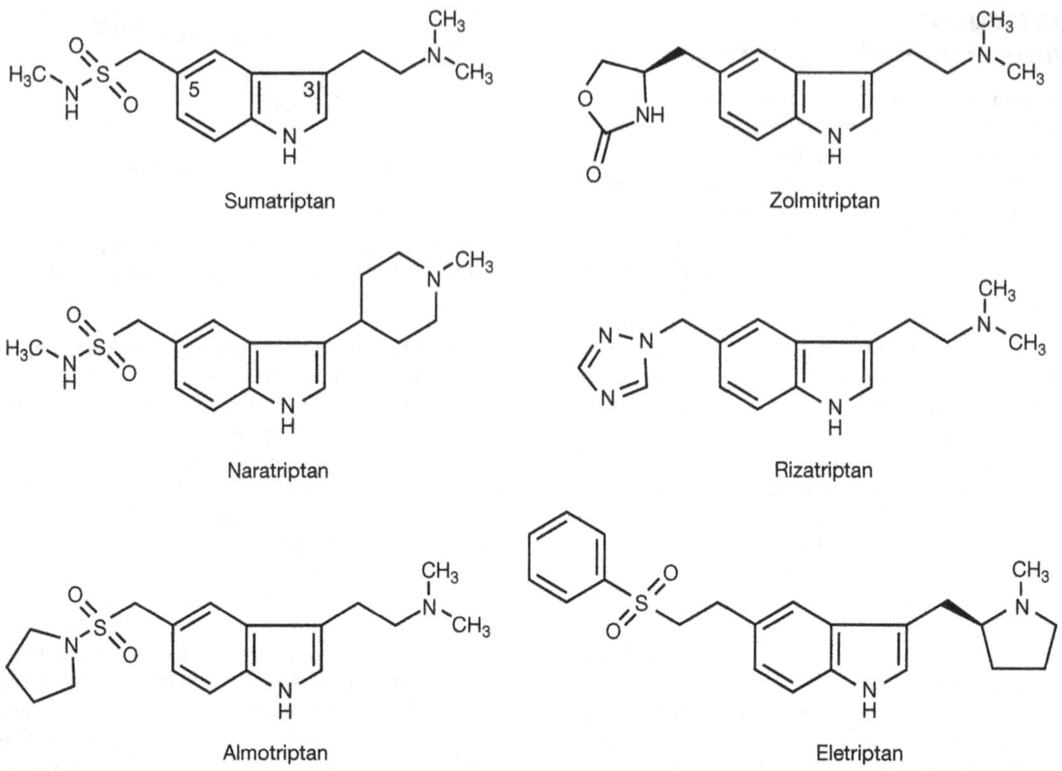

Figure 18.41 The triptans.

improved to around 97% via the subcutaneous route. Approval for additional triptans reflected improved characteristics such as oral bioavailability and potency. Structural modifications included a change in the geometry and polarity of the exocyclic ring and modified flexibility by introducing either a methylene of ethylene linker at the 5 position.

Description and preparations

Sumatriptan can be found as the free base but is most commonly prepared as the succinate salt. Dosages depend on the route of administration.

- Sumatriptan succinate tablets (50 and 100 mg). Adult dose 50–100 mg, maximum of 300 mg within 24 hours.
- Sumatriptan succinate subcutaneous injection (12 mg/mL). Adult dose 6 mg. Maximum of 12 mg within 24 hours.
- Sumatriptan base nasal spray (20 mg/0.1 mL actuation). Adult dose 6 mg. Maximum of 12 mg within 24 hours.

Zolmitriptan shows increased oral bioavailability (40%) and also forms an active, demethylated secondary amine metabolite.

- Zolmitriptan base tablets (2.5 mg) and orodispersible tablets (2.5 and 5 mg). Adult dose 2.5 mg, Maximum of 12 mg within 24 hours.
- Zolmitriptan base nasal spray (5 mg/0.1 mL actuation). Adult dose 5 mg. Maximum of 10 mg within 24 hours.

Naratriptan is a relatively long-acting triptan with a plasma half-life of around 6 hours (sumatriptan 1–2 hours) which also shows improved oral bioavailability (60–70%).

- Naratriptan hydrochloride tablets (2.5 mg). Adult dose 1.0–2.5 mg, Maximum of 5 mg within 24 hours.

Rizatriptan shows an oral bioavailability of approximately 45% and appears to be metabolised significantly by MAO-A.

- Rizatriptan benzoate tablets (5 and 10 mg) and benzoate oral lyophilisate (10 mg). Adult dose 10 mg, Maximum of 5 mg within 24 hours.

Almotriptan achieves 70–80% oral bioavailability.

- Almotriptan maleate tablets (12.5 mg). Adult dose 12.5 mg, Maximum of 25 mg within 24 hours.

Eletriptan has shown a fivefold improved potency, improved oral bioavailability (50%) and increased elimination half-life of approximately 4 hours when compared with sumatriptan.

- Eletriptan hydrobromide tablets (20 and 40 mg). Adult dose 40 mg, Maximum of 80 mg within 24 hours.

Buspirone and derivatives

The 5-HT_{1A} receptors play an important role in the modulation of serotonergic neurotransmission. These receptors are located presynaptically, for example with high density in the dorsal and median raphe nuclei, where they function as so-called somatodendritic autoreceptors, mostly on serotonergic neurons. The presence of 5-HT_{1A} is known to occur postsynaptically as well, particularly at high densities in limbic areas of the brain and cortical areas. The consequence of interacting with both receptors is a reduction of the firing rate via neuronal hyperpolarisation across the cell membrane. The 5-HT_{1A} receptor has also been found to impact on the regulation of depression, sexual behaviour, appetite and anxiety. A number of drugs with full or partial 5-HT_{1A}-agonist activities are known to display anxiolytic properties. Buspirone is such a derivative and it served as the prototype for a number of azapirone-type anxiolytics (Fig. 18.42). A characteristic feature is the presence of a pyrimidylpiperazine motif where a pyrimidine is connected to the N_1 of piperazine. The N_4 is attached to a tetramethylene spacer (or linker) that can be connected to a variety of imide-type structures. Buspirone, for example, is a 3,3-tetramethyleneglutarimide-containing analogue. A loss of affinity has been observed with analogues where the pyrimidine ring was replaced by other heterocyles such as tetrazole, pyridazine or pyrazine. A number of azapirones show binding affinities for dopamine D_2 and α_1 adrenoceptors as well and the development of selective 5-HT_{1A}-active drugs is a major area of interest. It has also been suggested that 5-HT_{1A}-receptor agonism may lead to increased dopamine release in the prefrontal cortex which may also be useful for the treatment of negative symptoms in schizophrenic patients. It would appear that modifications of the pyrimidylpiperazine can impact significantly on receptor affinity and hence this group may function as the pharmacophore. Selectivity, on the other hand, can vary and is influenced to some extent by the bulky imide-type substituent. Deviation from the tetramethylene pattern decreases 5-HT_{1A} activity as well. Replacement of the pyrimidine moiety with a phenyl ring yields arylpiperazines which often retain 5-HT_{1A} activity, depending on the exact nature of substituents on the benzene ring.

Description and preparations

Buspirone is available as the hydrochloride salt (5 and 10 mg tablets) and is often considered to be useful for generalised anxiety disorder (GAD). Anxiolysis does not coincide with benzodiazepine-like sedation. The remaining derivatives are currently not available in most countries although tandospirone appears to be approved in Japan. The development of ipsapirone has been discontinued and approval for gepirone for the treatment in depression is still being sought.

- Buspirone hydrochloride tablets. Adult dose >18 years 5 mg 2–3 times daily, may be increased up to 60 mg.
- Tandospirone citrate. Adult dose daily oral administration 30 mg in three divided doses, may be increased up to 60 mg.

An important concept for the development of new drugs is based on the idea that the combination of different pharmacophores can contribute to a combined pharmacological action. An example is illustrated in Figure 18.43.

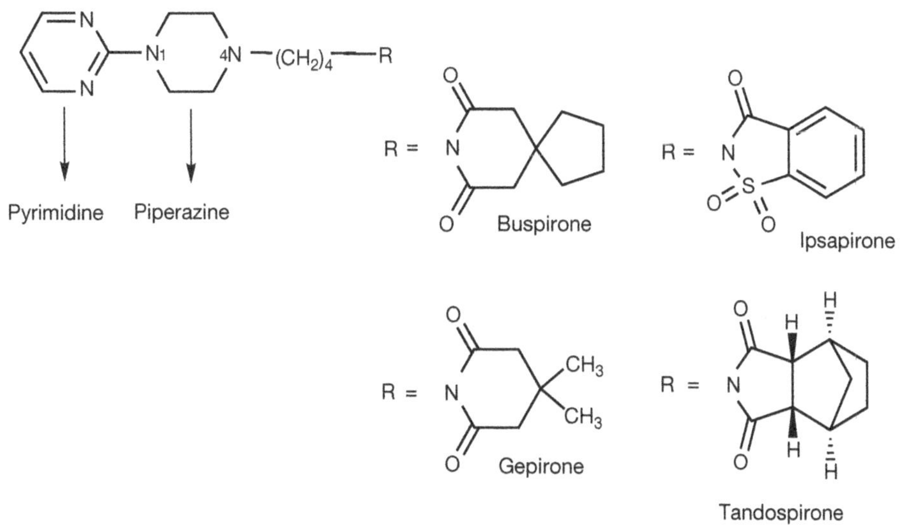

Figure 18.42 Pyrimidylpiperazines.

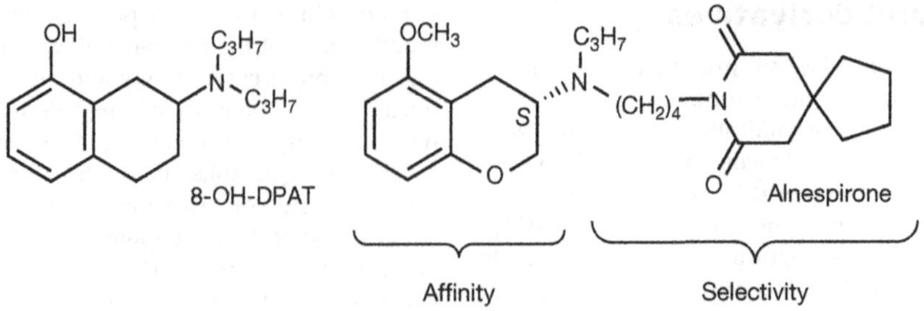

Figure 18.43 Alnespirone. A combination of two different pharmacophores to affect affinity and selectivity.

Alnespirone, when compared with buspirone, has been observed to display higher affinity and selectivity for the 5-HT_{1A} receptor. The presence of the aminobenzopyran moiety reflects the high-affinity element derived from 8-hydroxy-(2-*N,N*-dipropylamino)-tetraline (8-OH-DPAT) which is a full pre- and postsynaptic receptor agonist, commonly used as a pharmacological tool. Selectivity over dopamine D_2 and α_1 adrenoceptors was achieved by the introduction of the four methylene linker attached to the imide found in buspirone. Overall, the combination of both pharmacophore elements produced a full agonist at pre- and postsynaptic 5-HT_{1A} sites. The (*S*)-enantiomer was observed to be more potent than the (*R*)-enantiomer.

A large number of arylpiperazines are known to display affinities for the 5-HT_{1A}-receptor subtype with different selectivities for dopamine and adrenergic receptors. Replacement of the pyrimidine ring (found in azapirones) with an *ortho*-methoxylated benzene ring can result in the reversal of functional activity which provides selective 5-HT_{1A} antagonists (Fig. 18.44). The methylene spacer may vary between one and three. 5-HT_{1A} receptor antagonists are valuable pharmacological tools and a variety are also used as positron emission tomography (PET) radiotracers such as carbon-11 labelled WAY-100635 or ^{18}F-MPPF. Currently, there appears to be a need to explore the potential for clinically available derivatives. Antagonism at this receptor has also been suggested to play a potentially important role for the development of cognitive-enhancing drugs, for example, for the treatment of Alzheimer's disease.

Pindolol, based on the indole nucleus substituted on the 4 position, is a mixed β-adrenoceptor blocker and 5-HT_{1A} antagonist (Fig. 18.45). It is available as the racemic mixture and is normally used in the management of

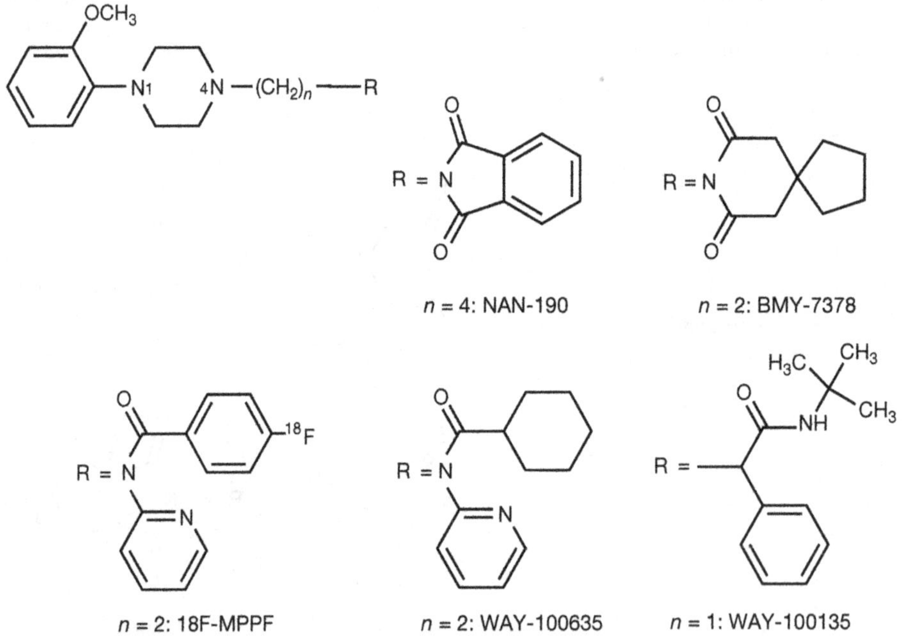

Figure 18.44 Arylpiperazines.

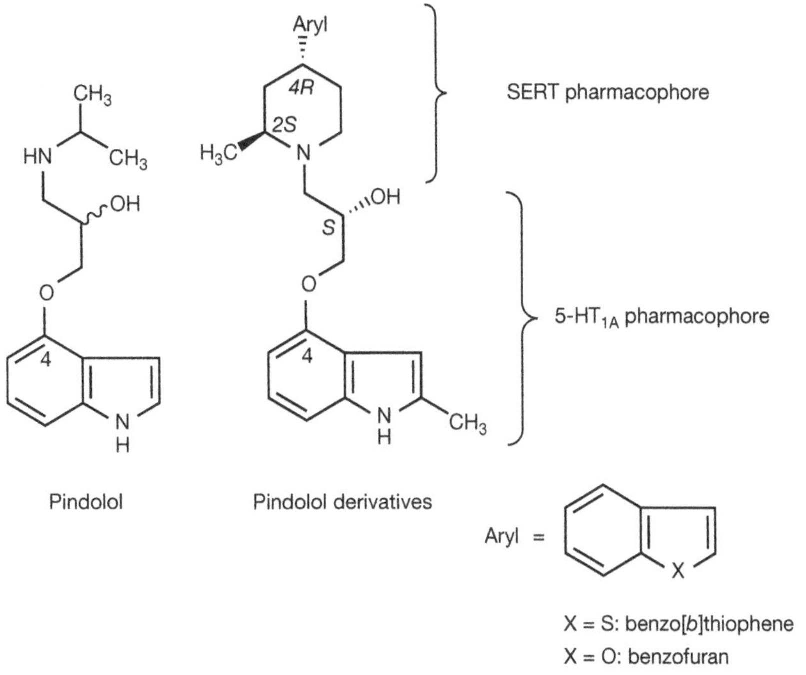

Figure 18.45 Pindolol derivatives.

hypertension and other cardiovascular conditions (up to 45 mg daily). The fact that pindolol also acts as a 5-HT_{1A} antagonist led to the observation that co-administration with SSRIs resulted in a shortened onset of therapeutic efficacy for the latter. As mentioned previously, SSRIs require several weeks of chronic administration in order to take effect, despite the fact that serotonin levels are increased immediately. Current knowledge suggests that increased availability of serotonin induced by reuptake blockage results in adaptive reduction of serotonergic activity by stimulation of 5-HT_{1A} receptor agonism and reduced cell firing rates. Chronic exposure to SSRIs would then lead to desensitisation of the somatodendritic autoreceptors, which results in the restoration of the firing rate, largely increased presence of serotonin and a reduction of depressive symptomatology.

In other words, 5-HT_{1A}-mediated presynaptic autoreceptor blockage is believed to prevent launching the negative 5-HT feedback on cell firing, hence resulting in fast-acting antidepressant activity. The consequence of this observation has been an intense search for novel drugs that combine both functions in one molecule, SERT blockage + 5-HT_{1A} antagonism, leading to so-called 'SSRI Plus' derivatives or 'enhanced SSRIs'. One example is shown in Fig. 18.45 where researchers at Lilly Research Laboratories reported on a variety of interesting in vitro activities based on (2*S*)-1-(2-methyl-1*H*-indol-4-yloxy)-3-((2*S*,4*R*)-4-aryl-2-methylpiperidinyl) propan-2-ols.

Antagonists at the 5-HT_{2A} receptor

The phenylpiperazine motif is also a feature of nefazodone and trazodone which show antidepressant activity, amongst other properties (Fig. 18.46). The phenyl ring carries a chlorine atom at the *meta*-position and the N_4 spacer is formed by a trimethylene chain, attached to a triazolone moiety. Nefazodone shares some aspects of TCA psychopharmacology because it displays some inhibition of NAT and SERT. Its strongest action, however, involves 5-HT_{2A} receptor antagonism and affinity for the α_1-adrenoceptors is also observed. Nefazodone has sometimes been referred to as a dual-action antidepressant (dominating SERT/5-HT_{2A} activity) but is currently not commonly prescribed due to cases of liver toxicity. Trazodone also shows antidepressant activity similar to TCA derivatives but causes marked sedation, possibly due to histamine H_1-receptor antagonism. Currently, the pharmacology does not appear to be fully understood but weak SERT inhibition, α_1-adrenoceptor affinity and 5-HT_{2A} antagonism appears to be involved.

A potent and highly selective 5-HT_{2A} receptor antagonist used for pharmacological studies is M100907 which is based on a piperidine ring flanked by a dimethoxylated benzene and a *para*-fluoro-substituted phenylethyl moiety. A structurally related derivative is ketanserin which carries a fluorobenzoyl and quinazolinedione component (Fig. 18.46). Ketanserin is a selective 5-HT_{2A} and α-adrenergic receptor antagonist. Interestingly, one of the most convincing arguments for the involvement of 5-HT_{2A}

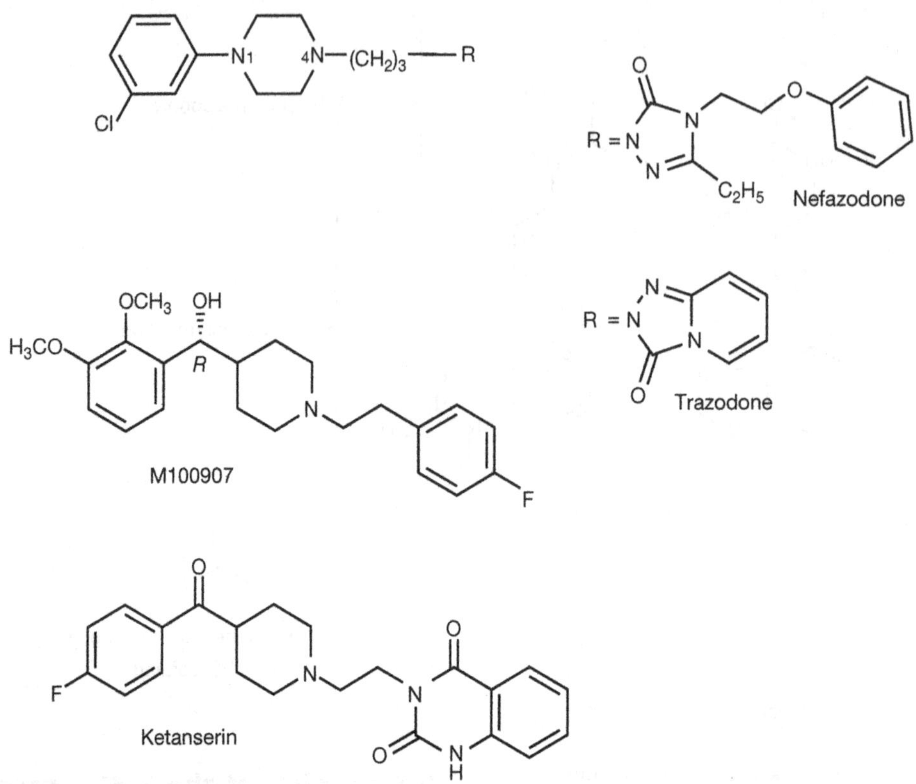

Figure 18.46 5-HT_{2A} receptor antagonists.

receptor agonism in the hallucinogenic activity of psilocybin in humans was provided by the observation of Swiss researchers that pre-administration of ketanserin abolished hallucinogenic effects. The typical antipsychotic haloperidol, a selective dopamine DA D_2-receptor antagonist, did not appear to reduce psilocybin-induced activity. Ketanserin inhibits serotonin-induced bronchoconstriction, platelet aggregation and vasoconstriction and is used for the management of hypertension. Ketanserin also displays high affinities for α-adrenergic and histamine H_1 receptors.

One reason for exploring the impact of 5-HT_{2A} antagonism on brain functioning is based on the recently developed idea that it plays a supporting role in antipsychotic pharmacotherapy. Traditionally, antipsychotic drug effects were predominantly correlated with dopamine D_2-receptor blockage. Conventionally, sufficient DA D_2-receptor occupancy has been determined to be of pivotal importance for antipsychotic drug action. At the same time, a dramatic occurrence of extrapyramidal symptoms is observed which can manifest in the formation of movement disorders. The combination of 5-HT_{2A} receptor blockade with weaker DA D_2-receptor antagonism is believed to reduce the extent of the movement-based side effect formation since a reduced DA receptor occupancy is often found to be sufficient to achieve the desired effects.

The combination of high affinity for 5-HT_{2A}, and potentially 5-HT_6 receptors, with higher selectivity for mesolimbic (and less nigrostriatal) dopamine neurons, is viewed as an important addition to the arsenal of antipsychotic drug therapy but some controversy still seems to exist on this topic. Involvement of the 5-HT_{1A} receptor is also thought to contribute to the overall impact of serotonergic neurotransmission on antipsychotic properties, leading to the desire to develop compounds which act as 5-HT_{2A}/DA D_2 antagonists/5-HT_{1A} partial agonists, generally referred to as 'atypical antipsychotics'.

Ritanserin (Fig. 18.47) acts as a potent but non-selective 5-$HT_{2A/2B/2C}$ antagonist with moderate affinities for dopamine receptors and appears to produce some reduction of schizophrenic core symptoms. It may also show antidepressant and anxiolytic properties. The antipsychotic effects could be improved by increasing the D_2/5HT_2 affinity ratio by structural modification, resulting in risperidone (Fig. 18.47).

The piperidine and side chain motif have been retained but both fluorophenyl groups have been replaced with a 1,2-benzisoxazole group. Haloperidol is a strong DA D_2-receptor antagonist that lacks significant serotonergic activity. It is a representative of the butyrophenone class of antipsychotics. Inspection of the risperidone structure

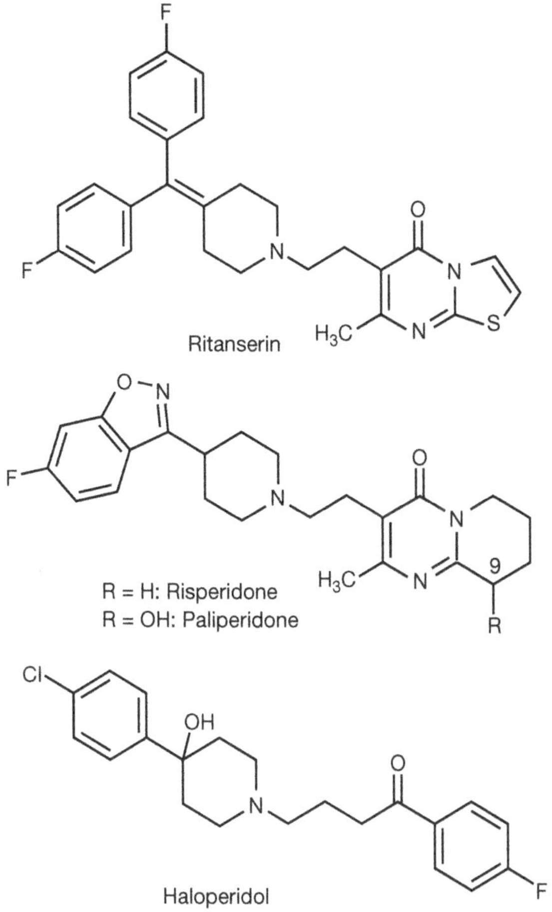

Figure 18.47 Antipsychotics with varying receptor profiles based on the piperidine motif.

shows that the butyrophenone component is still present in the form of a conformationally restricted version. Paliperidone is one major metabolite of risperidone (9-hydroxyrisperidone) and it represents an individually available drug as well. It has also been observed to act as an antagonist at α_1, α_2 and H_1 receptors.

Description and preparations

Risperidone free base preparations include film-coated tablets (1, 2, 3, 4 and 6 mg), orodispersible tablets (0.5, 1, 2, 3 and 4 mg), liquids at 1 mg/mL and depot preparations. Paliperidone is available as free base tablets (3, 6 and 9 mg), the hexadecanoate (palmitate) and extended release formulation using an osmotic-controlled release oral delivery system.

- Risperidone. Adult doses 4–6 mg daily in divided doses (psychosis), 1–6 mg once daily (mania).
- Paliperidone. Adult doses 3–6 mg daily.

Other commonly found atypical antipsychotics are displayed below. Sertindole and aripiprazole also belong to the arylpiperidine and arylpiperazine group (Fig. 18.48), whereas clozapine and derivatives carry the tricyclic structure similar to their antidepressant counterparts mentioned earlier. Note the presence of isosteric elements when comparing the structures.

Sertindole free base appears as film-coated tablets (4, 12, 16, 20 mg) but is less commonly prescribed due to the occurrence of cardiac arrhythmias and prolongation of the QT intervals. Aripiprazole is available in a variety of preparations such as tablets (5, 10, 15 and 30 mg), orodispersible tablets (10 and 15 mg), oral solutions (1 mg/mL) and injectables (7.5 mg/mL).

- Sertindole. Adult dose 12–24 mg daily in single dose.
- Aripiprazole. Adult oral dose 10–30 mg daily in single dose (schizophrenia, mania), 5.25–15 mg by intramuscular injection for control of agitation.

Clozapine (Fig. 18.49), a dibenzodiazepine, is used as tablets (25 and 100 mg) and appears as the free base. Olanzapine (Fig. 18.49) appears in a number of formulations including film-coated tablets (2.5–20 mg) and orodispersible tablets (5–20 mg). It can also be used as a powder for reconstitution. Zotepine (Fig. 18.49) is available as free base sugar-coated tablets (25–100 mg). Quetiapine (Fig. 18.49), on the other hand, is prepared as the fumarate salt and tablets range between 25 and 300 mg.

- Clozapine. Usual adult dose 200–450 mg daily (max. 900 mg) (schizophrenia), 25–50 mg (psychosis in Parkinson's disease).
- Olanzapine. Usual adult dose 5–20 mg daily (schizophrenia, mania), 5–10 mg by intramuscular injection for control of agitation.
- Zotepine. Usual adult dose 25–100 mg three times daily.
- Quetiapine fumarate. Usual adult dose 300–450 mg in two divided doses (max. 750 mg) (schizophrenia) and 400–800 mg for mania.

5-HT$_3$ receptor antagonists

The 5-HT$_3$ receptor subtype is the only representative within the serotonin receptor brigade that is not a GPCR. The 5-HT$_3$ receptor can be classified as a cation-selective ion channel that appears to share a large degree of homology with the nicotinic acetylcholine receptor. Five either homo- or pentameric subunits are observed to form the channel structure that is permeable to mono- and divalent cations. Currently, the most commonly employed drugs acting at the 5-HT$_3$ receptor are antagonists and are used for the treatment of nausea and vomiting induced by cytotoxic chemotherapy and radiotherapy, as well as prevention and treatment of postoperative nausea (presence of receptors in the area postrema). One additional

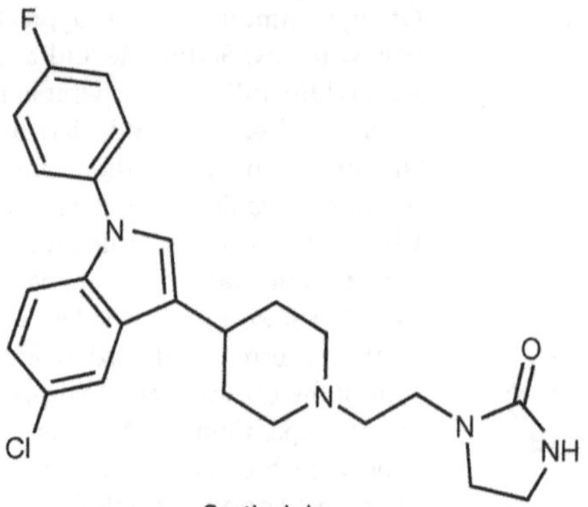

Sertindole

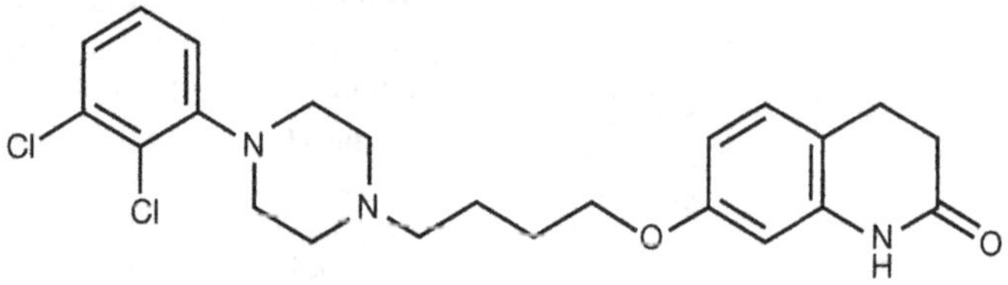

Aripiprazole

Figure 18.48 Other antipsychotics belonging to the arylpiperidine and arylpiperazine group.

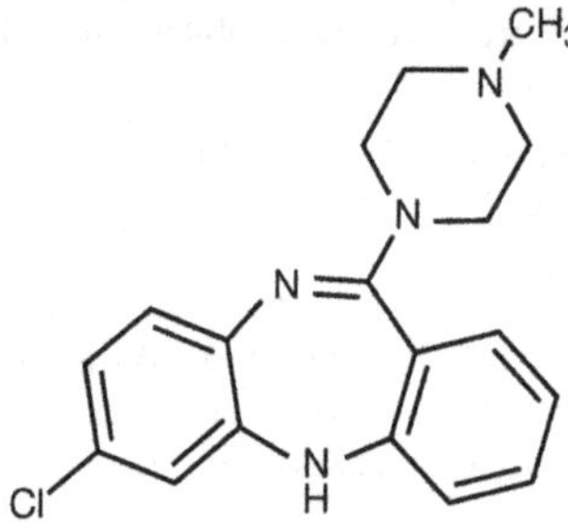

Clozapine

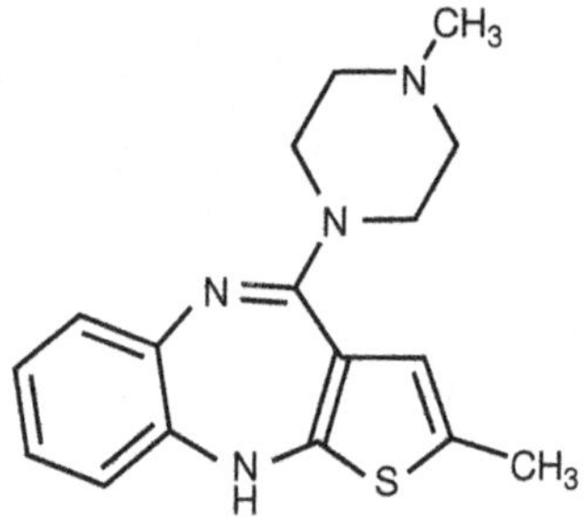

Olanzapine

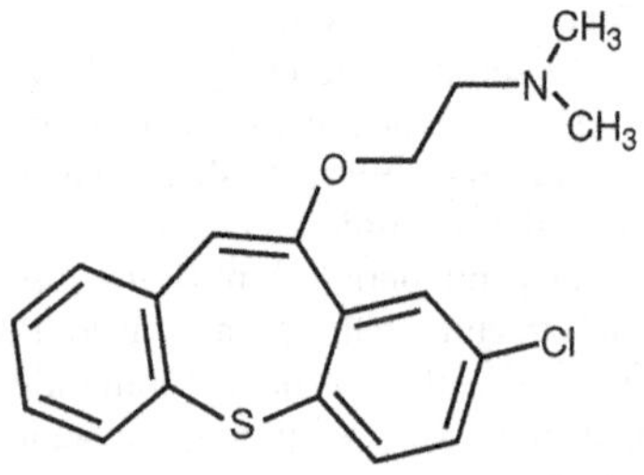

Zotepine

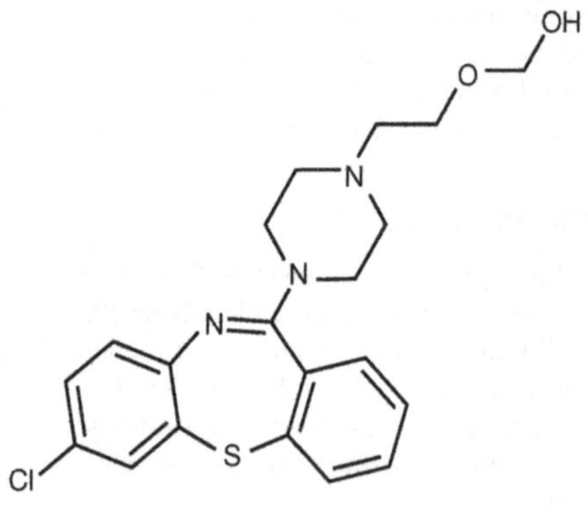

Quetiapine

Figure 18.49 Antipsychotics based on a dibenzodiazepine structure.

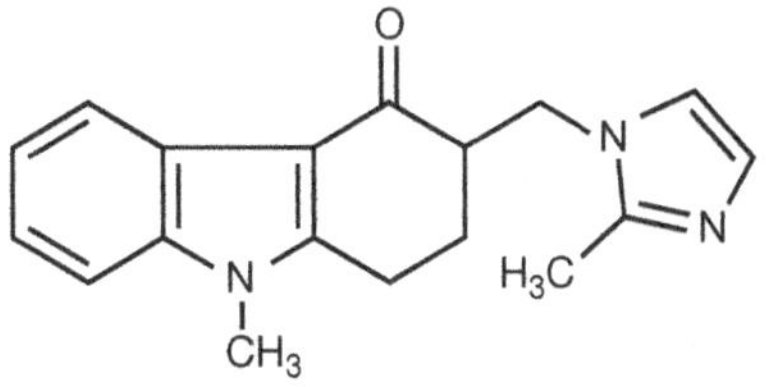

Ondansetron

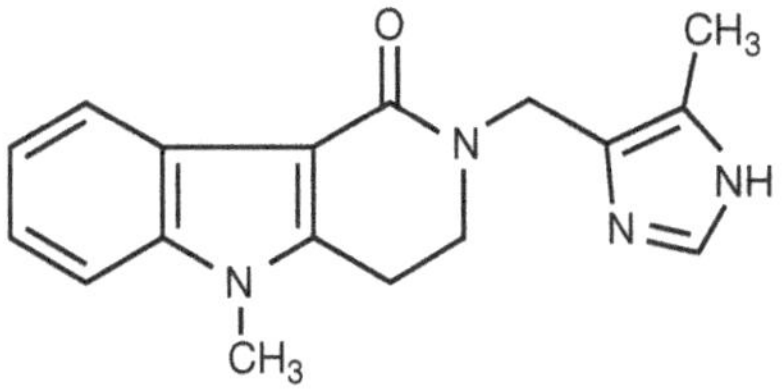

Alosetron

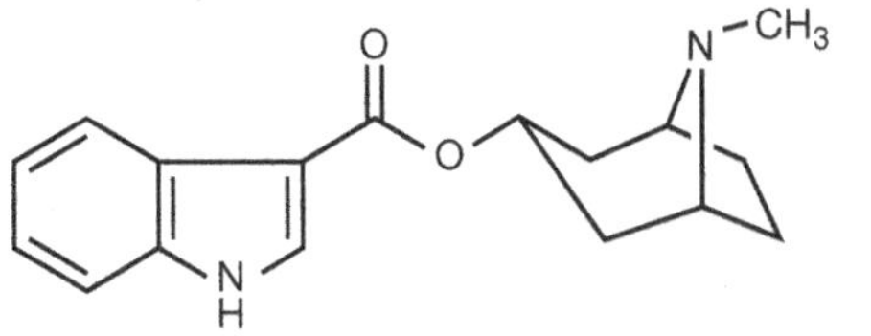

Tropisetron

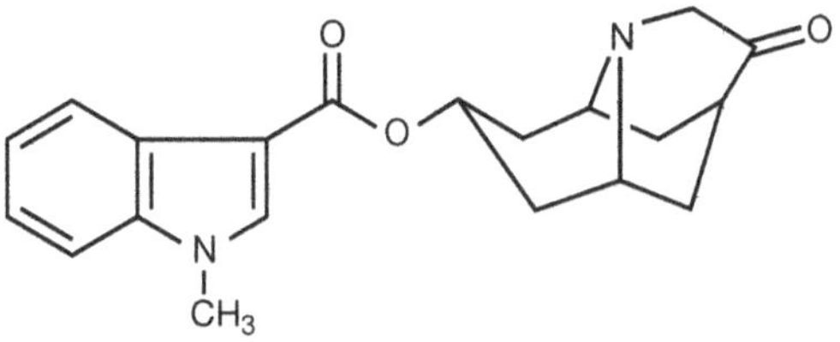

Dolasetron

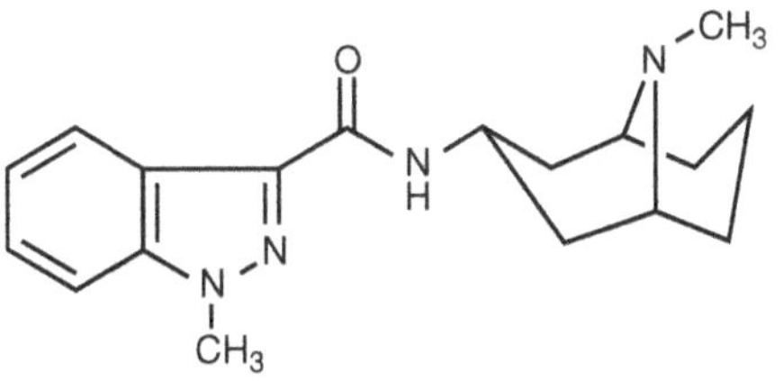

Granisetron

Figure 18.50 5-HT_3 receptor antagonists.

indication includes the treatment of the irritable bowel syndrome (IBS) with diarrhoea. The reason why these antagonists are contraindicated in patients with constipation is the fact that antagonism impacts on the colonic peristaltic reflex, reduces postprandial colonic motility and delays colonic transit.

Ondansetron was launched in 1990 and represented the first marketed drug in this class. Figure 18.50 indicates that the molecule is based on an imidazolyl tetrahydrocarbazolone motif. A variety of structural modifications led to reduced activity such as replacement of the indole with benzofuran or benzothiophen moieties. The carbonyl function also appeared to be important as the presence of an alcohol group or total reduction reduced potency dramatically. Alosetron represents a carbon-linked imidazole derivative which also includes an additional nitrogen atom in place of a carbon atom (Fig. 18.50). This resulted in higher binding affinities and longer duration of action. However, severe gastrointestinal adverse effects have been reported to occur, which led to withdrawal followed by reintroduction. A number of commonly prescribed antiemetics are based on molecules displaying the indole-3-carboxylate (e.g. tropisetron and dolasetron) or indazole-3-carboxamide (e.g. granisetron) nucleus (Fig. 18.50).

Description and preparations

Ondansetron has been described as the free base, hydrochloride salt and hydrochloride dihydrate and is available in a variety of formulations. These include hydrochloride tablets (4 and 8 mg) and solutions for injection (2 mg/mL), oral lyophilisates (4 and 8 mg), sugar-free syrup (4 mg/5 mL as hydrochloride) and suppositories (16 mg). Alosetron hydrochloride tablets (0.5 and 1 mg) are most commonly obtainable. Tropisetron is also available as the hydrochloride salt and comes either as capsules (5 mg) or as a solution for injection at 1 mg/mL. Dolasetron mesilate products are formulated as film-coated tablets (50 and 200 mg) and 20 mg/mL solution for injection. Granisetron is also available as the hydrochloride salt and appears as film-coated tablets (1 and 2 mg) and 1 mg/mL solution for injection and dilution.

- Ondansetron. Adult dose: 8 mg (orally) before treatment followed by 8 mg every 12 h. Rectal administration 16 mg daily intravenously 32 mg. Children: 5 mg/m^2 (intravenously) immediately before treatment and then 4 mg orally every 12 h. Alternatively, 100 µg/kg (maximum 4 mg) (over 2 years old).

- Alosetron hydrochloride. Adult dose 0.5–1 mg twice daily (severe diarrhoea, predominant irritable bowel syndrome in women).
- Tropisetron hydrochloride. Adult dose 2 to 5 mg intravenously; 5 mg orally.
- Dolasetron mesilate. Adult dosages: 1 hour before chemotherapy or within 2 h before surgery orally 100 mg. Intravenous injection 100 mg 30 min before chemotherapy. Treatment of postoperative nausea and vomiting, 12.5 mg via intravenous injection or infusion.
- Granisetron hydrochloride. Intravenous single administration (3 mg), maximum daily dose of 9 mg (adults). Orally up to 2 mg daily. Children: intravenous administration 10 to 40 µg/kg body weight, maximum of 3 mg daily.

SUMMARY

Around 10% of the total amount of serotonin is found in the CNS, and fundamental processes are driven and modulated by this neurotransmitter including mood, perception, cognition, and behaviour. Distinct, and sometimes only slight, chemical modifications of structural templates lead to a vast area of interaction with serotonergic neurotransmission, resulting in the development of pharmacologically diverse entities. In this chapter, the emphasis has been placed on antidepressants, hallucinogens and designer drugs, antimigraines, anxiolytics, antipsychotics and antiemetics.

Tricyclic antidepressants (TCAs) are represented by a central, seven-membered, non-aromatic ring that is flanked by two benzene rings where the dihedral angle (α) between the two benzene rings can impact on the extend of antidepressant activity. Several isosteric modifications retain antidepressant activity. Secondary amines appear to show higher selectivity for the noradrenaline reuptake transporter (NAT). Their tertiary counterparts tend to display a somewhat higher selectivity for the serotonin reuptake transport protein (SERT) while others are less selective (mixed SERT/NAT).

The first available monoamine oxidase inhibitors (MAOIs) had non-selective and irreversible properties. Apart from tranylcypromine, a number of developed MAOIs were hydrazine derivatives which included phenelzine and isocarboxazid. MAO-A and -B are pharmacologically distinguishable by their differential sensitivities towards clorgyline and selegiline. Introduction of reversible MAO-A inhibitors resulted in significantly improved safety during antidepressant therapy, particularly after introduction of the benzamide derivative called moclobemide.

Selective serotonin reuptake inhibitors (SSRIs) have become the tool for first-line therapy of depression. Among the most commonly used derivatives, a number of similar factors are shared such as pharmacophores, topological motifs and shapes, often referred to be the product of 'scaffold-hopping'. A number of SSRIs contain chiral centres which form the basis of enantioselective increase in potencies exemplified, for example, by the (*S*)-enantiomer of citalopram. Monoamine reuptake selectivities can sometimes be shifted by introducing minor structural modifications. For example, removal of the trifluoromethyl group on the *para* position of the phenoxy ring of fluoxetine and attachment of a methoxy group to the *ortho* position resulted in the discovery of nisoxetine, an effective NAT inhibitor (NARI). Another example of a dual SSRI/NARI is venlafaxine, an *N,N*-dimethylated and *para*-methoxy-phenylethylamine derivative, substituted with cyclohexanol at the β-position.

Hallucinogenic compounds can induce altered states of consciousness in humans, which means that they are characterised by their powerful impact on perception, mood and cognition. The structural backbone of the so-called 'classical' hallucinogens are represented by mescaline, *N,N*-dimethyltryptamine and lysergic acid diethylamide (LSD). The mescaline-type template is based on the 3,4,5-trimethoxyphenylethylamine structure. Another arrangement follows the 2,4,5-trisubstitution pattern which gives rise to the so-called 2C-X and 2C-T-X series where X refers to a large variety of alkyl, alkylthio and halogen substituents at the 4 position. Positions 2 and 5 are often occupied by methoxyl groups. The hallucinogenic amfetamines differ from their stimulant counterparts also by the presence of a similar 2,4,5-trisubstitution pattern. Attachment of a 3,4-methylenedioxy component to the methamfetamine structure gives MDMA (*ecstasy*), a derivative classified as an entactogen. Tryptamines are serotonin derivatives where psychoactivity is greatly affected by substitution on the indole ring, the side chain carbons and by alkylation of the side chain nitrogen. Lysergic acid diethylamide (LSD) is one of the most potent hallucinogens currently known. The active isomer carries the (5*R*,8*R*)-configuration and is called *d*-LSD. Epimerisation to the (5*R*,8*S*)-derivative gives the inactive iso-LSD. Several compounds alkylated at N(6) appear to result in derivatives with slightly higher potencies.

The triptan series refers to a class of drugs which act as selective 5-HT$_{1D/1B}$ receptor agonists and is used for the acute treatment of migraine attacks. Interestingly, a number of these compounds can be viewed as 5-substituted derivatives of the hallucinogenic N,N-dimethyltryptamine and examples include sumatriptan, zolmitriptan and rizatriptan.

A characteristic feature of azapirone-type anxiolytics is the presence of a pyrimidylpiperazine motif where a pyrimidine is connected to the N_1 of piperazine. The N_4 is attached to a tetramethylene spacer that can be connected to a variety of imide-type structures.

Buspirone, for example, is a 3,3-tetramethyleneglutarimide-containing analogue and acts as a 5-HT_{1A} agonist. On the other hand, SERT blockage + 5-HT_{1A} antagonism, ideally combined in one molecule, may show potential for the acceleration of antidepressant effects under SSRI treatment.

The phenylpiperazine motif is also a feature of several 5-HT_{2A} receptor antagonists such as nefazodone and trazodone. The phenyl ring carries a chlorine atom at the *meta*-position and the N_4 spacer is formed by a trimethylene chain, attached to a triazolone moiety. A potent and highly selective 5-HT_{2A} receptor antagonist used for pharmacological studies is M100907, which is based on a piperidine ring flanked by a dimethoxylated benzene and a *para*-fluoro-substituted phenylethyl nucleus. One of the most convincing arguments for the involvement of 5-HT_{2A} receptors in the hallucinogenic activity of psilocybin was provided when pre-administration of the 5-HT_{2A} receptor antagonist ketanserin abolished hallucinogenic effects in humans.

A number of so-called atypical antipsychotics, such as sertindole and aripiprazole, belong to the arylpiperidine and arylpiperazine group whereas derivatives such as clozapine and olanzapine share the dibenzodiazepine template.

Several 5-HT_3 receptor antagonists are used as drugs with antiemetic properties. Ondansetron represented the first marketed drug that is based on an imidazolyl tetrahydrocarbazolone motif. The carbonyl function appeared to be important in order to retain potency. Indole-3-carboxylates (e.g. tropisetron and dolasetron) or indazole-3-carboxamide derivatives (e.g. granisetron) are also available for the inhibition of this receptor subtype.

Q Self Test 18.4

Psilocybin is a major constituent of 'magic mushrooms'. What heterocycle is present in its structure?

A. Pyridine
B. Piperidine
C. Indole
D. Aziridine
E. Pyrrolidine

Q Self Test 18.5

Select the CORRECT statement regarding psilocybin:

A. The ring nitrogen is basic.
B. The ring nitrogen is neutral because its lone pair of electrons is part of the 10 π aromatic system.
C. The lone pair of electrons on the ring nitrogen is in an sp^2 hybridised orbital.
D. The side chain amine group will be neutral at pH 7.4.
E. The phosphoric acid group will be neutral at pH 7.4.

Q Self Test 18.6

Exposure of serotonin to monoamine oxidase A leads to oxidative deamination and formation of ammonia as a by-product. After consideration of the side chain substitution pattern of noradrenaline, which amine could be expected to form after conversion by this enzyme?

Q Self Test 18.7

The functional groups present in LSD are:

A. Amide and amine
B. Ester and amide
C. Amine and carboxylic acid
D. Amine and ester
E. Imine and carboxylic acid

Q Self Test 18.8

How many stereoisomers exist for the tricyclic antidepressant amitriptyline?

A. 0
B. 1
C. 2
D. 3
E. 4

Q Self Test 18.9

Select the INCORRECT statement regarding the bonding capability of the antipsychotic medicine risperidone (in the ionisation form drawn).

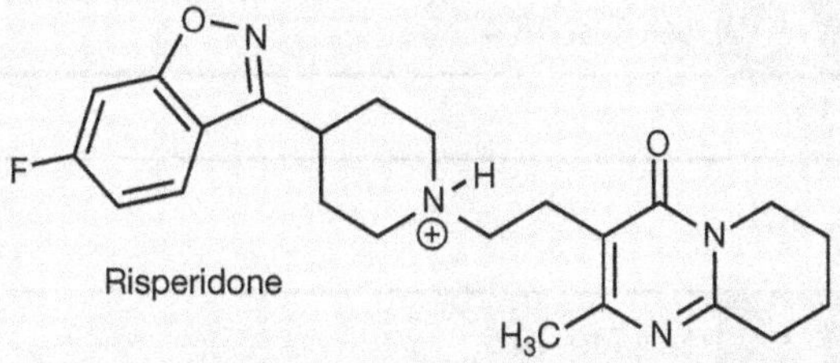

A. Risperidone has 1 hydrogen bond donor.
B. Risperidone has 6 hydrogen bond acceptors.
C. Risperidone could form an ionic bond with its receptor.
D. Risperidone could form a charge transfer (CT) complex with its receptor.
E. Risperidone has a good leaving group.

Q Self Test 18.10

Consider the structural presentations of compounds (1)–(3) shown below.
(a) Which compound would you expect to act as a stimulant, hallucinogen and entactogen?
(b) Which stereoisomer, (*R*) or (*S*), would you expect to show higher potencies?

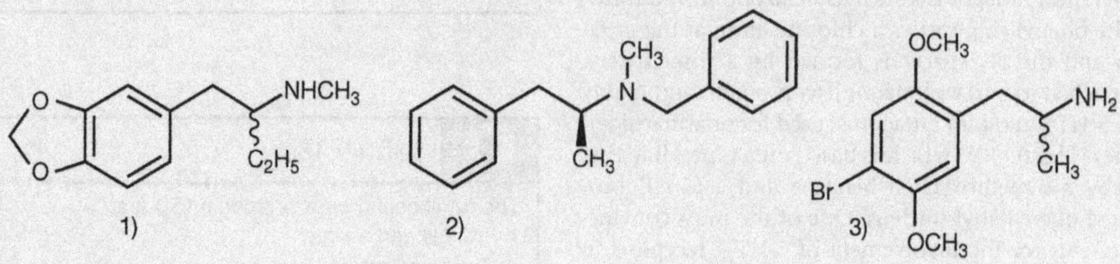

1) 2) 3)

A Self Test 18.1

A

A Self Test 18.2

B

A Self Test 18.3

E

A Self Test 18.4

C

A Self Test 18.5

C

A Self Test 18.6

N-Methylamine

A Self Test 18.7

A

A Self Test 18.8

A

A Self Test 18.9

E

A Self Test 18.10

(a) 1) Entactogen; 2) Stimulant; 3) Hallucinogen.
(b) 1) (*S*)-enantiomer; 2) (*S*)-enantiomer; 3) (*R*)-enantiomer

GENERAL READING

Abraham DJ, ed. *Burger's Medicinal Chemistry and Drug Discovery*. Vol. 6. Hoboken, USA: Nervous System Agents, John Wiley & Sons, Inc.; 2003.

Barnes NM, Sharp T. A review of central 5-HT receptors and their function. *Neuropharmacology*. 1999;38:1083–1152.

Bolasco A, Fioravanti R, Carradori S. Recent development of monoamine oxidase inhibitors. *Expert Opinion on Therapeutic Patents*. 2005;15:1763–1782.

Buschmann H, Holenz J, Párraga A, Torrens A, Vela JM, Díaz JL, eds. *Antidepressants, Antipsychotics, Anxiolytics: From Chemistry and Pharmacology to Clinical Application*. Weinheim, Germany: WILEY-VCH Verlag GmbH & Co. KGaA; 2007.

Carroll FI, Howard JL, Howell LL, Fox BS, Kuhar MJ. Development of the dopamine transporter selective RTI-336 as a pharmacotherapy for cocaine abuse. *AAPS J*. 2006;8:E196–E203.

Foley KF, Cozzi NV. Novel aminopropiophenones as potential antidepressants. *Drug Development Research*. 2003; 60: 252–260.

Howell LL, Kimmel HL. Monoamine transporters and psychostimulant addiction. *Biochem Pharmacol*. 2008; 75:196–217.

Hoyer D, Hannon JP, Martin GR. Molecular, pharmacological and functional diversity of 5-HT receptors. *Pharmacol Biochem Behav*. 2002;71:533–554.

Huang Y, Williams WA. Enhanced selective serotonin re-uptake inhibitors as antidepressants: 2004–2006. *Expert Opinion on Therapeutic Patents*. 2007; 17:889–907.

Jacobson KA, Gao ZG. Adenosine receptors as therapeutic targets. *Nat Rev Drug Discov*. 2006;5:247–264.

Kim DI, Deutsch HM, Ye XC, Schweri MM. Synthesis and pharmacology of site-specific cocaine abuse treatment agents: Restricted rotation analogues of methylphenidate. *J Med Chem*. 2007;50:2718–2731.

Nichols DE. Hallucinogens. *Pharmacol Ther*. 2004;101:131–181.

Rothman RB, Vu N, Partilla JS, et al. In vitro characterization of ephedrine-related stereoisomers at biogenic amine transporters and the receptorome reveals selective actions as norepinephrine transporter substrates. *J Pharmacol Exp Ther*. 2003;307:138–145.

Shulgin AT, Shulgin A. *PIHKAL*. Berkeley: Transform Press; 1991.

Shulgin AT, Shulgin A. *TIHKAL: The Continuation*. Berkeley, USA: Transform Press; 1997.

Tipton KF, Boyce S, O'Sullivan J, Davey GP, Healy J. Monoamine oxidases: Certainties and uncertainties. *Curr Med Chem*. 2004;11:1965–1982.

Youdim MBH, Bakhle YS. Monoamine oxidase: isoforms and inhibitors in Parkinson's disease and depressive illness. *Br J Pharmacol*. 2006;147:S287–S296.

Youdim MBH, Buccafusco JJ. Multi-functional drugs for various CNS targets in the treatment of neurodegenerative disorders. *Trends Pharmacol Sci*. 2005;26:27–35.

Youdim MBH, Edmondson D, Tipton KF. The therapeutic potential of monoamine oxidase inhibitors. *Nat Rev Neurosci*. 2006;7:295–309.

Chapter | 19 |

Drugs affecting haemostasis and thrombosis

David G Watson

CHAPTER CONTENTS

INTRODUCTION

SUMMARY OF PHARMACOLOGY

Haemostasis occurs in order to arrest the loss of blood from damaged blood vessels. In order to arrest bleeding a clot is formed, which is the end result of a cascade of events which involves a series of proteins in the blood including factors VII, VIIa, X, Xa, prothrombin and thrombin. The end result of the cascade is that the soluble protein fibrinogen is converted to the insoluble protein fibrin. The fibrin forms strands which encase various blood cells such as platelets and erythrocytes in a mesh forming a physical plug.

Thrombosis occurs when an unwanted clot is formed as a result of certain predisposing factors such as: injury to a blood vessel wall, altered blood flow (e.g. sitting for long periods on a journey), as a result of cardiac arrhythmias, altered blood coagulability which may be caused by pregnancy, oral contraceptives or may be inherited and due to arterial disease such as atherosclerosis. When such clots form they may travel to the heart, lungs or brain, rapidly causing damage and then death.

Treatment to promote haemostasis is rare but may be required when there is a congenital deficiency in a clotting factor such as in haemophilia, when it is difficult to staunch bleeding such as after surgery, and where there is vitamin K deficiency such as in neonates. In contrast, prevention and treatment of thrombosis is very common.

HAEMOSTATIC DRUGS

As fibrin is formed during the clotting cascade the fibrinolytic enzyme plasmin is formed in tandem and breaks down fibrin. Thus, if clot formation is defective, it is necessary to inhibit the action of plasmin. The amino acid lysine (Fig. 19.1) was observed to have antifibrinolytic activity and ϵ-aminocaproic acid (Fig. 19.1) was found to have even greater activity. Screening of analogues of ε-aminocaproic acid resulted in the discovery of tranexamic acid (Fig. 19.1), which is a potent inhibitor of the conversion of plasminogen into plasmin.

Plasmin is responsible for the breakdown of fibrin and is formed from plasminogen via the action of tissue plasminogen activating factor (TPA) which is a serine protease. TPA forms plasmin by cleaving plasminogen at the C-terminus side of a lysine residue. In common with all

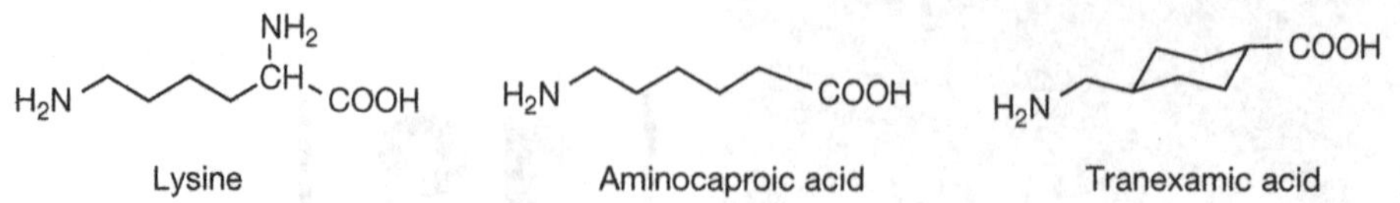

RPDFCLEPPYTGPCKARIIRYFYNAKAGLCQTFVYGGCRAKRNNFKSAEDCMRTCGGA
Aprotinin

Figure 19.1 Haemostatic drugs.

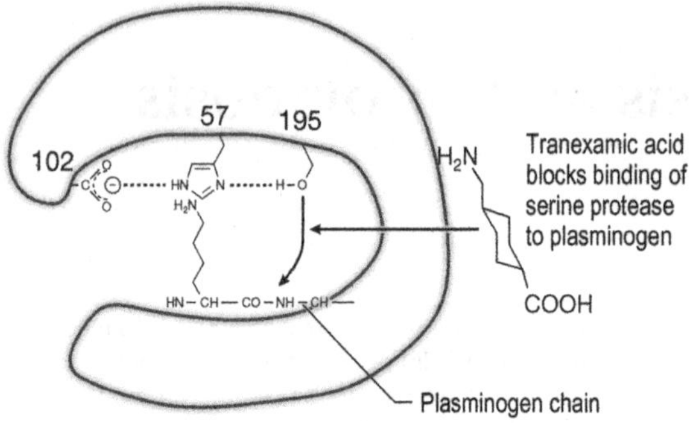

Figure 19.2 The active site of tissue plasminogen activating factor.

serine proteases, its mode of action is based on three key amino acid residues: glutamate 102, histidine 57 and serine 195 (Fig. 19.2). The serine is responsible for cleaving plasminogen next to a lysine residue; thus it is not surprising that lysine itself acts as a weak inhibitor of the enzyme. Tranexamic acid is structurally similar to lysine but obviously binds to the active site of the enzyme more tightly than lysine, and thus inhibits its ability to cleave plasminogen. It is only the trans-substituted isomer that is active as a haemostatic agent. The naturally occurring trypsin inhibitor aprotinin is also used as a haemostatic agent. It is a 58 amino acid protein and the commercial product is extracted from bovine pancreas. The inhibitory binding site of the protein is located around the lysine-alanine-arginine sequence outlined in red in Figure 19.1. There have been, as with many extracted proteins, concerns over contamination of aprotinin by other proteins such as prions.

INHIBITION OF THROMBOSIS

Oral anticoagulants

Coumarins are very common natural products and occur in a wide range of plant materials. The lead compound in the discovery of warfarin was dicoumarol (Fig. 19.3), which was isolated from mouldy hay. Warfarin was found to be more potent and have a quicker effect than dicoumarol and replaced it. Initially it was used as a rat poison but its usefulness as an anticoagulant was eventually realised. Warfarin is used in the form of its sodium salt in order to improve its water solubility. It takes about 72 hours to take effect since the body stores vitamin K, a lipophilic vitamin, efficiently and it takes time to deplete the reserves of the vitamin. Warfarin is the drug of choice as an anticoagulant but acenocoumarol and phenindione are sometimes used. The mechanism of action of warfarin is via interference with vitamin K recycling after vitamin K has acted as a co-factor in post-translational carboxylation of the various proteins involved in the clotting cascade (see Ch. 26). It acts as an inhibitor of vitamin K reductase which converts vitamin K epoxide back to vitamin K hydroquinone, which is the co-factor involved in post-translational carboxylation of glutamate. Within the reductase enzyme cysteine groups are responsible for carrying out the reduction of the intermediates in the vitamin K cycle. The exact mechanism by which warfarin inhibits the cycle is not known but its structure suggests that it may mimic transition states in the vitamin K cycle from vitamin K epoxide, the by-product of glutamate carboxylation, back to vitamin K hydroquinone, the co-factor utilised in glutamate carboxylation. It is very close in structure to possible intermediates in the conversion of both vitamin K epoxide to vitamin K quinone and then vitamin K hydroquinone (Fig. 19.4). Substrates are very tightly bound to enzymes in their transition state and transition state analogues bind in the same way but are unable to undergo the next step in the enzymatic transformation and are thus not released by the enzyme as the natural substrate would be. The list of drugs which interact either to reinforce the action of warfarin or to reduce its action is quite long. Drugs such as aspirin and other non-steroidal anti-inflammatory drugs increase the risk of bleeding if given during warfarin therapy. There is also concern that herbal remedies may contain coumarins which could interact with warfarin therapy. However, in order to be active, coumarins have to have a hydroxyl group in the 4 position as in the warfarin structure, and such coumarins are rarely if ever reported in properly stored plant materials. Since it is essential to hit the correct therapeutic window, i.e. not to over or under dose, warfarin levels have to be monitored frequently in the early days of treatment.

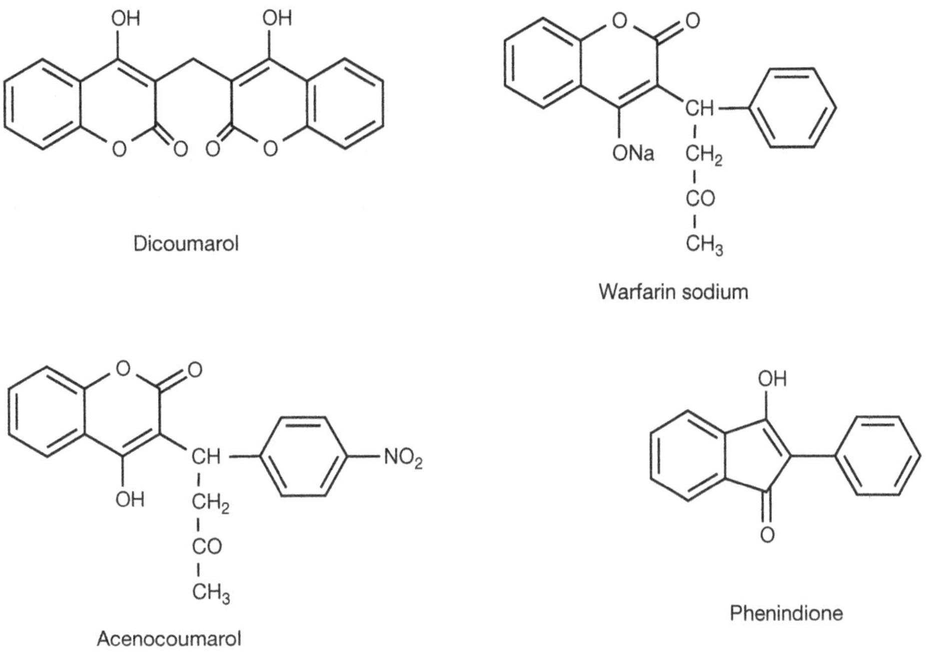

Figure 19.3 Oral anticoagulants.

Injectable antithrombotic agents

Heparin

Heparin was originally isolated from dog liver by aqueous extraction. The current commercial sources of heparin are mucosal tissues from animals such as cow lung or pig intestine. For this reason it is classed as a mucopolysaccharide. It is an extensively sulphated aminopolysaccharide having an average molecular weight (MW) of around 17 000. The structure shown in Figure 19.5 consists mainly of alternating glucuronic acid with some iduronic acid groups and 2-amino-2-deoxy glucose units which are 1-4 linked with occasional 1,6-chain branching. The polysaccharide chain is both *N*- and *O*-sulphated with the sulphate ester content being approximately 5.2 groups per tetrasaccharide unit. Heparin is in the form of its sodium salt and is highly water soluble. The sulphamate groups are very readily hydrolysed (Fig. 19.5), while sulphate groups are stable to stronger acidic conditions. Hydrolysis of the ester groups has been known to occur in intravenous infusions containing dextrose since acid compounds can be formed from dextrose upon autoclaving. The presence of the sulphate ester groups is required for activity. Figure 19.5 shows a pentasaccharide portion of the heparin polymer (fondaparinux-Enoxaparin) which was co-crystallised with antithrombin (AT) and was shown to interact with specific lysine and arginine groups of antithrombin. Each basic amino acid residue interacts with several of the sulphate and sulphamate groups. The binding of the pentasaccharide to AT changes its conformation and activates it towards inhibition of factor Xa. Factor Xa is also involved in the clotting cascade and thus low MW heparins are effective anticoagulants but do not promote the binding of AT to thrombin. The low MW heparins are more specific and thus have fewer side effects than heparin.

Heparin binds both to thrombin and AT at the same time and the basis of its action is this dual binding mechanism. The portion of heparin binding to thrombin is 5–6 residues in length and the interactions with the protein are similar to those shown for AT. It has been shown that the minimum length of sulphated polysaccharide required for binding to both AT and thrombin, and thus for thrombin inhibition, is seventeen residues.

Heparin and its low MW analogues are all poorly absorbed and unstable in the gut and have to be given by intravenous infusion or by subcutaneous injection.

In patients who are intolerant to heparin, a mixture of heparin, dermatant sulphate and chondroitin sulphate (Danaparoid sodium) may be used as an anticoagulant. The antithrombotic activity of other sulphated polysaccharides is well known. Recently (2008) there was some concern about contamination of heparin with oversulphated chrondroitin sulphate, which is believed to have led to a number of deaths in the USA. Simple analytical methods are not adequate for the quality control of

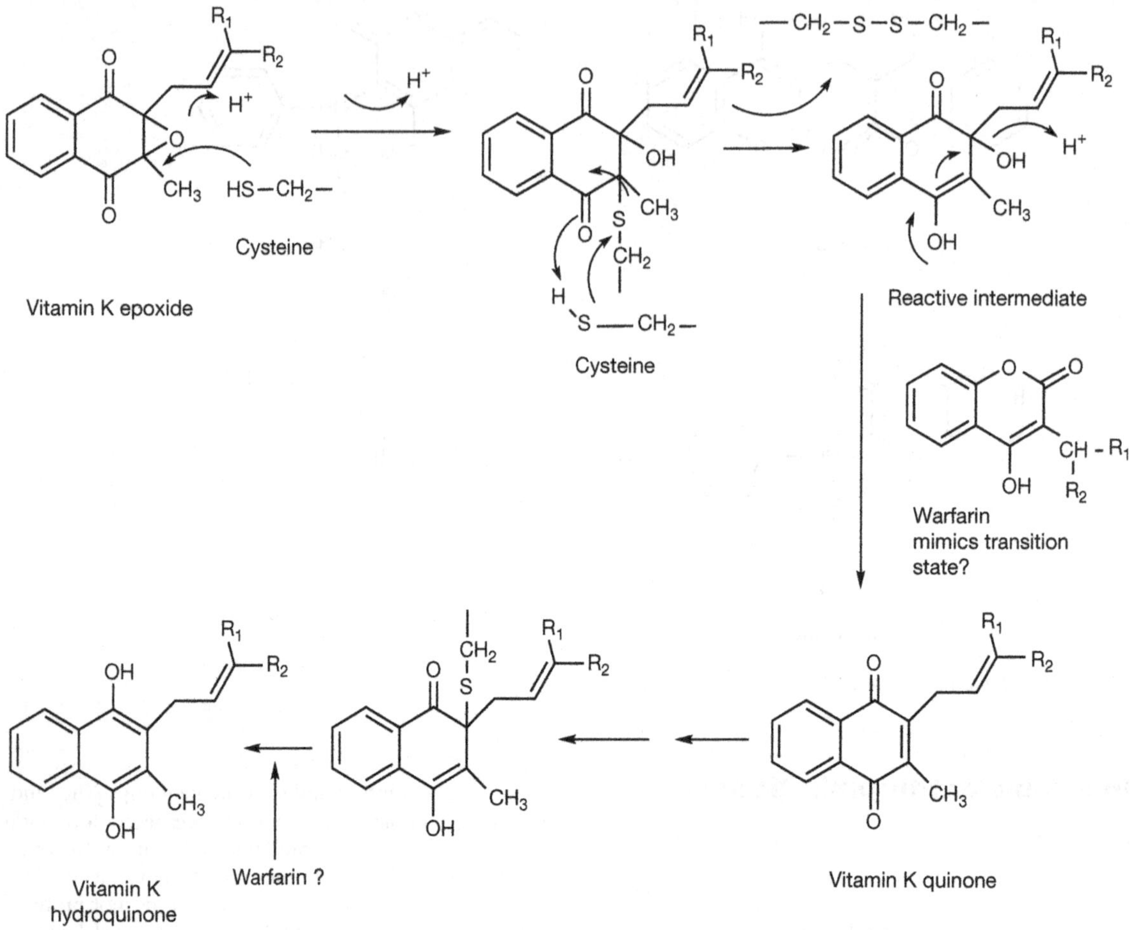

Figure 19.4 Vitamin K recycling with warfarin as a possible transition state mimic.

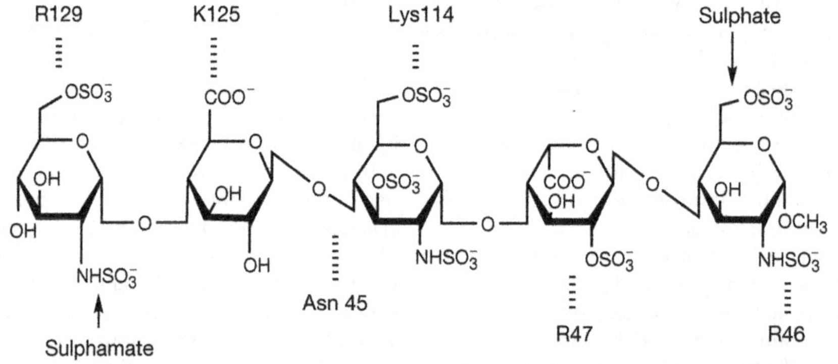

Figure 19.5 Interaction between basic residues in the structure of antithrombin and a heparin pentasaccharide.

complex substances such as heparin and thus the contamination was overlooked. More specific tests have now been introduced.

Protamine

A major hazard of heparin administration is haemorrhage, and heparin's action can be counteracted by injection of protamine. Protamines are arginine-rich proteins which are involved in DNA stabilisation during spermatogenesis. They are also used in certain formulations of insulin. The pharmaceutical material is derived from herring or salmon sperm or roe. Since these proteins are strongly basic and carry a net positive charge at physiological pH they effectively bind to the negatively charged groups of heparin and its low MW analogues, neutralising their antithrombotic activity.

Anticoagulants not exerting their effects via antithrombin

Hirudin is produced by the medicinal leech and may be extracted from its saliva. It is a 65 amino acid peptide. It is now expressed recombinantly in yeast cells and the recombinant product is almost identical to the naturally occurring protein. It acts directly on thrombin, binding to the active site of thrombin, and preventing the enzymatic cleavage of fibrinogen. It will bind both to free thrombin and to thrombin involved in complexes with fibrinogen. It has the advantage that it does not have the same side effect profile as heparin and thus can be used in heparin-intolerant patients. Bivalirudin is low MW (2180) synthetic peptide which mimics hirudin and binds to thrombin at the same site.

ANTIPLATELET DRUGS

Platelets are irregularly shaped blood cells which have an important role in the clotting mechanism. They release a number of different peptide growth factors including transforming growth factor and platelet derived growth factor and exert control over clot formation and tissue repair. A number of agents have been found to stimulate platelet aggregation including adenosine diphosphate (ADP), von Willebrand factor and collagen. If the levels of platelets are too high in the blood, clot formation is more likely to occur, and if the levels are too low bleeding is likely to occur. Antiplatelet drugs are directed at reducing the effects of platelets with regard to clot formation. A number of different drugs are used together without there being a common mechanism of action.

Aspirin

Aspirin has a direct effect on platelet aggregation through inhibiting the release of ADP by platelets. ADP plays a key role in promoting platelet shape change, which leads to their aggregation. Salicylic acid where the acetyl group of aspirin has been removed does not prevent platelet aggregation. It was eventually found that the basis of the action of aspirin was via the inhibition of cyclooxgenase-1 (COX-1) via acetylation of a serine residue in the protein, thus preventing the binding of arachidonic acid which is the precursor for the biosynthesis of thromboxane A_2 (see Chs 2 and 5), which is one of the principal promoters of platelet aggregation. The inhibition of COX-1 is irreversible and since platelets do not have a nucleus and hence cannot produce RNA for translation into protein. Thus the COX-1 present in the platelets cannot be replaced and knocking it out in the platelets produces long-term inhibition of platelet aggregation since the lifetime of platelets in the blood stream is 7–11 days. The obvious side effect is impaired clotting.

Clopidogrel

Clopidogrel undergoes metabolic activation to a reactive thiol (Fig. 19.6). The thiol reacts with a cysteine residue in P2Y12 protein in platelets, preventing its oligimerisation with other P2Y12 proteins which normally results in the formation of stable P2Y12 receptor complexes within a lipid raft. The P2Y12 receptor is responsible for binding ADP which is an important signalling molecule for platelet aggregation. Thus ADP activation of platelets is reduced.

Dipyridamole

Dipyridamole (Fig. 19.7) is an inhibitor of phosphodiesterase, which is responsible for the breakdown of cyclic AMP. Inhibition of cAMP breakdown in some way inhibits the effect of ADP binding to platelets. In addition. dipyridamole inhibits the breakdown of adenosine to adenine; thus the drug raises extracellular levels of adenosine. Adenosine is an inhibitor of platelet aggregation.

Glycoprotein IIb/IIIa antagonists

Glycoprotein (GP) IIb/IIIa receptors on the surface of platelets are important in the platelet aggregation process. These surface proteins are responsible for binding to fibrinogen, von Willebrand factor and fibronectin. Fibrinogen binding to the activated GP receptors is the final event in the clotting cascade and thus inhibitors of this process inhibit clotting in a very direct manner, whereas other antiplatelet agents only block a component in the process. These agents have become an important component in

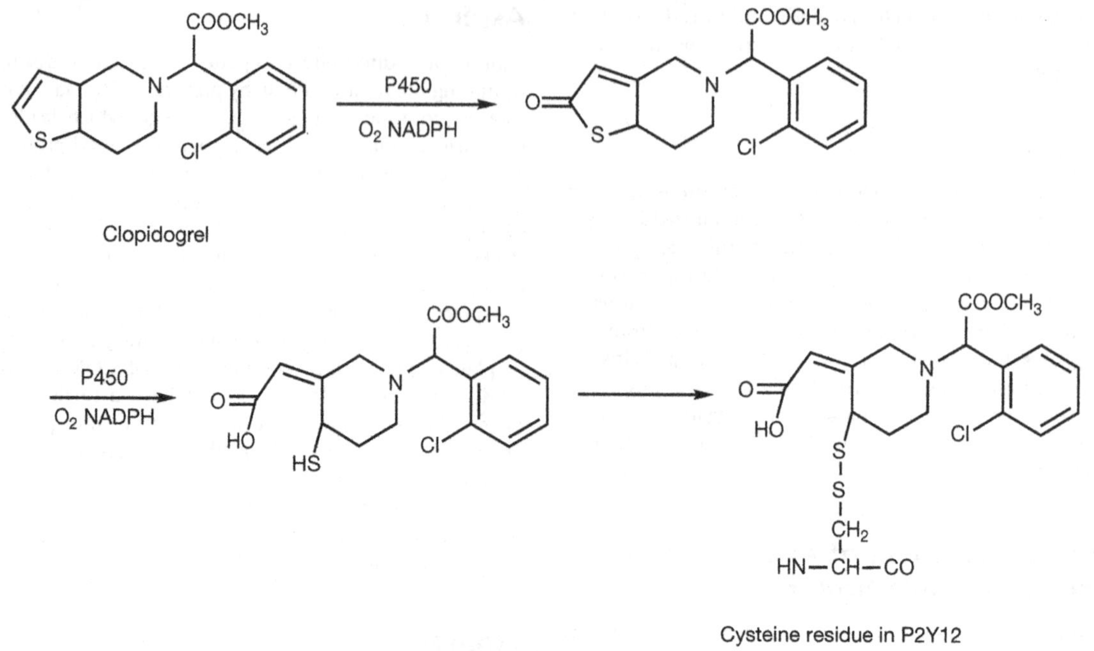

Figure 19.6 Metabolic activation of clopidogrel and its reaction with the P2Y12 protein.

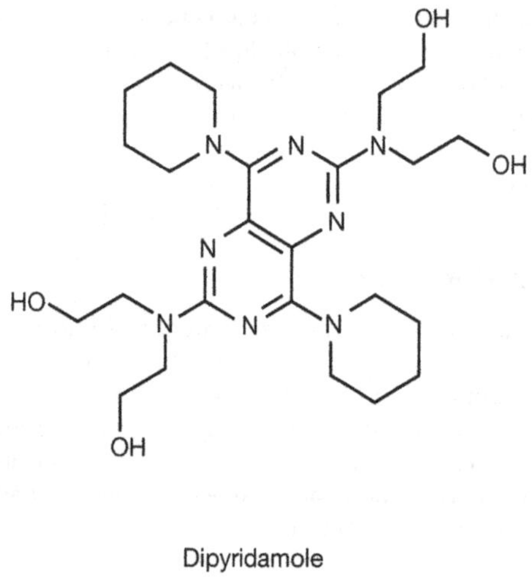

Figure 19.7 Dipyridamole.

percutaneous coronary interventions (PCI) which include angioplasty, insertion of stents and laser arterectomy. PCIs can result in tissue damage which can provoke restenosis and consequent increased risk of myocardial infarction. There are three drugs used as GP IIb/IIIa antagonists: tirofiban, eptifibatide (Fig. 19.8) and abciximab. Tirofiban (Fig. 19.8) is a peptomimetic drug. The recognition site in GP IIb/IIIa recognises a key amino acid sequence arginine-glycine-asparate (RGD) which enables it to bind to fibrinogen and thus promote platelet adhesion. Tirofiban mimics this sequence, binding to GP IIb/IIIa and thus blocking the binding of fibrinogen. Eptifibatide (Fig. 19.8) is a cyclic peptide which occurs naturally in snake venom and actually contains the RGD sequence. Abciximab is a Fab fragment (see Ch. 27) of a monoclonal antibody which is active against GP IIb/IIIa and thus blocks fibrinogen binding to this receptor. It is produced by transformed mammalian cell cultures. It also has some cross-reactivity against vitronectin receptors found on endothelial cells and b3 integrins found on leucocytes. Thus it exhibits additional anti-inflammatory effects. It may also have some activity against GP1b receptors, thus reducing the binding of von Willebrand factor and hence thrombin generation. Although abciximab only has a plasma half-life of 10 minutes, it reduces platelet aggregation for up to *ca.* 48 hours since it remains bound to platelets until they are removed from the circulation by senescence.

FIBRINOLYTIC DRUGS

Fibrinolytic drugs are all proteins which act to promote the formation of plasmin, which is the enzyme in the body responsible for breaking down fibrin, the protein

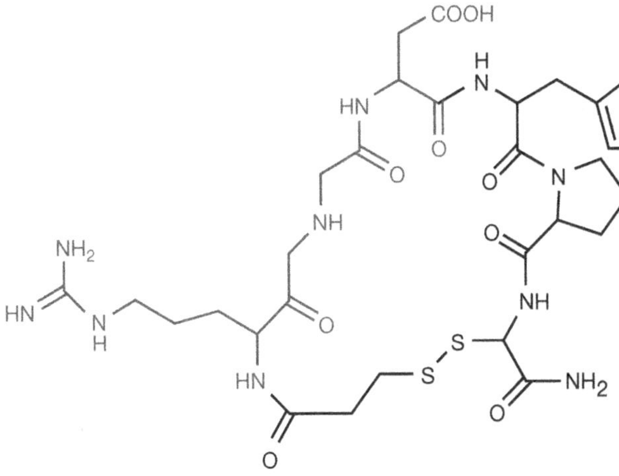

Eptifibatide

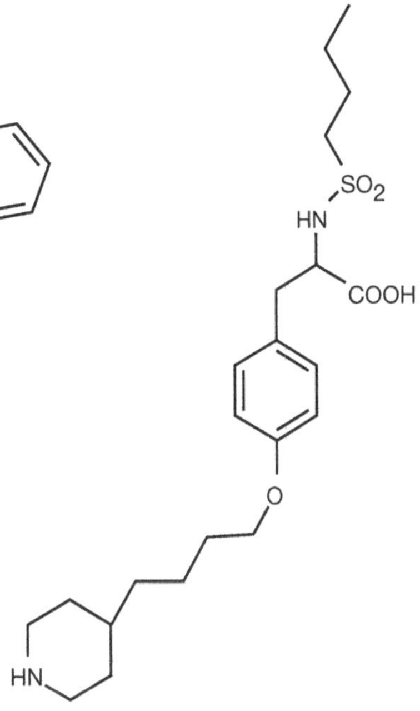

Tirofiban

Figure 19.8 Glycoprotein IIb/IIIa antagonists.

Serine protease

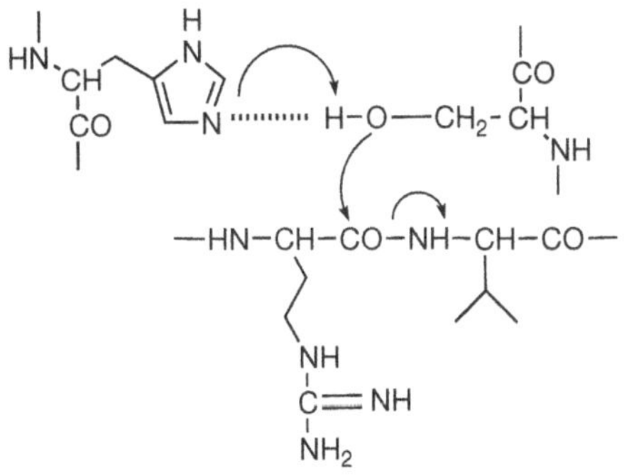

Plasminogen

Figure 19.9 Conversion of plasminogen into plasmin via the action of serine protease.

which binds together platelets to form a clot. Plasmin circulates in the body as the inactive protein plasminogen and is naturally activated in the body via the serine protease tissue plasminogen activating factor (TPA) to become active in clot digestion. TPA cleaves the plasminogen between an arginine and a valine residue (Fig. 19.9) to release the active form of the enzyme plasmin. Plasmin itself is also a serine protease. Thus recombinant TPA (see Ch. 27) can be infused into the body to dissolve clots. The glycosylation pattern of TPA governs its half-life in the body, and Reteplase® is a longer-acting version of the drug with a modified glycosylation pattern. Streptokinase is a bacterial protein and thus has the potential to cause allergic reactions and cannot be administered frequently. Unlike TPA, it is not an enzyme and activates plasminogen by binding to it and changing its conformation so that its active, serine protease, site becomes exposed and it can self-catalyse its conversion into plasmin. Urokinase is produced by cultures of human kidney cells and acts directly on plasminogen, converting it into plasmin. Its use in treating myocardial infarction is less well established than other agents.

PREPARATIONS OF HAEMOSTATIC AND THROMBOLYTIC DRUGS

- Tranexamic acid: tablets 500 mg and injection 100 mg/mL.
- Wafarin sodium: tablets 0.5, 1, 3 and 5 mg.
- Acenocoumarol: tablets 1 mg.
- Phenindione: tablets 10, 25 and 50 mg.
- Aspirin: tablets and dispersible tablets 75 mg.

- Clopidogrel: 75 mg tablets clopidogrel hydrogen sulphate.
- Heparin sodium or calcium: injection 1000, 5000 and 25 000 units/mL.
- Low molecular weight heparins: a range of injections between 6000 and 40 000 units/mL.
- Hirudins: bivalirudin 250 mg injection, lepirudin 50 mg injection.
- Protamine sulphate: injection 10 mg/mL.
- Abciximab: 2 mg/mL injection.
- Eptifibatide: 0.75 mg/mL infusion and 2 mg/mL injection.
- Tirofiban: 50 μg/mL infusion.
- Dipyridamole: 25, 100 and 200 mg tablets, 5 mg/mL injection.
- Alteplase: 10, 20 and 50 mg per vial for injection or intravenous infusion.
- Reteplase: 10 units per vial injection.
- Streptokinase: doses 100 000–1.5 million units per vial for injection.

ADDITIONAL READING

Davis CH, Deerfield D, Wymore T, Stafford DW, Pedersen LG. A quantum chemical study of the mechanism of action of vitamin K epoxide reductase (VKOR) II. Transition states. *J Mol Graph Model*. 2007;26:401–408.

Miner J, Hoffhines A. The discovery of aspirin's antithrombotic effects. *Tex Heart Inst J*. 2007;34:179–186.

Dansette PM, Libraire J, Bertho G, Mansuy D. Metabolic oxidative cleavage of thioesters: evidence for the formation of sulfenic acid intermediates in the bioactivation of the antithrombotic prodrugs ticlopidine and clopidogrel. *Chem Res Toxicol*. 2009;22:369–373.

Savi P, Zachayus J-L, Delesque-Touchard N, Labouret C, Hervé C. The active metabolite of clopidogrel disrupts P2Y12 receptor oligomers and partitions them out of lipid rafts. *PNAS*. 2006;103:11069–11074.

Johnson DJD, Li W, Adams TE, Huntington JA. Antithrombin–S195A factor Xa-heparin structure reveals the allosteric mechanism of antithrombin activation. *EMBO J*. 2006;25:2029–2037.

Carter WJ, Cama E, Huntington JA. Crystal Structure of thrombin bound to heparin. *J Biol Chem*. 2005;280:745–2749.

Mandava P, Thiagarajan P, Kent TA. Glycoprotein IIb/IIIa antagonists in acute ischaemic stroke current status and future directions. *Drugs*. 2008;68:1019–1028.

Chapter | 20 |

Drugs affecting the endocrine system

Jeffrey Stuart Millership

CHAPTER CONTENTS

INTRODUCTION

The endocrine system is a series of glands within the body including the hypothalamus, the pituitary, the thyroid, the parathyroids, the adrenal glands, the pineal gland, the pancreas and the reproductive glands (e.g. ovaries and testes) that controls many functions of the operation of the body. The endocrine system works alongside the nervous system to control many of the body's basic functions such as growth and development, homeostasis, energy levels, etc. The location of the glands within the body is depicted in Figure 20.1.

These glands are responsible for the production of hormones, which control many functions of the human system as indicated above. Hormones may be classified into three groups based loosely on their chemical structure:

- steroid hormones, e.g. corticosteroids, sex hormones
- amino acid-based hormones, e.g. thyroxine
- peptide hormones, e.g. insulin.

Under normal circumstances the body will control the levels of hormones by positive and negative feedback systems, although negative feedback is most common in the endocrine system and this can be exemplified by the thyroid hormones. The regulation of the secretion of the thyroid hormones (thyroxine, triiodothyronine) is controlled by the hypothalamic–pituitary axis. When there is a need for synthesis of thyroxine or triiodothyronine the hypothalamus secretes thyroid releasing hormone (TRH), which results in the pituitary gland secreting thyroid stimulating hormone (TSH), causing the pituitary gland to synthesise the thyroid hormones. These hormones are then transported in the bloodstream to their required sites of action. The hormones may be free or bound to transport proteins (e.g. thyroxine-binding globulin), and it is only the free form which is active. When the levels of these hormones approach the required levels once again, the negative feedback system switches on and causes the secretion of TRH to be switched off. Another feedback mechanism involving the endocrine system is associated with insulin production. Following the ingestion of food there will be an increase in the blood sugar levels. Within the endocrine system the pancreas responds to this by producing the hormone insulin. The insulin aids in the uptake of glucose into cells, thereby reducing the blood sugar levels. Once the blood sugar levels drop, the pancreas stops producing insulin.

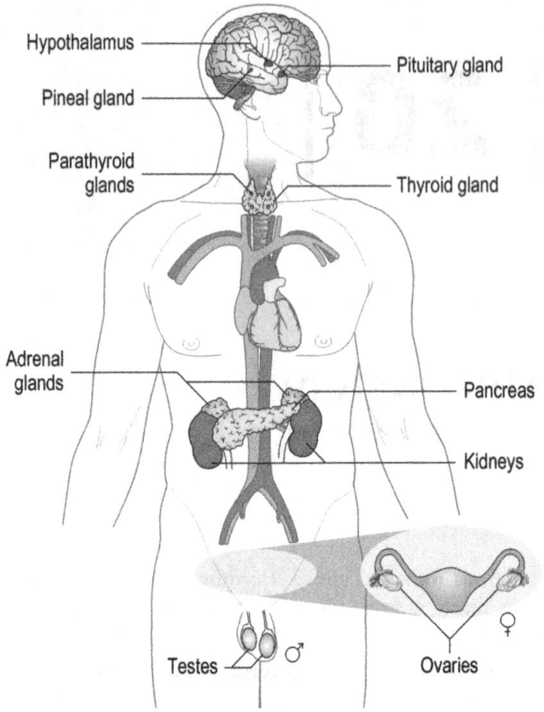

Figure 20.1 The endocrine system.

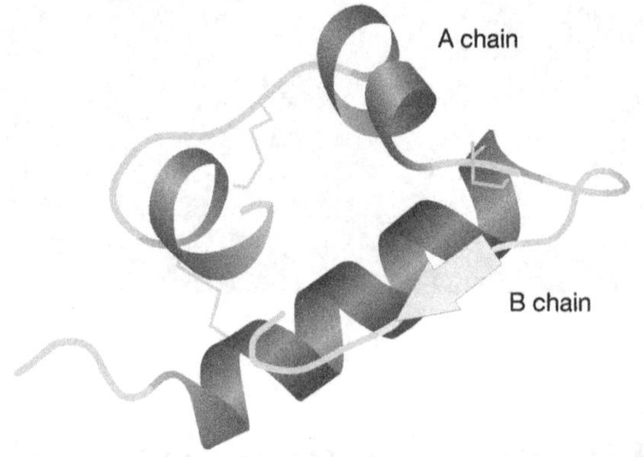

Figure 20.2 The 3-D structure of insulin.

DISEASES ASSOCIATED WITH THE ENDOCRINE SYSTEM

There are a number of disease states that are associated with the endocrine system. For example, hormones may be released in amounts that are too great or too small for the body to work normally. This situation is often referred to as hormone imbalance; however, other problems are associated with the endocrine system. Typical diseases associated with the endocrine system include hyperthyroidism and hypothyroidism, diabetes and osteoporosis. Additionally, in this chapter we will consider drugs that act on the endocrine system or drugs that are associated with problems related to this system. Details of drugs that are employed in the control of various aspects relating to the endocrine system will also be detailed. For instance, the utilisation of synthetic sex hormones for birth control will be dealt with.

Diabetes

As indicated above, the endocrine system includes the pancreas, which is responsible for the production of insulin. Insulin is a peptide hormone, with the human form comprising 51 amino acids within two chains (A and B), one of 30 amino acids and the other 21 amino acids. It has a molecular weight of 5808. The 3-D structure is shown in Figure 20.2. The B chain contains a larger region of α-helix.

Insulin is synthesised in the beta cells of the islets of Langerhans in the pancreas with the alpha cells producing glucagon, a second peptide hormone. The production of these two hormones controls the levels of blood sugar in the body. Whenever the level of sugar in the bloodstream is detected as being too high the pancreas releases insulin, which aids in the uptake of sugar by muscles, other cells and the liver, where it is stored as glycogen (a polymer containing large numbers of glucose units). When the pancreas detects that the blood sugar level is too low, it releases glucagon, which causes the breakdown of glycogen and the restoration of the normal blood sugar levels.

Diabetes or diabetes mellitus results in the body having too much sugar in the blood. It occurs in two main forms, type 1 or type 2 diabetes. Type 1 diabetes, previously referred to as early-onset diabetes, juvenile diabetes or insulin-dependent diabetes mellitus, is caused by the body being unable to produce insulin, whilst type 2 diabetes (adult-onset diabetes and non-insulin-dependent diabetes) results from the body not being able to produce enough insulin or not being able to utilise insulin properly.

The treatment of type 1 diabetes is the subcutaneous injection of insulin, as insulin cannot be administered orally because it would be broken down in the stomach due to the low pH. Initially, animal insulin was used in the treatment of diabetes, since bovine and porcine insulin are structurally similar to human insulin. Nowadays, most of the insulin used in the treatment of diabetes is human insulin produced via recombinant DNA (see Ch. 27). There are a number of insulin formulations available, e.g. short-, intermediate- or long-acting and biphasic (a mixture short- and intermediate-acting insulin), and these are described in more detail in Chapter 27. There is a range of therapy protocols indicated, based on the individual condition of the patient.

Treatment of type 2 diabetes is through a range of drugs with different modes of action. Two of the major classes are

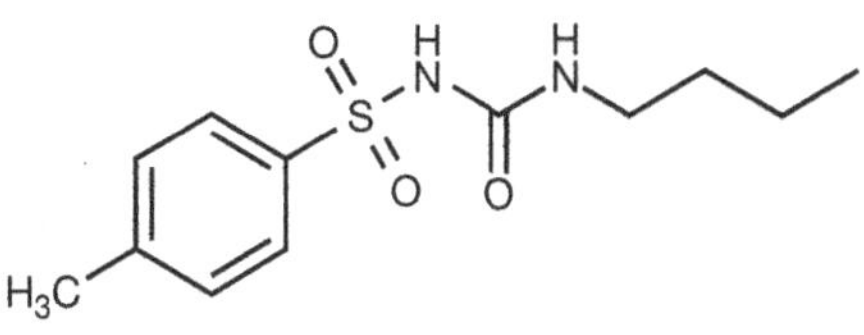

Tolbutamide

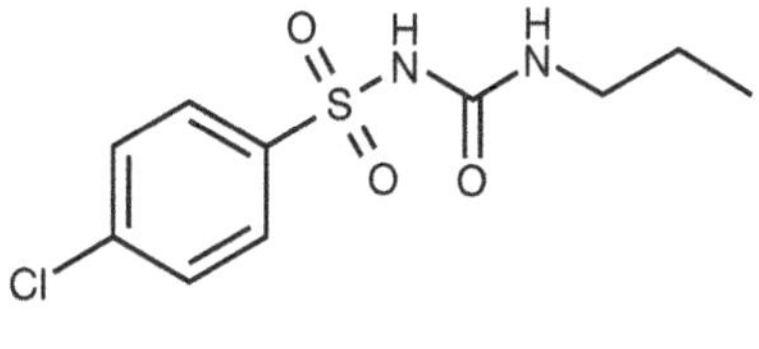

Chlorpropamide

Figure 20.3 Sulphonyl urea oral antidiabetic agents.

the sulphonylureas and the biguanides and these are used along with a number of individual compounds with a range of activities. The sulphonylureas are the oldest form of oral hypoglycaemic agents and work by stimulating the secretion of insulin in the pancreas. There are a large number of sulphonylureas that have been employed for this purpose and are nowadays classified as first and second generation (Fig. 20.3). The only first-generation sulphonylureas indicated in the BNF nowadays are chlorpropamide and tolbutamide (these are also discussed in Ch. 4).

The second-generation sulphonylureas are shown in Figure 20.4 and these compounds are considered to be

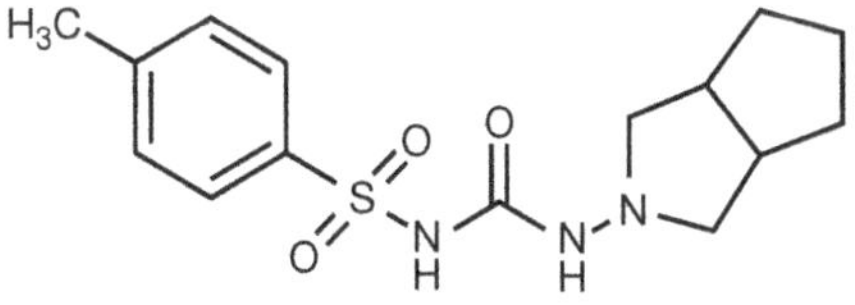

Gliclazide

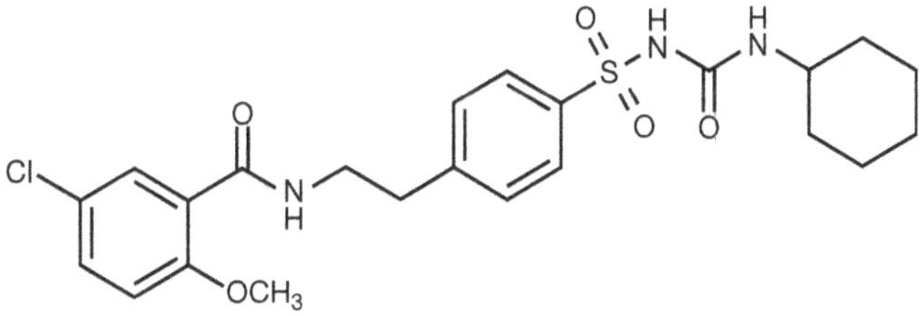

Glibenclamide

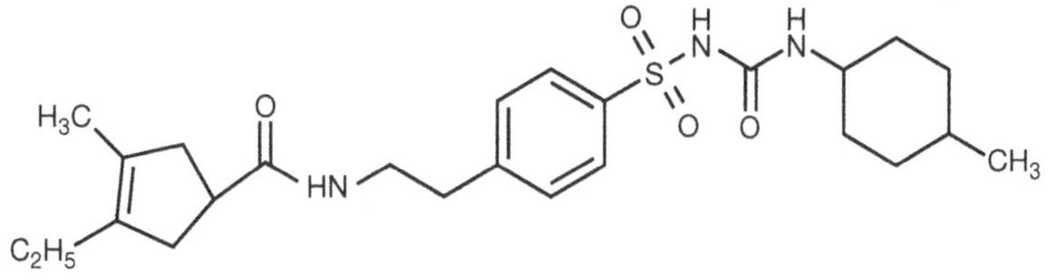

Glimepiride

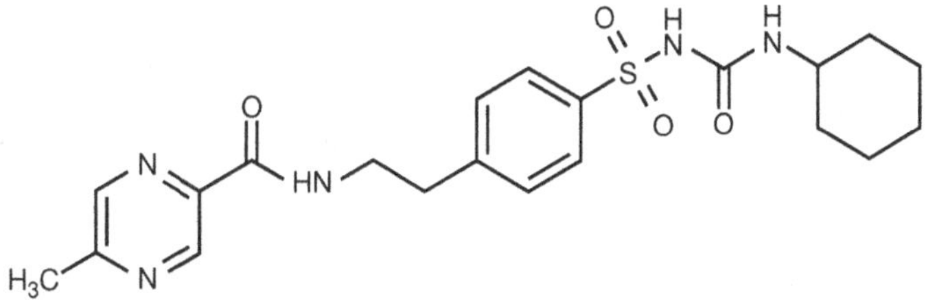

Glipizide

Figure 20.4 Second-generation sulphonylurea oral antidiabetic agents.

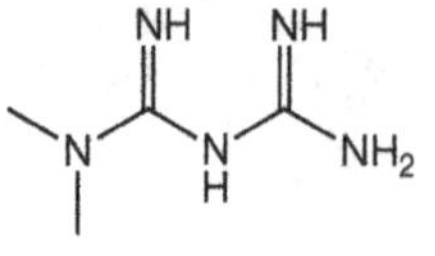

Figure 20.5 Metformin.

safer in that they have fewer side effects and are thought to be more effective than the older drugs.

The second class of compounds used are the biguanides and, although a number of these have been used in the past, several have been withdrawn due to side effects (lactic acidosis) and only one such agent, metformin (Fig. 20.5), is presently indicated in the UK. The mode of action of the biguanides still seems to be unclear but is reported to include decreasing the absorption of glucose and inhibiting hepatic glucose output.

A variety of other agents come under the heading of antidiabetic drugs and the list includes acarbose, nateglinide and repaglinide, pioglitazone and rosiglitazone, sitagliptin and vildagliptin, and exenatide (Fig. 20.6).

Acarbose is a synthetic oligosaccharide that was designed to reduce the rate at which enzymes in the intestine (alpha-amylase and alpha-glucosidase) break down carbohydrates. In doing so, acarbose slows down the release of sugar into the blood stream.

Pioglitazone and rosiglitazone are both classified as thiazolidenediones (based on the heterocyclic ring system in this group of drugs). This group of drugs is often banded under the heading 'glitazones'. This group of drugs is known to be useful in type 2 diabetes as they help in what is known as insulin resistance, in which the body produces insulin but cannot utilise it effectively to reduce blood sugar levels. These thiazolidenediones bind to peroxisome proliferator activated receptor-gamma (PPAR-γ) which is a nuclear receptor. In doing so, these drugs are involved in altering the transcription of several genes involved in glucose and lipid metabolism and energy balance. Consequently, the insulin resistance is reduced and the body can effectively deal with blood sugar.

Nateglinide and repaglinide are secretagogues in that they promote the secretion of insulin in the pancreas. These agents interfere with the beta cells in the islets of Langerhans and open the calcium channels in the cells, the increased calcium resulting in the enhanced insulin secretion.

Sitagliptin and vildagliptin belong to a new class of drugs known as dipeptidyl peptidase-4 (DPP-4) inhibitors. DPP-4 acts on two incretin hormones, namely glucagon-like peptide 1 (GLP-1) and glucose-dependent insulinotropic peptide (GIP), both of which are released in the intestine following food intake. They are able to stimulate the production of insulin, depending on the levels of glucose; however, they are both inactivated via the enzyme DPP-4. Sitagliptin and vildagliptin, as inhibitors of DPP-4, act by preventing the inactivation of GLP-1 and GIP.

Exenatide is a drug that is described as an incretin mimetic in that it has a strong structural resemblance to GLP-1. This drug is a synthetic peptide based on a hormone, exendin-4, found in the saliva of the Gila monster. Research on this peptide showed that it had properties similar to GLP-1. Now, GLP-1 cannot be administered to patients with type 2 diabetes since it is rapidly inactivated in the body by DPP-4, as indicated above. Due to the structural similarity between GLP-1 and exendin-4, it was investigated as a GLP-1 mimetic and shown to work effectively. It was also shown to have a considerably longer half-life than GLP-1 as it was not broken down by DPP-4 as quickly as the natural analogue.

Anti-obesity drugs

Obesity is defined as a body mass index greater than 30. Obesity may result via a variety of conditions but is, in some instances, closely associated with certain endocrine diseases such as diabetes. Obese people are advised to overcome their problem by means of appropriate dietary changes and an increase in physical exercise. However, when these do not work, drug treatment is necessary. Several drugs may be employed in these circumstances and fall into two types of anti-obesity drugs acting on the gastrointestinal (GI) tract and appetite suppressants.

Orlistat (Fig. 20.7) is the only GI tract drug indicated in the BNF, and is a lipase inhibitor, which reduces fat intake. This drug is a synthetic analogue of lipstatin which is a naturally occurring substance produced by *Streptomyces toxytricini*. Orlistat is an irreversible inhibitor of pancreatic and gastric lipases and as such it prevents these lipases from breaking down triglycerides into their absorbable form (free fatty acids and monoglycerols). The triglycerides are thus eliminated without absorption and thus there is a decreased dietary intake of fat.

In the BNF there are only two appetite suppressants (Fig. 20.8) indicated as anti-obesity drugs, namely Rimonabant and Sibutramine. Rimonabant has been marketed as an anti-obesity drug for several years in the UK, although it never received FDA clearance. It is a cannabinoid receptor antagonist, which blocks binding to neuronal CB1 receptors. This inhibition of binding of endogenous cannabinoids prevents an increase in appetite. This drug has recently had its market authorisation in the UK suspended due to concerns regarding psychiatric problems associated with its use.

Sibutramine (hydrochloride) is structurally related to the amfetamines, which were at one stage marketed as appetite suppressant drugs. These drugs were removed from the market due to their increased use as recreational drugs and because of the serious side effects of their use, e.g. tachycardia, hypertension and addiction. Sibutramine

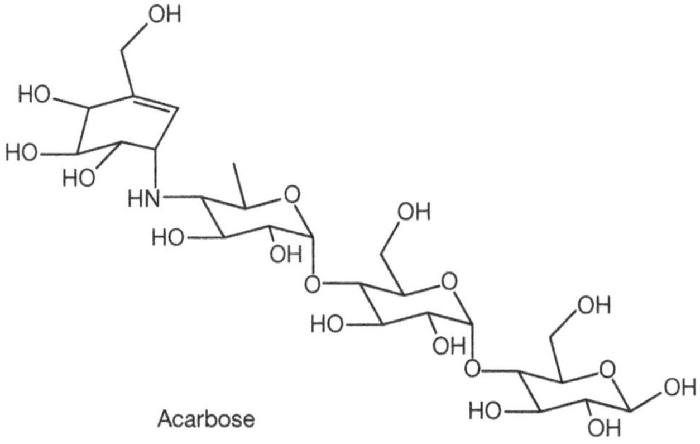

Acarbose

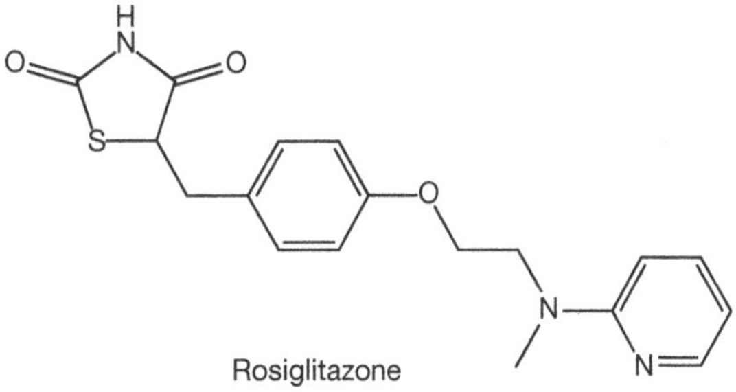

Rosiglitazone

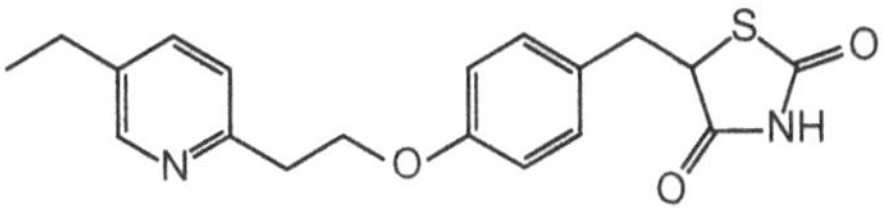

Pioglitazone

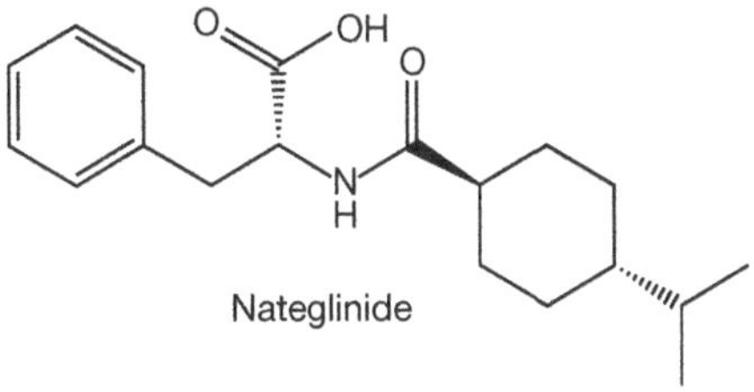

Nateglinide

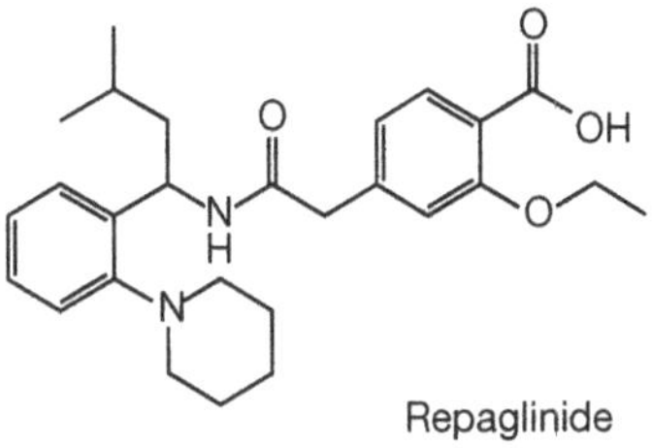

Repaglinide

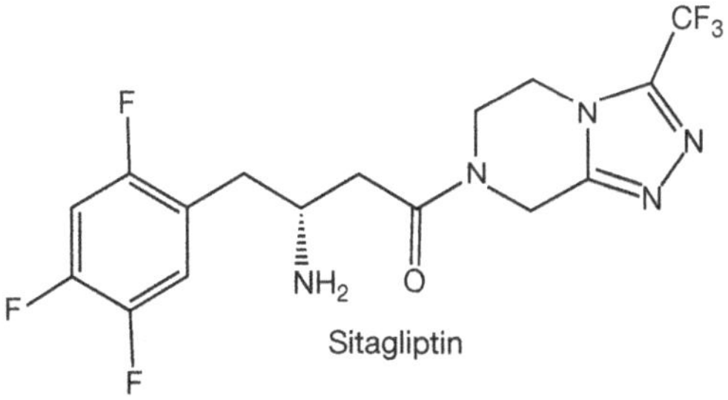

Sitagliptin

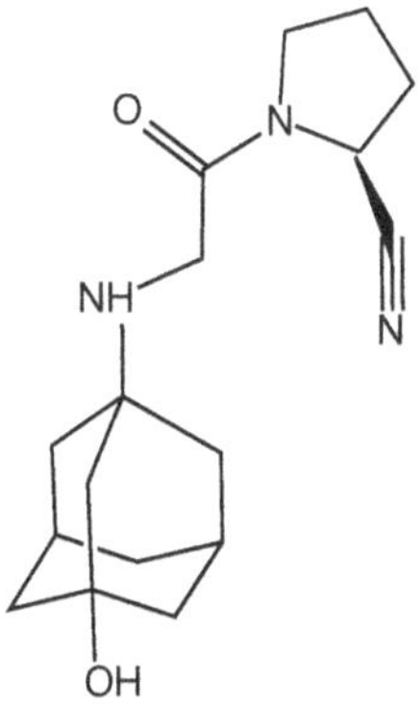

Vildagliptin

His-Gly-Glu-Gly-Thr-Phe-Thr-Ser-Asp-Leu-Ser-Luys-Gln-Met-Glu-
Glu-Glu-Ala-Val-Arg-Leu-Phe-Ile-Glu-Trp-Leu-Lys-Asn-Gly-Gly-
Pro-Ser-Ser-Gly-Ala-Pro-Pro-Pro-Ser-NH_2

Exenatide

Figure 20.6 Oral antidiabetic agents with miscellaneous modes of action.

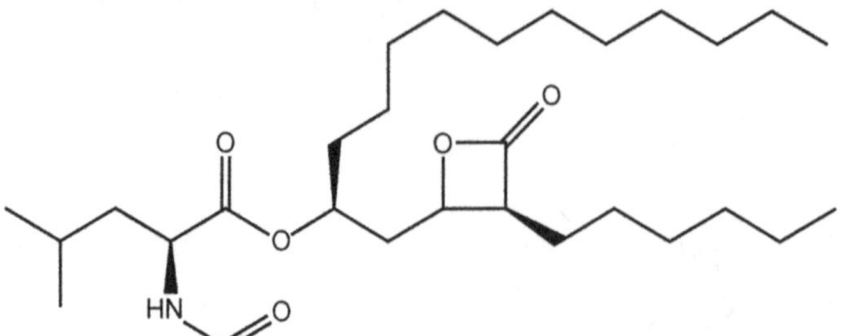

Orlistat

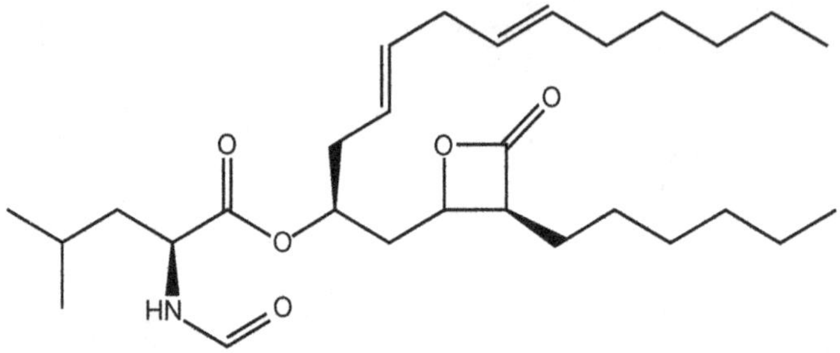

Lipstatin

Figure 20.7 Orlistat and lipstatin.

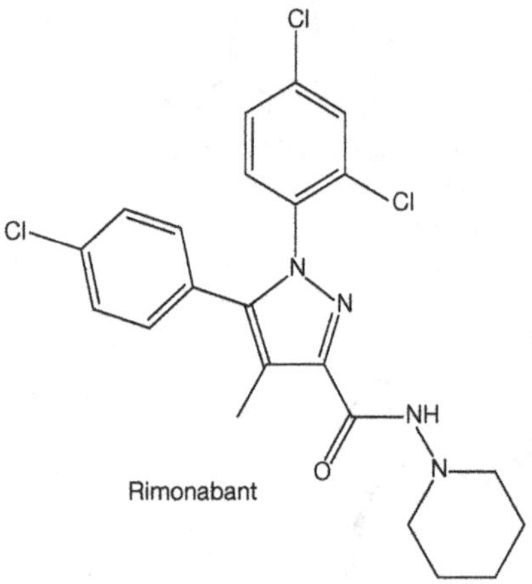

Rimonabant

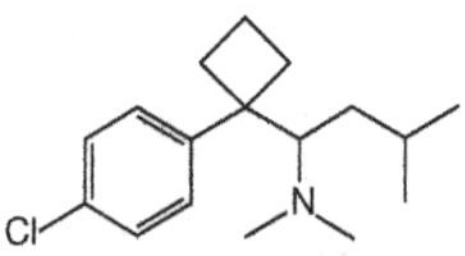

Sibutramine

Figure 20.8 Appetite suppressants.

is a serotonin and noradrenaline reuptake inhibitor, thereby promoting weight loss because of its ability to help patients feel that their hunger has been satisfied. It is also suggested that weight loss may be helped by the drug, increasing energy expenditure.

Thyroid hormones

The thyroid hormones, as indicated above, are amino acid-based hormones. The thyroid gland produces two main active thyroid hormones, thyroxine and triiodothyronine. When produced, these hormones circulate in the blood with the major fraction being bound to proteins which transport them throughout the body. However, these hormones are only active in the unbound form. The structures of the two hormones are shown in Figure 20.9.

The thyroid hormones (often referred to as T_3 and T_4) when released into the blood stream are transported throughout the body where they control metabolic processes in almost all cells in the body. T_3 is more active than T_4 by a factor of approximately 10. As one can observe, these two hormones contain iodine and it is the function of the thyroid gland to utilise dietary iodine in the conversion of tyrosine into monoiodotyrosine (MIT) and diiodotyrosine (DIT) (Fig. 20.10).

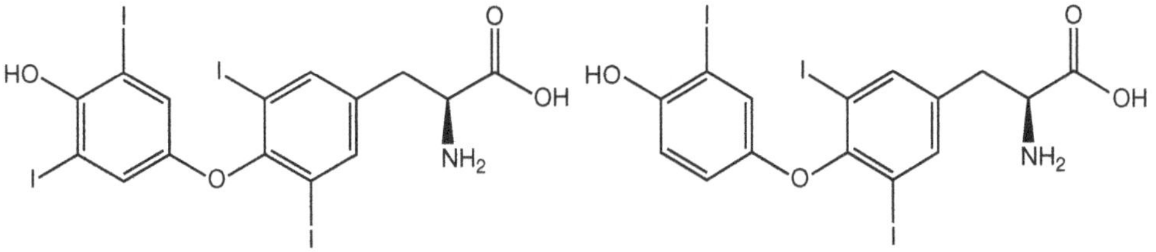

Thyroxine T_4 Triiodothyronine T_3

Figure 20.9 Thyroid hormones.

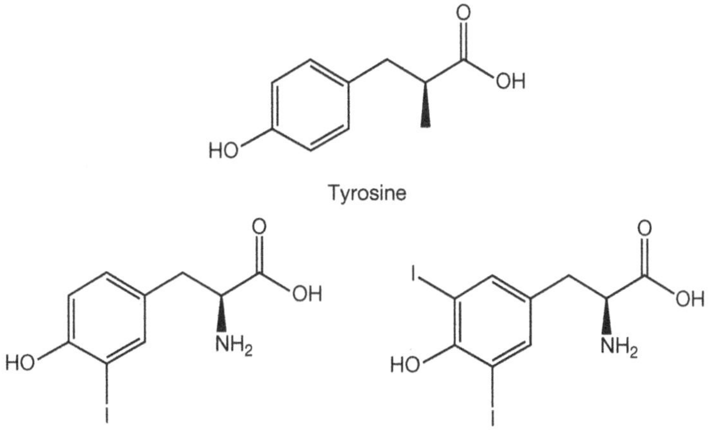

Tyrosine

Monoiodotyrosine MIT   Diiodotyrosine DIT

Figure 20.10 Tyrosine and iodotyrosines.

The linking of one molecule of MIT with one of DIT results in the formation of T_3, whilst two molecules of DIT combine in the formation of T_4. T_4 can also be converted into T_3 by the 5′-deiodinase enzyme system. Within the body, the control system associated with the production of these hormones is directed by TSH (thyroid stimulating hormone) and TRH (thyroid releasing hormone).

Within the thyroid system, disease states can lead to hypothyroidism and hyperthyroidism. Hypothyroidism results from abnormally low production of thyroid hormone in thyroid glands. The prevalence of this condition is reported as being between 2% and 5% of the world population, although a substantial number are in the subclinical category. Hypothyroidism is much more common in females than in males, and the frequency of the disease increases with age. The problem may arise due to an insufficient intake of iodine in the diet. It may be due to an inherited disorder (Hashimoto's thyroiditis) or it may be due to inflammation of the thyroid gland (lymphocytic thyroiditis). The conventional treatment for this condition is use of thyroid hormones levothyroxine sodium or liothyronine sodium (Fig. 20.11).

Hyperthyroidism results from an overactive thyroid gland producing excess amounts of thyroid hormones which circulate through the body. The thyroid hormones affect many cellular functions throughout the body and this excess results in increased metabolic activity leading to a variety of symptoms, the most common being increased heart rate, tremor, diarrhoea and weight loss. The treatment of hyperthyroidism involves the use of two drugs: carbimazole and propylthiouracil. Carbimazole is a prodrug that is converted into methimazole (Fig. 20.12), which is the active agent. Methimazole interferes by inhibiting the thyroid peroxidase system that is involved in the conversion of tyrosine into MIT and DIT, thereby preventing the synthesis of T_3 and T_4.

Propylthiouracil (Fig. 20.13) acts similar to methimazole in that it inhibits the thyroid peroxidase system. It also acts by inhibiting the enzyme 5′-deiodinase, which converts T_4 into the more active T_3 form.

It should also be noted that beta-blockers (e.g. propanolol) are indicated in hyperthyroidism for relief of some of the symptoms such as increased heart rate, tremor, etc.

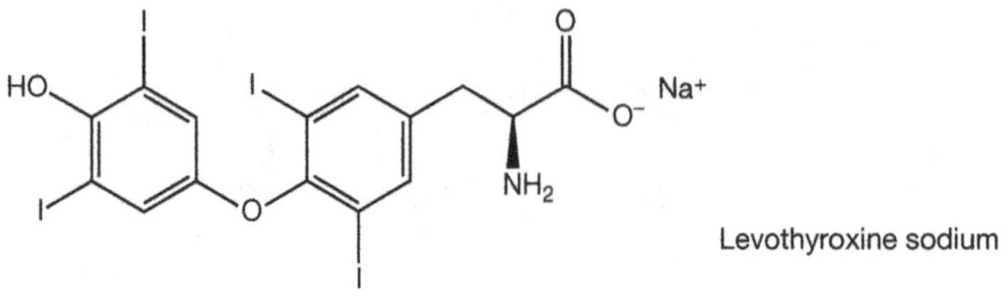

Figure 20.11 Compounds used in the treatment of hypothyroidism.

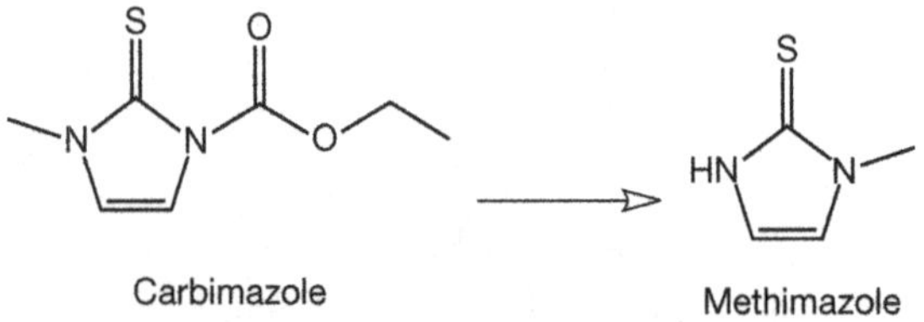

Figure 20.12 Conversion of the prodrug carbimazole into the active drug methimazole.

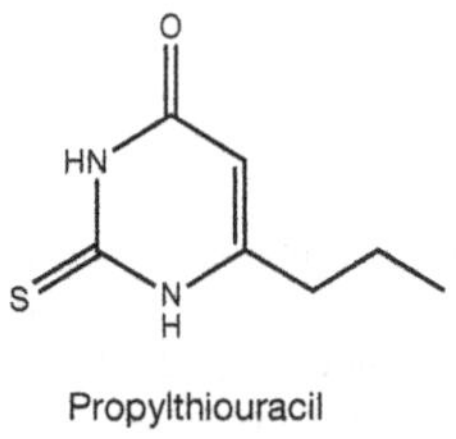

Figure 20.13 Propylthiouracil.

Glaucoma

Glaucoma is an eye condition in which the optic nerve becomes damaged due, in the main, to an increase in intraocular pressure (IOP). The increase in IOP results from problems with the eye's drainage system. In the eye, aqueous humour is found in the part of the eye in front of the lens, and this is continually produced in the ciliary body. Under normal conditions the aqueous humour is removed from the eye by means of drainage into the bloodstream through the trabecular meshwork and canal of Schlemm. In the normal forms of glaucoma these drainage systems become restricted or blocked and thus the IOP increases. There are several types of glaucoma: primary open-angle glaucoma (POAG) and closed-angle glaucoma (COAG) account for the majority of cases, although there are other types such as normal tension glaucoma, secondary glaucoma, paediatric glaucoma and acute glaucoma.

Primary open-angle glaucoma

In primary open angle glaucoma the drainage channels in the trabecular meshwork pathway become clogged. This prevents aqueous humour outflow and an imbalance occurs because fluid continues to be produced but is unable to drain away. This results in increased intraocular pressure (IOP). The intraocular pressure exerts force on the optic nerve at the back of the eye, resulting in damage, and can lead eventually to blindness.

Closed-angle glaucoma

In closed-angle glaucoma (angle-closure glaucoma) the angle between the iris and the cornea changes and completely restricts the drainage, resulting in a rapid increase in IOP and thus optic nerve damage.

There is no cure for glaucoma, although surgical procedures can be performed to relieve IOP. Treatment of glaucoma involves the use of drugs in order to reduce IOP and there are a number of different drug classes that might be employed. These are listed in Table 20.1.

The use of drugs in the treatment of glaucoma is designed mainly to reduce the production of aqueous humour or to improve the outflow of aqueous humour once produced. Beta-blockers commonly used for the treatment of glaucoma include betaxolol, carteolol, levobunolol, metipranolol and timolol (Fig. 20.14). This group of compounds acts by causing a decrease in production of the aqueous humour in the ciliary body.

Carbonic anhydrase (CA) inhibitors acetazolamide, brinzolamide and dorzolamide (Fig. 20.15) act through

Table 20.1 Details of drug classes used in the treatment of glaucoma

Drug class	Mode of action
Beta-blockers	Reduce the production of aqueous humour by blocking the messages which stimulate fluid production.
Carbonic anhydrase inhibitors	Produce a fall in pressure by suppressing production of aqueous humour.
Prostaglandin analogues	Increase the aqueous outflow from the eye.
Sympathomimetics	Decrease intraocular pressure by increasing the outflow of fluid. May be used in conjunction with a miotic.

inhibition of carbonic anhydrase in the eye. These compounds all have the typical primary sulphonamide group associated with CA inhibition (see Ch. 4). CA (probably CA II which is the predominant isoform in the eye) catalyses the formation of bicarbonate, which is involved in production of aqueous humour. The inhibition of this enzyme thus reduces the production of the aqueous humour and consequently results in a decrease in IOP.

Several prostaglandin $F_{2\alpha}$ ($PGF_{2\alpha}$) analogues have been developed for the treatment of glaucoma, including latanoprost, bimatoprost and travoprost (Fig. 20.16). These compounds are prodrugs of the active compounds that are hydrolysed to the active free acids. These compounds act by increasing uveoscleral outflow (drainage from the anterior chamber, through the ciliary body and choroids) of the aqueous humour from the eye. Although this process does occur normally it is a relatively minor pathway until promoted by these $PGF_{2\alpha}$ analogues. As indicated above, these analogues are prodrugs that are hydrolysed by ocular tissue, e.g. cornea. The prodrug portions of the compounds are highlighted in Figure 20.16.

Sympathomimetics and miotics (Fig. 20.17) have been used for the treatment of glaucoma although they are less widely used today given the advent of the drug classes reported above. The sympathomimetic dipivefrine is the dipivalyl prodrug of adrenaline. As such it is highly lipophilic, resulting in better penetration than adrenaline itself. The prodrug is hydrolysed by esterases in the aqueous humour. Adrenaline thus formed acts in a non-selective fashion on α and β adrenoreceptors, which can lead to opposing effects. However, the cumulative effect is to reduce the IOP. Brimonidine is a highly selective σ_2 agonist, which reduces IOP by reducing aqueous inflow and increasing uveoscleral outflow. Pilocarpine acts on a muscarinic receptor (M_3) on the iris sphincter muscle, which

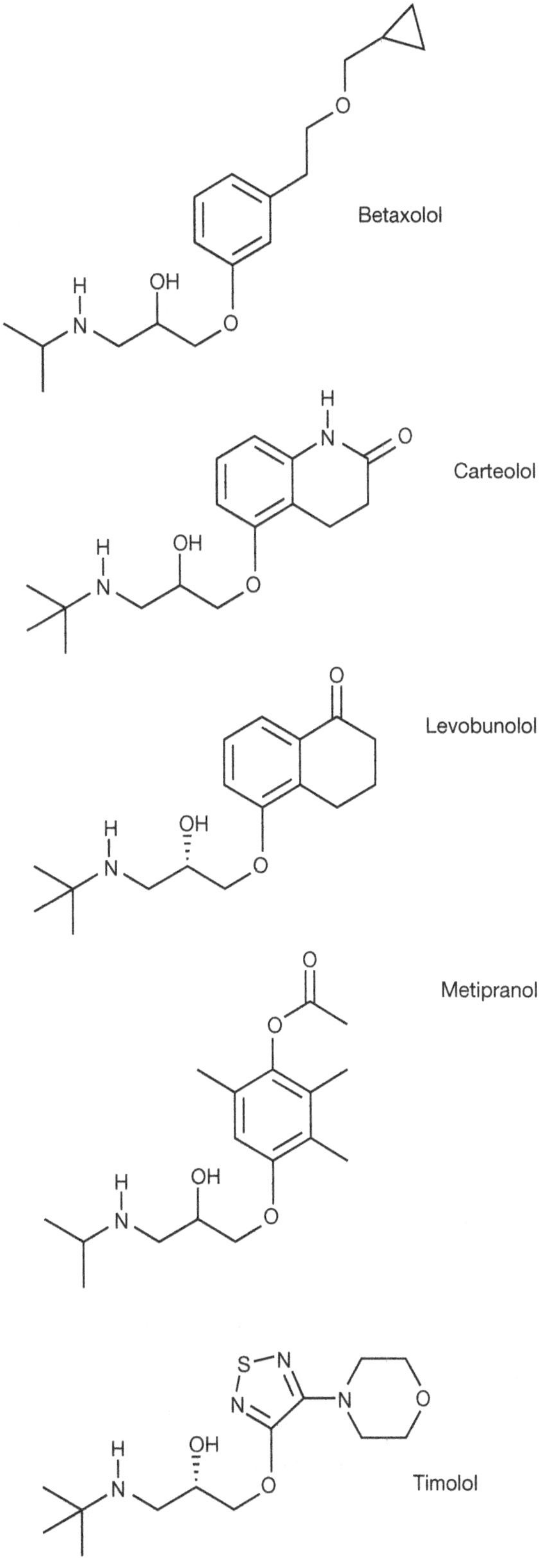

Figure 20.14 Beta-blockers used in the treatment of glaucoma.

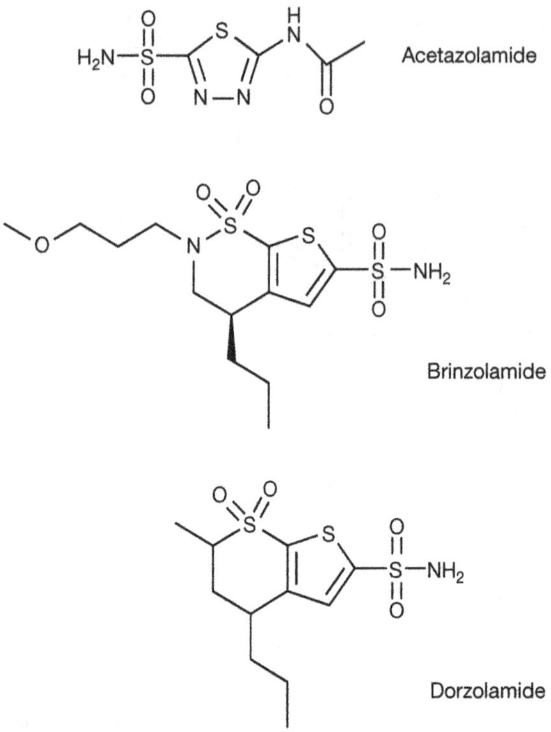

Figure 20.15 Carbonic anhydrase inhibitors used in treating glaucoma.

causes muscle contraction, resulting in the opening of the trabecular meshwork. This results in an increase in the rate at which aqueous humour leaves the eye, thereby reducing IOP.

STEROID HORMONES

One of the three classes of hormones is the steroid hormones. These hormones are synthesised in the adrenal glands and in the testes/ovaries. They are transported throughout the body where they control a variety of different physiological functions. The steroid hormones include the glucocorticoids (glucocorticosteroids) involved in metabolism, inflammation and stress; mineralocorticoids (mineralocorticosteroids) involved in control of water/salt balance; androgens, oestrogens and progestogens which are the sex hormones that are involved in the development of male and female secondary sexual characteristics and in reproduction.

Steroid biosynthesis

All of the steroid hormones are derived from cholesterol. Cholesterol biosynthesis is the major route through which

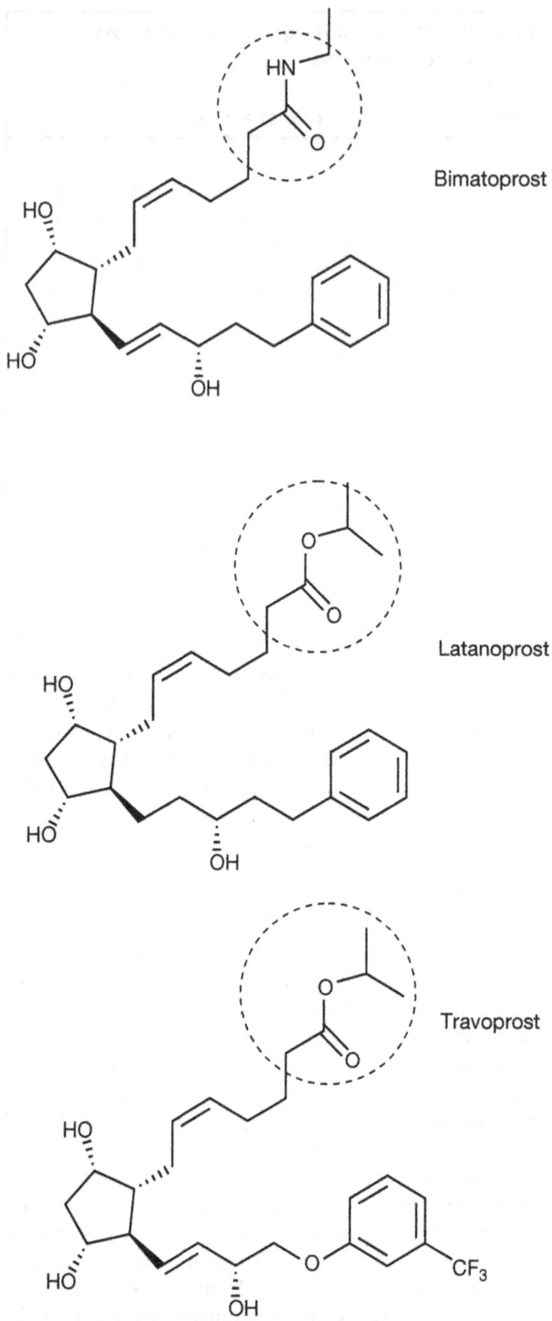

Figure 20.16 Prostaglandin ($PGF_{2\alpha}$) analogues used for the treatment of glaucoma (circled areas indicating prodrug moiety).

steroids (including steroid hormones) are formed in the body. Cholesterol biosynthesis proceeds initially via the mevalonic acid (mevalonate) pathway (Fig. 20.18). Two molecules of acetyl coenzyme A [acetyl CoA] combine to generate acetoacetyl CoA. This reacts with a

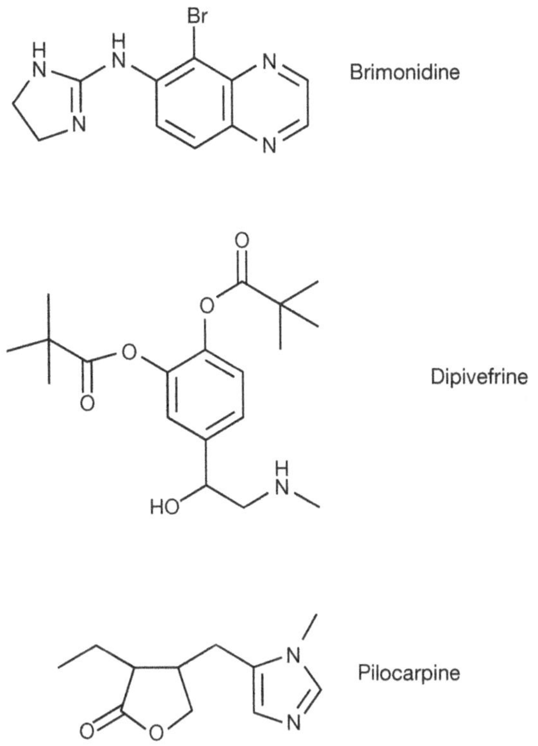

Figure 20.17 Structures of sympathomimetics and miotics used in the treatment of glaucoma.

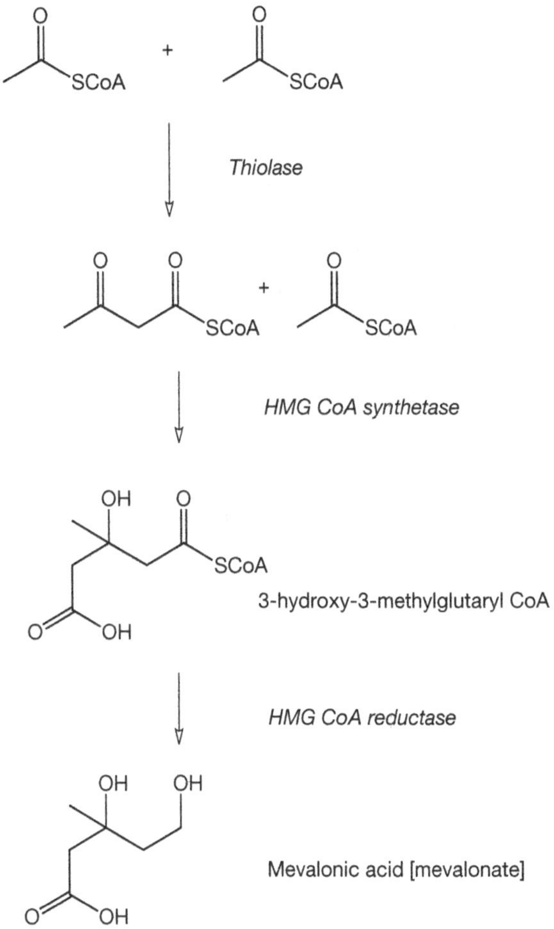

Figure 20.18 The initial steps in the biosynthesis of cholesterol leading to mevalonic acid formation.

further molecule of acetyl CoA to generate 3-hydroxy-3-methylglutaryl CoA (HMG CoA). HMG CoA is reduced by HMG CoA reductase to yield mevalonic acid. Note this last step is most important since it is the inhibition of this enzyme system which is the basis of the cholesterol lowering effect of statins.

The second step in the biosynthesis of cholesterol is the conversion of mevalonic acid into farnesylpyrophosphate (Fig. 20.19). This is initiated by phosphorylation of the mevalonic acid, followed by decarboxylation yielding isopentylpyrophosphate, which can reversibly isomerise to 3,3-dimethylallylpyrophosphate.

Condensation of this compound with one molecule of isopentylpyrophosphate results in the formation of geranylpyrophosphate, and addition of a second molecule of isopentylpyrophosphate yields farnesylpyrophosphate (Fig. 20.19).

The third phase of cholesterol biosynthesis (Fig. 20.20) involves the condensation of two molecules of farnesylpyrophosphate, yielding squalene via the enzyme squalene synthetase.

Squalene is essentially an open chain form of the steroid nucleus, which is converted into cholesterol via a number of steps involving the production of lanosterol. Figure 20.21 shows more clearly the cyclisation process in which squalene is firstly oxidised via squalene epoxidase to form 2,3-squalene epoxide. This then cyclises to produce the basic steroid nucleus, resulting in the formation of lanosterol. This is why all steroids have an oxygen atom at the 3 position.

Once formed, cholesterol may be utilised in the production of a variety of steroid hormones in the body. The numbering of the steroid nucleus in cholesterol (which is valid for all steroids) is shown in Figure 20.22 and this is followed with details of the major pathways to the steroid hormones (Figs 20.23, 20.24) whilst Figure 20.25 shows the formation of bile acids from cholesterol.

The biosynthetic pathway for the conversion of cholesterol into these compounds involves a range of enzymic systems, many of which are cytochrome P450 (CYP)

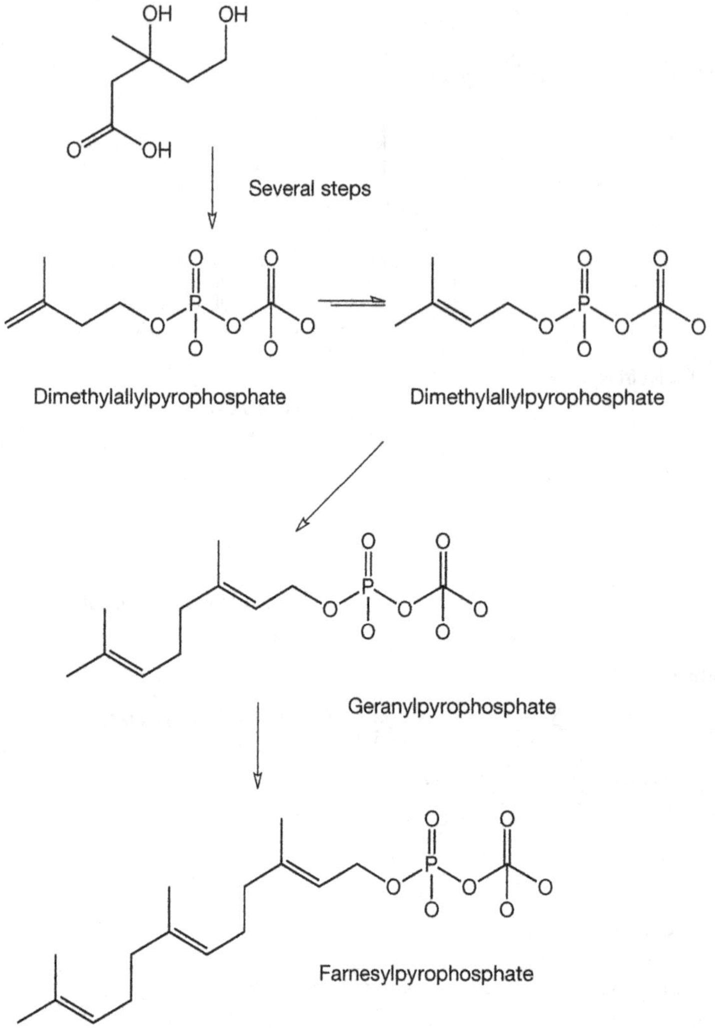

Figure 20.19 Formation of farnesylpyrophosphate.

enzyme systems. Thus, in the conversion of cholesterol into pregnenolone, CYP11A1 (the side chain cleavage enzyme or desmolase) is responsible for loss of the six carbon chain and the C_{20} ketone formation. Conversion of pregnenolone into androstenedione involves CYP17 (steroid 17-alpha-hydroxylase), which brings about the formation of the ketone at the C_{17} position. The oxidation of the 3-hydroxyl group occurs via the non-CYP enzyme 3-beta-HSD (3-beta-hydroxysteroid dehydrogenase). During this process the rearrangement of the 5,6 double bond occurs because of the formation of the energetically favourable ene-one system. The reduction of the C_{17} ketone to a hydroxyl group results in the formation of testosterone via 17-beta-HSD. Formation of estrone and estradiol involves the aromatisation of the A ring via CYP19 (aromatase) enzyme.

In Figure 20.24, the formation of the corticosteroids is outlined. The formation of progesterone results from the action of 3-beta-HSD on pregnenolone. The formation of cortisol from progesterone involves a series of three hydroxylation steps with hydroxylation of C17 (CYP17), hydroxylation of C21 (CYP21) and hydroxylation of C11 (CYP11B1). The biosynthesis of aldosterone shares two of the hydroxylation steps but in the final step formation of the C18 aldehyde function occurs via CYP11B2 (aldosterone synthetase).

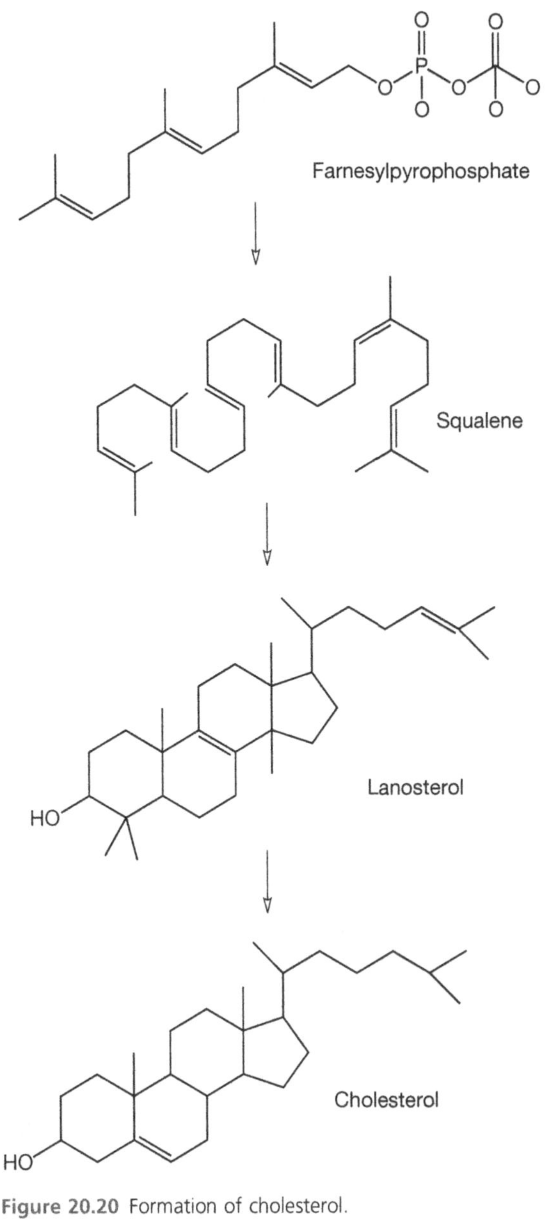

Figure 20.20 Formation of cholesterol.

The sex hormones

The three groups of sex hormones in the human body are the oestrogens and progestogens, often thought of as the 'female' sex hormones, and the androgens, the 'male' sex hormone. Despite being classified in such a way, these hormones are present in both males and females, although the levels present in the two sexes are somewhat different. These hormones are responsible for the development of secondary sexual characteristics (e.g. breast development, vaginal and uterine growth in females and penis development, growth of body and facial hair in males) and are vital for reproduction in both sexes.

As far as the endocrine system is concerned, these sex hormones are produced in the ovaries and testes (gonads) following events in the hypothalamus and the anterior pituitary gland. In the hypothalamus, messages received via feedback loops signal the need for the synthesis of these hormones and, as a result, it secretes gonadotrophin releasing hormone (GnRH). In the anterior pituitary gland, GnRH is responsible for stimulating the production of gonadotrophins, e.g. luteinising hormone (LH) or follicle stimulating hormone (FSH). These hormones travel to the ovaries and the testes where the production of oestrogens, progestogens and androgens occurs. As indicated above, these hormones are involved in the development of the secondary sexual characteristics and, during puberty, the development into the mature adult, and then subsequently influence the sexual functioning of adults in terms of spermatogenesis in males and the reproductive cycle in females. The general biosynthesis of the steroid hormones in the body is detailed in Figures 20.23 and 20.24 and the production of the main steroid hormones estradiol, progesterone and testosterone along with estrone outlines there. A third oestrogen, estriol, is derived from either estradiol via 16α-hydrolase or estrone, again via 16α-hydrolase, and then estradiol dehydrogenase.

During the female reproductive cycle which falls into two phases, the follicle cycle and the luteal cycle, the hormones FSH, LH, estradiol and progesterone are all involved in the various changes that occur over this period. FSH, as the name implies, stimulates the development of follicles in the ovary. As this process progresses, estradiol is secreted leading to an elevation of oestrogen levels. By means of a feedback loop, the production of FSH decreases and there is a corresponding increase in LH levels and at the midpoint of the cycle there is a sharp rise in its production leading to the release of an egg from the follicle (ovulation) into the fallopian tube. The second part of the reproductive cycle is known as the luteal phase in which the empty follicle changes into a corpus luteum, which secretes progesterone under the influence of LH. If the egg is not fertilised, the rising levels of progesterone result in the inhibition of GnRH, leading subsequently to a drop in progesterone levels and finally to menstruation. If the egg is fertilised, a set of different occurrences take place with the formation of human chorionic gonadotrophin (HCG), which enables the corpus luteum to survive and as such allows progesterone production to continue, thereby supporting the pregnancy.

In males, once again there are processes that involve FSH and LH that are involved in the production of testosterone and the production of sperm.

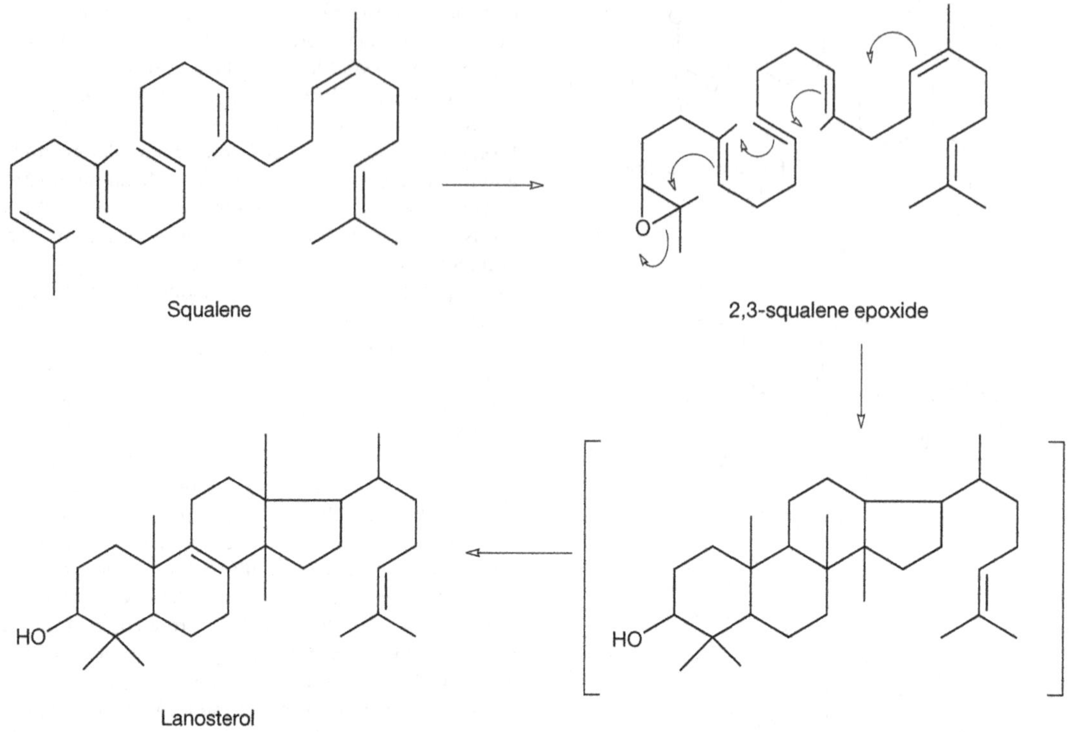

Figure 20.21 Conversion of squalene into lanesterol.

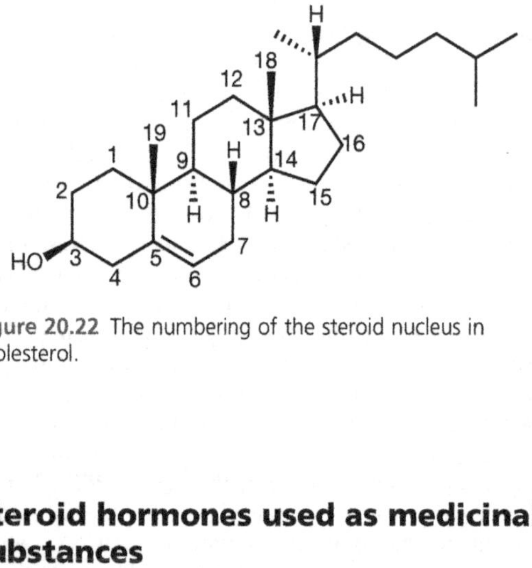

Figure 20.22 The numbering of the steroid nucleus in cholesterol.

Steroid hormones used as medicinal substances

There are numerous examples of the use of natural or synthetic steroids in a variety of medical areas that have gained importance. These include oral contraception, hormone replacement therapy, treatment for delayed puberty and muscle development, with the oral contraceptives one of the most well-known examples.

Development of oral contraceptives

Early work in the understanding of steroid hormones and how they work resulted in investigations of their use as contraceptive agents. It was soon shown that many of the naturally occurring compounds, when given parenterally, were active, but when administered orally were only weakly active. It was found that the compounds were absorbed reasonably well but were rapidly metabolised by the liver. In order to overcome these problems of rapid metabolism, a large number of derivatives were synthesised and tested. One of the most successful methods discovered was the introduction of an acetylene group at the 17 position of the steroid ring, for example in ethinyl estradiol (Fig. 20.26). This compound was easily synthesised by reacting estrone with potassium acetylide in liquid ammonia.

Further investigations resulted in the discovery that etherification of the 3-hydroxy group of ethinyl estradiol resulted in formation of potent orally active oestrogens such as mestranol (the 3-methyl ether) and quinestrol (the 3-cyclopentyl ether), although this is not now used in oral contraceptives (Fig. 20.27).

In a similar fashion to the oestrogens, synthetic progestogens were investigated and a large number were synthesised. One of the first to be used was ethisterone,

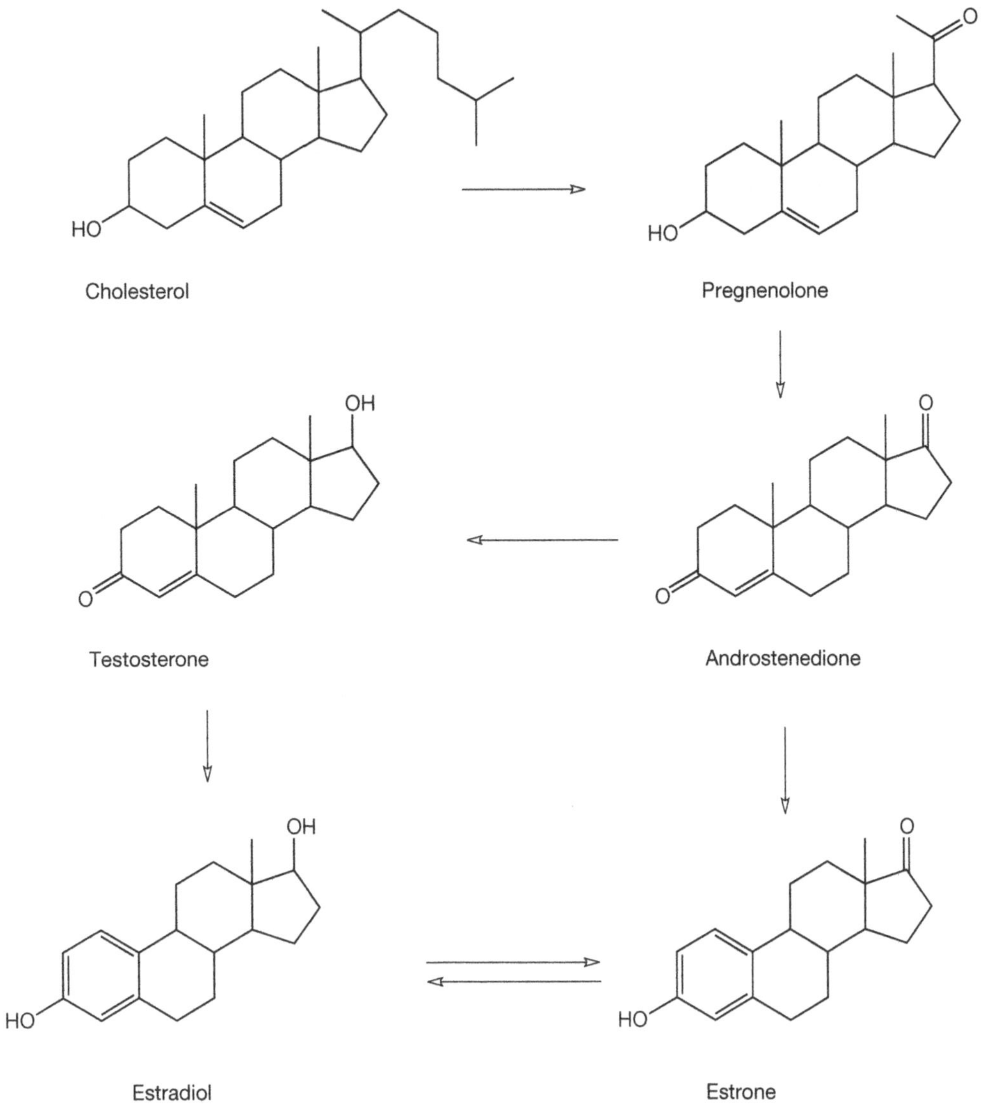

Figure 20.23 Biosynthesis of the sex hormones.

which once again incorporated an ethinyl group at the 17 position (Figs 20.28, 20.29, 20.30).

Since the early work in this area, there have been many compounds discovered that possess significant oral progestogenic activity. For example, it was discovered that removal of the C19 methyl group enhanced the activity, resulting in compounds such as norethindrone and norethinodrel. Also, compounds in which the 3-keto group is lost were also found to be useful progestogens.

There have been many developments in formulations used for oral contraceptives since the original studies. Nowadays, there are numerous products available such as the combined hormonal therapy (oestrogen plus progestogen) or the progestogen-only contraceptive. In some instances, the combined tablets contain fixed doses of the two components and others where the contents vary. There are also tablets containing lower than normal levels of the oestrogen because of the risk factors associated with circulatory disease. Most of the oral contraceptives available in the UK at present comprise estradiol in combination with one of the following: norethisterone, levonorgestrel, norgestimate, desogestrel, drospirenone, gestodene, as well as a product which contains mestranol with ethisterone. The progestogen-only pills available

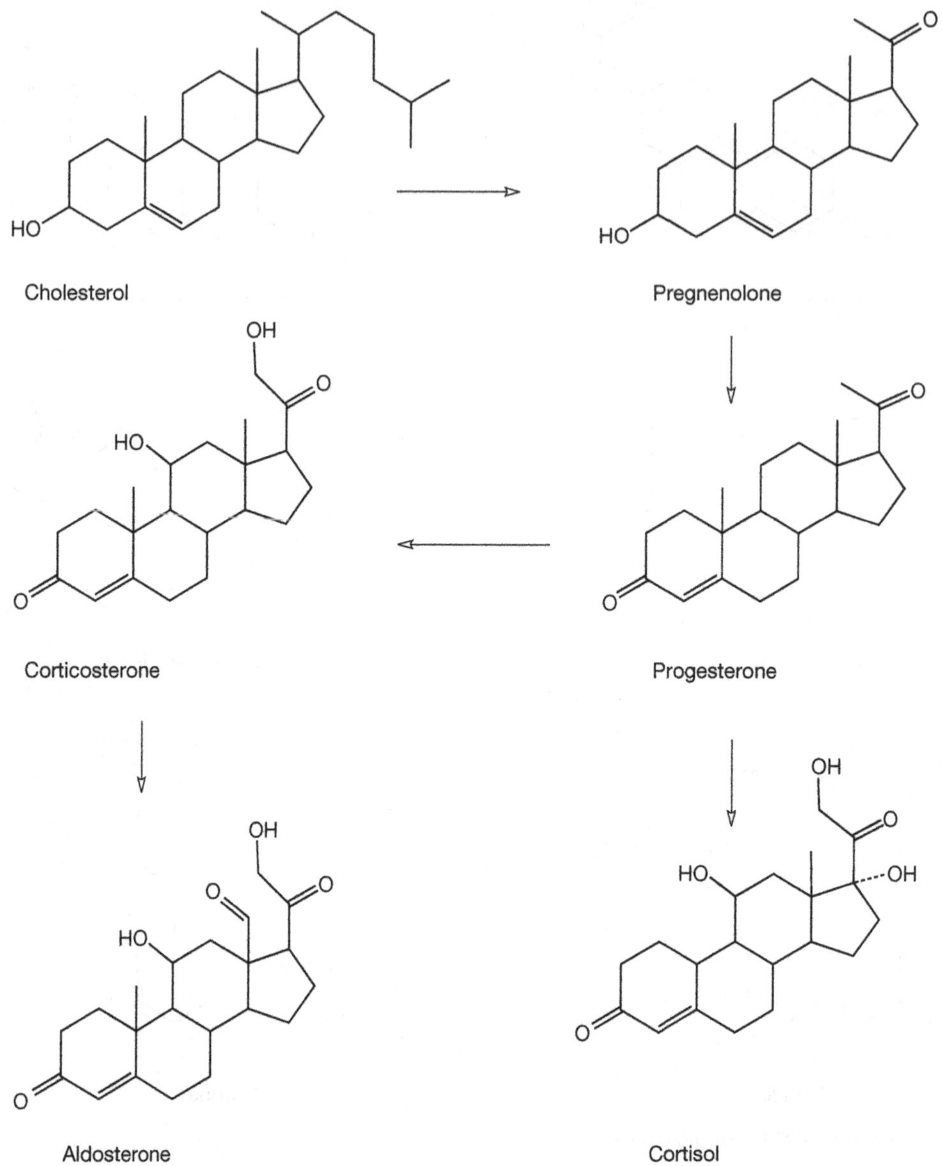

Figure 20.24 Synthesis of the mineralocorticosteroid and glucocorticosteroid hormones.

contain desogestrel, etynodiol diacetate, norethisterone or levonorgestrel. An emergency contraception product is also available which contains a high dose of levonorgestrel.

Hormone replacement therapy

In addition to their use as oral contraceptives, oestrogens and progestogen, either in combination or as oestrogens only treatments, have been used as hormone replacement therapy to alleviate the problems associated with the menopause. There are concerns about such treatments because of the side effects known to be associated with these products, e.g. increased risks (in some or both) of heart attack, stroke, blood clots, certain cancers, whilst both treatments seem to have a positive effect in relation to osteoporosis.

Male sex hormones

Anabolic or androgenic steroids are used for the treatment of a variety of conditions including their use in treating young males with delayed puberty, treating patients with

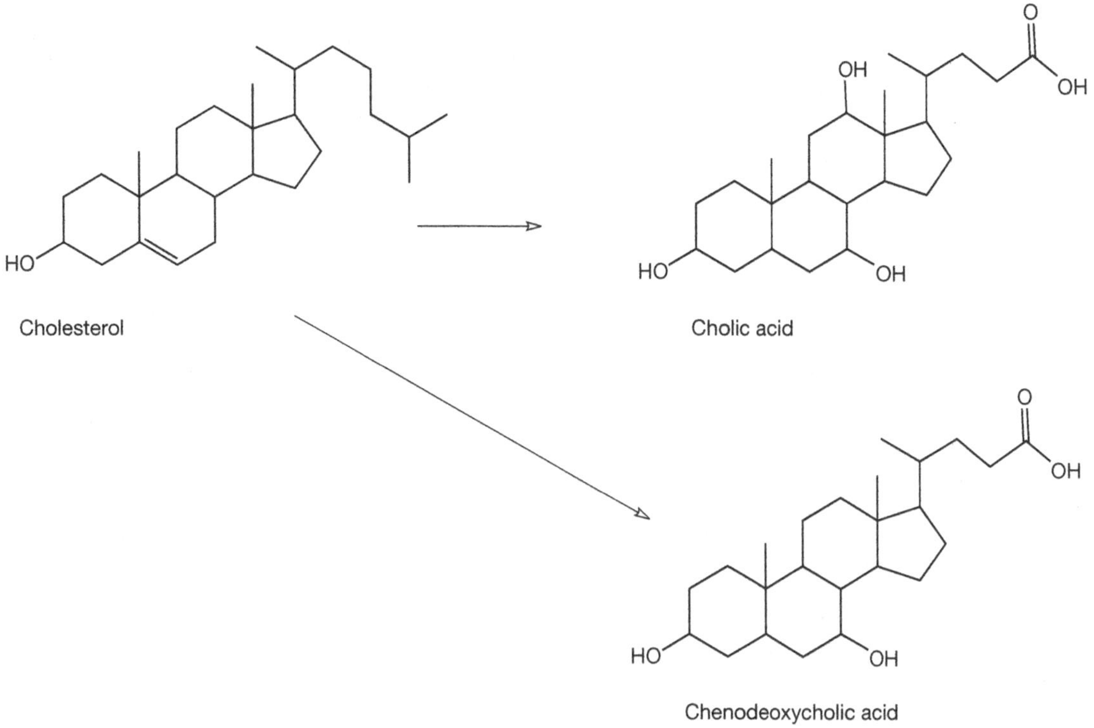

Figure 20.25 Biosynthesis of bile acids from cholesterol.

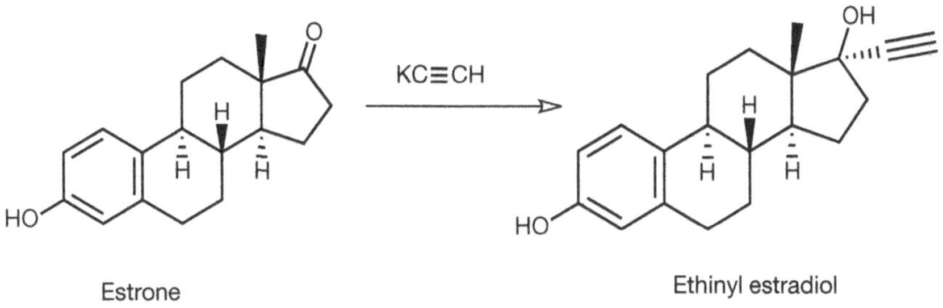

Figure 20.26 Synthesis of ethinyl estradiol from estrone.

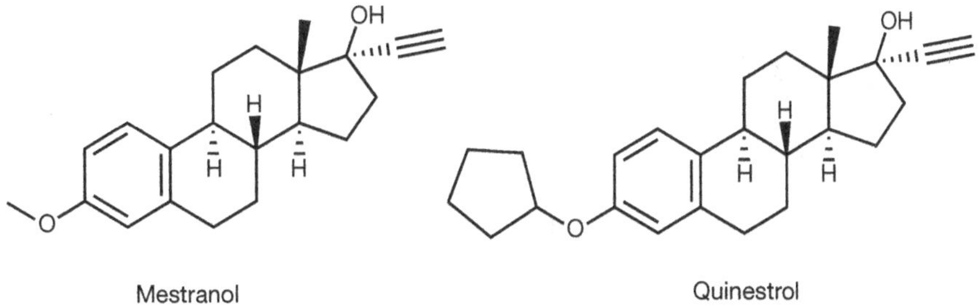

Figure 20.27 The structures of mestranol and quinesterol.

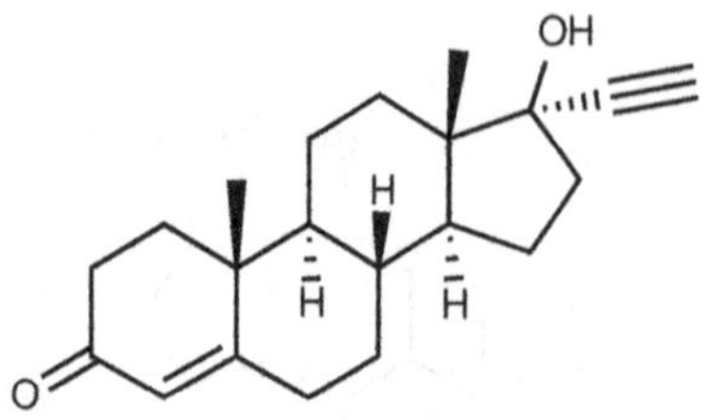

Figure 20.28 Structure of ethisterone.

severe weight loss due to some form of trauma or muscle wasting resulting from, for instance, HIV and in replacement therapy. In such circumstances the formulated product contains testosterone or testosterone esters such as the propionate, enantate [enenthate], undecanoate or mesterolone (Fig. 20.31).

In addition to the use of androgenic anabolic steroids for medical purposes, there is considerable interest in these compounds by sportsmen and women as performance-enhancing drugs. One of the most well-known cases involved Ben Johnson, who was found to have been taking stanozolol. Diana Modahl was found to have testosterone levels that were well above the allowed limits and also her testosterone/epitestosterone ratio was also high. However, when the reserve sample was tested it was discovered that there were difficulties with the sample and the case was dropped. Dwain Chambers was found to have taken tetrahydrogestrinone, and Greg Rusedski was found to have taken nandrolone. However, he was subsequently cleared because of what was thought to be a problem with supplements supplied by the Association of Tennis Players (and taken by a large number of tennis players who also proved positive) that appears to have been contaminated with this steroid.

The cyclist Floyd Landis was also found to have high testosterone/epitestosterone levels. The structure of some of these steroids is shown in Figure 20.32. Stanozolol and nandrolone have been used for conventional medical purposes and epitestosterone is the 17-hydroxy epimer of testosterone that is present naturally in the human body. These, along with many other anabolic steroids, have been used in sport and by bodybuilders on the basis that these compounds are capable of increasing muscle mass and increasing their competitive nature. The problem is that although the use of such compounds may be relatively safe at the levels used for conventional medical treatment, their use as performance-enhancing drugs often involves much higher doses, and it has been suggested that these doses may well lead to serious side effects such as hepatotoxicity, hepatitis and the risk of tumour growth.

Tetrahydrogestrinone achieved fame as one of the 'designer' steroids produced by the American company Bay Area Laboratory Cooperative (BALCO) in California. The chemists in the company studied known agents with anabolic activity to develop new agents that would be unknown to the drug testing laboratories. In the case of tetrahydrogestrinone, the chemists worked on the production of this designer drug based on knowledge of the activities of trenbolone and gestrinone (Fig. 20.33).

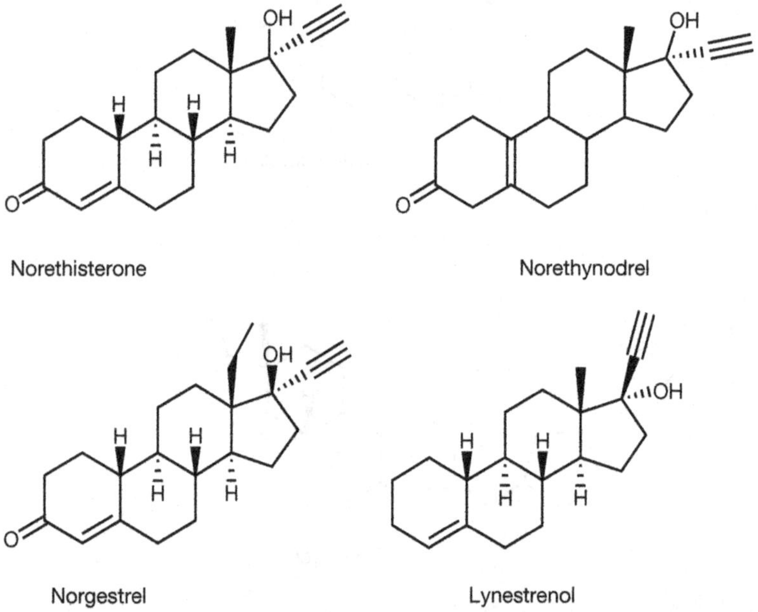

Figure 20.29 Synthetic progestogens.

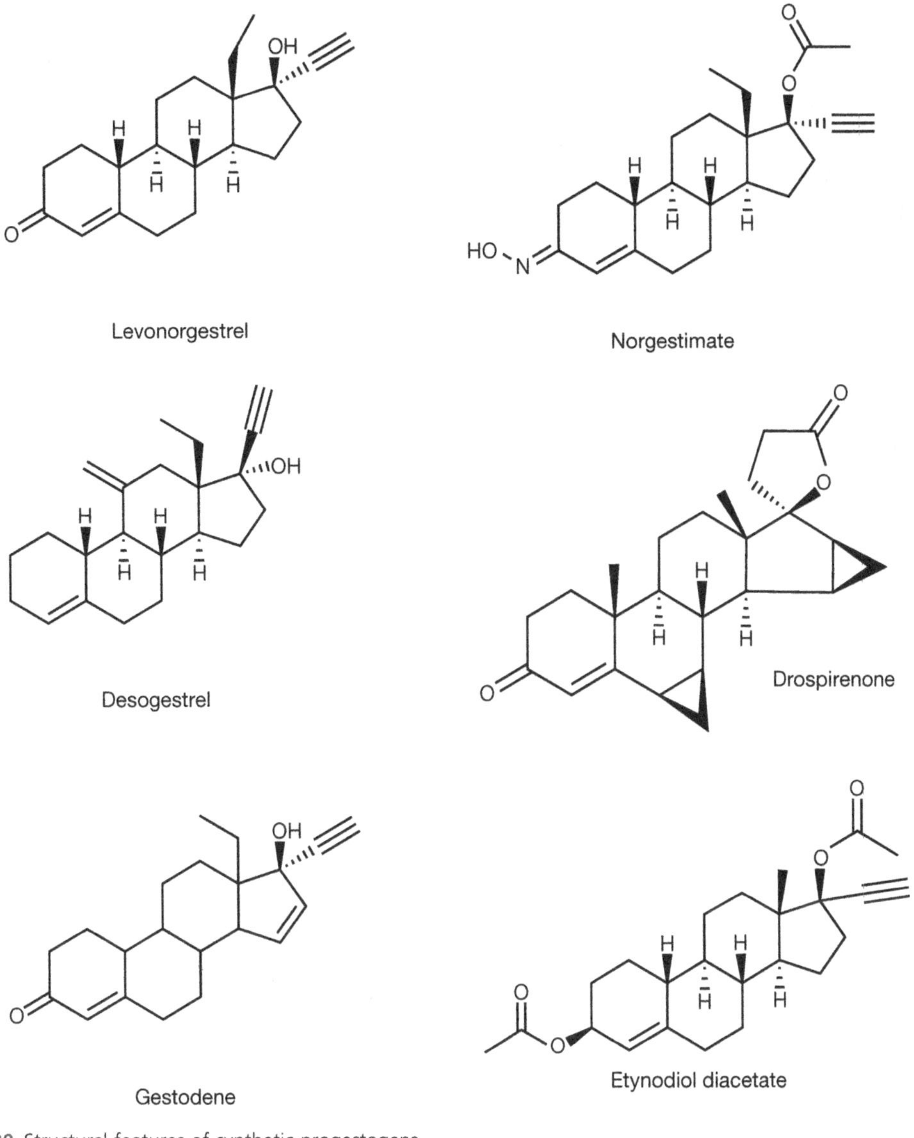

Figure 20.30 Structural features of synthetic progestogens.

The compound was synthesised by the palladium charcoal catalysed hydrogenation of the acetylenic group of gestrinone. This compound was used for a number of years by athletes and it was undetected for a number of years until a sample was sent to Don Catlin, the director of the drug testing laboratory at UCLA, who, along with his team there, developed analytical methodology for the detection and quantification of this steroid. There are likely to be more such 'designer' compounds emerging and thus there is a constant need for vigilance by the drug testing agencies.

One final area where steroids are used is as anti-androgens in the treatment of benign prostatic hyperplasia, prostate cancer and male hypersexuality. Dutasteride and finasteride (Fig. 20.34) are specific inhibitors of 5α-reductase, which is involved in the metabolism of testosterone. These two compounds are indicated for the treatment of benign prostatic hyperplasia, with finasteride also being indicated for male-pattern baldness.

Cyproterone acetate is an anti-androgen, which is indicated for the treatment of prostate cancer and male hypersexuality. It is an inhibitor of 21-hydrolase.

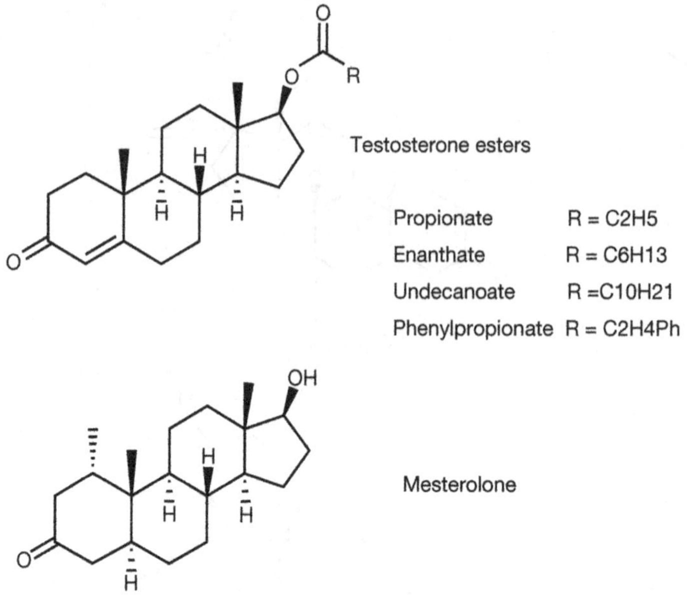

Figure 20.31 Structure of testosterone esters and mesterolone.

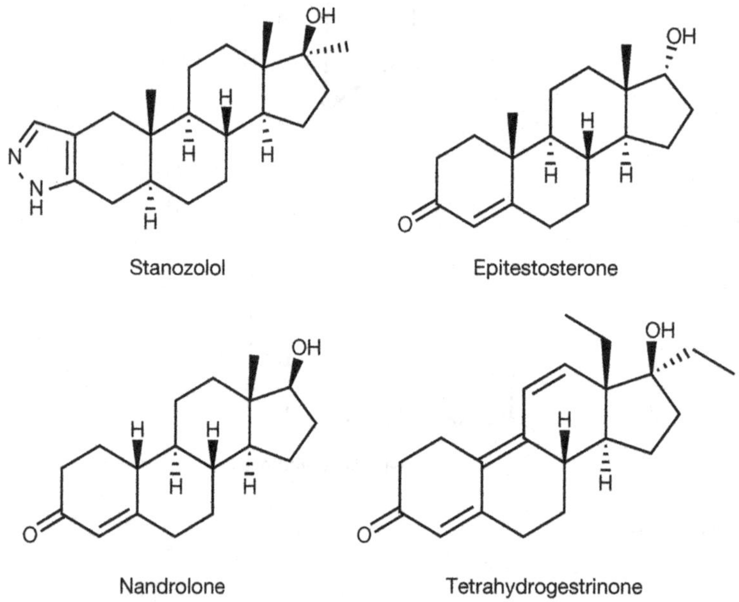

Figure 20.32 Structures of anabolic steroids associated with drug abuse in sport.

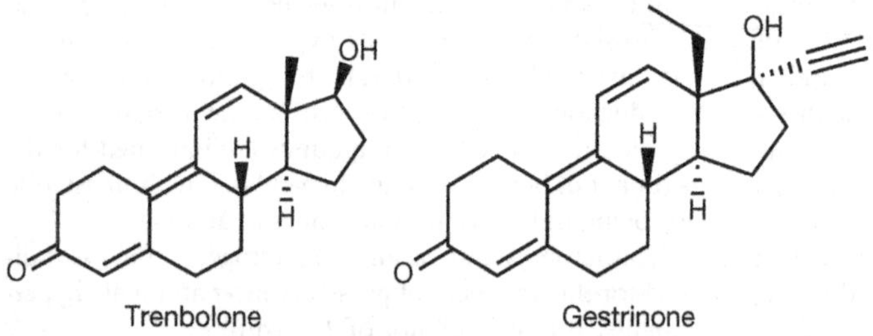

Figure 20.33 The structures of trenbolone and gestrinone.

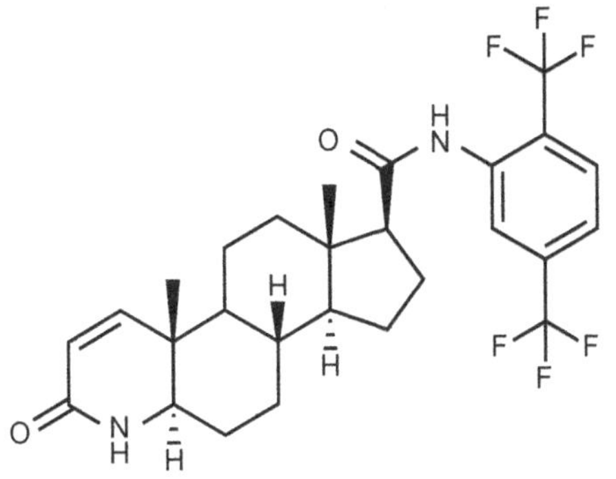

Dutasteride

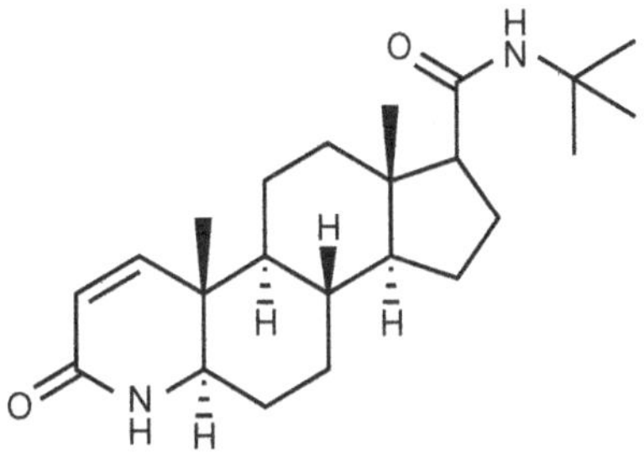

Finasteride

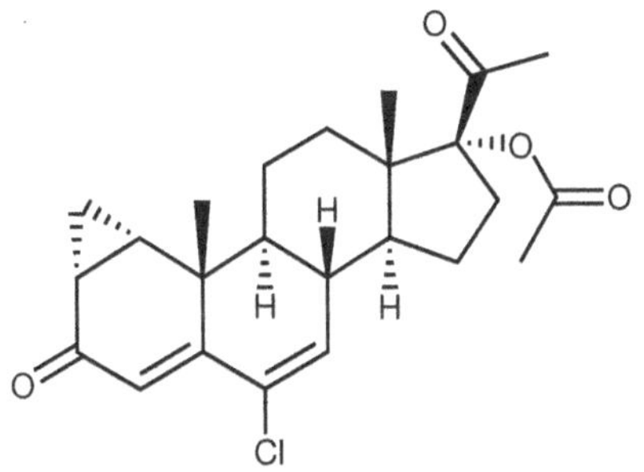

Cyproterone acetate

Figure 20.34 Anti-androgens dutasteride, finasteride and cyproterone acetate.

Glucocorticosteroids and mineralocorticosteroids

The glucocorticosteroids and mineralocorticosteroids are produced in the adrenal gland. The major glucocorticosteroids are cortisol (hydrocortisone), cortisone and corticosterosterone. The natural glucocorticosteroids are important because of their involvement in the control of metabolism of fats, carbohydrates and proteins (Fig. 20.35). Additionally, they play important roles in inflammation, the immune system and in the stress response. Production of these hormones is under the control of adrenocorticotrophic hormone (ACTH), which is secreted by the pituitary, and this influences the adrenal gland to produce cortisol, etc.

Synthetic glucocorticoids are indicated for a wide variety of conditions including rheumatoid arthritis, asthma, ankylosing spondylitis, lupus erythematosus, inflammatory bowel disease, dermatitis, allergic reaction, etc. These steroids are available in a variety of formulations allowing for oral, topical, inhalation and intravenous forms. Typical examples of synthetic glucocorticoids include betamethasone, cortisone acetate, deflazacort, dexamethasone, hydrocortisone, methylprednisolone and triamcinalone (Fig. 20.36). As can be seen, this group of compounds are structurally similar, with the modification of several positions having a major bearing on the activity. The introduction of unsaturation at C_{1-2} increases the glucocorticoid activity as does the ethyl group at C_{16}. The introduction of the fluorine atom increases glucocorticoid activity but also increases mineralocorticoid activity as well. Various other modifications have also been shown to have significant effects on the activity. For example, C21 ester formation and acetonide formation via C16, and 17 hydroxyl, as in triamcinolone acetonide, aids in the topical activity of these steroids through changes in the lipophilicity, improving absorption by the skin.

The main mineralocorticosteroid is aldosterone (see Fig. 20.24), which plays an important role in the renin-angiotensin system. As a result of various possible stimuli, e.g. hypotension, decreased sodium levels, etc., the renin-angiotensin system is activated and renin is produced, and this enzyme is responsible for the conversion of angiotensinogen into angiotensin. Angiotensin is responsible for the stimulation of the adrenals to produce aldosterone. Aldosterone is then responsible for the retention of

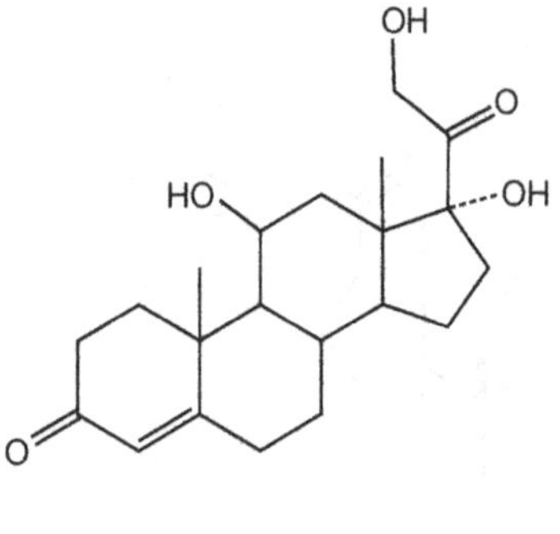

Cortisol (hydrocortisone)

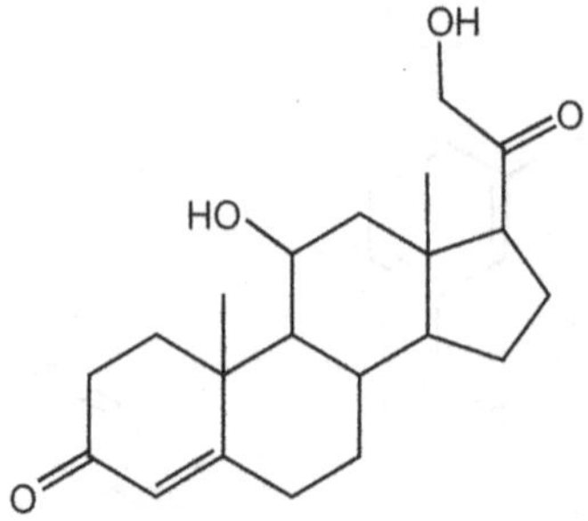

Corticosterone

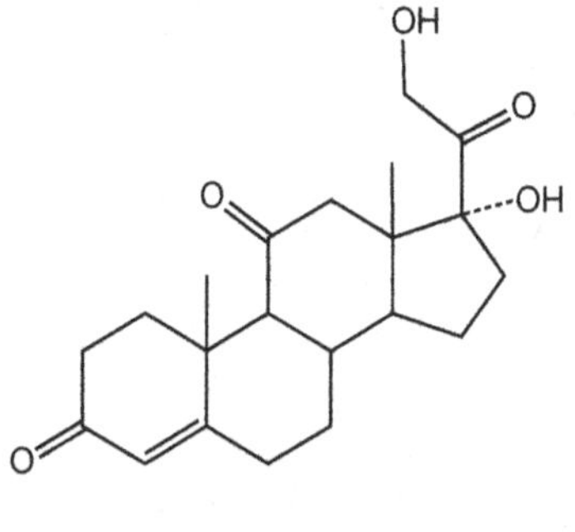

Cortisone

Figure 20.35 Corticosteroids.

sodium in the kidneys and an increase in fluid volume within the body. Unlike most steroids, it binds to membrane receptors rather than as part of a protein receptor complex to DNA. There are a number of disease states (hypoadrenalism, Addison's disease) where the adrenal glands fail to produce aldosterone (and cortisone), and replacement therapy is required. In the case of aldosterone, it is not possible for it to be used directly in replacement therapy because it is too unstable, and fludrocortisone acetate (Fig. 20.37) is used in its place.

Steroids used in the treatment of asthma

Asthma is a disease state in which the airways in the lungs become inflamed and narrow, thus causing difficulty in breathing. Reports suggest that in the UK and the USA approximately 7–10% of the population are in receipt of a prescription for asthma drugs. Asthma is a reversible condition whereby, in response to a trigger, the asthmatic attack is initiated; this trigger may be an allergen, an environmental trigger (chemical, vapour, tobacco smoke, etc.) or exercise. There are numerous drugs used in the treatment of asthma including inhaled and oral corticosteroids, β_2 agonists (both long acting (LABAs) and short acting), leukotriene modifiers and bronchodilators. In some instances, corticosteroids and bronchodilators are combined in an inhaler. Glucocorticosteroids are used in the treatment of asthma because of their anti-inflammatory activity. The structures of inhaled and oral corticosteroids used in this area are detailed in Figures 20.38 and 20.39.

The corticosteroids are active anti-inflammatory agents via their involvement in the arachidonic acid cascade, which leads to the formation of prostaglandins and leucotrienes which are responsible for the inflammatory response (see Ch. 2). The arachidonic acid is formed by the breakdown of phospholipid membranes, which is brought about by the enzyme phospholipase A_2. The corticosteroids are thought to be involved in the stimulation of the synthesis of proteins (lipocortins) that are able to inhibit the action of phospholipase A_2, thus reducing the production of arachidonic acid.

THE CARDIAC GLYCOSIDES

Cardiac glycosides, such as digoxin and digitoxin (Fig. 20.40), are indicated for the treatment of heart failure and supraventricular arrhythmias. These two

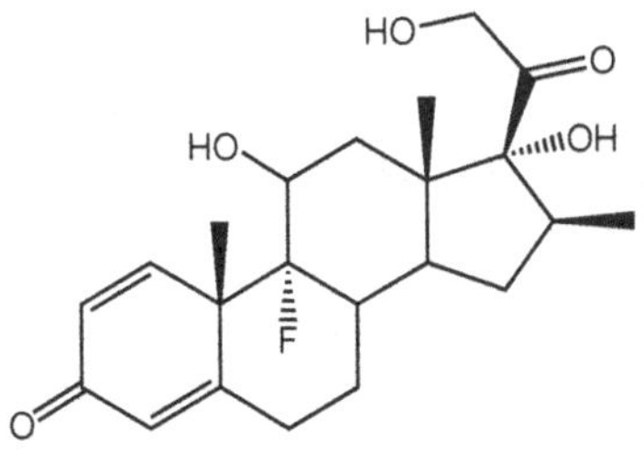

Betamethasone

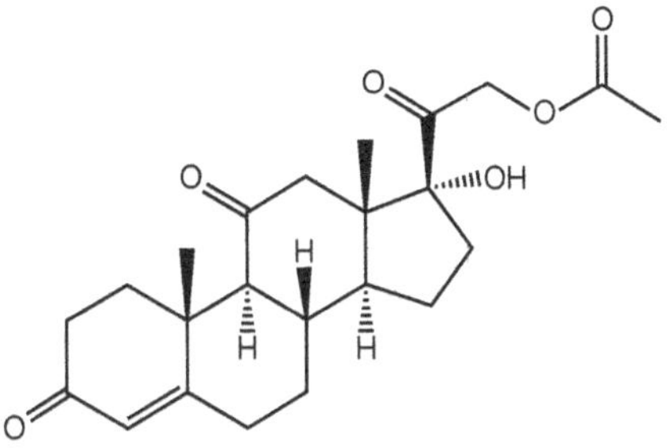

Cortisone acetate

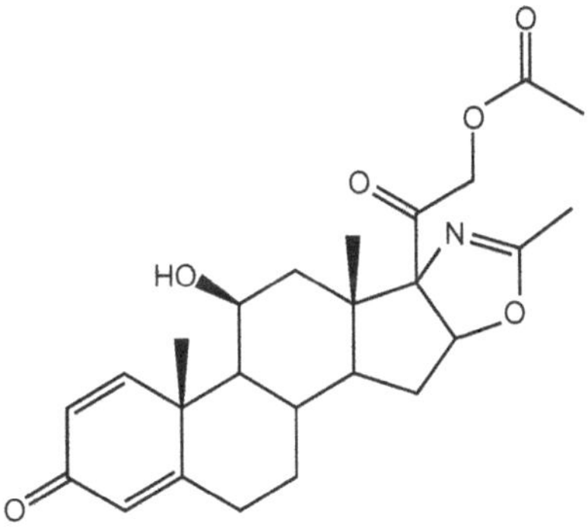

Deflazacort

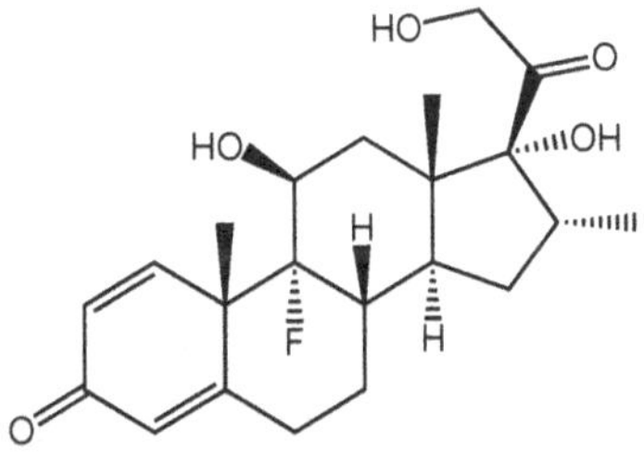

Dexamethasone

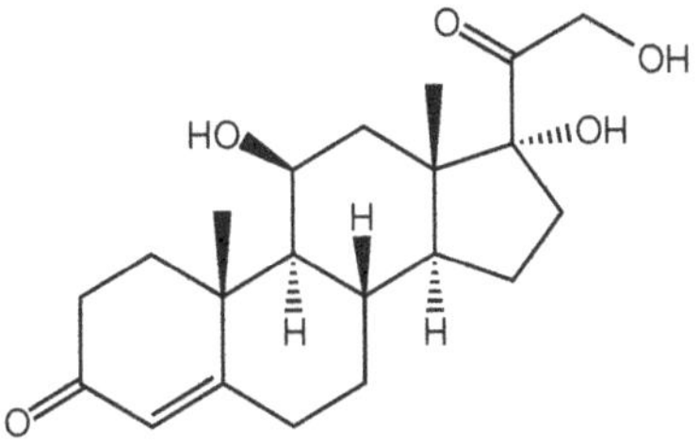

Hydrocortisone

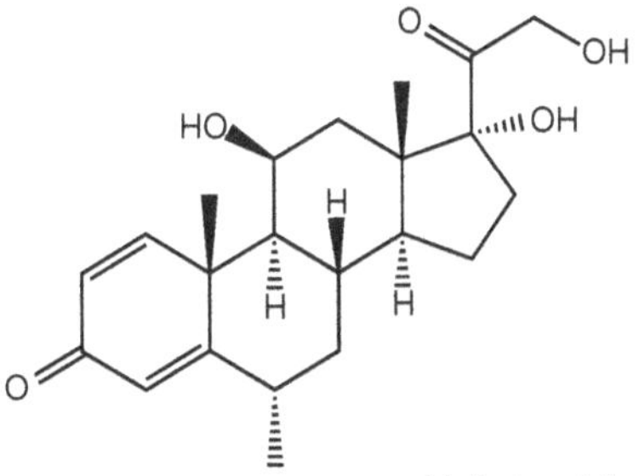

Methylprednisolone

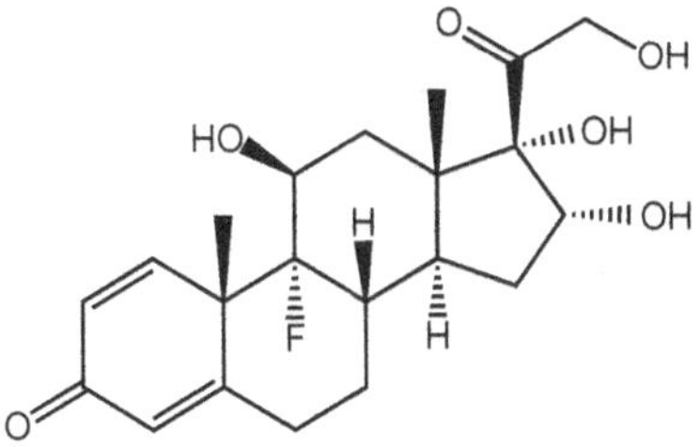

Triamcinalone

Figure 20.36 Synthetic glucocorticosteroids.

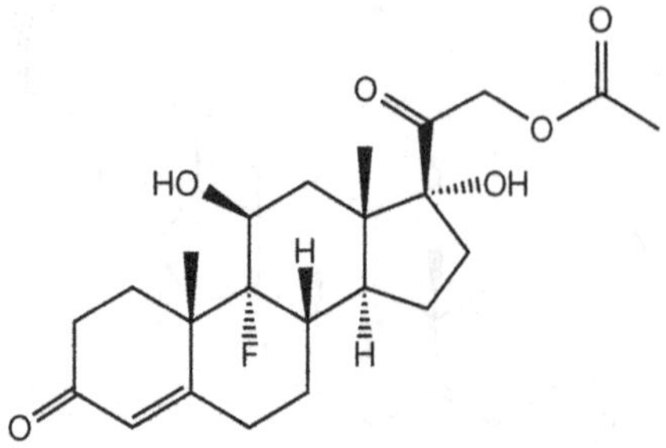

Figure 20.37 Fludrocortisone acetate.

compounds, which are naturally occurring compounds, are defined as glycosides since they are comprised of a sugar portion, the glycone moiety, and the aglycone portion, which in this case is a steroid (other glycosides exist, e.g. apterin which is a coumarin glycoside). These cardiac glycosides are obtained from species of digitalis, digoxin from *Digitalis lanata* and digitoxin from *Digitalis purpurea*. These compounds are cardenolides indicating that they contain an unsaturated butyrolactone ring system.

The mode of action of the cardiac glycosides is via their inhibitory action on the system Na-K-ATPase, which eventually results in increased intracellular calcium levels. These increased calcium levels result in a series of events that produce an increase in the strength of contraction of the heart (positive inotropic effect) and a reduction in the heart rate (negative chronotropic effect).

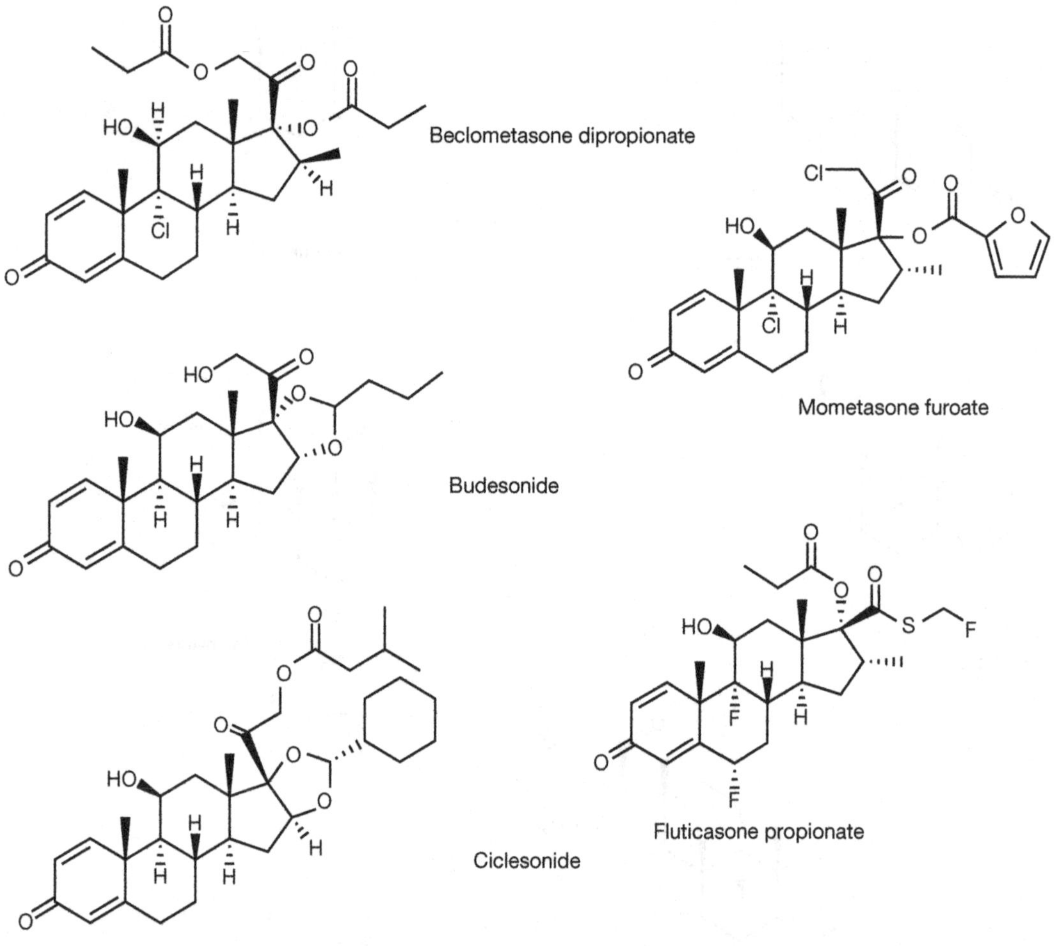

Figure 20.38 Inhaled steroids used in asthma treatment.

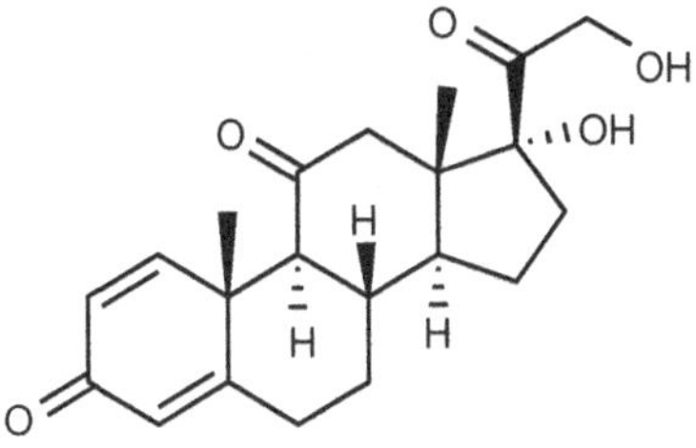

Prednisone

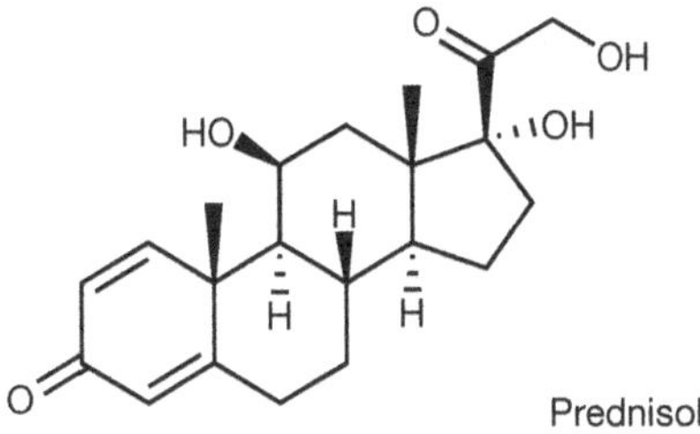

Prednisolone

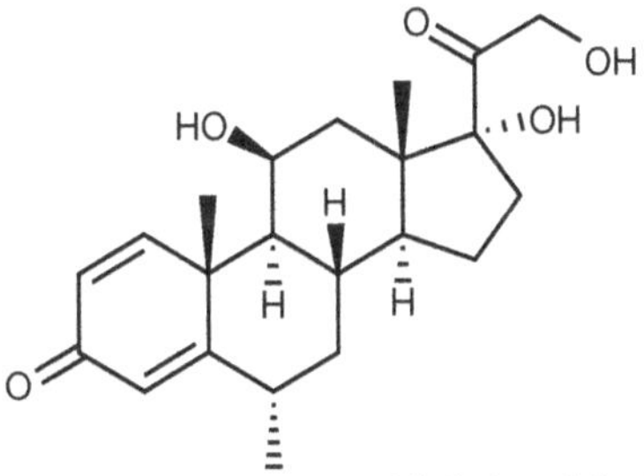

Methylprednisolone

Figure 20.39 Oral steroids used in asthma treatment.

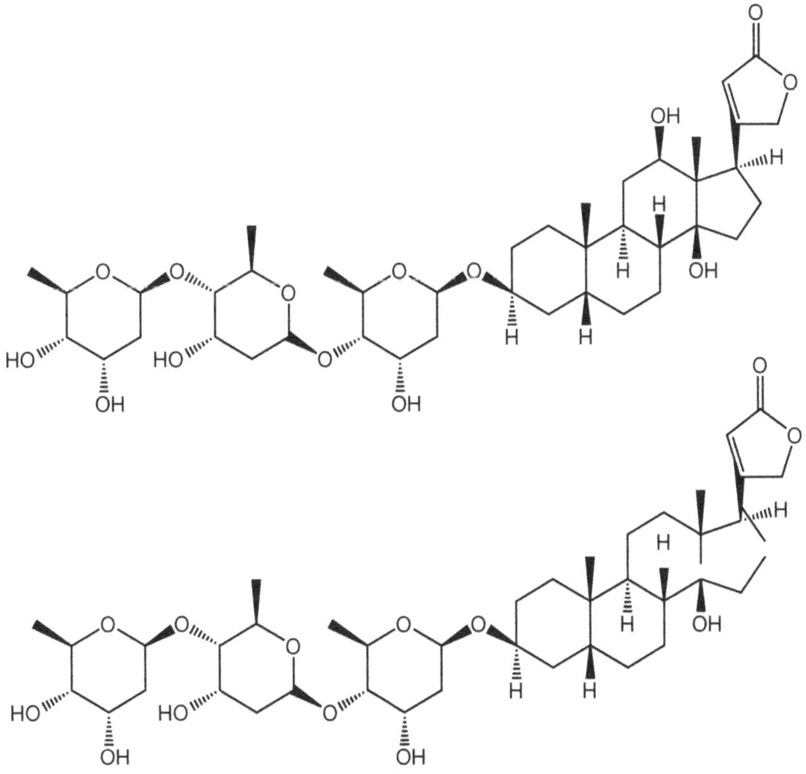

Figure 20.40 Cardiac glycosides.

FURTHER READING

General reading

Katz M, Gans EH. Topical corticosteroids, structure-activity and the glucocorticoid receptor: Discovery and development – A process of planned serendipity. *J Pharm Sci*. 2008;97(8): 2936–2946.

The endocrine system

http://www.vivo.colostate.edu/hbooks/pathphys/endocrine/index.html.

Steroidogenesis

http://www.vivo.colostate.edu/hbooks/pathphys/endocrine/basics/steroidogenesis.html.

Hormones of the reproductive system

http://users.rcn.com/jkimball.ma.ultranet/BiologyPages/S/SexHormones.html.

Inhaled anaesthetics

Campagna JA. Mechanisms of actions of inhaled anesthetics. *N Engl J Med*. 2003;348(21):2110–2124.

Epilepsy

http://www.pharmj.com/pdf/hp/200307/hp_200307_epilepsyaetiology.pdf.

http://www.pharmj.com/pdf/hp/200307/hp_200307_epilepsydrugtherapy.pdf.

Chapter 21

Anticancer drugs

David G Watson

CHAPTER CONTENTS

INTRODUCTION

Antineoplastic drugs have a major role in cancer treatment, sometimes alone and sometimes in conjunction with surgery or radiotherapy. The modern era of chemotherapy in cancer treatment began after the Second World War, following observations of the effects of nitrogen mustards, which had been developed as chemical warfare agents, on transplanted lymphomas in mice. The nitrogen mustards were the first drugs in the alkylating agent class of anticancer drugs and they were followed soon by antimetabolites, the first one of which was aminopterin, a folate antagonist. The antineoplastic drugs can be classified as follows: (1) alkylating agents, (2) antimetabolites, (3) natural products, (4) organometallic compounds, (5) hormones, (6) angiogenesis inhibitors, (7) signal transduction inhibitors, and (8) miscellaneous including biotechnologically produced drugs.

ALKYLATING AGENTS

Nitrogen mustards

Nitrogen mustards have the general structure shown in Figure 21.1. They form an aziridinium ion which is subject to attack by the nucleophilic positions within DNA bases. The positions within DNA which can be subject to attack include: N-2, N-3, O-6 and N-7 of guanine; N-1, N-3 and N-7 of adenine; O-6 of thymine; N-3 of cytosine and phosphate oxygen atoms (see Ch. 7). The availability of the lone pair on the nitrogen is critical for formation of the aziridinium ion and the nitrogen must have a p*Ka* of 6 or less so that the drug is largely un-ionised at pH 7.4. The low p*Ka* is ensured by the R groups, being electron withdrawing; in addition, the chloroethyl groups alone reduce the p*Ka* of the nitrogen. The damaged DNA formed by the cross-linking reaction shown in Figure 21.1 prevents cell division from occurring. This class of drugs relies on cancer cells being rapidly dividing in order to target them, but also targets other fast-growing cells such as white blood cells, resulting in

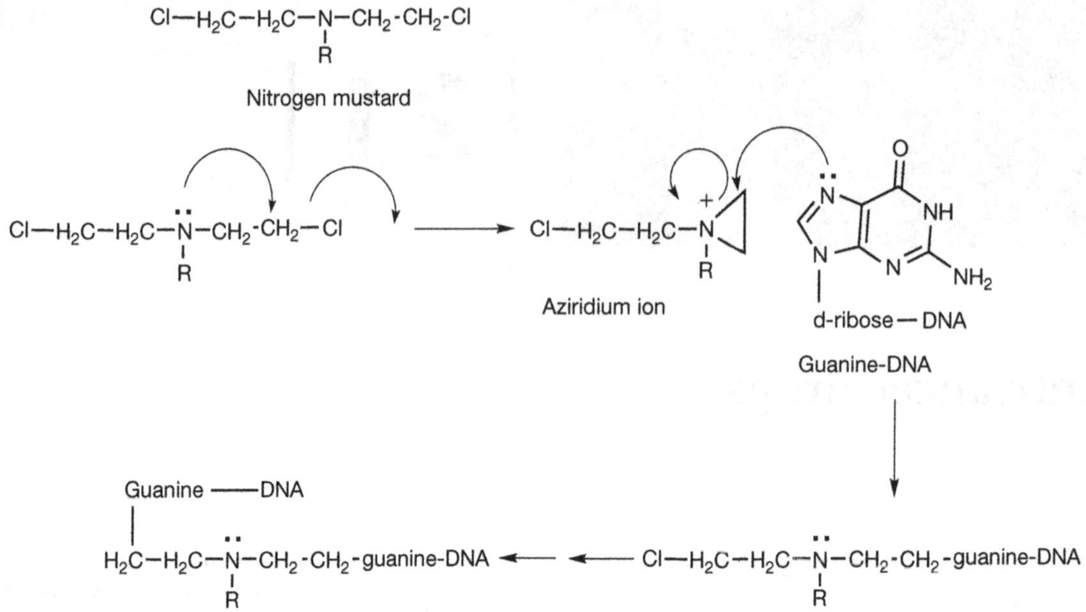

Figure 21.1 Mechanism of DNA cross-linking by nitrogen mustards.

myelosuppression. Nitrogen mustards include meclorethamine (less used because it is highly toxic and reactive) and chlorambucil and melphalan, where the reactivity of the nitrogen atom is reduced by the benzene ring withdrawing electrons, thus producing compounds which are slow alkylators (Fig. 21.2). In the case of melphalan there was a hope that it would be useful for targeting melanoma, since phenylalanine is a biosynthetic precursor of melanin; however, clinical data gave no indication of such targeting. This type of targeting is also used in the case of estramustine

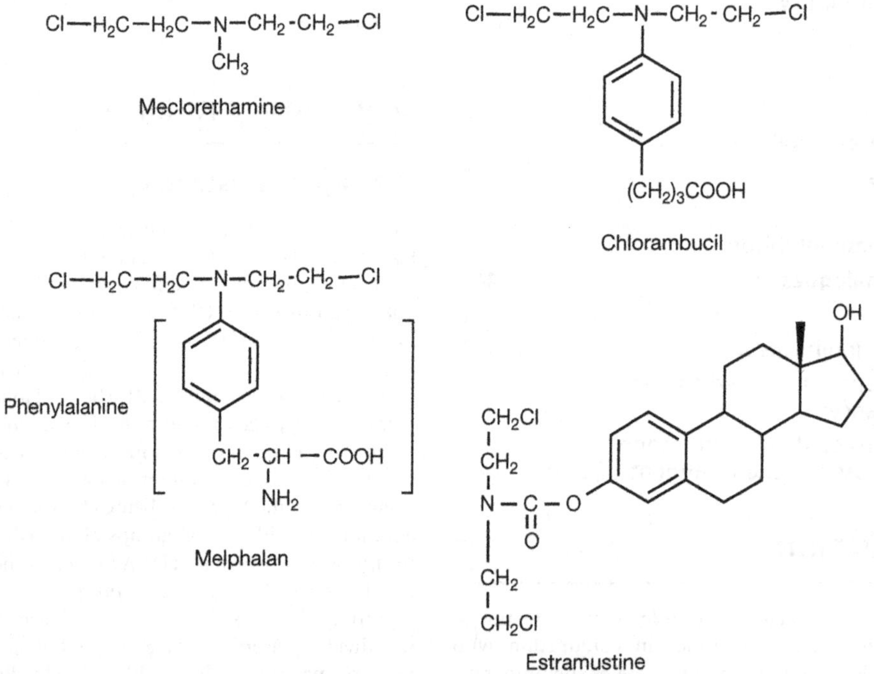

Figure 21.2 Slow alkylating anti-cancer drugs.

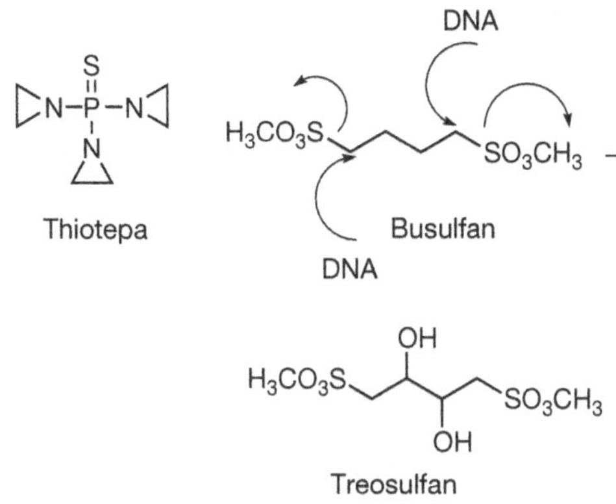

Figure 21.3 Mechanism of busulfan action.

phosphate, which is used to treat prostate cancer. In this case, the nitrogen mustard is linked to estradiol which has some effect in targeting the oestrogen-dependent tumour.

Other types of reactive alkylating reagents have been developed. Some of these have the aziridine ring already built into them such as thiotepa (Fig. 21.3), which is a slow alkylator, since the ring has to be activated by protonation before it will alkylate.

In busulfan (Fig. 21.3) it is the sulphonate group which is a good leaving group and which promotes alkylation of DNA. The four carbon atom spacing between the alkylating groups is optimal for cross-linking DNA strands. The mode of action of treosulfan is similar to that of busulfan.

Cyclophosphamide is closely related in its mode of action to the nitrogen mustards. It is a prodrug which is activated via the action of a P450 enzyme as shown in Figure 21.4.

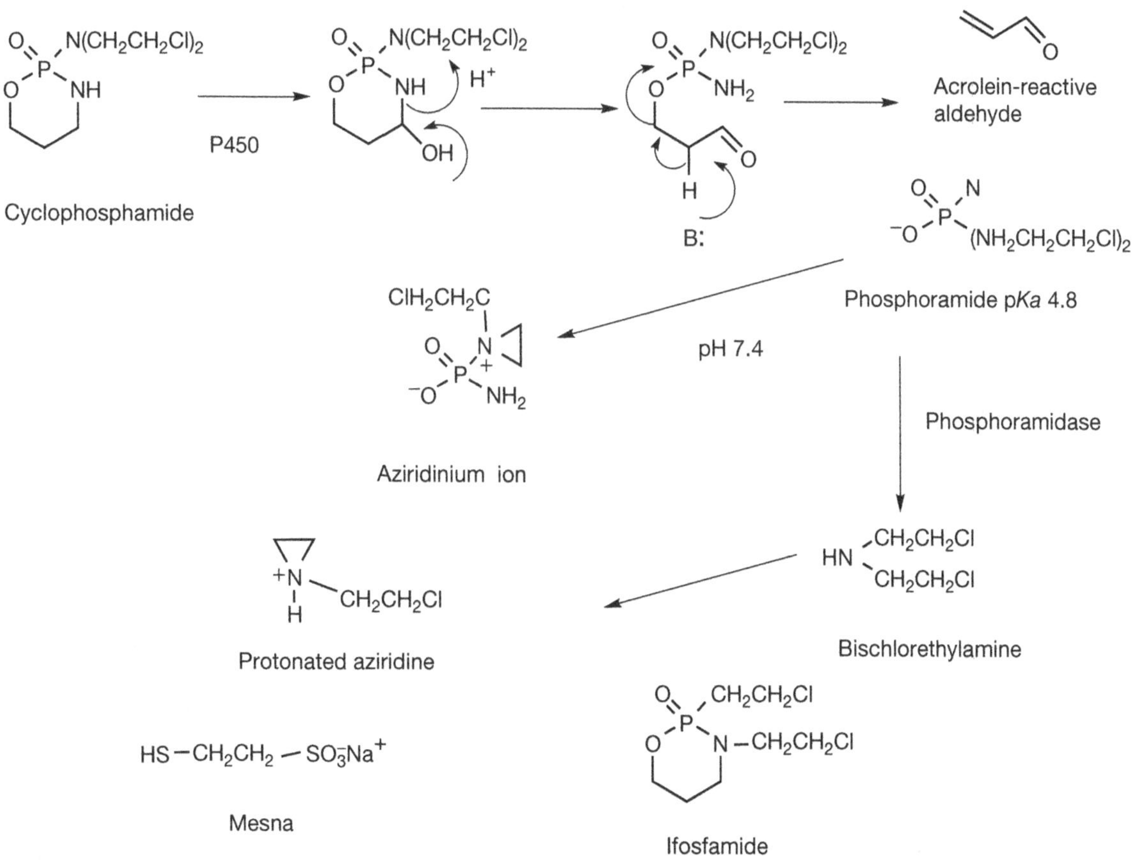

Figure 21.4 Mechanism of action of cyclophosphamide.

The product of the enzyme action then breaks down into a phosphoramide mustard and acrolein which may be responsible for some of the side effects of the drug. The side effects of acrolein can be reduced by co-administration of a sulfhydryl reagent such as mesna, which converts the acrolein into an inactive product. The phosphoramide metabolite is strongly acidic which means that it is completely ionised within cells and becomes trapped there. The phosphoramide is a reactive nitrogen mustard and can form the aziridinium ion which reacts with DNA bases as was shown in Figure 21.1. The selectivity for neoplastic cells may be due to their lower pH, which results in slower formation of the aziridinium ion and hence longer persistence of the trapped drug within the cells. Alternatively, neoplastic cells have high levels of phosphoramidases, which results in the formation of chloroethylamine which alkylates DNA via protonated aziridine.

Isophosphamide is an isomer of cyclophosphamide which is activated in a similar manner via a P450 enzyme. It is metabolised more slowly than cyclophosphamide, which may offer some advantages.

The final category of alkylating reagents is the nitrosoureas. The two commonly used drugs are carmustine and lomustine (Fig. 21.5). As shown in Figure 21.5 for lomustine, the nitrosoureas undergo spontaneous decomposition in an aqueous environment to produce two reactive species: a reactive diazohydroxide which can alkylate DNA and an isocyanate which is reactive towards amine groups within proteins.

Temozolomide is an alkylating agent but in this case the alkylating group is methyl. The methyl group derives from diazomethane which is produced by the spontaneous decomposition of the drug in an aqueous environment (Fig. 21.6). The diazomethane then reacts with the 7 position of guanine. However, resistant cells are able to repair DNA which has been damaged in this way, which limits the effectiveness of the drug. However, it is the standard treatment for brain tumours in combination with initial intensive radiotherapy.

Dacarbazine acts in a similar manner to temozolomide, generating diazomethane, but it requires metabolic activation by a cytochrome P450 enzyme before it hydrolyses.

Cisplatin (Fig. 21.7) behaves in a manner analogous to an alkylating agent in that it cross-links guanine nucleotides. The N7 positions of adjacent guanines on a single strand of DNA react with cisplatin. Cisplatin only has a short half-life in plasma since it is hydrolysed in water quite rapidly. Transplatin is less effective as a cytotoxic agent. In part this may be because it is less effectively taken up by cells but also it can only cross-link between two DNA strands which is less effective as a cytotoxic mechanism since the lesion is more readily repaired. Carboplatin is less reactive than cisplatin and has reduced renal toxicity in comparison with it, while remaining an effective cytotoxic. Oxaliplatin similarly has reduced toxicity and altered selectivity.

Preparations of alkylating agents

- Chlorambucil: Tablets 2 mg.
- Chlormethine hydrochloride: Injection 10 mg.
- Estramustine phosphate: Capsules 140 mg.
- Mephalan: Tablets 2 mg.
- Thiotepa: Injection 15 mg.
- Busulfan: Concentrate for i.v. infusion 6 mg/mL, tablets 2 mg.
- Treosulfan: Capsules 250 mg, injection 1 g and 5 g.
- Cyclophosphamide: Tablets 50 mg, injection 200 mg and 500 mg.
- Ifosfamide: Injection 1 g.
- Carmustine: Injection 100 mg, implant 7.7 mg.
- Lomustine: Capsules 40 mg.
- Dacarbazine: Injection 100 mg, 200 mg, 500 mg and 600 mg.
- Temozolomide: Capsules 5 mg and 20 mg.
- Carboplatin: Injection 10 mg/mL.
- Cisplatin: Injection 1 mg/mL and 50 mg for reconstitution.
- Oxaliplatin: Injection 50 mg and 100 mg for reconstitution.

Q Self Test 21.1

Draw the product that would result from the reaction between guanine and the following alkylating drugs.

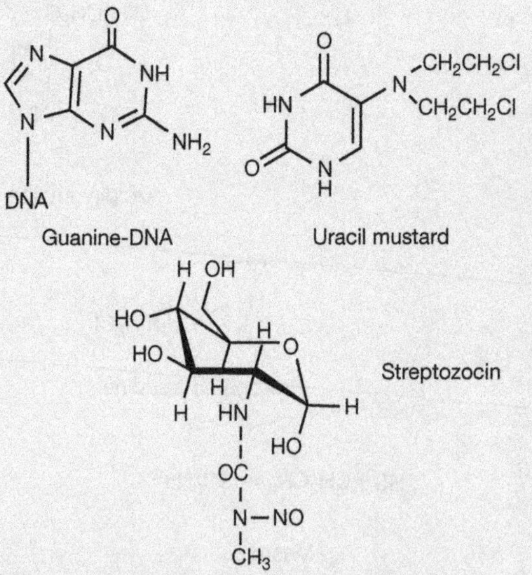

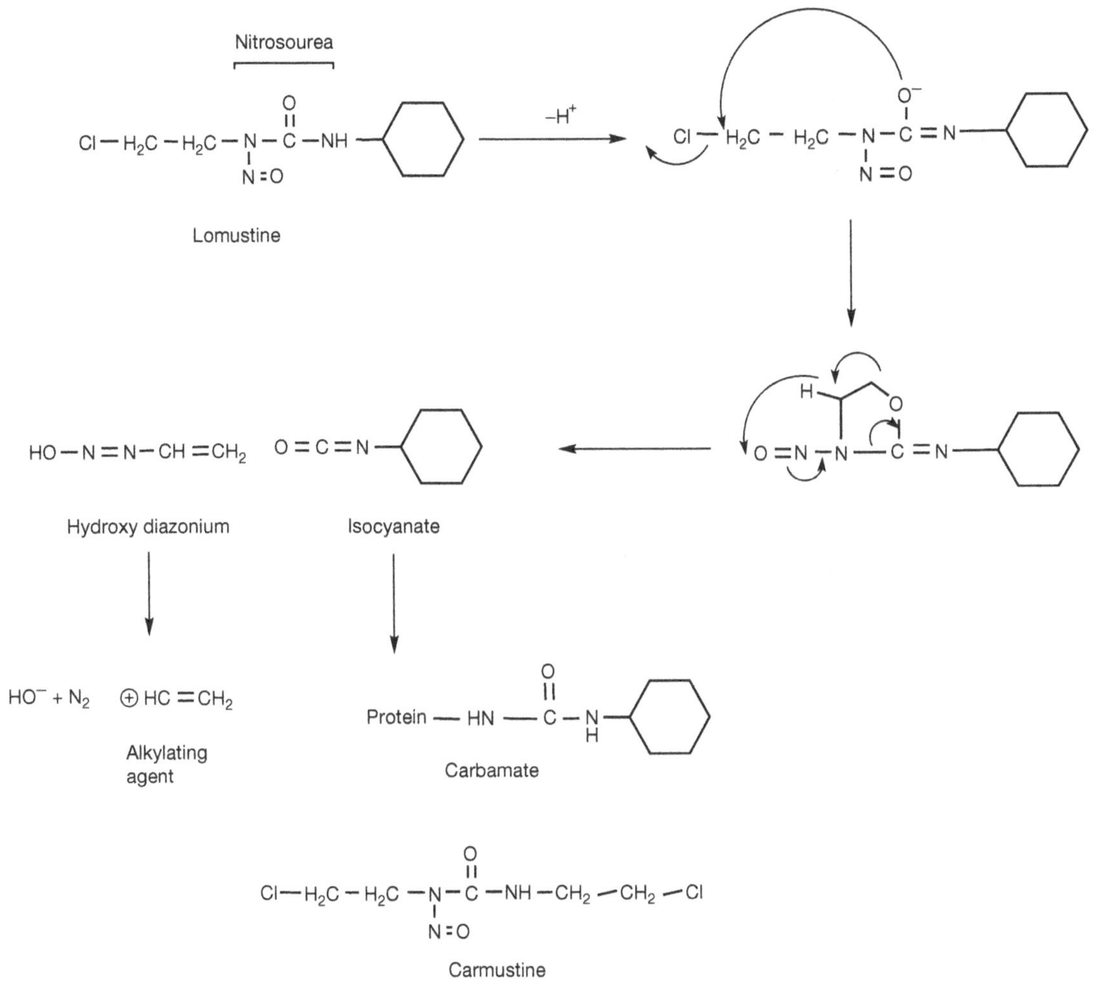

Figure 21.5 Mechanism of lomustine action.

ANTIMETABOLITES

Most antimetabolites are enzyme inhibitors and inhibit key enzymes involved in nucleotide synthesis by acting as false substrates. Mercaptopurine (Fig. 21.8) is one of the most effective drugs for treating childhood leukaemia. It is a prodrug and requires activation to form its ribosyl pyrophosphate derivative in order to become effective. The activated form of the drug inhibits several enzymes involved in nucleotide biosynthesis but the most important of these is phosphoribosyltriphosphate amidotransferase (PPAT). The reaction promoted by PPAT is the rate-limiting step in purine biosynthesis. The enzyme is subject to feedback inhibition by ATP, which binds to a specific site on the enzyme, and mecaptopurine ribosyltriphosphate produces inhibition by a similar mechanism. 2-Thioguanine is similar to mercaptopurine and probably acts via a similar mechanism, mimicking the feedback inhibition produced by GTP.

Pyrimidine antimetabolites act via the inhibition of the synthesis of pyrimidine nucleotides, particularly the inhibition of the biosynthesis of deoxythyminemonophosphate (dTMP). The biosynthesis of dTMP is shown in Figure 21.9. A nucleophilic SH group in thymidylate synthetase attacks carbon-6 in deoxyuridinemonophosphate, precipitating attack on the methylene bridge in 5,10-methylenetetrahydrofolate. The ternary complex then undergoes oxidative breakdown, releasing deoxythymidine monophosphate. In Figure 21.10 the same reaction is shown for the antimetabolite 5-fluorouracil (5-FU),

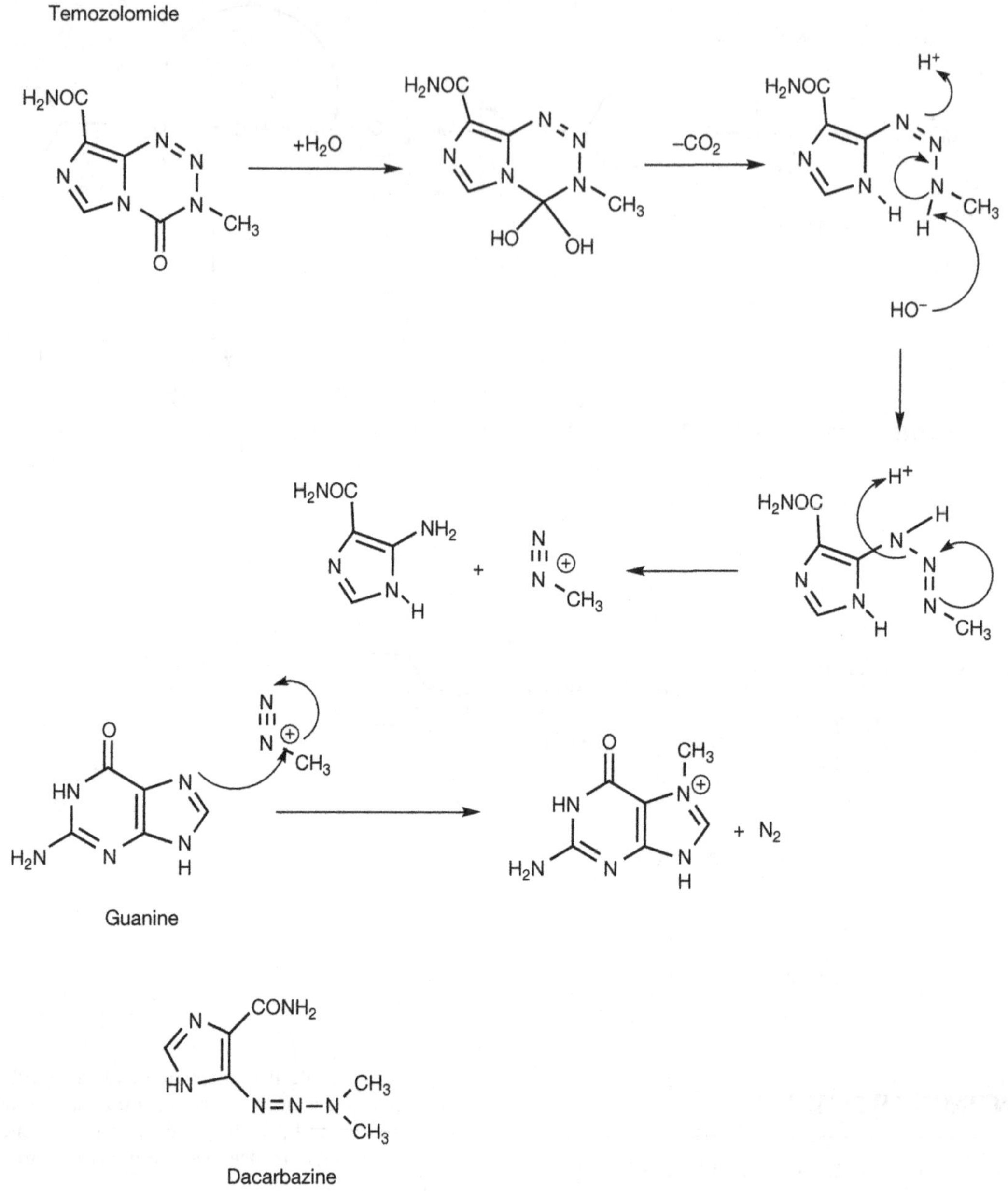

Figure 21.6 Mechanism of action of temozolomide.

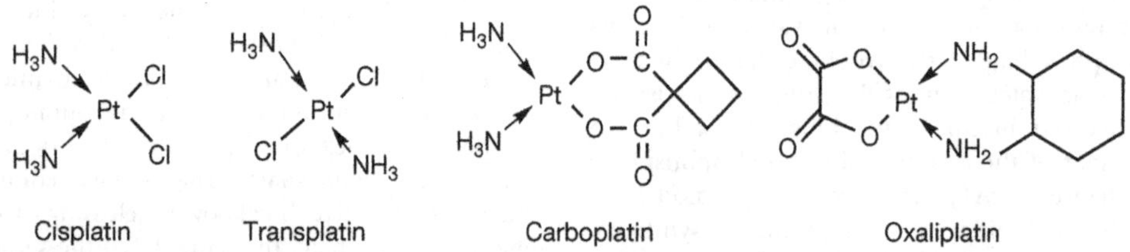

Figure 21.7 Platinum anticancer drugs.

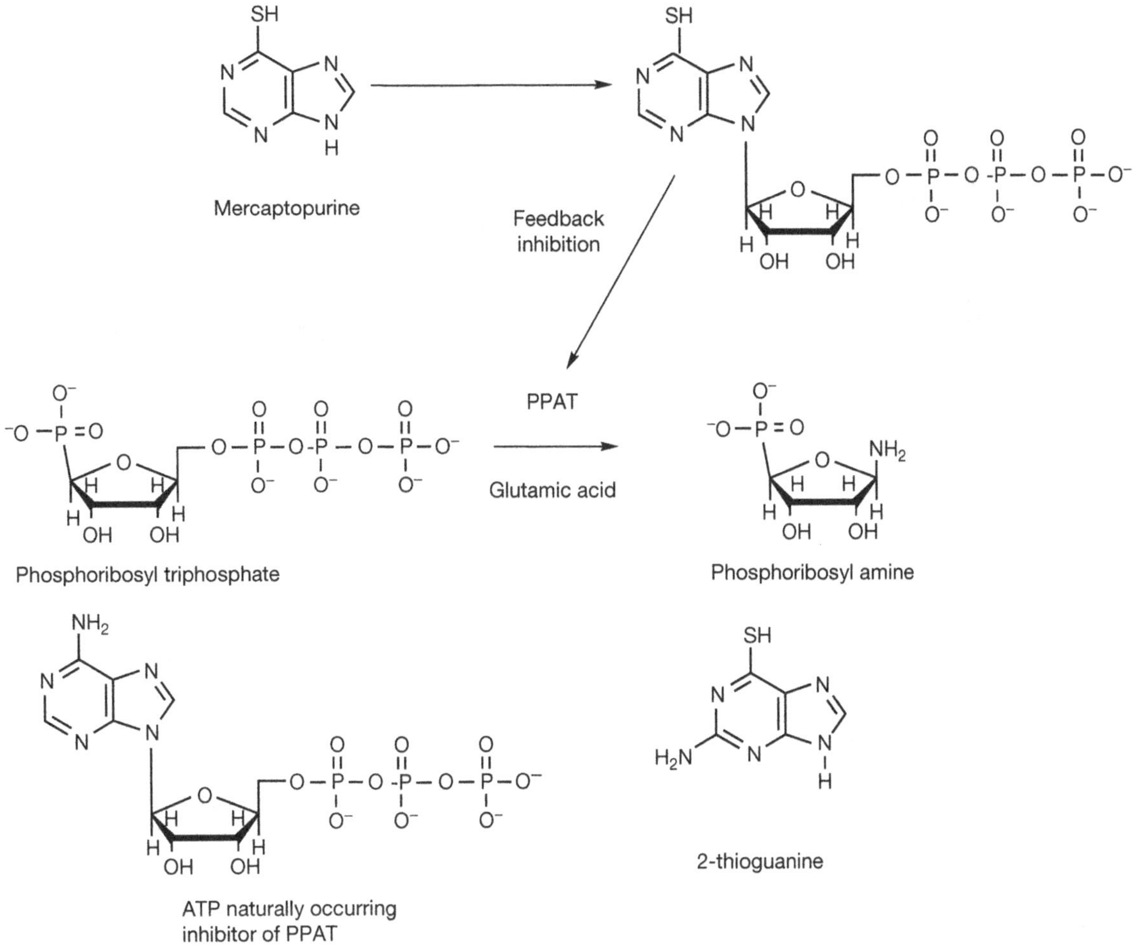

Figure 21.8 Purine antimetabolites.

which is converted to 5-fluorouridinemonophosphate, which forms a complex with 5,10-methylenetetrahydrofolate which *does not* break down to release deoxythymidine monophosphate and dihydrofolate, and this results in inhibition of DNA formation.

The oral bioavailability of 5-FU is variable due it being enzymatically reduced in the gut wall. Tegafur (Fig. 21.10) was developed as a prodrug of 5-FU with better oral bioavailability resulting from its resistance to reduction during absorption. It is slowly metabolised to 5-FU in the liver. Capecitabine is another prodrug of 5-FU which has improved oral bioavailability and is converted to 5-FU by three enzymes in the liver: carboxyesterase, cytidine deaminase and uridine phosphorylase. Apart from improved oral bioavailability, the drug has some selectivity for tumours expressing a high level of uridine phosphorylase activity.

A number of drugs have been targeted at DNA polymerase. The adenine analogue fludarabine (Fig. 21.11) binds to DNA polymerase and ribonucleotide reductase, thus interfering with DNA synthesis. Cladribine is similar in structure to fludarabine but is much more toxic. It acts by inhibiting enzymes involved in DNA repair. The potential for interfering with ribonucleotide reductase arises from the replacement of ribose with its epimer arabinose. Thus the 2′ position can not be reduced as shown in Figure 21.11 for ribose. Cytarabine is a pyrimidine nucleoside analogue. It is phosphorylated in cells and acts via inhibition of DNA polymerase and via incorporation into DNA and RNA, producing miscoding. It also incorporates arabinose in place of ribose and thus can interfere with ribonucleotide reductase. Gemcitabine is an analogue of deoxycytidine in which fluorine has been introduced into the sugar ring. Since fluorine is very similar in size to

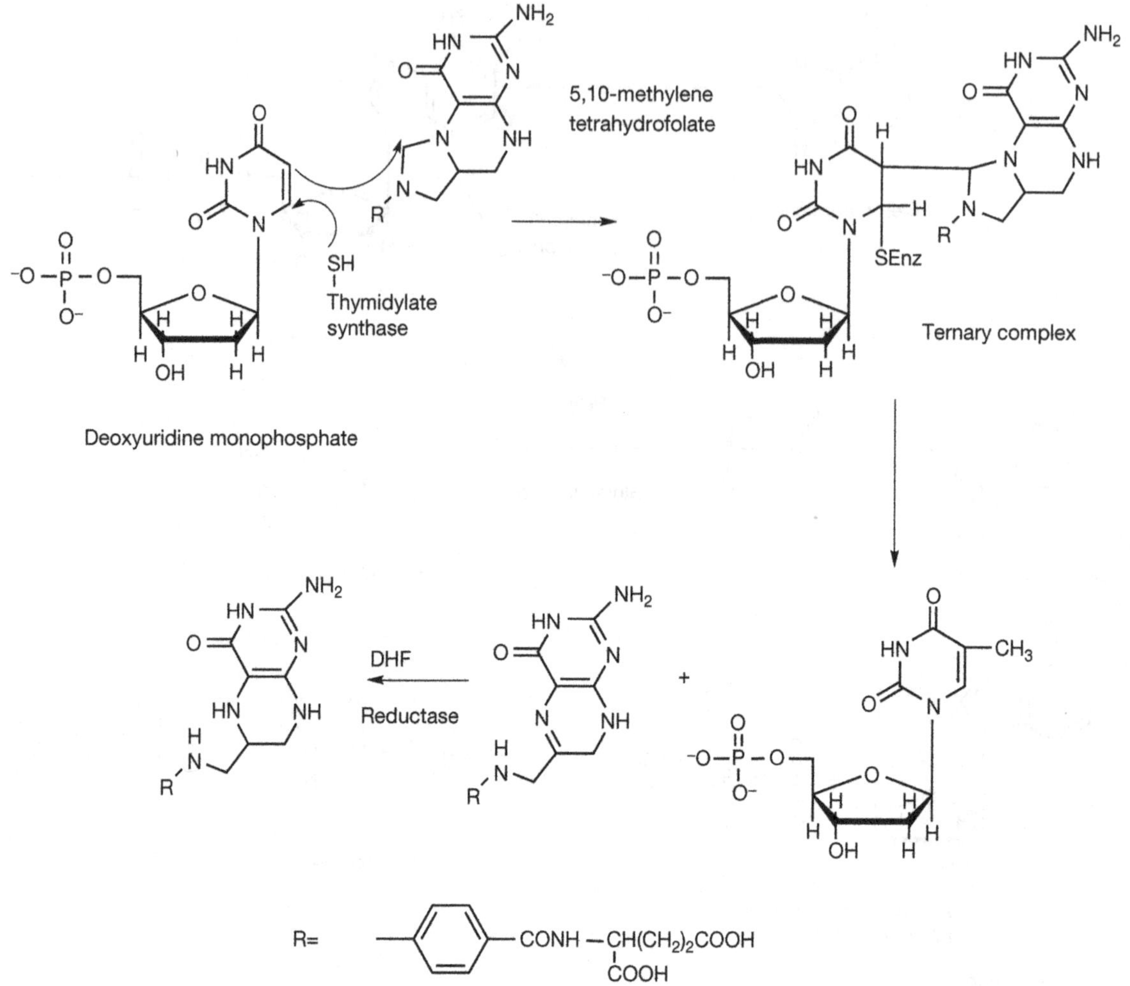

Figure 21.9 Biosynthesis of thymidine monophosphate.

hydrogen, it is a substrate for DNA polymerase and becomes incorporated into DNA, thus inhibiting DNA synthesis and, again, is an inhibitor of ribonucleotide reductase.

Pentostatin also belongs in the antimetabolite category although its mechanism of action is totally different from that of other antimetabolites. Pentostatin is a natural product isolated from the fermentation broth of *Streptomyces*. It is an example of a drug which is a transition-state analogue which is believed to mimic the transition state of 2-deoxyadenosine when it is being deamidated (Fig. 21.12). The conversion of 2-deoxyadenosine into 2-deoxyinosine is an important metabolic step in controlling DNA synthesis. If the conversion does not occur, 2-deoxyadenosine accumulates and is converted into its triphosphate (dATP), which is a potent inhibitor of ribonucleotide reductase. Inhibition of the formation of deoxyribonucleotides inhibits DNA synthesis. It is believed the transition state involved in the deamination of adenosine is as shown in Figure 21.12. Pentostatin resembles the transition of 2-deoxyadenosine deamination and thus binds to the deamidase enzyme, causing inhibition.

Antimetabolites interfering with the function of folic acid

Folic acid is the vitamin responsible for providing single carbon units in the biosynthesis of DNA and RNA bases (see Ch. 26). Interfering with the action of folic acid results in the inhibition of DNA biosynthesis and thus with cell proliferation. An important group of antimetabolites

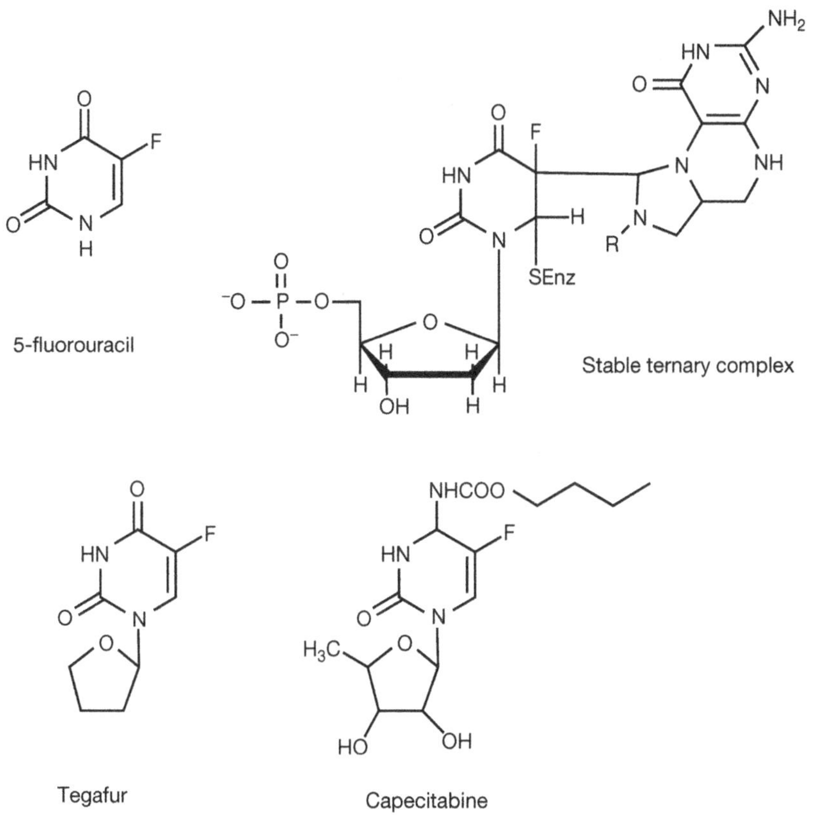

Figure 21.10 5-Fluorouracil and related drugs.

used in cancer chemotherapy interferes with the action of folic acid. Figure 21.13 shows the biosynthetic steps involved in the conversion of folic acid to methylene tetrahydrofolate, which is responsible for transferring a methylene unit to precursors of nucleic acid bases. DHF is generated during methylene transfer. Methotrexate is close in structure to folic acid. The presence of an additional amino group in the structure increases its basicity so that it is protonated at physiological pH, and this allows it to inhibit binding of DHF to the enzyme dihydrofolate reductase.

Methotrexate (Fig. 21.14) is often used in conjunction with calcium folinate which is injected 24 hours after administration of methotrexate in order to reduce its cytotoxic action to rescue normal cells while not reducing the cytotoxic effect on cancer cells. The selective toxicity of this combination for cancer cells rests on the fact that the normal cells are able to reduce the formyl group in folinate, yielding methylene THF, whereas the cancer cells are unable to complete this step. Raltitrexed inhibits the synthesis of nucleotides through a specific inhibition of thymidylate synthetase where it prevents the binding of the normal co-factor, methylene THF. Pemetrexed is a less specific inhibitor of folate action and acts on thymidylate synthetase, dihydrofolate reductase and formyl transferase.

Preparations of antimetabolites

- Mercaptopurine: Tablets 50 mg.
- Thioguanine: Tablets 40 mg.
- Fluorouracil: Capsules 250 mg, injections (fluorouracil sodium) 25 mg/mL and 50 mg/mL, cream 5% w/w.
- Tegafur with uracil: capsules 100 mg tegafur with 224 mg uracil.
- Capecitabine: Tablets 150 mg and 500 mg.
- Fludarabine: Tablets 10 mg, injection 50 mg.
- Cladribine: Injection 1 mg/mL.
- Cytarabine: Injections 20 mg/mL, 100 mg/mL and 50 mg per vial (encapsulated in liposomes).
- Gemcitabine: Injections 200 mg and 1 g.
- Pentostatin: Injection 10 mg.
- Methotrexate: Tablets 2.5 mg and 10 mg, injections 25 mg/mL and 100 mg/mL.
- Calcium folinate: Tablets 15 mg, injections 3 mg/mL, 7.5 mg/mL, 10 mg/mL.
- Ralitrexed: Injection 2 mg.
- Pemetrexed: Injection 500 mg.

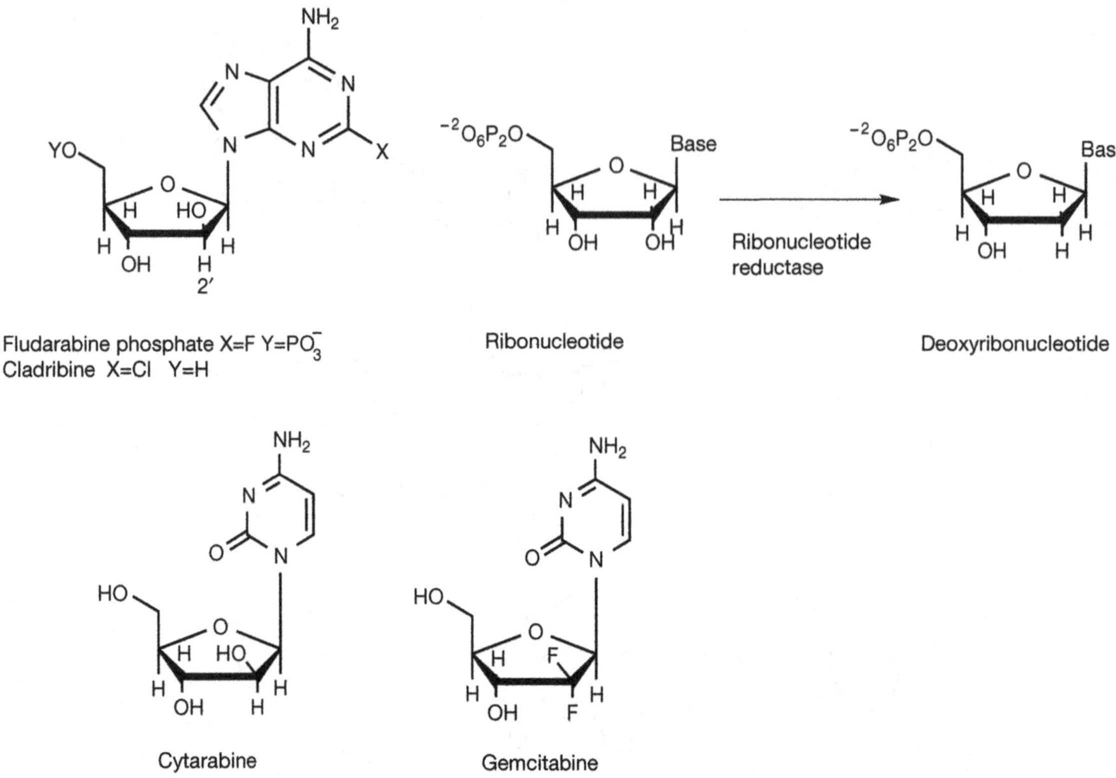

Figure 21.11 Antimetabolites interfering with DNA synthesis.

Q Self Test 21.2

Indicate which enzymes the antimetabolites shown below inhibit.
Draw the complex formed between trifluridine and the enzyme it inhibits.

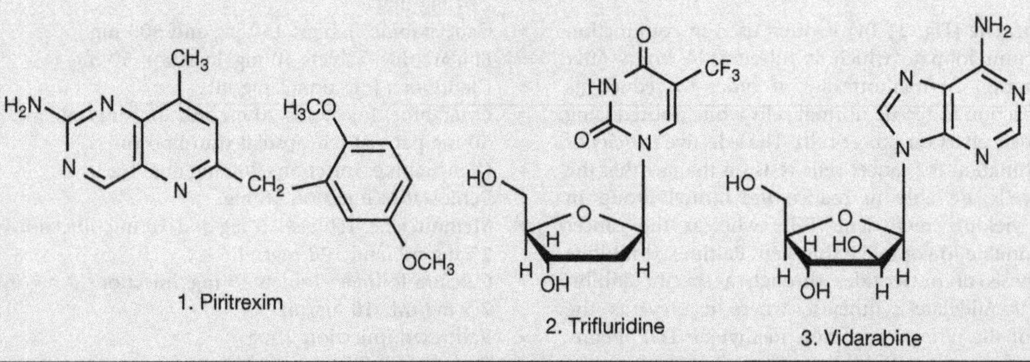

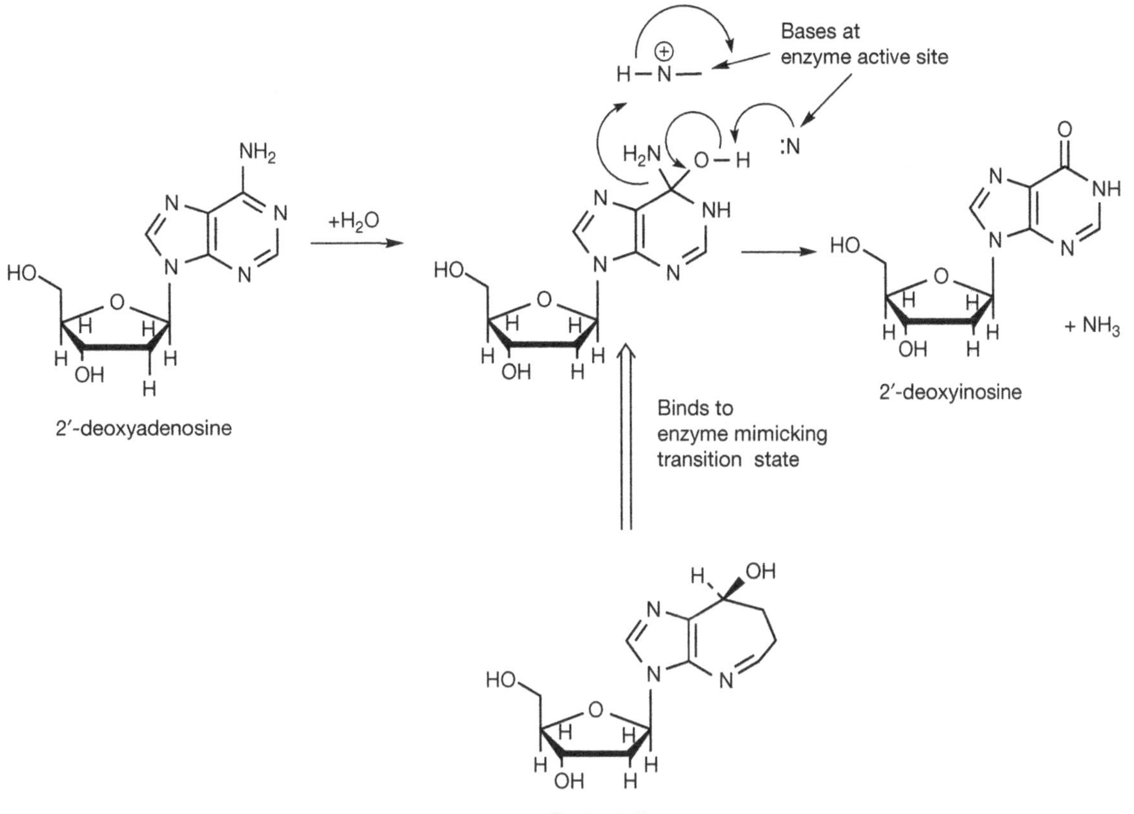

Figure 21.12 Mimicking of transition state of adenosine deaminase by pentostatin.

CYTOTOXIC ANTIBIOTICS

Daunorubicin (Fig. 21.15) was isolated from *Streptomyces peucetius*. It was found to be highly cytotoxic but its usefulness was limited by severe cardiotoxicity. The basis of the cytotoxic action of daunorubicin was found to be its ability to interacalate with DNA. Intercalation is a feature of flat aromatic and heteroaromatic molecules which bind perpendicular to the DNA axis. They are held in place by non-covalent charge transfer interactions (see Ch. 1) in combination with electrostatic and hydrogen bonding interactions. Intercalation causes distortion of the DNA structure by causing the base pairs to be pushed apart. It is more energetically favourable for pyrimidine-3′,5′purine sequences than purine-3′,5′pyrimidine sequences.

The structure of the complex formed between daunorubicin and DNA determined by X-ray diffraction indicates that the daunorubicin forms a complex with GC sequences in DNA. The daunorubicin molecule is orientated at *ca.* 90° to the long axis of the GC base pair. It interacts with GC pairs both above and below it in the helix (Fig. 21.16). The sugar ring attached to the molecule sits in the minor groove of the DNA.

Daunorubicin may prevent DNA replication via two mechanisms. It may inhibit the action of topoisomerase II which causes double-stranded breaks in the sugar phosphate backbone of the DNA allowing conformational change within coiled DNA (see Ch. 7). It is not clear exactly how the intercalated drug inhibits replication but part of the process involves a ternary complex formed between DNA, the daunorubicin and topoisomerase II. However, another component in the mechanism of action is oxygen-dependent DNA damage. This might be due to the enzymatic reduction of the daunorubicin which can occur followed by the production of superoxide which can generate reactive hydroxyl radicals. The process can be promoted by the presence of the ferrous ion (Fig. 21.17). The hydroxyl radicals can cause strand breaks in DNA. The generation of reactive hydroxyl radicals is probably the mechanism that causes the severe cardiotoxicity of daunorubicin and related drugs.

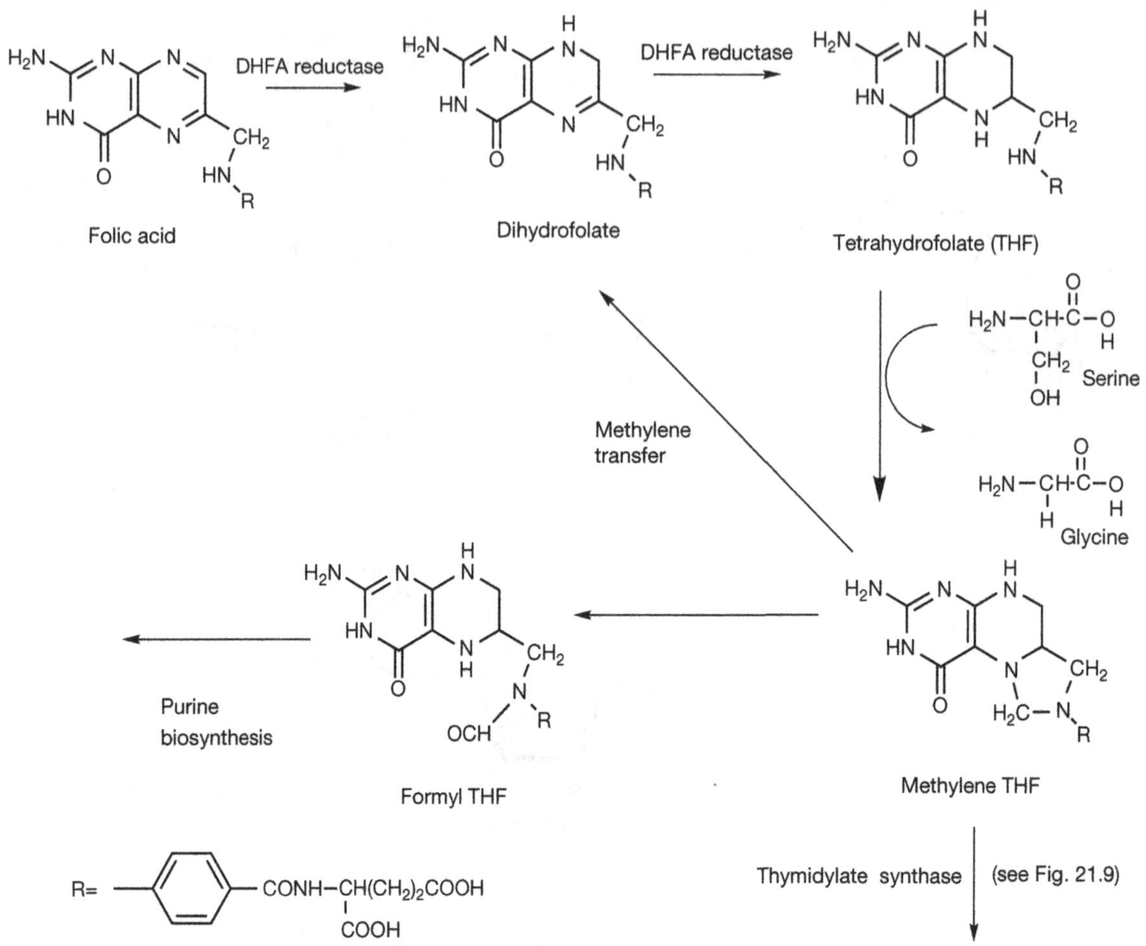

Figure 21.13 Inhibition of DHF by methotrexate.

Another possible mechanism of DNA damage is by alkylation with daunorubicin which is promoted via a two electron oxidation (Fig. 21.18) where an adduct is formed between DNA and the drug. Apart from daunorubicin, there are three other similar antibiotics commonly used in cancer chemotherapy: doxorubicin, idarubicin and epirubicin (see Fig. 21.16). Their mode of action is the same as that of daunorubicin. Mitomycin-C is another antitumour antibiotic and it acts in a similar manner to the anthracylines. It functions as a prodrug which is activated via reduction to a semi-quinone which rearranges to form an alkylating agent. An advantage of bioreductive activation is that this means that the drug is targeted at solid tumours which are hypoxic at their centre.

Mitoxantrone (see Fig. 21.16) is a synthetic compound which is related in structure to the anthracycline antibiotics. It acts via a similar mechanism to the anthracyclines but it has a slightly higher reduction potential than these drugs and thus does not generate reactive oxygen species to the same extent. Its primary mode of action is via intercalation with DNA and consequent interference with topoisomerase II. The amine side chains may bind with the phosphate backbone of the DNA. The cardiotoxic side effects of mitoxantrone are lower than those of the anthracylines.

PLANT DERIVATIVES

The search for anticancer compounds from natural sources can be dated back at least as far as the Ebers papyrus in 1550 BC. The use of plants in folk remedies can provide a lead for discovery, although in many cases the therapeutic indication which led to an interest in the plant was not anticancer activity.[1]

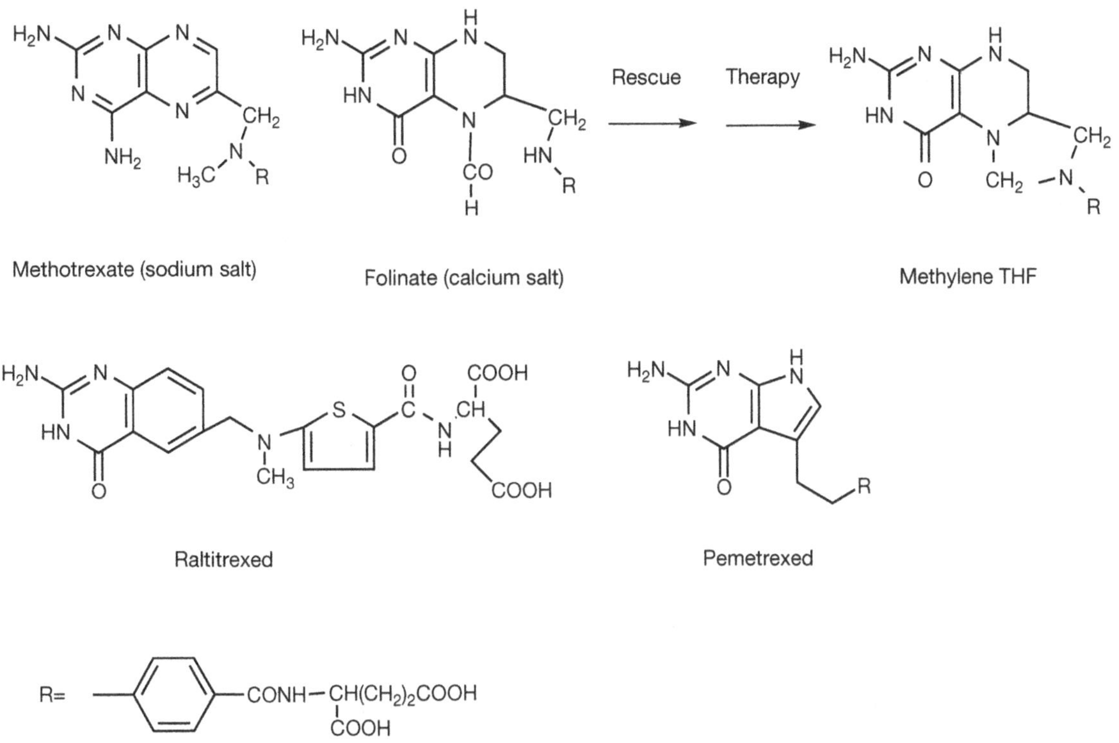

Figure 21.14 Antimetabolites interfering with folate function.

Vinca alkaloids

The Madagascar periwinkle (*Catharantheus roseus*) has a reputation in folk remedy in the treatment of diabetes. When the antidiabetic activity of extracts was tested in rats it was found that the rats succumbed to infection due to the death of white blood cells. The alkaloids vincristine and vinblastine (Fig. 21.19) were found to be responsible for the cytotoxicity of the plant extracts.[2] The compounds work by inhibiting the formation of microtubules which must be formed as part of the cell division process. Figure 21.20 illustrates the process of mitosis where tubulin fibres attach themselves to chromatids formed from DNA replication within the cell and separate the genetic material into two halves which will form the genetic material in the nucleus of the two daughter cells produced. In order for the cell division process to occur, the microtubules undergo both elongation and depolymerisation so that the cell division process can move from the metaphase to the anaphase. Since the vinca alkaloids exhibit general toxicity via inhibition of cell division, they cause myelosuppression which affects the rapidly proliferating white blood cells the most. Even though the structures of the alkaloids are very similar, they exhibit a different spectrum of activities. Vincristine is more effective against Hodgkin's disease and paediatric solid tumours than adult solid tumours. Vinorelbine is a semi-synthetic analogue of the Vinca alkaloids and is most effective against non-small cell lung, breast and ovarian cancer.

Vinca alkaloid preparations

- Vinblastine sulphate: Injection 1 mg/mL.
- Vincristine sulphate: Injection 1 mg/mL.
- Vindesine sulphate: Injection 5 mg/vial.
- Vinorelbine tartrate: Injection concentrate 10 mg/mL.

Taxanes

The discovery of taxol originated from a screening programme instituted in 1960 by the US national cancer institute. One of plants screened was the Pacific yew tree *Taxus brevifolia* where extracts were found to have in vitro cytotoxic activity against tumour cells. Initially, there was a lack of interest in the compound since it was only found in very small amounts in *T. brevifolia* but eventually better sources were found in other *Taxus* species. Figure 21.21 shows the important structural features for taxol which contribute to its activity. As with the Vinca

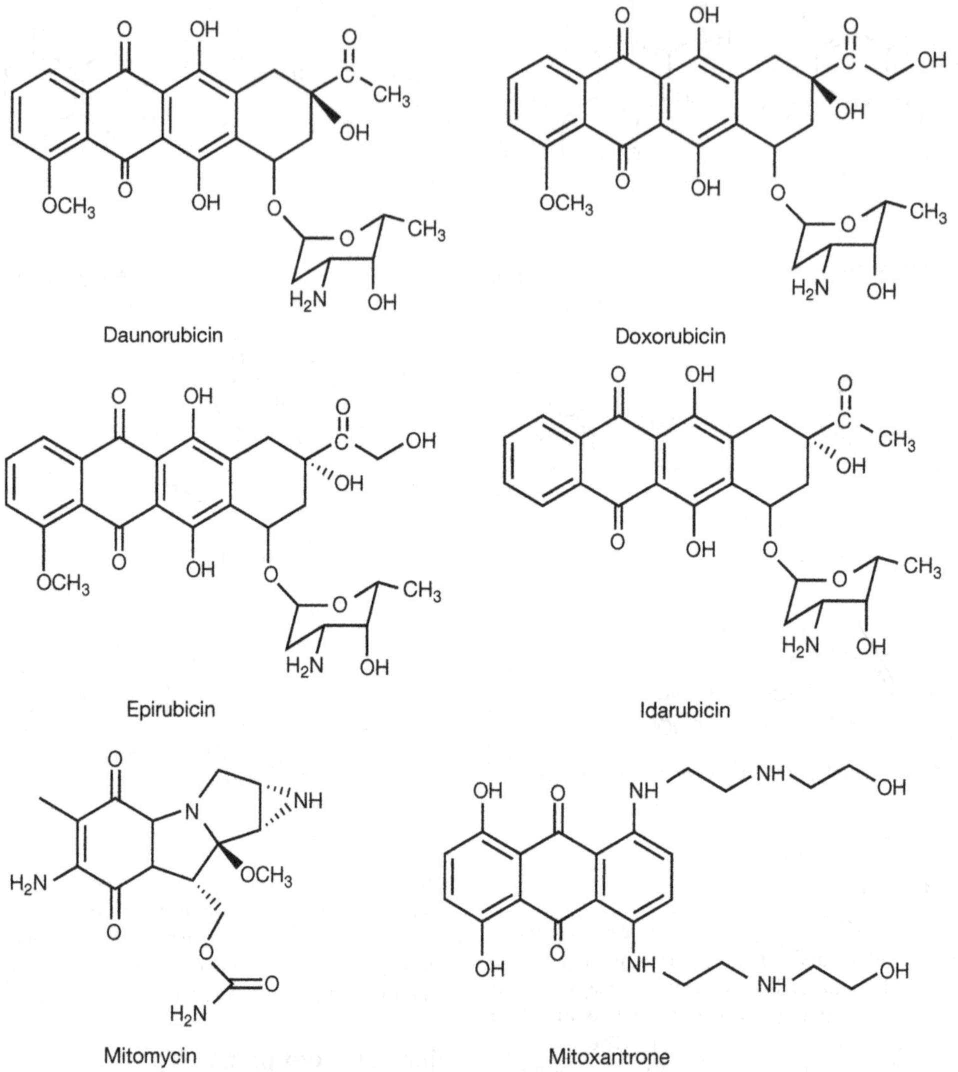

Figure 21.15 Cytotoxic antibiotics.

alkaloids there is little rationale for its particular activity against tubulin. As indicated in Figure 21.20, it acts in a different manner to the Vinca alkaloids in that it binds to tubulin and promotes its polymerisation rather than inhibiting it. However, in the course of promoting polymerisation, it reduces the flexibility in the tubulin structure which is required for elongation of the tubulin fibres. Taxol promotes lateral contacts within the tubulin dimer at the expense of longitudinal contacts which normally promote the elongation of the microtubule and which are essential for completion of the cell division process.[3] Taxol (paclitaxel) is poorly water soluble and therefore it has to be formulated in polysorbate or polyoxyl castor oil which can cause hypersensitivity. Docetaxel (Fig. 21.21) is a semi-synthetic analogue of taxol which has better water solubility and is also more potent than taxol. Research is ongoing into finding a potent water soluble derivative of taxol but so far none of the candidate compounds has a product license.

Taxol preparations

- Paclitaxel: 6 mg/mL concentrate for intravenous infusion.
- Docetaxel: 40 mg/mL concentrate for intravenous infusion.

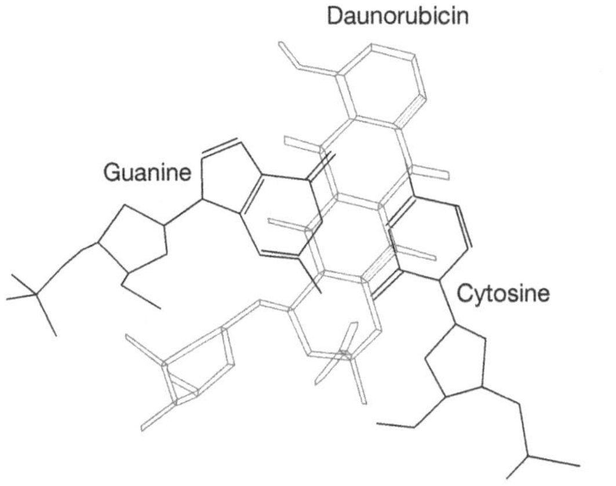

Figure 21.16 Interaction of daunorubicin with a GC base pair.

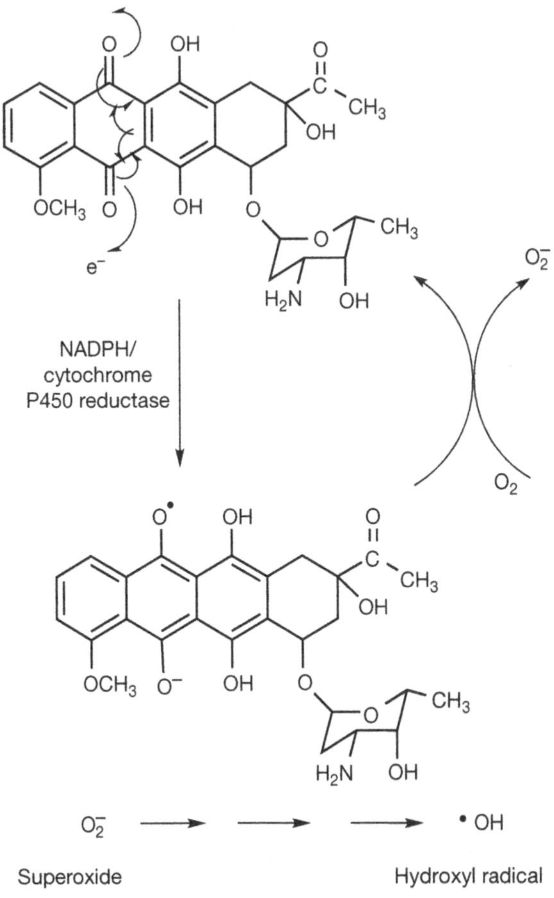

Figure 21.17 Mechanism of hydroxyl radical generation by daunorubicin.

Topoisomerase inhibitors

The podophyllotoxin (Fig. 20.22) was isolated from the American mandrake (*Podophyllum pelatum*), which had been traditionally used by American Indians as a laxative and anthelmintic, in 1880. It was subsequently shown to be a potent cytotoxic agent but was too toxic for use in cancer chemotherapy. Chemists at Sandoz in the 1950s further investigated *Podophyllum* species for analogues of podophyllotoxin. This eventually led to the development of the semi-synthetic compounds tenipinoside and etoposide (Fig. 21.22). These agents are topoisomerase II inhibitors. Teniposide is more cytotoxic than etoposide although it is not orally bioavailable.[4]

If the DNA in chromosomes were stretched out to its full length it would be far too long to fit into a cell. Thus the DNA helix coils up rather like the twisted cord of a telephone receiver where the torque due to the twist of the flex makes it twist round itself. This supercoiling can be either clockwise or anticlockwise (positive or negative). Replication of the DNA can only occur when it is negatively supercoiled, and topoisomerases such as topoisomerase II can break the double-stranded DNA and reform the strands to convert a positive strand into a negative strand (Fig. 21.23). In addition, DNA cutting is required to resolve tangles in the DNA during chromosome replication.

Mutations in topoisomerase genes are fatal to cells and likewise drugs which inhibit topisomerase activity. Etoposide and teniposide act by binding to the covalent topoisomerase/DNA complex, formed by reaction of the phosphate groups in DNA with a tyrosine residue in the enzyme, and stabilising it so that the DNA break is not repaired. This inhibits DNA replication, and thus cell division, and leads to cell death. Etoposide and teniposide are used to treat lymphomas, acute leukaemia, testicular cancer, small cell lung cancer, ovarian, bladder and brain cancers.

Camptothecin (Fig. 21.24) was isolated from the Chinese tree *Camptotheca acuminate* during screening for sterols which could be employed in the synthesis of cortisone. It was found to be cytotoxic but was unfortunately too toxic to be clinically useful. Rings A–D are essential for anticancer activity. The lactone ring E is essential for activity and the hydroxyl substituent in this ring at position 20 is also essential for activity and cannot be substituted by another element. For highest activity, the configuration at the 20 position must be S, the R isomer is up to 100 times less active. Modifications of the A and B rings can improve activity. Camptothecin inhibits topoisomerase I which has a similar type of activity to topoisomerase II except that it promotes single-strand breaks in DNA. Through its action in inhibiting topoisomerase I, camptothecin promotes fragmentation of chromosomal DNA. The toxicity

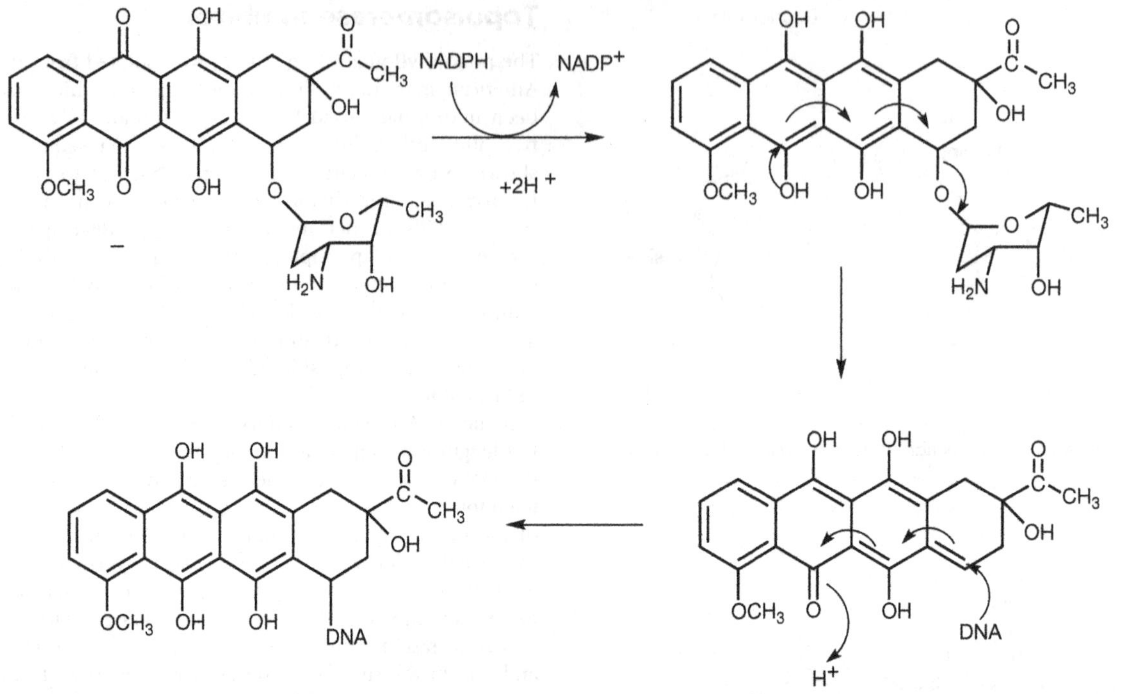

Figure 21.18 Alkylation of DNA by daunorubicin.

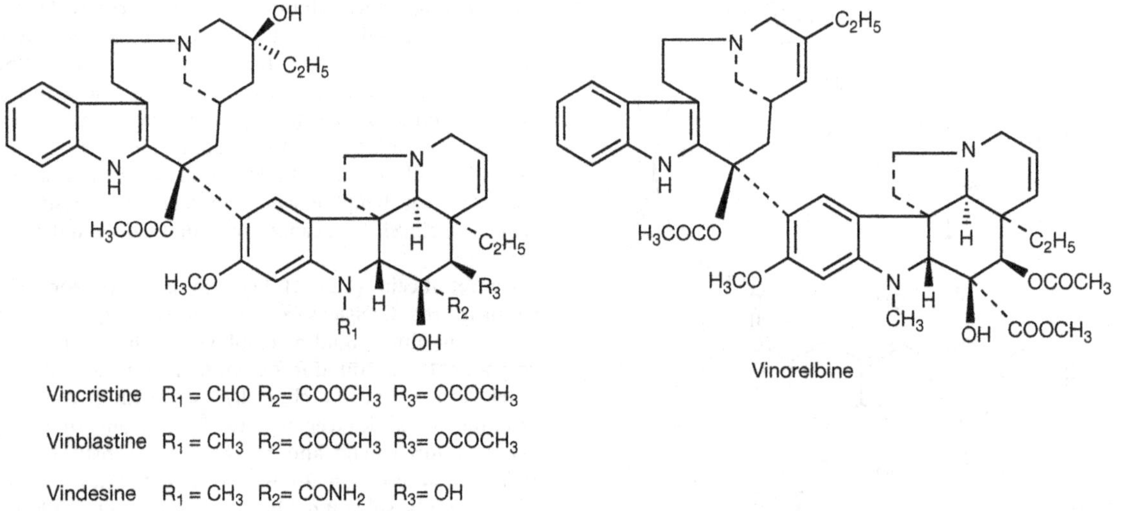

Figure 21.19 Vinca alkaloids.

of camptothecin was reduced by modification of rings A and B. Irinotecan and topotecan (Fig. 21.24) are clinically licensed analogues of camptothecin and have better water solubility than camptothecin. Irinotecan is a prodrug in which the ester linkage to the A ring has to be hydrolysed before it displays cytotoxicity. Irinotecan is used to treat metastatic colorectal cancer and topotecan is used to treat ovarian cancer. As a class of agents, camptothecin analogues show good promise for further development.

Figure 21.20 Meta and anaphases in cell division where polymerisation and depolymerisation of the protein tubulin is essential to the process.

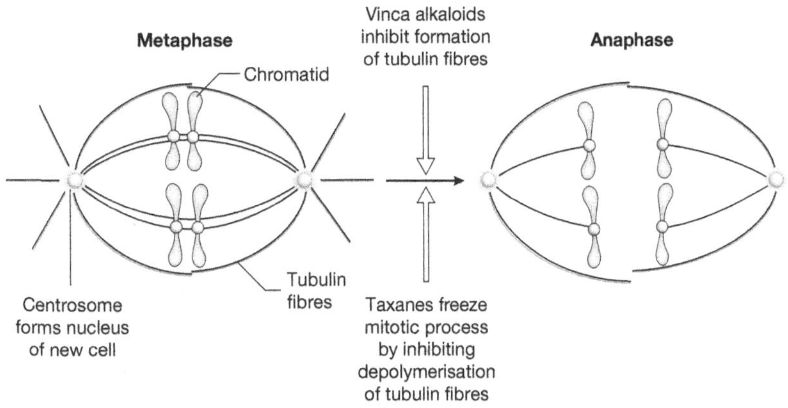

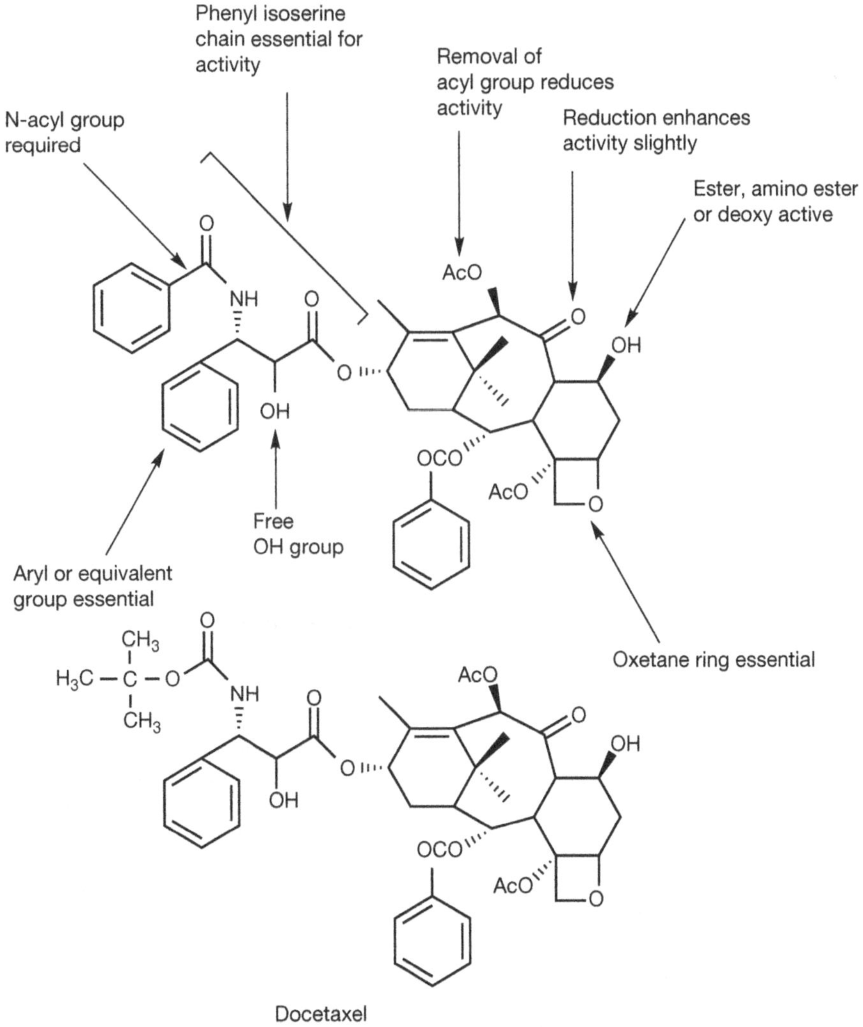

Figure 21.21 Structurally important features of taxol and docetaxel.

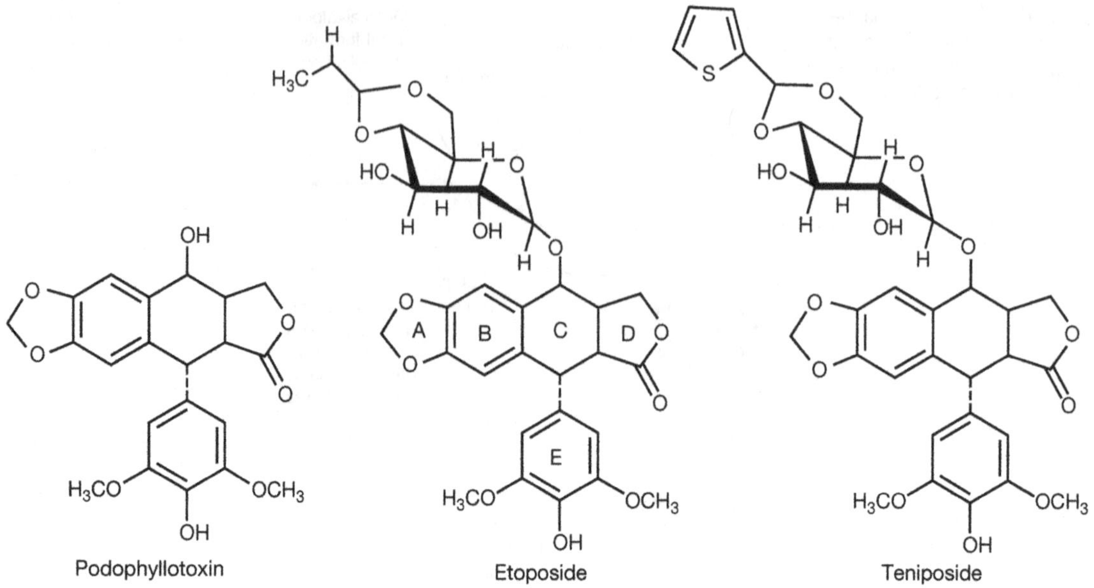

Figure 21.22 Podophyllotoxin and topoisomerase II inhibitors derived from it.

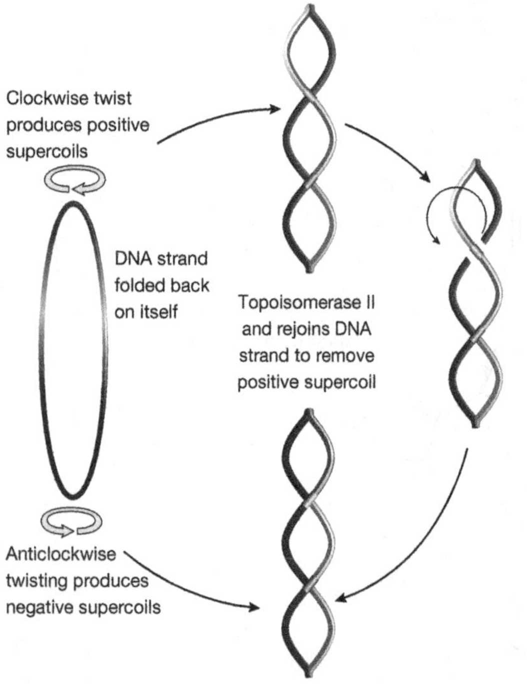

Figure 21.23 Conversion of positive to negative supercoils by the action of topoisomerase II.

Topoisomerase inhibitors

- Etoposide: Concentrate for i.v. infusion 20 mg/mL.
- Etoposide phosphate: 100 mg reconstitution as injection.
- Etoposide: Capsules 100 mg and 50 mg.
- Irinotecan: Concentrate for i.v. infusion 20 mg/mL.
- Topotecan hydrochloride: 1 mg or 4 mg per vial for reconstitution for i.v. infusion.

NEW TARGETS

Imatinib

Protein kinase inhibitors (PKIs) provide a promising therapeutic strategy for cancer chemotherapy.[5,6] Phosphorylation of proteins is a universal mechanism for the control of many cellular processes. The phosphorylation of proteins occurs when the γ-phosphate group of ATP is transferred to either tyrosine or serine/threonine within proteins. One family of enzymes catalyses tyrosine phosphorylation and another serine/threonine phosphorylation. Tyrosine phosphorylation is up-regulated in tumour cells and thus provides a selective target for therapy. Although there are numerous protein kinase structures, they have some features in common and the active site of the enzyme consists

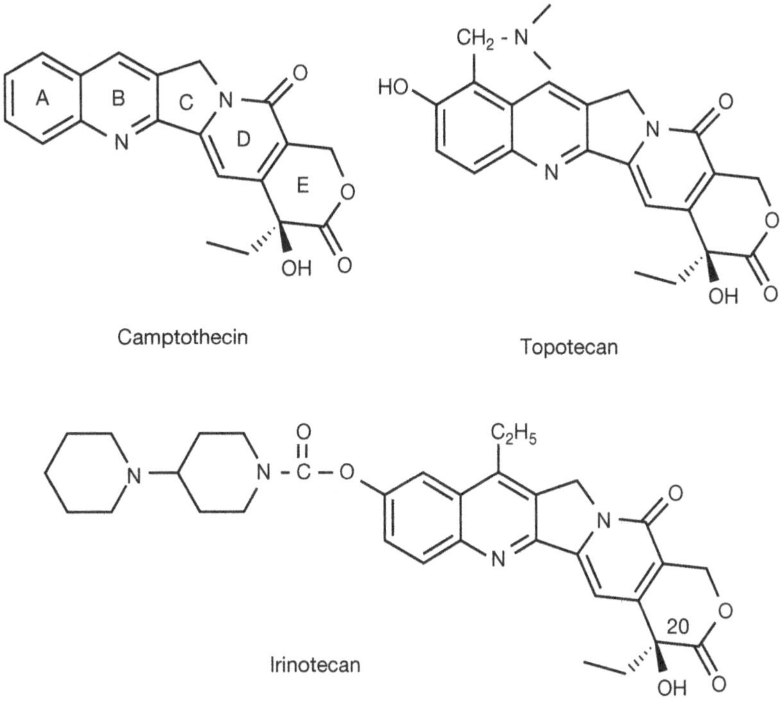

Figure 21.24 Camptothecin and its analogues.

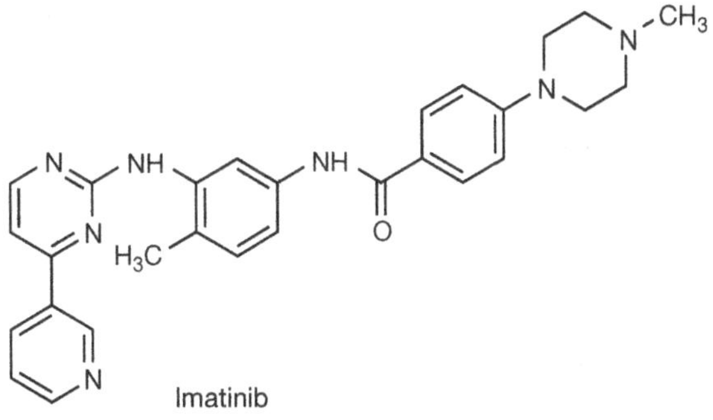

Figure 21.25 Protein kinase inhibitor imatinib.

of two domains which hinge together in order to bind ATP. The majority of PKIs inhibit the binding of ATP to its binding site within the enzyme. However, the only licensed PKI, imatinib (Fig. 21.25) was discovered by development of lead compound discovered in a random screen. Imatinib inhibits protein kinase activity by binding to the enzyme so it becomes conformationally immobilised and is not itself able to undergo the phosphorylation required to activate it. The particular protein kinase targeted by imatinib is BCR-ABL protein kinase, which is an oncogene protein which enhances cell growth rates and resistance to apoptosis. This oncogene is found in 95% of patients with chronic myeloid leukaemia (CML). Imatinib has minimal effects on normal cells and is very effective in the selective treatment of CML. There are some indications of resistance occurring via mutations in BCR-ABL, and new analogues of imatinib are being developed in order to counteract these. In addition to inhibiting BCR-ABL, imatinib inhibits the c-KIT and PDGFR protein kinases which are dysregulated in gastrointestinal stromal tumours, and the drug is also being used to treat this tumour.

Protein kinase inhibitors

- Imatinib mesilate (Glivec): Tablets 100 mg and 400 mg.

HORMONE ANALOGUES

Cancers such as breast cancer and prostate cancer are associated with hormonal imbalances. Various hormone antagonists and inhibitors of hormone biosynthesis are used in cancers in which hormone activity is a component in the disease.

Tamoxifen

The tamoxifen structure (Fig. 21.26) was derived from the observation made in 1937 that triphenylethylene had

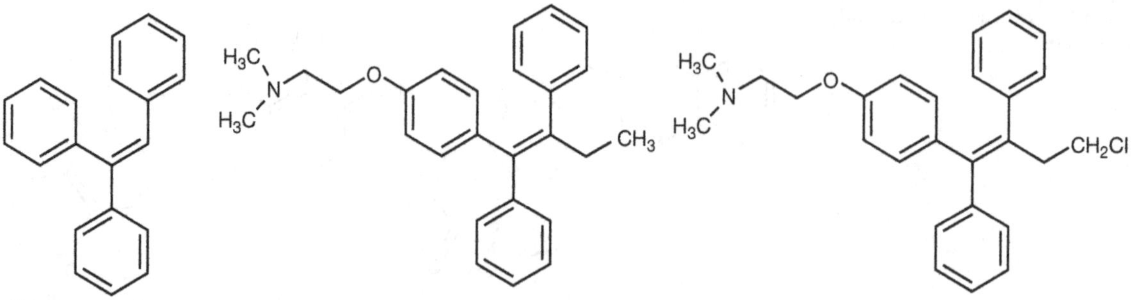

Triphenylethylene Tamoxifen Toremifene

Figure 21.26 Oestrogen receptor modulators.

DNA binding region

RY**CAVCNDYASGYHYGVWSCEGCKAFFKRSIQGHNDYMCPATNQCTID**
KNRRKSCQACRLRKCYEVGMMKGGIRKDRRGGRMLKHKRQRDDGEGRGEVGSAGDM

Oestrogen binding region

RAANLWPSPLMIKRSKKNSLALSLTADQMVSALLDAEPPILYSEYDPTRPFSEA
SMMGLLTNLADRELVHMINWAKRVPGFVDLTLHDQVHLLECAWLEILMIGLVW
RSMEHPGKLLFAPNLLLDRNQGKCVEGMVEIFDMLLATSSRFRMMNLQGEEFV
CLKSIILLNSGVYTFLSSTLKSLEEKDHIHRVLDKITDTLIHLMAKAGLTLQQQHQR
LAQLLLILSHIRHMSNKGMEHLYSMKCKNVVPLYDLLLEMLDAHRLHA

Figure 21.27 Part of the amino acid sequence of the oestrogen receptor showing the cysteine-rich helices (in bold) that bind zinc and the oestrogen binding region.

weak oestrogenic activity. Tamoxifen was synthesised in 1962 and consisted of two geometrical isomers. It was found that while the Z-isomer functioned as an agonist at the oestrogen receptor, the E-isomer was an antagonist, and during the 1970s was adopted for the treatment of oestrogen-dependent breast cancer. In fact, subsequently it has been discovered that the action of tamoxifen is tissue dependent and, although it functions as an antagonist (modulator) in uterine tissue where it acts at the oestrogen-α receptor, in bone it functions as an agonist where it is binding to the oestrogen-β receptor.[7,8]

Like all steroids (apart from aldosterone), oestrogen binds to a hormone receptor which controls gene expression by binding to DNA. This type of receptor interacts with a variety of lipophilic molecules including vitamin D, retinoic acid, thyroxine and some prostaglandins. Figure 21.27 shows the primary sequence of part of the oestrogen receptor. A highly conserved domain of *ca.* 70 amino acids is present in all steroid receptors and forms two helices. Each helix contains four cysteine residues and four of these residues at the N-terminus of each helix which contains two zinc-binding Cys_2–Cys_2 sequence motifs. The structure consists of two helices perpendicular to each other. A zinc ion, coordinated by four conserved cysteines, holds the base of a loop at the N-terminus of each helix. This structural domain seems to be a general structure for protein–DNA recognition. The ligand binding region is composed of a long sequence of amino acids over 250 residues in length and oestrogen binds in this region, causing conformational change in the receptor and subsequent receptor dimerisation (Fig. 21.28). Following this, binding of the receptor to DNA occurs, which triggers off the gene transcription which, in the context of breast cancer, triggers of cell proliferation. Binding of an antagonist (or, more strictly, modulator) such as tamoxifen to the receptor blocks the conformational change which would normally be induced by oestrogen and thus blocks dimerisation and binding to DNA (Fig. 21.28). Toremifene is structurally close to tamoxifen and has the same mode of action.

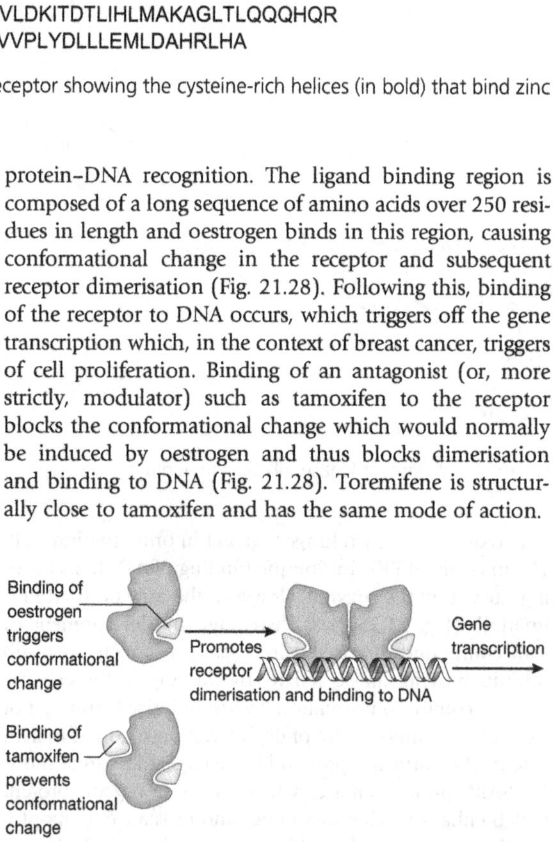

Figure 21.28 Dimerisation of the oestrogen receptor.

> **Q** Self Test 21.3
>
> List the basic amino acids (see Ch. 6) in the basic region of the oestrogen receptor (bold in Fig. 21.27) which is an important component in the receptor binding region.

Aromatase inhibitors

Oestrogens have a pivotal role in the development of breast cancer and 70% of breast cancers have been found to produce oestrogens in vivo. Drugs such as tamoxifen, discussed earlier, are active against breast cancer via blocking oestrogen receptors. The action of aromatase converts androstene dione to oestrogen (Fig. 21.29). The enzyme carrying out this conversion is a cyp450 which has the enzyme cyp450 reductase as a co-factor and oxidises the 19 methyl group through to formaldehyde. An aspartate (D309), histidine (H480) and a serine residue are involved in removing the first proton from ring A, and the second proton is removed by the cyp450 haem group, resulting in the formation of the estrone aromatic ring (Fig. 21.29).

The earliest aromatase inhibitor was aminoglutethimide (Fig. 21.30) which was originally synthesised as an

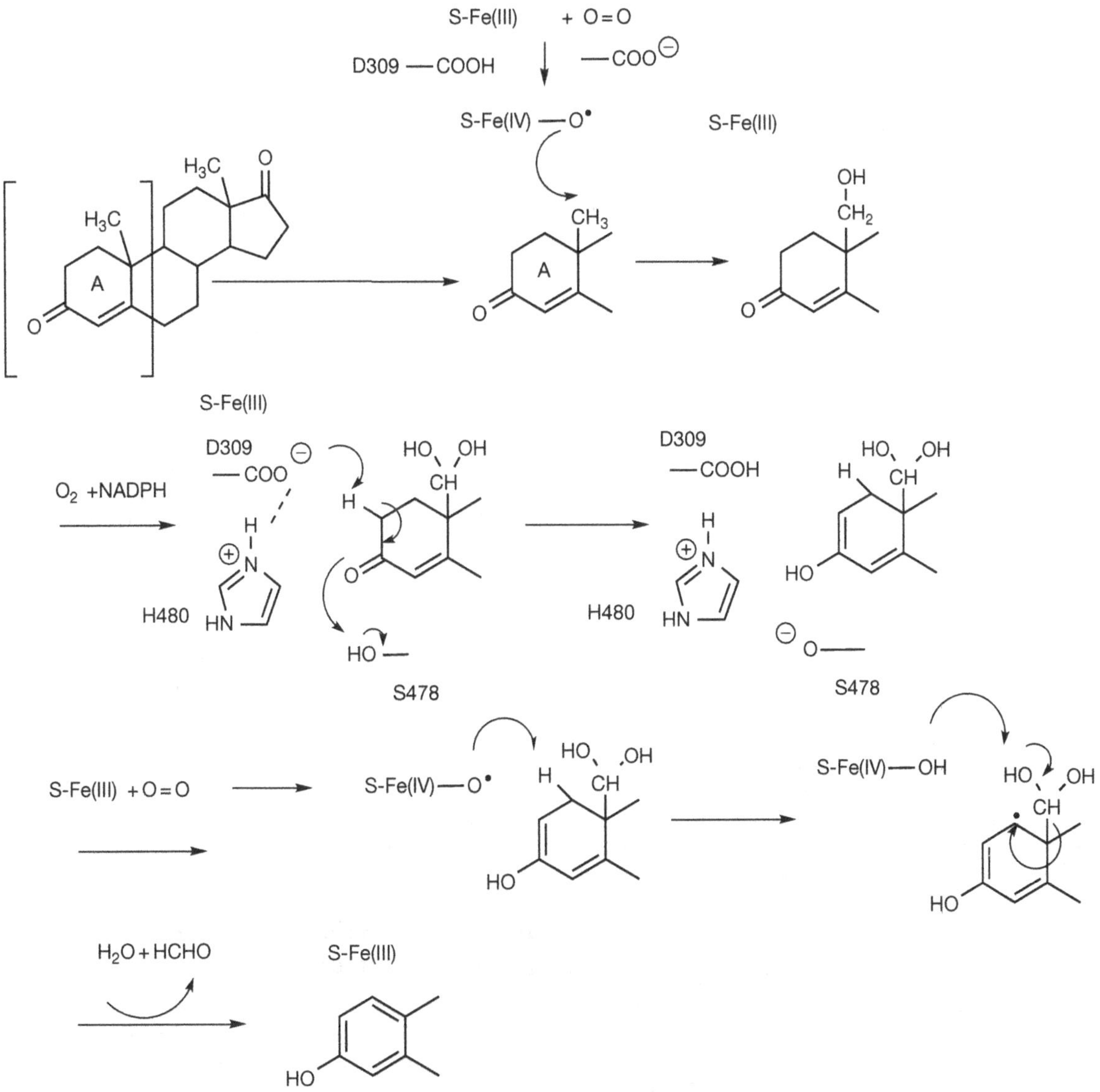

Figure 21.29 Conversion of ring A in androstene dione to an aromatic ring.

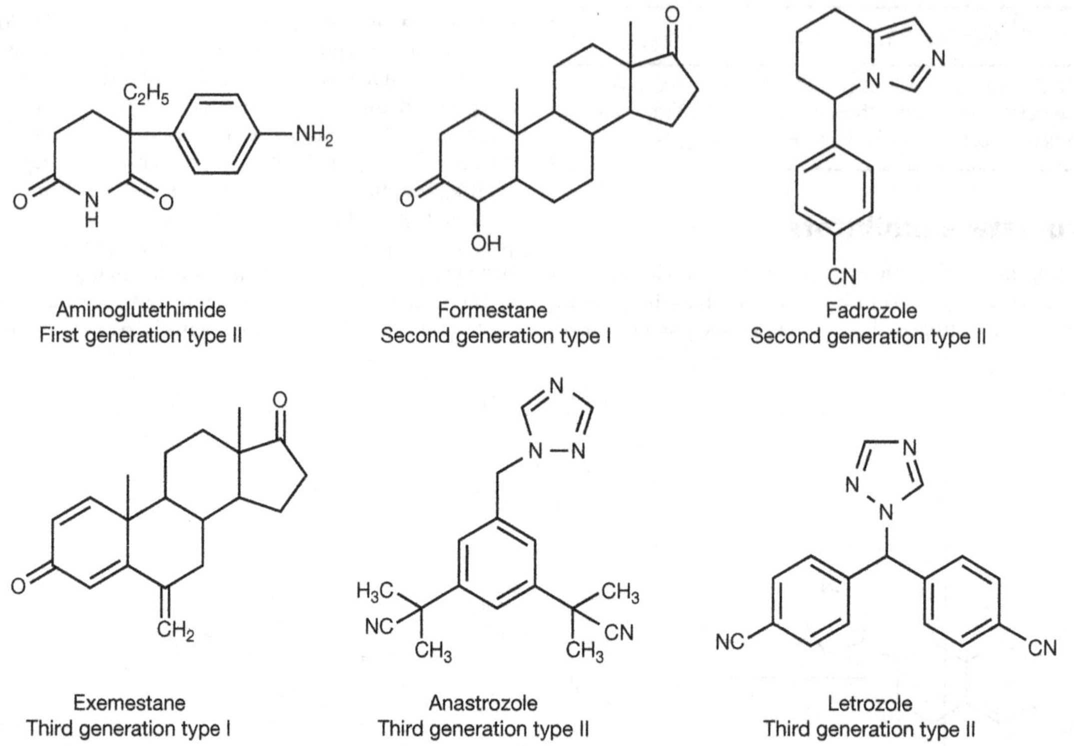

Figure 21.30 Aromatase inhibitors.

anti-epileptic drug. However, the observation was made subsequently that it produced side effects similar to the symptoms of Addison's disease. Addison's disease results from a deficiency in steroid hormones, in most cases due to the deficiency of various enzymes in the biosynthetic pathway producing steroid hormones. Aromatase inhibitors can be divided into two classes: those binding to active site of the aromatase enzyme by competing with androstene dione (type I inhibitors), and those binding to the haem group (type II inhibitors). Aminoglutethimide belongs to the latter category and is rather non-specific in which haem-containing enzymes it targets. Thus it produces a general deficiency in steroid hormones, which has to be compensated for by co-administration with a corticosteroid such as dexamethasone. Various other drugs have been produced including later-generation type II inhibitors and type I inhibitors. The aromatase inhibitors on the market are shown in Figure 21.30. It is easier to model the interaction of the type I inhibitors with the enzyme active site rather than interaction with the haem group.

Figure 21.31 shows the proposed interaction between exemestane and the aromatase enzyme.[9] The structure of exemestane is close to that of androstenedione and it fits the active site of the enzyme very closely, interacting with the lipophilic phenylalanine and isoleucine side chains and hydrogen bonding to serine 478. However, because of the extra double bond, it cannot complete the aromatisation reaction. It has been suggested that exemestane is a suicide inhibitor which reacts with the aromatase enzyme and this may occur via a reactive species generated at the C-19 position which would normally be eliminated upon formation of an aromatic ring. Release of the androstenedione substrate from the enzyme depends on the removal of the C-19 methyl group.

The third-generation type II aromatase inhibitors interact with the iron in the haem ring of the Cyp450. This prevents the haem group from reacting with oxygen and thus blocks hydroxylation of the C-19 methyl group. In the case of anastrozole, apart from the primary interaction of the molecule with the haem group, the binding to the active site is reinforced by hydrogen bonding between a threonine at position 310 and the triazole ring and between one of the CN groups in the molecule and asp 309.

Hormone analogues used to treat prostate cancer

Like breast cancer, prostate cancer is driven by a steroid hormone, in this case testosterone, and treatments block the effects of testosterone. The disease can be treated surgically by orchidectomy but the alternative front-line treatment is to use analogues of the peptide hormone

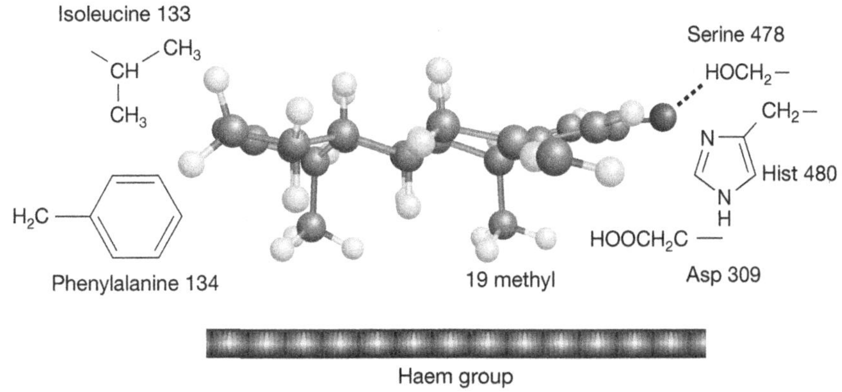

Figure 21.31 Interaction exemestane with the active site of the aromatase enzyme.

gonadorelin (gonadotrophin releasing hormone, GnRH). This decapeptide has the amino acid sequence shown in Figure 21.32 with the unusual pyroglutamate residue at its N-terminus. It is responsible for releasing gonadotrophins, which have a range of actions including promoting testosterone production. The normal mode of action is for GnRH to be released by the body in pulses so that the receptor is not continuously exposed to the hormone. Testosterone production is suppressed by the use of GnRH agonists which, somewhat counterintuitively, due to the sustained circulating levels used, eventually cause down-regulation of receptor activity by overstimulation. In the initial phase of the treatment there is an increased production of testosterone, which may cause a flare-up in the cancer which is managed by using testosterone antagonists (see below). There are four commonly used GnRH agonists: buserelin, goserelin, leuprorelin and triptorelin. They are all modifications of the basic GnRH structure where the sixth amino acid from the N-terminus has been substituted with a D-amino acid, either tBu-serine, leucine or tryptophan, and the C-terminus has either an ethylamide or a diazane group.

Thus the structures of the agonists are very similar to that of GnRH where the N-terminus and C-terminus residues are conserved across many species. The GnRH receptor is a transmembrane G-coupled receptor and, as is the case with all of these receptors, is activated by several points of contact with its natural ligand. The gonadorelin analogues all bind more strongly to the receptor than GnRH and cause its activation. The GnRH analogues all have to be given by injection but there is the option of formulations designed to provide depot administration or an implant which release the hormone over several weeks.

The flare effect of the GnRH analogues is managed by using antagonists of testosterone. In addition they are used as treatments on their own to directly block the action of testosterone. The three commonly used analogues are shown in Figure 21.33. Cyproterone acetate

pyroGlu-His-Trp-Ser-Tyr-Gly-Leu-Arg-Pro-Gly $CONH_2$.

Gonadorelin

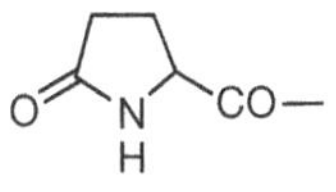

Pyroglutamate

pyroGlu-His-Trp-Ser-Tyr-tBuDSer-Leu-Arg-Pro$CONHC_2H_5$

Buserelin

pyroGlu-His-Trp-Ser-Tyr-tBuDSer-Leu-Arg-Pro$CONHNHCONH_2$

Goserelin

pyroGlu-His-Trp-Ser-Tyr-DLeu-Leu-Arg-Pro$CONHC_2H_5$

Leuprorelin

pyroGlu-His-Trp-Ser-Tyr-DTrp-Leu-Arg-Pro$CONHC_2H_5$

Triptorelin

Figure 21.32 Gonerelin analogues used in the treatment of prostate cancer.

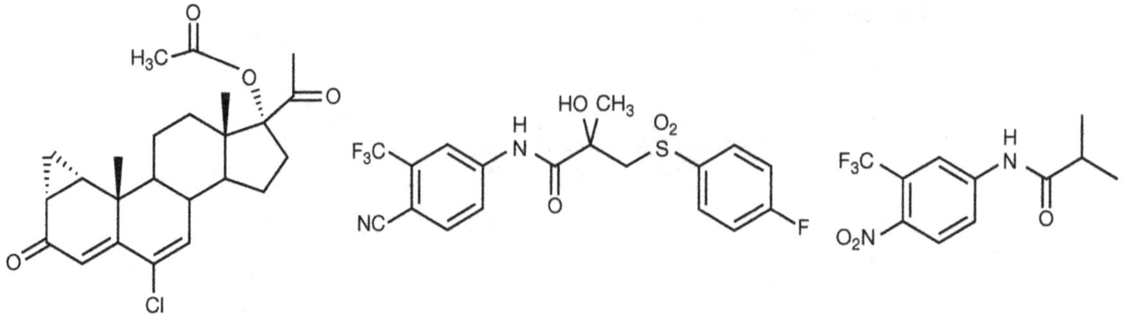

Cyproterone acetate Bicalutamide Flutamide

Figure 21.33 Anti-androgens used in the treatment of prostate cancer.

(CA) is a steroid analogue based on the structure of progesterone and, in addition to binding to the testosterone receptor, it also has some activity at the corticosteroid receptor and at the progesterone receptor. Despite being a much bulkier molecule than testosterone it binds strongly to its receptor and a co-crystallisation of CA with the cloned receptor has elucidated its binding mode.

Figure 21.34 shows the interactions of CA with a number of amino acids in the receptor forming a hydrogen bond network with arginine and glutamine residues and having a van der Waals interaction between the chlorine in the structure and a phenylalanine residue.[10] Although CA binds strongly to the receptor it does not activate it. The bulky acetate group displaces a leucine residue in the protein causing a conformational change without activating the receptor.[11] In bicalutamide the CN group interacts with the hydrogen bonding network in the receptor in the same way as the carbonyl group of CA. The rest of the structure destabilises with normal structure of the receptor, thus binding without activation. In flutamide, the CN group is replaced by a nitro group.

Q Self Test 21.4

Suggest how the flutamide analogue R3 might disrupt the conformation of the AR. The active enantiomer of R3 is shown. What is its absolute conformation?

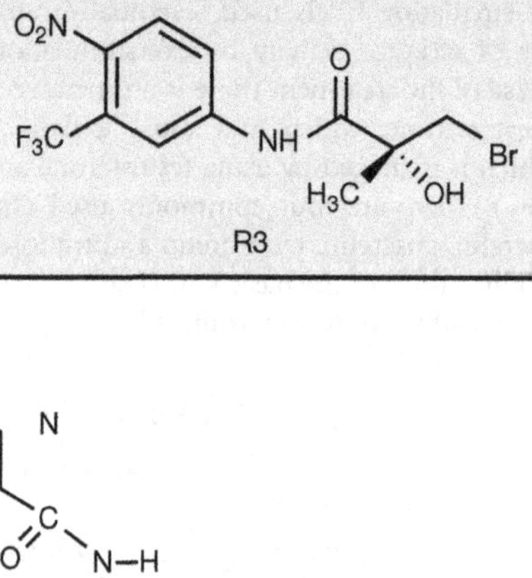

R3

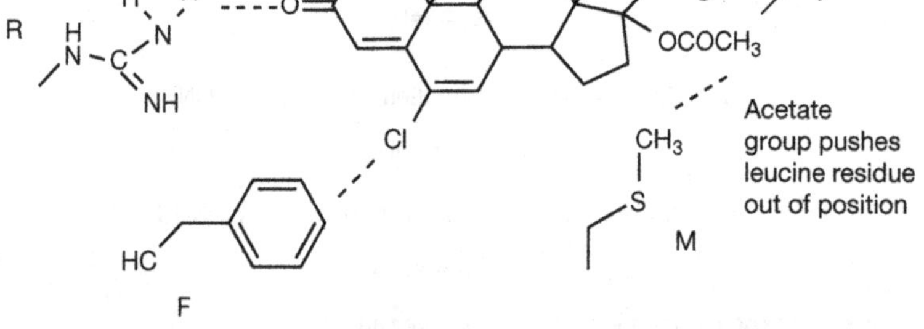

Figure 21.34 Binding of cyproterone acetate to the androgen receptor.

Preparations containing hormone analogues used in the treatment of cancer

Breast cancer

- Anastrolozole: Tablets 1 mg.
- Exemestane: Tablets 25 mg.
- Fulvestrant: Oily injection 50 mg/mL.
- Letrozole: Tablets 2.5 mg.
- Tamoxifen citrate: Tablets 10 mg and 20 mg, oral solution 10 mg/5 mL.
- Toremifen citrate: Tablets 60 mg.

Prostate cancer

- Bicalutamide: Tablets 150 mg.
- Buserelin acetate: Injection 1 mg/mL, 100 μg metered nasal spray.
- Cyproterone acetate: Tablets 50 mg.
- Flutamide: Tablets 250 mg.
- Goserelin acetate: Implant 3.6 mg and 10.8 mg.
- Leuprorelin acetate: Microsphere formulation for subcutaneous injection 3.75 mg and 11.25 mg.
- Triptorelin acetate: Injection 4.2 mg and 3.75 mg.

A Self Test 21.1

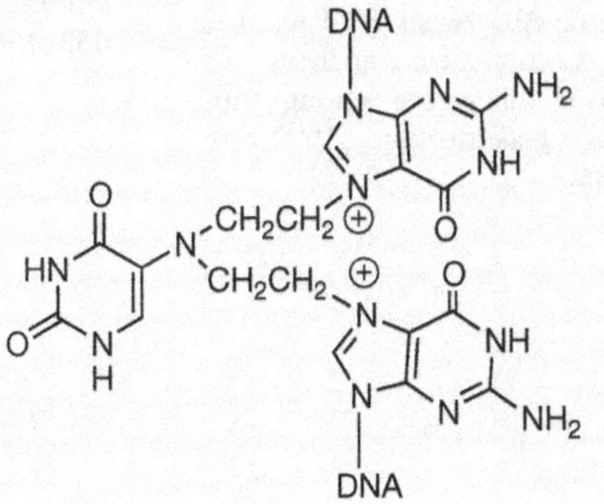

A Self Test 21.2

1. Dihydrofolate reductase 2. Thymidylate synthetase.
3. Ribonucleotide reductase.

A Self Test 21.3

4 Lysines, 7 arginines, 1 histidine.

A Self Test 21.4

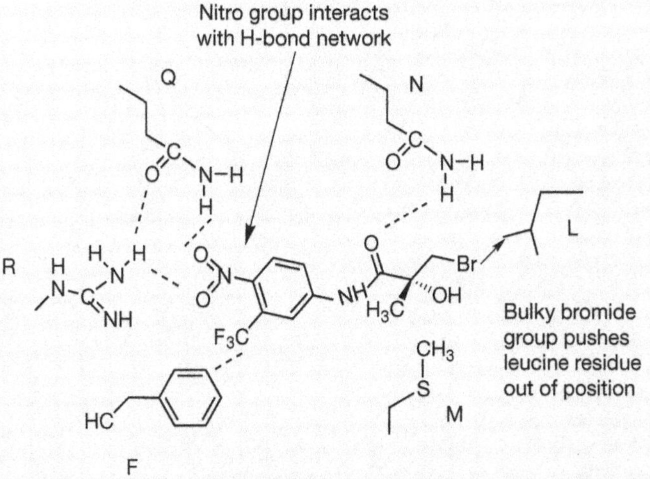

REFERENCES

1. Srivastana V, Negi AS, Kumar JK, Gupta MM, Khanuja SPS. Plant based anticancer molecules: Chemical and biological profile of some important leads. *Bioorg Med Chem.* 2005;13:5892–5908.
2. Hait WH, Rubin E, Alli E, Goodin S. Tubulin targeting agents. Update on Cancer Therapeutics.
3. Fiser SBH, Orr GA. Insights into the mechanism of microtubule stabilization by Taxol. *Proc Natl Acad Sci.* 2006;103:10166–10173.
4. Montecucco A, Biamonti G. Cellular response to etoposide treatment. *Cancer Lett.* 2006.
5. Scapin G. Structural biology in drug design: selective protein kinase inhibitors. *Drug Discov Today.* 2002;7:601–611.
6. Arora A, Scholar EM. Role of tyrosine kinase inhibitors in cancer therapy. *J Pharmacol Exp Therap.* 2005;315:971–979.
7. Schwabe JWR, Neuhaus D, Rhodes D. Solution structure of the DMA-binding domain of the oestrogen receptor. *Nature.* 1990;348:458–461.
8. McDonell DP. The molecular determinants of estrogen receptor pharmacology. *Maturitas.* 2004;48:S7–S12.
9. Wijayaratne AIL, Nagel SC, Paige LA, et al. Comparative analyses of mechanistic differences among antiestrogens. *Endocrinology.* 1999;140:5828–5840.
10. Bohl CE, Wu Z, Miller DD, Bell CE, Dalton JT. Crystal structure of the T877A human androgen receptor ligand-binding domain complexed to cyproterone acetate provides insight for ligand-induced conformational changes and structure-based drug design. *J Biol Chem.* 2007;282:3648–13655.
11. Bisson WH, Abagyan R, Cavasotto CN. Molecular basis of agonicity and antagonicity in the androgen receptor studied by molecular dynamics simulations. *J Mol Graph Model.* 2008;27:452–458.

Chapter | 22 |

Antimicrobial chemotherapy

CHAPTER CONTENTS

SECTION A – ANTIBIOTICS

Justice Nii Addy Tettey

INTRODUCTION

Antibiotics are generally products, or modifications thereof, of microbial metabolism that at low concentrations kill or inhibit the growth of other microorganisms. The observation that fungi and yeast could produce substances capable of destroying other bacteria was made by Vuillemin at the end of the nineteenth century and led to the concept of *antibiosis* (anti – against; bios – life). The microorganisms from which useful antibiotics have been obtained include fungi

(*Penicillium, Cephalosporium* and *Micromonospora*) and bacteria (*Bacillus* and *Streptomyces*). The discovery of penicillin by Alexander Fleming in 1928 marked the beginning of antimicrobial chemotherapy in the modern era. This serendipitous discovery was followed by the introduction of the sulphonamides (1932), cephalosporins (1940s), macrolides (1952), vancomycin (1956), quinolones (1962) fluorinated quinolones (1980s) and quite recently linezolid (2000).

The fundamental basis of antimicrobial chemotherapy is *selective toxicity*. This is achieved by exploiting structural and biochemical differences between a mammalian host and the causative microorganism. Some of the biochemical and structural differences which have been exploited to produce useful antibiotics include cell metabolism, cell wall synthesis, protein and nucleic acid synthesis. Antibacterial agents may be bacteriostatic or bactericidal and may have either a narrow spectrum (affecting few species or genera) or broad spectrum (affecting both Gram-positive and Gram-negative bacteria) of activity. In this chapter, the antibacterial agents are discussed based on their mechanisms of action, such as the effects on bacterial cell wall synthesis, cell metabolism, protein synthesis and nucleic acid synthesis. Other antibiotics in current use, which exert their action by entirely different mechanisms, are also described.

INHIBITION OF CELL WALL SYNTHESIS

Unlike eukaryotic cells, prokaryotic cells possess a cell wall which maintains cell integrity and offers protection from the harsh environments in which they exist. The bacterial cell wall conforms to two basic designs which can be distinguished by the Gram stain, i.e. Gram negative and Gram positive. In both designs, the bacterial cell wall is made up of peptidoglycan which consists of the saccharides N-acetylglucosamine (NAG) and N-acetylmuramic (NAM) linked together by peptide bonds to confer mechanical strength. These peptide bonds are formed between the pentaglycine of one saccharide chain with the penultimate *D*-alanine of another chain, leading to the loss of a terminal alanine. The production of the cell wall in bacteria involves multiple processes such as the partial assembly of cell wall components within the cell, transportation of the partially assembled components across the cell membrane to the cell wall (transglycosylation), assembly into the cell wall and finally cross-linking of the polysaccharide chains. Due the absence of the cell wall in eukaryotes, the interference with the various processes involved in cell wall synthesis serve as useful targets for achieving antibiosis. Commonly used antibiotics such as the β-lactams (penicillins, cephalosporins, carbapenems and monobactams) and vancomycin, which inhibit the synthesis of the cell wall, have a specific effect on one or more of the processes involved in cell wall synthesis.

In 1929, Fleming reported the inhibition of the growth of staphylococci by a rare strain of mould, *Penicillium notatum*. The isolation and identification of the active substance, benzylpenicillin (Penicillin G), was achieved at Oxford University by Florey and Chain towards the end of the Second World War. The penicillin nucleus, with the characteristic β-lactam ring, was isolated in 1959 by Batchelor and co-workers and serves as the precursor for many semi-synthetic penicillin derivatives. The natural penicillins (Penicillin G and phenoxymethylpenicillin (Penicillin V)) are obtained through fermentation processes. The semi-synthetic analogues have mostly been produced using 6-aminopenicillanic acid (6-APA) which is derived from the natural penicillins by selective hydrolysis of the amide side chain while avoiding hydrolysis of the intrinsically more labile β-lactam ring. The selective hydrolysis of the natural penicillins to 6-aminopenicillanic acid has been achieved by the use of penicillin amidases/acylases (Fig. 22.1).

The β-lactam group of antibiotics remains one of the most important and widely used therapeutic agents. The clinically important groups include the penicillins, cephalosporins, carbapenems and monobactams. These compounds derive their classification from the β-lactam moiety which is invariant in their structures and also accounts for their antibacterial activity. The generic structures of the β-lactam antibiotics are shown later on in this chapter.

Multiple enzymes are involved in the synthesis of the bacterial cell wall. The β-lactam antibiotics bind to several of these enzymes, which are collectively called penicillin binding proteins (PBP) and inhibit the cross-linking of the peptidoglycan strands. The most important PBP, transpeptidase, is involved in the final cross-linking step in cell wall synthesis. The cross-linking of the bacterial cell wall involves the formation of new peptide bonds between the pentaglycine of one saccharide chain with

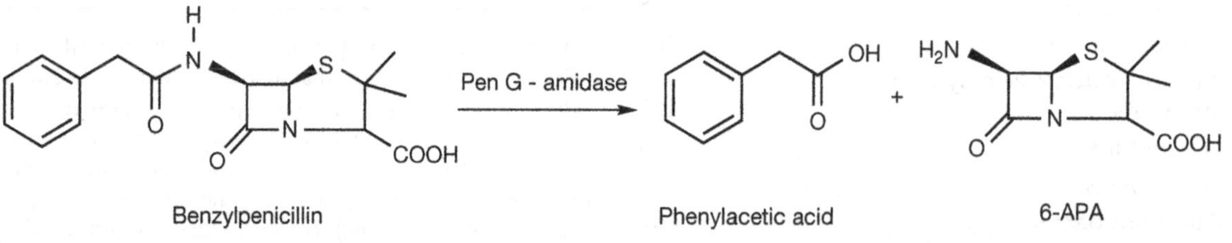

Figure 22.1 Enzymatic hydrolysis of benzylpenicillin to 6-APA.

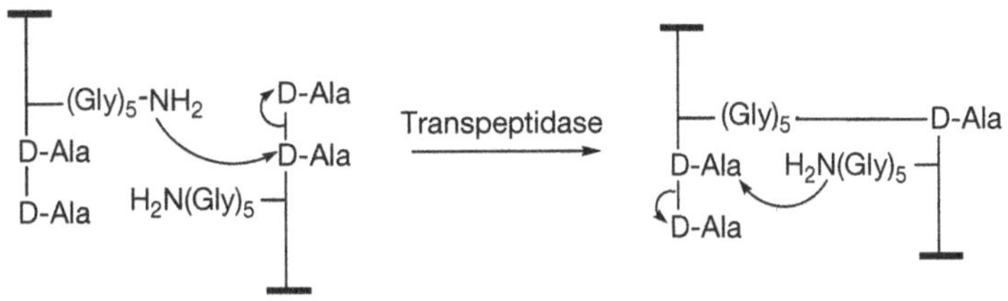

Figure 22.2 Cross-linking of bacterial cell wall by formation of new peptide bonds.

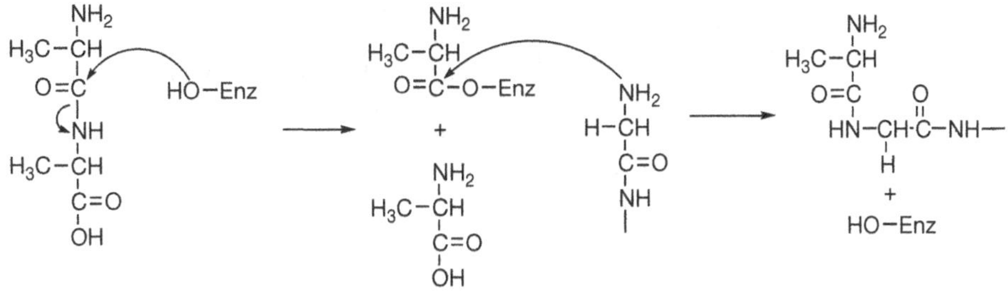

Figure 22.3 The action of transpeptidase in promoting cell wall cross-linking.

the penultimate *D*-alanine of another chain (Fig. 22.2), leading to the loss of the terminal alanine.

The transpeptidase enzyme participates in the reaction as above and effectively attacks the sensitive amide linkage of the D-alanyl-*D*-alanine terminated peptides. The transpeptidase enzyme is regenerated after it has facilitated the peptide bond formation between the carbonyl of the penultimate *D*-alanine group and the N-terminus of glycine (Fig. 22.3).

However, the structure of the penicillin (and other β-lactams) resembles the D-alanyl-*D*-alanine moiety (Fig. 22.4) and can therefore react with the transpeptidase enzyme to form a covalent ester bond.

The acylated enzyme formed by reaction with the β-lactams does not react as readily with nucleophiles as the activated complex formed with D-Ala-D-Ala. Therefore, the transpeptidase enzyme is inactivated, resulting in the inhibition of further cross-linking of the bacterial cell wall. This triggers a sequence of events including the release of bacterial autolysin and eventually results in cell death. The β-lactams are therefore bactericidal.

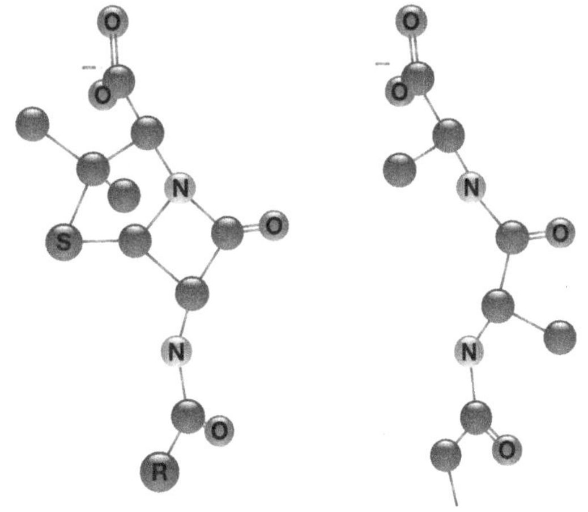

Figure 22.4 Structural similarity between the penicillin molecule and D-alanyl-*D*-alanine.

STRUCTURE–ACTIVITY RELATIONSHIPS OF THE PENICILLINS

It is evident from the spatial orientation of the penicillin molecule relative to the D-alanyl-*D*-alanine moiety that an intact β-lactam ring is required to maintain structural similarity and therefore competition for the active site of the transpeptidase enzyme. The parent 6-aminopenicillanic acid moiety is invariant in all the penicillins (Fig. 22.5) and allows only two points for chemical modification; the side chain (R) attached to the amino group on *C-6* and the carboxyl group on *C-3*.

The nature of the side chain (R) determines the hydrophilic/hydrophobic balance of the molecule, the antibacterial spectrum and chemical properties such as instability to acids and β-lactamases – the bacterial defence mechanism. The carboxyl group is a site for salt formation and facilitates the formation of Na, K and Ca

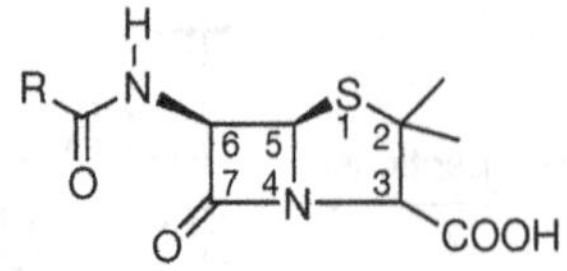

Figure 22.5 Generic structure of the penicillins.

salts. The free carboxyl group is required for activity and therefore non-degradable moieties, such as amides and esters, lack antibacterial activity in vitro. Prodrugs, which are rapidly degraded in vivo to release the active penicillin, are formulated to overcome problems with oral bioavailability. Slow-release parenteral dosage forms are achievable by ester formation at the carboxylic acid group or by ion pair formation or by ester formation. Procaine penicillin and benzathine penicillin represent the former type and bacampicillin the latter.

REACTIVITY OF THE β-LACTAM RING

Amide resonance is responsible for the lower susceptibility of carbonyl groups to nucleophilic attack. In a normal amide, the planar arrangement of the O, C and N atoms is generally assumed to be necessary for effective delocalisation of the nitrogen lone pair and therefore exists in the stable canonical forms shown in Figure 22.6.

The ring strain caused by the orientation of the β-lactam in the penicillin molecule affects this resonance stabilisation

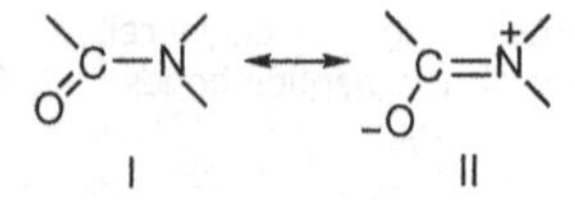

Figure 22.6 Resonance stabilisation of planar amides.

and results in a greater probability of canonical form I. The corollary is that the electron-deficient carbon is more susceptible to nucleophilic attack. Such attack leads to disruption of the C–N bond, dissimilarity of the resulting molecule to D-alanyl D-alanine, and subsequently loss of antibacterial action. For example, in dilute alkali solutions, the nucleophilic attack on the electro-deficient *C-7* carbon in the penicillin molecule leads to rapid hydrolysis to penicilloic acids (Fig. 22.7).

Other important reactions of the β-lactam antibiotics, such as attack by bacterial lactamases and reaction with penicillin-binding proteins (e.g. transpeptidase enzyme), proceed via an identical mechanism of nucleophilic attack on the *C-7* carbon.

Penicillins are also unstable in acidic solutions although the degradation proceeds by a different mechanism from that of alkaline hydrolysis. In aqueous acid, the oxygen of the *C-7* carbonyl becomes protonated (Fig. 22.8). The neighbouring carbon (*C-7*) is rendered more electron deficient and therefore more susceptible to nucleophilic attack. This leads to the formation of penicilloic acids. The acylation of the 6-amino group of the penicillins is an essential feature for antibacterial activity. However, the oxygen in the amide side chain can interact

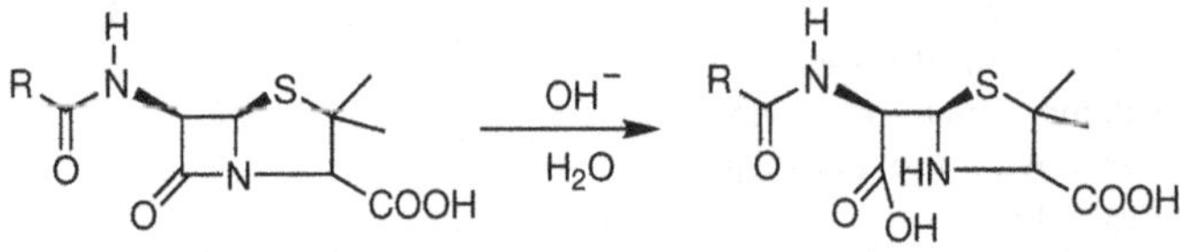

Figure 22.7 Alkaline hydrolysis of the β-lactam ring.

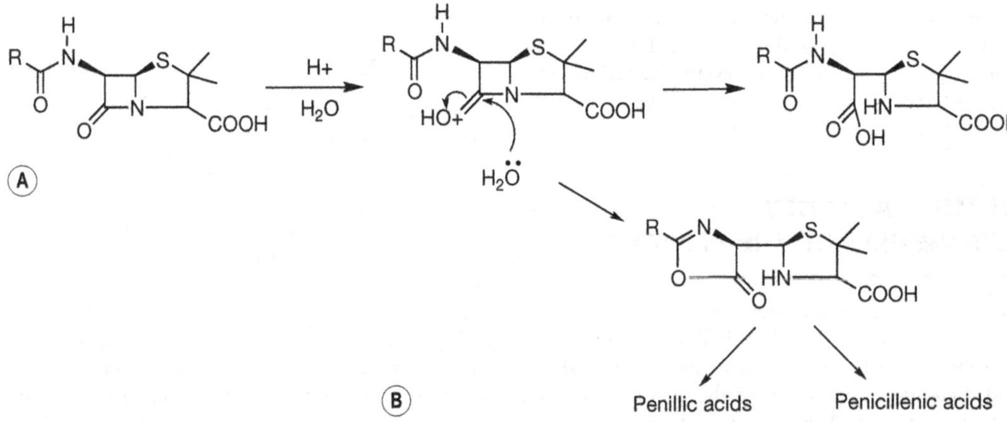

Figure 22.8 Degradation of the penicillins in acidic media.

with the electro-deficient carbon of the β-lactam ring in what is referred to as *neighbouring group participation*. This yields an intermediate product which leads to the formation of penillic and penicillenic acids (Fig. 22.8).

This mechanism explains the instability of penicillins such as Penicillin G in the acidic environment of the stomach. Substituents at the C-6 position in penicillins affect both the carbonyl carbon and the nitrogen of the β-lactam ring inductively. The attachment of an electron withdrawing group such as an amino group results in the reduction of the net negative charge on the oxygen in the β-lactam ring. This subsequently slows down the conversion from state A to B. In addition, the use of an electron withdrawing group at the R position reduces the effect of neighbouring group participation since the net negative charge of the oxygen is reduced, rendering its interaction with the C-7 carbonyl improbable.

CLASSIFICATION OF THE PENICILLINS

The penicillins can be classified on the basis of their antibacterial activity (broad spectrum, narrow spectrum), method of production (natural or semi-synthetic) and based on their stability/instability to bacterial β-lactamases. ·

Naturally occurring penicillins

Benzylpenicillin ((6R)-6-(2-phenylacetamido) penicillanic acid, Penicillin G (Fig. 22.9)) and phenoxymethyl penicillin ((6R)-6-(2-phenoxyacetamido) penicillanic acid, Penicillin V) are naturally occurring penicillins produced by strains of *Penicillium notatum*. The β-lactam ring in Penicillin G is susceptible to hydrolysis by bacterial β-lactamases and is also unstable in acidic or alkaline environments, as explained before. The instability in an acidic environment makes Penicillin G unsuitable for oral administration and it is therefore formulated as the freely soluble sodium and potassium salts for parenteral administration.

Penicillin G is administered either as an intramuscular injection or as a slow intravenous infusion. Due to the high water solubility of the potassium and sodium salts

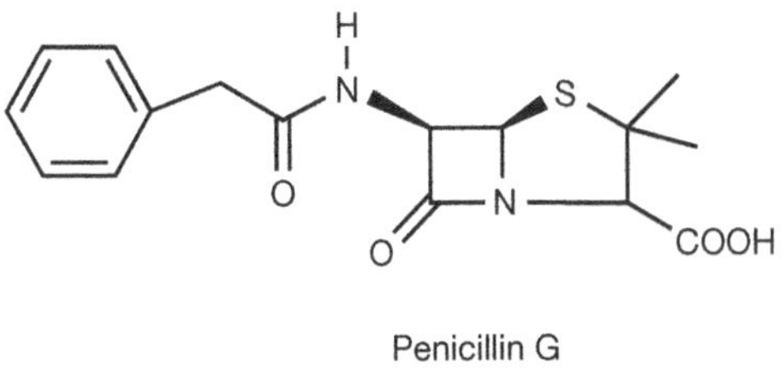

Penicillin G

Figure 22.9

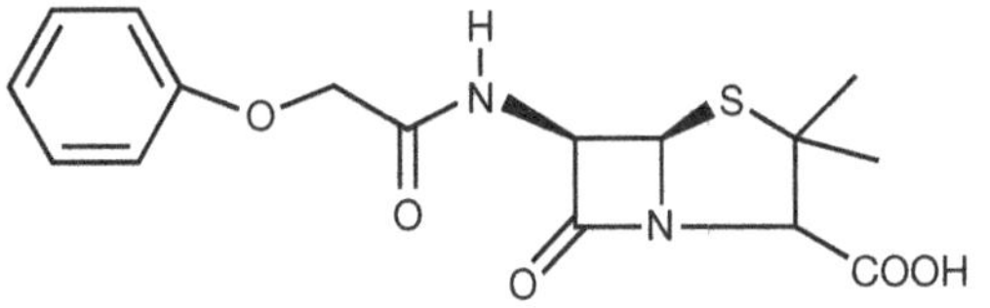

Penicillin V

Figure 22.10

of Penicillin G, it is rapidly absorbed from intramuscular sites and frequent dosing is required to maintain therapeutic concentrations. The adsorption of benzylpenicillin can be delayed by producing derivatives of reduced solubility. Procaine penicillin, an equimolar salt of procaine and penicillin, occurs as white crystals or microcrystalline powder with reduced water solubility. It is therefore suitable for use in intramuscular depot preparations, providing therapeutic concentrations of Penicillin G to inhibit sensitive organisms for up to 24 h. Benzathine penicillin, which has poorer aqueous solubility, is also used in intramuscular depot preparations. It is prepared by the reaction of dibenzylethylene diamine with penicillin G in a 1:2 ratio and provides therapeutic concentrations for up to 120 h when administered by deep intramuscular injection.

In Penicillin V (Fig. 22.10), the additional electro-withdrawing effect of the phenoxy substituent, as opposed to the phenyl in Penicillin G, reduces the propensity of the β-lactam ring to undergo acid-catalysed hydrolysis. This makes it possible to administer Penicillin V orally.

Penicillin G and Penicillin V are both too lipophilic to penetrate the Gram-negative bacterial cell wall, labile to β-lactamase inactivation and are therefore classified as narrow-spectrum antibiotics susceptible to β-lactamase inactivation. The natural penicillins are generally indicated for infections caused by Gram-positive organisms including most anaerobes. They are ineffective against *Pseudomonas aeruginosa*.

β-Lactamase stable penicillins

Bacteria produce hydrolytic enzymes called β-lactamases which are serine hydrolyase enzymes (penicillinases and cephalosporinases) which hydrolyse the β-lactam ring. The subsequent loss of resemblance to the D-alanyl-*D*-alanine results in the loss of antibacterial activity. The naturally occurring penicillins are hydrolysed by Gram-positive β-lactamases and this led to the design of compounds resistant to β-lactamases. The addition of a bulky carbocyclic or heterocyclic aromatic ring directly to the carbonyl moiety, substituting the amino group on 6-aminopenicillanic acid, causes steric hindrance around the sensitive carbonyl of the β-lactam ring. This effect either slows down the rate of hydrolysis or results in the

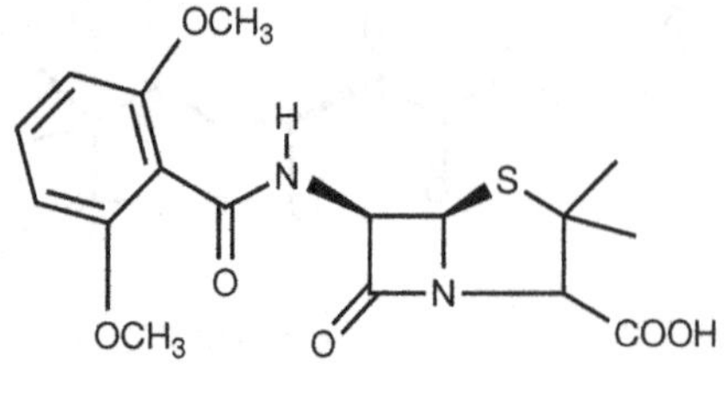

Methicillin

Figure 22.11

loss of affinity for the active site of the β-lactamase enzyme. The design of β-lactamase stable penicillins led to methicillin (Fig. 22.11).

Methicillin has lost its clinical significance due to the high incidence of resistant *Staphylococcus aureus* infections. The use of heterocyclic substituents, based on isoxazolyl, led to the development of the penicillins cloxacillin and flucloxacillin (Fig. 22.12).

The isoxazolyl penicillins are highly lipophilic and therefore do not penetrate the Gram-negative bacterial cell wall. They are classified as narrow-spectrum penicillins stable to Gram-positive β-lactamases. These penicillins can be administered orally because of their stability in acid. Members of this class of antibiotics are preferred for treatment of staphylococcal infections of the skin and soft tissue. The isoxazolyl penicillins are prepared as sodium salts and available as capsules, intramuscular and slow intravenous infusions, elixirs and syrups.

Broad-spectrum penicillins

The antibacterial spectrum of the penicillins depends on their ability to cross the bacterial cell wall. However, structural differences exist in the composition of the cell wall in Gram-negative and Gram-positive bacteria and result in marked differences in permeability. The naturally occurring penicillins are too lipophilic to penetrate the outer lipoprotein/liposaccharide layers of the cell walls of Gram-negative bacteria and are therefore classified as narrow-spectrum (active against mostly Gram-positive bacteria) antibiotics. The Gram-negative bacterial cell wall contains hydrophilic protein channels called *porin trimers* that allow the passage of hydrophilic substances of molecular weight not exceeding 600 Daltons. This observation led to the synthesis of the aminopenicillins, such as ampicillin and amoxicillin (Fig. 22.13), which are active against both Gram-negative and Gram-positive bacteria.

The general design of the aminopenicillins is based on the substitution of an amino group on the α-carbon of Penicillin G. This lowers the lipophilicity of the naturally occurring penicillins and facilitates penetration of the Gram-negative cell wall via the porin trimer. The electron withdrawing property of the amino group confers acid stability on the aminopenicillins and hence the successful design of oral dosage forms. Amoxicillin is prepared as the sodium salt for parenteral use (i.m./i.v.) and as the trihydrate for capsules and paediatric suspensions. Ampicillin is used as the sodium salt in parenteral preparations, trihydrate for capsules, but also as the unmodified compound for capsules and oral suspensions.

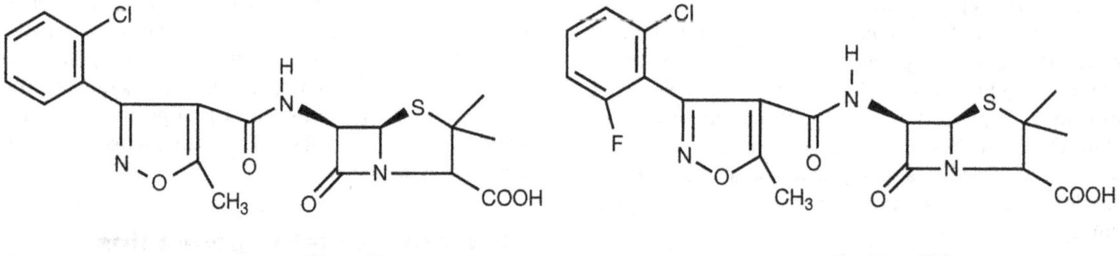

Figure 22.12

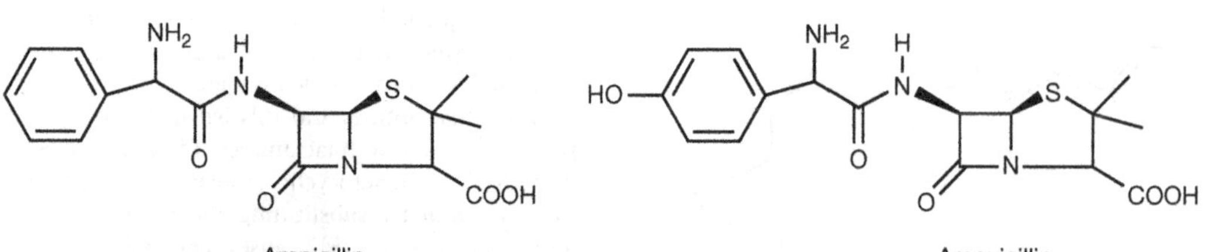

Figure 22.13

Figure 22.14 β-lactamase enzyme inhibitors.

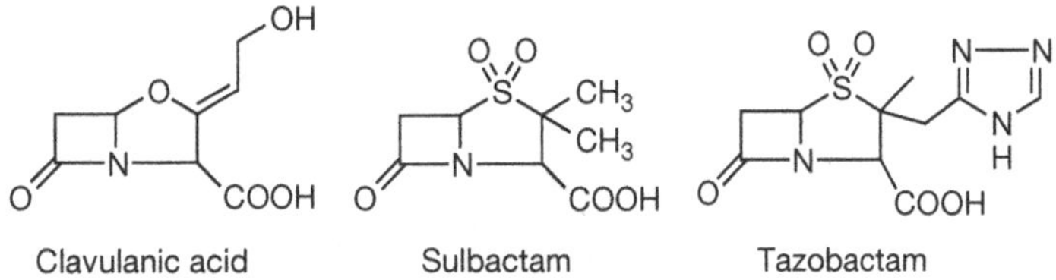

The aminopenicillins are, however, not stable to bacterial β-lactamases. Several steps have been taken to extend their activity to β-lactamase-producing organisms and these include co-formulation with β-lactamase stable penicillins and the use of β-lactamase inhibitors.

Combination treatments often involve the use of broad-spectrum penicillin and β-lactamase-stable penicillin. Clinically useful combinations include ampiclox® (ampicillin and cloxacillin) and magnapen® (ampicillin and flucloxacillin). These combinations are usually indicated for infections caused by susceptible organisms where a mixed infection is present and includes penicillin-resistant staphylococci.

The alternative to combination treatments is the use of β-lactamase enzyme inhibitors such as clavulanic acid, sulbactam and tazobactam (Fig. 22.14), which bear structural resemblance to the β-lactam antibiotics and subsequently compete for the active site of the β-lactamase enzyme.

The initial interaction between the hydrolytic enzyme and the inhibitor involves the attack on the electro-deficient β-lactam carbon. With the β-lactam antibiotics, the attack on the carbon leads to the disruption of the C–N bond and subsequent loss of antibacterial activity. The β-lactamase enzyme is regenerated after disruption of the β-lactam ring. With the β-lactamase inhibitors, a subsequent attack by the nucleophiles at the active site of the β-lactamase enzyme results in the formation of a second bond between the enzyme and inhibitor. This increased interaction prevents the regeneration of the β-lactamase enzyme, leading to its inactivation (Fig. 22.15).

This concept has been applied successfully to the development of broad-spectrum antibiotics suitable for use in infections involving β-lactamase-producing organisms. A clinically useful example is co-amoxiclav which is a mixture of amoxicillin (as the trihydrate or sodium salt) and clavulanic acid (as potassium clavulanate) and is available as oral (tablet, oral suspension) and parenteral (intravenous infusion and injection) preparations.

The oral bioavailability of ampicillin (approx. 30%) is less than that of amoxicillin (approx. 70–90%). The absorption of ampicillin following oral administration has been enhanced by the formation of suitable prodrugs. At intestinal pH, ampicillin exists as a zwitterion. The conversion of ampicillin into an ester (R = degradable ester group, Fig. 22.16) suppresses zwitterion formation and presents ampicillin as a simple base, which would be 10–50% un-ionised at intestinal pH and subsequently undergo passive absorption.

However, the penicillins require a free carboxylic acid moiety at C-3 and therefore ester groups used in suppressing ionisation must be readily degradable to facilitate

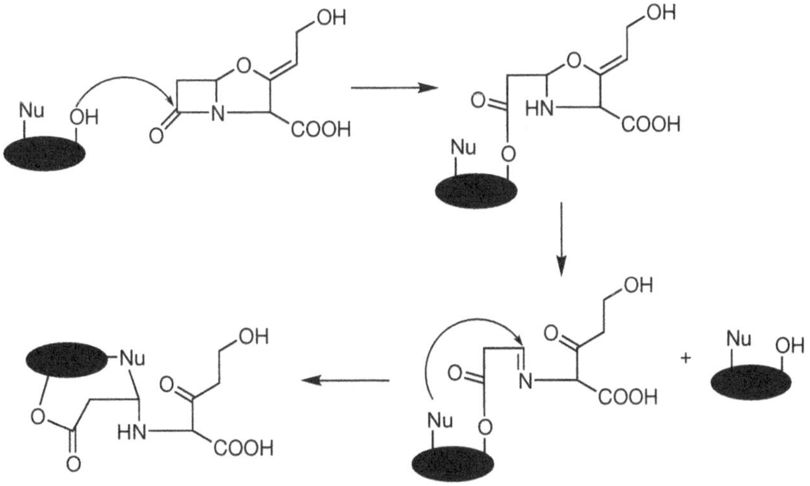

Figure 22.15 Irreversible inactivation of β-lactamases by formation of two covalent bonds between the enzyme and inhibitor.

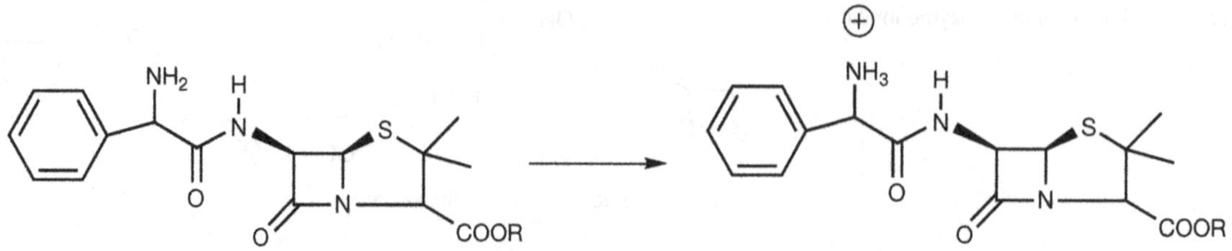

Figure 22.16 Suppression of zwitterion from ampicillin.

activity. Suitable prodrugs have been developed using acyloxymethyl esters (bacampicillin and pivampicillin) and phthalidyl esters (talampicillin). Prodrugs of ampicillin based on acyloxymethyl ester formation undergo rapid hydrolysis in vivo after or during passage through the intestinal mucosa, leading to the liberation of free active ampicillin (Fig. 22.17).

Talampicillin, which is based on a phthalidyl ester, liberates the active compound (ampicillin) with the formation of phthaldehydic acid (Fig. 22.18).

Antipseudomonal penicillins

The Gram-negative bacteria *Pseudomonas aeruginosa* stands out as a difficult organism due to its resistance to the activity of antibiotics. Modification of the structure of the 6-APA to achieve improved permeability of the Gram-negative cell wall and specificity for pseudomonal penicillin binding proteins (PBP) has been achieved with the synthesis of the carboxypenicillins and the acylureido penicillins.

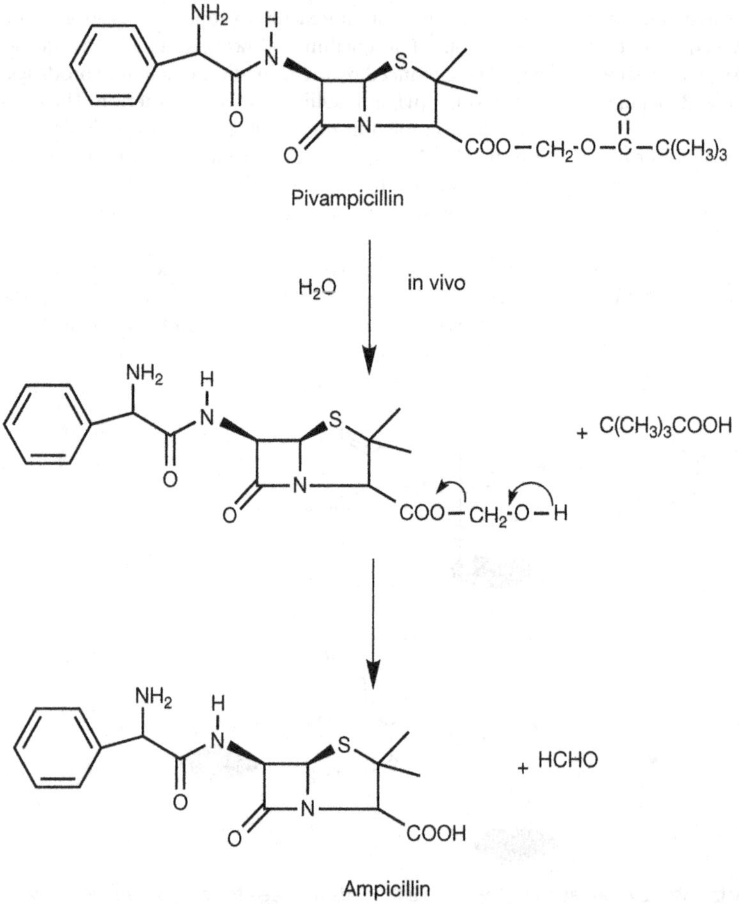

Figure 22.17 In vivo hydrolysis of pivampicillin to yield ampicillin.

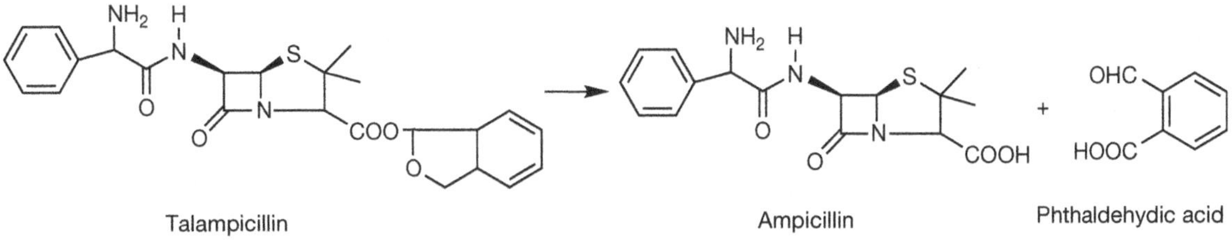

Figure 22.18

The addition of carboxylic, sulfanic or sulphonic acid groups to the α-carbon of the amide side chain improves the antipseudomonas activity in vitro. The first clinically useful antipseudomonal carboxypenicillin was carbenicillin (Fig. 22.19).

Carbenicillin is used by itself or in combination with gentamicin for the treatment of infections by sensitive strains of *Pseudomonas aeruginosa*. The replacement of the phenyl moiety with 3-thienyl groups to produce ticarcillin leads to an increase in antipseudomonal activity. However, the carboxy penicillins show diminished activity against streptococci and enterococci due to reduced binding to the PBPs.

The acylureido penicillins are derivatives of ampicillin designed to improve the penetration of the outer membrane of the *Pseudomonas* cell. The clinically useful ones are azlocillin and piperacillin (Fig. 22.20).

Although the carboxy and acylureido penicillins are active against *Pseudomonas*, they are still susceptible to inhibition by bacterial β-lactamases. Most of the antipseudomonal penicillins are now used in combination with β-lactamase inhibitors to improve their activity against susceptible β-lactamase-producing organisms. Some clinical examples are Tazocin® (Tazobactam (sodium salt) + Piperacillin (sodium salt)), Timetin® (Clavulanic acid (potassium salt) + Ticarcillin (sodium salt)). The antipseudomonal penicillins are presented as parenteral preparations because of their instability in acidic conditions.

Cephalosporins

The introduction of the cephalosporins was a result of investigations in the mid-1940s by Giuseppe Brotzu who discovered that *Cephalosporium acremonium*, isolated for a sewage outfall, inhibited the growth of several bacterial species including *Salmonella typhus*. The prototype of the cephalosporins, cephalosporin C, was subsequently

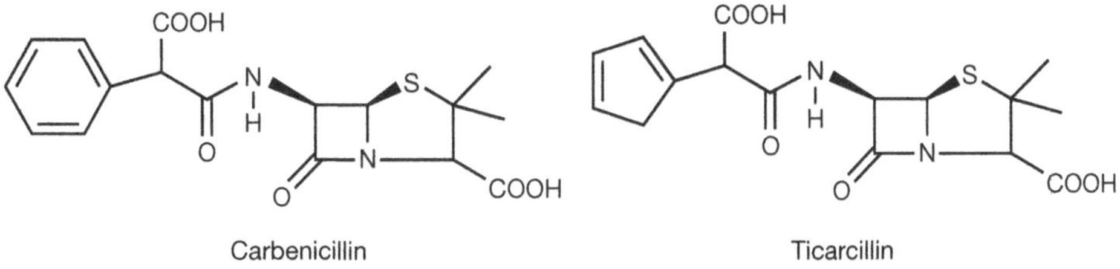

Figure 22.19

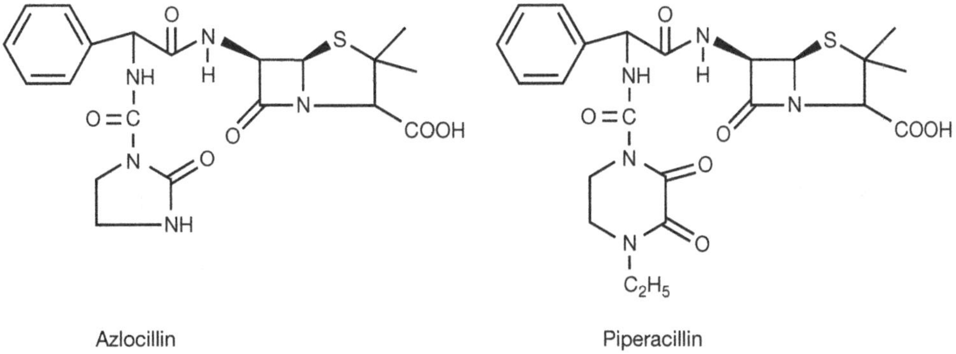

Figure 22.20

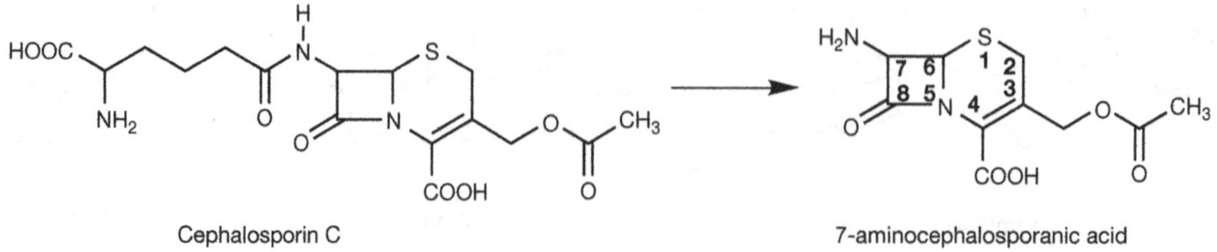

Figure 22.21

isolated by Abraham and Newton. The enzymatic removal of the side chain in cephalosporin C, analogous to the removal of the benzyl group in Penicillin G, produces 7-aminocephalosporanic acid (7-APA; Fig. 22.21). 7-APA is the key intermediate in the synthesis of most of the present-day cephalosporins and can also be produced through chemical synthesis.

Although the cephalosporins have a similar chemical mechanism of action as the penicillins, the presence of a six-membered ring rather than a five-membered ring in the penicillins relieves ring strain and renders the cephalosporins less chemically reactive. However, upon attack of the *C-8* carbonyl by nucleophiles, suitable substitutions at *C-3* can act as an electron sink (Fig. 22.22) and increase the reactivity of the β-lactam ring. The acetoxy substituent extending from the dihydrothiazine ring in cephalosporin C and cephalothin is a classical example.

The cephalosporins are classified as first-, second- or third-generation agents. They differ in terms of antibacterial spectrum, stability to bacterial β-lactamases and pharmacokinetics. As a therapeutic group, the cephalosporins are not absorbed from the gut unless they possess a phenylglycine-like moiety on the α-carbon of the side chain. Examples of cephalosporins with this feature are cefalexin, cefadroxil and cefaclor. Cephradine is an exception and features a cyclohexadienyl substituent.

First-generation cephalosporins

First-generation agents possess potent activity against Gram-positive bacteria but only moderate potency against Gram-negative bacteria. They have no activity against *Pseudomonas aeruginosa.* The first-generation agents suitable for oral administration include cefalexin, cefadroxil and cephradine (Fig. 22.23).

Cephalothin (Fig. 22.24) represents a first-generation agent which is suitable for parenteral administration. These parenteral forms are characterised by the presence of an acetoxymethyl group extending from the dihydrothiazine ring which, as discussed above, increases the reactivity of the lactam ring.

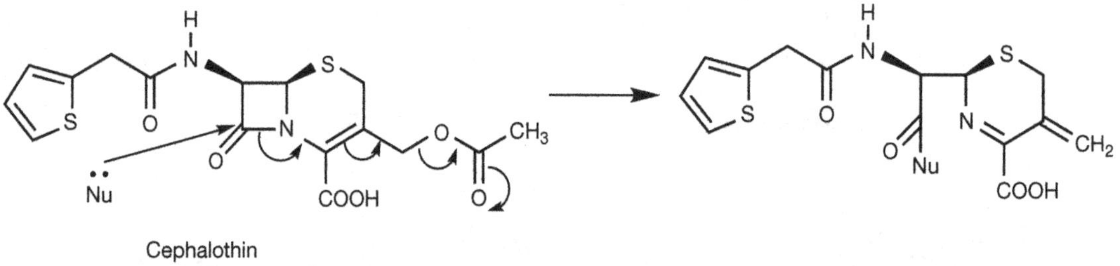

Figure 22.22 Increased reactivity of the cephalosporin ring.

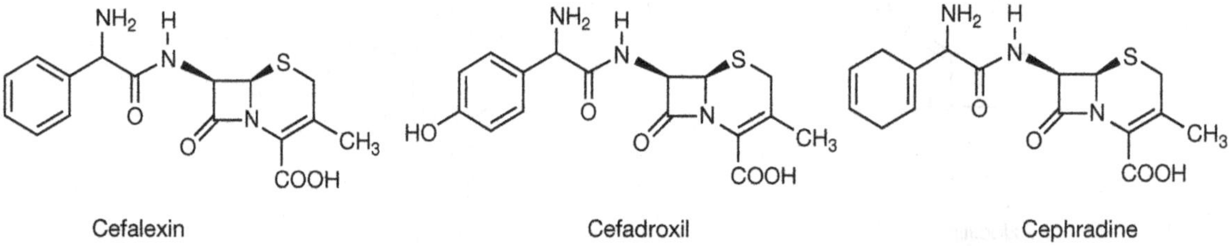

Figure 22.23

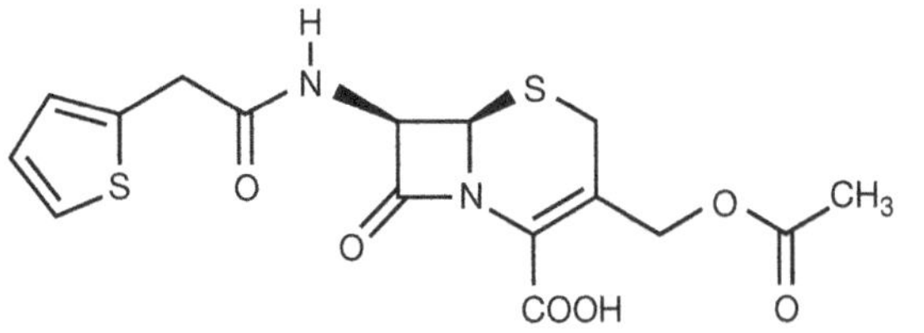

Cephalothin

Figure 22.24

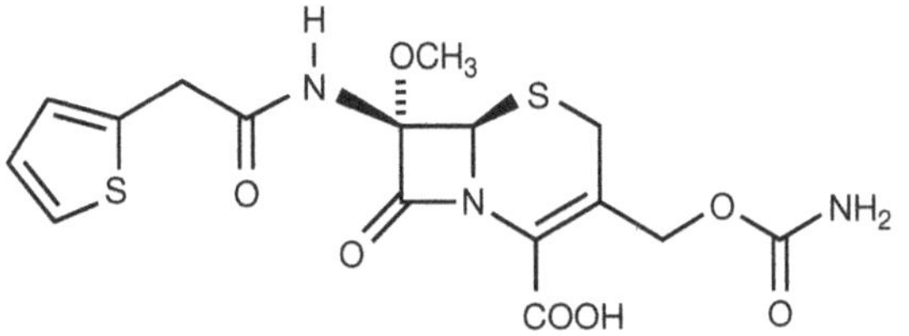

Cefoxitin

Figure 22.26

Second-generation cephalosporins

The second generation of cephalosporins possess an extended spectrum of antibacterial activity compared to the first-generation agents. They are active against Gram-negative pathogens such as *Escherichia coli* and some species of *Klebsiella*, *Proteus* and *Neisseria gonorrhoea*. They are, however, ineffective against *Pseudomonas*. Cefaclor represents an example of an orally active second-generation agent. Most of the second-generation cephalosporins are parenteral agents with a nitrogen-rich heterocyclic moiety extending from the dihydrothiazine ring. A clinically useful example is cefamandole (Fig. 22.25).

The cephamycins, a class of cephalosporins obtained from *Streptomyces* sp., display broad-spectrum antibacterial activity and stability to β-lactamases. The cephamycins contain a methoxyl substituent on the β-lactam ring and the shielding effect makes the ring less susceptible to lactamase attack. A clinically useful semi-synthetic analogue of cephamycin is Cefoxitin (Fig. 22.26).

Perhaps one of the most successful second-generation cephalosporins is cefuroxime (Zinacef®) (Fig. 22.27). Cefuroxime is stable to bacterial β-lactamases and can be administered either parenterally or orally as its acetoxyethoxy ester cefuroxime axetil (Zinnat®).

Third-generation cephalosporins

The third-generation agents display a broader spectrum of antibacterial activity compared to the first- and second-generation cephalosporins. Although these agents display enhanced activity against Gram-negative bacteria they are generally not clinically effective against *Pseudomonas*. The third-generation agents have high β-lactamase resistance and this is attributed to the acylamino side chain. The useful clinical examples are cefotaxime and ceftizoxime (Fig. 22.28).

Ceftriaxone has a long elimination half-life and therefore allows once-a-day dosing. Some third-generation agents are active against *Pseudomonas aeruginosa* and include the clinically useful agent ceftazidime (Fig. 22.29).

Newer agents such as cefepime referred to as fourth-generation cephalosporins (Fig. 22.30), possess a quaternary nitrogen and have improved activity against *Pseudomonas*.

The complete structure activity evaluation of all the existing cephalosporins is beyond the scope of this chapter. However, there are some generalisations:

- Newer generations have more Gram-positive activity than preceding generations.
- Increase in Gram-negative activity results in a decrease in Gram-positive activity.
- The frequency of dosing generally decreases with increasing generation.
- The total daily dosage is similar within a generation.

Carbapenems

The prototype of the carbapenems, thienamycin, was isolated in 1976 by Kahan and co-workers from *Streptomyces cattlea*. Unlike the other β-lactam antibiotics, the carbapenems possess an exocyclic sulphur atom. The series allows chemical modification at the position marked **R** in Figure 22.31.

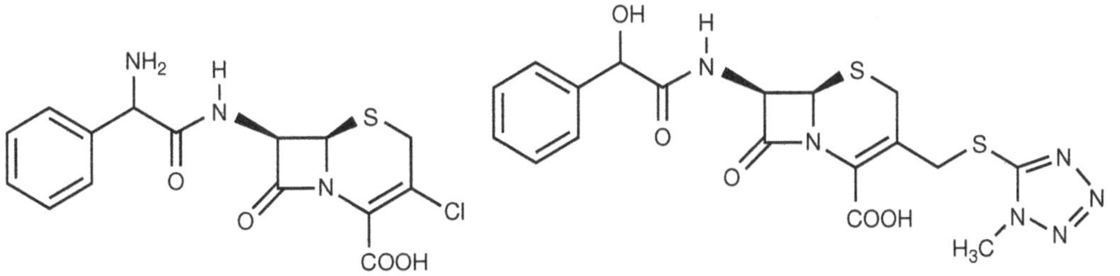

Cefaclor

Cefamandole

Figure 22.25

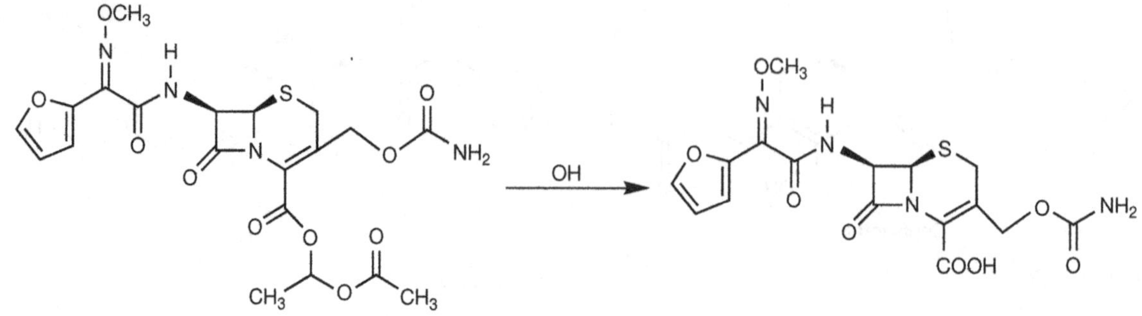

Cefuroxime axetil   Cefuroxime

Figure 22.27

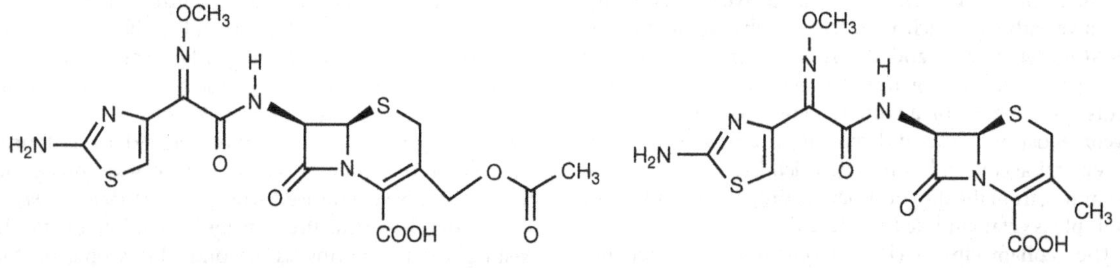

Cefotaxime   Ceftizoxime

Figure 22.28

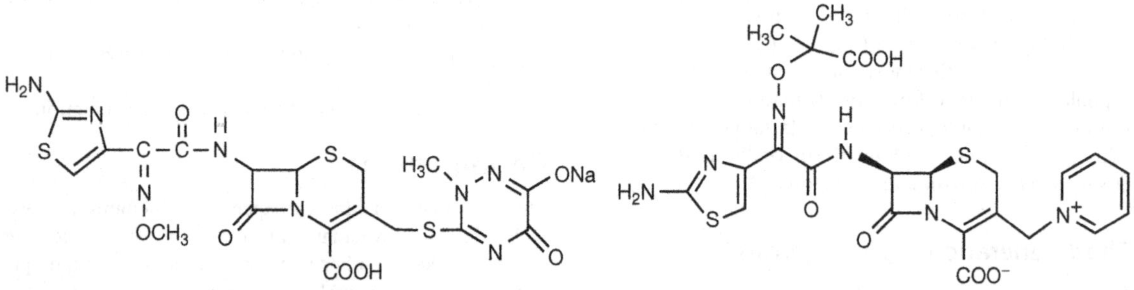

Ceftriaxone   Ceftazidime

Figure 22.29

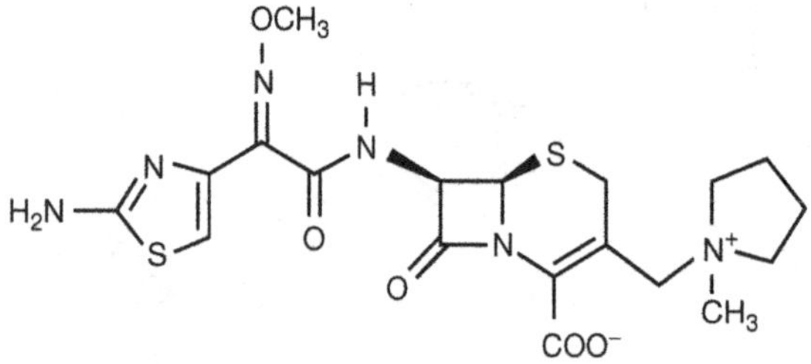

Cefepime

Figure 22.30

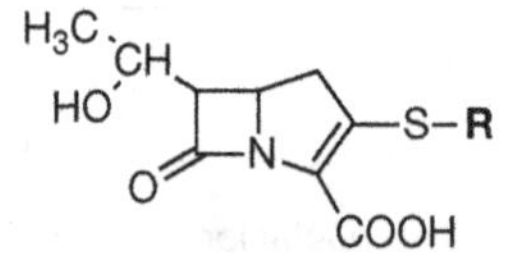

Figure 22.31 Generic structure of carbanapenems.

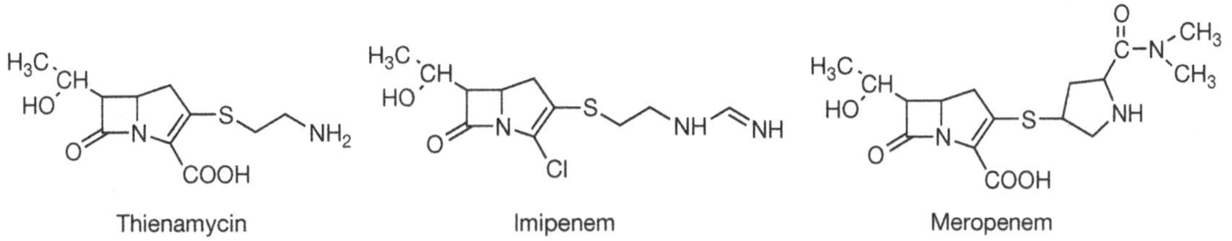

Figure 22.32

Thienamycin (Fig. 22.32) is a potent broad-spectrum antibiotic with β-lactamase inhibiting properties. This compound could not be marketed because of chemical and biological instability. The molecule was prone to inactivation in concentrated solutions due to the nucleophilic attack of the terminal primary amine group on the β-lactam ring.

In 1985, the self-inactivating property of thienamycin was overcome by the use of a terminal imino functionality which is less nucleophilic. Imipenem (Fig. 22.32) has a broad spectrum of activity and is administered by deep intramuscular injection or as an intravenous infusion. Renal dehydropeptidase 1, an enzyme present in the kidney, attacks and inactivates imipenem. This problem has been overcome by the co-administration of imipenem with cilastatin, a renal dehydropeptidase 1 inhibitor. Meropenem (Fig. 22.32), an analogue introduced in 1996, is stable to the action of renal dehydropeptidase 1 and is also administered by deep intramuscular injection or as an intravenous infusion. Since the discovery of thienamycin in 1976, only parenteral analogues have been successfully used clinically because the carbapenem structure is unstable in both the stomach and intestine.

Monocyclic β-lactam (monobactams)

The monobactams are β-lactam antibiotics which contain only one cyclic ring (Fig. 22.33). Unlike the other β-lactams, the monobactams are active almost entirely against Gram-negative bacteria. The general monobactam structure allows for structural alteration at a single locus (R). The only clinically useful example is aztreonam (Fig. 22.34).

Although the monobactams bear a structural similarity to the penicillins, clinical hypersensitivity reactions in penicillin-sensitive patients is rare. It is indicated for Gram-negative infections including *Pseudomonas aeruginosa*,

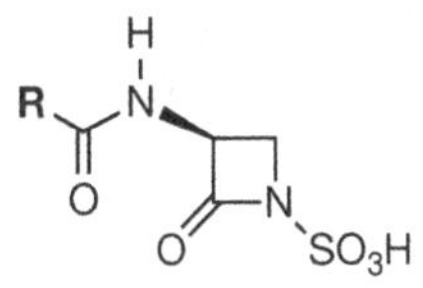

Figure 22.33

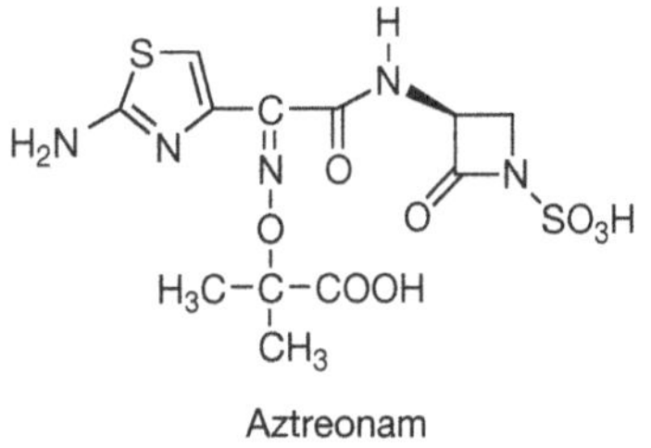

Figure 22.34

Haemophilus influenzae and *Neisseria meningitides* and administered by deep intramuscular injection or as an intravenous infusion.

Other inhibitors of cell wall synthesis

Vancomycin, a mucopeptide produced by *Streptomyces orientalis*, was first isolated from soil samples in 1956. It is bactericidal and acts by inhibiting cell wall replication. Vancomycin interacts with *D*-alanine and prevents the reaction of transpeptidase with the latter in the final stages of cross-linking. Due to its large size, vancomycin cannot enter the porin channels in Gram-negative bacteria and is therefore only effective in Gram-positive infections. It remains one of the few agents active against MRSA.

INHIBITION OF BACTERIAL CELL METABOLISM

The exploitation of subtle differences between the cellular metabolism in bacteria and mammalian host presents a niche for achieving selective toxicity. One such difference which has been exploited successfully to produce a useful class of antibiotics is the difference in the synthesis of tetrahydrofolate. Both bacterial and mammalian cells require folate in the form of tetrahydrofolate as a co-factor for thymidylate synthesis. Mammalian cells are incapable of synthesising folate and have specialised mechanisms for transporting folate from the diet into cells. On the contrary, most bacterial cells do not possess a similar transport mechanism and are incapable of utilising

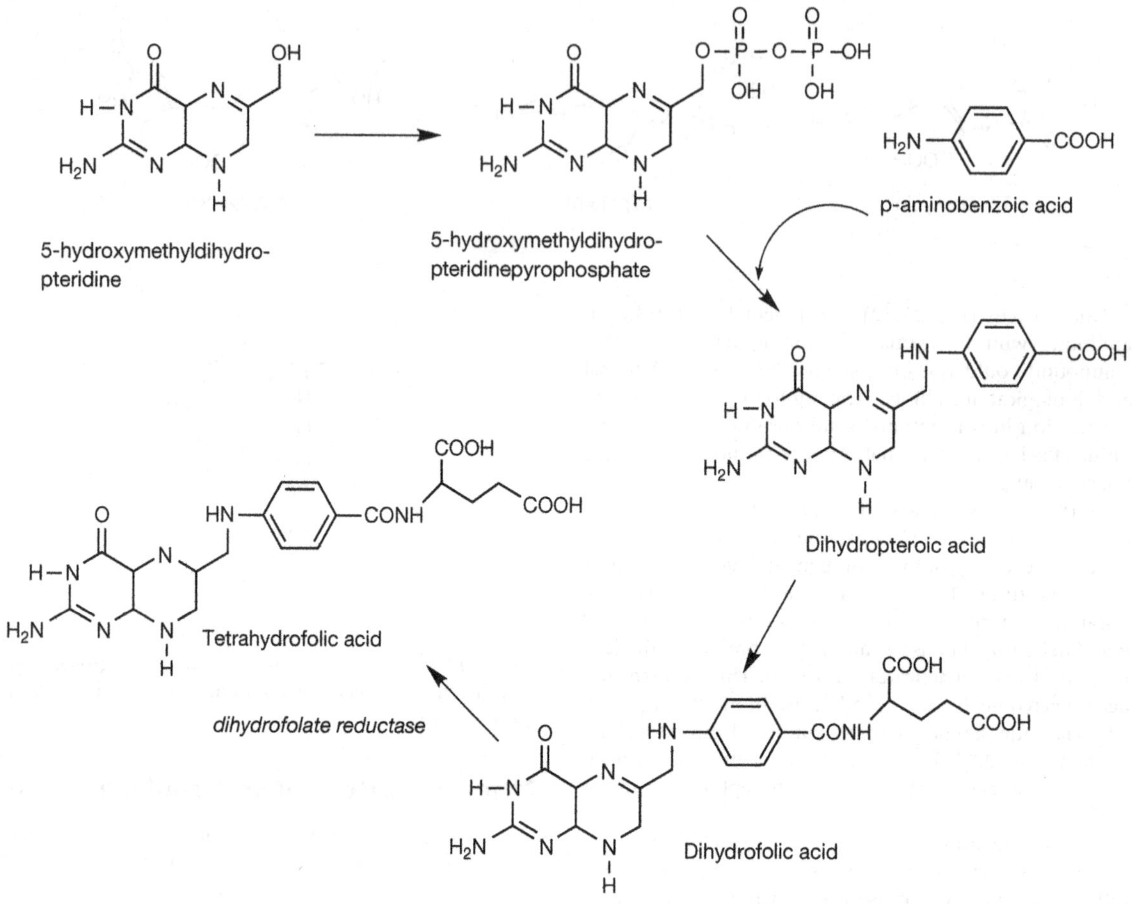

Figure 22.35 Inhibition of folate biosynthesis.

preformed folate. Bacteria therefore have to synthesise their own dihydrofolate and require endogenous p-aminobenzoic acid as a precursor (Fig. 22.35).

In 1931, Gerhard Domagk and co-workers found that the azo dye sulfamidochrysoidine (Prontosil Red®) was effective against virulent strains of *Streptococci pyogenes* in infected mice. The antimicrobial activity was later found to be due to its reduced metabolite, sulfanilamide (Prontosil white; Fig 22.36). Sulfanilamide forms the prototype of this class of synthetic antibacterial agents known as the *sulphonamides*.

Sulphonamides

Following the introduction of the sulphonamides in clinical use, the antibacterial activity was found to be inhibited by the presence of pus. This inhibitory effect of pus was found to be due to the presence of the structurally similar p-aminobenzoic acid (PABA): a compound which is also present in folic acid. This led to the observation that the sulphonamides competed with PABA, leading to the disruption of folate synthesis and cessation of bacterial growth. The importance of the sulphonamides in

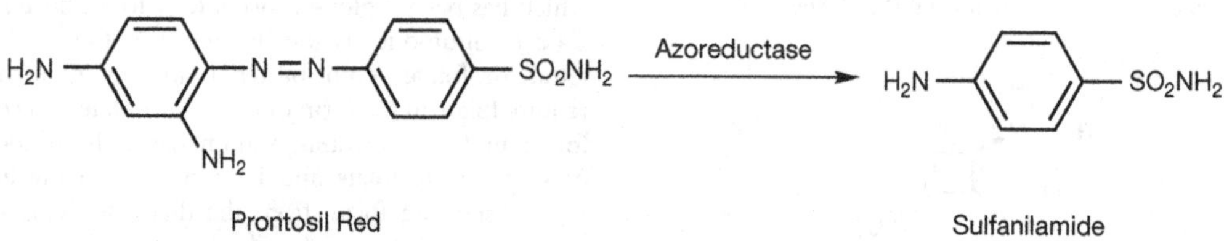

Figure 22.36 Action of azoreductase on Prontosil Red.

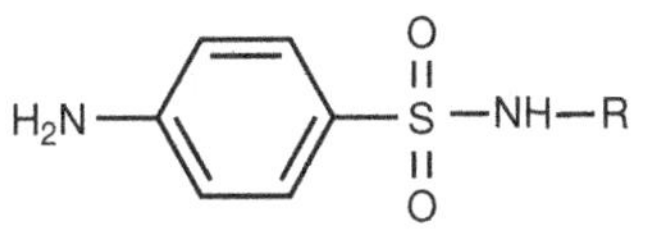

Figure 22.37 General structure of the sulphonamides.

present-day therapeutics has decreased due to the increase in bacterial resistance. Also, the typical side effects of sulphonamide therapy such as Stevens-Johnson syndrome, renal failure and blood dyscrasias are reasons why less toxic and more active alternatives such as the penicillins are preferred in practice.

The evaluation of the antibacterial activity of the sulphonamides stems from a general structure (the nitrogen of the sulphonamido group is designated N^1 and the nitrogen of the *p*-amino substituent is designated N^4) with certain provisions (Fig. 22.37):

- Antibacterial activity requires the presence of a primary amine and sulphonamido substituents placed *para* to each other on the aromatic ring.
- The sulphonamido group must be present as a secondary amine.
- Substitution of the *p*-amino group leads to loss of antibacterial activity. However, substituents on the *p*-amino group, which readily degrade in vivo to release the free amino group, have been employed with success. For example, succinyl sulfathiazole undergoes enzymatic degradation in vivo to yield the active sulfathiazole with a free primary amine moiety.
- The *R* substituent represents the only possible moiety that can be altered in the generic sulphonamide structure without impairing antibacterial activity.

The first generation of sulphonamides was characterised by the tendency to crystallise in the kidney due to their insolubility. This is the result of strong intermolecular hydrogen bonding. This problem was aggravated by the metabolism of the N^4-amino moiety to the less soluble acetyl derivative. The precipitation of the low solubility N^4-acetyl metabolites results in crystalluria. Fortunately, the R group in the general structure of the sulphonamides can be modified to overcome the problem of insolubility. The sulphonamides are acidic (proton donor) compounds and this is due to the electron withdrawing sulphonyl moiety that stabilises the anion formed after the loss of hydrogen (Fig. 22.38).

The prototype sulphonamide, sulfanilamide has a p*Ka* of 10.4. Substitution of an electron withdrawing group at the R position increases the acidity (decreased p*Ka*) of the sulphonamido N–H. Subsequently, compounds with a p*Ka* of 6–7 will be ionised at physiological pH (7.4) and can be useful in the treatment of systemic infection with decreased risk of crystalluria. This principle has been applied in the design of sulfadimidine (p*Ka* 7.4) and sulfadiazine (p*Ka* 6.5) (Fig. 22.39) by the addition of the electron withdrawing 4,6,-dimethylpyrimidine and pyrimidine, respectively.

Sulfadimidine is indicated for the treatment of upper and lower respiratory infections, urinary tract and genital tract infections. It is formulated as the sodium salt for parenteral administration. Sulfadiazine is indicated for the

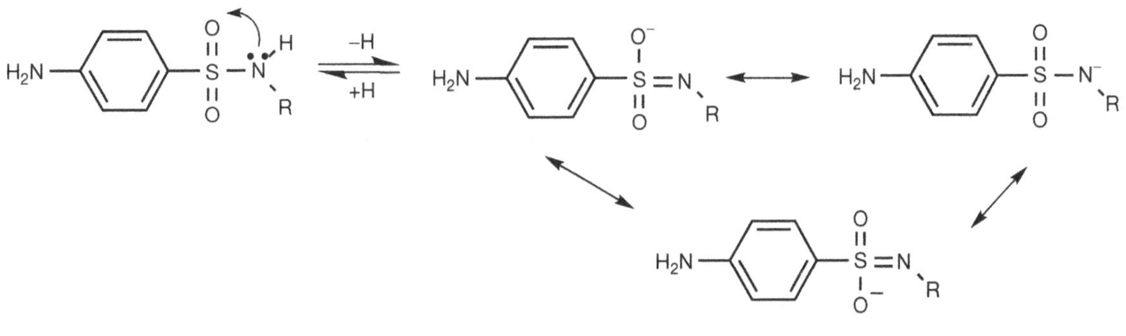

Figure 22.38

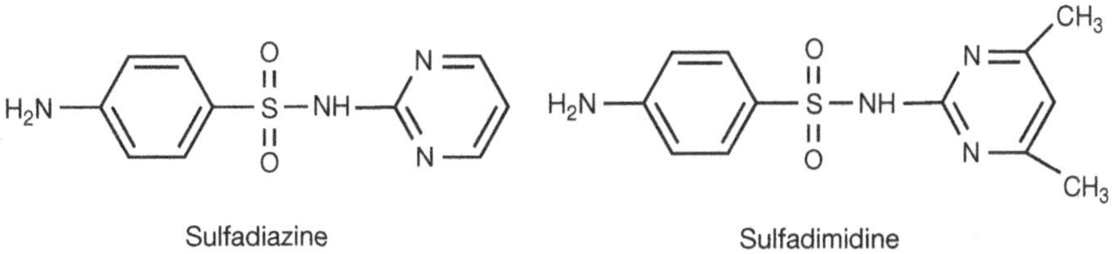

Figure 22.39

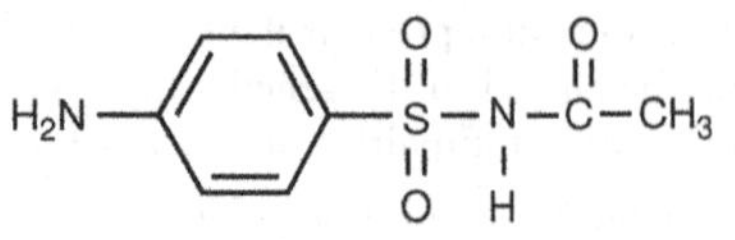

Figure 22.40

prevention of rheumatic fever recurrence and is formulated as the sodium salt for injection or as sulfadiazine tablets.

Although the addition of an electron withdrawing group results in increased ionisation at physiological pH, the downside is that complete ionisation of a sulphonamide will result in rapid excretion, requiring frequent administration, and therefore rendering it unsuitable for systemic administration.

A typical example is sulfacetamide (Fig. 22.40) which possesses a carbonyl substituent directly attached to the sulphonamido nitrogen. The reduced p*Ka* (5.4) means it is 99.9% ionised at physiological pH. The potentially rapid excretion of sulfacetamide has limited its use to the treatment of ocular infections, such as conjunctivitis, caused by susceptible organisms. It is formulated as the sodium salt and used as a 10–30% w/v ophthalmic solution.

Even at optimal p*Ka*, regular dosing is required to maintain therapeutic concentrations because of the rapid excretion of sulphonamides. The renal excretion of the sulphonamides can be reduced by increasing the degree of protein binding. The substituent at R can be selected to increase the degree of protein binding and therefore slow down the rate of excretion since only unbound drug is filtered through the glomerulus. Substitution of a methoxyl group on the heterocyclic ring results in an increase in protein binding as in sulfametopyrazine (Fig. 22.41) and yields longer-acting sulphonamides with the advantage of less frequent administration. Sulfametopyrazine remains useful in the treatment of urinary tract infections and chronic bronchitis and may be administered at a dose of 2 g once weekly. However, toxic effects due to accumulation are more likely to occur with these longer-acting sulphonamides.

The sulphonamides have been used in the treatment of intestinal infections. Substitution of the aniline N^4 with a succinyl group produces an acidic compound which is fully ionised at intestinal pH and is therefore not appreciably absorbed into the bloodstream. Slow enzymatic hydrolysis of the product in the intestine releases the free primary amine group which is essential for activity. This concept of prodrug design has been exploited in the synthesis of succinyl-sulfathiazole (p*Ka* 4.5) from sulfathiazole (p*Ka* 7.1) (Fig. 22.42).

The importance of the sulphonamides has decreased as a result of increased bacterial resistance and they have been replaced by compounds with higher therapeutic indices and activity. The biosynthetic pathway for tetrahydrofolate provides an additional point for selective attack on bacteria. The conversion of dihydrofolic acid to tetrahydrofolate (coenzyme F) requires dihydrofolate reductase. Trimetoprim (Fig. 22.43), a sulfone, is structurally similar to dihydrofolate (see Fig. 22.35) and therefore competitively inhibits the formation of tetrahydrofolate, ultimately affecting the biosynthesis of proteins and nucleic acids.

Due to a mutation in the human genome, trimetoprim inhibits bacterial dihydrofolate reductase but not mammalian dihydrofolate reductase. Trimetoprim has therefore been used in combination with the sulphonamides to provide synergism in activity while reducing the toxicity potential of the individual compounds. A useful clinical example is co-trimoxazole, which is a compound formulation of trimetoprim and sulfamethoxazole.

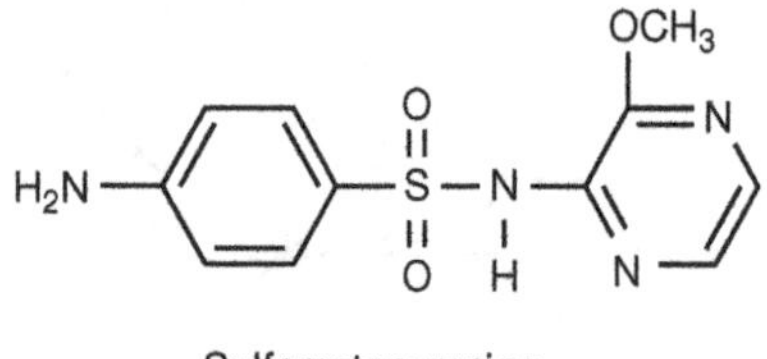

Figure 22.41

Bacterial protein synthesis inhibitors

The mechanism(s) through which both eukaryotes and prokaryotes synthesise protein for various cell activities are generally universal. However, differences exist in the ribosomes, the multi-macromolecular complexes in which decoding of the genetic information for the synthesis of proteins occurs. Bacterial ribosomes have a sedimentation coefficient of 70S and dissociate reversibly into 50S and 30S subunits. Mammalian ribosomes exhibit a sedimentation coefficient

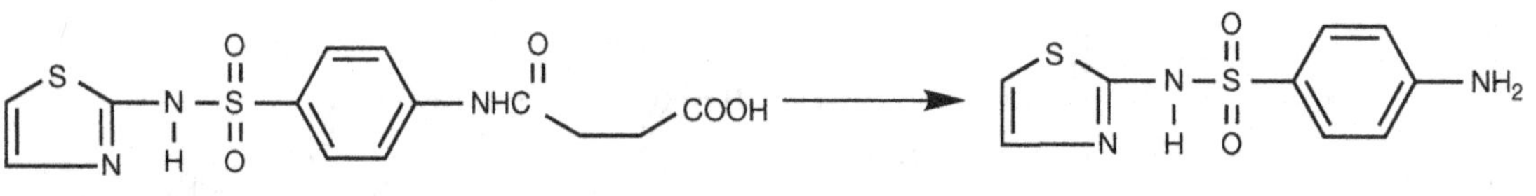

Figure 22.42 Conversion of succinyl-sulfathiazole to sulfathiazole.

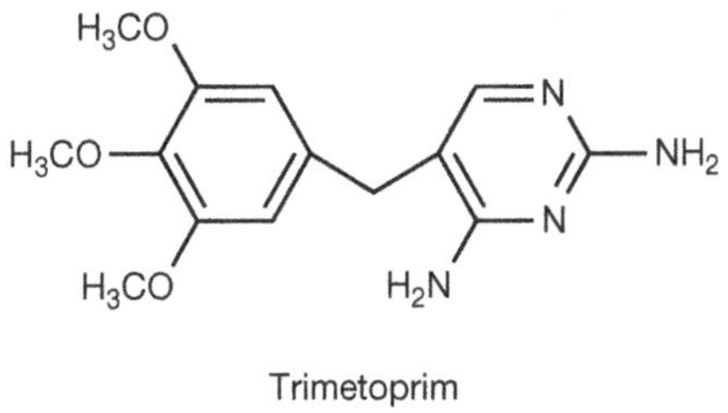

Figure 22.43

of 80S and are composed of 60S and 40S subunits. Most antibiotics which affect bacterial protein synthesis have an affinity or specificity for the 70S and or its subunits. The major class of antibiotics which selectively interfere with protein synthesis on 70S ribosomes include the aminoglycosides, macrolides, tetracycline, licosamides, chloramphenicol and the aminocyclitols.

Aminoglycosides

The aminoglycosides are products of actinomycetes or a semi-synthetic derivative. The first aminoglycoside, streptomycin, was isolated by Selman Walksman in 1944 from *Streptomyces griseus*. This group of broad-spectrum antibiotics includes kanamycin, gentamicin, amikacin, netilmicin, tobramycin and neomycin and are used primarily in the treatment of Gram-negative infections. The aminoglycosides have specificity for the 30S subunit of the bacterial 70S ribosome. Binding to the 30S subunit results in interference with the initiation of protein synthesis and misreading of mRNA.

The work on the mode of action of these drugs is largely concentrated on streptomycin, which has been shown to bind to a specific protein in the 30S subunit of bacterial ribosomes. This event inhibits protein synthesis and/or causes the production of defective proteins which results in cell death.

Macrolides

These antimicrobial agents are derived from the actinomycetes. The prototype macrolide, erythromycin, was isolated in 1952 by McGuire and co-workers from *Streptomyces erythreus*. Other clinically useful examples which are semi-synthetic analogues of erythromycin are clarithromycin and azithromycin. The compounds are so named due to the presence of a 14-member *macrocyclic lactone* ring. The large lactone rings are linked through glycoside bonds with amino-sugars. The macrolides bind to the 23S mRNA molecule in the 50S subunit and inhibit the translocation step in bacterial protein synthesis. The modification of erythromycin to clarithromycin and azithromycin improves acid stability and therefore facilitates improved absorption in the stomach.

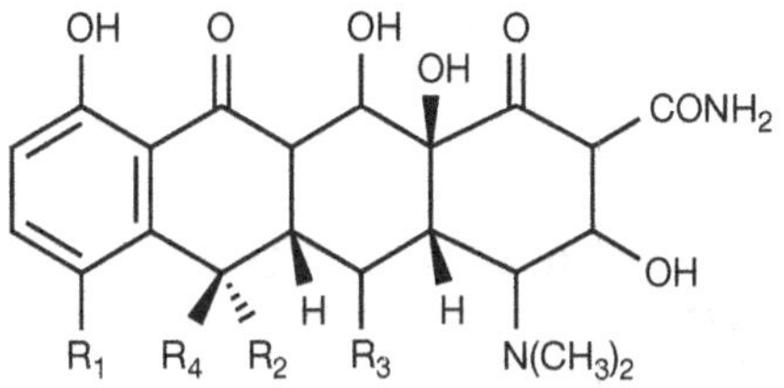

Figure 22.44

Tetracyclines

The tetracyclines are derived from *Streptomyces* and have a broad spectrum of activity which includes rickettsial and chlamydial infections. The first tetracycline, chlortetracycline (Aureomycin) was discovered by Benjamin Duggar in 1948. They are characterised by 4-fused rings with a vast array of substitutions (Fig. 22.44). The commonly used tetracyclines which bear the general structure below include chlortetracycline (7-chlorotetracycline, R_1=Cl, R_2=OH, R_3=H, R_4=H), tetracycline (R_1=H, R_2=OH, R_3=H, R_4=CH_3), and doxycyline (R_1=H, R_2=H, R_3=OH, R =CH_3).

These differ little in antibacterial activity and are distinguished by their pharmacokinetic behaviour. Minocycline (R_1=$N(CH_3)_2$, R_2=H, R_3=OH, R_4=H) shows a broader spectrum of antibacterial activity. The tetracyclines act by blocking the binding of aminoacyl tRNA to the A site on the ribosome. The tetracyclines subsequently inhibit protein synthesis at the small ribosomal subunits of both the 70S (prokaryote) and 80S (eukaryote) ribosome. However, an active transport system for the tetracyclines in bacteria means effective concentrations are achieved in the bacterial cells but not in mammalian cells. The tetracyclines are presented as capsules and tablets for oral use.

Oxazolidiones

The oxazolidiones, of which linezolid is the prototype, are the synthetic antibiotics indicated for the treatment of methicillin resistant *Staphylococcus aureus* (MRSA) infections.

Linezolid (Fig. 22.45) exerts its antibacterial action by binding to the 23S ribosomal RNA of the 50S subunit.

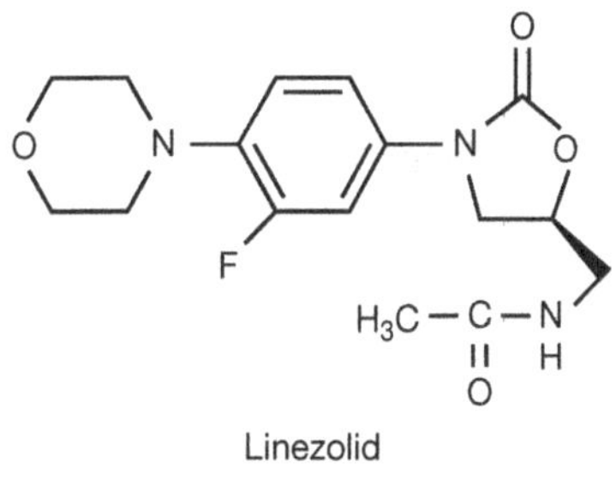

Figure 22.45

The oxazolidione represent a fairly recent addition to the arsenal of antibacterial agents, and research to produce useful analogues is in progress.

BACTERIAL NUCLEIC ACID SYNTHESIS INHIBITORS

Chemotherapeutic agents which selectively affect the synthesis of DNA and/or RNA in bacterial cells can block the growth of these organisms, leading to rapid death. The quinolones and the rifamycin derivatives are nucleic acid synthesis inhibitors which are selectively active against prokaryotes.

Quinolones

The quinolones are synthetic antibiotics which trace their origin to a concerted effort by scientists to synthesise novel antimalarial agents. In 1962, nalidixic acid (Fig. 22.46) was isolated from the by-products of chloroquine synthesis.

Nalidixic acid is indicated for the treatment of urinary tract infections. The success of nalidixic acid in the 1960s led to the synthesis of other analogues of comparable activity such as cinoxacin and acrosoxacin. Information gleaned from the activity of several synthesised quinolones indicates that the following structural requirements are essential for activity:

- A small group such as an ethyl, methoxyl, cyclopropane or methylamine group at *N-1*. The substitution also influences aqueous solubility and the spectrum of antibacterial activity.
- A carboxyl group at *C-3*.

Several important observations have been made regarding the substitution pattern(s) in the A-ring (pharmacophore) and in the B-ring. In general, the A-ring facilitates entry into the bacteria, fluorine substitution at *C-6* increases antibacterial activity while a piperazine at *C-7* confers antipseudomonal properties. Substitutions on the B-ring have little effect on antibacterial activity. Based on the increased activity due to fluorine substitution at *C-6*, Bayer produced the first marketed fluoroquinolone, ciprofloxacin. This was followed by other clinically useful analogues such as ofloxacin, norfloxacin, perfloxacin (Fig. 22.47), levofloxacin and grepafloxacin.

The fluorinated quinolones are generally more potent and less toxic than the first-generation agents. Agents containing a piperazine group at the C-7 position, such as ciprofloxacin and norfloxacin, are useful in the treatment of pseudomonal infections. The fluoroquinolones inhibit bacterial topoisomerase II (predominantly) and topoisomerase IV.

Rifamycins

The rifamycins belong to a class of naturally occurring highly substituted derivatives of naphthalene called

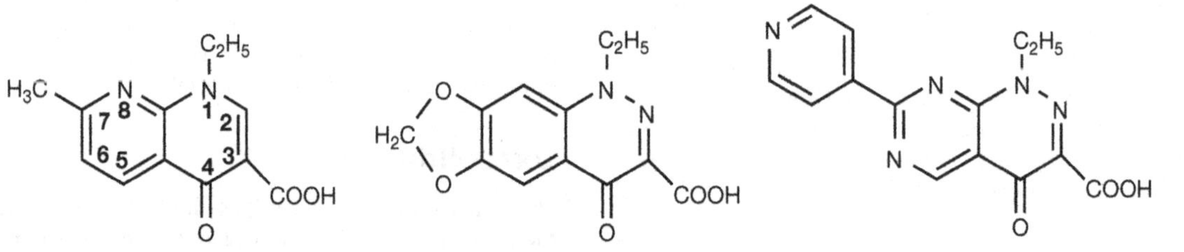

Figure 22.46

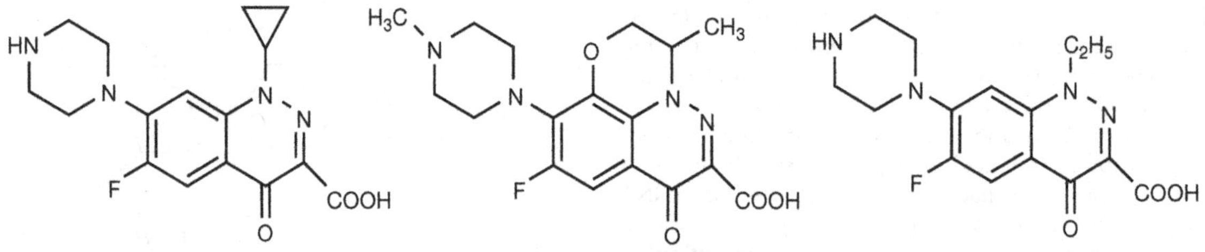

Figure 22.47

ansamycins. These compounds are the products of the *Streptomyces*. The prototype rifamycin B was isolated from *Streptomyces mediterranei* and a series of chemical modifications led to rifampicin, which is active against Gram-positive bacteria (including *Mycobacterium tuberculosis*, see Section B) and some Gram-negative bacteria. Rifampicin acts specifically on the bacterial RNA polymerase and is inactive against mammalian RNA polymerase and DNA polymerase. This class of compounds inhibits bacterial mRNA synthesis by binding to the beta subunit of the polymerase and subsequently blocking the entry of the nucleotide required to activate the polymerase.

OTHER ANTIBACTERIAL AGENTS

Chloramphenicol

Chloramphenicol was originally obtained from *Streptomyces venezuela* but is now produced by chemical synthesis. Although it has a broad spectrum of activity, it is rarely used systemically due to a high incidence of aplastic anaemia.

The compound has two asymmetric centres (Fig. 22.48) but only diastereoisomer the R,R-isomer demonstrates significant antibacterial activity. Chloramphenicol binds to the 50S subunit and inhibits the bacterial enzyme peptidyl transferase. This prevents the growth of the polypeptide chain during protein synthesis.

Clindamycin and lincomycin

These antibiotics have limited use because of their serious side effects. They bind exclusively to the 50S subunit of 70S ribosomes and the binding site is related in some way to those for erythromycin and chloramphenicol since erythromycin can displace bound lincomycin, and lincomycin inhibits chloramphenicol binding.

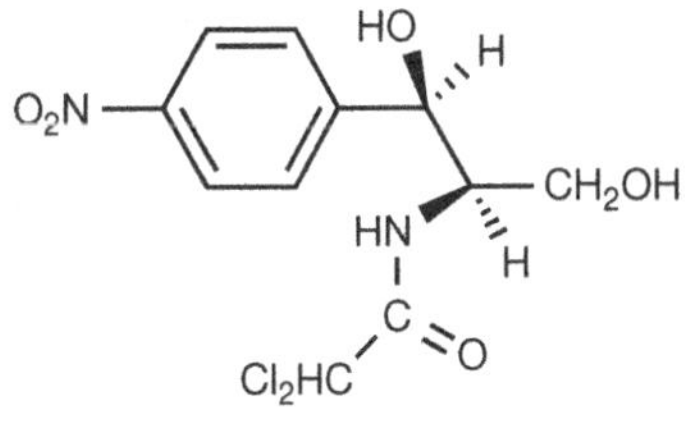

Figure 22.48

PENICILLIN HYPERSENSITIVITY

A major adverse effect associated with the penicillins is the development of IgE type 1 or accelerated immunological reactions. These allergic reactions develop rapidly after administration and the manifestations may range from harmless exanthemas to anaphylactic reactions. Anaphylactic reactions occur in about 0.015–0.045% of patients and can be fatal in 10% of these cases. The β-lactams such as penicillins and cephalosporins may form drug–protein conjugates directly due to their inherent reactivity (Fig. 22.49). The β-lactams can react with lysine groups on proteins to form the penicilloyl/cephalosporyl group, which is the major antigenic determinant.

Once they are covalently bound to a macromolecular carrier, they exist in the form of a hapten, and the bound penicillins subsequently participate in immunological reactions. Penicillenic acid, which is one of the degradation products of the penicillins, is also highly reactive and is much more immunogenic than penicillin itself. The hypersensitivity reactions occur when patients with preformed specific IgE antibodies to the penicilloyl/cephalosporyl group, which are bound to mast cells and circulating basophils, are exposed to the haptenic structures. This leads to the release of inflammatory mediators. It is estimated that 8% of patients develop allergic reactions to penicillin. On the contrary, 5% develop reactions to the cephalosporins and this has been attributed to the lower chemical reactivity of the parent cephalosporanic acid molecule. The penicilloyl/cephalosporyl moiety may be introduced into humans as a result of previous therapy, contamination, exposure to residues of penicillins/cephalosporins in vaccines and meat from drug-treated livestock. Mouldy food can serve as a good source of traces of penicillins. In addition, immunologically competent macromolecular impurities in penicillin preparations formed by polymerisation react with proteinaceous material in the fermentation medium or amidases from the cleavage of the side chain.

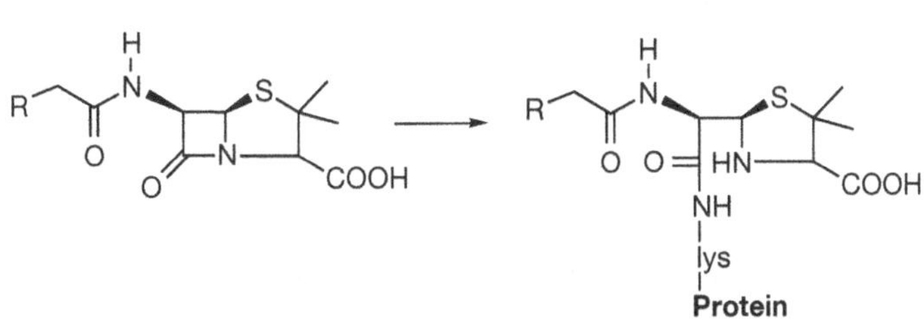

Figure 22.49 Formation of penicillin drug protein conjugate.

SECTION B – ANTITUBERCULOSIS DRUGS

Geoffrey Coxon

INTRODUCTION

Tuberculosis (TB) is a disease that has plagued mankind for centuries, dating as far back as ancient Egyptian times, and is caused by a slow-growing type of bacterium called *Mycobacterium tuberculosis.* The disease is spread by coughing, talking, spitting and sneezing, which spread the mycobacteria through the air in tiny aerosolised droplets of water which are inhaled into the lungs. The bacteria are then engulfed by macrophages in the air sacks of the lungs, called the alveoli, where they replicate and can spread throughout the body. Although 95% of the bacteria are killed in the lung, the remaining bacteria can continue to grow if untreated, or remain dormant for years before being reactivated. The primary location of the disease called pulmonary TB is in the lungs, where bacterial growth destroys tissue, making it very hard for the patient to breathe, resulting in death. It is in the lungs where the disease is most contagious but symptoms can also include meningitis, legions on the skin and degradation of the heart, bones and intestines, which makes treating the disease and choosing the correct drug regimens very difficult.

TB was much more prevalent in the past than it is today and has caused the deaths of around one billion people over the last two hundred years. Improvement of sanitation and living conditions have been significant factors in reducing cases of TB, but the introduction of chemotherapy in the 1950s has been instrumental in fighting this age old adversary. In recent years, however, the disease has made a strong resurgence and now infects approximately one-third of the world's population and causes 8 million new cases of TB each year, resulting in around 2 million deaths worldwide. The resurgence has been caused due to three main reasons. First, the chemotherapy used to attack the complex and robust bacteria is not very efficacious by modern drug standards and has to be given as a precise combination over a period of months in order for it to be effective. Second, poor compliance leads to drug-resistant strains of the mycobacterium which are not susceptible to the current cocktail of drugs available. This leaves the pharmacist and doctor faced with the option of administering other non-tuberculosis-specific and potentially toxic antibiotics to treat the disease as a last resort, the failure of which will almost certainly result in the death of the patient. Last, there is also a strong epidemiological coexistence between TB and HIV, as patients who are immunocompromised readily contract the disease which has led to approximately one-third of all AIDS-related deaths resulting from TB infections.

The disease, and the bacterium which is the cause, are vastly complex and symptoms can vary enormously, which makes its treatment difficult. For example, a patient may have open cavities or lesions that are teaming with the bacteria which the drugs can not easily eradicate. There are other problems associated with killing the bacterium using the available drugs, which mostly kill the bacteria only when they are growing. In this case, the drugs have to penetrate a very complicated mycobacterial cell wall which is sometimes described as 'waxy' because of its complex fatty acid barrier which makes getting a drug molecule into the cytoplasm extremely difficult. Additionally, after treatment, the bacteria that are not killed outright can lie in a dormant state, waiting to be reactivated. These bacteria are called 'persistors' and the reason for reactivation is not understood, which makes destroying them very difficult. It is therefore vitally important that all of the growing bacteria are killed in the first instance to destroy as many bacteria as possible, which will also help prevent drug resistance from occurring, which is proving to be a major problem in developing countries.

TB is treated in two phases. There is an *initial phase* and a *continuation phase* and depending upon the patient's ability to comply with the drug regimen, these phases may be carried out either unsupervised or supervised. The latter is known as DOT (directly observed treatment), where the drugs are given to the patient three times per week in order to maintain the strict regimen that must be observed.

During the initial phase there is the concurrent use of at least three drugs for 2 months, which is designed to reduce the bacterial population as rapidly as possible in order to prevent resistance. These drugs are generally given as a combination preparation, or 'triple therapy', unless one of the component drugs cannot be given because of intolerance or potential drug resistance. The three drugs normally used in combination are isoniazid (INH), rifampicin (RIF) and pyrazinamide (PZA) which in combined tablet form are known as Rifater®. Ethambutol (EMB) is now also used during the initial phase. Streptomycin (SM) may be used in cases where resistance to INH has been established before treatment begins but is rarely used in the UK where, due to its potentially toxic nature, it is only available for named patients. Treatment may be extended but only in cases of meningitis or for resistant strains, which may also require modification of the regimen.

Traditionally, TB drugs are generally considered to be either first-line or second-line. The first-line drugs exhibit superior efficacy with acceptable toxicity, whereas the second-line drugs have either less efficacy, increased side effects or both. Discussed below are the main drugs used to treat TB, although others such as kanamycin, amikacin and thioacetazone may also be used. It is important to note that no new drug has been specifically designed and introduced to treat TB since rifampicin in 1962, which indicates the difficulty in discovering new agents and highlights how, by modern standards, these drugs are relatively poor.

FIRST-LINE DRUGS

As discussed earlier, one of the main reasons it is hard for drugs to destroy *M. tuberculosis* is because it has a complex and almost impermeable cell wall. In recent years, the sequencing of the genome of *M. tuberculosis* has furnished medicinal chemists with a plethora of new, specific and validated targets which may be exploited to design more drugs to fight growing and drug-resistant bacteria. Moreover, the mechanism of action of many of the existing drugs designed in the 1940s and 1950s has been established, giving us more information on how best to use the current medicines.

Isoniazid

Isoniazid (INH) (isonicotinic acid hydrazide, Fig. 22.50) was discovered via a purely synthetic strategy in the quest to find a new agent to combat the disease. It is bacteriostatic at concentrations of 0.025–0.05 μg/ml in vitro but at higher concentrations is bactericidal. This is a prodrug and requires activation before destroying the bacteria, which it does by inhibiting a ketoenoylreductase enzyme known as InhA. This enzyme catalyses the last of four steps involved in the 2-carbon elongation cycle of fatty acid biosynthesis. INH is first activated by the catalase-peroxidase enzyme katG which oxidises the isonicotinic acyl group of the molecule to either an isonicotinic acyl anion or radical. These forms then react with either an NADH radical or anion whilst in the active site of InhA to form an isonicotinic acyl-NADH complex. This new molecule is then tightly bound to the active site of the enzyme, thus preventing access of the natural enoyl-AcpM substrate which stops the production of mycolic acids and hence the biosynthesis of the cell wall of the bacteria.

Resistance to INH generally occurs when the drug is administered alone for 3 months and is caused mainly by the absence of the gene encoding the catalase-peroxidase *katG*, which prevents activation of the drug. Mutations in InhA have also been identified and postulated as a reason for resistance to the drug.

INH is well absorbed orally or intramuscularly and distributes well throughout the body, and its metabolism occurs initially by liver *N*-acetyltransferase. This means that patients who are poor acetylators can experience toxicity problems, as acetylation of INH is first required before the hydrolysis can occur and the drug cleared by the kidneys.

Ethambutol

Ethambutol (EMB, Fig. 22.50), chemical name (*S*,*S*′)-(+)-2,2′-(ethylenediimino)di-1-butanol, exhibits bacteriostatic activity against *M. tuberculosis* in vitro or in macrophages at 1 μg/mL. Stepwise resistance of the drug occurs when the drug is administered alone but cross-resistance with other antimicrobials is rare, so its principle role is as a companion drug to prevent resistance.

EMB inhibits the polymerisation of the cell wall arabinan component of the mycolylarabinogalactan and lipoarabinomannan, which are integral structural polysaccharides. It is believed that it may specifically target the arabinosyl transferase enzyme embB with only the (*S*,*S*′)-diasteromer binding to the active site, which is supported by the fact that the (*R*,*R*′)-diastereomer is inactive.

Approximately 80% of EMB is absorbed orally and is well distributed throughout the body, including the central nervous system, before being metabolised to inactive metabolites which are readily excreted in urine. The major toxic effect of the drug is neuropathy resulting in visual problems when a patient has insufficient renal

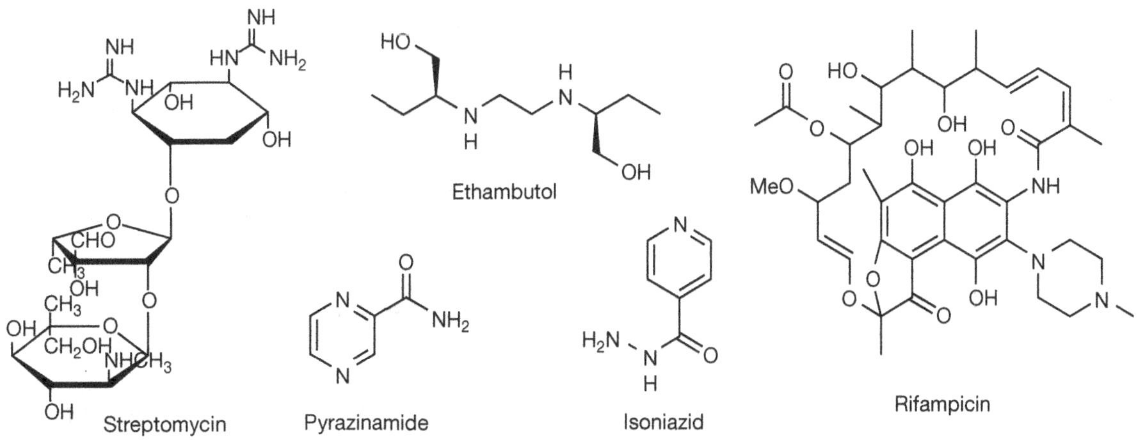

Figure 22.50

activity and in some cases infrequent hypersensitivity reactions occur, which include dermatitis, arthralgias and fever.

Pyrazinamide

Pyrzinamide (PZA, Fig. 22.50) is a synthetic analogue of nicotinamide, is bactericidal against growing bacteria, and is unconventional in the fact that it has high sterilising activity in vivo and is responsible for shortening the therapy to 6 months. It is most active at acidic pH in vitro, which is similar to the environment found intracellularly in phagolysosomes, which may account for its high sterilising activity, but it shows no activity at physiological pH. The exact mechanism of action of this is unclear. However, it is known that PZA is a prodrug which requires activation to pyrazinoic acid (POA) by the PZase/nicotinamidase enzyme. In this form, and at low pH, the protonated POA can bring protons into the cell, which causes cytoplasmic acidification resulting in the de-energising of the cell because of a collapse in proton motive force which effects membrane transport. It is also known that resistance to PZA rapidly evolves if the drug is used alone and is associated with mutation in the *pncA* gene which encodes the PZase/nicotinamidase enzyme.

PZA is well absorbed orally and distributes well throughout the body, reaching concentration levels above that needed to kill the tubercle bacilli. The peak plasma concentrations are around 50 μg/mL, resulting in a half-life of the drug of 12–24 hours, which makes once-daily dosing practical. It is metabolised by the liver with metabolites, mainly POA, being excreted by the kidneys. The most common side effects with PZA are nausea and vomiting, and early trials with the drug resulted in the dose of the drug being lowered from 40–50 mg/kg/day to 20–35 mg/kg/day, indicating that dosages of the drug may need changing if liver and renal function are compromised.

Rifampicin

Rifampicin (RIF, Fig. 22.50) is a broad-spectrum semi-synthetic derivative of the complex macrocyclic antibiotic rifamycin B, produced by *Streptomyces mediterranei*, and is known as rifampin outside the UK. An important feature about RIF is that it is active against both actively growing and slowly metabolising non-growing bacilli. The latter feature is thought to be important in reducing the treatment from 12–18 months to 9 months.

RIF is bactericidal against *M. tuberculosis* at 0.005–0.2 μg/mL and works by inhibiting RNA synthesis by binding to the bacterial DNA-dependent RNA polymerase β-subunit encoded by the *rpoB* gene. Resistance occurs rapidly when used alone and arises because of a mutation in a defined 81-bp region of the *rpoB* gene and can cause cross-resistance to other rifamycins such as rifabutin and rifapentine, which have very similar structures. RIF is well absorbed orally, giving peak plasma concentrations of 7–8 μg/mL after a dose of 600 mg and distributes well throughout the body. Its lipophilic nature allows it to distribute throughout the central nervous system and penetrate phageosomes, and this makes it a good candidate to treat the meningitis form of the disease. It is deacylated to an active form which undergoes biliary excretion and enterohepatic recirculation and, due to autoinduction of RIF metabolism, biliary excretion increases with continued therapy. This means that plasma concentrations become maximal after six doses whether administered daily or twice weekly, whereby subsequent excretion of the drug takes place primarily to the gastrointestinal tract, with lesser amounts in urine.

Streptomycin

Streptomycin (SM) is an aminoglycoside antibiotic isolated from the bacteria *Streptomyces griseus* and was introduced in the 1940s as the first drug to reduce TB mortality. Importantly, SM is traditionally known as a first-line drug. However, because it is available only as a named drug, it may more accurately be classed a second-line drug. Due to its hydrophilic nature owing to the presence of several hydroxyl groups and two guanidine groups, this drug is poorly bioavailable orally and has to be administered by an intramuscular injection and is virtually excluded from the central nervous system. A dose of 1 g yields peak plasma concentrations of 25–45 μg/mL, which is more than enough for the drug to be inhibitory, which can be achieved at levels of 0.4–10 μg/mL. It is bactericidal against *M. tuberculosis* in vitro but is inactive against intracellular tubercle bacilli, and resistance develops rapidly when it is given alone.

The drug works by interfering with protein synthesis, as it inhibits the initiation of mRNA translation which leads to misreading of the genetic code, ultimately damaging the cell membrane. The main site of action is in the small 30S subunit of the ribosome, specifically at ribosomal protein S12 (*rpsL*) and 16S rRNA (*rrs*) in the protein synthesis. The mutations in *rpsL* and *rrs* give rise to SM resistance and, as other aminoglycoside antibiotics such as kanamycin, amikacin, viomycin and capreomycin are inhibitors of protein synthesis, cross-resistance can be a problem. The toxicity of SM is like that of the other aminoglycosides but with less renal and acoustic toxicity (affects the hearing).

SECOND-LINE DRUGS

Second-line anti-TB drugs are generally used when the first-line drugs are ineffective due to resistance or patient intolerance. They are all less efficacious than the first-line drugs and generally exhibit more toxic effects to the patient.

Ethionamide and protionamide

Ethionamide and protionamide (Fig. 22.51) are very similar in structure and action to INH and they are also prodrugs that undergo catalase-oxygenase activation to inhibit the enzyme inhA, thus preventing the synthesis of mycolic acids and consequently inhibiting cell wall biosynthesis. Resistance also occurs by mutation of the oxygenase enzymes and inhA and it is tuberculostatic at 0.6–2.5 μg/mL, making it less potent than INH. It is well absorbed orally and well distributed throughout the body, and is metabolised by the liver with metabolites excreted *via* the kidney. However, ETH and PTH also interfere with INH acetylation, which can cause gastrointestinal side effects leading to poor compliance.

Cycloserine

Cycloserine (Fig. 22.51) possesses a broad range of anti-mycobacterial activity and inhibits *M. tuberculosis* at 5–20 μg/mL, again by preventing cell wall biosynthesis. It works by mimicking *D*-alanine which is the natural substrate for the enzyme *D*-alanine racemase (Alr) and *D*-alanine: *D*-alanine ligase (Ddl), thus preventing the synthesis of the mycolyl peptidoglycan. Alr serves to convert *L*-aniline to *D*-alanine and mutations in the active site of this enzyme have been proposed to be responsible for the resistance of CS. CS is readily absorbed orally and widely distributed amongst tissues before being excreted by the kidneys, with little of the drug being metabolised. It is one of several alternatives for re-treatment regimens or for treatment of primary drug-resistant TB, although it has poor activity against MDR-TB strains.

Para-aminosalicylic acid

Para-aminosalicylic acid (Fig. 22.51) is bacteriostatic against *M. tuberculosis* and is not completely absorbed orally due to its hydrophilic nature, as dictated by the functional groups attached to the benzene ring. A 4-g dose will yield plasma concentrations of 70–80 μg/mL, from which about 85% of the absorbed drug will be excreted in the urine as various degradation products. It is thought that PAS works by inhibiting a dihydrofolate reductase (DHFR) or the salicylate kinase enzyme Dhbe, which is responsible for synthesising iron-regulating molecules called siderophores which are necessary for the bacteria to survive, although it has been suggested that they also interfere with folic acid metabolism.

Quinolones

The first of the 'quinolone' drugs, nalidixic acid (Fig. 22.51), was obtained in the early 1960s during the manufacture of chloroquine and since then many fluorinated derivatives have been synthesised and evaluated as anti-TB drugs showing bactericidal activity. Ciprofloxacin, ofloxacin and levofloxacin (the S(−) form of ofloxacin) are the best studied of the quinolones and work by inhibiting DNA synthesis targeting the DNA gyrase A and B

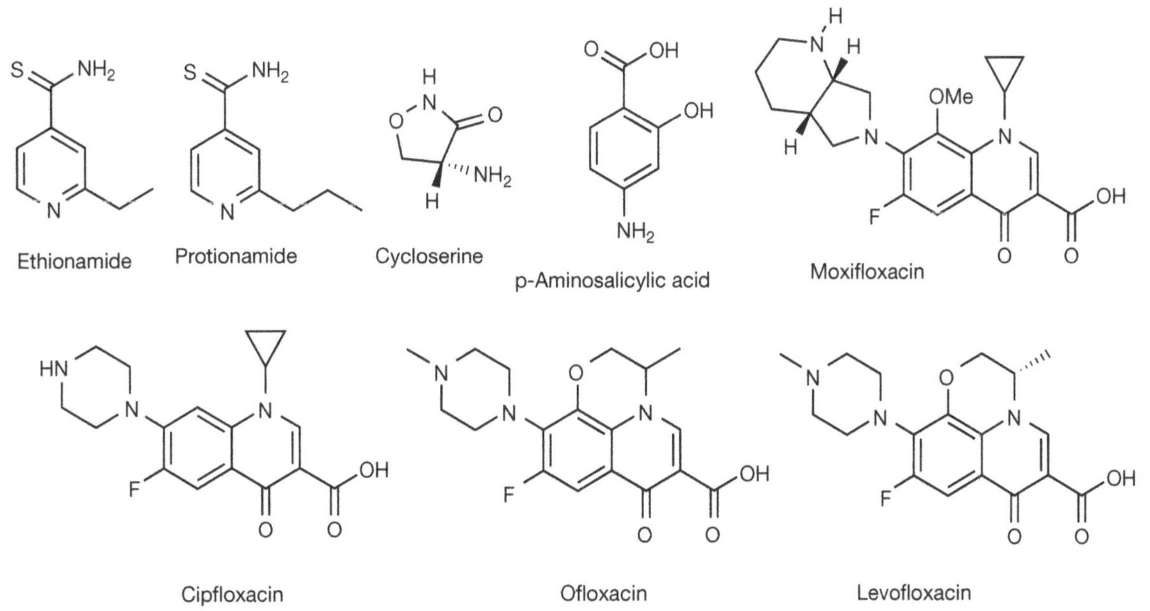

Figure 22.51

subunits at concentrations well within the achievable plasma levels. It can be seen that the structures of the quinolones are very similar, with only small differences based around a central quinolone pharmacophore which have been designed to increase binding to the gyrase enzyme and improve the druglike properties of the molecule or reduce toxic effects. Resistance to the FQs has been found to occur when they are administered on their own. However, ofloxacin, in combination with other second-line drugs, may be used as a treatment for resistant TB. The use of these drugs is still being investigated and, indeed, new drug molecules are being evaluated and tested to treat the disease in the future, with the best example being that of the diarylquinolone R207910.

Chapter | 23 |

Antiviral drugs

Simon P Mackay, David G Watson

CHAPTER CONTENTS

INTRODUCTION

In patients who are not immunocompromised, most virus infections are overcome by the host's immune system, and are resolved without treatment. Thus other than alleviation of some of the more uncomfortable symptoms such as aching muscles, headaches and congestion direct treatment of the virus is not necessary. Specific treatments for viral infections in the immunocompromised are available, such as HIV or herpes virus infections, hepatitis and influenza. The role of vaccines in such treatments is not covered in this chapter. Here we are concentrating on the role of drugs in the alleviation of viral infections. Before discussing particular diseases and their treatments, it would be appropriate to remind ourselves of what we are combating, namely the causative organisms of the infections in question. The following section is a synopsis of viral biology.

VIRUSES

Viruses are obligate intracellular parasites that can infect all life forms. They contain either an RNA or DNA genome surrounded by a protective, virus-coded protein coat. Viruses have both an extracellular and an intracellular existence. In the extracellular form, the virus particle (virion) is the structure by which the virus genome is carried from the cell from which it has been reproduced to an uninfected cell. The genome contains the code for the proteins and enzymes required to construct a new virion from the infected cell. The basic structure of two common types of virus particles is illustrated in Figure 23.1.

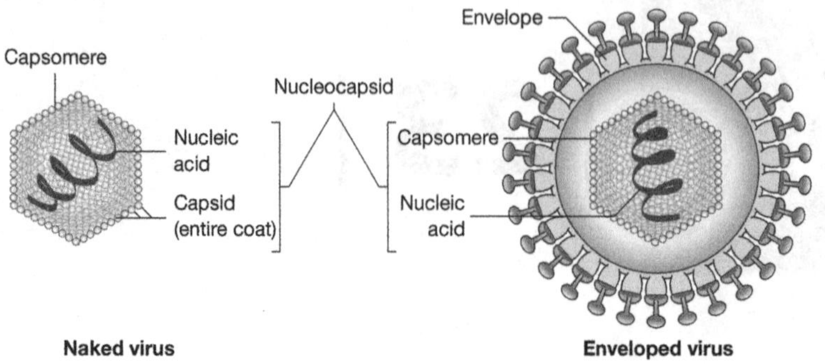

Figure 23.1 Structural features of naked and enveloped virus particles.

The capsid is composed of one or more individual proteins, known as structural subunits, which are arranged in a precise and highly repetitive manner around the nucleic acid. The small genome size of most viruses limits the number of proteins manufactured. A few viruses contain only one protein in their capsid, but most viruses have several chemically distinct kinds of subunits. The subunits form higher assemblies called capsomeres. The capsomere structure is formed and maintained by non-covalent intermolecular forces. It is the capsomere structure that is observed with the electron microscope. The combined assembly of the nucleic acid and the capsid is referred to as the nucleocapsid.

Certain viruses have more complex structures in which the nucleocapsid is enclosed in an envelope (Fig. 23.1). During envelope biosynthesis, the virus uses lipids derived from the host membrane to create the lipid bilayer prior to incorporating virus-specific proteins, usually glycoproteins, into the membrane. The envelope controls viral specificity and certain aspects of cellular penetration.

Viral multiplication in humans

The multiplication cycle of all viruses exhibits several common features (Fig. 23.2). A short period after infection has occurred only small amounts of parenteral infectious material can be detected in the host. This interval is known as the eclipse phase. At this point replication has been initiated but progeny viruses have not been released from infected cells. This is followed by the maturation phase, an interval in which the viral progeny accumulate in the host cell at an exponential rate. Host cells infected with lytic viruses terminate their metabolic activity and viral production stops. The viral numbers start to slowly fall. Host cells infected with non-lytic viruses may, in contrast, continue to synthesise viruses indefinitely. Mature viruses that are released from the host cell are able to infect further host cells. The reproductive cycle of viruses ranges from around 6–8 hours (e.g. picornaviruses), to greater than 72 hours (e.g. certain herpes viruses). The viral yield from an infected cell ranges from several thousand copies (e.g. poxvirus) to greater than 100 000 copies (e.g. poliovirus).

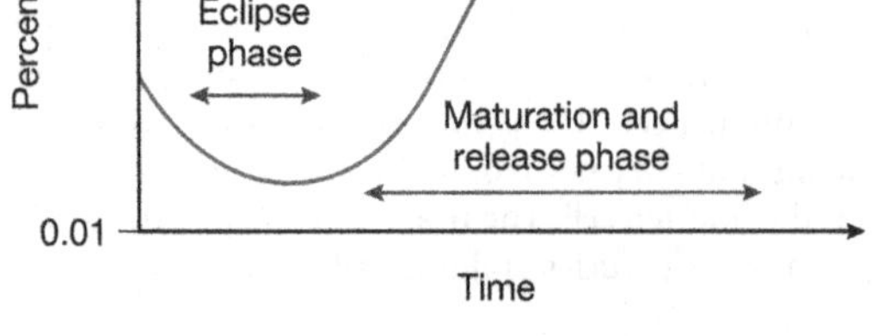

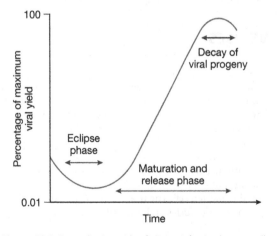

Figure 23.2 Reproductive cycle of viruses infecting human cells.

Consequences of a viral infection

Epidemiological studies have indicated that viral infections are the most common cause of acute disease that does not require hospitalisation in developed countries, the most common being upper respiratory tract infections. In contrast, viral infections such as measles, mumps, rubella and rotavirus infections, which cause diarrhoea, are important causes of infant mortality, whilst the viral infection HIV remains a major cause of adult mortality and morbidity in developing countries. Host cells that allow viral replication are termed permissive. The production of infective progeny usually results in host cell death. For this reason, the infections are termed cytocidal (or cytolytic).

The viral infection process

In order to infect a cell, a virus must attach itself to the cell surface and penetrate into the cell. Once internalised, the virus must become sufficiently uncoated to make its genome accessible to host biosynthetic machinery so that transcription and translation can proceed to produce new viruses (Fig. 23.3).

1 Attachment

Attachment of the virus to the host cell membrane is through the specific binding of a virus protein (termed the

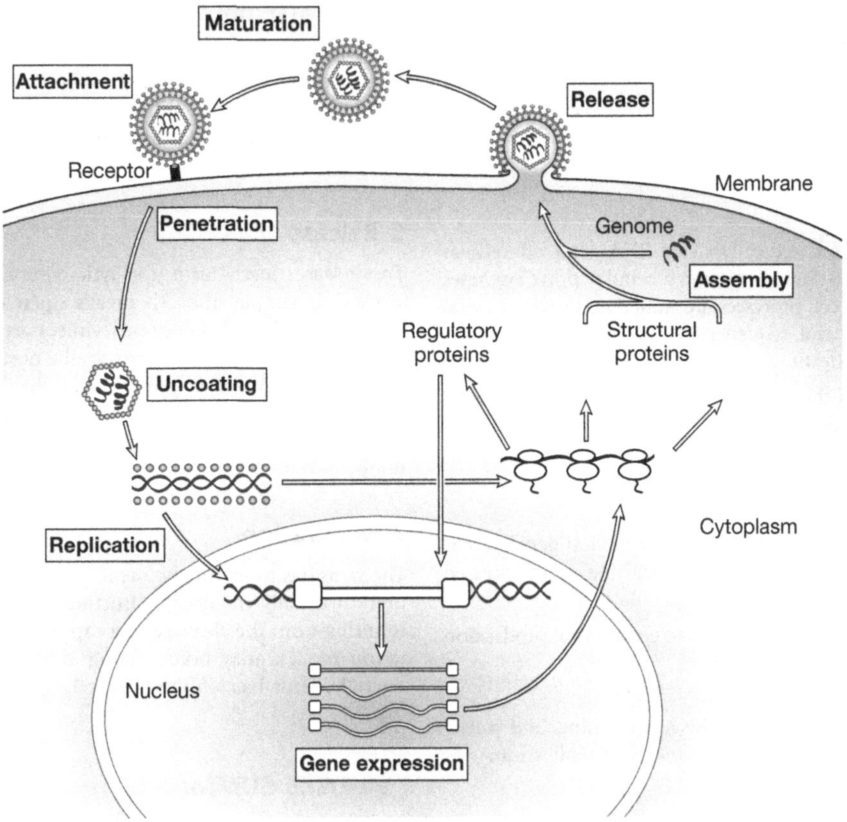

Figure 23.3 The infection cycle by which a virus enters a host cell and utilises host cellular machinery to reproduce itself.

anti-receptor) to a receptor on the host cell membrane surface. The anti-receptors are distributed throughout the viral surface. Complex viruses, such as the herpes simplex virus or poxvirus, may possess more than one type of anti-receptor. The majority of host receptors involved in the attachment process are glycoproteins, but other cell membrane constituents such as sialic acid and heparin sulphate have been identified. Attachment appears primarily to be dependent on electrostatic interactions that are temperature and energy independent. The susceptibility of a host cell to a particular virus is therefore dependent on whether it expresses a receptor that would enable the virus to attach via its specific anti-receptor. This is why viral infectivity is often limited to a particular cell type and cells lacking specific receptors are resistant. For example, a glycoprotein called gp120 on the surface of the human immunodeficiency virus (HIV), the cause of AIDS, specifically binds to the CD4 molecule found on certain human T lymphocytes. Cells that do not have surface CD4 molecules generally cannot be infected by HIV. In immunoresistant individuals, attachment is blocked by antibodies that bind to the viral or cellular receptor sites involved, which have been raised by the host's immune system as a response to the infection or prior immunisation.

2 Penetration

Penetration occurs almost instantaneously after attachment between the receptors. It involves energy-dependent mechanisms, the most common of which is receptor-mediated endocytosis, the process by which many hormones and toxins enter cells. The virion is endocytosed and contained within a cellular cytoplasmic vacuole called an endosome. In the case of viruses that penetrate as a consequence of fusion of their envelopes with the plasma membrane, for example, herpesviruses, the envelope remains in the cell membrane and the nucleocapsid enters the cytoplasm. Fusion of viral envelopes with host cell membrane requires the interaction of specific viral proteins in the envelope with proteins in the host cell membrane.

3 Uncoating

Uncoating is a general term applied to the events occurring after penetration which enables the viral genome to be expressed. In most cases the virus disassembles either spontaneously or with the aid of host cell enzymes until only the viral nucleic acid remains. A key step in uncoating is the acidification of the content of the endosome to a pH of about 5, owing to the activity of a proton pump present in the surrounding membrane. The low pH causes rearrangement of coat components, in order to expose normally hidden hydrophobic sites, which then bind to the lipid bilayer of the membrane, causing the extrusion of the viral core into the cytosol.

4 Replication

Pathogenic viruses, either DNA or RNA, shut off cellular protein synthesis and disaggregate cellular polyribosomes so that the host cell processes are shifted exclusively to viral synthesis. A general sequence of events can be observed during viral replication:

- Synthesis of the RNA or DNA genome of the virus
- Integration of the viral genome into the host genome in the cell nucleus
- mRNA production (transcription)
- Protein synthesis (translation).

The viral proteins synthesised once the viral genome has become integrated into the host genome and expressed have three main functions:

- Modify host cell metabolism to ensure viral production
- Facilitate genome replication
- Facilitate viral assembly.

Viruses can be either DNA or RNA containing, and consequently employ different mechanisms of replication.

DNA viruses

The viral genome is coded for by the same nucleic acids as the host (DNA). After integration of the viral DNA into host DNA by the viral integrase enzyme, transcription occurs in the nucleus and translation in the cytoplasm. Generally, transcription of the viral DNA into mRNA is by the host RNA polymerase systems. The translation of the viral mRNA of early proteins is the key initial step in viral DNA replication to establish the replicatory process. After DNA synthesis, the remainder of the genome is transcribed into late messengers. Regulation is carried out by proteins present in the virions, or specified by viral genes transcribed and translated by the cellular host.

RNA viruses

In order to replicate the RNA viral genome, the viral RNA can act directly as the mRNA and be translated to form viral proteins. Alternatively, in the case of retroviruses, which are unique in that their genomes are transcribed into DNA from RNA by an RNA-directed DNA polymerase or reverse transcriptase, so called because information is going from RNA into DNA, which is the opposite to the conventional process of transcription (DNA into mRNA). Once transcribed into DNA, it is integrated into the cellular DNA by the viral integrase enzyme. Transcription of the viral genome by the cellular RNA polymerases yields the viral molecules that end up in virions.

5 Viral assembly

The viral proteins and genome are assembled to form the nucleopcapsid structure of a mature virion. The viral assembly can occur at different intracellular sites: in the cytoplasm, in the nucleus or on the inner surface of the cell membrane.

6 Release

The release mechanism for lytic viruses (most naked viruses) is simple: the cell breaks open (lyses) and the viruses are released. Enveloped viruses acquire their lipid membrane coat as the virus crosses the host cell membrane by a process known as budding. Budding is controlled by the virus and involves the physical interaction of the capsid proteins with the inner surface of the host cell membrane. Budding may or may not result in host cell death.

7 Maturation

The virus has to mature before it becomes infectious. Maturation usually involves a structural change to the virus resulting from the cleavage of a capsid protein. The maturation process may occur during viral assembly or later once the virus has left the host cell.

VIRUSES SUMMARY

- DNA viruses: Viral DNA becomes incorporated into host cell DNA and codes for RNA which in turn codes for the structural proteins and enzymes that the virus required to reproduce itself. (Examples: herpesviruses (chickenpox, shingles, cold sores/genital herpes), glandular fever, adenovirus).
- RNA viruses: Viral RNA enters the cell and uses the cell's machinery to produce the proteins and enzymes that the virus requires to reproduce itself. (Examples: influenza, measles, mumps, rubella, colds, meningitis, rabies, yellow fever).
- RNA retroviruses: The virus contains a reverse transcriptase enzyme which makes a DNA copy of viral RNA. The viral DNA becomes incorporated into the host cell nucleus and produces viral proteins and enzymes.
- The virus life cycle is as follows: (a) attachment to host cell surface at receptor or other cell surface macromolecule; (b) penetration via pinocytosis; (c) uncoating of viral DNA or RNA; (d) formation of viral proteins and enzymes; (e) replication by synthesis of copies of viral DNA/RNA; (f) assembly of viral structural proteins to form virus particles (virons); and (g) release of virons from cell.
- Any of the stages (a)–(g) can be targeted by drugs but in practice stage (e) is most commonly targeted. Vaccination aims to prevent viruses from even reaching stage (a) by promoting their destruction in the blood stream.

ANTIVIRAL DRUGS

Introduction

Antiviral drugs are among the most recently developed drugs and perhaps more than any other group of drugs are rationally designed. The strategies for halting viral replication are limited and the most common strategy is to inhibit replication of viral DNA using analogues of DNA bases which become incorporated into viral DNA and prevent thus inhibit its production. Thus the window for therapeutic intervention is relatively narrow since the drugs are also likely to interfere with the production of human DNA because the enzymes used by the virus and host to activate nucleosides and incorporate them into DNA are very similar. The other major class of antiviral drugs are protease inhibitors which are specifically concerned with inhibition of protein processing by the HIV virus.

HIV infections

Since the early 1980s, acquired immunodeficiency syndrome (AIDS) has evolved into a worldwide epidemic. Death is not caused directly by the virus, the human immunodeficiency virus (HIV), but the severe impairment of the immune system that is a consequence of the viral infection results in infection by opportunistic pathogens which ultimately kill the host. Glycoprotein spikes on the protein coat of the HIV virus have a high affinity for CD4 receptors mainly found on the surface of helper T lymphocytes, but also present in macrophages, dendritic cells, and neuroglial cells. All of these are involved in the immune response. The HIV-CD4 complex penetrates the infected host cell by endocytosis and then the virus replicates and destroys the host cell. Virus is then released into the circulation. The diagnostic 'CD4 cell count' drops as the infection spreads, ultimately destroying the host cellular immune system. In 1983, the causative strain responsible for this process, HIV-1, was isolated independently by two groups, and, in 1986, a genetically distinct virus, HIV-2, which occurs in different geographic locations (West Africa) was isolated. When reverse transcriptase activity was detected in a sample of lymph tissue from a patient at risk of AIDS, HIV was confirmed as a retrovirus. This means it contains RNA rather than DNA, and hence it must form viral DNA if it is to take over control and replicate inside the host cell. Once inside the host cell, the protein coating is removed from the HIV, releasing its RNA. The viral enzyme known as reverse transcriptase then transcribes this RNA into a DNA copy, forming a RNA-DNA hybrid. The RNA component of this hybrid is destroyed in the presence of ribonuclease H, leaving the DNA strand to replicate and form double-stranded DNA. This double-stranded DNA enters the nucleus of the host cell and is inserted into host DNA by the viral integrase enzyme. The host DNA now acts as the vector for the regeneration of new viral DNA, which is packaged by structural proteins coded for by the viral DNA, and released from the cell when it lyses.

For viral DNA synthesis and integration following retroviral infection, the genes of the retroviral genome are expressed together as a fusion protein. This multi-domain precursor is then processed by a viral protease enzyme at specific sites to the mature proteins essential for HIV multiplication. These enzymes are reverse transcriptase, integrase, (more) HIV protease and structural internal proteins of the new virion. All these catalytic proteins are potential targets for drugs to inhibit the viral replication process in this devastating disease. For an animated description of the HIV replication cycle, see http://www.hopkins-aids.edu/hiv_lifecycle/hivcycle_txt.html.

Reverse transcriptase (RT) inhibitors

Nucleoside reverse transcriptase inhibitors (NRTIs)

Screening of the NCI drugs database in the 1980s identified several compounds capable of preventing HIV replication in vitro, and one of these, 3′-azido-3′-deoxythymidine (AZT or zidovudine, Fig. 23.4) was the first drug to be used for the treatment of AIDS. In January 1986, a double-blind clinical trial began on 282 patients. After 16 weeks, the monitoring board stopped the trial when it had become apparent that amongst those receiving the drug, 1 out of 145 had died, compared with 16 deaths amongst those receiving a placebo. Supplies of zidovudine were released for treatment on a named-patient basis, with the FDA granting registration the following spring. Several trials confirmed that zidovudine used on its own delayed death by 12 months. If therapy was initiated before AIDS developed, it typically delayed onset of AIDS by 12 months.

Zidovudine (AZT)

Zidovudine inhibited RT, but treatment was of limited efficacy, mainly because of dose-limiting side effects caused by affects against host metabolism, and the development of

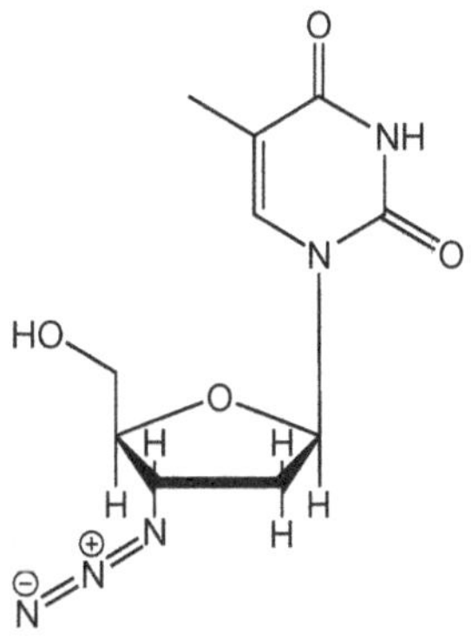

Figure 23.4 Zidovudine.

resistance by the virus. However, the principle that RT could be a target against the disease was established, and indicated the need for novel antiretroviral agents that could be developed with two primary objectives in mind:

- Administration at doses over long periods of time to allow recovery of the host immune systems required a review of host toxicity.
- Action against a variety of targets within the virus was needed to overcome the development of resistance within the virus.

Before considering the mode of action of these NRTIs, we may need to remind ourselves of the mechanism by which nucleic acid polymerase enzymes work to produce new DNA or RNA strands. This is described in Chapter 7.

Mechanism of inhibition of RT by NRTIs

For zidovudine to act as an inhibitor of RT, it must first be converted to the monophosphate by thymidine kinase, which in turn is more slowly converted to the triphosphate by thymidylate kinase (Fig. 23.5). The bulk of the azido group is believed to interfere with the activity of thymidylate kinase, thereby slowing the rate of phosphorylation. By occupying the active site of these kinase enzymes, zidovudine also slows the generation of the endogenous thymidine triphosphate, therefore lowering the reservoir of thymine base substrates for chain elongation. This is not the main mechanism of action, however. The zidovudine triphosphate is incorporated in the viral DNA chain in place of thymidine (the base it is an analogue of) and no more nucleotides can be added since the azido group is non-nucleophilic, and blocks the creation of further phosphodiester linkages which are needed to continue with the elongation of the nucleic acid chains (Fig. 23.6). Thus, reverse transcriptase is inhibited because it cannot conjugate further nucleotides onto the 3′-end of the new chain. Zidovudine triphosphate also affects mammalian DNA polymerase, for which it has one hundredth the affinity of that for viral reverse transcriptase. This causes considerable toxicity, notably dose-dependent suppression of bone marrow, resulting in anaemia and leucopenia which causes treatment to be abandoned by many patients.

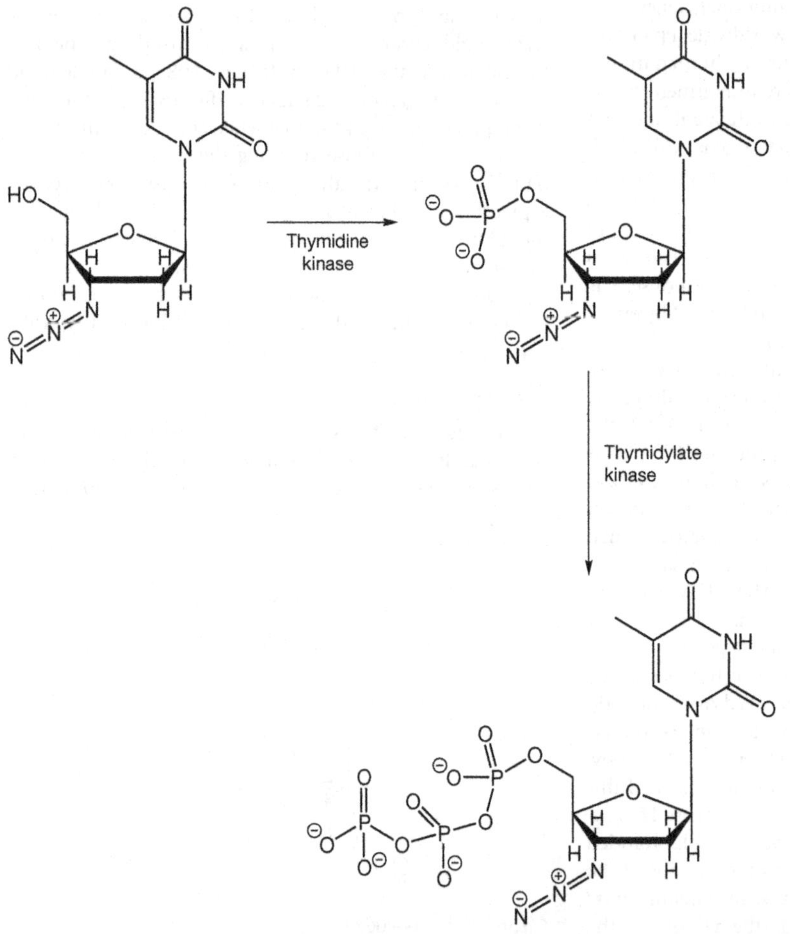

Figure 23.5 Conversion of zidovudine to its active triphosphate form.

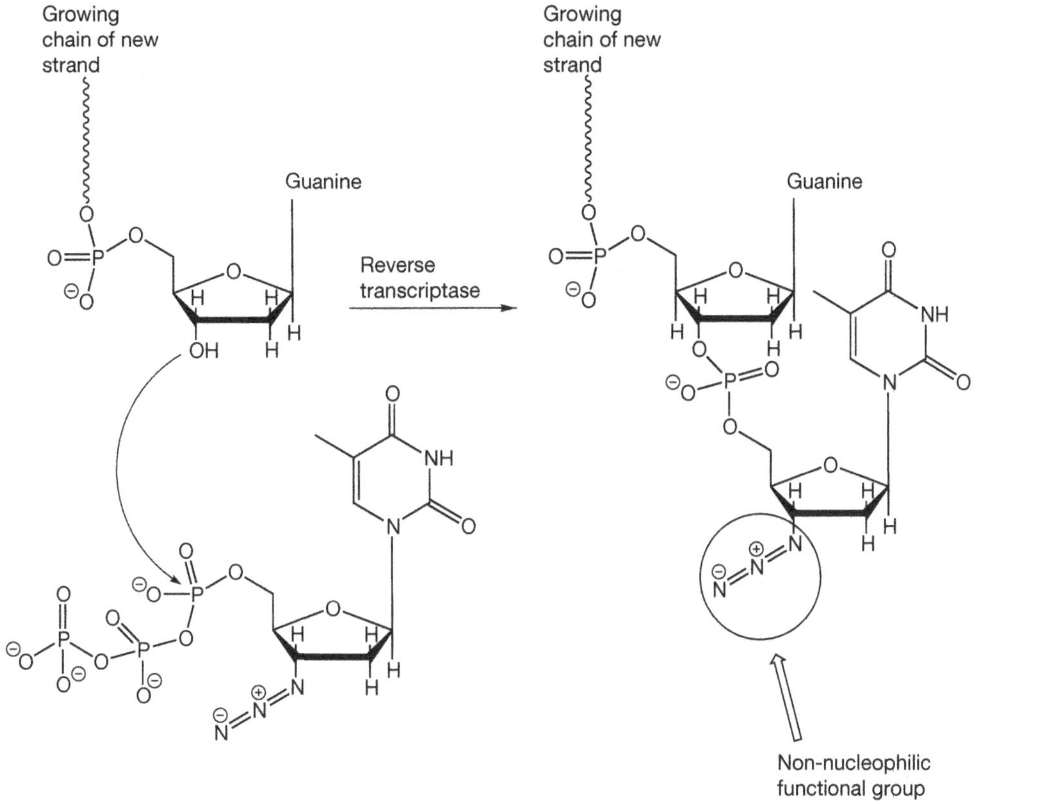

Figure 23.6 Zidovudine cannot be conjugated with further nucleotides because the 3′-azido group is non-nucleophilic, and will not displace biphosphates from incoming triphosphate substrates.

Following on from zidovudine, a number of other NRTIs have been produced (Fig. 23.7). Zalcitabine is a NRTI analogue of cytidine, and its triphosphate prevents nucleic acid chain extension because absence of the 3′-hydroxy group on the sugar ring stops formation of the phosphodiester linkages which are needed for the completion of nucleic acid chains. Stavudine acts in a similar manner. Zalcitabine is used for treatment of HIV infection when therapy with zidovudine has failed or has produced unacceptable toxicity. Lamivudine, another cytidine analogue (formerly known as 3TC), slows the reproduction of HIV by inhibiting reverse transcriptase in a similar way; it is further distinguished by the fact that it is an L-nucleoside (based on a modified L ribose molecule). Currently, there is research going on into the use of L-nucleosides as antiviral agents since they have been found to retain antiviral activity but are less toxic with respect to incorporation into the host DNA. Abacavir has been found to be a very effective reverse transcriptase inhibitor. It is an analogue of guanosine but participates in the same type of chain termination reactions as the thymidine and cytosine analogues. Didanosine is an analogue of dexoyadenosine, which, again, causes chain termination in DNA synthesis by the virus.

Preparations

- Zidovudine: Capsules 100 mg. Oral solution 50 mg/ 5 mL. Injection 10 mg/mL. Tablets 300 mg. Tablets 300 mg zidovudine and 150 mg lamivudine.
- Zalcitabine: Tablets 375 micrograms and 750 micrograms.
- Stavudine: Capsules 15 mg. Oral solution 1 mg/ml.
- Lamivudine Tablets 150 mg. Oral solution 50 mg/ 5 mL and 25 mg/5 mL. Tablets 100 mg.
- Abacavir: Tablets 300 mg. Oral solution 20 mg/mL. Tablets with abacavir 300 mg, zidovudine 300 mg and lamivudine 150 mg.
- Didanosine: Tablets 25 and 200 mg. Capsules 125, 200, 250 and 400 mg.

Non-nucleoside reverse transcriptase inhibitors (NNRTIs)

The idea behind NNRTIs started at the beginning of the 1990s with the discovery of 1-(2-hydroxyethoxymethyl)-6-(phenylthio)thymine (HEPT) and tetrahydroimidazo [4,5,1-jkj][1,4]benzodiazepine-2(1H)-one and -thione

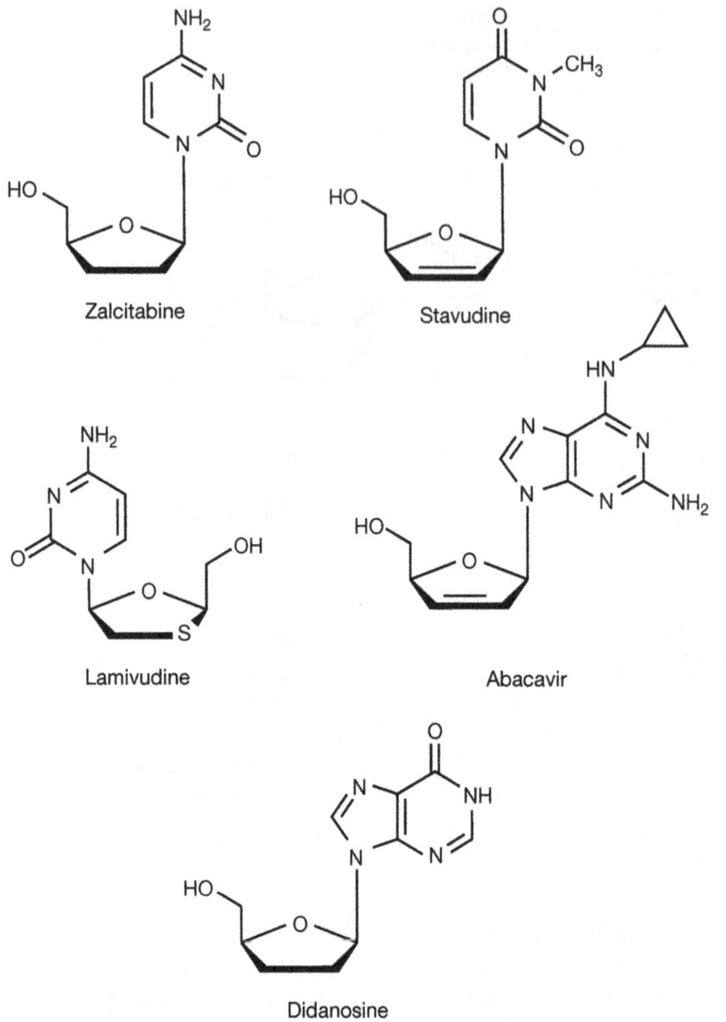

Figure 23.7 Other NRTIs.

(TIBO) as specific HIV-1 inhibitors, targeted against HIV-1 RT. These three compounds had a unique specificity against HIV-1, but were inactive against HIV-2 or any other retrovirus, and they acted through the inhibition of RT. However, although the interaction was specific to RT with the consequent prevention of viral replication, they did not act at the substrate binding site associated with the NRTIs. Whereas the latter, following their intracellular phosphorylation, act as competitive inhibitors by interacting at the site where the natural nucleotide substrates bind and subsequently prevent chain elongation by incorporation into the nucleic acid, NNRTIs block the HIV-1 RT mechanism through binding to an allosterically located, non-substrate binding site. The NNRTI binding site is functionally and spatially associated with the substrate binding site, but is distinct (0.1 nm away), and through a cooperative mechanism, binding with the NNRTI site produces a conformational change in the enzyme that locks it into an inactive conformation that is unable to perform the catalytic event of elongating the new viral nucleic acid. Since HEPT and TIBO were discovered, a variety of NNRTIs have been licensed for treating HIV infection. Whilst they and the new classes currently undergoing clinical trials can be considered structurally and chemically diverse, they occupy the same binding site that causes a repositioning of the catalytic residues that locks the enzyme in its inactive conformation. Structural modelling studies have demonstrated that, despite their diverse structures (Fig. 23.8), the positions and conformations adopted by the NNRTIs, when bound to HIV-1 RT seem to be quite similar. For example, TIBO and nevirapine maintain a 'butterfly' shape that roughly overlay each other and appear to stack with π-electron aromatic side-chain residues that line the pocket (Fig. 23.9), and whilst

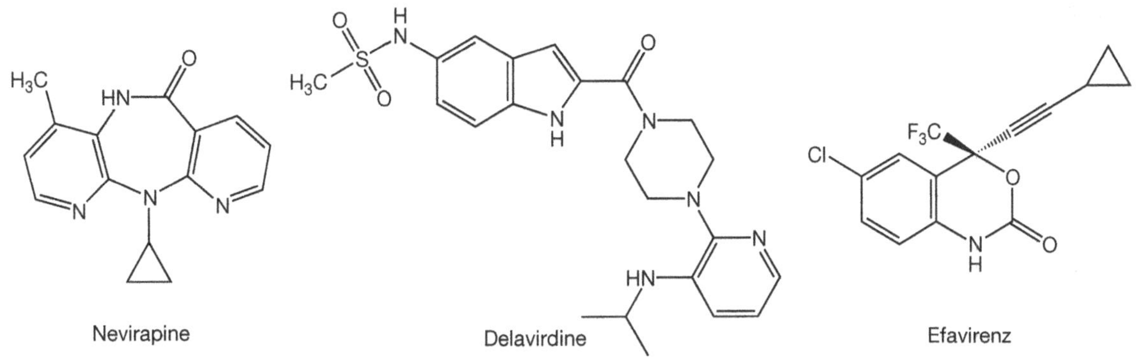

Figure 23.8 Examples of NNRTIs illustrating structural diversity.

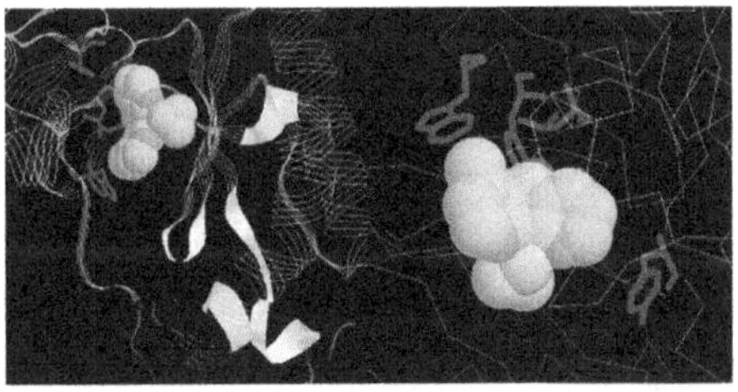

Figure 23.9 Two representations of nevirapine binding to the NNRTI allosteric site.

delavirdine occupies the same pocket, the complex is stabilised quite differently by hydrogen bonding to the Lys 103 and hydrophobic contacts with Pro 236.

Preparations

- Efavirenz: Capsules 50, 100 and 200 mg. Tablets 600 mg. Oral solution 30 mg/ml.
- Nevirapine: Tablets 200 mg. Suspensions 50 mg/5 mL.

HIV protease inhibitors

A key step in the establishment of infection is the processing of the fusion proteins that produce the enzymes required for the reverse transcription of the viral RNA into DNA. If the fusion protein is not hydrolysed into its active constituents, the enzymes required to initiate reproduction of the viral genome are halted. Workers at Roche in 1987 discovered that HIV retroviral proteases contain a highly conserved Asp-Thr-Gly motif, which had a similar catalytic mechanism to cellular aspartic proteases. Most aspartic proteinases belong to the pepsin family, which includes digestive enzymes such as pepsin and chymosin as well as lysosomal cathepsins D and processing enzymes such as renin, and certain fungal proteases. Crystallographic studies have shown that these enzymes are bilobed molecules with the active site located between two homologous lobes. Each lobe contributes one aspartate residue of the catalytically active diad of aspartates. These two aspartyl residues are in close geometric proximity in the active molecule; one aspartate has a p*Ka* of 4.5, whereas the second one has an unusually low p*Ka* of 1.2 (influenced by the protein environment), making it a very strong acid. These differences in p*Ka* values means that one residue can act as a proton donor, whilst the other is a proton acceptor, and through the involvement of a water molecule, can achieve acid- and base-catalysed hydrolysis at the same time (Fig. 23.10). In contrast to serine and cysteine proteases, catalysis by aspartic proteinases does not involve a covalent intermediate, although a tetrahedral intermediate exists. The nucleophilic attack is achieved by two simultaneous proton transfers: one from a water molecule to the diad of the two carboxyl groups, and a second one from the diad to the carbonyl oxygen of the substrate with the concurrent CO–NH bond cleavage. This general acid–base catalysis, which may be called a 'push-pull' mechanism, leads to the formation of a non-covalent neutral tetrahedral intermediate.

When the first inhibitors for this protease were developed, very little was known about the enzyme other than its aspartate-catalysed mechanism of action: there was no crystal structure to propose inhibitors based on modelling, and differences with the host proteases were unclear. All that was known was that the HIV protease was a much smaller enzyme than the equivalent host aspartate proteases (around 100 amino acids as opposed to 200), and was able to cleave substrates N-terminal to proline residues, and since mammalian proteases were unable to carry out such cleavages, the possibility of selectivity for the virus over the host arose. Additionally, even before the protease had been isolated, a study of peptides obtained from infected cells suggested that the Met-Met and Tyr-Pro sites were the likely positions of cleavage in the fusion protein.

The approach taken was not unlike that used in designing the ACE-inhibitors and on previous attempts to design inhibitors of renin, another protease enzyme. Given that

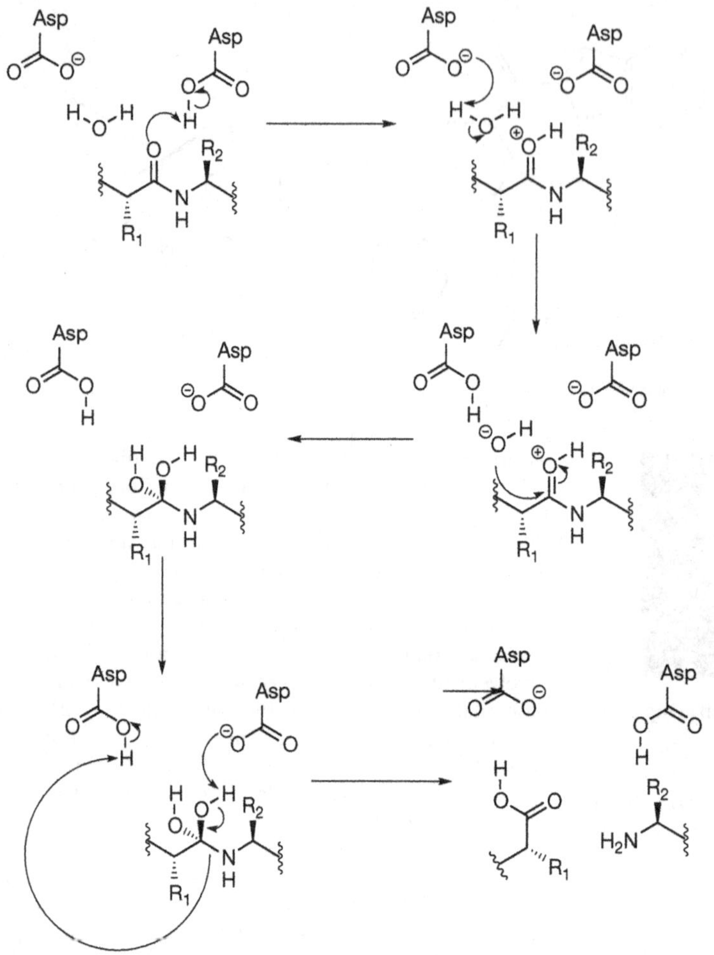

Figure 23.10 Mechanism of action of aspartate proteases, showing the generation of a tetrahedral unstable transition state through the addition of a water molecule to the amide bond where cleavage takes place.

Tyr-Pro had been identified as a cleavage site for the HIV protease, the rationale for inhibitor design was based around the Phe-Pro or Tyr-Pro motif, given the specificity of the enzyme in hydrolysing between these residues. To establish the activity of inhibitors, rather than using the HIV fusion protein itself in the assay (expensive and difficult to isolate at the time), a series of peptides that contained the Tyr-Pro cleavage consensus sequence were prepared, with the N- and C-termini protected to prevent cleavage by exopeptidases that were present in the partially purified enzyme preparation from an *Escherichia coli* vector. The hexapeptide, succinyl-Ser-Leu-Asn-Tyr-Pro-Ile-isobutylamide was used as the substrate for all routine screening assays in the Roche inhibitor design project (Fig. 23.11).

As mentioned above, aspartic proteases hydrolyse peptides and proteins through the addition of water to the target amide bond, and the reaction proceeds via an unstable tetrahedral transition state. In order to progress a reaction, enzymes, being catalysts, are known to undergo conformational changes to facilitate the stability of the transition state to lower the activation energy of the reaction from reactants to products. The design of 'transition-state' inhibitors is a commonly used strategy, because compounds that resemble transition states, but are within themselves stable, bind very tightly to the active site of the enzyme, lock it in its intermediate conformational state, dissociate very slowly and act as efficient inhibitors. Within the HIV protease project, of the possible transition-state mimetics that were chemically stable, the reduced amide ketomethylene derivatives and hydroxyethylamines were deemed the most appropriate, and were incorporated into an Asn-Phe-Pro motif that resembled the substrates. The most potent inhibitors from this series (Compounds 1–4) were found to be the hydroxyethylamines, with an IC_{50} of 140 nM (Fig. 23.12). Although this was impressive, greater potency was required for clinical evaluation, so a move away from peptide motifs through a systematic structure–activity relationship modification program was initiated.

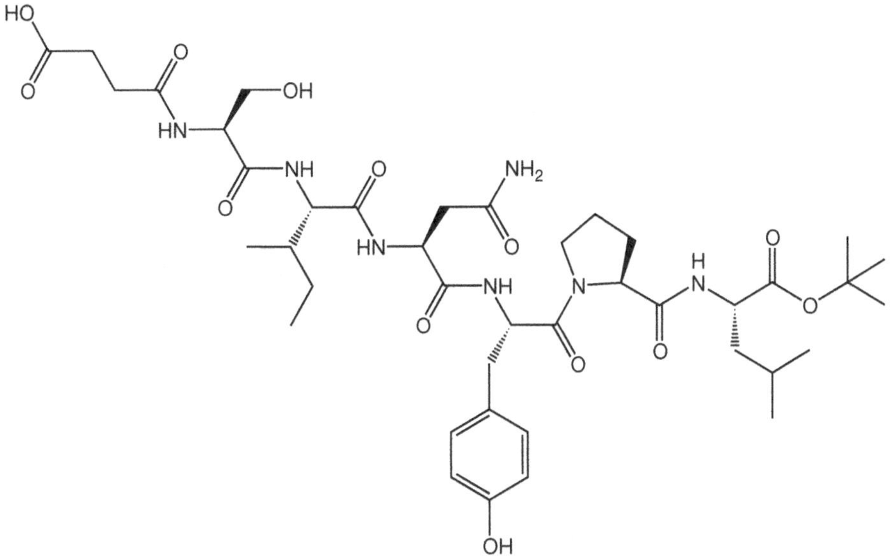

Figure 23.11 The peptide substrate Succinyl-Ser-Leu-Asn-Tyr-Pro-Ile-isobutylamide used to assay the effectiveness of inhibitors against HIV protease.

In order to examine the effect of size, protected smaller dipeptides (see Figs 23.5, 23.6) showed much reduced activity compared with the tripeptide equivalents (see Figs 23.3, 23.4), while addition of residues to the N-terminus (see Figs 23.7, 23.8), the C-terminus (see Figs 23.9, 23.10), or both ends of the molecule (see Figs 23.11, 23.12) gave no improvement in activity or potency (Fig. 23.13).

At the C-terminus, medium-sized lipophilic residues appeared to be preferred, with little difference between esters and amides. The t-butyl amide group was chosen as the C-terminal residue for subsequent compounds on the basis of metabolic stability (see Fig. 23.13), amides being more stable than the corresponding esters (see Figs 23.3, 23.4 and Fig. 23.14). Replacement of the N-terminal benzyloxycarbonyl group by smaller non-aromatic groups, such as acetyl or t-butoxycarbonyl reduced activity, but introduction of bicyclic aromatic groups such as β-napththoyl or quinoline-2-carbonyl (see Fig. 23.14) led to compounds with significantly improved activity.

The most dramatic changes in activity were seen with modifications to the proline residue – ring size was found to be very important for activity – replacing a 5-membered ring with a 4-membered ring (see (Fig. 23.15) abolished activity, whilst incorporation of a 6-membered ring improved potency 12-fold (see Figs 23.15, 23.16). Replacement of proline by two fused 6-membered rings led to the greatest enhancement activity, and the S,S,S-decahydroisoquinoline carboxylic acid was the best replacement of proline of all (see Fig. 23.17). Within the series of compounds prepared, the order of potencies against the virus also paralleled the enzyme-inhibitory potency, which indicated good cellular penetration across lipid membranes, an essential characteristic for any effective drug. The first compound to be marketed in the USA based on this research programme, in December 1995, was Roche's saquinavir (Fig. 23.15). A dose of 600 mg is administered three times a day by mouth in combination with a reverse transcriptase inhibitor such as lamivudine, or with both an NRTI and an NNRTI.

The establishment of the structure of HIV protease was determined by X-ray crystallography by a Merck team in the United States. As expected, the active site lay at the junction of two lobes joined like butterfly wings, which enabled researchers to design inhibitors of HIV protease based on molecular modelling studies. Saquinavir is rapidly metabolised, disappearing from the body in about 90 minutes. Abbott's ritonavir (Fig. 23.16) is longer lasting and need only be administered twice daily. It was the first protease inhibitor to be licensed in the UK. Merck's indinavir is less protein bound and so penetrates tissues more effectively than the first two drugs. It is administered three times a day by mouth. All compounds contain the essential hydroxyethylamine transition-state motif essential for effective inhibition of HIV protease.

A number of other protease inhibitors (Fig. 23.16) have been developed in the last few years with the aim of improving pharmacokinetic profile. One of the first of these was amprenavir, which does not contain peptide bonds which slows down its clearance from the body. Its pharmokinetics are further improved when it is administered as its phosphate prodrug fosamprenavir. Lopinavir was also developed to give improved pharmacokinetics. Its effectiveness is improved by co-administration with

Compound	Structure	IC_{50} (nM)
1	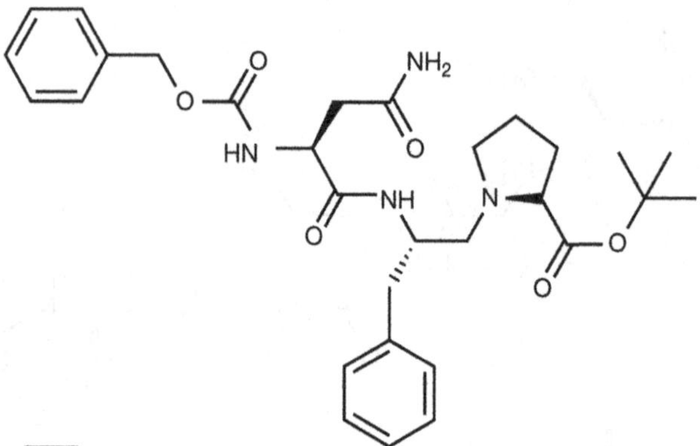	50 000
2	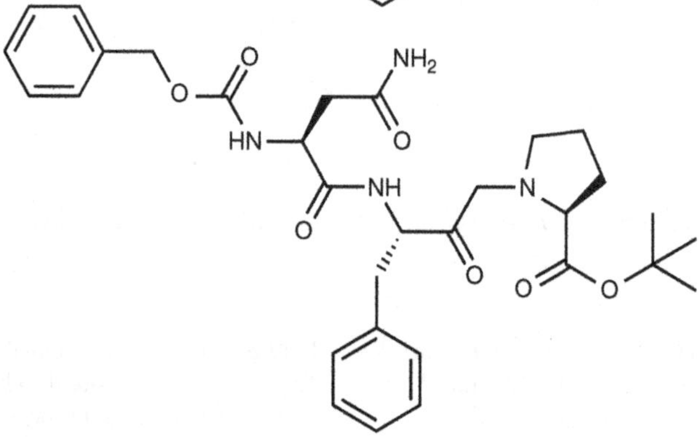	870
3	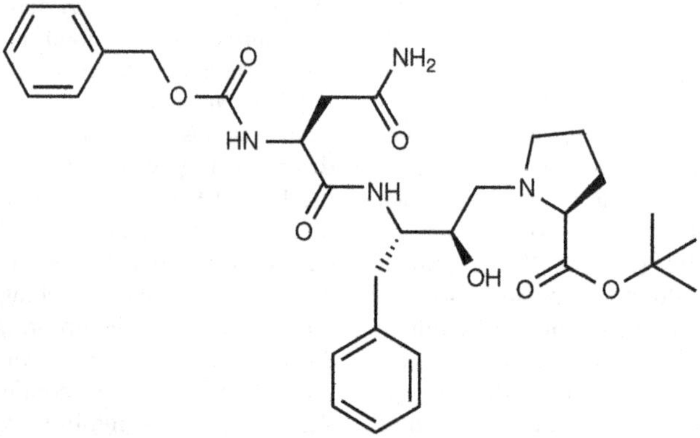	300
4	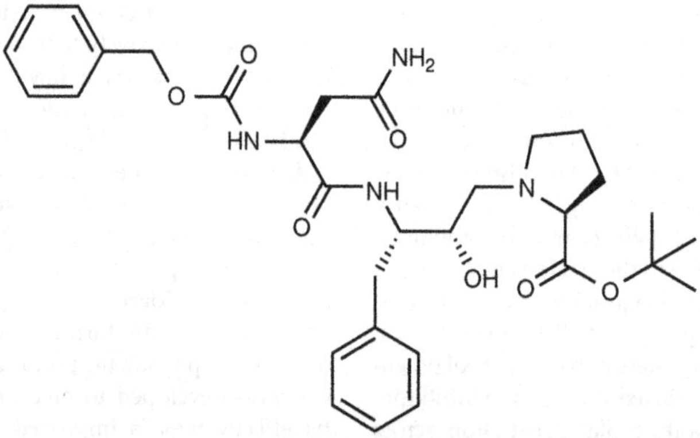	140

Figure 23.12 Comparison of the first transition-state mimetics based on the Asn-Phe-Pro substrate motif.

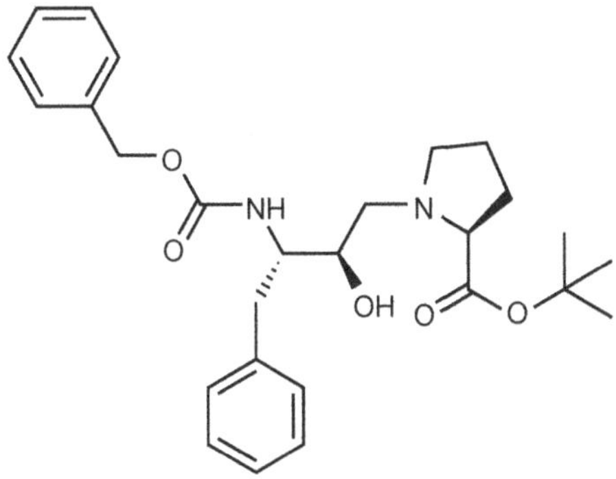

Compound 5 30 000 nM

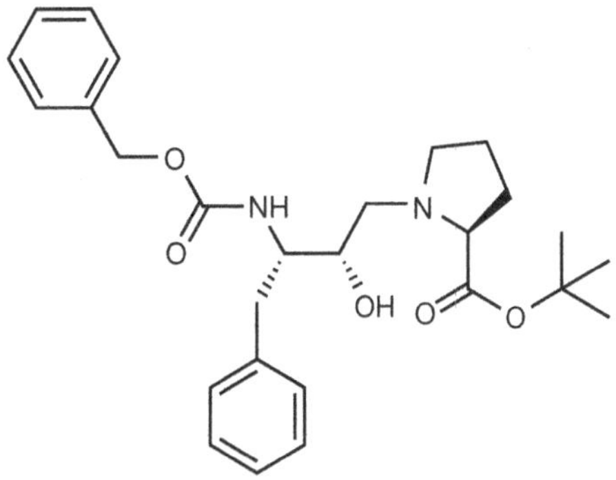

Compound 6 6500 nM

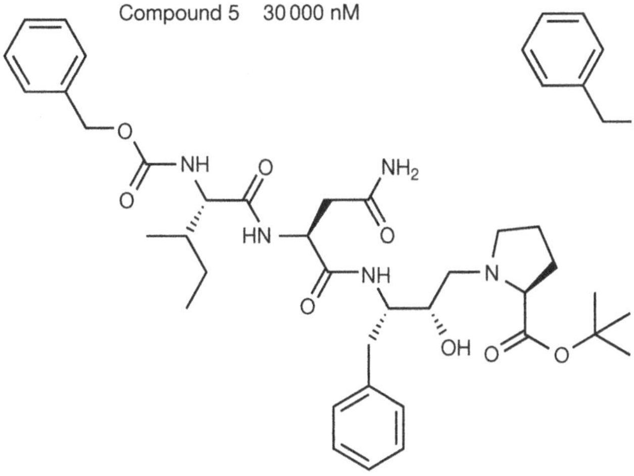

Compound 7 1100 nM

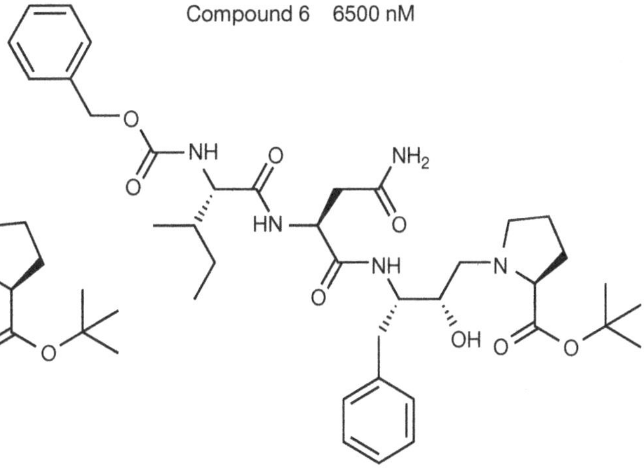

Compound 8 600 nM

Figure 23.13 The effect of inhibitor size on potency, comparing dipeptides, tetrapeptides and pentapeptides to the optimum tripeptides.

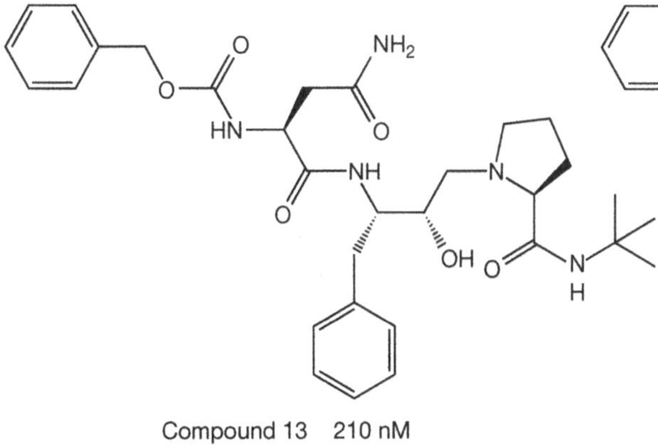

Compound 13 210 nM

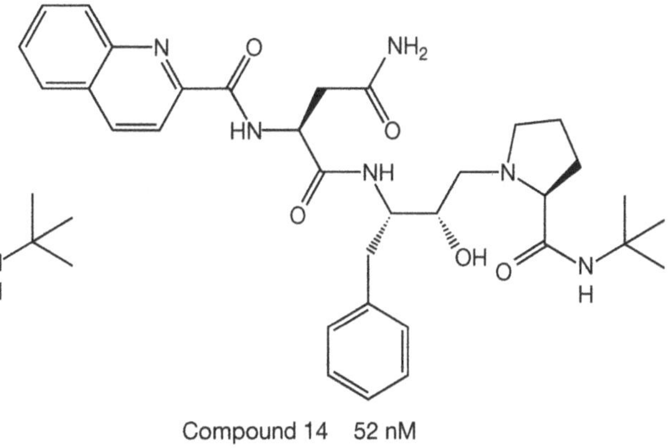

Compound 14 52 nM

Figure 23.14 The effect of changing C- and N-terminal protecting groups on potency.

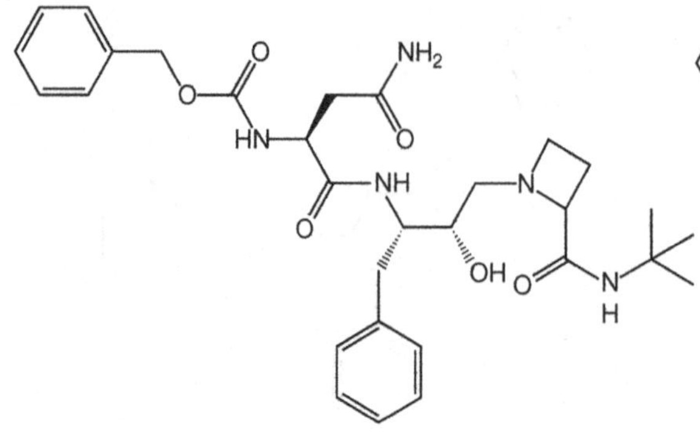

Compound 15 Inactive

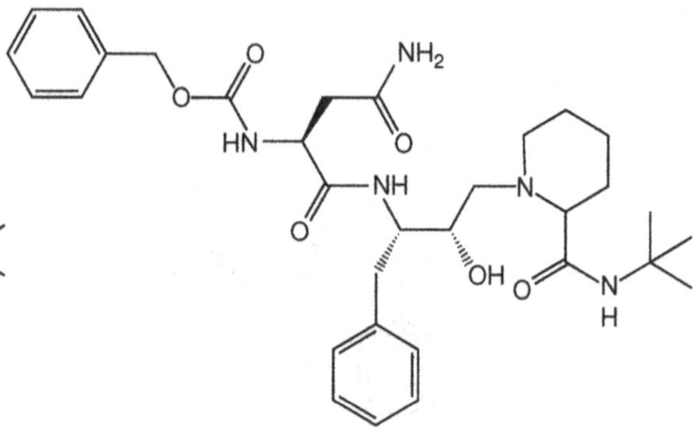

Compound 16 12 nM

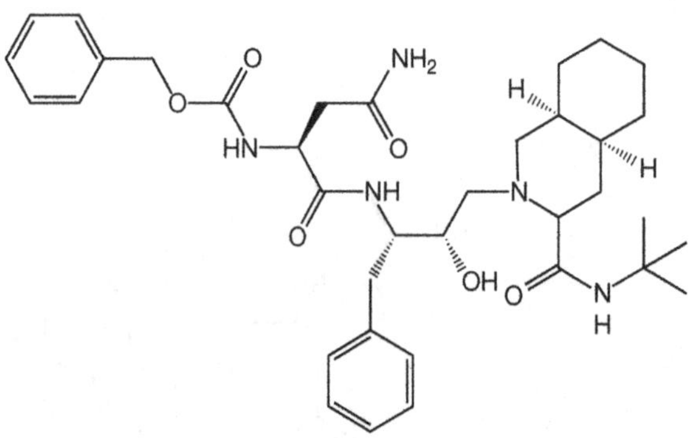

Compound 17 2.7 nM

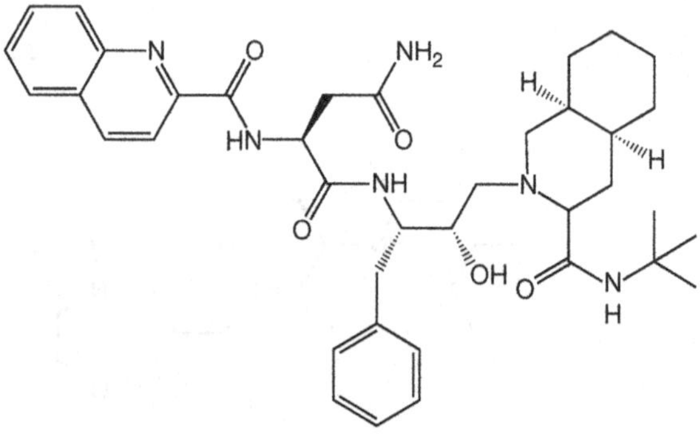

Saquinavir <0.4 nM

Figure 23.15 The effect of substituents on potency, with saquinavir, the most potent, being marketed.

ritonavir, which is a potent inhibitor of cytochrome P450. A serious side effect of protease inhibitors is elevation of cholesterol and lipid levels in the body. This may be due to the proteases inhibiting enzymes which are involved in lipid metabolism. Atazanavir has both improved pharmacokinetics enabling it be administered once a day and it has less effect on patient's lipid profiles. Clinical trials have shown that these protease inhibitors, when used in combination with an NRTI and an NNRTI, dramatically reduce the HIV viral load. In such a combination, indinavir, for example, was so effective that after treatment it proved impossible to detect virus in 85% of patients. Since an estimated 10^{12} viruses are estimated to be formed daily before treatment, this is remarkable. As a consequence, AIDS can now be held at bay for many years if chemotherapy is continued. The cost of treatment is very high and in many parts of the world it is quite unaffordable, and so patients continue to die of AIDS. The recent supply of generic forms of the anti-HIV medicines to sub-Saharan Africa, where AIDS is an epidemic, bodes well for people suffering from this disease, but strict compliance with the dose regimens must be adhered to if drug resistance by the virus is to be prevented.

Preparations

- Ritonavir: Capsules 100 mg. Oral solution 400 mg/5 mL.
- Saquinavir: Capsules 200 mg.
- Indavir: Capsules 200 mg.
- Amprenavir: Capsules 50 mg. Oral solution 15 mg/mL.
- Fosamprenavir: Tablets 700 mg. Oral solution 50 mg/mL.
- Lopinavir with ritonavir: Capsules lopinavir 133.3 mg, ritonavir 33.3 mg. Oral solution lopinavir 400 mg/5 mL and ritonavir 100 mg/5 mL.
- Atazanavir: Capsules 100, 150 and 200 mg.

ANTIRETROVIRAL THERAPY AND DRUG RESISTANCE

Hitting different targets in the HIV replication cycle by using combination therapy can result in a greater than 10 000-fold reduction in the viral load being achieved. Under such conditions, sustained suppression of the virus in the plasma does not necessarily eliminate it from the protected

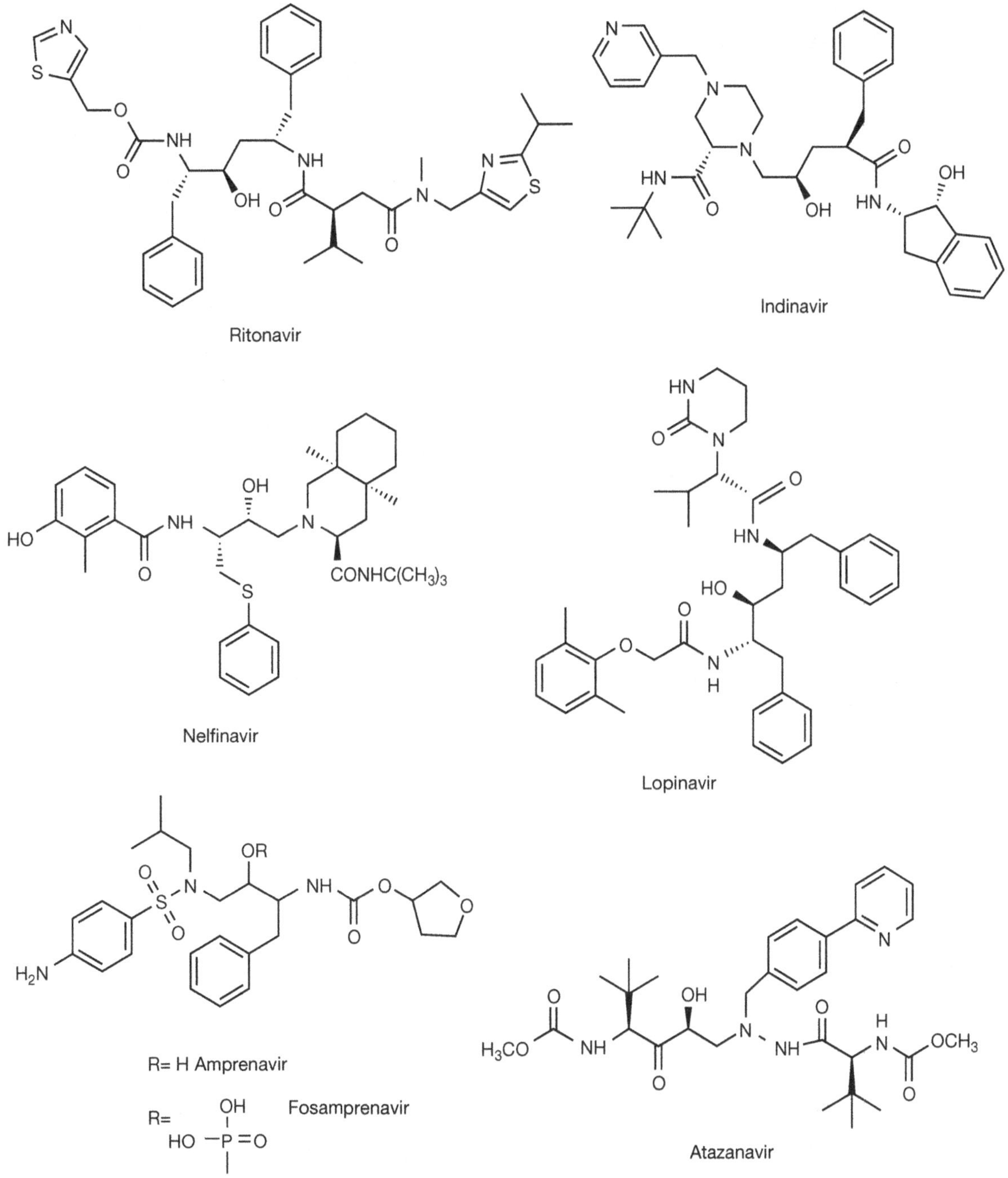

Figure 23.16 Further development of protease inhibitors.

sanctuaries such as the CSF and the lymph nodes, where drugs penetrate less readily. Consequently, drug resistance is an inevitable development of the incomplete suppression of the replication of the causative organism, and under such conditions, mutations in the viral genome that produce enzymes resistant to inhibition will arise. Specific mutations that allow for viral survival and drug resistance are generally due to amino acid residues in either RT or HIV-protease which will enable catalysis to continue, whilst hindering the binding of the drug to the target.

Herpes, varicella zoster, cytomegalovirus, hepatitis

Figure 23.17 shows some antiviral drugs related to the purine base guanosine. These drugs work by blocking the synthesis of viral DNA or by becoming incorporated into viral DNA, thus preventing its transcription. In living systems, the triphosphate of guanosine becomes incorporated in a DNA strand linked to the strand via its 5′ and 3′ positions (Fig. 23.18). Two such DNA strands give the DNA double helix.

Aciclovir

In 1975, at the Wellcome Laboratories in the USA, researchers in the course of screening analogues of guanine arabinoside found that an acyclic derivative, aciclovir, had outstanding activity against the herpes virus. It is administered to treat superficial herpes simplex infections such as cold sores (by topical application) and genital herpes (by oral administration), or for treating life-threatening herpes varicella-zoster (chickenpox) infections in immunocompromised patients. Its safety has resulted in it being available over the counter for the treatment of cold sores.

Aciclovir was one of the first antiviral drugs. As can be seen from its structure in Figure 23.17, it lacks a hydroxyl attached to the 3′ carbon and thus, when it becomes incorporated into a DNA strand, it prevents it from extending further. In addition, it remains bound to the viral DNA polymerase enzyme, preventing it from synthesising further DNA. Its therapeutic selectivity is based upon two factors: (1) herpes simplex virus (HSV) and varicella-zoster virus (VZV) express high levels of thymidine kinase (see Fig. 23.2), and (2) aciclovir has a greater affinity for the viral DNA polymerase than the DNA polymerase present in human cells. Aciclovir is used to treat herpes simplex virus. It has low toxicity but a narrow spectrum of activity and is only used in the treatment of genital and labial herpes and varicella-zoster (shingles) infections. Valaciclovir is prodrug of aciclovir, containing a readily cleavable ester group, which has an improved oral availability of 54% compared with 20% for aciclovir. Like many of the antiviral nucleosides, infusions of the drug are formulated as the strongly alkaline sodium salt (Fig. 23.19). Aciclovir and its analogues do not cure viral infection, but do effectively suppress the replication of viruses. Thus, patients should be warned that cold sores will reappear in the future and further medication will be necessary. It should be noted that aciclovir is only effective when administered at the onset of infection. The selectivity of aciclovir is enhanced by the very fact that once it is phosphorylated in the virally infected cell, it becomes too polar to diffuse out of the cell.

Preparations of aciclovir

- 200, 400 and 800 mg tablets. Intravenous infusion of the sodium salt of aciclovir 25 mg/mL. Cream 5% w/w. Eye ointment 3% w/w. 500 mg tablets (valaciclovir).

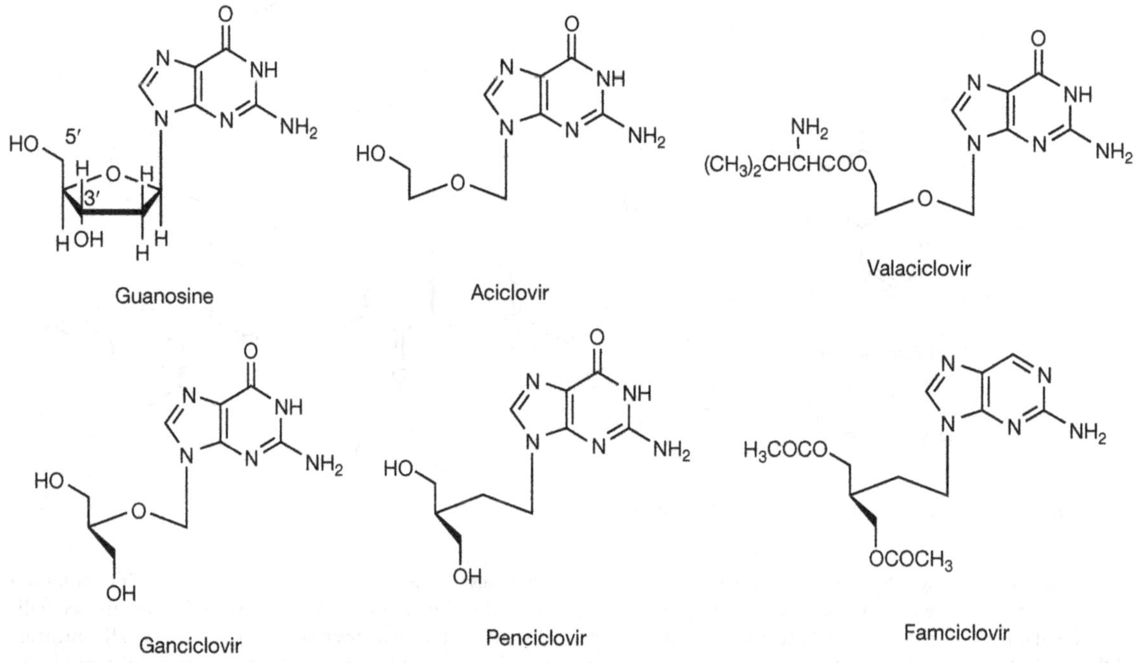

Figure 23.17 Analogues of guanosine used in antiviral therapy.

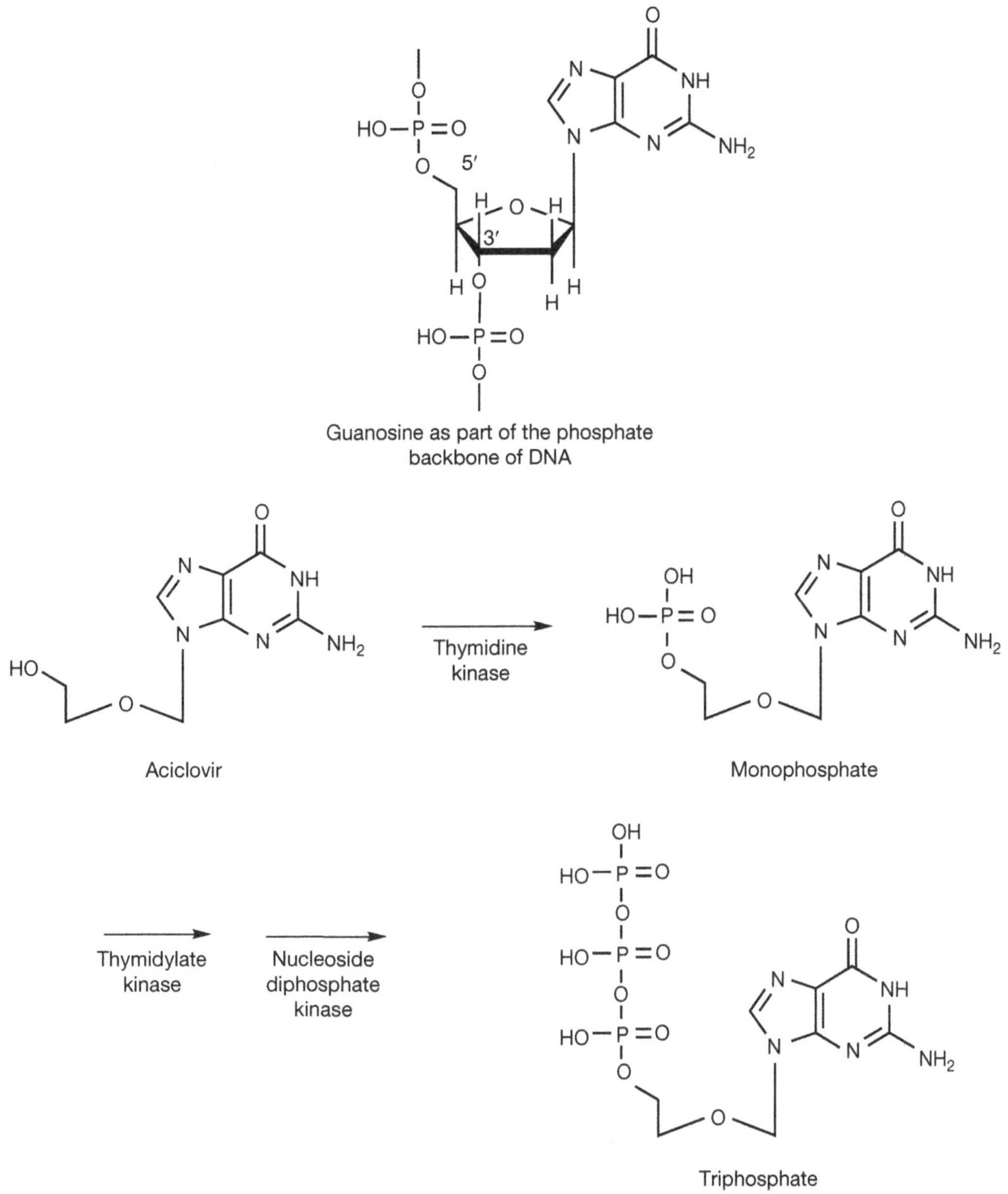

Figure 23.18 Mechanism of inhibition of DNA replication by aciclovir.

Ganciclovir

The structure of ganciclovir (Fig. 23.17) is closely related to that of aciclovir. Ganciclovir has the equivalent of 3′ and 5′ hydroxyl groups within its structure and thus, unlike aciclovir, it can become incorporated into DNA and thus has a broader spectrum of activity. The absence of a 5-membered ribose or deoxyribose sugar to maintain the structural rigidity of the sugar-phosphate backbone of the newly synthesized nucleic acid means that its structure becomes non-functional as a template for further replication or transcription. Ganciclovir is effective against HSV and VZV but it is also effective against cytomegalovirus (CMV). Ganciclovir is more readily phosphorylated in CMV-infected cells by a kinase encoded by the viral DNA, and the drug is then converted to its triphosphate by enzymes within the infected host cell. The triphosphate is a selective inhibitor of the formation of viral DNA by competitive inhibition of the incorporation of guanosine triphosphate into DNA or through itself becoming

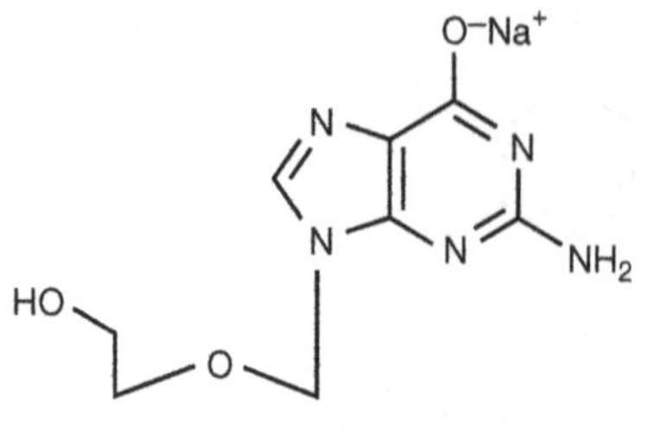

Figure 23.19 Sodium salt of aciclovir.

incorporated into DNA, thus preventing viral replication. Since the drug can become incorporated into human DNA, it is very toxic and can cause myelosuppression. The drug is only recommended for use for the treatment of CMV in immunocompromised patients. Ganciclovir has poor oral bioavailability and is administered by intravenous infusion as the strongly alkaline sodium salt; thus infusion has to be carried out slowly. Ganciclovir is also available in the form of its ester valine ester, valganciclovir (cf. aciclovir), which has better oral bioavailability.

Ganciclovir preparations

- Infusion 500 mg for reconstitution. Eyedrops 0.15% w/v for treatment of herpetic keratitis. Tablets 450 mg (valganciclovir).

Penciclovir and famciclovir

Penciclovir (Fig. 23.17) is closely related to ganciclovir in structure and has the same mechanism of action. Penciclovir has similar activity to aciclovir against herpes simplex infection. Its safety is similar to that of aciclovir due to its lack of effect on DNA synthesis in uninfected cells. A closer structural similarity to deoxyguanosine makes penciclovir a superior substrate in comparison to aciclovir for viral thymidine kinase, resulting in an enhancement of phosphorylation. This is offset by reduced activity of penciclovir triphosphate as an inhibitor of DNA synthesis. It has poor oral bioavailability and is used in the form of a cream (1% w/w) to treat labial herpes. Famciclovir (Fig. 23.17) is a prodrug of penciclovir which has good oral bioavailability (73%) and is deacetylated and oxidised (aldehyde oxidase) in the liver to penciclovir. The toxicity of famciclovir is low. It is administered three times a day by mouth, whereas treatment of herpes with aciclovir by the oral route requires five daily doses.

Preparations

- Penciclovir 1% w/w cream.
- Famciclovir 150 mg tablets.

Cidofovir

Cidofovir (Fig. 23.20) is a phosphonic acid derivative and is not susceptible to hydrolysis by cellular enzymes. It does not require initial phosphorylation by thymidylate kinase for activation and is converted by cellular kinases to its diphosphate derivative which acts as a competitive inhibitor for the incorporation of deoxcytosine triphosphate into DNA. It may become incorporated into DNA itself, causing chain termination. It is also used in the treatment of CMV in AIDS patients.

Preparations

- Infusion 75 mg/mL.

Adefovir

Like cidofovir, adefovir (Fig. 23.20) is a derivative of phosphonic acid and acts via a similar mechanism. It is used to treat chronic hepatitis B which has become resistant to the antiretroviral drug lamivudine.

Preparations

- Tablets 10 mg.

Foscarnet sodium

Foscarnet sodium (Fig. 23.20) mimics pyrophosphate and inhibits the binding of nucleoside triphosphates to DNA polymerase. Thus it has a relatively broad spectrum of activity, but is used to treat CMV and herpes in AIDS patients. Since it has a different mode of action from drugs such as aciclovir, it can be used in combination with them to increase the effectiveness of treatment. Since it forms insoluble salts with bases it is incompatible with basic drugs such as pentamidine and vancomycin, which may be used to treat secondary infections in AIDS.

Preparations

- Intravenous infusion 24 mg/mL.

Idoxuridine

Idoxuridine (Fig. 23.20) was a very early viral antimetabolite which is incorporated into DNA in place of thymidine. It was believed to be of value in treating ocular herpes simplex but is currently regarded as being ineffective both for this and for treatment of the skin.

Preparations

- 5% w/v in DMSO for treatment of cold sores.

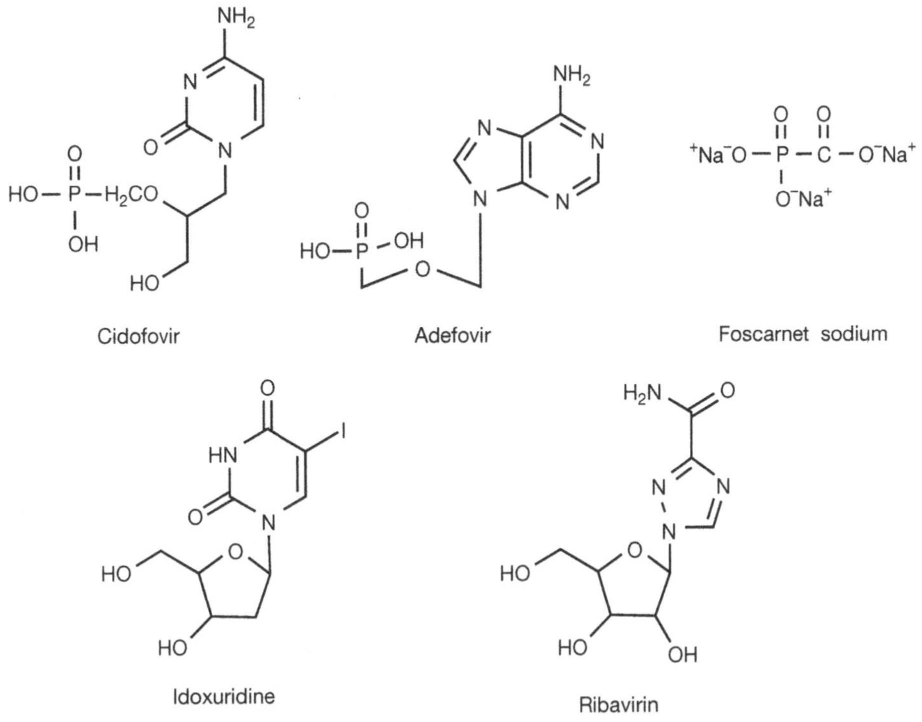

Figure 23.20 Cidofovir, adefovir, foscarnet sodium, idoxuridine and ribavirin.

Ribavirin

Respiratory syncytial virus (RSV) is a major cause of mortality in young infants and the elderly. The mechanism of action of ribavirin is not entirely clear although it is probable that it acts as an inhibitor of inosine dehydrogenase which is involved in the introduction of a carbonyl group into the inosine structure en route to the synthesis of guanosine triphosphate (GTP). GTP is required for viral RNA transcription. Ribavirin may also interfere with the action of the viral RNA polymerase. There is some debate over the effectiveness of ribavirin in treating RSV. It is also used in combination with interferon in the treatment of hepatitis C. RSV is also treated with monoclonal antibody therapy and this is discussed in the Chapter 26.

Preparations

- Tablets and capsules 200 mg. 6 g vials for reconstitution in water (300 mL) for delivery by nebuliser.

INFLUENZA CHEMOTHERAPY

Influenza is one of the most deadly infectious diseases. For many outbreaks, it is the old or very young who are at risk of death, but lethal mutants of the virus can arise such as the outbreak in 1918 which killed more than 50 million people worldwide, more than the First World War. Even in an average year, 500 million people are affected by influenza and hundreds of thousands die. Thus health authorities are keen to avoid a recurrence of the 1918 pandemic. In fact, some aspects of the 1918 epidemic are now manageable since the complication of pneumonia which was responsible for many deaths in that pandemic is now more readily treatable. There are three types of influenza: A, B and C. Type A is the most common source of epidemics and pandemics and it is highly genetically variable. Every so often the type A virus manages to completely reorganise its genetic make-up so that the human immune system is not able to recognise it. The best way to protect against influenza is by vaccination but this only applies to established strains of the virus. Since a vaccine for a new strain takes 6 months to produce, an alternative line of defence is important. The first chemotherapeutic agent against flu was amantadine (Fig. 23.21) which was a serendipitous rather than a rational discovery. Amantadine and the related compound rimantadine (Fig. 23.21) have activity against the early stages of influenza. They are believed to interfere with the M2 transmembrane ion channel protein in the virus and inhibit uncoating of the virus which must occur before the viral DNA can be integrated into the host cell nucleus. The compounds have some use in prophylaxis

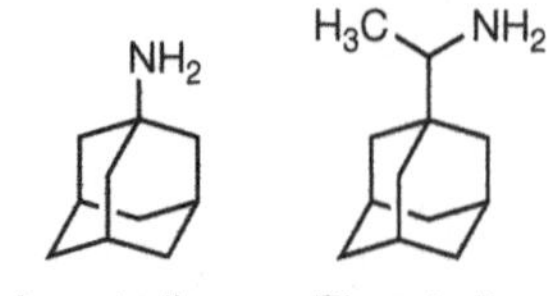

Figure 23.21 Amantadine.

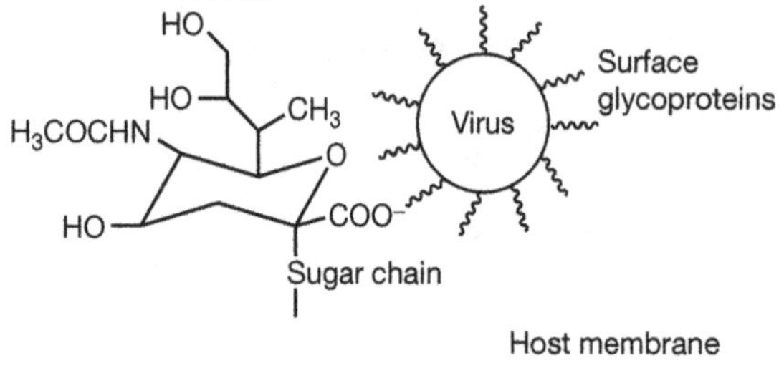

Figure 23.22 Binding of influenza virus to sialic acid.

but resistance develops readily and the two drugs have CNS side effects.

The influenza virus enters the host cell by initially binding, via its cell surface glycoproteins, to receptors bearing sialic acid residues on the surface of the host cell (Fig. 23.22). It then inserts a short fusion peptide into the host cell membrane which triggers fusion of the viral and host cell membranes (endocytosis). The virus then accomplishes the other steps in its reproduction cycle and the new viruses produced then leave the host cell by budding off the cell surface. However, the sialic acid residues on the cell surface which were useful for the initial attachment hinder the new viruses when it comes to leaving the host cell surface.

Thus the virus employs the enzyme neuraminidase (NA), which cleaves the negatively charged sialic acid residue off the host cell membrane (Fig. 23.23). The search for inhibitors of the viral NA began in the 1960s. Once the crystal structure for the viral NA was determined in the 1980s, more rapid progress in the rational design of an inhibitor was made. It was observed that within the enzyme site the OH group in the 4 position on the sialic was positioned near two negatively charged aspartic acid residues. When the 4 OH was replaced with a positively charged guanidine group, the strongly binding inhibitor zanamivir (Relenza) was produced. As might be judged from the structure, its oral bioavailability is poor, and it has to be administered via an inhaled aerosol since it also has only a short half-life in plasma. Oseltamivir was developed as an orally bioavailable NA inhibitor. The replacement of the glycol side chain with a more lipophilic hydrocarbon side chain did not reduce binding, and removal of the oxygen from the ring of the molecule improved stability in vivo. Zanamivir and oseltamivir are moderately effective in inhibiting influenza infection. Zanamivir taken prophylactically inhibits infection by 82% but this falls to 30% if it is taken after the onset of

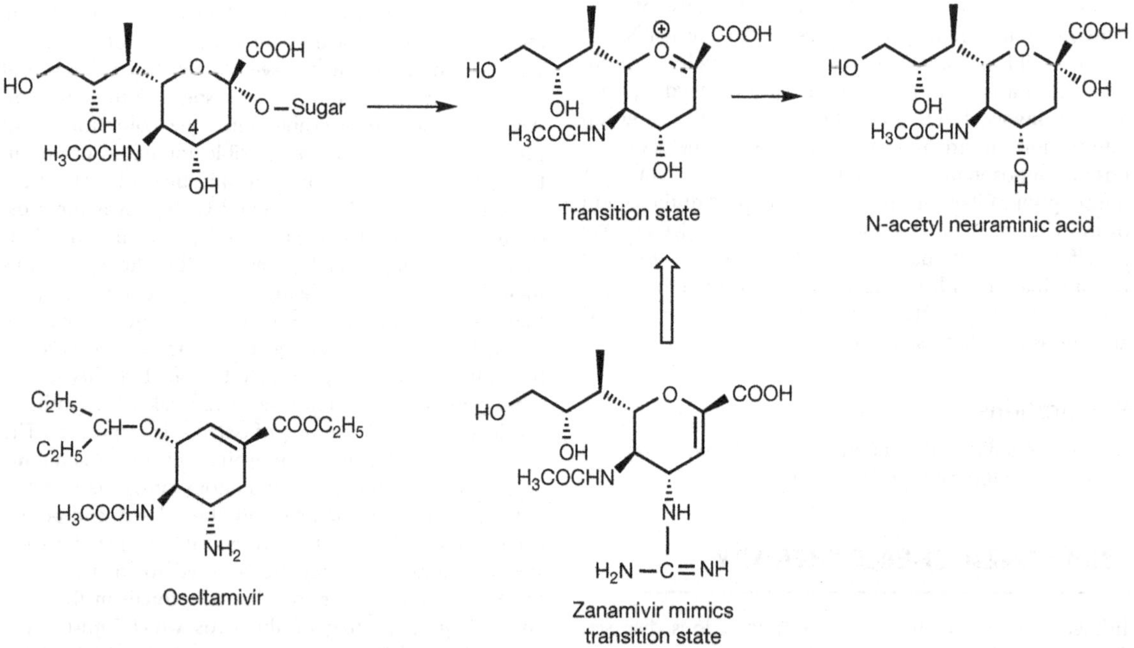

Figure 23.23 Mechanism of action of oseltamivir.

infection. The drugs are useful in preventing or treating influenza in the elderly and in infants.

There are a number of other potential targets in the life cycle of the influenza virus, such as the initial cell surface binding stage, but as yet there are no other drugs close to market.

Preparations

- Zanamivir: 5 mg blister packs for inhalation.
- Oseltamivir: Capsules 75 mg. Suspension 60 mg/5 mL.
- Amantadine: 100 mg capsules.

FURTHER READING

De Clercq E. Antiviral drugs in current clinical use. *J Clin Virol.* 2004;30(2):115–133.

De Clercq E. New approaches toward anti-HIV chemotherapy. *J Med Chem.* 2005;48(5):1297–1313.

Menendez-Arias L. Targeting HIV: antiretroviral therapy and development of drug resistance. *Trends Pharmacol Sci.* 2002;23(8):381–388 and references therein.

Tomasselli AG, Heinrikson R. Targeting the HIV-protease in AIDS therapy: a current clinical perspective. *Biochemica Biophysica Acta.* 2000;1477: 189–214.

Vacca JP, Condra JH. Clinically effective HIV-1 protease inhibitors. *Drug Discov Today.* 1997;7:261–272.

Herdewijn P. Structural requirements for antiviral activity in nucleosides. *Drug Deliv Today.* 1997;2:235–242.

Mathe C, Gosselin G. L-nucleoside enantiomers as antiviral drugs: A mini-review. *Antiviral Res.* 2006;71:276–281.

Luscher-Mattli M. Influenza chemotherapy: a review of the present state of art and of new drugs in development. *Arch Virol.* 2000;145:2233–2248.

Wade RC. 'Flu' and structure based drug design. *Structure.* 1997;5:1139–1145.

Wyde PR. Respiratory syncytial virus (RSV) disease and prospects for its control. *Antiviral Res.* 1998;29:63–79.

Chapter | 24 |

Antifungal chemotherapy

Alexander Balfour Mullen, David G Watson

CHAPTER CONTENTS

INTRODUCTION

Fungal microorganisms constitute one of the largest groups of living organisms on the planet, with around 75 000 species having been described and an estimated additional 1.5 million fungal species awaiting discovery. Although some fungal species are found in an aquatic environment most are terrestrial. The vast majority of fungi are saprophytic, i.e. they secure food by the extracellular digestion of dead organic matter, such as plants. In nature, the mineralisation of organic matter by fungi plays a pivotal role in ensuring a sustainable ecosystem. These eukaryotic microorganisms are extensively utilised within industry to provide a number of important chemicals or products, e.g. alcohol and bread (*Saccharomyces cerevisiae*), vitamin B_2 (*Ashbya gossypii*), the enzyme glucose oxidase used in diabetic test strips for monitoring glucose (*Aspergillus niger*), the enzyme rennin used in coagulation of milk during cheese making (*Mucor miehei*). In addition, many of the secondary metabolites originating from fungi have proved invaluable in the treatment of human infectious disease, e.g. griseofulvin (*Penicillium griseofulvum*) and β-lactam antibiotics such as penicillins and cephalosporins (*Penicillium chrysogenum* and *Cephalosporium acremonium*, respectively).

INCIDENCE OF FUNGAL INFECTIONS

Despite the large number of known fungal species, only around 300 species are recognised as being true or potential human pathogens. Most of these are opportunistic fungal pathogens responsible for relatively benign superficial or cutaneous infections (mycoses) in healthy humans, e.g. athlete's foot (*Trichophyton* species). There are, however, a relatively small number of pathogenic or opportunistic fungi that can cause life-threatening systemic mycoses, e.g. aspergillosis (*Aspergillus* species). In the past two decades, the incidence of these systemic mycoses has steadily risen due to advances in medical technology such as:

- improved recognition and diagnosis of fungal infections
- prolonged survival of immunocompromised patients with cancer, diabetes or AIDS
- increased numbers of patients undergoing invasive surgical procedures, e.g. organ transplantation, implantation of prosthetic devices
- medical therapeutics, e.g. availability of parenteral nutrition, peritoneal dialysis, haemodialysis and indwelling catheters.

ANTIFUNGAL CHEMOTHERAPY

Fungi, being eukaryotic cells, possess many of the cellular features observed in host mammalian cells. During the development of the early antifungal agents, limited knowledge of the fundamental differences between fungal and mammalian cell function meant that researchers were often trying to exploit relatively minor differences in fungal and mammalian biochemical pathways. As a result, early antifungal agents often had limited selectivity and/or an appreciable degree of host toxicity. Pertinent examples will be discussed later in the chapter. In recent years, an increased understanding of basic fungal and mammalian cell function has allowed pathways that are unique to fungi to be identified, and these are currently being exploited in the development of antifungal agents with high potency and specificity but with low host toxicity.

Inhibitors of DNA/RNA synthesis

The only drug used clinically in this class is flucytosine.

Flucytosine

This drug is largely active against yeasts and some *Aspergillus* species. Flucytosine is a pyrimidine analogue that is actively taken up into cells via the cell membrane enzyme cytosine permease, a natural transporter of cytosine, adenine, guanine and hypoxanthine (Fig. 24.1). Intracellular flucytosine is then converted by the enzyme cytosine deaminase into the antimetabolite 5-fluorouracil, thus it acts as a prodrug (the mechanism of its action is discussed in Ch. 21). The 5-fluorouridine triphosphate metabolite of 5-fluorouracil results in the formation of abnormal RNA, ultimately leading to disruption in protein synthesis. The 5-fluorodeoxyuridine monophosphate metabolite inhibits thymidylate synthase, an essential enzyme required for the formation of thymidine, one of the pyrimidine bases of DNA (see Ch. 21). The selective toxicity of flucytosine against fungal cells results from the absence or limited expression of cytosine deaminase within mammalian cells, which means that its toxicity is selective for these cells.

Intrinsic (natural) resistance or the development of resistance (acquired) to flucytosine during therapy is common; therefore susceptibility testing is recommended before and during therapy. Flucytosine is usually administered in conjunction with amphotericin B in the treatment of systemic candidiasis, cryptococcosis and torulopsosis. The combination of flucytosine and amphotericin B is synergistic. However, most filamentous fungi are resistant to flucytosine since they do not express cytosine permease or cytosine deaminase.

Description and preparations

Flucytosine is a white to off-white, crystalline powder, with a solubility of 1 g in 67 mL water at 25°C. Prolonged storage of aqueous flucytosine solutions at temperatures higher than 25°C can result in flucytosine decomposing to 5-fluorouracil, whilst storage below 18°C may result in drug precipitation. It has a low octanol/water partition coefficient. Flucytosine has two p*Ka* values of 2.9 (protonation of weak primary amine group attached to the ring) and 10.71 (deprotonation of amide nitrogen in position 1). Typical preparations include:

- Infusion bottles containing 2.5 g flucytosine in 250 mL isotonic sodium chloride solution. Adult dose: 200 mg/kg daily in four divided doses.
- Tablets (Europe) containing 500 mg flucytosine. Adult dose: 50–150 mg/kg daily in four divided doses.
- Capsules (USA) containing 250 mg or 500 mg flurocytosine. Adult dose: 50–150 mg/kg daily in four divided doses.

Pharmacokinetics

Flucytosine is usually administered intravenously over 20 to 40 minutes. Protein binding is low (approximately 2–4%) and volume of distribution is high (0.7–1 L/kg) with cerebrospinal fluid (CSF) concentrations comparable to serum concentrations. Approximately 90% of a drug dose is excreted unchanged in the urine. The drug has a half-life of 3–6 hours in adult patients with normal renal function. Patients with renal impairment should be given smaller doses which can be estimated according to their creatinine clearance. Only a small percentage of flucytosine is metabolised to 5-fluorouracil by the body, with an area under

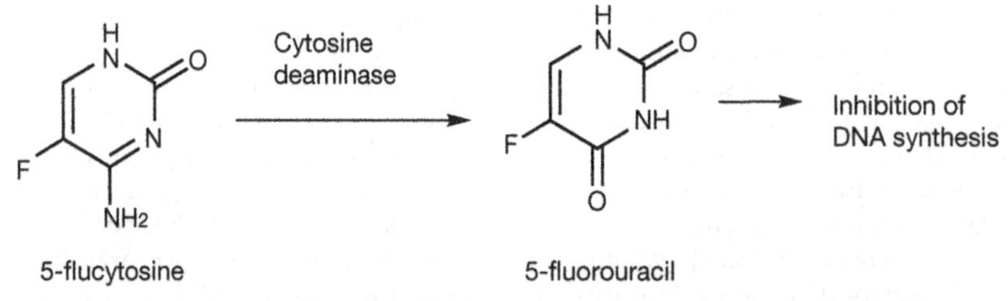

Figure 24.1 Selective conversion of flucytosine to the anti-metabolite 5-fluorouracil by fungal enzymes.

the curves (AUC) ratio of 5-fluorouracil to flucytosine of 4% being recorded. This may, however, explain why high doses of intravenous flucytosine can result in bone marrow suppression. Oral bioavailability of flucytosine is high, with bioavailability greater than 80% reported. Gastrointestinal microflora is capable of converting flucytosine to fluorouracil and it has been speculated that the oral route may therefore be associated with a greater risk of bone marrow toxicity.

Fungal resistance to flucytosine

The most common mechanism of intrinsic resistance is a decreased uptake of flucytosine by the fungus by a reduction in cytosine permease activity, which results in reduced concentrations of drug entering into the cell. The development of resistance to flucytosine during therapy may be a result of reduced expression of, or a deficiency in, an enzyme at any step in the intracellular metabolism of flucytosine. However, the most common resistance mechanisms observed in clinical isolates are due to either reduced cytosine deaminase or URPTase activity.

Microtubule inhibitors

Griseofulvin (Fig. 24.2) is the only drug in this class.

Griseofulvin

Dermatophyte fungi are moulds that specifically infect the keratinised layers of the skin by virtue of their ability to degrade keratin. Three genera, *Epidermophyton*, *Microsporum* and *Trichophyton*, are responsible for causing ringworm or tinea infections (dermatophytosis). Griseofulvin is used exclusively for the oral treatment of dermatophyte infections where topical therapies have failed or are inappropriate.

Griseofulvin is produced by various strains of *Penicillium griseofulvum*. It has a narrow spectrum of antifungal activity, being inactive against other important fungal pathogens such as *Candida* spp. and *Aspergillus* spp. It has no other antimicrobial activity.

Griseofulvin appears to be fungistatic, primarily exerting its antifungal activity by interacting with the microtubule proteins, α- and β-tubulin, thereby inhibiting the assembly of functional microtubules that comprise the spindle apparatus of the fungal cell. Disruption of the spindle apparatus inhibits mitosis and results in cell division arrest. The exact binding site of griseofulvin on the microtubules appears to be distinct from drugs such as colchicine and Vinca alkaloids (Ch. 21), and may account for its relatively selective toxicity against fungal cells. However, griseofulvin has been shown to be teratogenic (causing fetal abnormalities) in rats and has induced aneuploidy (abnormal numbers of chromosomes following cell division) in mammalian cells both in vitro and in vivo. For this reason griseofulvin should not be administered to pregnant women or women likely to become pregnant within 1 month of finishing treatment. In addition, males should not father children within 6 months of treatment.

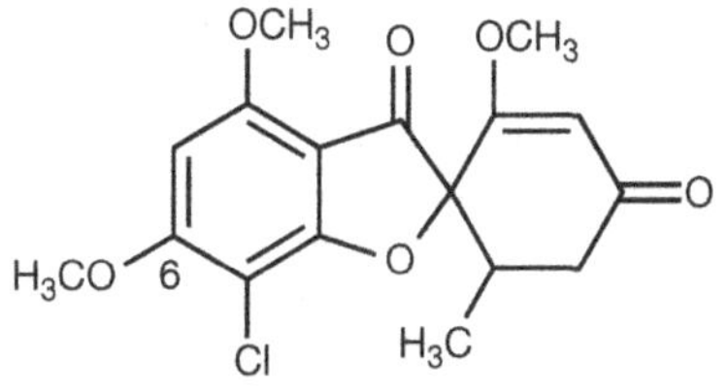

Figure 24.2 Griseofulvin.

Description and preparations

Griseofulvin is a white to creamy or yellowish white, odourless crystalline powder. It is practically insoluble in water, slightly soluble in methanol and ethanol, soluble in acetone and chloroform, and freely soluble in dimethylformamide and tetrachloroethane. Griseofulvin is stable at room temperature and to light exposure. Typical preparations include:

- A tablet containing 125 mg or 500 mg griseofulvin. Adult dose: 500–1000 mg daily as a single or divided dose for 2 weeks after visible signs of infection have disappeared.
- An oral suspension containing 25 mg/mL griseofulvin. Adult dose: 500–1000 mg daily as a single or divided dose for 2 weeks after visible signs of infection have disappeared.

Pharmacokinetics

The small intestine is the main absorption site of griseofulvin. Oral bioavailability is typically low, being less than 50%, and variable, but can be enhanced by administering griseofulvin with or immediately after a fatty meal. Oral bioavailability is also limited by the rate of drug dissolution and can therefore be enhanced by reducing drug particle size. For this reason most pharmacopoeias specify the particle size of griseofulvin powder, e.g. EP stipulates a particle size range of up to 5 μm in maximum dimension, with an occasional number of larger particles that exceeds 30 μm permitted. Following oral absorption, peak serum levels are observed after 4 hours. In plasma, around 84% of griseofulvin is bound to plasma proteins, predominantly albumin. Griseofulvin has a volume of distribution of 1.2–1.4 L/kg. The terminal half-life is extremely variable between subjects with a range of 9.5–21 hours reported. Griseofulvin is metabolised in the liver, with the major metabolite being 6-desmethylgriseofulvin or its glucuronide derivative. These metabolites have no residual antifungal activity. Around 50% of the metabolite is excreted in the urine with another 30% in the faeces.

> **Q** Self Test 24.1
>
> Draw the glucuronide metabolite of griseofulvin. Why is the drug converted to this metabolite by the body?

A significant proportion of griseofulvin accumulates in keratinous tissues, with concentrations exceeding plasma levels during therapy. However, concentrations rapidly fall after discontinuing therapy due to griseofulvin being excreted in sweat. The resulting high local keratinous tissue concentrations of griseofulvin facilitate its antifungal activity against dermatophyte infections. However, the speed at which griseofulvin accumulates into infected keratinous tissue is dependent on the thickness of keratin at the site of infection and therefore determines the duration of therapy. Infected hair or skin, having a relatively thin keratinous layer, responds to relatively short courses of treatment, typically between 4 and 6 weeks. In contrast, toe- or fingernails, with a thick keratin layer, require prolonged therapy of between 6 and 12 months.

Drugs that interfere with fungal cell membrane function

Sterol components of the fungal cell membrane play an important role in the normal functioning of the cell membrane by modifying its physical integrity. The major cell membrane sterol present varies among eukaryotes. For example, in plants β-sitosterol and stigmasterol are the major membrane sterols whilst in mammalian cells cholesterol is the most common sterol. As a consequence, individual eukaryotic species will possess slightly different biosynthetic pathways (enzymes) to allow manufacture of their preferred sterol. The importance of specific sterols to cell viability has resulted in many pharmaceutical companies directing resources to develop drugs that will specifically inhibit key stages in the fungal sterol biosynthetic pathway that are unique to, or sufficiently different from, the corresponding mammalian pathway. A summary of drugs interfering with fungal sterol biosynthesis is provided in Figure 24.3.

Polyene macrolide antifungal agents

Of the 200 different known polyene macrolides (large-ring lactones), only amphotericin B and nystatin (which is a mixture of related compounds the major component being nystatin A1) have an acceptable toxicity profile for clinical use as antifungal agents. The chemical structures of amphotericin B and nystatin A1 are shown in Figure 24.3.

Amphotericin B

This drug was initially isolated and characterised from *Streptomyces nodosus* in 1956. Amphotericin B has broad antifungal activity against a wide range of yeasts and moulds including *Aspergillus* spp., *Mucor* spp., *Candida* spp., *Cryptococcus neoformans* and *Histoplasma capsulatum*. It remains the drug of choice in the treatment of life-threatening systemic mycoses. In addition, it also has potent activity against *Leishmania* protozoa. It has no antibacterial activity.

Description and preparations

Amphotericin B is a yellow to orange, odourless powder. It is practically insoluble in water, ethanol and ether. It is slightly soluble in methanol and soluble in dimethylformamide, dimethylsulphoxide and propylene glycol. It has two p*Ka* values of 5.7 (carboxylic acid functional group) and 10 (amine functional group on aminosugar attached to macrolide ring through a glycoside linkage). At physiological pH it exists as a zwitterion in aqueous solution. The zwitterionic species can form head-to-tail dimers at concentrations above 1 μm and soluble high-order aggregates (micelles) above 10 μm. The seven conjugated double bonds in amphotericin B make the molecule prone to oxidation. Amphotericin B is therefore stored between 2° and 8°C in airtight containers and protected from light. In aqueous solution amphotericin B is inactivated by extremes of pH due to hydrolysis of the glycosidic linkage. It has a high octanol/water partition coefficient. Typical preparations include:

- A sterile lyophilised powder for intravenous infusion containing 50 mg amphotericin B, 41 mg sodium deoxycholate as a solubiliser and 20.2 mg sodium phosphate as a buffer (Fungizone®). Upon reconstitution with sterile water for injection a mixed micellar dispersion of amphotericin B and deoxycholate is formed. Adult dose: 1–1.5 mg/kg daily or on alternate days.
- A lozenge containing 10 mg amphotericin B. Adult dose, 10 mg four times a day.
- An oral suspension containing 100 mg/mL amphotericin B. Adult dose: 100 mg four times a day.
- A tablet containing 100 mg amphotericin B. Adult dose: 100–200 mg four times a day.

Pharmacokinetics

There is no systemic absorption of amphotericin B following oral administration in the form of a lozenge, tablet or suspension for the treatment of oral, perioral or intestinal fungal infections.

Intravenous administration of the conventional micellar dispersion (Fungizone®) diluted in 5% w/v dextrose is usually performed over 4 to 6 hours and results in amphotericin B becoming widely distributed throughout well-perfused tissues, particularly the heart, lung, liver and spleen. The high molecular weight of amphotericin B precludes its entry into the central nervous system (CNS). Following a single intravenous infusion it has

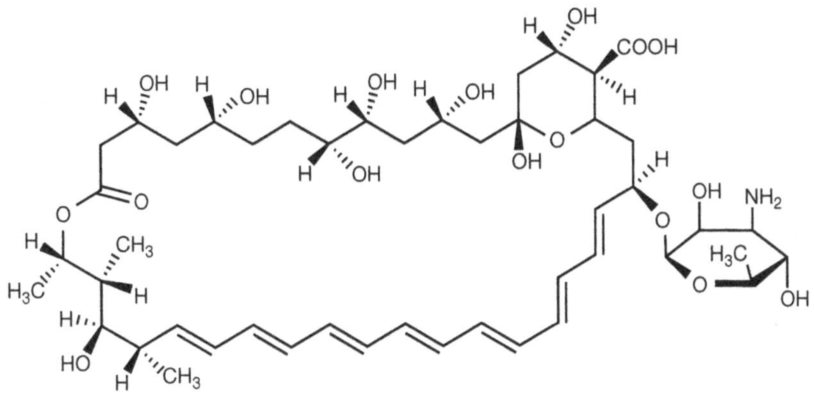

Amphotericin

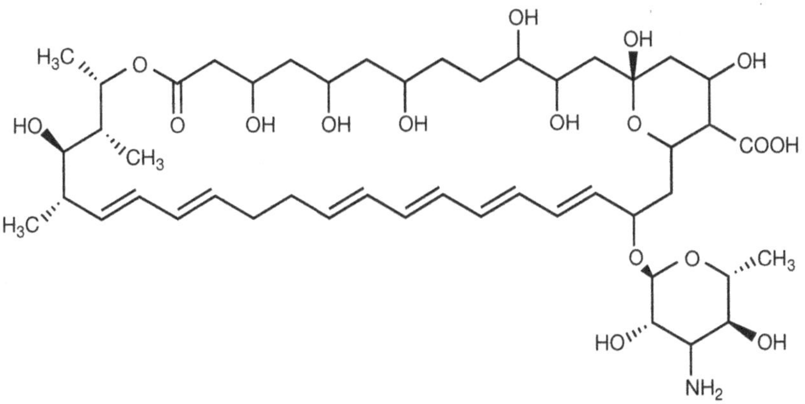

Nystatin A

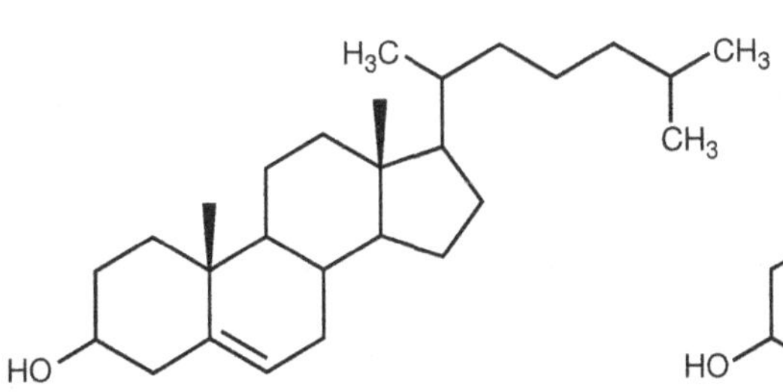

Cholesterol

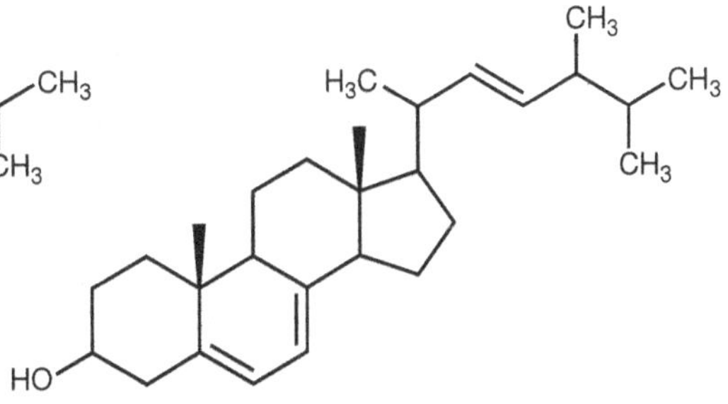

Ergosterol

Figure 24.3 Polyene macrolide antifungal drugs.

a volume of distribution of 4 L/kg and a half-life of 24–48 hours. Upon prolonged administration, the half-life increases to around 15 days. Amphotericin B is extensively protein bound in the plasma, mainly to β-lipoproteins. Amphotericin B does not appear to be metabolised in vivo and is slowly excreted by the kidneys.

Clinical toxicity of amphotericin B (Fungizone®)

The clinical usefulness of amphotericin B in the treatment of systemic mycoses is limited by its toxicity profile. Acute adverse reactions during and in the immediate post-infusion period include nausea, vomiting, headache, fever and chills. Thrombophlebitis at the infusion site is also a common problem. These acute reactions are dose related and can be ameliorated by pre-infusion administration of paracetamol, chlorphenamine and hydrocortisone. Chronic adverse reactions can include renal, cardiovascular and haematological toxicity. Of these, renal toxicity is the most clinically prevalent with over 80% of all patients receiving amphotericin B exhibiting some renal impairment. The extent of kidney impairment is dose related and often irreversible upon cessation of therapy.

Antifungal activity of amphotericin B

The antifungal activity and toxicity of amphotericin B is intimately related to its chemical structure. Amphotericin B is a surface-active molecule, possessing a hydrophilic (polyhydroxyl backbone on the macrolide ring plus the aminosugar moiety) and hydrophobic side (conjugated heptadiene system on the macrolide ring). Due to this surface activity, amphotericin B in aqueous solution can interact with the sterol component of biological membranes. This interaction is thought to increase membrane permeability through the formation of pores. The increased permeability results in the loss of intracellular protons, cations and small molecules such as amino acids and ultimately causes cell death. In addition, amphotericin B has immunomodulatory activity and can induce oxidative damage. The importance of these two mechanisms to the antifungal activity of amphotericin B remains to be determined.

Mammalian toxicity – molecular mechanisms

The selective toxicity of amphotericin B against fungal rather than mammalian cells is modest and arises from the higher binding affinity of amphotericin B for the main fungal membrane sterol, ergosterol, compared to the main mammalian sterol, cholesterol. This higher affinity is, however, relatively small, approximately 14 times greater for ergosterol compared to cholesterol, and partly explains the narrow therapeutic index of the drug. The similar binding affinities of amphotericin B for both sterols is not surprising given their similar molecular structure (Fig. 24.3).

As previously mentioned, amphotericin B can exist as a number of molecular species in aqueous solution depending on the local concentration of the drug. Upon intravenous administration of Fungizone®, the amphotericin B – deoxycholate micelle – dissociates. This results in high local concentrations of amphotericin B and as a consequence amphotericin B can coexist in the plasma as a number of species: in a monomolecular (uncomplexed) state, as a dimer or as soluble high-order complexes. All of these amphotericin B species are capable of interacting with ergosterol, but only the high-order complexes appear to have appreciable affinity for cholesterol. Therefore the rapid dissociation and release of amphotericin B from Fungizone® exacerbates toxicity by promoting the formation of high-order complexes.

Amphotericin B, when released from Fungizone®, can also associate with the cholesterol component of high density lipoprotein (HDL). Lipoproteins are lipid–protein complexes involved in the circulation and distribution of lipids in the body. The amphotericin B is subsequently transferred from HDL to low density lipoprotein (LDL) by a lipid transfer protein. The resulting amphotericin B-LDL complex can then enter mammalian cells expressing LDL receptors by the process of receptor-mediated endocytosis. Internalised amphotericin B is then capable of interacting with cholesterol present in the cell membrane. Therefore the natural biodistribution of amphotericin B contributes to its clinical toxicity profile.

Drug delivery technology – modulating the clinical profile of amphotericin B

The clinical disadvantages associated with the use of Fungizone® provided the impetus for the development of alternative delivery systems that had increased efficacy but reduced toxicity. Three alternative lipid-based amphotericin B delivery systems have subsequently been developed and introduced into clinical practice.

AmBisome®. This is a sterile lyophilised liposomal formulation. Each vial contains 50 mg amphotericin B, 194 mg hydrogenated soybean phosphatidylcholine, 84 mg distearoylphosphatidylglycerol and 52 mg cholesterol. Upon reconstitution with sterile water for injection, small unilamellar liposomes that have a mean diameter of 80–100 nm are formed. Adult dose: 1–3 mg/kg daily.

Amphocil®. This is a sterile lyophilised colloidal dispersion. Each vial contains 50 or 100 mg amphotericin B and sodium cholesterol sulphate approximately equimolar amount. Upon reconstitution with sterile water for injection it forms a colloidal dispersion. Adult dose: 1–4 mg/kg daily.

Abelcet®. This is a sterile aqueous suspension of a lipid-amphotericin B complex. Each 20 mL vial contains 100 mg amphotericin B, 30 mg/L α-dimyristoylphosphatidylglycerol, 68 mg/L α-dimyristoylphosphatidylcholine. Adult dose: 5 mg/kg daily.

Each of these formulations changes the in vivo pharmacokinetics of amphotericin B with the net result of minimising exposure of the kidneys to it and thus reducing the incidence of toxicity, particularly nephrotoxicity. The lipid-based delivery systems also enhance clinical efficacy by promoting the delivery of amphotericin B to organs where fungal infections commonly reside, e.g. liver and lungs. The severity and incidence of acute adverse reactions with these lipid-based formulations is also less compared to Fungizone®. The exact biodistribution of amphotericin B when administered as a lipid-based formulation appears to be formulation dependent. The reduced toxicity of the lipid-based formulations also appears to be a result of the slow release of amphotericin B from the formulations following administration. This ensures that low concentrations of amphotericin B are maintained in the plasma, thereby minimising the formation of the high-order complexes of amphotericin B that are especially toxic to mammalian cells. In addition, some of the delivery systems, e.g. AmBisome®, appear to reduce toxicity by restricting the formation of amphotericin B-LDL complexes.

Comparative studies of the lipid-based amphotericin B formulations with Fungizone® would appear to indicate that they are less potent on a weight-for-weight basis compared with amphotericin B. However, with the reduced toxicity profile of the lipid formulations, higher doses of amphotericin B can be tolerated by the patient, thereby offsetting any loss in drug potency experienced due to its formulation in a lipid delivery system.

Nystatin

This polyene macrolide antibiotic is isolated from *Streptomyces nourseri* and *S. albidus*. Nystatin is considered too toxic for parenteral administration. It is composed of a number of tetraene compounds (compounds that contain four conjugated double bonds), the principle component being nystatin A_1 (Fig. 24.3) which has a very similar structure to amphotericin B. Its use is mainly reserved for the treatment of oral, perioral, intestinal, vulvovaginal or cutaneous *Candida* spp. infections.

Description and preparations

Nystatin is a yellow to light brown hygroscopic powder with an odour characteristic of cereals. The activity of nystatin is unusual in that it is expressed in units. A number of similar standards coexist with the European Pharmacopoeia stating that potency is not less than 4400 IU per milligram. It is insoluble in ethanol, chloroform and ether. It is very slightly soluble in water, slightly soluble in methanol, and soluble in dimethylformamide. Nystatin is hygroscopic and prone to oxidation. It should be protected from light and stored between 2° and 8°C in an airtight container. Typical preparations include:

- A tablet containing 500 000 units of nystatin. Adult dose: 500 000–1 000 000 units every 6 hours.
- An oral suspension containing 100 000 units/mL. Adult dose: 1–5 mL four times a day.
- A topical cream/ointment/gel containing 100 000 units/g. Adult dose: apply to the affected areas two to four times a day.
- A vaginal pessary/cream containing 100 000 units/dose unit. Adult dose: 100 000–200 000 units per vaginum at night.

All nystatin preparations are well tolerated by patients. Very occasionally nausea, vomiting and diarrhoea are reported following oral administration and skin irritation following topical application. Commercial development of a parenteral liposomal formulation of nystatin is in progress for the treatment of systemic mycoses and it is anticipated that this will provide similar clinical benefits to those observed with AmBisome.

Pharmacokinetics

No clinically significant absorption into the systemic circulation occurs following administration of nystatin by any of the indicated routes.

Mode of action

Nystatin exerts its antifungal activity by the same mechanism as described for amphotericin B.

Azole antifungal drugs

This is the largest group of antifungal agents and they can be subdivided on the basis of their chemical structure into imidazoles and triazoles. The mode of action of all azole antifungals is identical in that they interfere with fungal sterol biosynthesis by inhibiting fungal cytochrome P450-Erg11p (also known in the nomenclature as lanosterol 14-α-demethylase or Cyp51p) which catalyses the reaction shown in Figure 24.4. This depletes the fungal plasma membrane of ergosterol, an essential membrane sterol, and concomitantly leads to the accumulation of 14-α-methylated precursors (the exact precursors reflect the unique biosynthetic pathway of individual fungal species). The net result is an alteration of plasma membrane fluidity and functional disruption of important membrane-bound enzymes such as chitin synthase and arrest of cell growth (fungistatic action) or cell death (fungicidal action).

Extensive research has been undertaken in order to understand the structure–activity relationship for the interaction between azole antifungals and cytochrome P450-Erg11p so that optimal activity can be realised against a wider spectrum of fungal pathogens and to address the issue of emerging (acquired) resistance to some of the pre-existing azole antifungal agents in current clinical usage.

At the active site within the cyp450 lies a protoporphyrin IX ring containing iron (III) where cyclic oxidation/reductions are performed. The azole antifungal agent has the ability to bind to this active site such that it prevents access, binding and subsequent transformation of the endogenous, 14-α-methylated sterol ligand.

The imidazole or triazole rings of the antifungal drugs orientate themselves perpendicular to the plane of the protoporphyrin ring, with the lone pair of electrons of the N3 or N4 atoms in the imidazole or triazole rings, respectively, becoming coordinated with the iron atom. The remainder of an individual azole molecule can interact with hydrophobic and aromatic residues within the substrate access channel of the apoprotein. As there is slight variation in the conformation of the active site and in the amino acid composition of the apoprotein between fungal species, this controls the potency and spectrum of antifungal activity of a given azole.

Inhibition of the Cyp450-Erg11p by an azole is non-competitive with respect to the endogenous substrate, leading to a greater disruption of the sterol metabolic

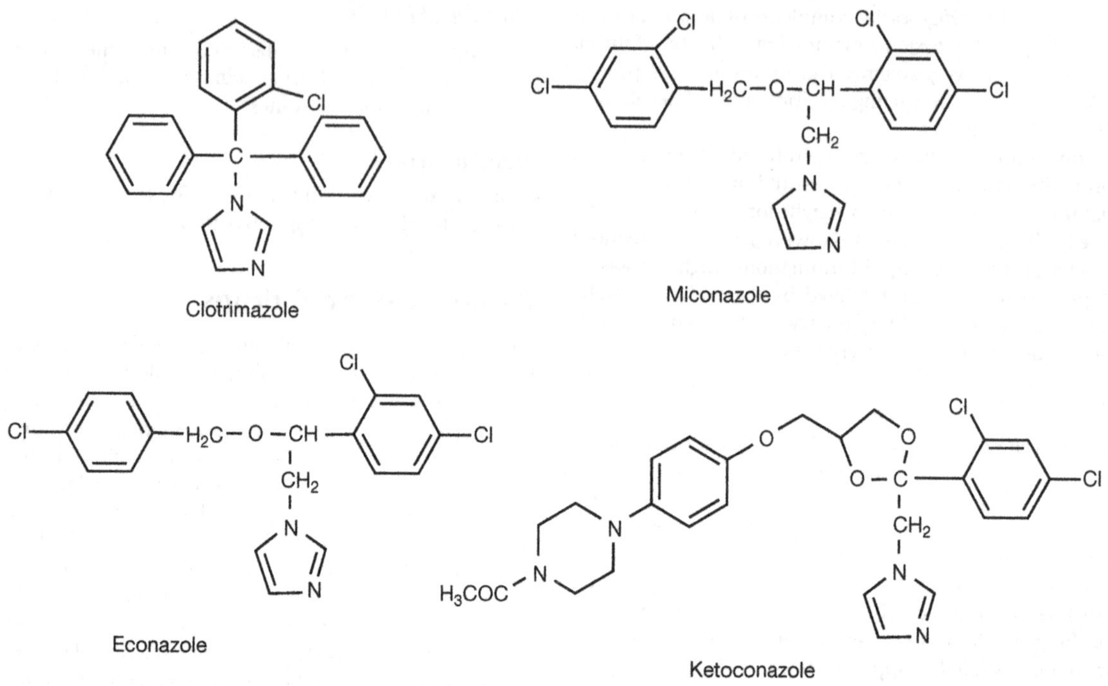

Figure 24.4 Imidazole antifungal agents.

pathway than that resulting from a competitive inhibitor. Correspondingly, as cyp450 is not a single enzyme, but consists of a family of closely related isoforms, this explains why all of the azoles, to a greater or lesser extent, can also interact with mammalian cyp450 enzymes, resulting in toxicity.

Imidazoles

Clotrimazole

Clotrimazole (Fig. 24.4) was the first compound of its class and was investigated in the early 1970s as a parenteral agent for the treatment of systemic mycoses. However, initial trials were discouraging. It became apparent that the primary limitation of clotrimazole administered by the parenteral route was that it induced the hepatic microsomal enzymes involved in its own metabolism. Therefore clotrimazole blood levels quickly became undetectable (i.e. below clinically active concentrations) soon after initiating therapy.

As a consequence of these preliminary studies, the systemic use of clotrimazole as an antifungal agent was abandoned and, instead, its use for the treatment of cutaneous and mucocutaneous infections was pursued. Clotrimazole administered by these routes proved highly successful and it remains a useful clinical agent for the treatment of yeast and dermatophyte infections.

Description and preparations

Clotrimazole is a white to pale yellow crystalline powder. It is a lipophilic substance with a reported logP value of 3.5. It is practically insoluble in water, and soluble in methanol, ethanol, methylene chloride, chloroform and acetone. It should be stored in an airtight container and protected from light. Typical preparations include:

- A cream containing 1% w/w clotrimazole for cutaneous and mucocutaneous application. Adult dose: application to the infected area two or three times a day, continuing for 14 days after all visible signs of infection have healed.
- As a powder containing 1% w/w clotrimazole for cutaneous application. Adult dose: application to the infected area two or three times a day, continuing for 14 days after all visible signs of infection have healed.
- As a spray or solution containing 1% w/w clotrimazole for application to hairy cutaneous areas. Adult dose: application to the infected area two or three times a day, continuing for 14 days after all visible signs of infection have healed.
- A cream containing 500 mg clotrimazole or a tablet containing either 100, 200 or 500 mg clotrimazole for vaginal administration. Adult dose: vaginal application of 500 mg clotrimazole (as cream or tablet) as a single dose at night or alternatively with the tablet formulation, 100 mg at night for six

consecutive nights or 200 mg at night for three consecutive nights. Studies indicate a single dose of 500 mg is as clinically effective, as the more prolonged courses and may aid patient compliance.

Pharmacokinetics

Less than 1% of clotrimazole enters the systemic circulation following topical application whilst between 3% and 10% of a dose has been reported to do so following vaginal administration. As a result, very little of an applied dose (typically <1%) enters into the systemic circulation. Additionally, with higher systemic doses achieved via vaginal application, the course duration 1–6 days, allied to low blood concentrations, is not enough to induce metabolism.

> **Q** Self Test 24.2
>
> Why does cutaneous, mucocutaneous and vaginal application of clotrimazole not induce hepatic microsomal enzymes?

Miconazole

Like clotrimazole, miconazole was originally developed as an intravenous and oral antifungal agent. The intravenous formulation was discontinued due to anaphylactic reactions associated with the injection vehicle excipient, polyoxyl 35 Castor Oil (Cremophor EL), used to enhance the solubility of miconazole. Unlike clotrimazole, repeated administration does not induce the hepatic microsomal enzymes involved in its own metabolism. Following oral administration, around 20% of a dose is systemically absorbed where it undergoes oxidative O-dealkylation and oxidative N-dealkylation prior to excretion (Fig. 24.5). Approximately 40% of the administered dose is excreted unchanged in the faeces. The faecal route of excretion for metabolites predominates over urinary excretion. Oral administration of miconazole has been observed to interfere with the metabolism of other therapeutic agents including phenytoin, warfarin and quinidine.

The use of miconazole is now restricted to the treatment of mucocutaneous, intestinal and vulvovaginal fungal infections. A similar range of preparations to clotrimazole are available for the treatment of these infections.

Econazole

Oral and intravenous routes of administration for the treatment of systemic fungal infection using econazole were abandoned when it became apparent that econazole was readily metabolised to inactive compound. Consequently, the clinical uses of econazole have been restricted to topical application like those of clotrimazole and miconazole.

Ketoconazole

When introduced in the early 1980s, ketoconazole (Fig. 24.4) was seen as a useful clinical development as it represented the first imidazole antifungal that had sufficient oral bioavailability to make it useful in the treatment of cutaneous (dermatophytic) and systemic (mycotic) yeasts, with weaker activity against a limited number of moulds (e.g. *Aspergillus* spp.) infections.

Description and preparations

Ketoconazole is a white to off-white crystalline powder. It is lipophilic with a reported logP value of 3.5. It is practically insoluble in water, sparingly soluble in ethanol, but soluble in methanol and methylene chloride. It should be protected from light.

Typical preparations include:

- A tablet containing 200 mg ketoconazole. Adult dose: 200 mg once a day with food, typically for 14 days or

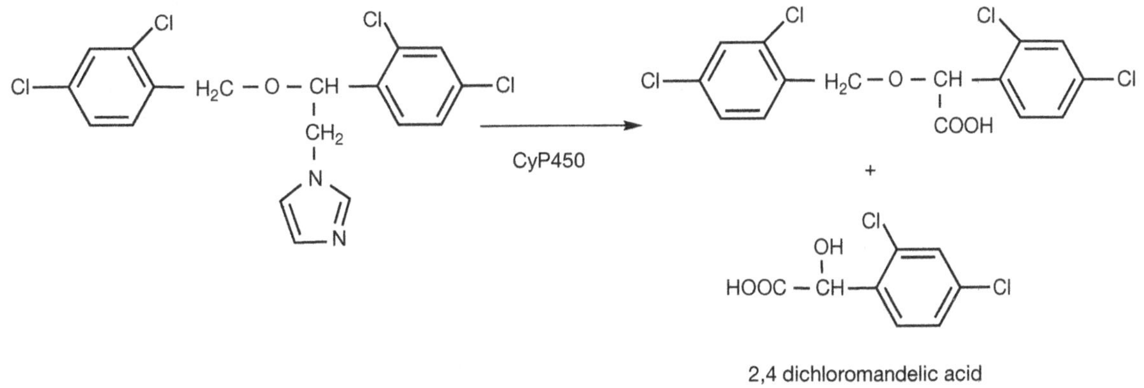

Figure 24.5 Cyp450 metabolism of miconazole.

for 7 days after clinical symptoms have resolved and microbial cultures are negative. The dose may be increased to 400 mg daily when initial clinical response is poor.
- A cream containing 2% w/w ketoconazole for cutaneous and mucocutaneous application. Adult dose: application to the infected area once or twice a day, continuing for a few days after all visible signs of infection have healed.
- As a shampoo containing 2% w/w ketoconazole for scalp application in the treatment of dandruff and seborrhoeic dermatitis. Adult dose: application to the scalp as a shampoo for 3 to 5 minutes before rinsing off. Repeat every 3 to 4 days for 2 to 4 weeks.

Pharmacokinetics

Following oral administration, approximately 75% of an administered ketoconazole dose is absorbed. However, there is considerable inter- and intrapatient variation, with oral absorption impaired when gastric acidity is decreased due to clinical pathology, e.g. achlorhydria, or due to concurrent administration of agents that decrease gastric acidity, e.g. antacids, H_2-receptor antagonists or proton pump inhibitors, or whether the patient is in a fed or fasted state (absorption is enhanced in the fed state).

Peak plasma levels occur around 2 hours after oral administration, with a terminal half-life of around 8 hours. Ketoconazole is extensively bound (>95%) to plasma proteins, mainly albumin, which results in relatively low free drug concentrations. Therefore, with clinical dosing schedules, ketoconazole tends to be fungistatic rather than fungicidal, which is a potential concern if the patient is immunocompromised. Ketoconazole is widely distributed throughout the body but penetration into CSF is low, excluding its use in the treatment of fungal meningitis.

Ketoconazole is extensively metabolised by the liver following gastrointestinal absorption into several inactive metabolites that are predominantly excreted through bile into the faeces. Only a small fraction of the drug or its metabolites are excreted unchanged in the urine. The major metabolic pathways identified for ketoconazole include oxidation, cleavage, degradation and scission of the imidazole and piperazine rings; oxidative O-dealkylation; aromatic hydroxylation and N-deacetylation. Experimentally, in isolated rat microsomes, the generation of N-deacetyl ketoconazole metabolites has been implicated in the hepatotoxicity that is occasionally associated with ketoconazole therapy. Oxidative attack by flavin-containing monooxygenases on the N-1 position of the N-deacetyl ketoconazole metabolite results in the generation of ring-opened dialdehydes that are cytotoxic.

Ketoconazole also suffers from a number of other clinical disadvantages. At daily doses greater than 400 mg, ketoconazole may reversibly inhibit endogenous steroid synthesis with resultant suppression of testosterone and cortisol and disruption of endocrine function. In addition, ketoconazole extensively interferes with the metabolism of many drugs including warfarin, ciclosporin, HMG-CoA enzyme inhibitors, HIV protease inhibitors and calcium channel blockers to name but a few. These limitations are primarily due to the relative lack of binding specificity that ketoconazole has between mammalian and fungal cyp450 enzymes, and this was an important determinant in the development of newer azole analogues that have greater selectivity and enhanced antifungal activity.

Triazoles

Fluconazole

Researchers at Pfizer sought to overcome the limitations of the existing imidazole antifungal compounds by developing analogues of tioconazole that had greater metabolic stability and which were less lipophilic, thereby improving oral bioavailability and delivering high plasma concentrations of unbound drug respectively. After 2 years of extensive research they concluded that the imidazole moiety, which was metabolically vulnerable, had to be replaced with something that had greater metabolic stability. Of the analogues that were synthesised, only one compound, UK-46245, containing a 1,2,4-triazoyl-1-yl group, showed promising activity, with antifungal activity being three times greater than the corresponding imidazole derivative in an in vivo model. Hypothesising that this was due to enhanced metabolic stability, the researchers replaced the metabolically vulnerable hexyl chain with a second triazole group to give compound UK-47265. This compound was a major breakthrough in that it proved to be up to 100 times more potent than ketoconazole, with excellent pharmacokinetic properties. However, during further development, the compound proved to have unacceptable hepatotoxicity and it was also teratogenic in rodents. Subsequent research demonstrated that a 2,4-difluorophenyl derivative, compound UK-49858, was devoid of hepatotoxicity and teratogenicity and retained the excellent antifungal activity and pharmacokinetic profile observed with compound UK-46245. UK-49858 was subsequently renamed as fluconazole (Fig. 24.6). The triazole ring may look strongly basic but, in common with many π-deficient rings (see Ch. 4), it is only very weakly basic with a p*Ka* value <2.

Fluconazole is fungistatic at therapeutic concentrations and has good activity against *Candida albicans* infections. However, some non-*albican Candida* species (e.g. *C. glabrata, C. parapsilosis, C. krusei* and *C. tropicalis*) are less sensitive to fluconazole. Fluconazole is active against *Trichophyton* spp, *Cryptococcus neoformans, Histoplasma capsulatum, Microsporum* spp. and *Epidermophyton* spp. Fluconazole, however, has no useful activity against moulds such as *Aspergillus* spp.

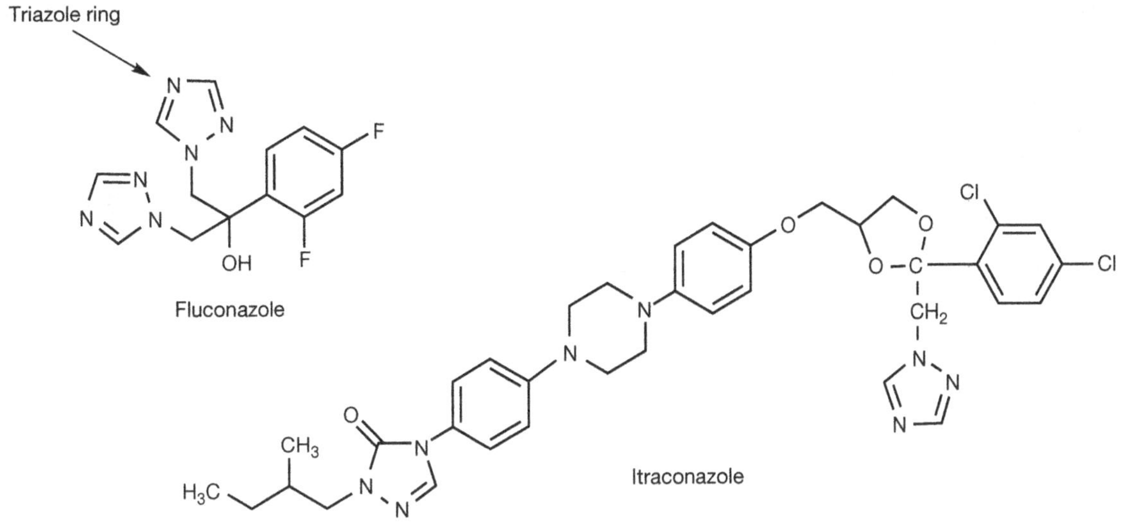

Figure 24.6 Fluconazole and itraconazole.

Description and preparations

Fluconazole is a white crystalline powder. It is reported to exist in three polymorphic forms and as a hydrate, with form III being used in clinical formulations. Fluconazole has moderate lipophilicity with a reported logP value of 0.5. Fluconazole is slightly soluble in water and propan-2-ol, sparingly soluble in ethanol and chloroform, soluble in acetone and freely soluble in methanol. Typical preparations include:

- a capsule containing 50, 150 or 200 mg fluconazole.
- a suspension containing 50 or 200 mg/5 mL fluconazole.
- an intravenous infusion containing 2 mg/mL fluconazole in 0.9% aqueous sodium chloride solution.

The adult dose is 50–400 mg once a day with dose and duration of therapy depending upon the clinical indication. Fluconazole has greater specificity than older imidazole compounds such as ketoconazole for fungal cyp450-Erg11p than mammalian cytochrome enzymes, so disruption of endogenous steroid production is not a clinical problem. Fluconazole, however, is still associated with a number of important cyp450-mediated drug interactions with drugs including coumarins, sulphonylureas, ciclosporin and antiretrovirals.

Pharmacokinetics

Fluconazole has good oral bioavailability irrespective of fed or fasted state, with greater than 90% of a dose being absorbed. Peak plasma levels are proportional to dose and are achieved within 1–2 hours of oral dosing. Plasma protein binding, half-life and the volume of distribution at steady-state are 10%, 25–30 hours and 0.55 L/kg, respectively. Fluconazole is found in body fluids such as saliva, breast milk and vaginal secretions at levels comparable to those in the plasma with CSF concentrations around 80% of plasma levels.

Only 11% of a dose is metabolised, with 6.5% being a glucuronide conjugate and 2% an N-oxide. The major route of elimination for fluconazole and its metabolites is renal excretion, with only 2% being excreted in the faeces.

> **Q Self Test 24.3**
>
> Draw the glucuronide and N-oxide metabolites for fluconazole. Explain why no dosage adjustment is required in the case of hepatic failure.

Itraconazole

Itraconazole is a structural analogue of ketoconazole in which the metabolically susceptible imidazole group has been replaced by a triazole moiety and the side chain has been further extended (Fig. 24.6). Its spectrum of antifungal activity is similar to that of fluconazole, but in addition it also has activity against *Aspergillus* spp. The extended side chain of itraconazole allows it to bind with greater affinity to the apoprotein structure of fungal cytochrome P450-Erg11p than ketoconazole, enhancing antifungal potency and, in parallel, reducing its affinity for mammalian cytochrome P450 enzymes involved in endogenous steroid biosynthesis. However, like ketoconazole, itraconazole still has the capacity to interfere with the metabolism of many important drug classes through interaction with cyp4503A4.

Description and preparations

Itraconazole is an odourless beige crystalline powder with a bitter taste. The racemate mixture of 4 diastereomers (2 enantiomeric pairs) is used in clinical formulations. Itraconazole is very lipophilic with a reported logP value of 5.7. Itraconazole is practically insoluble in water and very sparingly soluble in ethanol. Typical preparations include:

- a capsule containing 100 mg itraconazole coated on sugar spheres to facilitate drug dissolution.
- an intravenous infusion containing 10 mg/mL itraconazole. Itraconazole is maintained in aqueous solution by forming a molecular inclusion complex with hydroxypropyl-β-cyclodextrin.
- an oral solution containing 10 mg/5 mL itraconazole complexed with hydroxypropyl-β-cyclodextrin.

The adult dose is 100–200 mg once or twice a day with dose and duration of therapy depending upon the clinical indication.

Pharmacokinetics

The absorption of itraconazole from the gastrointestinal tract shows similar pH dependency as ketoconazole. The effect of fed and fasted states on oral absorption is formulation dependent with peak plasma levels doubled when capsules are taken with food and lowered by 25% when the oral solution is taken with food. Both formulations, however, have greater than 90% oral bioavailability with time to peak plasma concentration, plasma protein binding, terminal half-life and volume of distribution at steady-state values of 2–5 hours, 99.8%, 20–40 hours and 11 L/kg, respectively. Itraconazole also extensively accumulates in well-perfused organs such as muscle, lung, spleen, liver and kidneys. Itraconazole has unusual pharmacokinetics in that it preferentially accumulates in keratinous tissues of the hair, nails and skin, providing drug concentrations that are four- to tenfold higher than the corresponding plasma concentrations. This permits itraconazole to be administered in a discontinuous or 'pulsed' manner for 1 week out of every 4 weeks for 3 months in the treatment of fungal infections of the nails since high, sustained, concentrations are retained within these keratinous tissues. Itraconazole undergoes extensive phase I hepatic metabolism with greater than 30 metabolites identified, many of which are biologically active. The major metabolite is hydroxyitraconazole, where plasma concentrations are two to three times higher than those of itraconazole with comparable antifungal activity. Faecal excretion of itraconazole accounts for between 3% and 18% of the drug, with effectively none undergoing renal excretion. Around 40% of metabolites are excreted in the urine, with the remainder being excreted in the bile.

Interestingly, recent evidence suggests that the stereoisomers of itraconazole are preferentially metabolised to hydroxyitraconazole in humans by CYP3A4 enzymes. However, the resultant impact on itraconazole pharmacokinetics and/or pharmacodynamics and clinical efficacy as an antifungal agent remain to be established. However, the importance of stereochemistry on clinical antifungal activity is not surprising, given that the enzyme is constructed from L-amino-acids.

Second-generation triazole antifungals

Voriconazole

Voriconazole resulted from the continuing efforts of Pfizer scientists to retain many of the excellent clinical features of fluconazole whilst extending the spectrum of antifungal activity to include filamentous fungi. Early studies highlighted that the inclusion of a methyl group α to one of the fluconazole triazole groups increases potency against *Aspergillus fumigatus*. Subsequent experimentation demonstrated that replacement of one of the triazole rings with a 6-membered heterocyclic ring such as pyridine or pyrimidine, whilst retaining a methyl group α to the heterocyclic ring, further enhanced potency against *A. fumigatus*. The inclusion of fluorinated pyridine or pyrimidine analogues also enhanced antifungal activity, by reducing the susceptibility of the heterocyclic rings to metabolic oxidation, thereby enhancing their half-lives. On the basis of potency and better solubility profile the fluoropyrimidyl analogue was selected for further evaluation. Antifungal testing of individual diastereomers, isolated using a combination of chromatography and recrystallisation following salt formation with the optically active (1R)-10-camphosulfonic acid, indicated that antifungal activity resided almost entirely with the (2R, 3S) enantiomer, compound UK-109496, which was renamed as voriconazole (Fig. 24.7).

Voriconazole exhibits broad-spectrum activity against a wide range of clinically important fungal infections such as *Candida* (including fluconazole-resistant species such as *C. glabrata* and *C. krusei*), *Aspergillus*, *Scedosporium* and *Fusarium* spp. and atypical pathogens including *Acremonium*, and *Chyrsosporium* spp. It has no useful activity against zygomycetes such as *Mucor* or *Rhizopus* spp.

Description and preparations

Voriconazole is non-hygroscopic white to light-coloured crystalline powder. Voriconazole is lipophilic with a reported logP value of 2.6. Voriconazole is a weak base that has a maximum aqueous solubility of 2.7 mg/mL at pH 1.2. It is soluble in methanol and ethylacetate. Typical preparations include:

- a tablet containing either 50 mg or 200 mg voriconazole.
- a lyophilised powder containing 200 mg voriconazole which, when reconstituted with 19 mL water for injection, provides a 10 mg/mL solution that can be further diluted prior to administration as an intravenous infusion. Voriconazole is maintained in

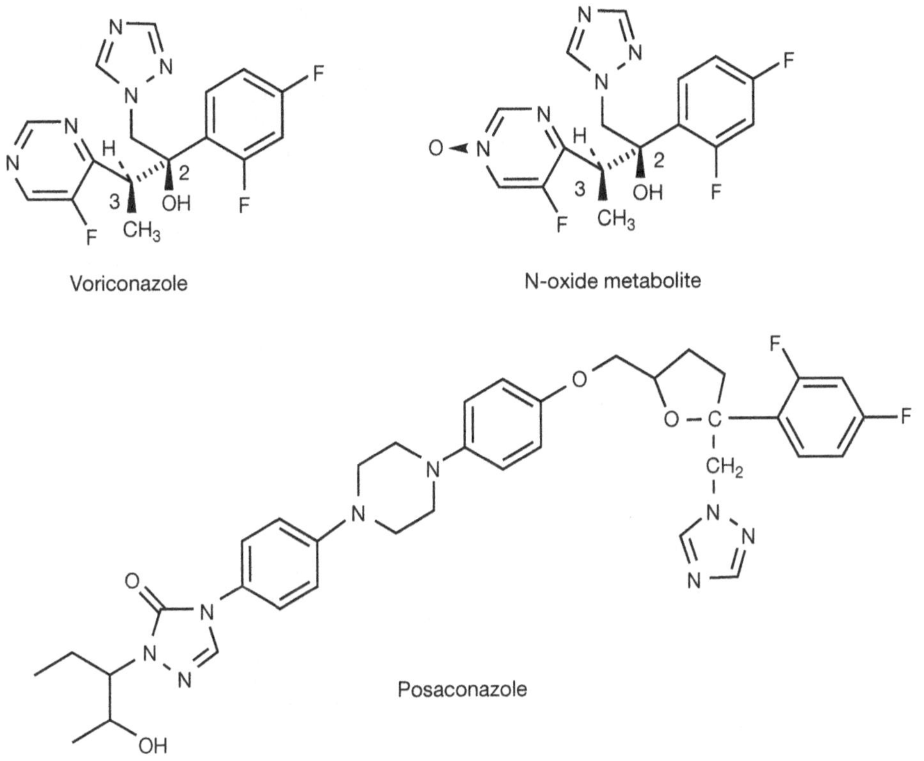

Figure 24.7 Second generation triazole antifungals.

aqueous solution following reconstitution by formation of a molecular inclusion complex with sulfobutyl ether β-cyclodextrin sodium.

- a powder for oral suspension which, when reconstituted, provides 40 mg/mL voriconazole.

The adult oral dose is 400 mg every 12 hours on the first day of therapy before reducing to 200 mg every 12 hours (or 300 mg every 12 hours if inadequate clinical response) on subsequent days. Tablets should be administered at least 1 hour before, or 1 hour after food, with the oral suspension administered at least 1 hour before or 2 hours after food. Intravenous therapy is initiated at 6 mg/kg every 12 hours on the first day of therapy before reducing to 4 mg/kg every 12 hours on subsequent days. Duration of therapy is dependent upon clinical and mycological response.

Pharmacokinetics

The absorption of voriconazole following oral administration is independent of gastric pH with oral bioavailability being around 96% when taken 1 hour before food. The time to peak plasma is 1–2 hours. During multiple dosing regimens, time to peak plasma and AUC are reduced by 34% and 24%, respectively, when administered with high-fat meals. Plasma protein binding is modest at 58% compared to the rest of the triazole family of antifungal agents and this partly explains the relatively high volume of distribution at steady-state of 4.6 L/kg observed during voriconazole therapy. Voriconazole therefore is extensively distributed in all tissues including the cerebrospinal fluid.

The major route of elimination of voriconazole is hepatic metabolism, followed by renal excretion. Voriconazole is a substrate for the three enzymes, CYP2C19, CYP2C9 and CYP3A4. The major metabolite of voriconazole results from N-oxidation of the fluoropyrimidyl moiety, and accounts for 72% of circulating metabolites (Fig. 24.7). The N-oxide metabolite of voriconazole has no useful antifungal activity. In vivo studies indicate that the polymorphic enzyme CYP2C19 is significantly involved in voriconazole metabolism. Consequently 2–5% of Caucasians and blacks and 15–20% of Asian individuals who are functionally deficient or absent in this enzyme can be expected to be poor metabolisers of voriconazole. In these individuals the AUCs are approximately four times higher than subjects who are homozygous extensive metabolisers. Heterozygous extensive metabolisers have AUCs that are twofold higher than the homozygous extensive metabolisers.

In vitro studies indicate that CYP2C19 and CYP2C9 are high-affinity, low-capacity enzymes, whilst CYP3A4 has a low affinity and high capacity for voriconazole. This explains the observation that voriconazole pharmacokinetics are non-linear due to the fact that it can readily saturate the high-affinity, low-capacity enzymes and this results in a disproportionate increase in bioavailability observed with increasing dose. For example, increasing the oral dose from 200 mg twice a day to 300 mg twice a day has been reported to produce a 2.5-fold increase in the $AUC_{0-\infty}$. The terminal half-life of voriconazole is dependent on dose but has been reported to be around 6 hours following a 200-mg oral dose.

The oral dose of voriconazole does not have to be adjusted in patients who have renal impairment. However, intravenous administration of voriconazole should be avoided in these patients as the carrier vehicle sulfobutyl ether β-cyclodextrin sodium can accumulate in these patients. Dosage adjustment is required in patients who have chronic hepatic impairment. As voriconazole is a substrate for a number of cytochrome P450 enzymes, a number of clinically important drug interactions occur with drugs including ciclosporin, tacrolimus, phenytoin, warfarin, HIV protease inhibitors and non-nucleoside reverse transcriptase inhibitors.

Posaconazole

Posaconazole is a structural analogue of itraconazole with an extended spectrum of antifungal activity in which the dichlorophenyl- and dioxolane moieties of itraconazole has been replaced by difluorophenyl- and tetrahydrofuran moieties (Fig. 24.7). Posaconazole is synthesised solely as the (R, R, S, S) enantiomer. In comparative in vitro studies it was the most potent of the clinically available azoles and, unlike other azoles, it also has useful activity against zygomycetes. This extended spectrum of antifungal activity is thought to arise from the long side chain of posaconazole occupying a specific channel within the cypP450-Erg11p that is not utilised by fluconazole or voriconazole.

Description and preparations

Posaconazole is white to off-white crystalline powder. Posaconazole is a lipophilic substance with an aqueous solubility of less than 2 μg/mL. Three polymorphic forms of posaconazole have been identified but the three-step synthetic process is controlled to constantly produce form I. Prototype tablet and capsule formulations of posaconazole were abandoned in favour of an oral suspension with superior bioavailability. The ready-to-use oral suspension contains 40 mg/mL which is micronised posaconazole in order to increase its surface area and thus bioavailability. There is at present no parenteral formulation of posaconazole available although a water-soluble ester prodrug (carboxylate ester of posaconazole with γ-butyric acid phosphate) has undergone evaluation.

The adult oral dose is 400 mg every 12 hours with a meal or with 240 mL of a nutritional supplement. In adults who cannot tolerate a meal or a nutritional supplement, the dose should be modified to 200 mg every 6 hours. Duration of therapy is dependent upon clinical and mycological response.

Pharmacokinetics

The absorption of posaconazole following the recommended oral administration schedule is slow with a median time to peak plasma of 5 hours. The effect of food on oral absorption is pronounced, with bioavailability around 2.6 times and 4 times greater when administered with a non-fat meal/nutritional supplement or high-fat meal (≈ 50 g fat), respectively, when compared to the fasted state. The pharmacokinetics of posaconazole remains linear following single or multiple doses of up to 800 mg when taken with a high-fat meal. Steady-state pharmacokinetics are typically achieved after 7–10 days multiple dosing. Posaconazole has a large apparent volume of distribution at steady-state of 1774 L with greater than 98% protein bound, predominantly to serum albumin.

The overall metabolism of posaconazole is limited in comparison to other azole antifungals and predominantly mediated through phase 2 biotransformations via UDP-glucuronosyltransferase pathways. Posaconazole does not appear to be as extensively metabolised as other azole antifungal agents by cytochrome P450 enzymes with oxidative and cleavage products and their subsequent glucuronidation and sulfation derivatives being minor metabolites. These metabolites undergo renal excretion and account for approximately 14% of an administered dose. Over 70% of an administered dose undergoes faecal excretion, with around 66% of the excreted material being posaconazole, presumably due to it being a substrate for intestinal P-glycoprotein.

Posaconazole is also different from other azole antifungal agents in that the plasma concentration of the parent compound exceeds those of its metabolites over its dosing schedule. However, the clinical relevance of this observation has yet to be determined.

No dosage adjustments are required on the basis of age, gender, race or renal function although dosage adjustments may be required in individuals with severe hepatic impairment. However, posaconazole is known to interact with a number of other clinically used drug substances. Posaconazole is an inhibitor of CYP3A4 at clinical dosages resulting in elevated plasma levels of drugs extensively metabolised by this enzyme, e.g. terfenadine, quinidine, HMG-coenzyme A inhibitors, non-nucleoside reverse transcriptase inhibitors and calcium channel blockers. In addition, inhibitors or inducers of UDP-glucuronosyltransferase pathways or P-glycoprotein may result in increased or decreased plasma concentrations of posaconazole, respectively.

Like other clinically available azole antifungal agents, co-administration with H_2-antagonists or proton pump inhibitors reduces bioavailability as a consequence of a reduction in gastric acidity.

Ravuconazole

Ravuconazole is currently progressing through clinical trials. It has an identical pharmacophore to voriconazole and as such has a very similar spectrum of antifungal activity to voriconazole. In preclinical models, ravuconazole has demonstrated that it is extensively distributed in tissues, including the CNS, and has an extensive plasma half-life. Oral and parenteral (as a water soluble di-lysine phosphoester prodrug) formulations are being evaluated in phase II studies in humans.

Miscellaneous antifungal drugs

Naftifine (Fig. 24.8) was discovered during random screening for antifungal action and it was found to inhibit ergosterol biosynthesis via blocking epoxidation of squalene, which is an early step in ergosterol biosynthesis. Naftifine was only found to be suitable for topical use; therefore numerous analogues were prepared, resulting in terbinafine (Fig. 24.8) which was found to orally active.

Terbinafine

Description and preparations

Oral dosage 250 mg per day.

- Tablets 250 mg terbinafine hydrochloride.

Amorolfine

Amorolfine (Fig. 24.8) is an inhibitor of Δ14 reductase, which is one of the steps in the conversion of lanosterol to ergosterol. It is used topically for the treatment of fungal nail infections.

Description and preparations

- Cream 0.25% w/w.
- Nail lacquer 5% w/v.

Drugs that interfere with fungal cell walls

Echinocandins

The fungal cell wall is an obvious therapeutic target due to its absence in mammals. However, the development of effective clinical chemotherapeutic agents that interfere with the synthesis, structure or function of fungal cell walls has been complicated due to diverse interspecies differences in the chemical composition of fungal cells walls, with notable intraspecies variation also observed due to cell wall remodelling in response to changes in environment (e.g. apical hyphal growth in moulds) or reproductive requirements (e.g. budding in yeasts). Major components of all fungal cell walls include polysaccharide biopolymers based on glucose (β-1, 3 and β-1, 6 glucans), mannose (mannans) or N-acetyl-D-glucosamine (chitin) with glycoproteins also present. Each of these components contributes to the overall architecture and function of the fungal cell wall.

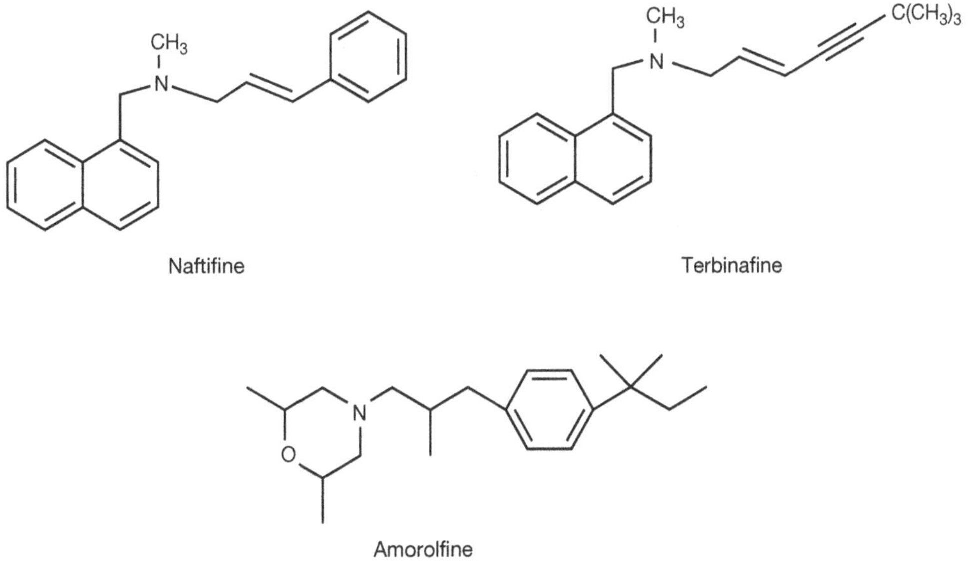

Figure 24.8 Drugs that interfere with fungal cell walls.

The first class of antifungal agents to enter into clinical practice that interfere with the fungal cell wall were the echinocandins.

The echinocandins are amphiphilic cyclic hexapeptides with an N-linked acyl lipid side chain. Original members of the class were isolated from a number of *Aspergillus* species. Early studies undertaken with echinocandin B established that these natural products had potent activity against *Candida* species but had the significant disadvantage of only being active by parenteral administration and causing erythrocyte lysis. This led to analogues of echinocandin B being synthesised in an attempt to identify structure–activity relationships for this class of agent that would retain antifungal activity but have minimal mammalian toxicity. Structural modification was divided into two parts: modification of the peptide nucleus, and modification of the fatty acid side chain. As can be seen from continuing development of drugs in this field, there is a constant battle between microbes and humans.

A Self Test 24.1

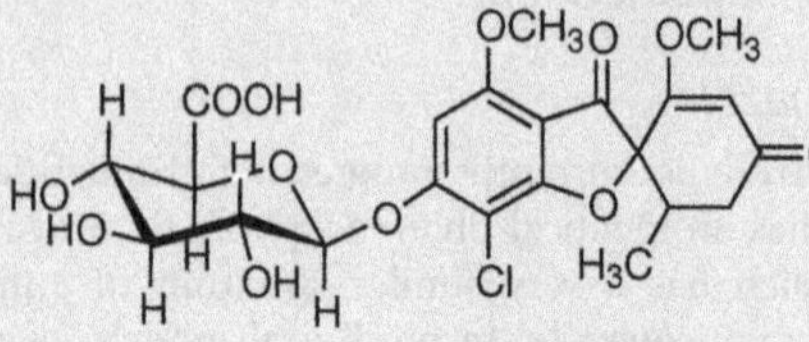

Griseofulvin

A Self Test 24.2

The levels entering the circulation are too low to induce metabolism.

A Self Test 24.3

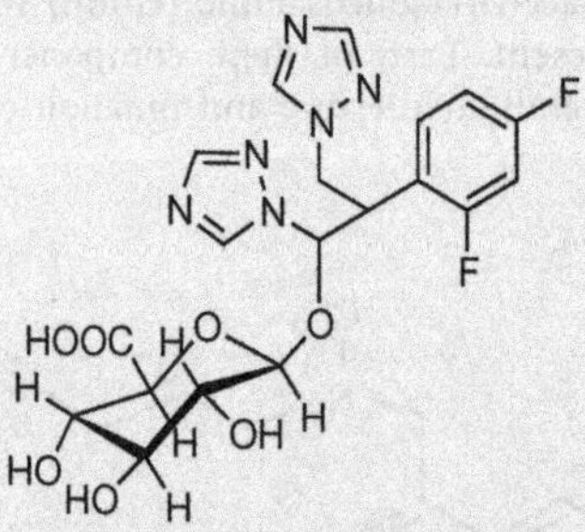

Glucuronide

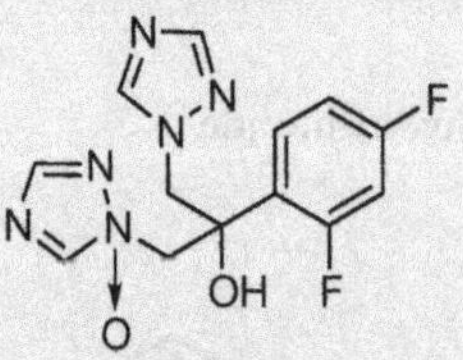

N-oxide (most likely position)

Dosage adjustment in case of hepatic failure is not required since elimination of the drug is not greatly dependent on hepatic metabolism.

Chapter | 25 |

Antiparasitic drugs

David G Watson

CHAPTER CONTENTS

INTRODUCTION

Most of the drugs used to treat parasitic diseases were developed over 50 years ago and the more recent developments of this type of drug have been in antimalarial drugs, since malaria is the disease which is most likely to affect travellers from the West to tropical regions. Thus many other parasitic diseases remain poorly treated because these diseases affect poorer countries which cannot afford to pay for expensive new treatments. An obvious solution to such diseases would be to vaccinate, but parasites have complex life cycles and thus it is difficult to design vaccines which promote immunity to the various stages. In addition, parasites can vary their surface antigens, which can render vaccines ineffective. Many parasites have developed mechanisms for reducing the immune response of the host by producing compounds which cause immunosuppression. It is likely, as developing countries become wealthier, that more effective and less toxic drugs will be developed to treat parasitic diseases. However, at the moment, many antiparasitic drugs are quite toxic and have to be administered using complex dosage regimens.

MALARIA

Isoquinolines and related compounds

Malaria is a protozoal organism; more specifically it belongs to the sporozoan (spore forming) subclass of protozoa. These organisms are all animal parasites, whereas the majority of protozoa are not. Protozoa are single-celled organisms and generally have the complex life cycle of the malaria parasite, where they have to exist in various forms in the animal host and then transfer from the animal host to an insect vector. In the case of malaria, the insect vector is the *Anopheles* mosquito. There are four common forms of the causative agent of malaria: *Plasmodium falciparum*, which is very common and causes a severe form of the disease, and *P. vivax*, *P. ovale* and *P. malariae*, which cause less severe forms of the disease.

Table 25.1 Malaria life cycle in the human and the drugs used to treat the various stages

Stage	Treatment
Sporosites transmitted by mosquito bite transfer to the liver within 30 minutes.	No effective drug treatment although vaccination may eventually be effective.
The parasite develops over 10–14 days into schizonts.	Primaquine, tafenoquine.
After this time liver cells rupture, releasing motile form of the parasite the merozoite which passes into the blood stream and enters red cells. The stage for prophylactic intervention.	Chloroquine, mefloquine, proguanil, pyrimethamine, dapsone and doxycycline.
The parasite enters the red blood cell and matures into a schizont over 48 hours and the cell ruptures and releases merozoites after this time to infect further red blood cells. This gives rise to the acute form of the disease with its typical tertian pattern of the production of fever every third day.	Quinine, mefloquine, chloroquine, halofantrine, pyrimethamine, proguanil, atovaquone, atemether, arteflene and artesunate. Tetracycline and doxocycline are used in combination with some of these drugs.
Mosquito bite results in transmission of the disease and some drugs are effective in blocking transmission.	Primaquine, proguanil and pyrimethamine.

The disease is estimated to cause 300 million acute cases each year which result in 1 million deaths. The life cycle of the malaria parasite in humans is summarised in Table 25.1 along with the drugs which are used to treat the various stages. Quinine was one of the earliest effective drug treatments to emerge from a period of nearly 2000 years during which most medical practice was based on the Ancient Greek medical theories involving balancing the four humours, which resulted in treatments such as blood letting which generally made the patient worse. The fact that patients died did not have an influence on medical theory and a modification of such medieval practices did not occur until at least the middle of the nineteenth century. However, some effective treatments did emerge during this period, and one of these was cinchona bark, which originates from Peru and was first used to treat malarial fever around 1630. The South American Indians originally used it to treat shivering brought on by cold water following swimming across a river and this was presumably because of its ability to promote blood circulation. Thus to some extent its use to treat malaria was based on a misconception that the shivering brought on by malaria had the same origin as the effects of cold water. The bark was introduced into Europe, where malaria was then endemic around this time and water extracts from the bark were used to treat malaria (plus presumably diseases producing similar symptoms) until the nineteenth century.

Quinine was isolated from extracts from the bark and by 1826 industrial scale production of the drug was underway. This led to the new conception in therapeutics that knowing the precise dose of a therapeutic agent was important. Although the active principal in the bark was isolated, the actual causative agent of malaria was not identified until around 1880 when the presence of the parasites in blood cells was recognised by microscopical examination, and this was followed shortly afterwards by the observation that quinine acted by damaging the parasites. Figure 25.1 shows the structure of quinine which was elucidated in 1944. Although quinine looks like a DNA intercalator, its likely mechanism of action, according to recent research, in common with that of chloroquine (Fig. 25.1; discussed below), is as an inhibitor of the disposal of haem by the parasite.

Paul Erlich pioneered the use of dye stuffs as drugs at the end of the nineteenth century. He observed that dyes had a particular affinity for certain structures within tissues. Dyes with a basic functionality were able to penetrate the brain or fatty tissue, whereas dyes with an acidic functionality were not. The testing of dyes led to the evolution of a number of different drugs. With regard to antimalarials, the observed effectiveness of the dye methylene blue against malaria led to testing of a series of compounds where the methyl group in methylene blue was replaced with a longer side chain. Eventually, the quinoline compound pamaquin was arrived at, remarkably close in structure to quinine considering that the structure of quinine was not known at this point. The isoquinoline compound chloroquine was synthesised in 1934, although not adopted until after the Second World War. It was the most effective antimalarial compound synthesised until that point and has remained the front line of defence against malaria. It is still effective against benign malaria although many strains of *P. falciparum* have developed resistance against it. Chloroquine appears to have the structure of a DNA intecalator with a flat planar structure bearing a side chain that can interact with the DNA phosphate backbone. However, chloroquine does not

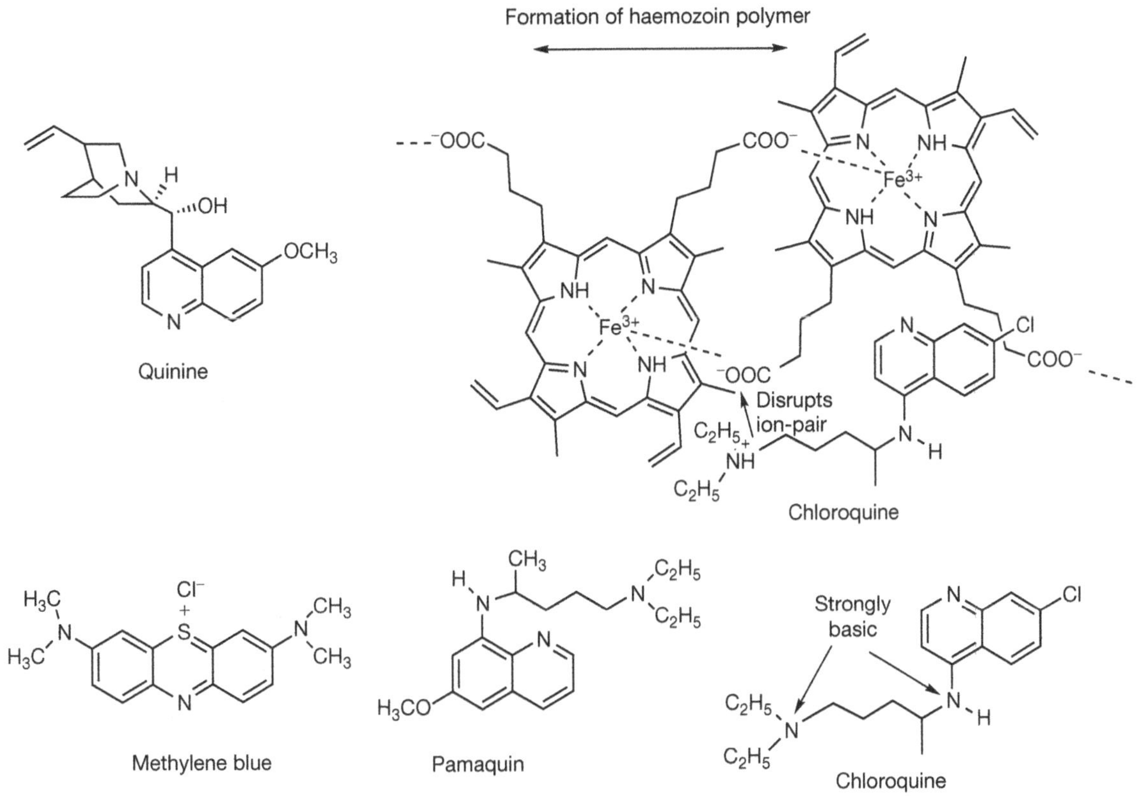

Figure 25.1 Quinine and chloroquine and the disruption of the formation of haemazoin.

appreciably accumulate in the nucleus of the parasite and, although it does have DNA intercalating properties, its mode of action is altogether different. Chloroquine is effective against the erythrocyte stage of the infection where the *Plasmodium* digests the red blood cell protein haemoglobin in a digestive vacuole to provide its main source of amino acids. In the process, the parasite produces haem as a toxic by-product which can destroy the organism by generation of reactive oxygen species if not neutralised.[1–3] In order to detoxify haem, the parasite forms crystals of a polymeric form of haem known as haemazoin which forms in the parasite. This by-product of malaria was recognised as early as the eighteenth century, when a black pigment was observed to accumulate in the liver and spleen of people who had died from malaria. Chloroquine has two strongly basic centres with p*Ka* values around 10. However, like all diamines, protonation of one centre weakens the basicity of the other. Thus one of the basic centres is incompletely ionised at physiological pH and its accumulation in the more acidic vacuole of the parasite is probably favoured. Its structure has the exact geometry required to inhibit the formation of haemazoin, thus generating levels of free haem which are toxic to the parasite. Resistance to chloroquine is due to the parasite resisting its uptake. The need to form haemazoin represents a very useful but, surprisingly, neglected drug target and there is a renewed interest in developing drugs to exploit it. Other isoquinoline drugs have been developed over the past 60 years. Primaquine was adopted for use in the 1940s and is very effective against benign malaria. Mefloquine (Fig. 25.2) is closer in structure to quinine and was developed in the 1960s. It was useful in treating resistant forms of malaria but resistance has also developed in this case. Mefloquine has been found to act via inhibition of haemazoin formation as have halofantrine and lumefantrine (Fig. 25.2), which have been used to treat resistant malaria, the latter in combination with artemether.

Primaquine[4] and tafenoquine, a recently developed analogue undergoing clinical trials, are 8-aminoquinolines, unlike chloroquine and mefloquine which are 4-subsituted aminoquinolines, and they have a different mode of action against the parasite being effective against the liver stage of the parasite in the treatment of benign malarias. Primaquine is only fully effective if given in combination with chloroquine or quinine, and these combinations are also effective against the erythrocyte stage of the infection. Its mechanism of action is not fully

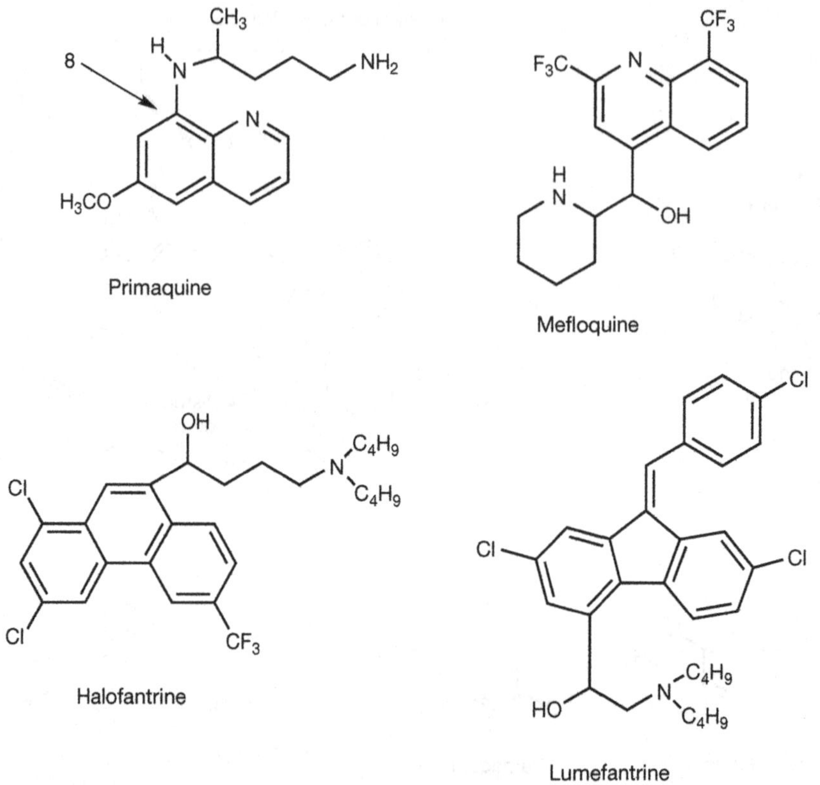

Figure 25.2 Antimalarial drugs.

known. However, as a drug, it produces oxidative stress which can result in methaemoglobinaemia which is caused by oxidation of the iron in haem. Primaquine is extensively metabolised and among its metabolites are hydroxylated metabolites (Fig. 25.3) which could potentially give rise to the classically reactive quinone methide species observed in the case of paracetamol overdose (see Ch. 5). It is possible that it is this type of compound which is responsible for the toxicity of the drug. The reason for the potentiation of primaquine by chloroquine is unclear. However, in the red blood cell, chloroquine also potentiates oxidative stress which may promote formation of the reactive species generated from primaquine. Normally, this is not a desirable property of a drug.

Artemisinin and its analogues

Artemesinin (Fig. 25.4) is a recent addition to the range of drugs available for treating malaria.[5] However, it has been used to treat malaria for over 2000 years in China. It is

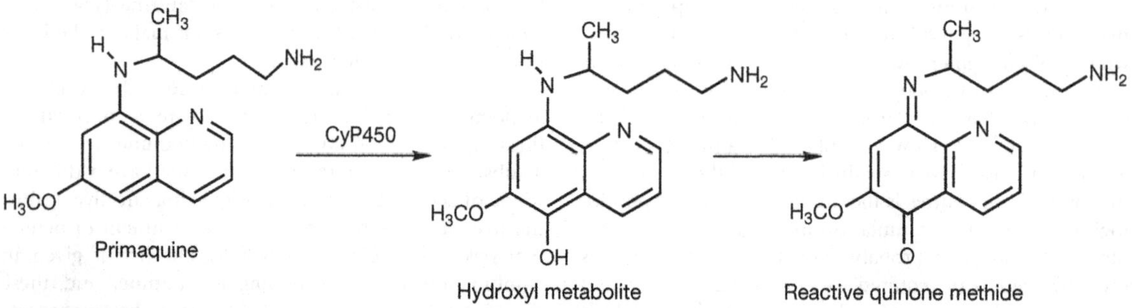

Figure 25.3 Metabolism of primaquine to a reactive metabolite.

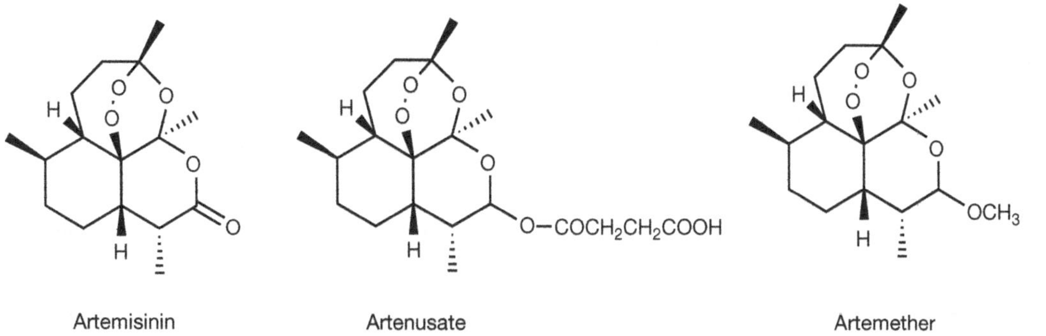

Figure 25.4 Artemisinin and its analogues.

present in extracts from the common plant *Artemisia annua*. The drug has a very short duration of action and poor bioavailability but is very effective. Thus it is given in combination with other drugs, particularly lumefantrine. The properties of artemisinin have been improved by the production of analogues such as artesunate (a water-soluble prodrug) and artemether (Fig. 25.4). These drugs also have a short duration of action but have better bioavailability than artemisinin. The mechanism of action is not fully known but since the drug is a peroxide it is naturally unstable and will break down to give ROS. Since the *Plasmodium* accumulates iron in its digestive vacuole, this provides an ideal environment for artemisinin and its analogues to break down in a generate ROS. Thus the toxicity of the drugs may be due to species such as hydroxyl radicals. In the absence of the peroxide bridge there is no antimalarial activity. Since the molecules are unstable, they have a short duration of action and drugs with an extended duration of action such as lumefantrine are used in combination to follow up the initial effects of artemisinin and its analogues. Artemisinin along with quinine is the treatment of choice for the most severe form of malaria, cerebral malaria.

Inhibitors of folic acid biosynthesis

Proguanil emerged out of a screening programme undertaken during World War Two as an effective antimalarial compound. It is an effective malaria prophylactic and is a prodrug, being metabolically converted from a biguanide compound to a 1,3,5-triazine derivative cycloguanil, the active form of which bears a resemblance to folic acid, and it thus acts as a dihydrofolate reductase (DHFR) inhibitor (Fig. 25.5). Cycloguanil is a bioisotere of pyrimethamine which also acts as a DHFR inhibitor and is used as an antimalarial drug. Resistance to these

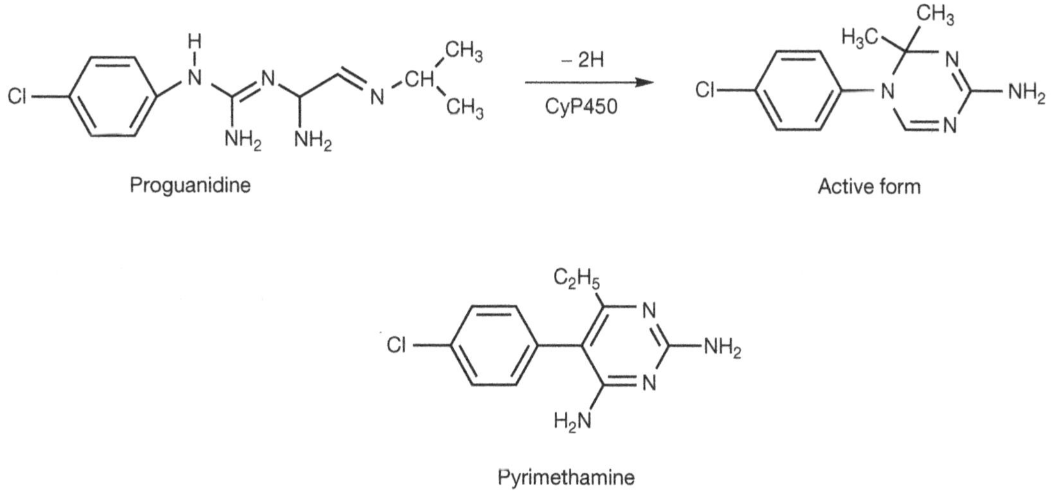

Figure 25.5 DHFR inhibitors.

inhibitors has developed where the DHFR enzyme is altered so that it has less affinity for the inhibitors.

Pyrimethamine is usually given in combination with sulfadoxine (Fig. 25.5) which, like many sulphonamide antibacterial compounds, is an inhibitor of the biosynthesis of dihydropteroate which is a precursor of folic acid. Unlike humans, plasmodia synthesise folic acid rather than absorb it from the environment. It is used for prophylaxis rather than treatment.

Miscellaneous drugs

Atovaquone (Fig. 25.6) was developed in the 1980s out of a screening programme sponsored by the Wellcome trust.[6] It is a naphthoquinone and is believed to interfere with the respiratory chain because of its similarity to ubiquinone (Fig. 25.6). Atovaquone binds to the cytochrome bc_1 complex which is responsible for transferring electrons from ubiquinol to cytochrome c and thus oxidising it to ubiquinone, which acts as an electron acceptor. The binding of atovaquone to cytochrome b disrupts this process and thus inhibits respiration. Resistance has developed to the drug via alteration in the binding site, thus reducing the affinity of the enzyme for the drug. Atovaquone is combined with proguanil in tablets.

Antimalarial preparations

- Chloroquine sulphate injection 54.5 mg/mL.
- Chloroquine phosphate tablets 250 mg.
- Chloroquine phosphate syrup 80 mg/5 mL and 68 mg/mL.

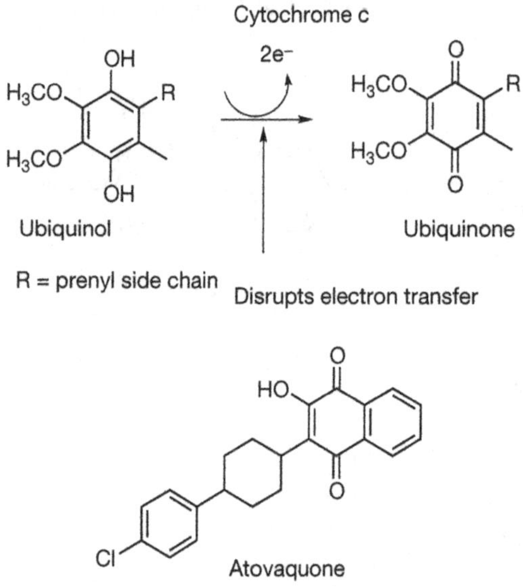

Figure 25.6 Mechanism of action of atovaquone.

- Chloroquine phosphate (250 mg), proguanil hydrochloride (100 mg) tablets.
- Mefloquine hydrochloride tablets 250 mg.
- Primaquine phosphate tablets 7.5 or 15 mg.
- Proguanil hydrochloride tablets 100 mg.
- Proguanil hydrochloride 100 mg, atovaquone 250 mg tablets.
- Pyrimethamine 25 mg tablets.
- Pyrimethamine 25 mg, sulfadoxine 500 mg tablets.
- Quinine sulphate tablets 200 and 300 mg.
- Quinine dihydrochloride injection 300 mg/mL.
- Aremether 20 mg, lumefantrine 120 mg tablets.

TRYPANOSOMIASIS

Trypanosomiasis, and leishmaniasis discussed below, are also caused by protozoa. Unlike malaria, this class of protozoa live in a range of organisms including mammals, plants and insects. They are motile, having a single flagellum and they also have a characteristic mitochondrial structure called a kinetoplast.[7] Trypanosomes are transmitted to humans via the bite of the tsetse fly (African sleeping sickness caused by *Trypanosoma brucei*) or indirectly via the bite of the assassin bug (*Trypanosoma cruzi* which causes Chagas' disease found in South America). Like malaria, trypanosomes have a complex life cycle and *T. brucei* has two stages in the human host and four stages in the tsetse fly. The stages of trypanosomes in a mammalian host are simple compared to malaria in that they simply live in physiological fluids including blood and lymph rather than moving between liver and blood cells. As with all tropical diseases, drug development has been slow and vaccine development difficult since the parasite can easily change its surface antigens.

Pentamidine was developed 70 years ago and its development was based on the misapprehension that reducing blood glucose levels could be a way of controlling trypanosome infections. It has been observed that compounds containing the guanidine moiety such as Synthalin® could act as oral antidiabetic agents reducing blood sugar levels. Analogues of Synthalin® were found to act as trypanocides and this led to the development of pentamidine. Pentamidine, in fact, has a completely different mechanism of action to that originally proposed. When trypanosomes are exposed to pentamidine (Fig. 25.7) it accumulates in the kinetoplast, which is rich in DNA.[8] Pentamidine has the classic structure of a DNA minor groove binder in that it can wind its structure around the DNA minor groove with the strongly basic guanidine groups in its structure binding to the phosphate groups of the DNA backbone. The width of the minor

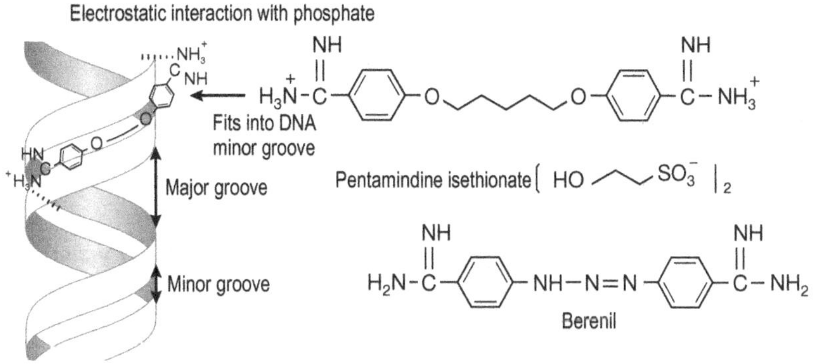

Figure 25.7 Antitrypanosomal DNA minor groove binders.

groove is determined by the base pairing in the DNA and pentamidine binds to an AATT sequence. The drug accumulates in the kinetoplast, which is rich in DNA containing AT sequences, and prevents replication of its DNA. Berenil, which is used in treating cattle suffering from African sleeping sickness, also works according to the same principal.

Pentamidine is a strongly basic drug with a p*Ka* value of around 10, and thus it is not absorbed orally and has to be given by injection. Thus far, no successful prodrug has been designed for it. It is used for treating African sleeping sickness. The side effects are severe and it is not completely effective at producing a cure.

Suramin (Fig. 25.8) arose out of the early twentieth-century experiments with dyes as therapeutic agents. Studies of the antitrypanosomal activities of these compounds resulted in the introduction of suramin in 1920 and it remains the first choice for prophylaxis of African trypanosomiasis.[9] It is a high molecular weight, highly polar polyanionic compound; thus has poor oral bioavailability and has to be administered via injection. Its use is limited by the fact that is cannot penetrate the central nervous system (CNS) and is thus not able to treat advanced stages of the disease. Its mechanism of action is not exactly known, but in general it binds strongly to proteins and thus inhibits a wide range of enzymatic processes.

The late-stage CNS stage of African sleeping sickness is treated with melarsoprol. Arsenic, like a number of toxic elements, has a very long history of medical use and arsenate salts were viewed by the Victorians as a tonic. Potassium arsenate (Fowler's solution) was used in the nineteenth century to treat malaria. David Livingstone, who explored much of central Africa during the mid-nineteenth century, recommended Fowler's solution as a treatment for sleeping sickness. Pioneering work by Ehrlich in the late nineteenth century led to the development of organic arsenicals which had better bioavailability. Acetarsol (Fig. 25.8) was the first of these compounds to be widely used in the treatment of syphilis. Melarsoprol was introduced in 1949 as a less toxic alternative to earlier arsenical treatments. It is only used to treat advanced sleeping sickness because of its toxicity. As the structure suggests, it has a strong affinity of thiol groups, and this may be the basis of its activity where it forms a complex with

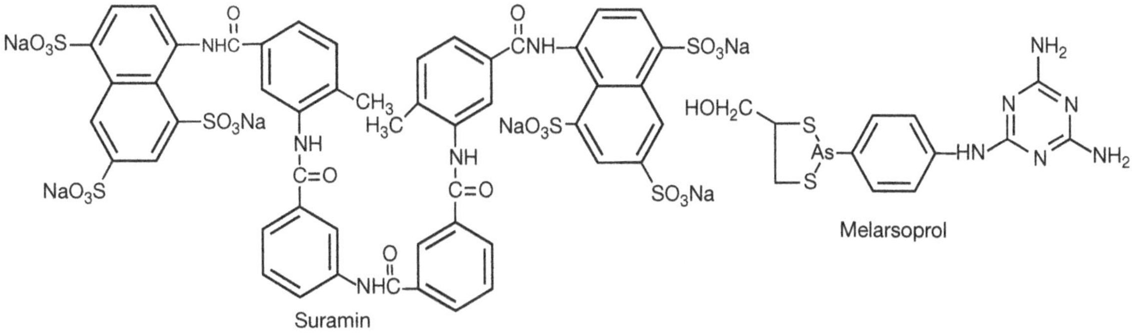

Figure 25.8 Suramin and melarsoprol.

trypanothione, which is an important antioxidant thiol present in trypanosomes. Melarseprol is rapidly metabolised in the body; thus it is one of its metabolites which exerts the therapeutic action. The drug is not orally bioavailable; thus it is given by intravenous injection.

The most recently introduced therapy for trypanosomiasis is eflornithine, which is a difluoromethyl analogue of the amino acid ornithine. It was designed as a potential antitumour drug but proved ineffective for this because of the rapid turnover rate of human ornithine decarboxylase. It is a suicide inhibitor of the enzyme ornithine decarboxylase (ODC) which is involved in the biosynthesis of the polyamine putrescine (Fig. 25.9). The drug is more effective at inhibiting the production of putrescine in trypanosomes than in humans because the turnover rates of ODC are slower in the parasite. Thus the drug is therapeutically efficacious, particularly in combination with melarsoprol. However, the parasites can readily acquire resistance, and a number of mechanisms have been proposed for this including reduced uptake of the drug. African trypanosomiasis infection rates are as high as they were in the 1920s before the era of modern drugs; resistance to existing drugs is an increasing problem and there is a need for new affordable drug treatments.

The effects and treatment of Chagas' disease, which is due to *Trypanosoma cruzi*, are somewhat different from those of African sleeping sickness. The disease can be symptomless for long periods and thus may be overlooked. If left untreated, it can result in severe damage to the heart and the digestive system. The two drugs used to treat Chagas' disease are benzindazole and nitrofurtimox (Fig. 25.10).[10] Benzindazole exerts its action via the generation of electrophilic metabolites by the reductive processes of the cell which result in the formation of nitroso and hydroxylamine compounds. These reactive compounds react with the thiol defensive compounds in the cells, such as glutathione and trypanothione (which is a defensive compound specific to trypanosomes and leishmania). Depletion of the thiol defensive systems renders the parasite vulnerable to oxidative stress. The reactive intermediates also tend to react with proteins and lipids in the parasite. Nitrofurtimox works in a similar way except that in this case intermediate reactive compound is a nitro anion radical compound which causes the generation of the superoxide radical via a redox cycling reaction with molecular oxygen. The superoxide radical depletes the thiol defense system and also reacts with lipids and proteins. The drugs are generally quite effective although resistance has been reported.

Antitrypanosomal preparations

The treatment of trypanosomiasis is specialised; thus no preparations are listed in the BNF.

LEISHMANIASIS

Leishmania parasites are close relatives of trypanosomes. They are transmitted to the host via the bite of the sandfly and in the mammalian bloodstream they inhabit neutrophils and then macrophages as way of avoiding the host's immune response. Leishmaniasis is the only protozoal disease to be endemic in Europe, occurring mainly in Southern Europe. The most common forms of the organism are: *Leishmania major*, *L. tropica*, *L. aethiopica*, *L. mexicana* and *L. braziliensis*, which causes the cutaneous form of the disease, and *L. donovani* which causes the visceral form of the disease. The disease affects around 12 million people worldwide and, in the case of visceral leishmaniasis, the mortality rate is around 90% in the absence of treatment. There are only four treatments for the disease, two of which are based on antimony.[11] Antimony has a long history as a drug and antimony compounds were used to treat syphilis and other infections from the Middle Ages until the early nineteenth century. The main form of antimony used in therapy was antimony potassium tartrate and, after the success of organic arsenicals in treating infectious disease at the beginning of the twentieth century, there was a revived interest in antimony. Initially, antimony potassium tartrate, a complex between antimony (III) and tartaric acid was used in treating leishmaniasis but then further organic derivatives were developed, although these were not as

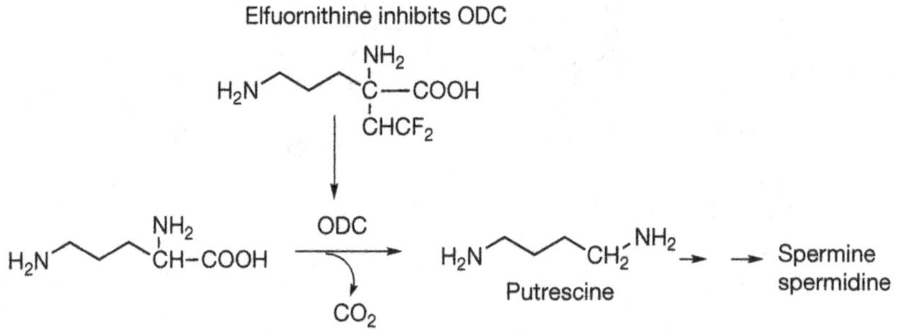

Figure 25.9 Mechanism of action of eflornithine.

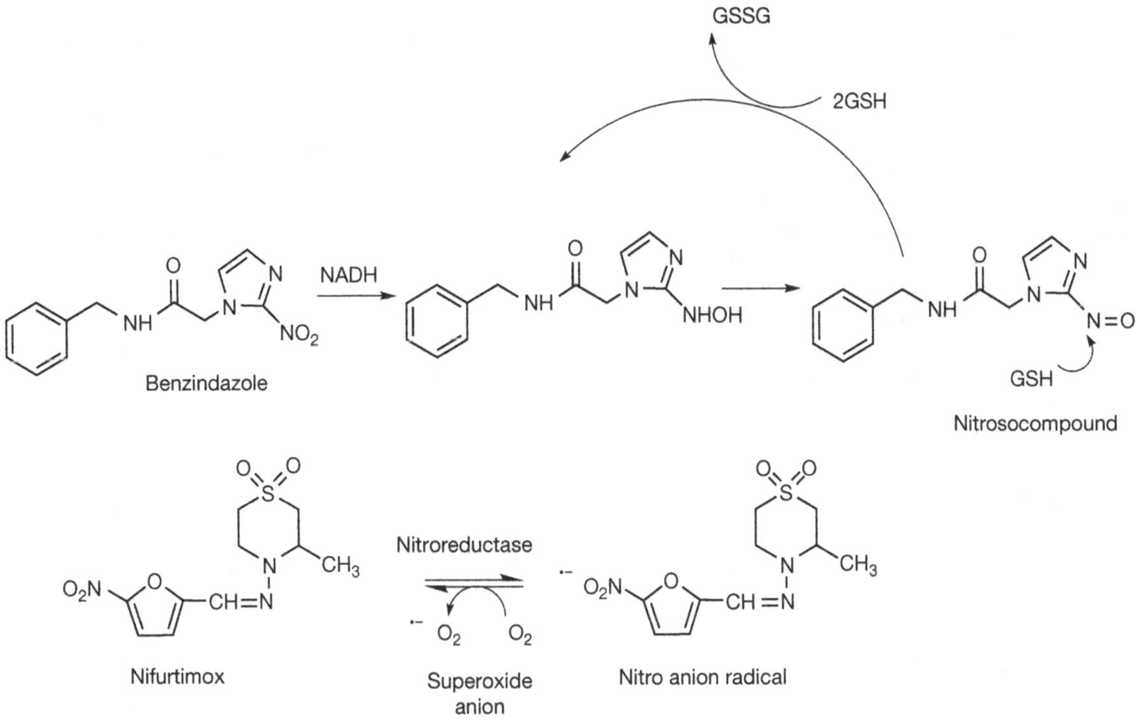

Figure 25.10 Mechanism of action of nitrofurtimox.

successful in reducing irritation as they had been in the case of arsenicals. In 1935, sodium stibogluconate (Fig. 25.11), which is a complex between antimony (V) and gluconic acid, was introduced and was found to be less toxic than the antimony (III) complexes while still being an effective drug. Along with sodium megluminate (Fig. 25.11), it remains the principal treatment for leishmaniasis. The drugs are administered by infusion, have severe side effects, and are also poorly defined in chemical composition, consisting of a mixture of complexes rather than the single structures shown in Figure 25.11.

The antifungal drug amphotericin (see Ch. 24) is also used in treating advanced cases of leishmaniasis. Recently, an alkylphospholipid miltefosine has been licensed in India and Germany for treatment of cutaneous leishmaniasis and is better tolerated than the other drugs used in therapy. However, it remains to be seen if this drug is fully effective.

Antileishmanial preparations

- Sodium stibogluconate 100 mg/mL infusion.

TOXOPLASMOSIS

Toxoplasmosis is caused by a protozoa, *Toxoplasma gondii*. However, in this case, the disease transmission is via environmental contamination. The parasite's primary host is

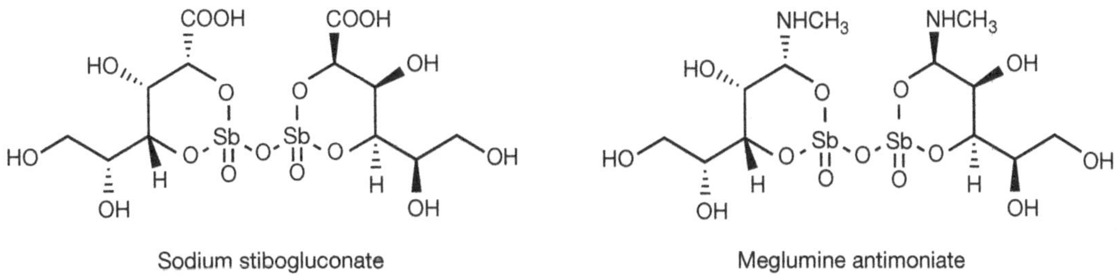

Figure 25.11 Antimonial drugs.

the domestic cat, and humans can pick it up via contact with cat faeces, but it can also be picked up from contaminated drinking water or raw or partially cooked meat. The parasite localises itself in the form of cysts in either muscular or neural tissue. Up to one-third of the world's population may carry the disease. Unlike other protozoal diseases, toxoplasmosis is not life threatening except in immunocompromised individuals. The symptoms of acute infection are flulike but the infection can be latent and can be transmitted from a mother to her unborn child. The disease is often self-limiting but, if treatment is required, the combination of pyrimethamine and sulfadoxine described above for treating malaria is the first choice. The macrolide antibiotics clindamycin and spiramycin (see Ch. 22) are also used in treatment but only in serious cases because of their severe side effects.

GIARDIASIS

Giardiasis is caused by the flagellate protozoa *Giardia lamblia*. The parasite is transmitted by contaminated food or water and is the most common cause of 'backpacker's diarrhoea'. The disease may run its course but, if treatment is required, metronidazole is most commonly used. The structure of metronidazole was based on azomycin (Fig. 25.12), which is a natural product isolated from *Streptomyces* bacteria, that was found to be effective against *Trichomonas* (see below) but was too toxic for general use. Analogues of azomycin were synthesised, of which metronidazole (Fig. 25.12) was the most effective against *Trichomonas*. Subsequently, it was found that the drug was effective against a range of infections including *Giardia*, amoebic dysentery, dental infections and *Helicobacter pylori*. In general, metronidazole works well on infections which occur in an anaerobic environment. Tinidazole is sometimes used as an alternative to metronidazole. It has a longer half-life in the body and can treat some infections which are resistant to metronidazole. Its mechanism of action is essentially as described for benzindazole, above, where a complex series of reductions, partly summarised in Figure 25.13, takes place, favoured by the reductive (anaerobic) environment of the target organism.[12,13] DNA is the target of the reactive species generated and the major damage appears to occur in the AT regions of DNA and results in release of thymine and thymidine from DNA strands. It has been proposed that the radical nitro anion is the species responsible for producing the DNA damage.

Several reactive intermediates have been proposed as being formed during metronidazole reduction but none has been characterised. The effectiveness of the drug is lower if the environment of the target organism is to some extent aerobic, and this is attributed to the presence of oxygen causing the reactive intermediates to decompose via an alternative route. Some research work has focused on making analogues which are more resistant to deactivation by exposure to an aerobic environment.

Mepacrine (Fig. 25.14) can be used in resistant giardiasis. This drug was developed during the Second World War to treat malaria but has been re-introduced to treat giardiasis and is also the subject of research into the treatment of Alzheimer's disease. Albendazole may also be used as an alternative and is described below under the treatment of nematode infections.

TRICHOMONIASIS

Trichomoniasis is the most common protozoal infection in developed countries with an estimated 180 million infections annually. It is produced by the flagellated protozoan *Trichomonas vaginalis*. Many infections are asymptomatic. The infection occurs in women where the parasite survives in the anaerobic environment of the vagina. If the infection

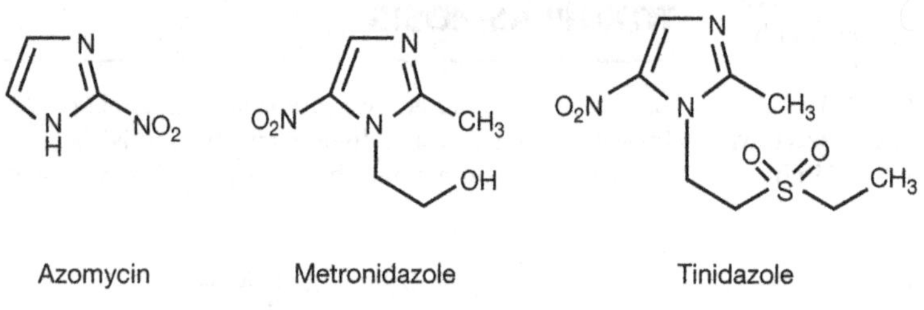

Figure 25.12 Drugs for treating giardiasis.

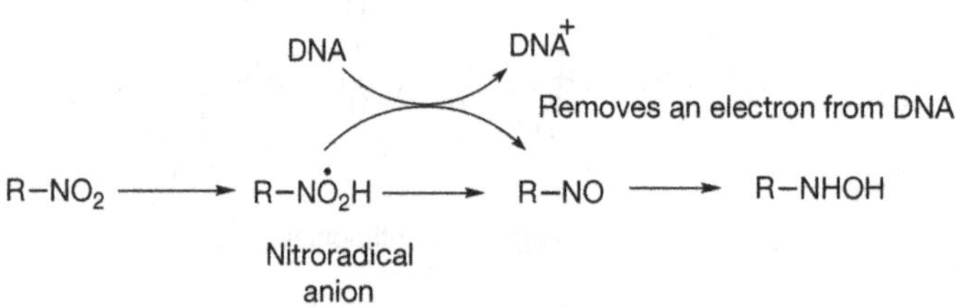

Figure 25.13 DNA damage produced by reduced nitro products of metronidazole.

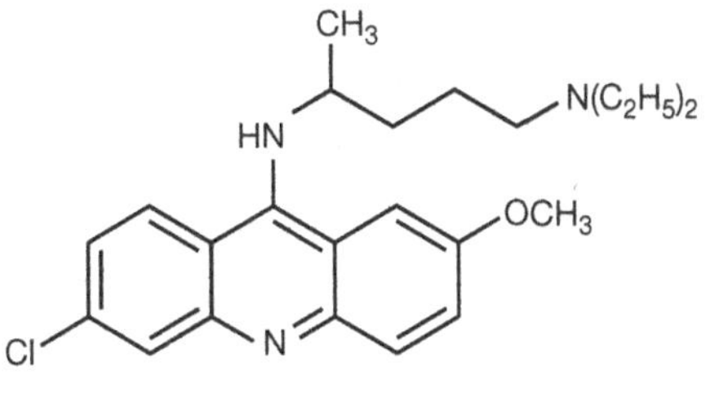

Figure 25.14 Mepacrine.

is not treated it can cause preterm delivery and a high infant mortality rate. In addition, it can predispose an individual to HIV infection and cervical cancer. The infection is effectively treated with metronidazole or tinidazole.

Preparations for the treatment of giardiasis and trichomoniasis

- Mepacrine hydrochloride tablets 100 mg.
- Metronidazole tablets 200, 400 and 500 mg.
- Suspension 200 mg/5 mL.
- Intravenous infusion 5 mg/mL.

PNEUMOCYSTIS PNEUMONIA

Pneumocystis carinii was originally thought to be a protozoan but has been reclassified as a yeast-like fungus. The organism is not naturally pathogenic in humans but can infect immunocompromised patients such as those suffering from AIDS or patients taking immunosuppressive medication. The preferred treatment is the folate inhibitor combination of cotrimoxazole in high dosage. For prophylaxis against pneumocystis, two formulations have been specifically prepared: atovaquone suspension (atovaquone is described under antimalarial drugs), and pentamidine isetionate which is prepared in the form of the nebuliser solution for inhalation. The inhaled drug is easier to administer and better tolerated than the infusion of the drug.

Preparations for the treatment of pneumocystis

- Atovaquone suspension 750 mg/5 mL.
- Pentamidine isetionate 300 mg/bottle.

ANTHELMINTICS

Anthelmintics are a major therapeutic area in the treatment of domestic and farm animals, and the range of preparations is wider for the treatment of animals than humans. In human therapy there is a small range of generally effective therapies. The drug of choice for the treatment of threadworm, hookworm, whipworm and roundworm is mebendazole (Fig. 25.15). Mebendazole was synthesised since it was originally proposed that analogues of benzimidazole (Fig. 25.15) might be able to mimic adenine (Fig. 25.15) and thus act as an antimetabolite inhibiting synthesis of DNA. Mebendazole was the most metabolically stable of the analogues studied and has proved to be very effective against a variety of helminths. It is, in fact, a spindle toxin like some of the anticancer drugs such as the *Vinca* alkaloids (see Ch. 24). Like colchicine, albendazole prevents the separation of chromosomes during cell division by inhibiting the extension of microtubules (Fig. 25.15).[14] Elongation of the microtubules is required in order to drive the divided chromosomes (chromatids) apart to form two new nuclei. The target cells of the drug are the intestinal cells of the helminth and once these cells cease to divide the parasite cannot absorb nutrients and dies. Albendazole (Fig. 25.16) is also a benzimidazole compound. It is more commonly used in treating animals than humans, probably because of habit and concern that it might have more genotoxic potential, as is mebendazole. Albendazole is a prodrug and the active form of the drug is regarded as being the (+) sulphoxide metabolite (Fig. 25.16), which has a longer half-life in the body than the parent drug and also a longer half-life than mebendazole. This may be the critical factor in the use of albendazole to treat hyatid disease in humans, which is caused by

Figure 25.15 Inhibition of microtubule growth by mebendazole.

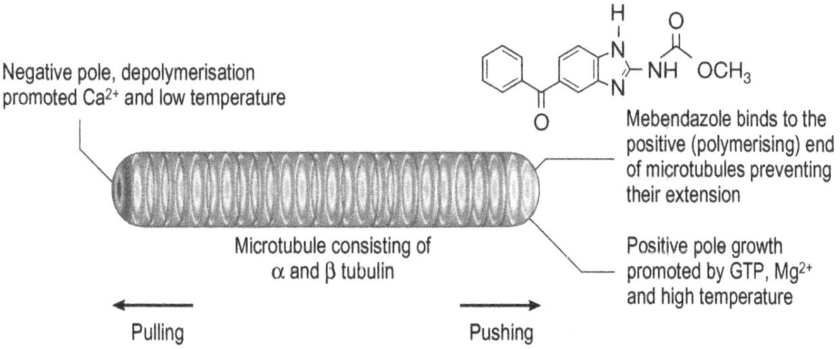

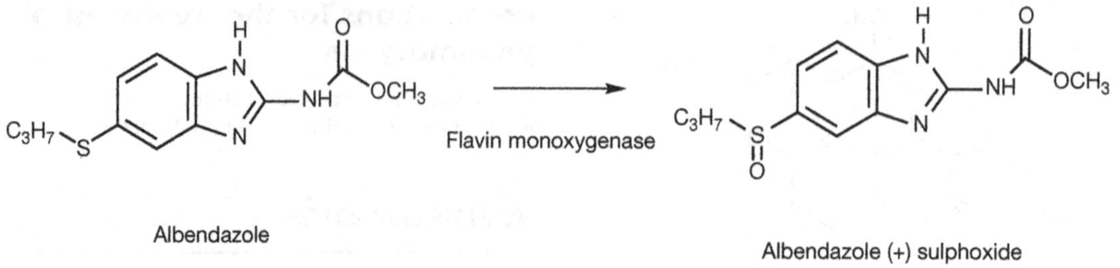

Figure 25.16 Metabolic activation of albendazole to its (+) sulphoxide.

the accumulation of cysts containing the larvae of the tape worm *Echinococcosis granulosis* in the lung.

Piperazine (Fig. 25.17) acts at the same receptor as γ-aminobutyric acid (GABA). It is readily absorbed by parasitic worms and causes paralysis by acting at the GABA ligand-gated chloride channel of nematode muscle. Since it is a diamine it is highly charged at stomach pH and thus readily passes into the lower intestine, giving it a chance to reach the site where intestinal worms reside.

Praziquantel (Fig. 25.17) was developed in the 1970s and is the preferred treatment for schistosomiasis, which is a disease caused by the fluke *Schistosoma*. The vector for the disease is a water snail which releases an infective stage (cercariae) of the fluke into the water from which it can penetrate through the skin of the host and into the bloodstream. The parasite migrates to the liver where it matures into an adult male or female worm. The worms then migrate to the mesenteric venules of the bowel where they pair up, and eggs are produced which circulate back to the liver or penetrate through the blood vessel walls into the bowel or bladder where they are excreted. Schistosomiasis is the second most damaging disease economically in developing countries after malaria. Praziquantel appears to act via increasing the permeability of the worm tegument to Ca^{2+} causing muscle contraction. Its exact mode of action is unclear although the action of the drug results in the antigenic components of the parasite being exposed to the host's immune system. Thus the immune system also has a role in the effectiveness of the drug. The effect of the drug is quite specific since, although praziquantel is sold as a racemate, only the (−) form of the drug is an effective schistosomocide. There is a move to use the enantiomerically pure (−) form since, when used at half the dose of the racemate, it has the same cure rate and fewer side effects. Although the structure of praziquantel is quite amenable to structure–activity relationship (SAR) studies, these have not been carried out. Resistance to the drug is currently not extensive. It is an inexpensive drug and a single oral dose can effect a cure rate of 60–90%. Praziquantel is also used against tapeworm infections.

Levamisole (Fig. 25.17) was discovered in a general screening programme at Janssen. It is an effective treatment for roundworm. It works via its action on nicotinic receptors on muscle cells at the same site of action as acetylcholine, where it acts as an agonist causing depolarisation of the muscle cell, causing an efflux of Na^+ and K^+ and hence contraction. At higher doses, since it is a large organic cation, it causes ion channel blockage of the non-specific Na^+ and K^+ ion channels in the muscle cells and hence paralysis.

Ivermectin (Fig. 25.18) is used to treat onchocerciasis, which is a disease caused by a nematode which is transmitted via the bite of a black fly. The bite injects the larvae under the skin of the host where they mature into adults in nodules, thus evading the host's immune system. The adults mate and produce larvae which are responsible for the strong inflammatory response of the host which causes acute dermatitis, and if the larvae migrate into the cornea of the eye this causes blindness – 'river blindness'.

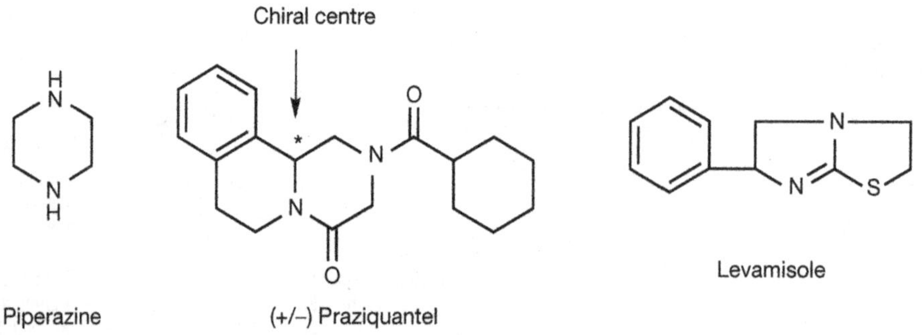

Figure 25.17 Piperazine, praziquantel and levamisole.

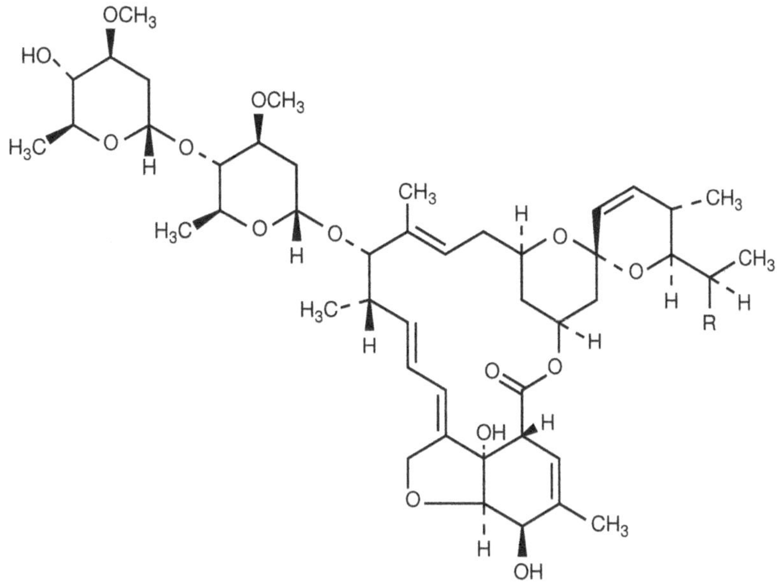

Figure 25.18 Ivermectin.

R = C_2H_5 ivermectin B_1a
R = CH_3 ivermectin B_1b

Eighteen million people are infected with the disease and it is the cause of 300 000 cases of blindness. Ivermectin is a semi-synthetic analogue of a macrolide antibiotic abamectin, isolated from the soil bacterium *Streptomyces avermitilis*, which was chemically reduced to give ivermectin. Ivermectin acts on the parasite muscle by causing opening of a glutamate-gated ion channel, causing a change in the permeability to chloride and hence paralysis. The drug is very effective, with a single dose providing protection for 6–12 months.

REFERENCES

1. Egan TJ. Haemozoin formation. *Mol Biochem Parasitol.* 2008;157:127–136.
2. Egan TJ. Haemozoin (malaria pigment): a unique crystalline drug target. *Targets.* 2003;2:115–124.
3. Sullivan DJ. Theories on malarial pigment formation and quinoline action. *Int J Parasitol.* 2002;32:1645–1653.
4. Vale N, Moreira R, Gomes P. Primaquine revisited six decades after its discovery. *Eur J Med Chem.* 2008;1–17.
5. Golsener J, Waknine JH, Krugliak M, Hunt NH, Grau GE. Current perspectives on the mechanism of action of artemisinins. *Int J Parasitol.* 2006;36: 1427–1441.
6. Kessl JJ, Meshnick SR, Trumpower BL. Modeling the molecular basis of atovaquone resistance in parasites and pathogenic fungi. *Trends Parasitol.* 2007;23:494–501.
7. Simpson AGB, Stevens JR, Lukes J. The evolution and diversity of kinetoplastid flagellates. *Trends Parasitol.* 2006;22:168–174.
8. Wilson WD, Tanious FA, Mathis A, et al. Antiparasitic compounds that target DNA. *Biochimie.* 2008;90:999–1014.
9. Brigotti M, Alfieri RR, Petronini PG, Carnicelli D. Inhibition by suramin of protein synthesis in vitro. Ribosomes as the target of the drug. *Biochimie.* 2006;88:497–503.
10. Maya JD, Cassels BK, Iturriaga-Vásquez P, et al. Mode of action of natural and synthetic drugs against *Trypanosoma cruzi* and their interaction with the mammalian host. *Comp Biochem Physiol A.* 2007;146:601–620.
11. Amatoa VS, Tuon FF, Bacha HA, et al. Mucosal leishmaniasis. Current scenario and prospects for treatment. *Acta Trop.* 2008;105:1–9.
12. Boiani L, Aguirre G, Gonzalez M, Cerecetto H, et al. Furoxan-, alkylnitrate-derivatives and related compounds as anti-trypanosomatid agents: Mechanism of action studies. *Bioorg Med Chem.* 2008;16:7900–7907.
13. Edwards DI. Reduction of nitroimidazoles in vitro and DNA damage. *Biochem Pharmacol.* 1986;35:53–58.
14. Martin RJ. Modes of action of anthelmintic drugs. *Vet J.* 1997;154:11–34.

Chapter | 26 |

Vitamins and minerals

David G Watson

CHAPTER CONTENTS

VITAMINS

Introduction

To some extent this chapter is distinct from the rest of the book in that vitamins are not, in most cases, really drugs and as a group their chemistry is diverse. Thus they do not have common modes of biological action and there is no clear progression in their development as therapeutic agents. However, vitamin and mineral supplements, after pain killers and skin treatments, are the third highest selling over-the-counter medicines. For certain vitamins, e.g. vitamin C and vitamin E, there is an interest in the efficacy in disease prevention. The chemistry and biochemistry of vitamins, in its own right, is very interesting and has some bearing on the actions of a number of drugs.

The word vitamin stems from the term 'vital amine' which arose from the discovery of one of the first vitamins, the amine thiamine (vitamin B_1). Thiamine is an amine, which is not true of all vitamins, but the name vitamin was generally adopted. A vitamin can be defined as an organic compound present in the diet in small amounts which is essential for the normal physiological functioning of the organism but which cannot be synthesised by the organism. Absence of the vitamin leads to clear symptoms of deficiency. A balanced diet should provide enough vitamins but there is some support for the view that certain vitamins can be used in amounts larger than the recommended daily amount (RDA) as therapeutic agents or for prophylaxis, e.g. large doses of vitamin C for treating colds or vitamin D for prevention of osteoporosis.

Since a balanced diet should provide for most vitamin requirements, it is debatable whether vitamin supplements are required other than in situations where there is likely to be deficiency such as vitamin B_{12} to supplement a vegan diet or folate during pregnancy. However, there are indications that in some cases vitamins can be used as medicine. The other issue that arises in these cases is whether or not large doses of vitamins are toxic, and in some cases this is the case. It is highly unlikely that moderate supplementation of the diet with multivitamins will do any harm and may be quite beneficial, certainly in the case of antioxidant vitamins such as C and E. But, as with any medicine, it would be preferable not to take large doses for long periods. Treatment of an acute condition, such as the use of large doses of vitamin C to treat a cold after its onset, for a short period, is the best use of these supplements.

Drug treatment can cause depletion of certain vitamins and minerals and Table 26.1 summarises the effects of various drugs on normal levels of nutrients. Thus vitamin supplementation may be recommended when someone is taking a vitamin-depleting drug for a long period.

Table 26.1 Effects of drugs on vitamins and minerals in the body

Drug	Effects
Antacids (aluminium hydroxide, sodium bicarbonate)	Reduces calcium, copper and folic acid absorption
Gentamicin	Interferes with potassium and magnesium function
Tetracycline	Binds to calcium
Phenobarbital, phenytoin, primidone	Affects vitamin D and vitamin K function
Aspirin	Folate, iron and vitamin C function
Corticosteroids	Affects calcium function.
Colchicine	Vitamin B_{12} absorption
ACE inhibitors	Bind zinc and this may be responsible for affecting the sense of smell and taste
Furosemide	Depletes calcium, magnesium and potassium
Cimetidine and ranitidine	Affect vitamin B_{12} absorption
Chlorpromazine	Affects riboflavin absorption
Alcohol	Depletes vitamin C and thiamine

Vitamin A

RDA 0.8 mg.

Dietary sources (% RDA per 100 g in brackets)

There are relatively few rich dietary sources of vitamin A and it can be obtained mainly from green and yellow vegetables and liver. Sources include: beef liver (4000%), red peppers (3000%), carrots (1500%), butter (500%), eggs (300%), pumpkin (200%), peach (150%) and beans (25%).

It is absorbed directly in the form of retinol esters from liver, butter and eggs and the esters are converted to free retinol by esterases in the body. Plant foodstuffs such as carrots and spinach contain vitamin A in the form of carotene (provitamin A) and this is converted in the body to retinol via the action of beta carotene dioxygenase which produces two molecules of retinal from each molecule of beta carotene. It exists in a number of different forms (vitamers; Fig. 26.1).

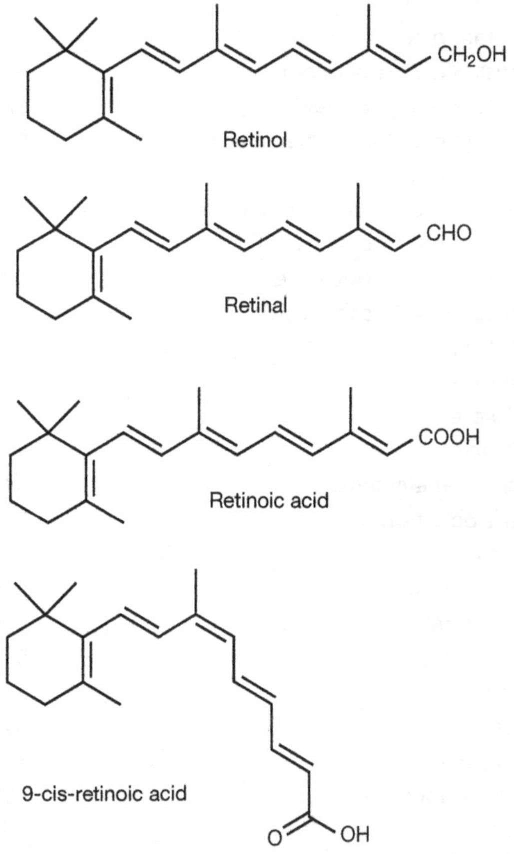

Figure 26.1 Biologically active forms of vitamin A.

Chemistry and biological functions

Role in the visual process

Vitamin A is crucial for the functioning of the visual process. It is bound to the visual protein rhodopsin and its interconversion between its cis and trans forms triggers the visual process (Fig. 26.2). Vitamin A in the form of retinal forms a Schiff's base with a lysine residue in opsin, the visual pigment protein, and at the same time undergoes isomerisation from the all trans form to yield a cis configuration at the 11 position (Fig. 26.2). The vitamin A protein complex absorbs light in the 400–600 nm region and this causes it to revert to the all trans form; thus the light energy is converted to molecular motion. The all trans retinal protein complex is unstable and slowly dissociates.

Retinoids

Dietary vitamin A gives rise to a number of important biologically active metabolites known as the retinoids. The most important forms of these are the all trans form and the 9-cis form of retinoic acid (Fig. 26.1). Retinoids have a wide range of biological activities and have effects on embryonic development, spermatogenesis, regulation of immune function, bone metabolism and differentiation of epithelia. They mediate these effects via specific retinoid receptors which are similar to the nuclear steroid binding receptors in that they directly affect DNA transcription. Since retinoids have been found to exert effects on cell differentiation they have been tested as anticancer drugs along with synthetic analogues. Retinoids show some promise in a number of types of cancer but their use is limited by high levels of toxicity. Vitamin A has also been used in the treatment of skin diseases such as acne.

Symptoms of deficiency

Vitamin A is stored effectively by the body, particularly the liver, because of its high degree of lipophilicity. This means that symptoms of deficiency are slow to manifest. The only unequivocal signs of deficiency are xerophthalmia (drying of the conjunctiva and the eyeball) and nyctalopia (night blindness). Other symptoms are very generalised, including drying of the skin and mucous membranes. In some parts of the world, particularly India and Africa, vitamin A

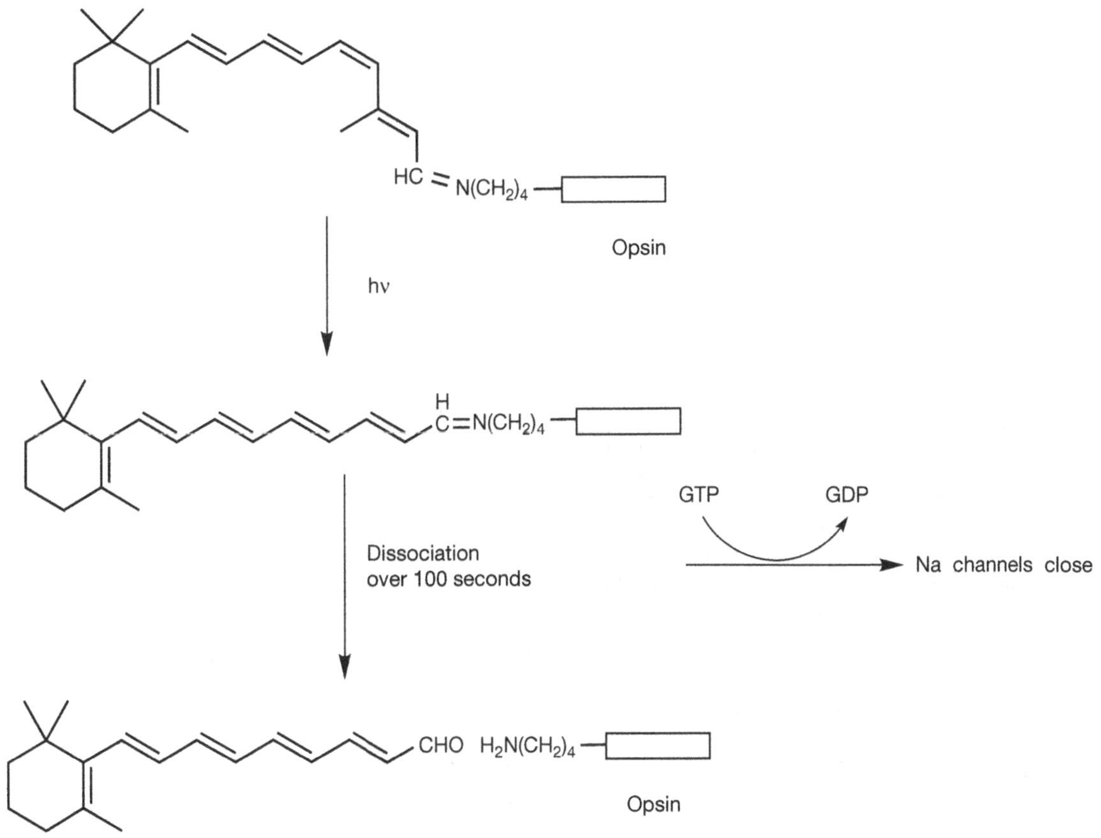

Figure 26.2 Vitamin A in the visual process.

deficiency does occur and it is estimated that 250 000 to 500 000 children a year go blind as a result of vitamin A deficiency caused by malnourishment.

Toxicity

Vitamin A deficiency is unlikely where a balanced diet is consumed. There is probably greater risk from toxicity due to taking too much vitamin A. Persistent large excesses of vitamin A, >1000 × RDA, have to be taken for toxicity to manifest, although the threshold for toxicity is given as *ca.* 4 × RDA. This is the narrowest margin between RDA and toxicity for any vitamin. Symptoms of toxicity include: the skin flaking, alopecia, conjunctivitis, nausea, dizziness, loss of muscular coordination and brittle bones. Extreme intoxication produces liver failure and death.

Vitamin B_1 (thiamine)

RDA 1.2 mg.

Dietary sources (% RDA per 100 g in brackets)

Most foods contain a low concentration of thiamine. The most important dietary sources are: Brewers yeast (1500%), pork (120%), whole wheat and other whole grains (70%) pork liver (60%), oatmeal (70%), peas (30%), asparagus (25%) and salmon (25%) (Fig. 26.3).

Biological functions

Vitamin B_1 gave rise to the science of nutrition when it was discovered that populations consuming a diet of polished rice where the outer husk of the rice had been removed suffered from the disease beriberi, which could be reversed when diet was improved. Vitamin B_1 was eventually isolated from yeast extract in 1932 and characterised. Like the rest of the B vitamins, it is very water soluble; thus excess thiamine is not retained to any great extent by the body although the thiamine required for physiological function is retained by binding to proteins. It has an essential role in metabolism of glucose, catalysing the decarboxylation of pyruvic (Fig. 26.4) and α-ketoglutaric acid plus a number of other substrates. Following decarboxylation of pyruvate the remaining acetate group is transferred to lipoic acid and then to acetyl CoA. Thiamine may have a role in neurotransmission although the biological nature of that role is not entirely clear. It has been found in synaptosomal membranes and nerve stimulation has been found to result in a release of thiamine.

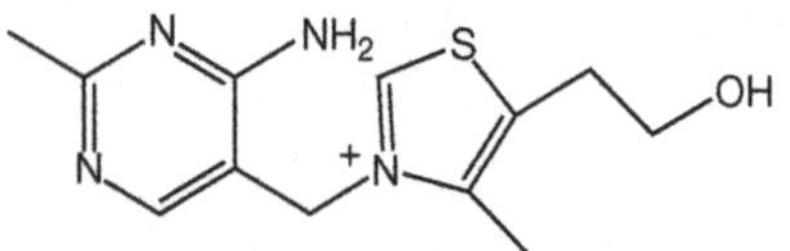

Figure 26.3 Vitamin B_1.

Symptoms of deficiency

Symptoms of deficiency include: anorexia, cardiac enlargement, muscular weakness (symptoms of beriberi) and neurodegeneration. Excessive alcohol consumption appears to have an effect on thiamine status, contributing to its damaging effects, and thiamine deficiency resulting from alcohol abuse can give rise to psychosis. Since thiamine is very water soluble, diuretics may also produce thiamine deficiency, and haemodialysis may produce deficiency. Some foodstuffs including tea, coffee and raw fish contain factors that antagonise the activity of thiamine.

Possible therapeutic indications

It has been observed that high thiamine intake is associated with a lower likelihood of developing cataract. Trials assessing the benefit of thiamine supplementation in arresting the progression of Alzheimer's disease indicated that there was no benefit. There was no strong evidence for thiamine being beneficial in treating heart disease or cancer. There have been reports that thiamine can increase mental acuity. Thiamine supplementation at 25–50 mg per day has been reported to be effective in reducing mosquito bites, although 2 weeks of supplementation are required to produce an effect. Another study found thiamine to be ineffective as an insect repellent.

Toxicity

Thiamine is not particularly toxic because of its rapid rate of excretion. However, very large doses of thiamine are toxic and doses of 1000 × RDA may be fatal.

Vitamin B_2 (riboflavin)

RDA 1.2 mg.

Dietary sources (% RDA per 100 g in brackets)

Meats, dairy products and green vegetables are the most important sources. Bioavailability is greater from animal products. Good sources include: beef liver (300%), cheese (35%), eggs (25%), pork (25%), lamb (25%) broccoli (20%) and asparagus (20%) (Fig. 26.5).

Biological function

Riboflavin is another highly water-soluble vitamin and was isolated from yeast extract in 1933. It has a bright yellow colour and excess vitamin is rapidly excreted in the

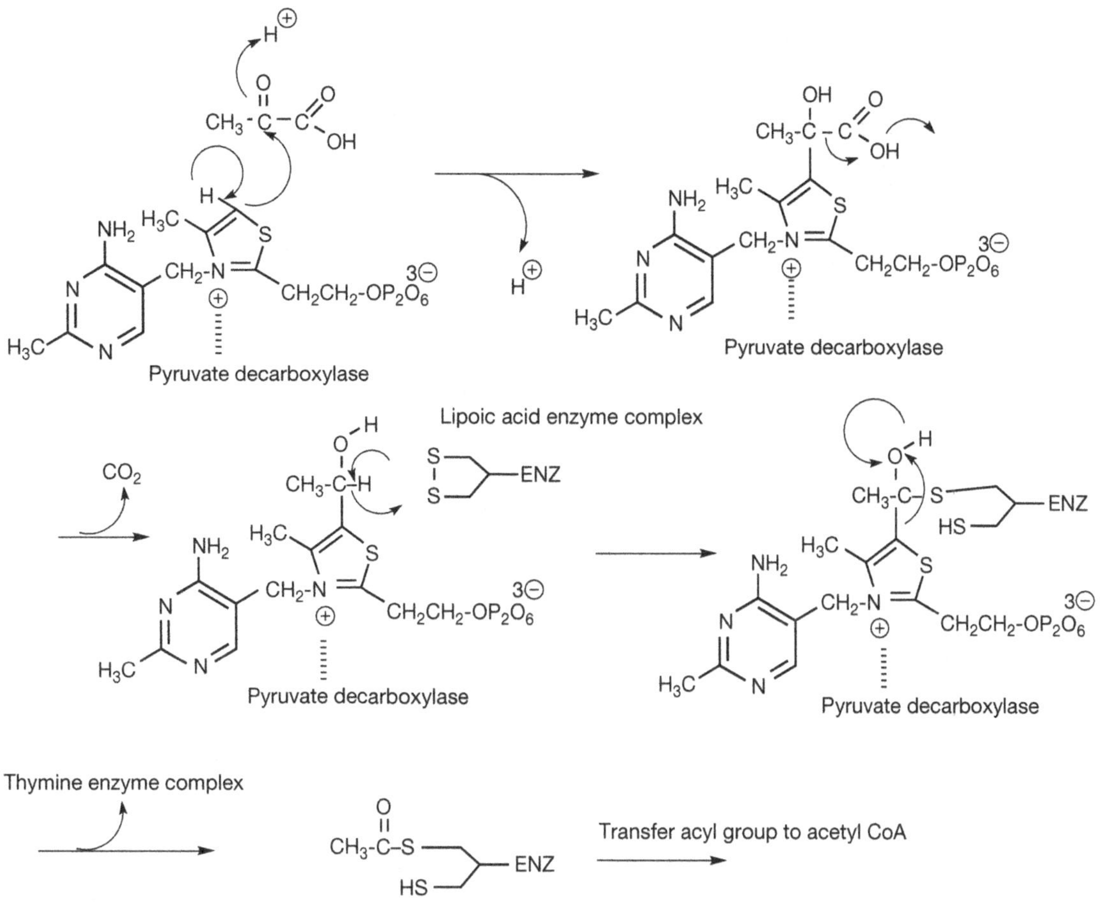

Figure 26.4 Decarboxylation of pyruvic acid with thiamine as co-factor.

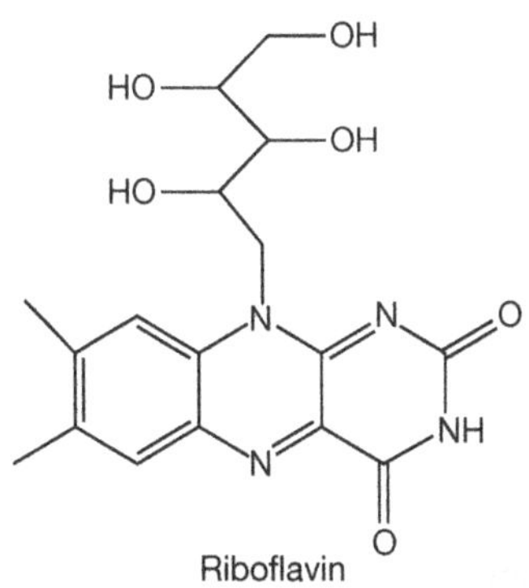

Figure 26.5 Riboflavin.

urine, turning it bright yellow. Riboflavin is incorporated into flavin adenine dinucleotide (FAD) which is an essential co-factor of flavoproteins, which are involved in biological oxidation and reduction and are required for the metabolism of carbohydrates, amino acids and lipids. Figure 26.6 shows the oxidation of succinic acid to fumaric acid which uses FAD as a co-factor. The $FADH_2$ formed then enters the terminal respiratory chain where eventually the 2H atoms are converted into H_2O.

Symptoms of deficiency

Many tissues are affected by riboflavin deficiency (ariboflavinosis). Riboflavin deficiency requires 3–4 months of deprivation to manifest and symptoms include lesions on the lips, inflammation of the tongue, lowered levels of white and red blood cells, excessive sensitivity to pain and vascularisation of the cornea. Deficiency also results in decreased conversion of tryptophan into niacin. A test for deficiency is to measure glutathione reductase levels, which are depressed when riboflavin levels are low as are xanthine oxidase levels. There is a link between riboflavin deficiency in pregnancy and the development of pre-eclampsia. However, supplementation with riboflavin in a trial indicated that there was no effect on the prevention of pre-eclampsia. Alcoholics are at increased risk of riboflavin deficiency as

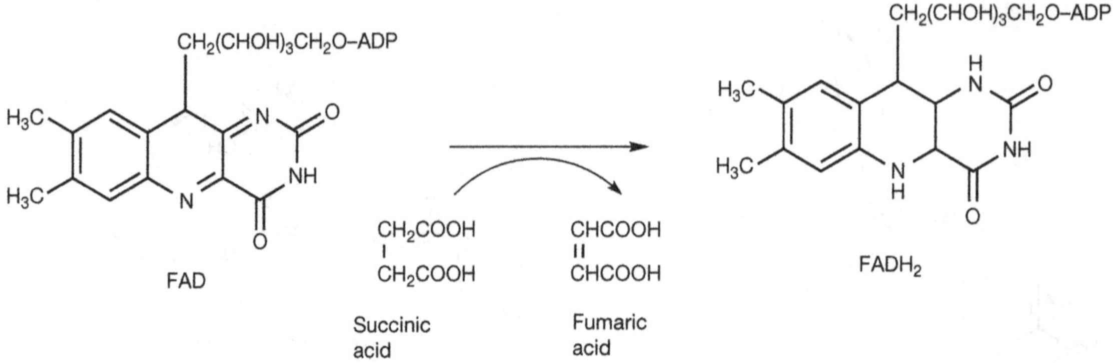

Figure 26.6 Oxidation of succinic acid with FAD as co-factor.

are anorexics and lactose intolerant subjects who may not consume dairy products, which are good sources of riboflavin. Physically active people such as athletes may have an extra requirement for riboflavin.

Therapeutic indications

Riboflavin may have some role in the prevention of migraine in combination with other drugs. There is some evidence that riboflavin may be able to prevent cataract formation and for this reason the RDA for elderly people may be set at 1.7 mg per day.

Toxicity

The toxicity of riboflavin is very low, partly because its absorption by the oral route is very poor. There has been no upper limit established for toxicity although, obviously, intravenous administration has potential to cause toxicity.

Vitamin B_5 (pantothenic acid)

RDA 5 mg.

Dietary sources (% RDA per 100 g in brackets)

The most important dietary sources are meats and some vegetables: pork liver (150%), kidney (80%), eggs (60%), peanuts (60%), wheat bran (60%), mushroom (40%), lentils (30%), broccoli (25%) and avocado (25%) (Fig. 26.7).

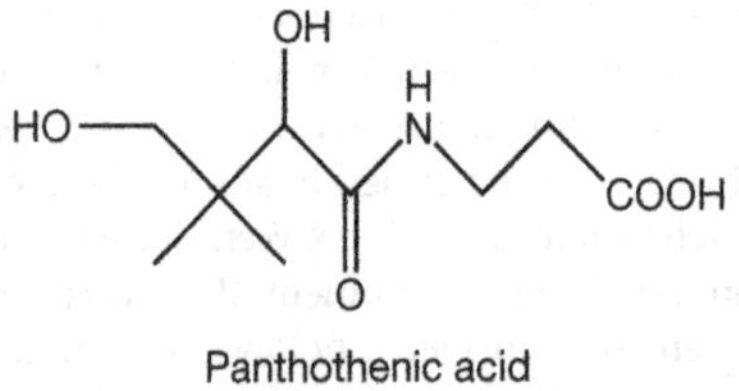

Figure 26.7 Pantothenic acid.

Biological functions

Vitamin B_5 is a component of co-enzyme A (CoA) which is required for the biosynthesis of fatty acids and lipids; the synthesis of cholesterol and metabolism involving acetylation.

Symptoms of deficiency

Deficiency is only observed in severe malnourishment and would be difficult to distinguish from the general debility produced by malnutrition.

Therapeutic indications

Administration of pantothenic acid orally and application of pantothenol ointment to the skin have been shown to promote wound healing in animals. However, few data exist in humans to support these findings. A pantothenic acid derivative called pantethine has been reported to have a cholesterol lowering effect.

Toxicity

The toxicity of pantothenic acid is very low with doses of up to 10 g/day having little adverse effects.

Vitamin B_6

RDA 1.2 mg.

Dietary sources (% RDA per 100 g in brackets)

Vitamin B_6 is widely distributed in foodstuffs, occurring mainly in meats and whole grains. Pyridoxine is more bioavailable from meat. Sources include: liver (80%), walnuts (70%), chicken (30–60%), tuna (40%), beef (30%), spinach (25%), whole wheat (25%), potatoes (20%), cauliflower (20%) and eggs (15%) (Fig. 26.8).

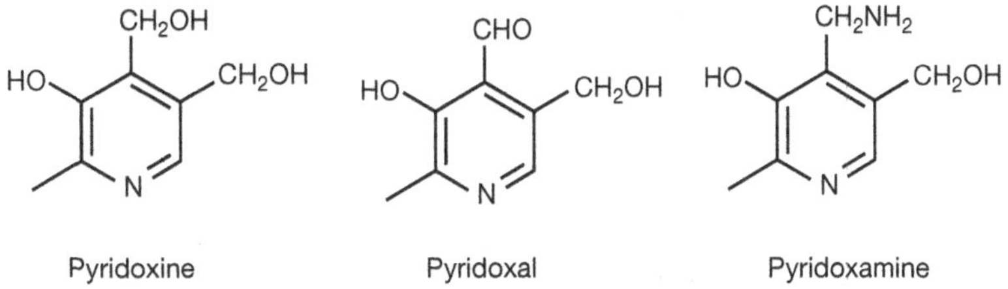

Figure 26.8 Forms of vitamin B_6.

Biological functions

Pyridoxine is the most key of all co-enzymes. It is involved in decarboxylation reactions which are required in the synthesis of neurotransmitters such as serotonin, noradrenaline, dopamine and γ-aminobutyric acid (GABA) from amino acids. It is involved in transamination reactions which are required for synthesis of amino acids from keto-acids and in elimination where, for instance, an amino group is removed from an amino acid. It is also involved in racemisation where the stereochemistry at a chiral centre is reversed. Figure 26.9 shows reaction mechanisms for decarboxylation with vitamin B_6 as the co-factor. The vitamin is activated by conversion to its phosphate ester. It has been said that nature created pyridoxine for the delight of organic chemists who enjoy pushing electrons around. This is amply illustrated in Figure 26.9 and these are only two of pyridoxine's reactions! Various explanations exist as to how it exerts its co-enzyme activity, and some mechanisms protonate the pyridine nitrogen. This is unlikely at physiological pH since its p*Ka* value is <5.0. The phenolic group is quite acidic and the most stable intermediates are as shown in Figure 26.9, where a linear conjugated system is formed yielding a reactive ortho quinone methide intermediate. The ortho quinone methide of pyridoxine has been observed to be formed in aqueous solution by photochemical reaction. This possible reaction might give some concern with regard to liver toxicity if large doses of pyridoxine are taken as a vitamin supplement.

Pyridoxine is involved as a co-factor coenzyme in about 100 enzyme systems. Thus, in addition to the reactions mentioned above, it is required for: glycogen phosphorylase, which catalyses the release of glucose from stored glycogen, haemoglobin biosynthesis, the generation of glucose from amino acids (gluconeogenesis), the biosynthesis of niacin from tryptophan and nucleic acid biosynthesis.

Symptoms of deficiency

Severe deficiency of pyridoxine is uncommon. Alcoholics are thought to be most at risk of vitamin B_6 deficiency due to low dietary intake and impaired metabolism of the vitamin. General symptoms of deficiency include sleeplessness, nervous disorders, dermatological symptoms, depression and anaemia. Abnormal electroencephalogram patterns have been noted in some studies of vitamin B_6 deficiency.

Possible therapeutic indications

Pyridoxine has been proposed a treatment for elevated levels of homocysteine, which is believed to be involved in the aetiology of coronary artery disease. There is some evidence that it promotes turnover of homocysteine. There is evidence that it can improve immune function in the elderly when administered at levels about 2–3 × RDA. There is some evidence that pyridoxine supplementation may improve cognitive function in the elderly although not mood. There is some evidence that pyridoxine may reduce the risk of kidney stone formation. Pyridoxine has been used for many years in the treatment of morning sickness and there is some evidence that it is effective when used at levels of 25 mg every 8 hours. It has been used in treating premenstrual syndrome and there is some evidence that it is effective. It is recommended that pyridoxine supplementation is used with drugs such as isoniazid and penicillamine that deplete its levels. Large doses (0.1–1 g) have been used in the treatment of schizophrenia and it has been found that pyridoxine can interfere with the actions of LDOPA and phenytoin.

Toxicity

Pyridoxine is not particularly toxic, and even where massive doses (>2 g/day) were taken there was merely some evidence of lack of muscular coordination (ataxia) and loss of motor control (muscle spasm/twitch). There is some evidence that pyridoxine can cause sensory neuropathy and for this reason it is recommended that it is not taken in doses >100 mg per day.

Vitamin B_{12} (cyanocobalamin)

RDA 0.0015 mg.

Dietary sources (% RDA per 100 g in brackets)

Vitamin B_{12} is synthesised by bacteria in the guts of animals; thus animal tissues are the main source. Dietary sources include: beef liver (8000%), beef kidney (2500%), trout (500%), herring (300%), eggs (80%), cheese (50–100%), chicken (30%) and milk (30%). Grains and fruits do not contain vitamin B_{12}.

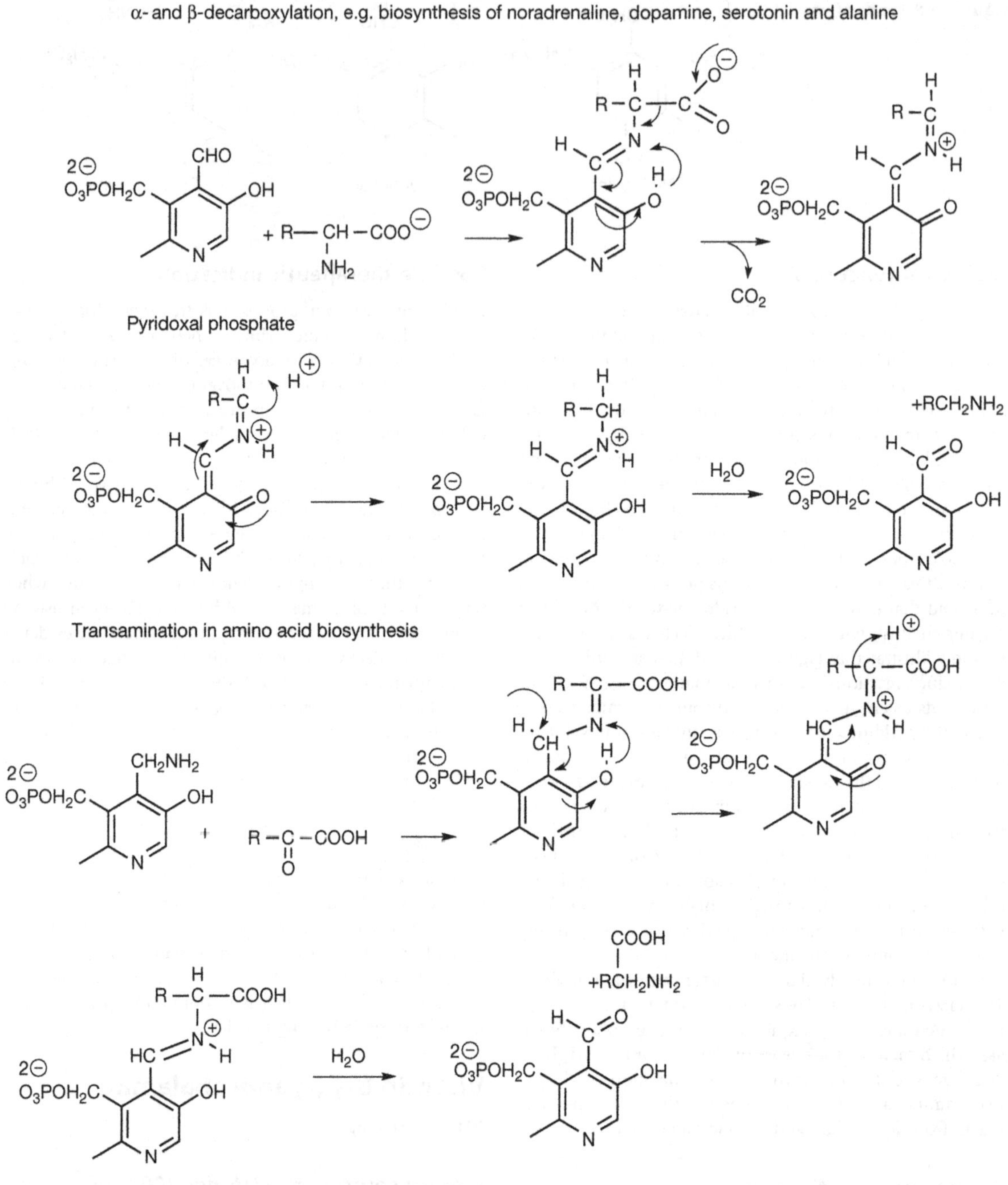

Figure 26.9 Mechanisms of decarboxylation and amination catalysed by pyridoxine.

Biological functions

There are a number of closely related forms of vitamin B_{12} of which cyanocobalamin is one (Fig. 26.10). Cyanocobalamin is the synthetic form of the vitamin which is given in supplements; however, in the body the active form of the vitamin either has a methyl group in place of the CN ion (methylcobalamin) or deoxyadenosine (5′-deoxyadenosylcobalamin). Vitamin B_{12} is essential for the correct functioning of the brain and nervous system and for haemoglobin synthesis. Some of the effects

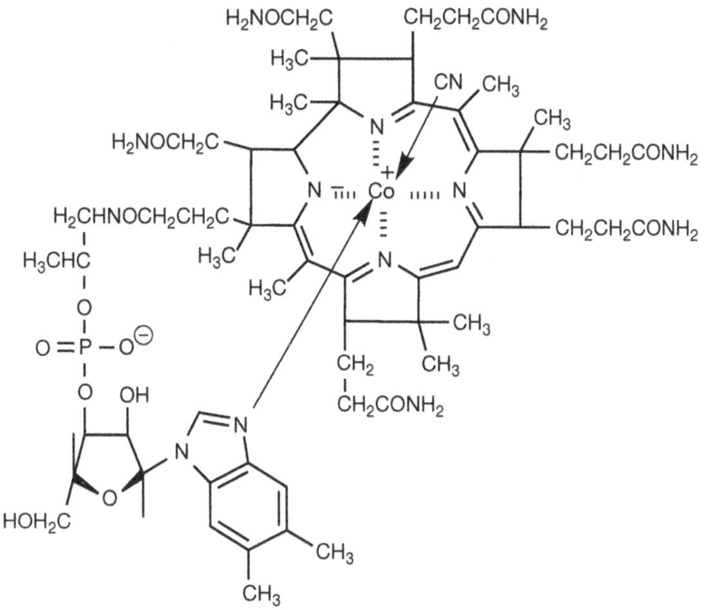

Figure 26.10 Cyanocobalamin.

of B_{12} deficiency can be removed by supplementation with folic acid since vitamin B_{12} deficiency results in loss of folate due to it accumulating as methyl tetrahydrofolate. Methylcobalamin is required for the function of the folate-dependent enzyme, methionine synthase, which is required for the synthesis of methionine, from homocysteine (Fig. 26.11). Methionine in turn is required for the synthesis of S-adenosylmethionine, a methyl group donor used in many biological methylation reactions including methylation of purines and pyrimidines.

Reduced levels of methionine synthase can lead to an accumulation of homocysteine which has been linked to cardiovascular disease.

Vitamin B_{12} is also required by the enzyme that catalyses the conversion of L-methylmalonyl-CoA to succinyl-CoA. This biochemical reaction plays an important role in the production of energy from fats and proteins, particularly the metabolism of branch chain amino acids such as leucine. This reaction requires the deoxyadenosine form of B_{12}. The reaction is shown in Figure 26.12, where the adenosine cobalamin allows a rearrangement of the methylmalonyl CoA to succinyl CoA. Succinyl CoA is also required for the synthesis of haemoglobin. Vitamin B_{12} deficiency is characterised by elevated levels

of methylmalonyl CoA in blood, although this is not a definitive test for it.

Symptoms of deficiency

Since B_{12} only occurs in meat, deficiencies are likely to result from a strict vegetarian diet containing no animal products. Vitamin B_{12} deficiency is also estimated to affect 10–15% of individuals over the age of 60. Vitamin B_{12} is absorbed from the small intestine as a complex with a protein called intrinsic factor (IF). The most common cause of vitamin B_{12} deficiency is pernicious anaemia which is an auto-immune disease where the cells of the stomach become inflamed and do not secrete the required amounts of acid and enzymes to release vitamin B_{12} from food. In addition, antibodies to IF further prevent B_{12} absorption. The condition is treated with high doses of vitamin B_{12} supplements or by intramuscular injection of vitamin B_{12}. A similar condition occurs in the elderly where there is malabsorption of vitamin B_{12} from food due to decreased secretion of stomach acid. This condition is easier to treat with supplementation since IF levels are still normal. Symptoms include megaloblastic anaemia, neuropathy, memory loss and abnormalities of lipid metabolism.

Tetrahydrofolate $-CH_3 + HS-(CH_2)_2-\overset{\overset{\displaystyle NH_2}{|}}{CH}-COOH \longrightarrow H_3CS-(CH_2)_2-\overset{\overset{\displaystyle NH_2}{|}}{CH}-COOH$

Homocysteine Methylcobalamin Methionine

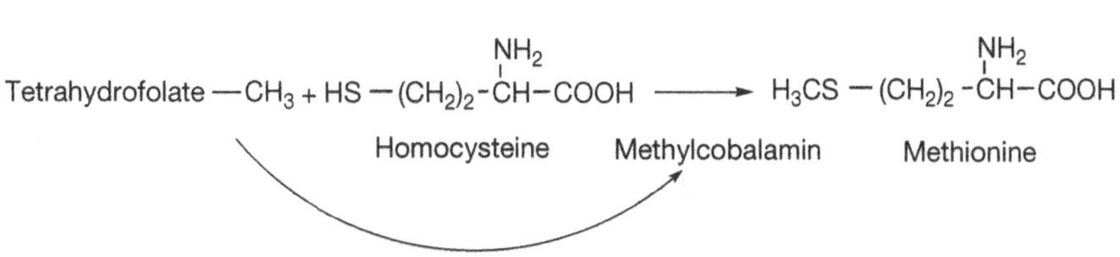

Figure 26.11 Methylation of homocysteine with methylcobalamin as co-factor.

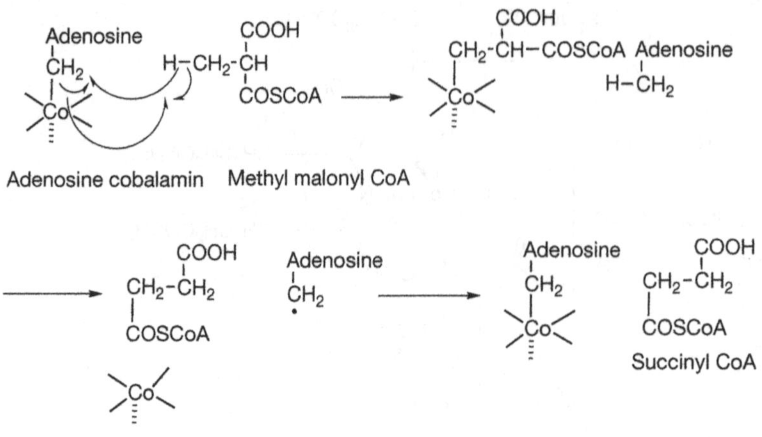

Figure 26.12 Rearrangement of methylmalonyl CoA catalysed by vitamin B_{12}.

Therapeutic indications

With folic acid vitamin B_{12} has been shown to reduce levels of the cardiac risk factor homocysteine in plasma. It is not clear if a reduction homocysteine does lower the risk of heart disease. There is some indication that vitamin B_{12} can decrease the risk of cancer but it is difficult to differentiate its effects from the effects of folate metabolism. It is important that vitamin B_{12} intake is adequate during pregnancy to reduce the risk of the neural tube defects developing in the unborn child. Thus vitamin B_{12} is an important supplement for vegans and the infants of vegan mothers where they are breast fed. Extensive research has been conducted into whether or not vitamin B_{12} supplementation can prevent the development of Alzheimer's disease; however, the trials thus far are inconclusive.

Toxicity

Vitamin B_{12} has no appreciable toxicity and dietary levels several hundred times RDA are safe, probably because the levels of vitamin which can be absorbed are rapidly exceeded.

Vitamin C (ascorbic acid)

RDA 40 mg.

Dietary sources (% RDA per 100 g in brackets)

Vitamin C is lost on storage and lost to a great extent in cooking where it dissolves in the cooking water; thus it is provided most effectively by raw fruits and vegetables and their juices. Sources include: rosehips (2500%), green pepper (250%), blackcurrant (250%), broccoli (200%), Brussels sprouts (200%), watercress (150%), strawberry (120%), oranges/lemons (100%), apple (15%).

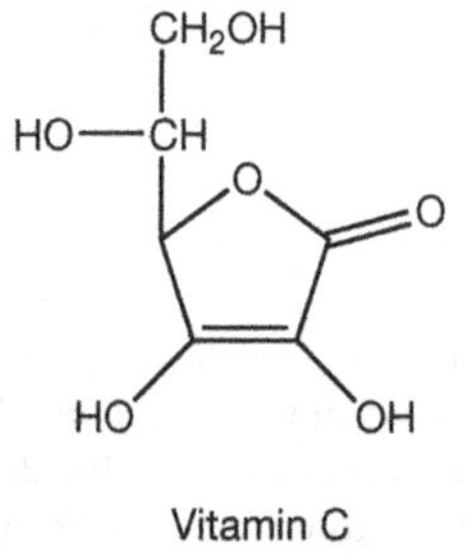

Figure 26.13 Vitamin C.

Biological functions

Vitamin C (Fig. 26.13) deserves a book in itself since so much research has been conducted into it over the years. Most living organisms produce vitamin C and thus do not require it as a vitamin; however, primates, guinea pigs, bats and birds require vitamin C as a vitamin. It has many biological functions. It is essential for the biosynthesis of the protein of connective tissue, collagen, since it is a cofactor for the hydroxylation of proline residues of procollagen in order to form the connective tissue protein collagen (Fig. 26.14). It is not possible to write a completely satisfactory mechanism for this reaction but it is known that Fe^{2+}, ketoglutaric acid and molecular oxygen are involved in the initial reaction which is catalysed by proline hydroxylase. Ketoglutaric acid is decarboxylated to succinic acid and this results at the same time in the hydroxylation of proline and the oxidation of Fe^{2+} to Fe^{3+}. The evidence seems to point to a role for ascorbic acid after the event in reducing Fe^{3+} back to Fe^{2+}. Figure 26.14 shows the equation for the reduction of Fe^{3+} to Fe^{2+} but even this is a simplification. The hydroxylation of procollagen to collagen results in the H-bonding of the collagen chains to each other, thus producing a material which on a weight-for-weight ratio is stronger than steel. Vitamin C is involved in a series of

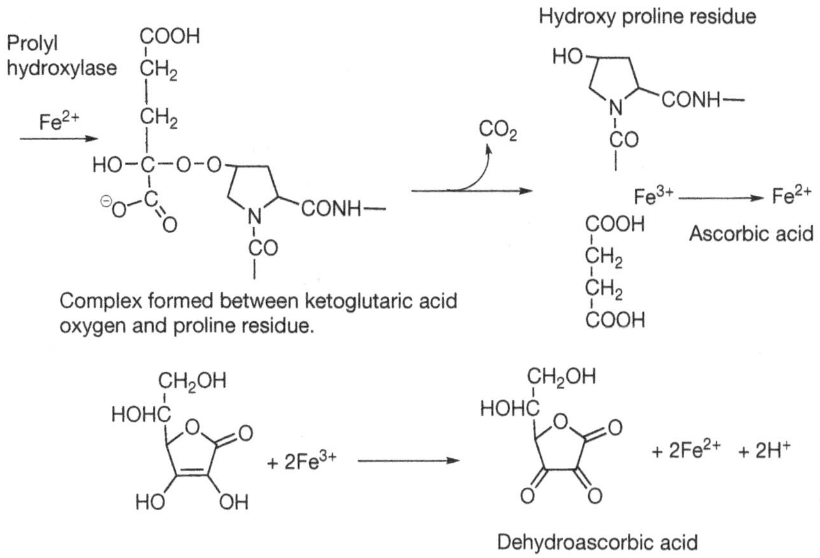

Figure 26.14 Hydroxylation of proline residues to produce collagen.

reactions which require hydroxylation including: the biosynthesis of noradrenaline, serotonin and carnitine, the metabolism of cholesterol to bile acids and oxidative metabolism of many drugs.

Other roles of vitamin C include: the oxidative degradation of the amino acid tyrosine, enhancing the absorption of iron from foods, antihistamine effects through increasing histamine degradation rates, immunostimulating effects through increasing neutrophil activation, stimulating IgG and IgM formation and protecting essential proteins against damage by neutrophils. A very important biological role for vitamin C is in the reduction of the oxidised form of vitamin E so that vitamin E can preserve its role in protection of biological membranes from oxidation (Fig. 26.15).

Symptoms of deficiency

The most obvious symptom of vitamin C deficiency is scurvy, which is due to defects in collagen formation causing impaired wound healing, haemorrhage and weakening of the gums and cartilage. Mild vitamin C deficiency manifests as fatigue and anorexia, and may be associated with hypercholesterolaemia and increased risk of heart disease. Smoking and alcohol consumption reduce vitamin C levels in plasma.

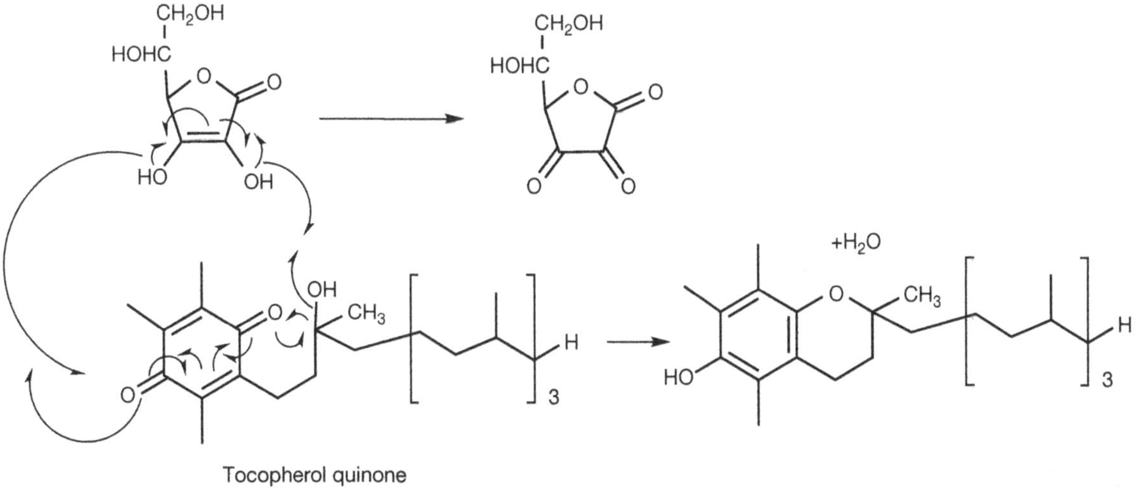

Figure 26.15 Reduction of tocopherol quinone by vitamin C.

Possible therapeutic indications

Vitamin C is the most widely studied vitamin in terms of therapeutic activity. Despite the fact that doses of vitamin C of 100–150 mg/day result in tissue saturation, higher intakes can result in increases in concentrations in extracellular fluids such as plasma with associated pharmacologic activity. The main problem with most evidence for vitamin C efficacy in disease prevention is that many studies report positive results based on dietary consumption of vitamin C where other compounds absorbed from fresh fruit and vegetables may also have a preventative role.

Extensive studies have been made of the role of vitamin C in preventing heart disease. A very large pooling of data indicated that when vitamin C was taken as a supplement at >700 mg/day there was a 25% reduction in the chance of getting coronary heart disease (CHD). Treatment with high doses of vitamin has consistently proved that vitamin C enhances blood vessel dilation in patients with atherosclerosis.

The role of vitamin C in the prevention and treatment of cancer has been studied for many years. Very early work was conducted by Linus Pauling at Vale of Leven hospital in Scotland in which positive claims that were made could never be reproduced. The theory behind cancer prevention is that high levels of the vitamin enhance collagen biosynthesis which helps to contain tumours; however, there is no reason to suppose the high levels of vitamin C lead to higher levels of collagen synthesis. There is some evidence for the prevention of cancer by vitamin C, particularly in the case of stomach cancer.

The role of vitamin C in prevention and treatment of the common cold has been extensively studied. In this case, doses of 1–5 g per day may be taken. Controlled studies appear to indicate only small effects although a study involving people at peak fitness including athletes and skiers found that vitamin C supplementation reduced the incidence of colds by 50%. Also, a long-term trial over 5 years in Japan found that supplementation at 500 mg daily reduced the incidence of colds by 66%. The means of administration may be critical, and localised administration via lozenges and hence buccal absorption may be most effective.

Toxicity

The toxicity of vitamin C is very low and doses of 10 g/day appear to be quite safe. The major concern at high doses is the risk of the formation of calcium oxalate kidney stones and it might be wise not to take calcium supplements with vitamin C. The increase of oxalate levels, even at high doses, only increases by about 50%. The evidence for rebound effects where, following withdrawal of high-dose therapy, vitamin C levels fall and for in vivo mutagenicity is not conclusive. The worst effects of vitamin C at high dose appear to be GI disturbances and diarrhoea.

Vitamin D (ergocalciferol)

RDA 0.01 mg.

Dietary sources (% RDA per 100 g in brackets)

Vitamin D is found largely in fish and to a lesser extent in other animals and very little in plants. Often, foods contain added vitamin D. Sources include: cod liver oil (250%), sardines (40%), herring (10%), salmon (10%), chicken (2%), butter (1%) and spinach (0.01%) (Fig. 26.16).

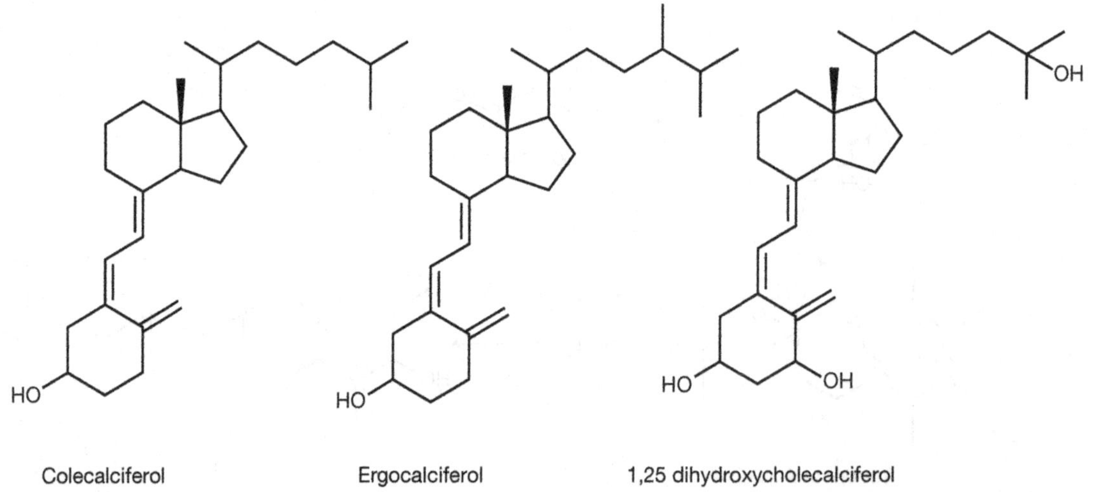

Figure 26.16 The most common forms of vitamin D.

Biological functions

Vitamin D is not strictly a vitamin because it can be made by the body if sufficient sunlight is available. If sunlight is of only low intensity, vitamin D deficiency can occur. The action of sunlight is required to convert 7-dehydrocholesterol into vitamin D via a photochemical reaction (Fig. 26.17). Thus, for people in far northern or far southern latitudes, absorption of vitamin D from the diet is necessary.

Vitamin D is composed of a number of related structures but the two most prominent members of the family are colecalciferol and ergocalciferol, which is formed from ergosterol rather than 7-dehydrocholesterol. Colecalciferol is transformed into the most active form of the vitamin, 1,25-dihydroxycholecalciferol, by hydroxylation at the 25 position in the liver and finally at the 1 position in the kidneys.

1,25-Dihydroxycholecalciferol, together with the peptide hormones calcitonin and parathyroid hormone, functions to regulate calcium and phosphate homeostasis. Vitamin D acts like a steroid hormone binding to receptor proteins and then to DNA, triggering the transcription of calcium-binding proteins. These binding proteins are involved in uptake of Ca^{2+} from the intestine, its resorption by the kidney and its binding by bone. These proteins are also involved in phosphate absorption from the intestine.

Symptoms of deficiency

In the absence of the formation of vitamin D via the action of sunlight, it has to be absorbed from restricted dietary sources; thus deficiency can occur. Even with mild vitamin D deficiency, loss of calcium from the bone can occur to compensate for reduced calcium absorption from the diet. This increases the risk of osteoporosis. Severe vitamin D deficiency in children results in rickets, where the bones of the growing child become bowed. Despite addition of vitamin D to foodstuffs, rickets is still reported from cities around the world. Vitamin D deficiency in adults results in a proneness to fractures in adults (osteomalacia) and also manifests as muscle weakness. There are a number of risk factors for vitamin D deficiency: infants who are exclusively breast fed and are not exposed to sunlight, people with dark skin, the elderly, people with Crohn's disease and obesity.

Therapeutic indications

There is some evidence that vitamin D in the form of colecalciferol taken at a level >800 IU is effective in reducing the risk of bone fractures in the elderly when taken with calcium supplementation at >1 g per day. Vitamin D can promote cell differentiation and there is some evidence from epidemiological studies that vitamin D is effective in reducing the incidence of some cancers, including gastrointestinal, prostate and breast cancer. Vitamin D has been shown to modulate T-cell response and thus may have an effect on autoimmune diseases, and there is some evidence to support this.

25-(OH)-vitamin D has shown some potential for the treatment of psoriasis.

Toxicity

At high levels (>100 × RDA) vitamin D causes hypercalcaemia, which can result in deposition of calcium phosphate in soft tissues such as heart and kidney. Certain patients are at higher risk of suffering from hypercalcaemia, including those suffering from hyperparathyroidism, sarcoidosis, tuberculosis and lymphoma. Although vitamin D is potentially toxic it can be regarded as being safe at levels <500 μg per day. Certain drugs including phenytoin, carbemazepam and ketoconazole can reduce vitamin D levels. Patients taking digitalis are more sensitive to the effects of hypercalcaemia.

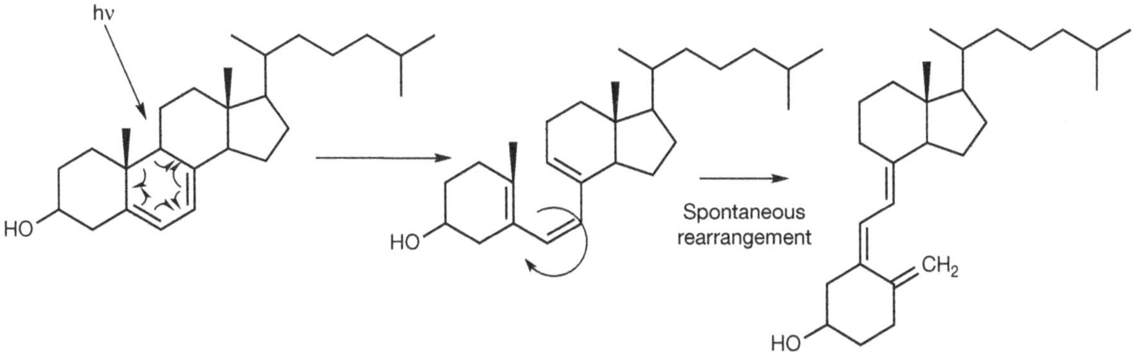

Vitamin D

Figure 26.17 Photochemical conversion of 7-dehydrocholesterol into vitamin D.

Vitamin E (tocopherols)

RDA 10 mg.

Dietary sources (% RDA per 100 g in brackets)

The main dietary sources are vegetable oils and, to a lesser extent, grains and nuts.

Sources include: wheat germ oil (1000%), peanut oil (100%), olive oil (80%), coconut oil (10%), maize (10%), whole wheat (10%) and oats (8%) (Fig. 26.18).

Biological functions

Vitamin E exists as eight different closely related structures, four tocopherols and four tocophertrienols. Alpha-tocopherol is regarded as being the most important in humans. Whereas vitamin C functions as an antioxidant in an aqueous environment, vitamin E acts to protect lipophilic structures such as the phospholipids which make up cell membranes from oxidation. Fatty acids containing double bonds are prone to damage via peroxidation. Figure 26.19 shows the action of vitamin E in terminating free radical-generated peroxidation of an unsaturated fatty acid. If the radical were not quenched,

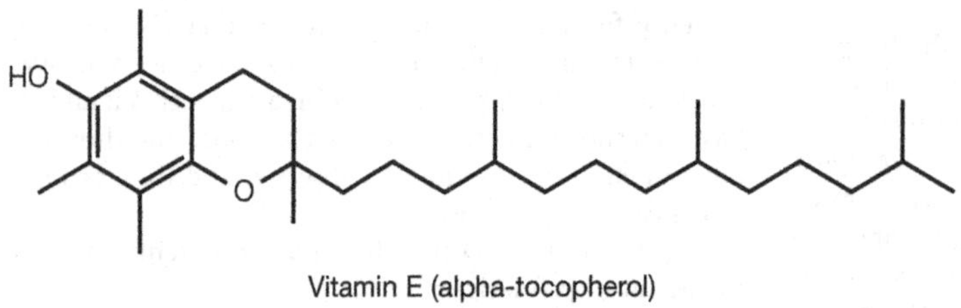

Figure 26.18 Vitamin E.

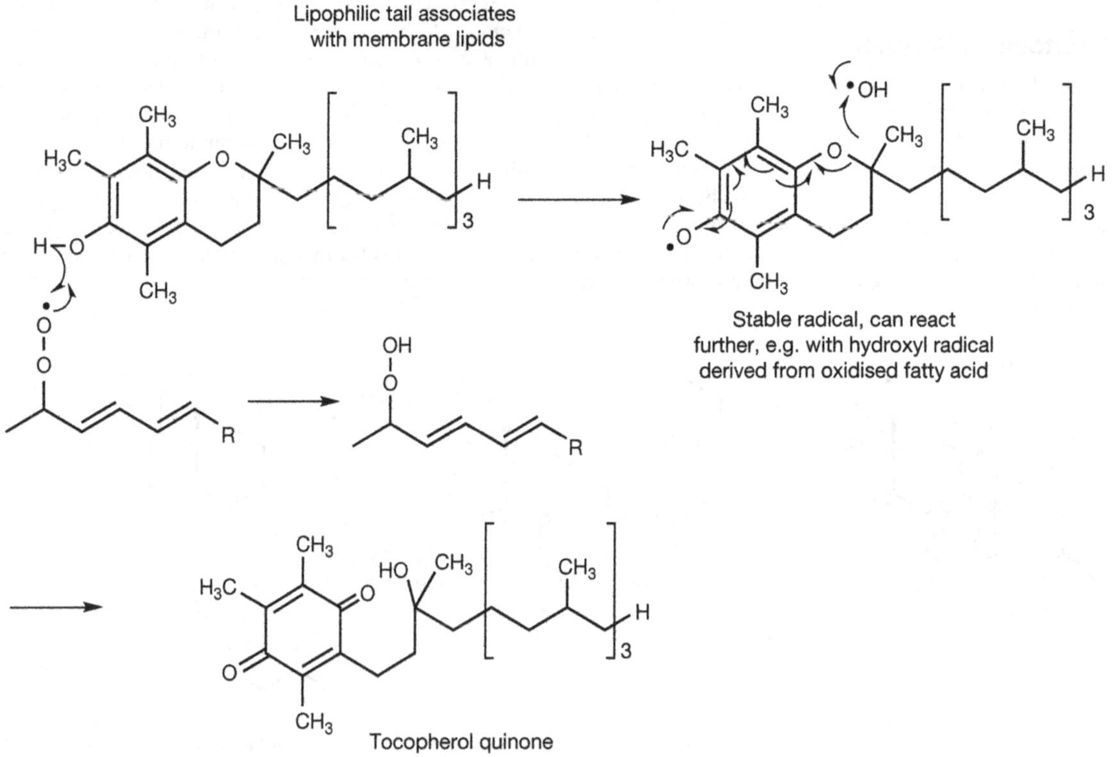

Figure 26.19 Termination of the propagation of oxidative damage to membrane lipids by vitamin E.

it would go on to initiate a chain reaction, damaging the membrane. The radical formed by vitamin E is quite stable and unreactive but can go on to react with a second radical such as hydroxyl (the most reactive of all radicals) to form tocopherol quinone. Vitamin E can be regenerated from tocopherol quinone by vitamin C as shown in Figure 26.15 or by another reducing compound such as glutathione. Many reactive oxygen species (ROS) are generated in the body and vitamin E plays an important role in protecting the body against them. A number of other roles have been identified for vitamin E including immune modulation and inhibition of platelet aggregation.

Symptoms of deficiency

Since vitamin E is lipophilic and thus efficiently stored by the body, acute deficiency is rarely observed. In conditions where there is malabsorption of fat, vitamin E deficiency may be observed. Deficiency of vitamin E is associated with loss of membrane function and this may be associated with: impaired balance, peripheral neuropathy, muscle weakness and damage to the retina.

Possible therapeutic indications

Several large studies have shown that adequate vitamin E intake or supplementation may reduce the risk of developing heart disease. However, there was no evidence that the vitamin reduced the likelihood of those with heart disease dying. There is some evidence that vitamin E can boost immune response in the elderly. There is no strong link between vitamin E supplementation and reduction of breast or lung cancer; however, there is strong evidence that vitamin E can reduce the incidence of prostate cancer. There is some evidence for effectiveness in treatment of diabetes and in reducing risk of developing dementia in the elderly. A number of studies have examined the effects of vitamin E on Parkinson's disease and there is evidence that it can play a preventative role. Since vitamin E may be oxidised to a quinine, which can act as an antagonist of vitamin K, in a manner similar to warfarin, people taking anticoagulants should not take high doses of vitamin E.

Toxicity

Vitamin E is one of the least toxic vitamins and is safe up to at least 100 × RDA (LD_{50} values in rats are 2 g/kg). The greatest risk in susceptible individuals is of haemorrhage due to vitamin K antagonist effects. However, at very high doses, vitamin E can antagonise other fat-soluble vitamins such as A and D.

Vitamin K

RDA 0.07 mg.

Dietary sources (% RDA per 100 g in brackets)

Green leafy vegetables are the major sources, while fruits are poor sources. Spinach (300%), cauliflower (250%), broccoli (200%), cabbage (200%), lettuce (150%), beef liver (100%), wheat bran (100%) and oats (100%) (Fig. 26.20).

Biological functions

Vitamin K is a co-factor for glutamyl carboxylase, which is responsible for the post-translational carboxylation of glutamyl residues in the clotting factors II, VII, IX and X (Fig. 26.21). The introduction of carboxyl groups into these proteins allows them to bind calcium, which is part of the clotting process. The anticoagulant drug warfarin interferes with the recycling of vitamin K epoxide back into its naphthoquinone form, resulting in a reduction in vitamin K levels and thus reduced tendency for clot formation. Paradoxically, vitamin K is also required for the anticlotting proteins, protein C and protein S. Vitamin K is also required for the activation of the calcium-binding proteins matrix gla protein and osteocalcin which are required for bone mineralisation. Like many vitamins, there are several structurally related forms of vitamin K.

Symptoms of deficiency

The symptom of vitamin K deficiency is increased risk of haemorrhage, ease of bruising, nose bleeding and blood in the urine. In infants, vitamin K deficiency may result in intracranial bleeding. Vitamin K deficiency is rare in adults although vitamin K status is assessed in the newborn and in the USA a routine injection of vitamin K is recommended for newborn babies, particularly premature babies where the vitamin K cycle may not be fully established. Human breast milk is relatively low in vitamin K. There has been some controversy over whether or not childhood leukaemia can be linked to injection of newborns with vitamin K, but a large retrospective study found no link. Certain drugs such as warfarin, sulphonamides and cephalosporins can affect vitamin K function.

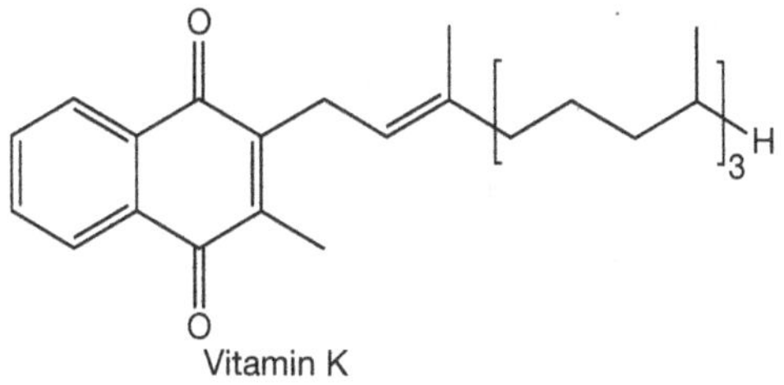

Figure 26.20 Vitamin K.

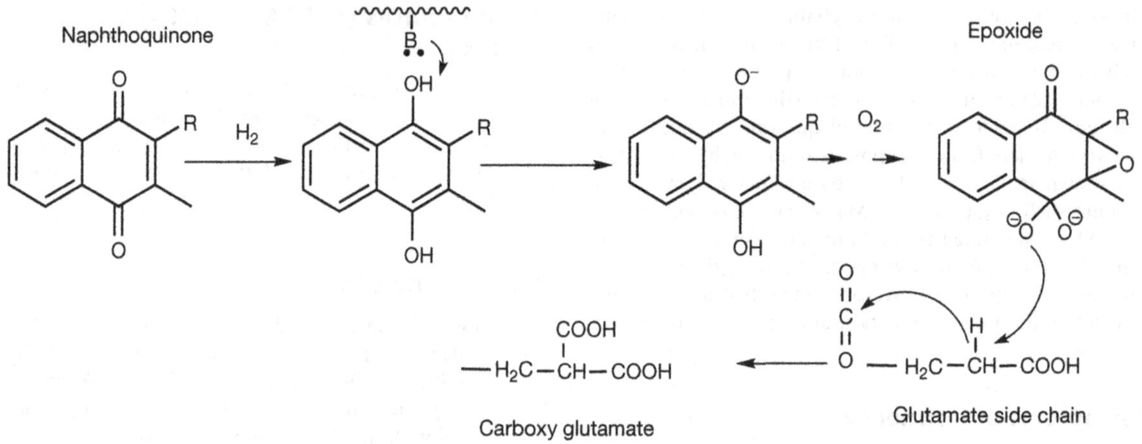

Figure 26.21 The role of vitamin K as a co-factor in the carboxylation of the glutamate side chain in clotting proteins.

Therapeutic indications

There is no strong evidence for vitamin K supplementation reducing the incidence of bone fracture in the elderly although there is some evidence that long-term therapy with anticoagulants such as warfarin can reduce bone density. There some evidence that vitamin K deficiency may promote calcification of atherosclerotic plaques through reducing the protective role afforded by carboxylated matrix gla protein.

Toxicity

Vitamin K has low toxicity, although a synthetic analogue menadione has been shown to cause jaundice and cell membrane damage when given by injection.

Biotin

RDA 0.07 mg.

Dietary sources (% RDA per 100 g in brackets)

Liver, nuts and eggs are the most important food sources for humans. Bioavailability is very variable. Sources include: molasses (150%), brewers yeast (100%), soybeans (100%), wheat bran (50%), walnuts (50%), peanuts (50%), oats (30%), eggs (15%) and cauliflower (15%) (Fig. 26.22).

Biological functions

Biotin is a di-alkyl urea and is a co-factor in four key carboxylase enzymes which are involved in fatty acid biosynthesis and amino acid metabolism. In order to function as a co-factor, biotin has to be linked covalently to the enzyme via a lysine group. It then functions as a carrier for a carboxyl group which is attached to a weakly basic urea nitrogen in the co-factor via reaction with carbonyl phosphate. Figure 26.23 shows the carboxylation of acetyl CoA by acetyl CoA carboxylase to form malonyl CoA; this is a crucial step in fatty acid biosynthesis. The other carboxylations which biotin participates in are the carboxylations of pyruvyl CoA (required in the formation of glucose from amino acids and fatty acids), propionyl CoA (required in the catabolism of amino acids and cholesterol) and methyl crotonyl CoA (required in the catabolism of leucine).

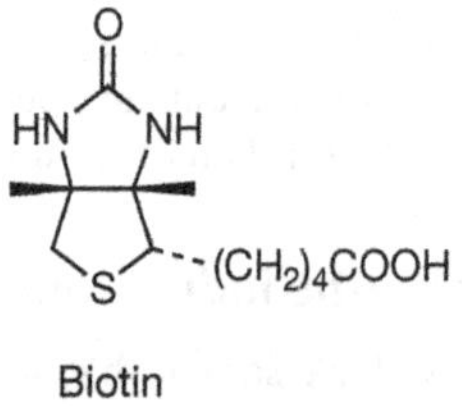

Figure 26.22 Biotin.

Biotin is also used in the modulation of histone activity. Histones are a family of proteins responsible for packaging DNA in order to form chromosomes. It is believed that attachment of biotin (biotinylation) helps reduce the binding of histones to DNA, thereby allowing DNA replication to occur.

In vitro biotinylation of amine and sulphhydryl groups within proteins is used as a method for tagging proteins in biochemical studies.

Symptoms of deficiency

Few cases of biotin deficiency have been reported in humans. There are some rare congenital disorders of biotin metabolism. However, it has been shown to occur

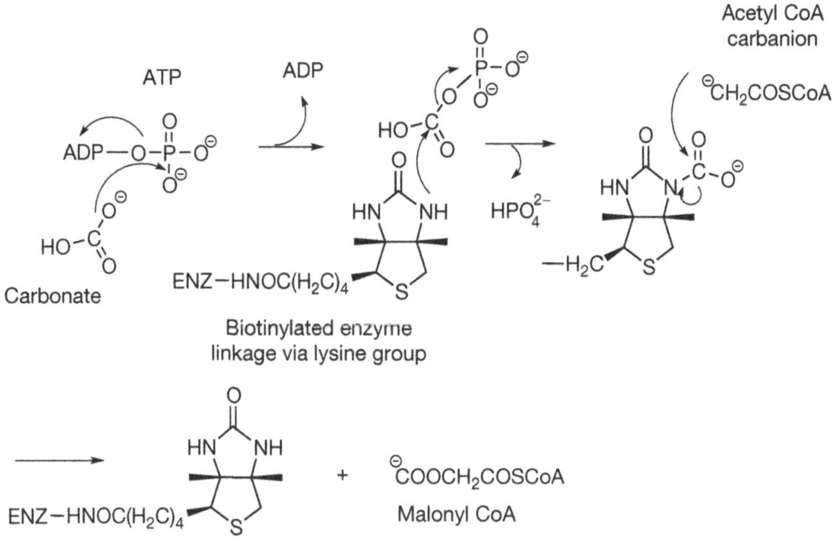

Figure 26.23 Carboxylation of malonyl CoA.

following extended consumption of raw eggs since egg white contains a protein avidin which binds to biotin and prevents its absorption. Cooking of eggs denatures the avidin. Symptoms of deficiency include: hair loss, a red rash on the face, unusual fat distribution and general depression and lethargy.

Therapeutic indications

Two rare hereditary disorders of biotin metabolism have been identified; these can both be treated by supplementation with high-dose biotin. There may be an increased requirement for biotin during pregnancy where cells are rapidly dividing and there is an increased requirement for DNA replication. Anticonvulsant medication used in treating epilepsy may deplete biotin. There is some evidence that biotin stimulates glycogen synthesis and thus may be useful as a supplement for diabetics. A number of trials indicated that biotin might be useful as a treatment for brittle nails. Biotin has been used for treating seborrhoeic dermatitis in infants.

Toxicity

The toxicity of biotin is low and doses of up to 200 mg per day are tolerated by those with hereditary disorders in biotin metabolism and doses of 5 mg per day have tolerated long term by non-deficient subjects.

Folate

RDA 0.2 mg (0.4 mg in pregnancy).

Dietary sources (% RDA per 100 g in brackets)

Folate is widely distributed in foodstuffs but is unstable to cooking and has reduced bioavailability in fruits and vegetables. Sources include: brewers yeast (800%), beef liver (100–500%), broccoli (100%), spinach (50%), Brussels sprouts (50%), peas (50%), wheat bran (40%), bananas (25%), oranges (15%) and tomatoes (15%) (Fig. 26.24).

Biological functions

Folic acid is important for the production of new cells and thus is particularly important during pregnancy. Its importance stems from its role as and acceptor/donor of one carbon unit which is a biochemical process required during DNA and RNA synthesis. In order to accept one carbon unit, folic acid is transported into the cell and trapped there by polyglutamylation. It is then reduced to tetrahydrofolate which can accept one carbon unit from

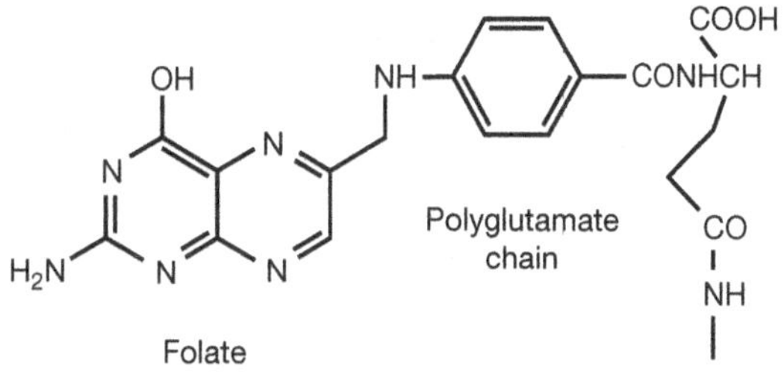

Figure 26.24 Folate.

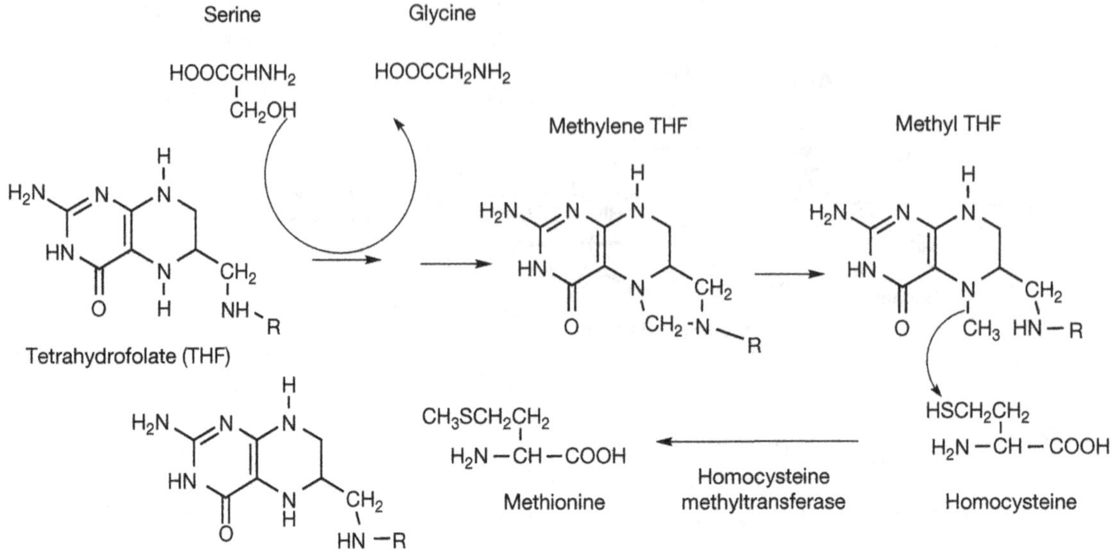

Figure 26.25 Methylation of homocysteine with methyl tetrahydrofolate as the co-factor.

several sources. Figure 26.25 shows the donation of a methyl group from methyltetrahydrofolate to homocysteine; the methyl unit is derived from serine, which is the most commonly used primary source of methyl groups. Tetrahydrofolate is involved in the methylation of some of the purines and pyrimidines used in DNA biosynthesis, including thymidine and all of the purines.

Figure 26.26 shows the role of formyl THF in the biosynthesis of inosine monophosphate which is subsequently elaborated to yield the purine bases used in DNA and RNA biosynthesis. Formyl THF, also known as leucovorin, is used to mitigate the myelosuppressive effects of methotrexate used in cancer chemotherapy which inhibits dihydrofolate reductase, thus reducing the levels of the various single carbon transfer forms of tetrahydrofolate.

Symptoms of deficiency

Folate deficiency can occur in alcoholics, pregnancy and dietary insufficiency. Deficiency results in changes in the red and white blood cells. Changes in the red blood cells lead to the same symptoms as pernicious anaemia which are observed in vitamin B_{12} deficiency. Increased levels of folate are required during pregnancy, lactation and rapid growth.

Therapeutic indications

Folate supplementation is often given in pregnancy where its deficiency can lead to birth defects resulting from defects in neural tube development such as spina bifida, anencephaly and encephalocele. The critical point where adequate folic acid levels are required is between 21 and 27 days post-conception where most women do not realise they are pregnant. Fortification of foodstuffs with folic acid has reduced the incidence of spina bifida greatly and it is recommended that women of childbearing age should take supplements of folic acid at 400 μg per day. There is no strong evidence that folic acid can reduce the risk of developing heart disease although it can reduce the levels of the risk factor homocysteine in plasma. Folate may reduce the risk of developing colorectal cancer and breast cancer although supplementation with high levels of folic acid may actually accelerate tumour growth. Supplementation may also be important in the elderly who exhibit depressed levels of folate, and adequate levels of folate may be important in reducing the risk of developing Alzheimer's disease.

Toxicity

The toxicity of the vitamin is low and it is safe up to at least 10 × RDA even in pregnant women. There is a risk that taking folic acid supplements may mask some of the effects of vitamin B_{12} deficiency without solving the underlying problem, thus resulting in neurological damage. Some drugs and xenobiotics reduce folate utilisation including ethanol, aspirin, ibuprofen, trimethoprim, pyrimethamine, phenytoin and phenobarbital.

Niacin

RDA 17 mg.

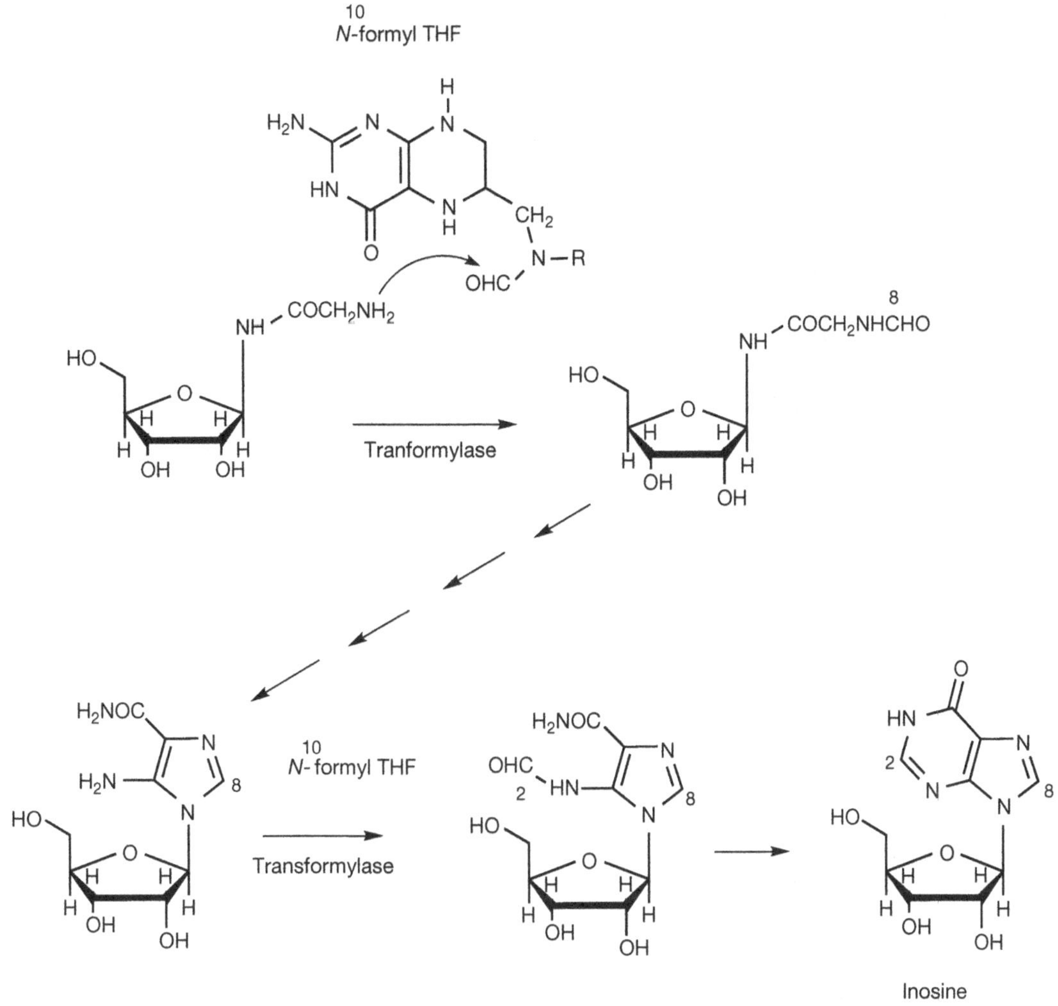

Figure 26.26 The role of formyl tetrahydrofolate in the synthesis of purines

Dietary sources (% RDA per 100 g in brackets)

Niacin is widely distributed in foodstuffs and can also be derived from tryptophan and thus the tryptophan content of food is also an important source. Sources include: brewers yeast (300%), peanuts (100%), tuna (75%), wheat bran (50–200%), chicken (30–80%), mushrooms (25%), brown rice (25%) and peppers (20%) (Fig. 26.27).

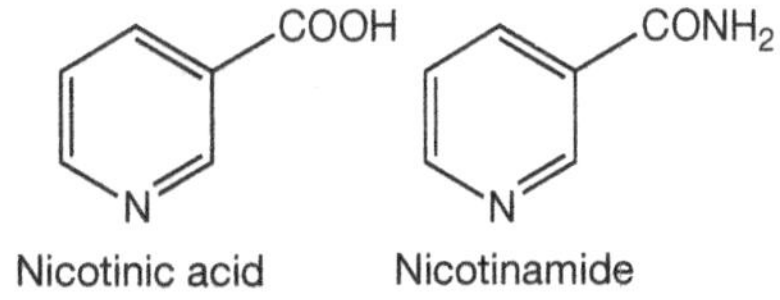

Figure 26.27 Forms of niacin.

Biological functions

Niacin in the form of nicotinamide functions as an essential component of the enzyme co-factors NAD(H) and NADP(H) which are involved in approximately 200 enzyme reactions. NADH is involved extensively in energy metabolism where glucose in metabolised to produce ATP, the main energy storage molecule in the body. NAD and NADH function as a redox pair, where in some cases NADH acts as a reducing agent and in other cases NAD acts as an oxidising agent. This is illustrated in Figure 26.28 which shows the maleate-aspartate shuttle which is required to effectively transport NADH through the inner membrane of the mitochondrion, which is impermeable to NADH, into the mitochondrial matrix where it can enter the electron transport chain which

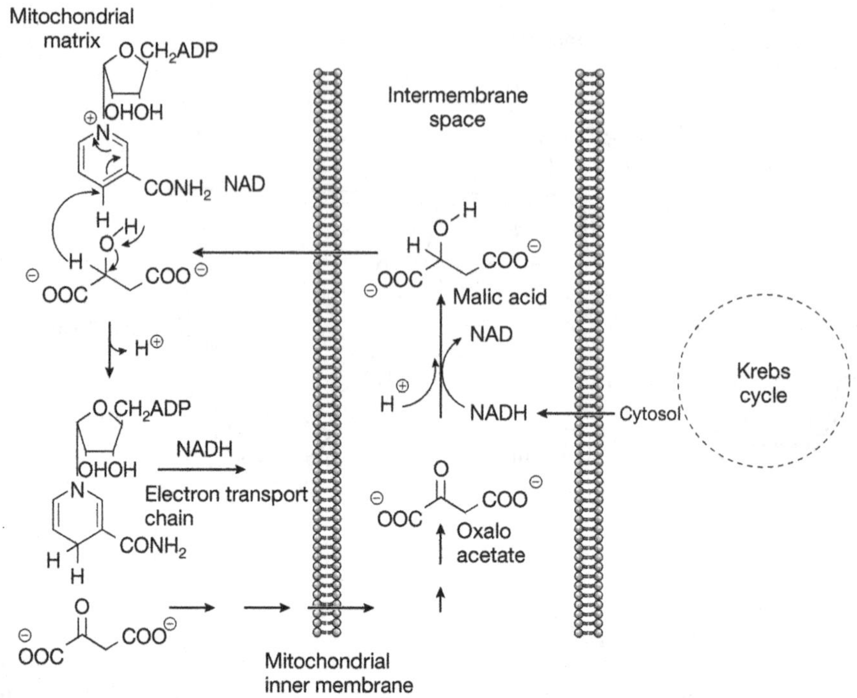

Figure 26.28 Oxidation and reduction by NAD and NADH in the maleate–aspartate shuttle.

results in the production of ATP. To achieve this, NADH produced in the cytosol by the Krebs cycle is used to reduce oxaloacetate to malic acid in the intermembrane space which is then transported into the mitochondrion where it is then oxidised by NAD to produce NADH.

Although NADPH only differs from NADH by addition of a phosphate group, it is used for different purposes, being used purely for reduction, not oxidation, and thus it is used in anabolic processes such as synthesis of fatty acids. In addition to redox reactions, NAD fulfils another important function which is in the transfer of the ADP-ribose portion of the molecule to a protein substrate, releasing nicotinamide as a side product. The ADP-ribose is attached to glutamate, aspartate or arginine side chains. This process has an important role in cell signalling. A number of bacterial toxins are ADP-ribosyl tranferases; for instance, cholera toxin ADP-ribosylates G-proteins, which provokes high levels of fluid secretion in the gut and thus life-threatening diarrhoea.

Symptoms of deficiency

The most marked indication of niacin deficiency is pellagra, where the skin is reddened as if sunburned on exposed surfaces along with cracking and shedding of the skin, inflammation of the tongue and diarrhoea. Pellagra was quite common in previous centuries in areas where the staple cereal was maize because although niacin is present in corn it is not readily bioavailable from this source. Niacin can also be synthesised by the body from dietary tryptophan although the conversion is not that efficient.

Therapeutic indications

There is some evidence that niacin can reduce the incidence of cancers of the mouth and throat. Niacin has been used to protect β-cells in the pancreas in insulin-dependent diabetics and has been reported to increase insulin sensitivity. The effects of niacin in lowering cholesterol and low density lipoprotein have been studied extensively. High doses up to 1 g per day are required but the evidence for effectiveness is not wholly conclusive. There is some evidence that high doses of niacin improve survival rates in HIV infection. In conjunction with tryptophan, niacin has been used to treat depression.

Niacin has been used to stimulate tooth eruption and gastric motility.

Toxicity

The vitamin is safe to at least 10 × RDA. However, high doses can produce side effects including flushing, hives and GI discomfort and even liver toxicity. High doses of nicotinamide are generally better tolerated than high doses of nicotinic acid.

ESSENTIAL ELEMENTS

Introduction

The major elements used in bulk by organisms are: hydrogen, sodium, potassium, magnesium, calcium, carbon, nitrogen, oxygen, phosphorus, sulphur and chlorine.

In addition, there are a number of essential trace elements which include: iron, copper, zinc, nickel, manganese, chromium, molybdenum, boron, silicon, selenium, iodine and fluorine. For some organisms vanadium is required. It is possible that tungsten, arsenic, tin and bromine may also possibly be essential trace elements.

Sodium

RDA 1600 mg.

Dietary sources

Most foodstuffs.

Biological functions

Osmotic control and maintenance of blood volume, conduction of electrical impulses, stability of DNA and membranes. Potassium is more much more abundant within cells and sodium is confined to extracellular fluids.

Symptoms of deficiency

Sodium deficiency is rare under normal circumstances but where excessive loss of sodium chloride through perspiration occurs salt intake may have to be increased. It also has to be replaced when electrolytes are lost through diarrhoea and vomiting.

Therapeutic indications

Sodium deficiency is corrected by infusions in severe cases or using oral rehydration salts to replace sodium lost by vomiting or perspiration. Extensive studies have been made on the effect of salt intake on blood pressure; however, the actual effects of a reduction in the diet remain controversial. Excessive sodium levels have been linked to hypertension but this is probably only in a subpopulation of susceptible individuals.

Toxicity

Ingestion of excessive amounts of salt results in nausea, vomiting, diarrhoea and abdominal cramps.

Potassium

RDA 3500 mg.

Dietary sources

Dried apricots, prunes, banana, baked potatoes, spinach.

Biological functions

Similar roles to sodium. Important for maintaining low blood pressure.

Symptoms of deficiency

An abnormally low plasma potassium concentration is referred to as hypokalaemia. Hypokalaemia results most commonly from loss of potassium as a result of prolonged vomiting, the use of some diuretics, some forms of kidney disease and metabolic disturbances. Symptoms of hypokalaemia include fatigue, muscle weakness and cramps, and intestinal paralysis. Acute hypokalaemia may result in cardiac arrhythmias that can be fatal.

Therapeutic indications

High dietary potassium has been linked to lower blood pressure, and dietary supplementation with moderate amounts of potassium has been found to lower blood pressure. Many drugs have effects in either raising or lowering potassium levels in the body. Levels are raised by digoxin, trimethoprim-sulfamethoxazole, ibuprofen, ACE inhibitors, angiotensin receptor blockers, spironolactone and heparin. Levels of potassium are lowered by diuretics, corticosteroids pseudoephedrine, some penicillins, carbenoxolone, caffeine and theophylline.

Toxicity

Excessive potassium levels can lead to cardiac arrest. People on non-steroidal anti-inflammatory drugs, ACE inhibitors and potassium-sparing diuretics should seek medical advice before taking potassium supplements.

Calcium

RDA 800 mg (children 400–600 mg).

Dietary sources

Milk, cheese, broccoli, kale, sweet potatoes, canned salmon with bones, sardines, calcium fortified orange juice.

Biological function

Calcium is the positively charged equivalent of phosphate, producing mechanical effects within organisms. Thus potassium causes vasoconstriction and vasodilation. When a muscle fibre receives a nerve impulse, ion channels in the muscle cell open, allowing calcium ions to enter the cell, which results in displacement of calcium ions stored within the cell, and finally binding of the calcium ions to proteins in the cell that cause the cell to contract and thus produce muscle movement. Calcium binds to negatively charged groups on proteins, particularly glutamate, causing the conformation of the protein to change as shown in Figure 26.29. The effectiveness of calcium in this type of activity relates to its high charge density and relatively large atomic radius so that it can interact with several carboxylate groups. The ability of calcium to bind to proteins and change their shape also is important in other protein systems apart from muscle cells. Thus calcium binds to enzymes which are involved in phosphorylation and de-phosphorylation, not actually at the active site but influencing the effect of the active site on the substrate (allosteric binding). The role of calcium in blood clotting and bone mineralisation has been discussed under vitamin K and vitamin D, respectively.

Symptoms of deficiency

Low blood levels of calcium are often associated with malfunction of the parathyroid gland but this is rarely due to calcium deficiency in the tissues since the skeleton contains large amounts of reserve calcium. Other causes include alcoholism, low magnesium intake and vitamin D deficiency. Low calcium levels cause muscular twitching and in the extreme case tetany. Calcium intake may be of concern in the elderly if not enough dairy products are being consumed, and also in vegans. High-fibre diets can reduce calcium absorption.

Therapeutic indications

It is recommended that elderly people increase their calcium intake to prevent osteoporosis. Calcium has been implicated in the prevention of colon cancer through helping in the elimination of bile acids and fat from the colon.

Toxicity

Excessive consumption of calcium can cause kidney stones and constipation.

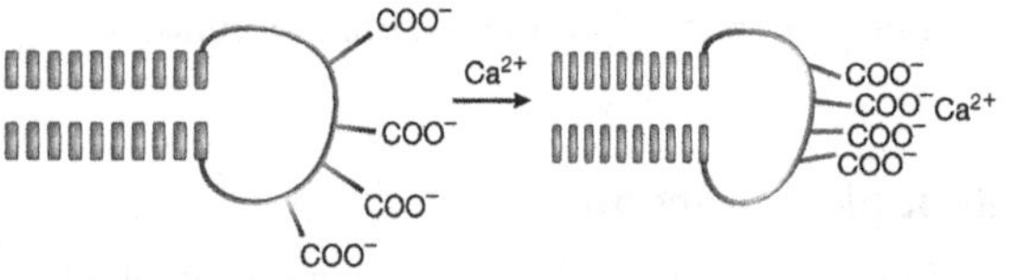

Figure 26.29 The action of calcium in trigger proteins. The binding of the calcium ion to the negatively charged carboxyl groups causes the protein to change shape and the helices to contract.

Magnesium

RDA 300 mg.

Dietary sources

Brown rice, avocados, spinach, haddock, oatmeal, baked potatoes, broccoli, yoghurt, bananas.

Biological roles

The magnesium ion has the highest charge density of any element used in biology (charge/atomic radius). Magnesium is strongly associated with di- and triphosphates which are highly negatively charged and can balance the high positive charge on the magnesium. This makes magnesium the most important cation at the active site of enzyme reactions involving phosphorylation/de-phosphorylation. Thus Mg^{2+} has an important role in stabilising and energising biomolecules containing phosphate groups such as ATP, GTP, DNA, RNA, phospholipids and polysaccharides such as phosphoinositols. For example, in the active site of a kinase (phosphorylating enzyme) the transfer of the phosphate group is assisted by Mg^{2+} moving away from ATP, thus destabilising it and facilitating transfer of a phosphate group to the substrate (Fig. 26.30) Thus it has a role in the energetic processes of the cell. It also has a role in cell division through its effects on DNA and RNA replication and it is involved in cholesterol biosynthesis though its association with pyrophosphate in isopentenyl pyrophosphate.

Symptoms of deficiency

Low magnesium levels can increase muscular cramp and muscle weakness and cause changes in heart muscle. Magnesium deficiency can occur in alcoholism, in association with gastrointestinal disorders, after treatment with diuretics and as a result of severe renal disease.

Therapeutic indications

There is some evidence that low serum magnesium levels are associated with the development of hypertension. There is a clear therapeutic use for high-dose magnesium infusions in the treatment of the life-threatening condition pre-eclampsia, characterised by seizures, which can occur during pregnancy. This has been the treatment of choice for many years and it is believed that the Mg^{2+} relieves cerebral blood vessel spasm. This is possibly the reason why there is some evidence that Mg^{2+} may be an effective treatment for migraine headaches. It also has been used to prevent ventricular arrhythmia. High levels of calcium intake can result in magnesium depletion.

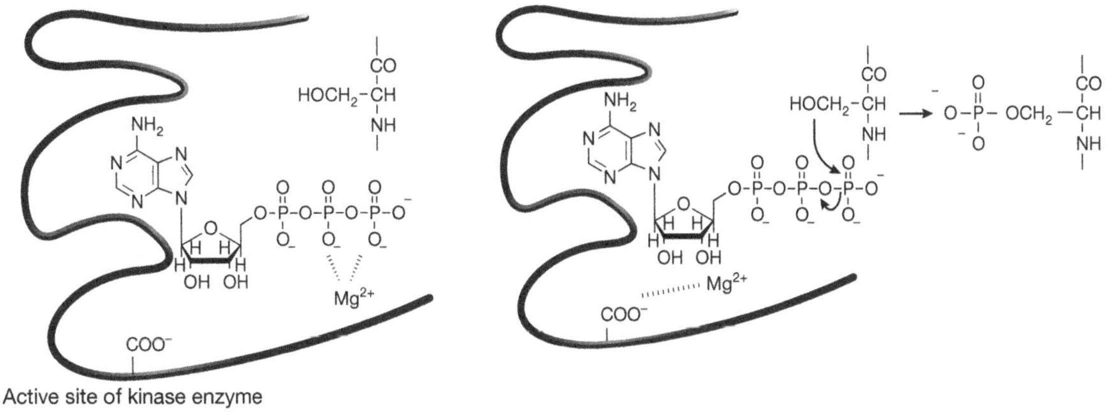

Figure 26.30 Role of magnesium in controlling the stability of ATP at the active site of a kinase. Mg moves away from ATP, destabilising it and making it more susceptible to nucleophilic attack by serine.

Toxicity

High levels of Mg^{2+} should not be taken by those with kidney conditions.

Iron

RDA 9 mg (men) 15 mg (women).

Dietary sources

Beef, baked potatoes, soybeans. Iron is only absorbed efficiently from meat in its haem form. Plants generally contain organic substances which complex with iron, reducing its bioavailability.

Biological functions

The main role of iron is as part of the haem molecule which becomes incorporated into a variety of haem proteins which are involved in oxygen carrying, oxidation and peroxidation reactions and in the transfer of electrons. The haem unit is bound into the active site of the enzyme by a sulphur atom attached to either a methionine or cysteine residue. Figure 26.31 shows the action of the haem unit within a cytochrome P450 (CyP450) enzyme. CyP450 enzymes are the most important enzymes in phase I metabolism of drugs and xenobiotics and also in the synthesis of hormones such as the steroid hormones.

Symptoms of deficiency

Iron deficiency is the most common nutrient deficiency in the world. Iron deficiency manifests as hypochromic anaemia where the red blood cells are pale in colour and this manifests as pale skin, tiredness, headache and palpitations. People most at risk of iron deficiency include: babies between the ages of 6 months and 4 years; adolescents, particularly adolescent girls who have commenced menstruation; pregnant women; people with gluten intolerance; vegetarians because of the low levels of iron in vegetables compared with meat; and athletes.

Therapeutic indications

Bleeding haemorrhoids, frequent nose bleeds, heavy menstruation and ulcers can all cause iron deficiency and such deficiencies can be aggravated by poor diet. Iron in its ferrous sulphate form may be the best absorbed. Iron supplementation is recommended for pregnant women.

Toxicity

A daily intake of iron of >25 mg per day for an extended period may cause undesirable side effects. Symptoms of iron poisoning include diarrhoea, vomiting and shock. When iron tablets are taken, they are best taken with food to reduce stomach upset.

Zinc

RDA 9 mg.

Dietary sources

Oysters, beef, lamb, eggs, whole grains, nuts and yoghurt.

Biological functions

Zinc (Zn^{2+}) is the mineral equivalent of vitamin C in that it appears to have many functions and can almost be regarded as a hormone. Its role in biology is due to a combination of the fact that it binds readily to a variety of

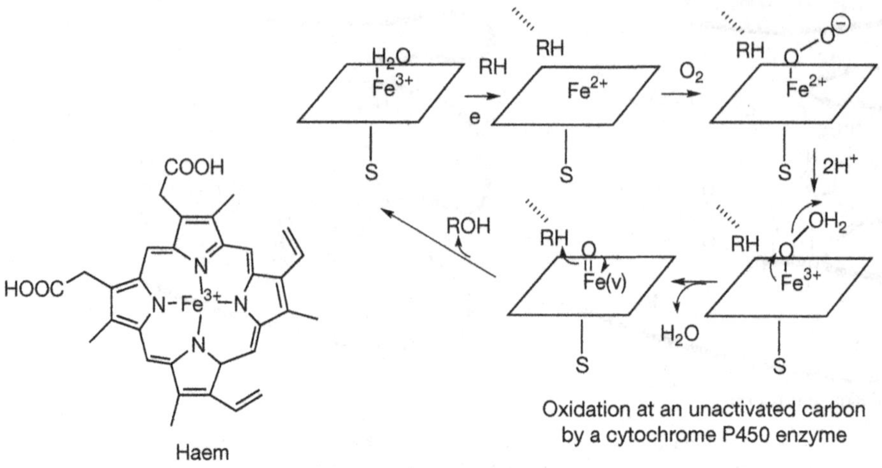

Figure 26.31 The function of the haem unit in a cytochrome P450 monoxygenase enzyme.

ligands and is capable of rapid off/on ligand exchange. Zinc is present at the active sites of hydrolytic enzymes: proteases, nucleotidases, collagenase. Figure 26.32 shows the proposed mechanism for zinc at the active site of a peptidase enzyme, e.g. carboxypeptidase, which hydrolyses terminal amino acids in proteins. At the active site of the enzyme zinc binds to water, making the water more basic so that it can attack the peptide bond. This type of mechanism is used in all the hydrolytic activities of zinc enzymes. Zinc is also involved in many of the enzymes associated with DNA synthesis: RNA polymerase, reverse transcriptase, tRNA synthetase. It is also involved with other key enzymes: carbonic anhydrase, alcohol dehydrogenase and phospholipase C.

Zinc cross-links proteins in a manner similar to S–S bridges. For example, insulin may be formulated as its zinc complex in order to produce a slow-release form of the drug. In the body, this cross-linking results in the formation of zinc fingers in receptor proteins which are important binding sites for hormones such as corticosteroids.

Symptoms of deficiency

These include impaired immunity, weight loss, loss of taste and smell, loss of appetite, skin rashes and depression. Some people may be borderline zinc deficient. Accelerated rates of wound healing and improved appetite and taste acuity occurred when these people were

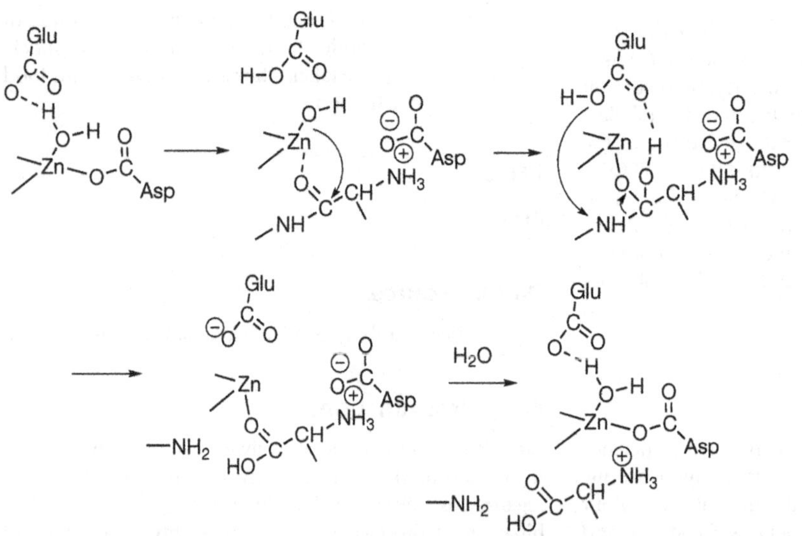

Figure 26.32 The role of zinc at the active site or a peptidase.

supplemented with zinc. Zinc deficiency may occur in pregnant women, young children and strict vegetarians.

Therapeutic indications

Zinc supplementation has been proposed to be useful in accelerating development in premature babies. Zinc is important for male fertility. Zinc has effects on the immune system and it has been shown that zinc in combination with oral rehydration therapy decreases duration and severity of acute childhood diarrhoea which affects over 3 million children in developing countries each year. Zinc lozenges have been used in treating the common cold but there is no strong evidence that they are effective; combining zinc with vitamin C may be more effective. Zinc may have some effect in promotion of wound repair. Its oxide, of course, has been used for many years in creams for treating nappy rash and in calamine lotion where it shows antipruritic properties.

Toxicity

Large amounts of zinc (2000 mg) cause vomiting. Even taking >30 mg daily can interfere with copper absorption. Taking supplements of >15 mg per day for prolonged periods would not generally be advisable. Zinc nasal sprays for treating colds should be avoided since they can cause a loss of the sense of smell.

Copper

RDA 2 mg.

Dietary sources

Oysters, nuts, seeds, cocoa powder, beans, whole grains, mushrooms.

Biological functions

In some senses enzymes with copper at their active sites act in an opposite manner to those with zinc at their active sites. Copper-based enzymes are responsible for carrying out oxidation reactions which lead to formation of organic structural polymers such a collagen and melanin (responsible for protection against UV radiation). Copper-based enzymes have two copper atoms in the Cu(I) oxidation state at their active site to which molecular oxygen becomes bound. Figure 26.33 shows the action of the copper-based enzyme tyrosinase which oxidises the amino acid tyrosine to produce dopachrome, the precursor of the melanin pigments.

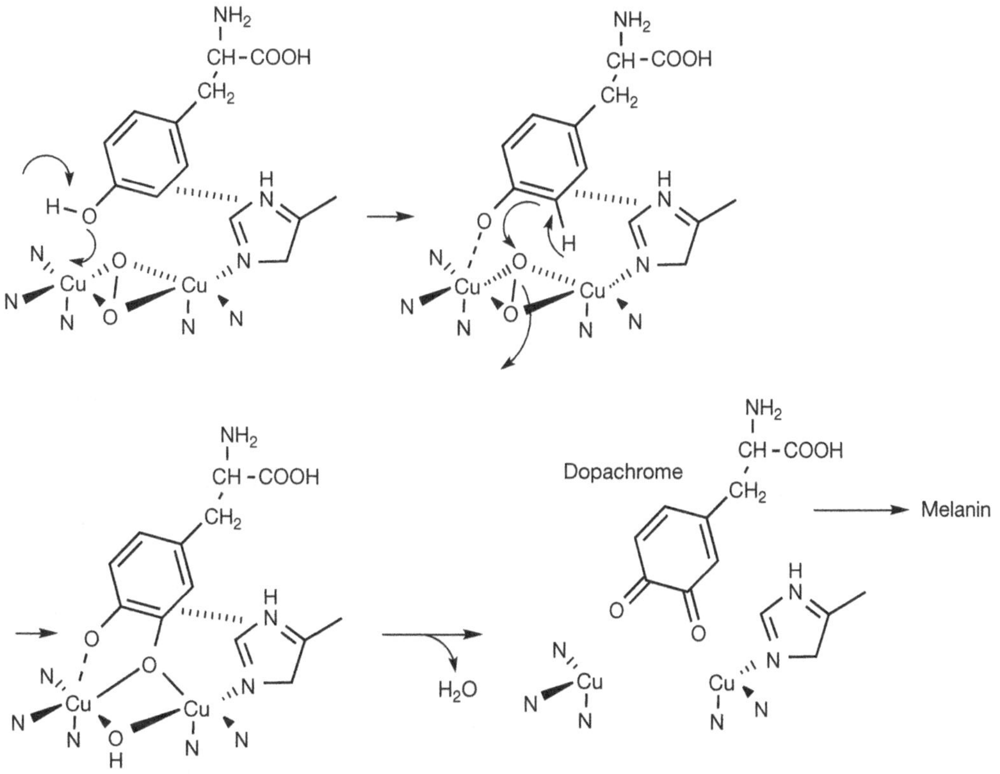

Figure 26.33 Oxidation of tyrosine to dopachrome by tyrosinase.

Copper is also present in amine oxidase which terminates the action of many nitrogenous drugs and neurotransmitters such as adrenaline by converting them to aldehydes and also in enzymes which reduce O_2 to H_2O, thus protecting cells against oxidation.

Symptoms of deficiency

Copper-deficient animals have weakened hearts and blood vessels and bone defects similar to those observed in osteoporosis.

Therapeutic indications

Dietary copper deficiency is rare, although both zinc and ascorbic acid can interfere with copper absorption.

Toxicity

Copper in large amounts >20 mg is poisonous. There should be no need to take supplement with more than 3 mg of copper per day.

Manganese

RDA 2.5 mg.

Dietary sources

Pineapple juice, wheat bran, wheat germ, whole grains, seeds, nuts, cocoa, shellfish, tea.

Biological functions

Manganese is involved in carbohydrate, lipid and protein metabolism and is required for the synthesis of glycoproteins and mucopolysaccharides such as hyaluronic acid. It is also involved in glucose metabolism. In plants, it is involved in the enzyme that splits water into oxygen and hydrogen.

Symptoms of deficiency

Animals which are manganese deficient have malformed bones which are similar to those observed in osteoporosis. They also have problems with their tendons.

Therapeutic indications

Manganese is widely distributed in food, and deficiency in humans is unlikely.

Toxicity

Amounts of manganese up to 10 mg daily have been found to be safe although there is little reason to take >3 mg. Industrial exposure to manganese has resulted in the production of symptoms similar to Parkinson's disease.

Cobalt

RDA Unknown.

Dietary sources

Dairy and other animal products.

Biological function

Cobalt occurs in vitamin B_{12} and this may be its only function. The free element appears to stimulate red cell formation although the mechanism for this is unknown.

Symptoms of deficiency

Cobalt deficiency in humans has not been observed.

Therapeutic indications

As for vitamin B_{12}.

Toxicity

No safe limit has been set for cobalt.

Chromium

RDA 0.1 mg.

Dietary sources

Brewers yeast, broccoli, ham, grape juice.

Biological functions

Chromium is involved in glucose metabolism and it appears to enhance the action of insulin. It is also involved in the action of a number of enzymes.

Symptoms of deficiency

Deficiency may be associated with glucose intolerance, which is associated with elevated cholesterol and glucose levels in plasma.

Therapeutic indications

Chromium is not common even in a balanced diet and thus supplements may be of value. It may benefit newly diagnosed diabetics who have mild glucose intolerance. It may also benefit those with low blood sugar levels since it promotes the action of insulin. Chromium is best absorbed in the form of its nicotinate or picolinate salts.

Toxicity

Amounts up to 1 mg per day have not been observed to exert toxic effects. The safety of dosages of 0.2 mg per day is well established. Chromium supplements may make insulin more effective in diabetics and thus care should be taken that too much insulin is not being taken.

Selenium

RDA 0.1 mg.

Dietary sources

Lobster, Brazil nuts, clams, crab, oysters and whole grains.

Biological functions

Selenium is involved in the protection of cells and membranes against oxidative damage and its action appears to be linked to the action of vitamin E. Selenium appears to have antiviral effects, for example on the AIDS virus. It is present in a number of proteins including glutathione peroxidase and in the form of the amino acid selenocystine.

Symptoms of deficiency

Dietary deficiencies have been associated with heart muscle damage.

Therapeutic indications

Environmental damage tends to reduce selenium levels in the soil and thus there is less selenium in the food chain. Selenium functions as an immunostimulant and antioxidant. It also binds toxic elements such as arsenic, cadmium and mercury. Supplements are best taken in the form of selenomethionine or selenocystine rather than selenite.

Toxicity

Selenium is toxic at 10–15 × RDA. One symptom of selenium toxicity is loss of hair and nails.

Molybdenum

RDA 0.5 mg.

Dietary sources

Beans, whole grains, cereals, milk, spinach.

Biological functions

Molybdenum is present in some enzymes, especially those required for purine metabolism, such as xanthine oxidase and metabolism of sulphur-containing compounds.

Symptoms of deficiency

Molybdenum deficiency is difficult to induce even in animals and no deficiency syndrome has been recognised in humans to date.

Therapeutic indications

There is little evidence of requirements for supplementation with molybdenum.

Toxicity

At levels 20 × RDA, it produces goutlike symptoms. Amounts >0.5 mg per day may interfere with copper metabolism.

Fluoride

RDA 2 mg.

Dietary sources

Fluoridated water, tea, canned salmon and mackerel.

Biological function

Cannot be regarded as essential although its incorporation into tooth enamel protects teeth from bacterial attack. Fluoride is also taken up by bone tissue, increasing its strength, although trials using it to treat osteoporosis have had mixed results.

Symptoms of deficiency

Not regarded as essential.

Toxicity

One cup of tea offers about 3 mg of fluoride. Up to 10 mg per day of fluoride is considered safe. Large amounts of fluoride may cause discolouration of teeth.

Chapter | 27 |

Biotechnologically produced products

David G. Watson

CHAPTER CONTENTS

PROTEINS AS DRUGS

Introduction

Proteins have been used successfully as drugs since the early twentieth century when insulin was first used to treat diabetes. The isolation of insulin was followed by the development of other protein drugs that were mainly extracted from animal tissues until the 1970s when smaller peptides, which had been discovered by extraction from animal tissues, became available via chemical synthesis. Table 27.1 lists some of these older protein drugs with their therapeutic actions.

In the case of small peptides with fewer than 20 amino acid residues, it is usually more economical to carry out chemical synthesis rather than to rely on biotechnology for production. Oxytocin with 9 amino acid residues is made synthetically. Calcitonin with 32 amino acid residues can be made synthetically but the rDNA product salcitonin (salmon calcitonin) is the main product in use. For peptides with more than 50 amino acid residues, it is unlikely that synthesis will ever compete with rDNA/biotechnological methods.

Disadvantages and advantages of protein drugs

After the difficulties of producing a drug using biotechnology have been overcome, there are other major difficulties in both registration and administration of the drug:

1. The drug may be contaminated by related biological materials such as DNA, viral protein and proteins from the cells used to produce the drug.
2. Analysis of macromolecules is difficult because of their complex structures. It would be very easy for small amounts of contaminating material to escape quality control procedures.
3. There are problems with the administration of peptide drugs since they have to be taken by injection. This limits market penetration since injection of drugs is acceptable for acute or life-threatening conditions but would not be popular as a long-term option for less serious conditions.
4. New drug delivery systems are being developed to produce nasal or pulmonary delivery, for example of calcitonin and insulin. However, no really successful system has been developed so far.
5. On the more positive side, about 68% of biotechnologically produced drugs reaching the stage of clinical trials are successful compared with <25% of drugs derived from chemical synthesis.
6. In the long term, peptide drugs will become more widely used therapeutic agents but at the moment the cost is prohibitive and also side effects of some of the drugs may be severe. The largest growth of licensed drugs in this area is in therapeutic monoclonal antibodies.

Production of peptide drugs by chemical synthesis

Automated peptide synthesis is quite routine now, although the expense of the reagents and difficulty of purification when more than 20 amino acids are incorporated into a peptide means that it is only viable for smaller peptides.

In order to synthesise a peptide, one end has to be protected so that the amino acid does not polymerise with itself. Also, if the side chain of the amino acid has an acidic or a basic group, it also has to be protected so that it does not become modified by the amino acid which is being added to extend the chain. The peptide is synthesised by protecting the carboxylic acid group of the first amino acid in the sequence by linking via esterification onto a resin (Fig. 27.1). The most commonly used resins these days are the Wang resins. The carboxylic acid ester is formed with a benzyl alcohol group which makes it a bit more labile than a link to an aliphatic alcohol. The amine group on each amino acid used in extending the chain is protected by a fluorenyloxy carbonyl (FMOC) group. This group can be removed in order to extend the chain using the base piperazine. If the amino acids contain side chains with either an acid or an amine group in them, e.g. lysine or glutamic acid, these groups are protected with either tertiary butyloxy carbonyl (tBOC) or by esterification with tertiary butanol, respectively. Importantly, the groups protecting the side chain are not removed by piperazine treatment and remain in place until the finished peptide is cleaved from the resin with trifluoroacetic acid which also removes the side chain protecting groups. As indicated above, this process is generally only viable for peptides with less than 20 amino acids. However, technology advances, and Roche have recently licensed Fuzeon™ which is a 36 amino acid synthetic peptide used in the treatment of AIDS. Figure 27.2 shows two examples of synthetic peptides used as drugs. Although these drugs are made by peptide synthesis methods, some of the amino acids have been modified so they are not entirely made up of naturally occurring amino acids. Octreotide is used to treat the symptoms produced by neuroendocrine tumours and also in reducing vomiting during palliative care. It is an analogue of somastatin, a tetradecapeptide

Table 27.1 Old peptide and protein pharmaceuticals

Peptide	Physical characteristics	Source	Therapeutic actions
Octreotide	8 amino acids synthetic somatostatin analogue	Chemical synthesis	Relief of the side effects produced by neuroendocrine tumours
Oxytocin	9 amino acids cyclic peptide	Chemical synthesis	Induction of uterine contractions to promote childbirth
Vassopressin and desmopressin	9 amino acids cyclic peptides	Chemical synthesis	Antidiuretic hormones used in treatment of diabetes insipidus
Tetracosactide	24 amino acids	Chemical synthesis	Used to test for adrenocortical insufficiency
Glucagon	30 amino acids	Bovine or porcine pancreas or synthetic	Reversal of insulin induced hypoglycaemia
Calcitonin	33 amino acids	Porcine thyroid, salmon or synthesis	Lowers plasma Ca levels in hypercalcaemia, treatment of Paget's disease
Insulin	51 amino acids Two chains linked by 2 S-S bridges	Bovine or porcine pancreas. *ca.* 98% pure	First used in 1922 to treat diabetes
Human growth hormone	191 amino acids	Human pituitary gland	Treatment of short stature resulting from deficiency of the hormone
Gonadotrophins	30 kDa	Relatively impure preparations extracted from human urine or placenta	Mainly used in the treatment of infertility in women associated with hypopituitarism
Streptokinase	46 kDa protein	Streptococci	First used in 1967 to dissolve blood clots
Albumin	67 kDa	Human blood	Replacement of human plasma proteins
Blood coagulation factors e.g. factor VIII	330 kDa	Human blood	Used to treat haemophilia
Vaccines	High molecular weight proteins	Infective organisms May be live but inactive pathogen, crude extract from dead pathogen or partly purified	Stimulation of the immune system to develop B-lymphocyte memory cells which recognise pathogen
Immunoglobulins	150 kDa or greater	Obtained from pooled human blood	Mixture of antibodies which can confer short-term resistance to a variety of pathogens, e.g. hepatitis A

which acts on the hypothalamus, inhibiting release of various hormones. It is used particularly to treat carcinoid tumour, which is a gastrointestinal tumour which secretes large amounts of serotonin. The tumour expresses somastatin receptors, and octreotide as a potent agonist for these receptors is effective in suppressing serotonin secretion. Lanreotide is another synthetic peptide which is used in treating carcinoid tumour and also thyroid tumours.

Buserelin is, again, a peptide-like structure with some natural and some unnatural amino acids in its structure. It is an agonist of gonadotropin releasing hormone and is used to treat prostate cancer (see Ch. 21) by suppressing the release of testosterone by the tumour. There are a number of other peptide analogues in the same category: goserelin, leuprorelin and triptorelin.

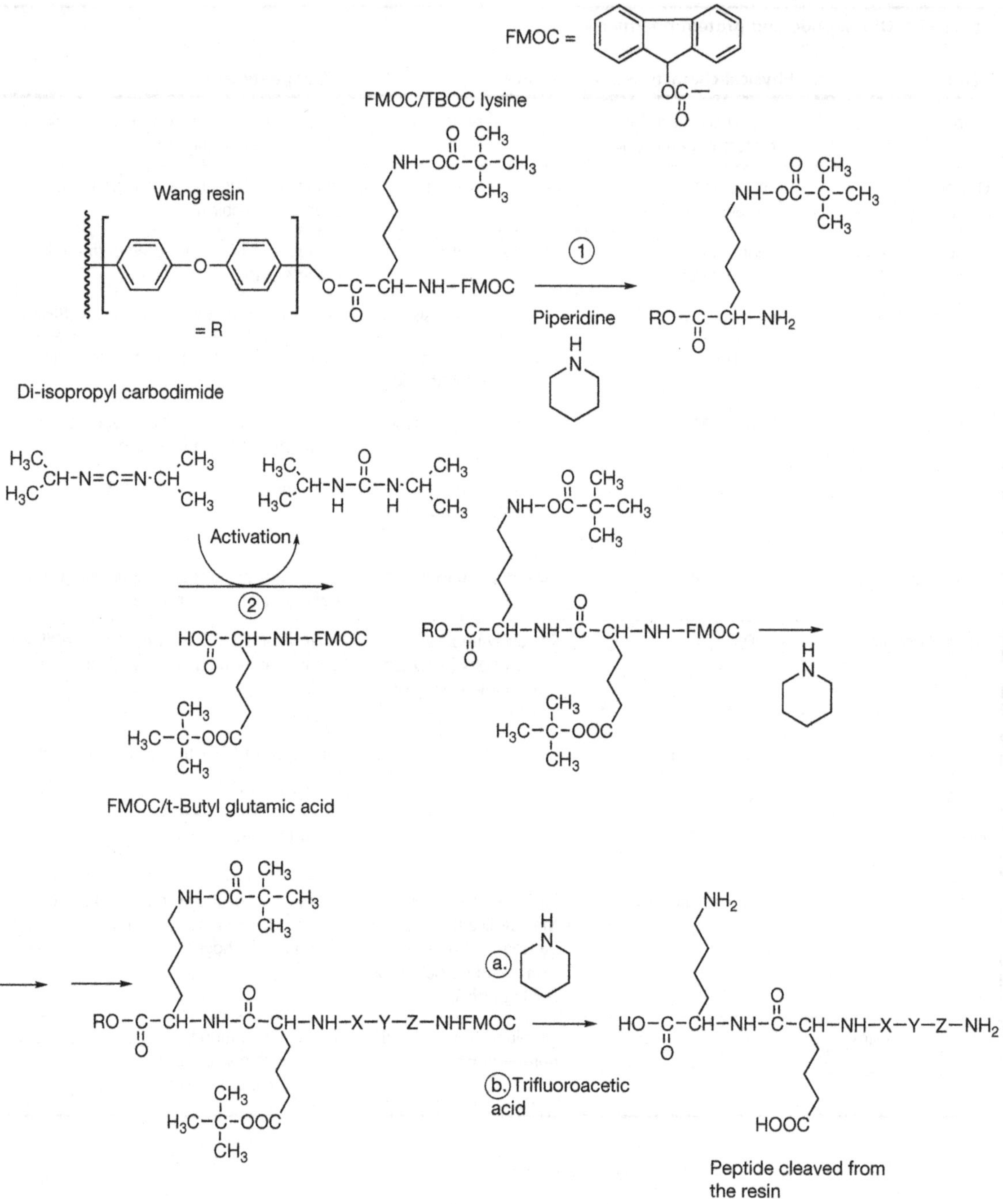

Figure 27.1 Typical procedure for resin-based synthesis of a peptide.

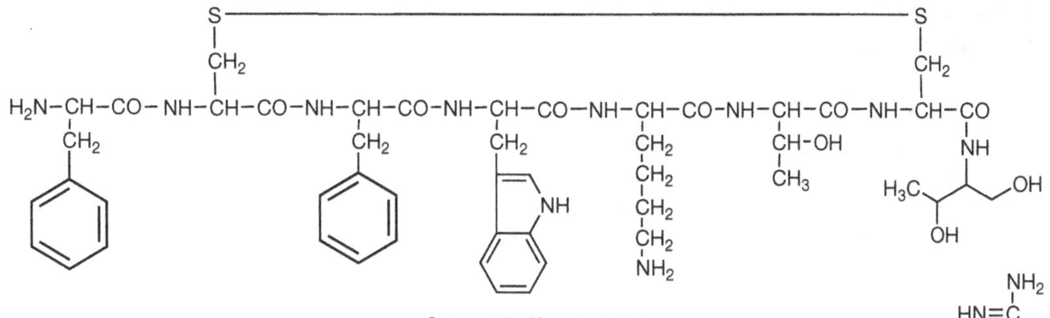

Octreotide (Sandostatin)

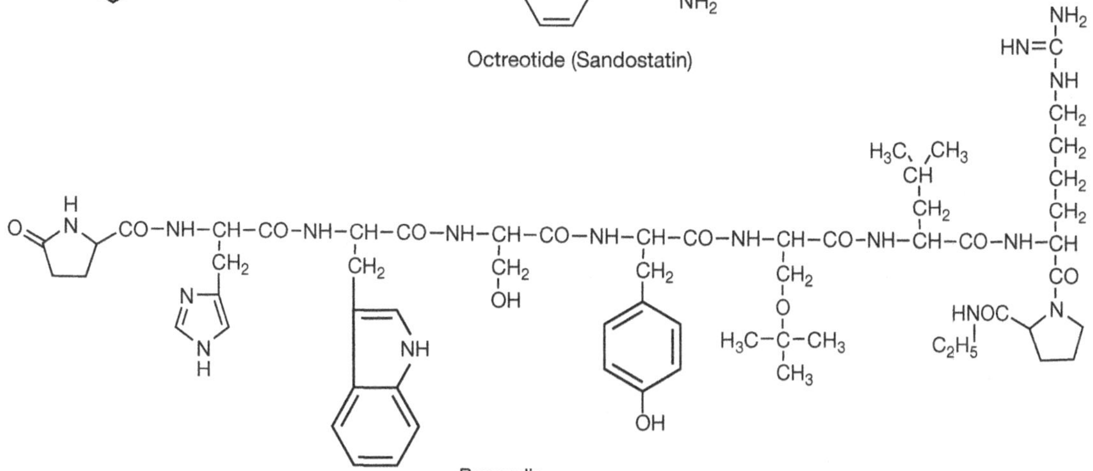

Buserelin

Figure 27.2 Synthetic peptide drugs.

> **Q Self Test 27.1**
>
> Draw the full structures of the synthetic peptide drugs lanreotide and goserelin.

Synthetic peptide drugs

Somatostatin analogues

- Octreotide: Octreotide acetate injection 50 μg/mL, 100 μg/mL, 200 μg/mL and 500 μg/mL. Depot injection as a microsphere suspension 10, 20 and 30 mg/vial.
- Lanreotide: Depot injection as microparticles 30 mg/vial, depot injection as gel 60 mg, 90 mg and 120 mg in prefilled syringe.

Gonadotrophin releasing hormone agonists

- Buserelin: Injection 1 mg/mL, nasal spray 100 μg per metered dose.
- Goserelin: Implants 3.6 mg and 10.8 mg (as acetate).
- Leuprolein: Depot injection as microsphere powder 3.75 mg/vial and 11.25 mg/vial.
- Triptorelin: Injection 4.2 mg/vial and 15 mg/vial. Depot injection 3.75 mg in prefilled syringe.

PRODUCTION OF PROTEIN AND PEPTIDE DRUGS BY GENETICALLY MODIFIED BACTERIA

Introduction

The technology for large-scale culture of bacteria is over 50 years old and bacteria can be cultured in stirred tank 'reactors' which may have a capacity of up to 10 000 litres. *Escherichia coli* is by far the most extensively used bacterium for the expression of rDNA. Human insulin (Humulin, Eli Lilly), the first biotechnologically produced peptide, was produced using transformed *E. coli* and this was quickly followed by the production of human growth hormone by this method.

Advantages of producing rDNA drugs in bacteria

1. Large-scale culture of bacteria is well established and the organisms are robust.
2. Bacteria multiply rapidly, reducing the danger of contamination by other organisms.
3. A rapid growth rate means a rapid product production.
4. Growth media for bacteria are simple and composed of cheap materials (e.g. molasses as a carbon source).

Disadvantages of the production of rDNA drugs in bacteria

1. The gene product is unstable in the host and may be degraded by proteases within the cells.
2. Post-translational modifications of the gene product are not carried out by bacteria. Thus glycosylation, phosphorylation and expression of secondary structure may not match those of the natural product. This may affect the efficacy of the drug and increase its antigenicity.
3. The gene product often accumulates in the cell rather than being excreted into the growth medium and thus the bacterial cells may require disruption before the product can be harvested. This increases purification difficulties since bacteria contain many other proteins that have to be removed before the product can be used.

Strategies for improving the production of rDNA drugs by bacteria

1. The gene coding for the desired peptide may be fused with one coding for another peptide; such hybrid proteins usually precipitate within the cell. This removes the possibility of degradation by proteases and simplifies purification because the cell may be disrupted and the hybrid protein separated by gradient centrifugation. The desired peptide may then be released from the fusion protein.
2. A gene coding for the excretion of the product into the growth medium may be inserted into the bacteria. This means that the product is removed from contact with bacterial proteases and separated from the bulk of bacterial proteins.

An example of the production of a rDNA drug by *E. coli*

Insulin is secreted by the pancreatic β-cells and is required for the synthesis of the glucose storage polymer glycogen and is also required for the entry of glucose into tissues. Reduced glucose entry into tissues is the major effect of insulin deficiency and this produces an increased level of glucose into the circulation due to inhibition of glycogen biosynthesis. The effects of glucose deficiency in tissues are: accelerated protein catabolism, accelerated lipid metabolism and decreased lipid synthesis. Increased glucose levels in plasma lead to hyperosmolarity and dehydration and some complications may arise from the reactivity of glucose itself. The effects of insulin deficiency can be eliminated by insulin injection.

Diabetes is the third leading cause of death in the USA. Treatment of diabetes with insulin began in 1921 following its discovery at the University of Toronto and, as a consequence, rather than facing certain death diabetics were able to have a normal lifespan. The early insulin preparations were crude extracts from animal pancreas. They tended to promote allergic reaction due to the presence of additional proteins and required frequent injection because of their low purity. Purification steps were later introduced involving alcohol/acid precipitation of the protein and later crystallisation as the zinc salt (the basic crystal form involves six insulin molecules and two zinc atoms). Modern extracted insulins are subjected to a chromatographic step, gel-filtration, in order to remove allergenic contaminating proteins. Human insulin produced by transformed *E. coli* became available in 1982.

THE STRUCTURE OF INSULIN

Insulin is a 50 amino acid protein which, unlike many peptides, is not glycosylated. It is produced naturally as three chains, the A, B and C chains. The C chain links the A and B chains and is removed by the body when the insulin is activated, leaving the A and B chains linked by two S–S bridges (Fig. 27.3). The metal ion zinc is also involved in stabilising the peptide, and insulin is stored in pancreatic β-cells as a hexamer complexed with two zinc atoms.

The need for biotechnologically produced insulins

There was a strong requirement for a good production process for insulin because:

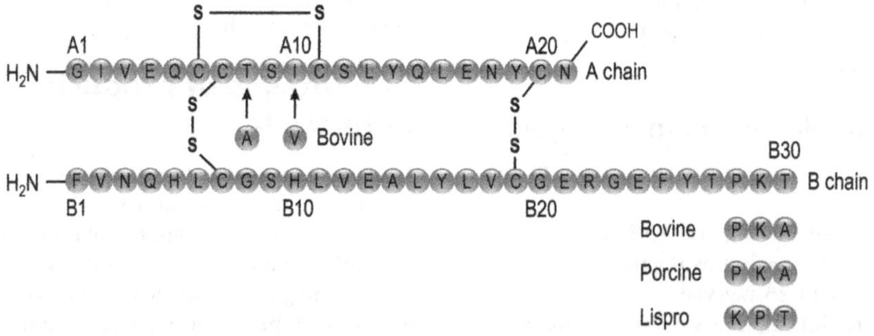

Figure 27.3 The structure of human insulin and animal insulins.

1. The number of diabetics is on the increase because it is safer for diabetic women to have children.
2. There are some problems with animal insulins. Since they are not identical to human insulins, they stimulate the immune system to produce antibodies to the insulin. This means that some of the insulin injected is destroyed by the body and the dosage has to be altered to compensate.
3. Animal insulins are contaminated with small amounts of related peptides such as glucagon and somastatin extracted from the pancreas.

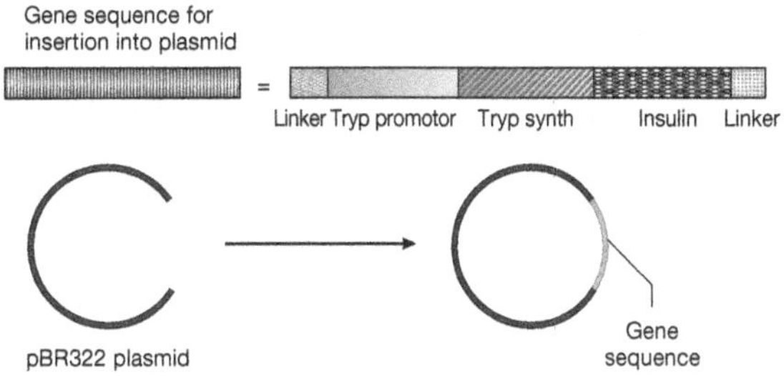

Figure 27.5 Construction of a gene sequence for the expression of insulin in *E. coli* and its insertion into a plasmid.

The biotechnological process leading to the production of human insulin

In the process used by Lilly, insulin is produced in the form of proinsulin as a fusion protein where it is joined to the protein tryptophan synthase via a terminal methionine. The tryptophan synthase is then removed by cleavage with cyanogen bromide. The proinsulin is then converted to insulin via treatment with a mixture of the protease enzymes trypsin and carboxypeptidase.

1. Human insulin was produced from mRNA isolated from the pancreas. The mRNA was translated into the cDNA coding for insulin using reverse transcriptase (translates RNA back into DNA) and DNA polymerase (Fig. 27.4).
2. The DNA was inserted into a plasmid pBR322 by cutting it open with restriction enzymes and inserting the DNA coding for proinsulin. To make the insertion, linkers have to be added to fit the DNA to the 'sticky' ends of the cut plasmid. The pBR322 plasmid is often used in genetic engineering because it carries ampicillin and tetracycline resistance genes which enable selection of transformed bacteria. Only the transformed *E. coli* survive the antibiotic treatment. In order to maximise production of insulin by transformed *E. coli* a promoter gene is included in the plasmid. Since insulin is manufactured by the β-cells in the pancreas and no other cells in the body, in common with all other genes, it is suppressed until it is triggered by a signal indicating that insulin formation is required. Rather than insert the natural trigger mechanism for insulin into the genetically engineered plasmid, an alternative promotor gene (the tryptophan synthetase operon which is triggered by low tryptophan levels) is used. This is located next to the insulin gene (Fig. 27.5) so that by the time a stop sequence in the DNA sequence is reached a hybrid protein has been produced consisting of tryptophan synthetase joined onto proinsulin.
3. The plasmid was then introduced into *E. coli* bacteria (Fig. 27.6), and single cells from the culture were isolated and grown to form clones on agar plates. The clones producing insulin were then selected using radiolabelled insulin antibodies that can map the position of the insulin-producing colonies on the plate by using a blotting technique where insulin antibodies are attached to a membrane which is then overlaid onto the plated colonies.
4. The clones producing proinsulin/tryptophan synthase are grown on a large scale (10 000 litres) and the proinsulin/tryptophan synthase is harvested. After the hybrid protein has been produced, the tryptophan synthetase has to be removed. This is done chemically using cyanogen bromide which cleaves selectively

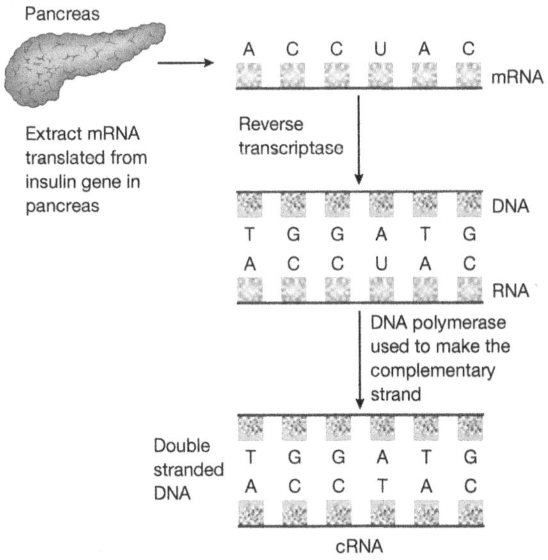

Figure 27.4 Production of cDNA coding for insulin.

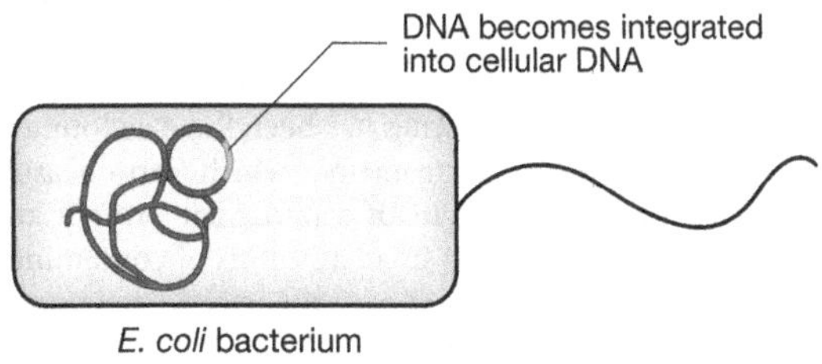

Figure 27.6 Introduction of a plasmid coding for insulin in *E. coli*.

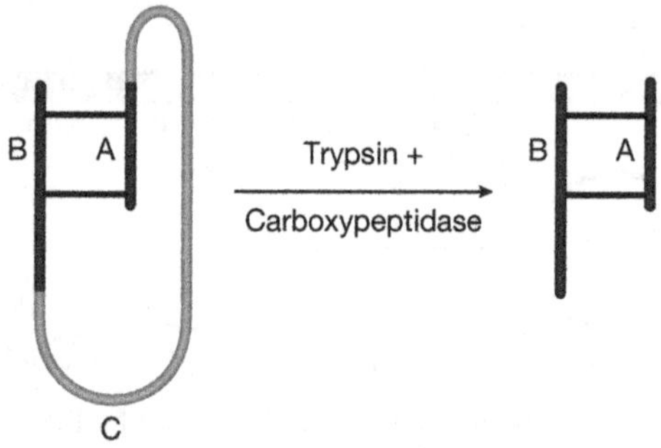

Figure 27.7 Removal of the C chain from proinsulin.

between the nitrogen terminal end of methionine and any adjacent amino acid (tryptophan synthetase is linked to proinsulin via a methionine residue at its N-terminus) and the C chain is then enzymatically removed using a combination of carboxypeptidase and trypsin to yield insulin (Fig. 27.7).

Quality control of recombinant insulin

Particularly stringent checks are needed to control the quality of the insulin produced because of the complexity of the molecule and the fact that it is derived from a biological system that could potentially be variable. High-performance liquid chromatography (HPLC) systems have to be capable of separating human insulin from the closely related animal insulins which differ from it by only one or two amino acids.

HPLC provides a highly specific technique which can distinguish between human insulin and animal insulins differing from it by one or two amino acids. In addition to making sure that the primary structure of the peptide is correct, the secondary structure of the peptide also has to be checked to ensure that it is correctly folded. This is carried out using a technique called circular dichroism which is related to the optical rotation technique used to determine the relative configuration (i.e. [+] or [−]) of small drug molecules. When the circular dichroism 'fingerprint' of a standard for insulin and a test sample of insulin are identical, they can be said to be arranged in three-dimensional space in the same way. The product is also quality controlled for biological activity by injection into a rabbit followed by the monitoring of blood glucose levels.

A major advance in simplifying quality control of biotechnologically produced drugs has been the development of electrospray mass spectrometry, which can measure exactly the molecular weight of a particular protein and also detect and characterise small amounts of contaminating proteins. Figure 27.8 shows the electrospray mass spectrum of human insulin.

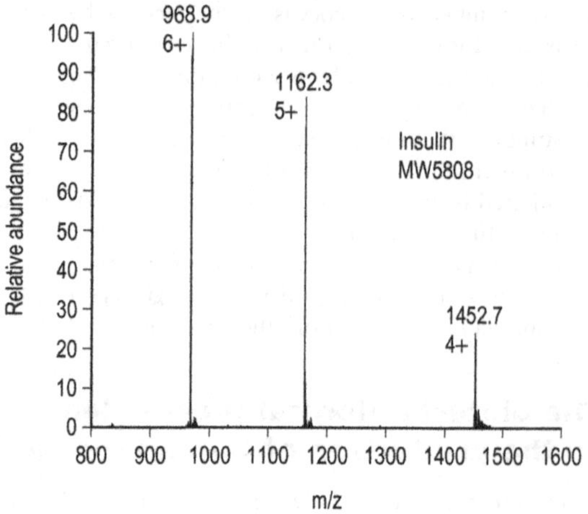

Figure 27.8 Electrospray mass spectrum of human insulin showing multiply charged ions. Insulin contains 6 basic centres: 2 × histidine, 1 × arginine, 1 × lysine and terminal amine groups on the A and B chains hence the 6+ ion. 6 × 968.9 −6 (for the 6 added protons) = 5808 which is the MW of human insulin.

Modern insulins

Formulation types

Recent developments in insulin presentation have been reviewed.[1] Initially, insulins were formulated in solution under acidic conditions in order to improve their stability. However, there was a tendency for the amide bond in the C-terminal asparagine residue to hydrolyse, with consequent loss of potency. As a result, the use of zinc to stabilise soluble formulations became common. The stability of such formulations is further enhanced by the presence of phenolic preservatives in the formulation which cause a change in the conformation of the zinc hexamers (Fig. 27.9) to render them even more stable.

Soluble insulins: contain a low concentration of zinc (0.01–0.04 mg/100 Units) and have a rapid action and relatively short duration (6–8 hours).

Isophane insulin: contains a low concentration of zinc (0.01–0.04 mg/100 Units) and is formulated with the

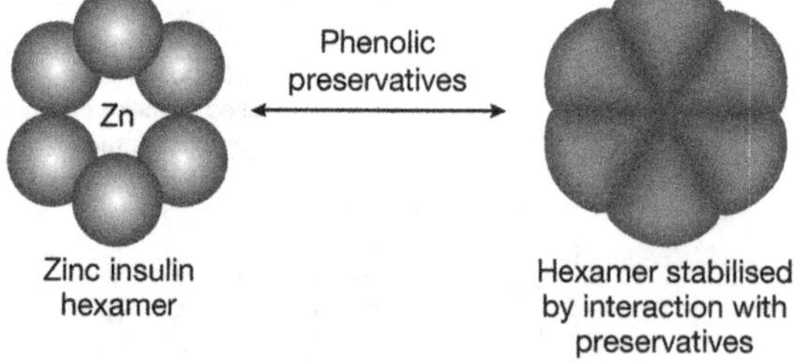

Figure 27.9 Insulin hexamers.

protein protamine that forms a complex with zinc/insulin, producing a formulation with a slow onset and long duration of action (18–24 hours).
Insulin zinc suspension (amorphous): contains a high concentration of zinc (0.12–0.25 mg/100 Units), producing a preparation with slow onset and a long duration of action (18–24 hours).
Insulin zinc suspension (crystalline): contains a high concentration of zinc (0.12–0.25 mg/100 Units) and the insulin is also in a crystalline form, producing a preparation with very slow onset and a very long duration of action (24–28 hours).
Biphasic insulin preparations: consist of mixtures of slow-acting insulin preparations and the rapid-action soluble insulin preparations.

Sources of insulin

Bovine insulin

Bovine insulin differs from human insulin by three amino acids (alanine for threonine A-chain 8, isoleucine for valine A-chain 10, alanine for threonine B-chain 30; see Fig. 27.3). Bovine insulin does promote antibody production to some extent and doses may need to be adjusted to compensate for this.

Porcine insulin

Porcine insulin differs from human insulin by one amino acid having alanine instead of threonine at B-chain 30 (see Fig. 27.3). The difference in structure from human insulin is not sufficient for antibody production to occur.

Human insulin types

- Human insulin (*emp*) is produced by the enzymatic removal of an octapeptide chain, including the B-chain 30 alanine, from porcine insulin and its replacement by a chemically synthesised octapeptide.
- Human insulin (*prb*) is produced as proinsulin in *E. coli* bacteria and then enzymatically and chemically treated to remove the C-chain.
- Human insulin (*pyr*) is produced as proinsulin in yeast and the C-chain is enzymatically and chemically removed.
- Human insulin (*crb*) is produced by expressing the A and B chain separately in *E. coli* and then combining them.

There has been some concern that human insulin is more likely to produce hypoglycaemic shock but, on the other hand, it is less likely to produce wasting away of fatty tissue at the injection site in comparison with animal insulins. Concern over the tendency of human insulin to produce hypoglycaemic shock has led to the production of analogues of human insulin that have fewer tendencies to cause this.

Human insulin analogues

Since insulin binds to its receptor as a monomer, any structural alteration which reduces insulin self-association results in more rapid action. Rapid-acting analogues were developed so that insulin could be injected immediately before a meal so that carbohydrate absorption and insulin action correlated more closely.

Rapid-acting analogues (reduced self-association)

- Lisproinsulin has the amino acids lysine and proline substituted at B28 and B29, respectively. It is produced from recombinant human insulin by replacing part of the B-chain with a synthetic peptide. This results in an insulin analogue that has less tendency to self-associate into hexamers but that is still active as an insulin. Thus lisproinsulin has a rapid onset of action and a short duration of action. The overall effect is of slightly less tendency towards hypoglycaemia since preprandial glucose levels in blood tend to be higher.
- Insulin Aspart is another rapid-acting insulin analogue produced from recombinant human insulin. In this case the B28, proline residue towards the terminus of the B chain is replaced by a negatively charged aspartate residue. The negative charge reduces the tendency of insulin to self-associate.
- Glulisine (Apidira) has B3 valine substituted with lysine and B29 lysine substituted with aspartic acid. Substitution of hydrophobic valine with polar lysine reduces self association and the addition of a carboxyl containing amino acid next to the carboxy terminus also reduces self-association.

Long-acting insulins

In recent years, analogues of insulin with modified structures have been produced which have prolonged duration of action, thus reducing the need for frequent injection.

- Insulin Detemir is an insulin analogue with increased duration of action mediated via increased binding to serum albumin. Serum albumin has a slow rate of clearance from the blood and thus acts as a reservoir for the insulin analogue. The affinity for albumin is promoted by removing the terminal (B30) threonine from insulin and acylating the B29 lysine with the fatty acid tetradecanoic acid (Fig. 27.10). The modified insulin thus has increased affinity for albumin which is a lipophilic protein. In addition, this analogue exhibits lowered immunoreactivity.
- Insulin Glargine uses another approach promoting self-association of the insulin at physiological pH by changing its pI value. The pI value of a protein is the pH where it is neutral, i.e. the charge on the amine groups in the protein exactly balances the

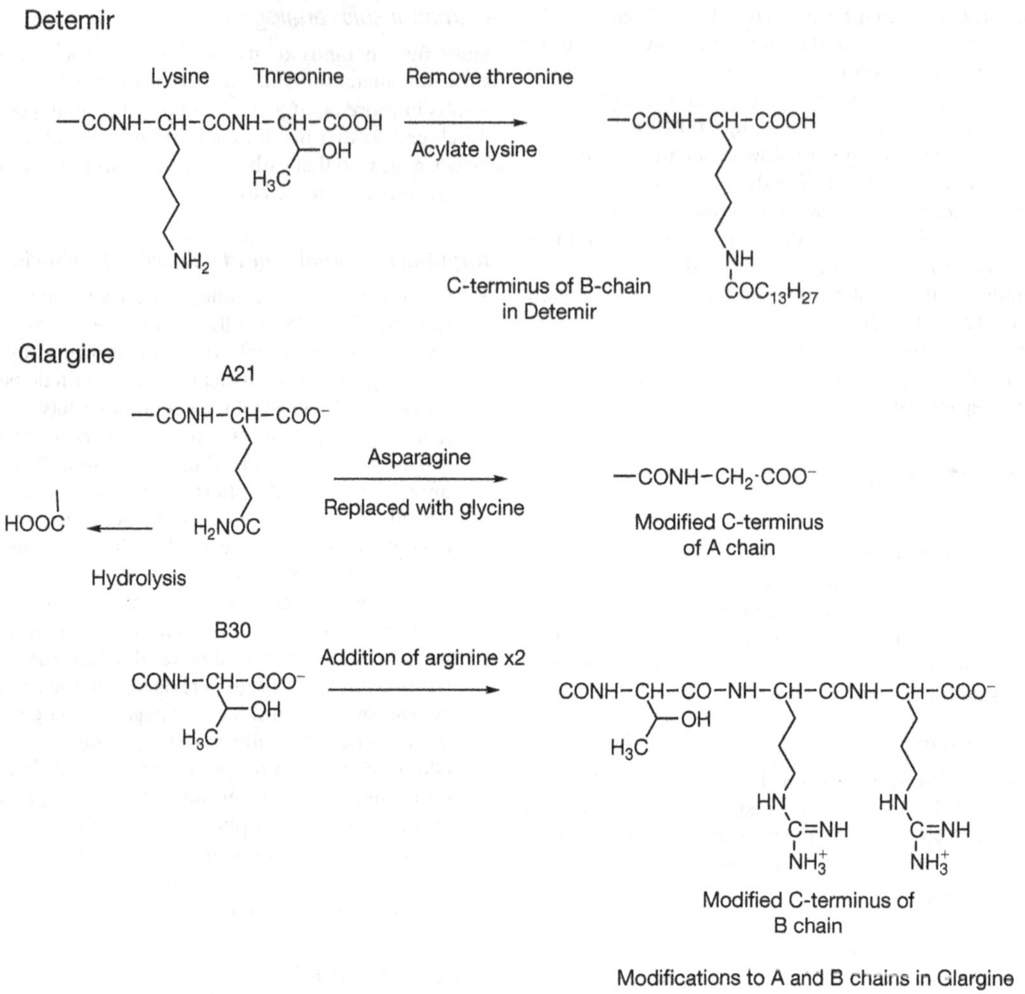

Figure 27.10 Modifications in long-acting insulins.

charge on the acidic groups, and at this pH a protein has a tendency to precipitate out of solution due to reduced solubility. Native insulin has a pI value of 5.7 and thus is negatively charged at physiological pH (7.4) and thus has no tendency to precipitate. Insulin Glargine has two arginine residues added at the C-terminus of the B-chain (Fig. 27.10). The addition of these two basic amino acids raises the pI value of the insulin to 6.7. This is sufficiently close to physiological pH for the insulin to precipitate following subcutaneous injection, forming a depot. In addition, asparagine at the C-terminus of the A chain is replaced by glycine, reducing the likelihood of chemical degradation which might cause cross-linking with the modified C-terminus of the B chain (Fig. 27.10). Insulin Glargine has a duration of action of 24 h.

Insulin formulations

Rapid acting

- Purified bovine insulin: 100 units/mL.
- Purified porcine insulin: 100 units/mL.
- Human (pyr) insulin: 100 units/mL.
- Human (prb) insulin: 100 units/mL.
- Human (crb) insulin: 100 units/mL.
- Human (crb) insulin for inhalation: 1 and 3 mg blister.
- Insulin Aspart: 100 units/mL.
- Insulin Glulisine: 100 units/mL.
- Insulin Lispro: 100 units/mL.

Long/Intermediate acting

- Insulin Detemir: 100 units/mL.
- Insulin Glargine: 100 units/mL.

Q Self Test 27.2

1. Write an equation for the hydrolysis of the amide bond in asparagine at the the C-terminus of the A chain in insulin.
2. One of the quality control checks used for insulin is to carry out a tryptic digest of insulin and examine the pattern of peptides produced. Trypsin is an enzyme that hydrolyses peptide bonds at the C-terminus side of lysine (K) or arginine (R). Using the structure of insulin shown in Fig. 27.3, draw the amino acid sequence of the peptide which would be released by trypsin from the C end of the B-chain of human insulin.
3. The basic amino acids are lysine (K), ariginine (R) and histidine (H). How many positive charges can insulin accommodate?
4. The acidic amino acids are aspartic acid (D) and glutamic acid (E). Taking an average p*Ka* value of 3 for the acids and 8 for the bases, what is the approximate pI value for insulin (easier than it seems)?

- Insulin zinc suspension. Bovine insulin: 100 units/mL.
- Isophane insulin. Bovine, porcine or human insulins with protamine: 100 units/mL.
- Protamine/zinc insulin: 100 units/mL.

Biphasic insulins

- Biphasic Insulin Aspart: 30% insulin Aspart/70% insulin Aspart protamine 100 units/ml.
- Biphasic insulin Lispro: (a) 25% insulin Lispro/75% insulin Lispro protamine. (b) 50% insulin Lispro/ 50% insulin Lispro protamine.
- Isophane insulins: a range of insulins based on either human or porcine insulins is available in which protamine is added to produce between 50% and 85% complexation with the insulin.

HUMAN GROWTH HORMONE

Human growth hormone (HGH) is secreted by the pituitary gland and plays a key role in somatic growth through its effects on the metabolism of proteins, carbohydrates and lipids; it stimulates cell proliferation at growth plates in bones by direct binding to receptors in these tissues. It is present at high levels in children and also becomes elevated in response to exercise. Low levels of HGH are associated with obesity. HGH also increases calcium absorption by the gut, increases glomerular filtration and stimulates erythrocyte production by bone marrow. HGH is well established for the treatment of short stature in children. It is being tested in a number of other applications including: osteoporosis, renal failure, treatment of severe burns and wound healing. Intranasal delivery is being evaluated. Side effects are infrequent, although the safety of the product is not absolutely established.

HGH was originally extracted from the pituitary gland of human cadavers and the extracted product was found in some cases to produce the Creutzfeld-Jacob disease, which is caused by a prion protein. HGH is a 191 amino acid non-glycosylated protein. The amino acid sequences vary greatly between species and non-primate growth hormones have little activity in man. The commercial products are produced by transformed *E. coli*: Genotropin™ (Pharmacia), Humatrope™ (Lilly), Norditropin™ (Novo Nordisk), NutropinAq™ (Ipsen) and Zomacton™ (Ferring) or mammalian cultures Saizen™ (Serono). All of the commercial products are chemically equivalent.

Human growth hormone antagonists

Pegvisomant is a mutated form of HGH.[2,3] The protein is altered so that it functions as an antagonist of HGH by binding strongly at one binding site of the HGH receptor but only weakly at the other binding site (Figs 27.11, 27.12).

In order to achieve the reduced binding to the HGH receptor, 8 amino acids at the binding site were altered. In addition, the protein is PEGylated at 4-6 lysine residues (Box 27.1). One of the amino acids replaced at binding site 1 was a lysine residue. This was carried out in order to ensure that the presence of PEG did not reduce the binding of the protein to the receptor to a great extent. Additionally, a lysine amino acid was introduced at binding site 2, thus increasing the likelihood of PEGylation at this site with consequent reduced binding affinity. The presence of PEG at the other positions reduces the overall binding affinity of the protein but greatly increases in circulating half-life compared with HGH. Pegvisomant thus functions as an antagonist of HGH and is used to treat acromegaly.

Colony stimulating factors

Granulocyte colony stimulating factor (G-CSF) is a haemopoietic growth factor which is involved in promoting the differentiation of stem cells formed in the bone marrow into granulocytes (neutrophils, basophils, eosinophils) which are responsible for killing bacteria in the blood. It is used to rectify myelosuppression in patients undergoing cancer chemotherapy where white cells in the blood are depleted by the chemotherapeutic agent. The protein occurs either as a 174 or a 180 amino acid protein. The commercial product filgrastim (Neupogen™) is produced in non-glycosylated form by transformed *E. coli*. Pegfilgrastim is a PEGylated version of the protein

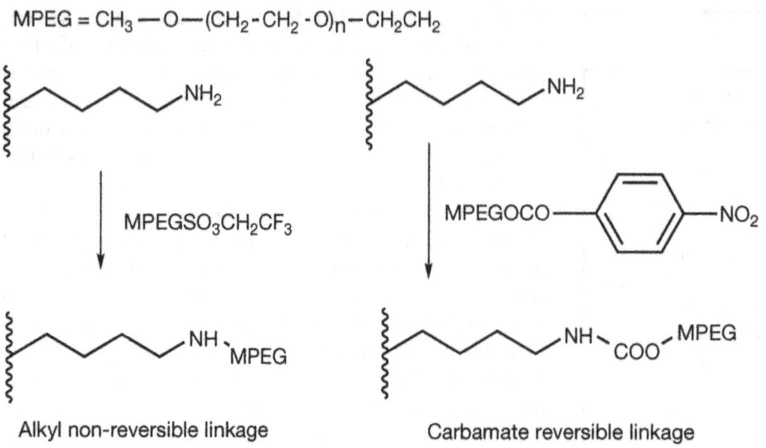

Figure 27.11 Reversible and irreversible PEGylation.

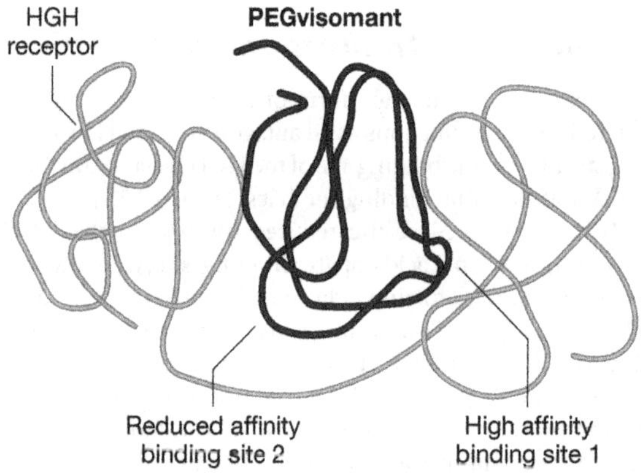

Figure 27.12 Binding of Pegvisomant.

which has an increased circulating half-life, reducing the necessity for daily injections. Lenograstim is another form of G-CSF produced by CHO cells; unlike filgrastim it is glycosylated and is slightly more potent.

C-GSF in the BNF

- Filgrastim 300 µg/mL.
- Lenograstim 105 or 263 µg/mL.
- Pegfilgrastim 10 mg/mL.

Interferons and other cytokines

Interferons (IFNs) are a group of inducible cytokines which have antiviral properties. IFN-α and -β are inducible in several cells while IFN-γ is produced by T lymphocytes.

Box 27.1 PEGylation

Reaction of proteins with polyethylene glycol (PEGylation) is of increasing importance for manipulating the pharmacokinetics of therapeutic proteins.[2] The polyethylene glycol chains are largely linear polymers around 12 kDa; however, the use of branched chains is becoming more common. PEG chains are very bulky because of the water associating with them and thus shield sites of proteins which might cause immunogenic reaction or be susceptible to proteolytic degradation. PEGylation generally results in increased circulating half-life for a therapeutic protein. The disadvantage of PEGylation is that it can reduce the activity of the therapeutic protein by preventing it binding efficiently to its site of action. The PEGs used are usually methylated at one end to avoid producing reagents reacting at both ends which would crosslink the protein. The PEGs can either be linked by a strong covalent bond which is not easily reversible, e.g. C–N, or via a linkage such as carbamate which is reversible (Fig. 27.11). Reversible linkages are used where the presence of the PEG chain reduces the activity of the protein. These chains are removed by enzymatic hydrolysis in the body. Lysine residues are a popular target for modification because they are both reactive and common in proteins.

α-Interferon

Recombinant α-interferon$_{2a}$ (Roferon-A, Roche) is produced in the form of a 165 amino acid protein that is unglycosylated. The drug is used to treat Kaposi's sarcoma and also hepatitis B and hepatitis C. Interferon α_{2a} (IntronA, Schering-Plough) has similar indications. It is produced by genetically transformed *E. coli*. It is also produced in a PEGylated form in order to increase its circulating half-life.

β-Interferon

Interferon-β_{1b} is an 18.5 kDa protein that is produced commercially using genetically transformed *E. coli*. The gene inserted into the *E. coli* was originally isolated from human fibroblasts and was engineered so that a cysteine residue present at position 17 was replaced by a serine residue which improves its stability during synthesis in *E. coli*. The commercial product, Betaferon® (Schering), is predominantly used for the treatment of relapsing-remitting multiple sclerosis. The discovery of its use in MS therapy was based on the unproven theory that MS might have a viral aetiology. Interferon β_{1a} is produced by CHO cells (Avonex®, Biogen). It is identical to human interferon β and has similar indications to betaferon. Rebif™ is a differently formulated version of interferon β_{1a}.

γ-Interferon

γ-Interferon is produced in the form a of a 140 amino acid single-chain polypeptide γ-Interferon$_{1b}$. It occurs naturally in a glycosylated form but the commercial product is unglycosylated and is expressed in *E. coli*. It is used in the treatment of chronic granulomatous disease and severe malignant osteoporosis where it is believed to increase the activity of phagocytic cells.

Interleukin-2

Interleukin-2 is a 15.5 kDa protein which stimulates the production of T lymphocytes. The protein occurs naturally in glycosylated form but the unglycosylated form is also active. The commercial product is produced in the unglycosylated form by genetically transformed *E. coli*. The drug is used to treat metastatic renal cell carcinoma.

Cytokine preparations in the BNF

- α-interferon (IntronA™, Roferon-A™, Viraferon™): preparations between 6 and 50 million units/mL.
- Pegylated α-interferon (Pegasys™, Pegintron™, ViraferonPeg™): preparations between 50 and 180 micrograms.
- β-interferon (Avonex™, Rebif™, Betaferon™): preparations between 22 and 300 micrograms.
- γ-interferon (Immukin®, Boehringer): 200 micrograms/mL.
- Interleukin-2 (Proleukin™): 18-million unit vial.

PRODUCTION OF PEPTIDE DRUGS BY ANIMAL CELL CULTURES

Introduction

Animal cells are capable of producing peptides which are closer to naturally occurring human peptides, i.e. they are capable of carrying out post-translational modifications of proteins such as glycosylation, phosphorylation and alterations in the tertiary structure of the protein. It is not always necessary to insert rDNA into animal cells to get them to express a required protein. A line of cells in culture may naturally produce the protein or the cells may be stimulated to produce the protein, e.g. using a virus. This means that the techniques to stimulate peptide production by animal cells are more diverse than those used for production using *E. coli*.

Post-translational modification

In animals, once the protein has been synthesised within the endoplasmic reticulum, it must be folded correctly, sorted and finally transported. Proteins that are secreted by a cell or are incorporated into the cell membrane undergo five principal types of modification: the formation of disulphide bonds, proper folding of the protein, addition and modification of carbohydrates, specific proteolytic cleavages, and formation of multiple chain proteins. Proteins that have not been assembled properly are likely to be enzymatically degraded. In bacterial cells, the formation of disulphide bonds may not occur correctly. In a protein containing several cysteine residues a number of permutations of S–S bond formation are possible and a mammalian cell production system is more likely to produce the correct combination of S–S bonds. It is possible to refold the protein post-production but there is no guarantee that the correctly folded protein can be easily produced. Often, the most critical modification, which mammalian cells are required for, in order to obtain full biological activity for a biotechnologically produced protein, is the post-translational glycosylation of a protein. This is not always critical for the biological activity of the protein but, where it is required, the protein must be expressed in mammalian cells. The sugar chains on proteins are fairly small, up to *ca.* 15 monosaccharide units in the most complex cases. Such short chains of sugar units are known as oligosaccharides. The glycoside chains are either O-linked, linked to serine of threonine side chains, or N-linked to the amide nitrogen of asparagine. There are principally eight sugars involved in building the oligosaccharide chains. These are: glucose, galactose, mannose, fucose, xylose, N-acetylglucosamine, N-acetylgalactosamine and neuramic (sialic) acid (Fig. 27.13). Small variations in such chains can produce large differences in the way that the body responds to a protein. For instance, variation in a single residue in a glycoside chain within the glycoproteins in the membrane of erythrocytes determines blood group. Thus the immune system of people who cannot synthesise the A or B antigens will destroy erythrocytes which contain the antigen which is not present in their cells. People with the O blood group can safely donate to people with A and B antigens since the O antigen lacks the extra sugar present in the A and B antigens and thus does not trigger an immune response.

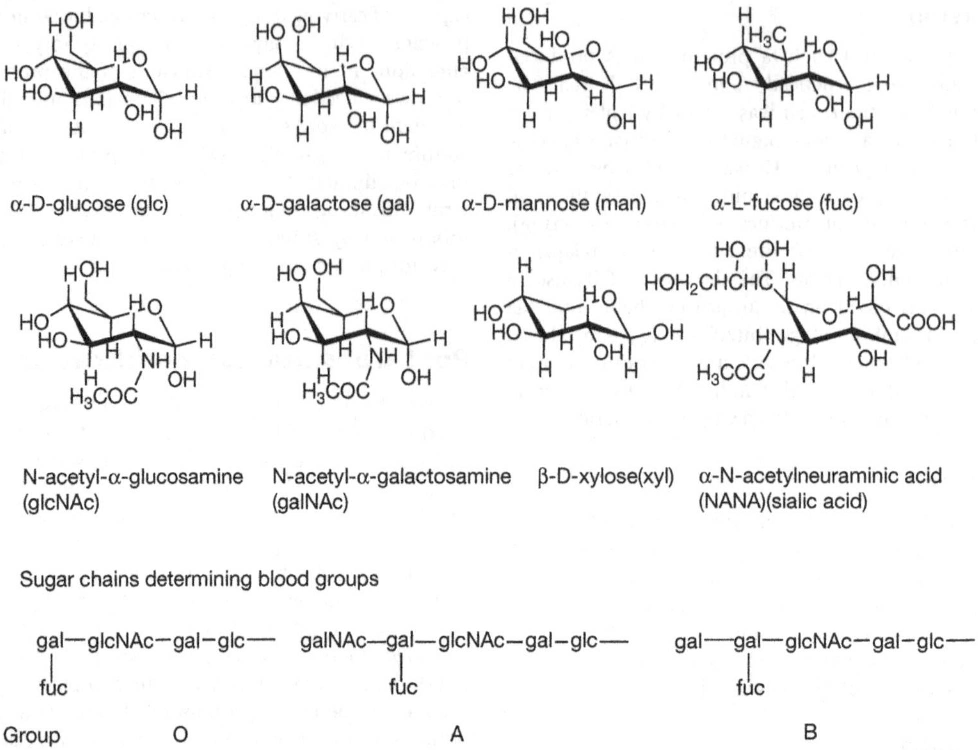

Figure 27.13 Monosaccharides commonly found in oligosaccharide chains in glycoproteins and glycosidic determinants of blood groups.

For biotechnologically produced mammalian proteins such as erythropoietin and tissue plasminogen activating factor the correct glycosylation pattern is essential for activity.

Advantages of producing peptides using animal cell cultures

1. Post-translational modifications of the product are likely to be made, thus resulting in a final product similar to the natural human peptide. The means that the peptide will have the correct secondary and tertiary structure and be glycosylated and phosphorylated in the same or in a similar manner to the natural material. These factors determine the location, antigenicity and longevity of the drug in vivo.
2. Animal cell cultures are less likely to degrade the peptide after it has been produced.

Disadvantages of producing peptides using animal cell cultures

1. The cultures are slow growing and can only be cultured at low cell density.
2. The growth medium requires expensive vitamins and co-factors as well as serum that is difficult to standardise.
3. The complexity of the growth medium and the slow growth of the cells render contamination with microorganisms more likely.
4. Animal cells are fragile and cannot be readily cultured in stirred fermentors that produce high shear stresses.
5. Some animal cells are anchorage dependent and have to be grown on surfaces, thus limiting the type of system that can be used to grow them.

Strategies for improving the production of peptides by animal cell cultures

1. Recent developments have produced higher-density cultures and have simplified the growth media.
2. New types of fermentor have been developed such as the air lift fermentor where a stream of air effects mixing and aeration or systems where the cells are immobilised in foams and the growth medium is allowed to percolate through, removing the product from the cell matrix.
3. Anchorage-dependent cells may be grown in suspension on microcarrier beads of diameter 150–200 μm.

An example of the production of a peptide drug by animal cell cultures in detail

Introduction

Erythropoietin (EPO) is produced mainly by the kidneys and acts on stem cells in the bone marrow, stimulating mitosis of erythroid progenitor cells (Fig. 27.14). It increases red cell production in response to reduced oxygen delivery to the kidney. Thus administration of the drug can correct anaemia caused by EPO deficiency such as occurs in chronic renal failure (CRF). There are many causes of CRF and to date the only means of correcting it are either transplantation or dialysis. A major side effect of the disease is anaemia that is due to EPO deficiency. This is caused in part by dialysis. Prior to the advent of biotechnologically produced EPO the only means of treating the anaemia associated with CRF were frequent blood transfusions or the administration of anabolic steroids; both methods of treatment have attendant risks and side effects. EPO is highly effective in correcting anaemia and eliminates the need for transfusions. The therapeutic goal is a haematocrit (packed red cell volume) of >0.3. Side effects are generally not serious but may include: exacerbation of hypertension; extracorporeal blood clotting; iron deficiency; seizures; flulike syndromes and headache. The most commonly reported side effect is exacerbation of hypertension and this may be treated with antihypertensive drugs. EPO is an ideal drug of abuse in sport since it raises red blood cell levels yet is very difficult to distinguish from the EPO that is naturally present. However, variations exist in the glycosylation pattern between the natural and the biotechnologically produced drug and these can be used for detection of this form of drug abuse.

The structure of EPO

EPO is a 166 amino acid glycoprotein that is heavily glycosylated (almost 50% of the molecular weight [MW] is due to glycosylation) and it has a molecular weight of 34 kDa. Glycosylation is essential for biological activity, and removal of terminal sialic residues from the glycan chains in the protein greatly reduces its half-life in the body. Animal cells have to be used in the production process in order to make a product with the correct glycosylation pattern.

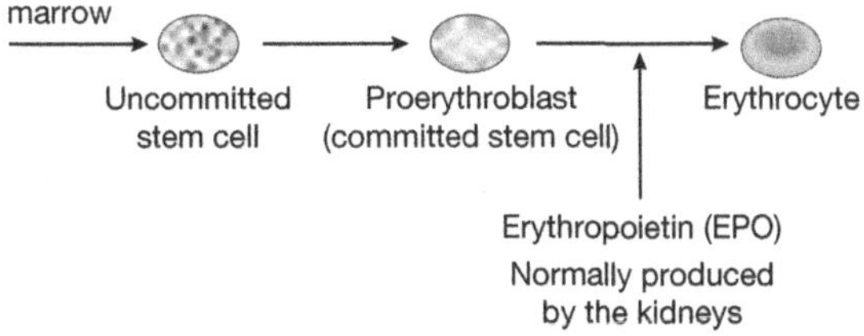

Figure 27.14 The action of EPO in stimulating red blood cell production.

The need for biotechnologically produced EPO

1. The levels of human EPO in blood and urine are too low for it to be obtained from these sources.
2. Given the complications of blood transfusions as a means of treating anaemia, despite its cost, EPO is a much better alternative.

The biotechnological process leading to EPO production

1. The first step was to characterise the primary structure of EPO. This enabled the design of DNA oligonucleotide probes to pick out the DNA sequences which could be linked to the amino acid sequences present in the gene for EPO. The DNA coding for EPO was isolated from human liver DNA using radiolabelled oligonucleotide probes in order to detect the fraction containing the EPO gene. The genetic material was then broken down into small pieces using restriction enzymes and the pieces were amplified by incorporation into bacteriophage which were then cultured with *E. coli* (Fig. 27.15) and finally the EPO gene was isolated using oligonucleotide probes.
2. An expression vector was designed incorporating: a promoter sequence (cf. insulin production), the isolated EPO gene and the gene for the enzyme dihydrofolate reductase (DHFR) (Fig. 27.16).
3. The vector was then used to transform a culture of Chinese hamster ovary (CHO) cells (Fig. 27.17). The dihydrofolate reductase gene enables selection of the transformed cells since the untransformed CHO cells lack this gene and thus cannot grow in a growth medium lacking certain amino acids. High-yielding cells were selected and cloned and are the commercial source of the drug.

A commercial supply of EPO was first produced by Amgen. The two products sold in the UK are Eprex® (Jannsen-Cilag) and NeoRecormon (Roche). These products are almost identical in structure, having the same amino acid sequence but very slight differences in glycosylation pattern. A version of EPO which is more extensively glycosylated called Darbepoetin is also sold by Amgen. The increased level of glycosylation gives this version of EPO a longer circulating half-life which means that it does not have to be administered as frequently.

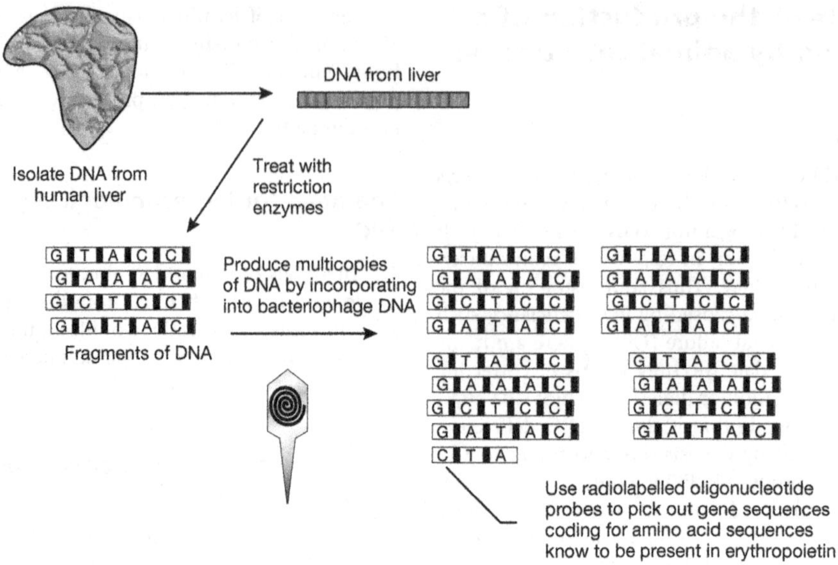

Figure 27.15 Isolation of the gene coding for EPO from human liver.

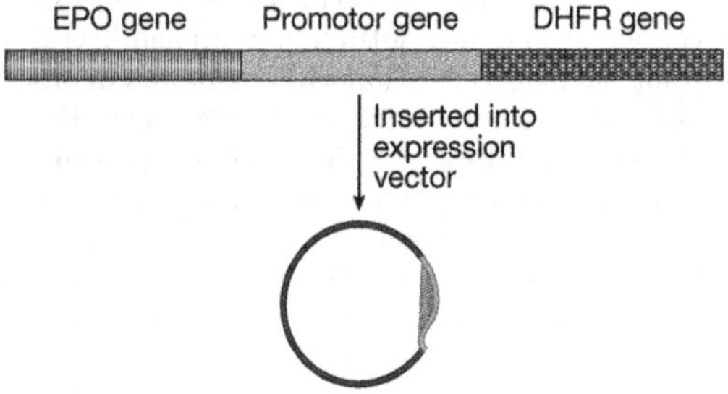

Figure 27.16 Gene sequence used for EPO expression.

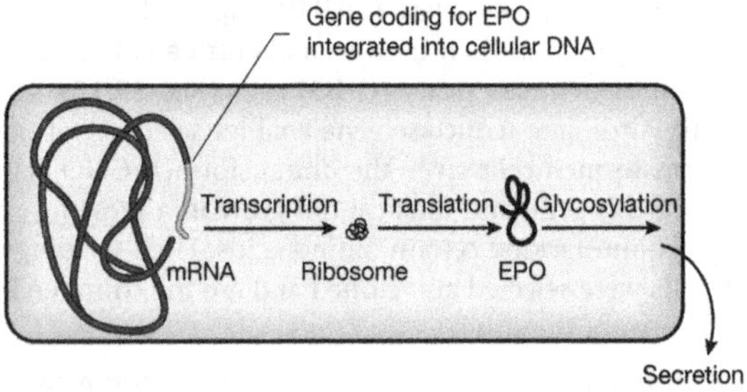

Figure 27.17 Production of EPO by CHO cells.

Other rDNA drugs produced using animal cell culture

Tissue plasminogen activator (TPA)

Tissue plasminogen activator (TPA) is a 527 amino acid serine protease glycoprotein with a molecular weight of 64 kDa. About 8% of the MW is due to carbohydrate. The gene has been expressed in both *E. coli* and CHO cells. The commercial products Alteplase® (Genentech) and Tenecteplase® (Boehringer Ingleheim) are produced by CHO cells. Related products include Reteplase® (Roche) which is expressed in *E. coli* and only contains part of the TPA structure but is equally effective. Different products may have different glycosylation patterns but such variations do not greatly affect biological activity.

TPA is the most important physiological activator of plasminogen, the clot-dissolving enzyme. It is locally released from blood vessels and binds to the fibrin clot with simultaneous binding of plasminogen, and this results in the digestion of the clot.

1. TPA is used in acute myocardial infarction (MI) and coronary thrombosis. With rapid intervention, it has been shown to reduce hospital 21-day mortality by 50% when used to treat MI.
2. TPA is also under clinical trials for the treatment of unstable angina, ischaemic stroke, acute stroke and pulmonary embolism. A major competitor of TPA is streptokinase, which is a bacterial enzyme. This compound is cheaper and may be more effective than TPA in some respects although there is a higher risk of allergenic response.

There is a danger of haemorrhage although contraindications are well established as being: a history of cerebrovascular accident, internal bleeding, and severe uncontrolled hypertension. TPAs with varying glycosylation patterns are being produced in order to try to reduce some of the side effects of the drug and in order to increase the plasma half-life of the drug so that it can be administered as a bolus injection rather than by continuous infusion.

Factor VIII, factor VII[a] and factor IX

Factor VIII is a complex of proteins involved in the blood-clotting cascade that results in the production of fibrin. A genetic abnormality resulting in a lack of factor VIII production results in haemophilia. The protein prepared by fractionation from human plasma is still extensively used but recombinant forms are also now available. The most important elements in the structure of factor VIII are two protein chains of 80 kDa and 90 kDa which are glycosylated to various extents. The two commercially available products are: Recombinate® (Baxter Health Care) which is prepared using genetically transformed CHO cells, and Kogenate® (Bayer/Miles) which is prepared using transformed baby hamster kidney cells. Recombinant versions of the blood-clotting proteins factor VIIa and factor IX are now also available.

Etanercept

Etanercept (Enbrel™) is used in the treatment of rheumatoid and psoriatic arthritis. It is produced using CHO cells. The protein acts as a soluble version of the tumour necrosis factor (TNF-α) receptor, TNF is involved in the pathology of rheumatoid arthritis (RA) and psoriasis. The soluble receptor binds to TNF before it can bind to TNF receptors on the inflammatory cells within the body, thus interrupting the inflammatory cascade.

Anakinra

Anakinra (Kineret™) provides another strategy for the treatment of RA. It is a recombinant version of the native interleukin-1 (IL) receptor antagonist IL-1Ra. IL-1 may have an even greater role than TNF-α in promoting RA through inhibiting proteoglycan synthesis and stimulating bone resorption. There is evidence to suggest that an imbalance between IL-1 and IL-1Ra exists in the rheumatic joint. Recombinant IL-1Ra differs from native IL-1Ra in that it has a methionine residue at its N-terminus.

Growth factors

Growth factors are involved in tissue repair (Box 27.2) and are a potentially exciting class of drugs. They include: epidermal growth factor (EGF); fibroblast growth factor (FGF); platelet derived growth factor (PDGF); transforming growth factor (TGF) and insulin like growth factor (IGF).

The only agent that has made it to the market is PDGF, which produces a chemotactic response in fibroblasts and smooth muscle, is an attractant for inflammatory cells and induces collagen synthesis. PDGF is available as a gel Regranex® for use in the treatment of diabetic foot ulcers where it promotes wound healing.

Box 27.2

The following events occur in response to injury of tissue:

Inflammatory cells rush to the site of the wound; platelets are deposited and blood coagulates and forms a temporary covering (PDGF).

Granulocytes, monocytes and lymphocytes next appear to scavenge damaged tissues.

Fibroblasts appear and begin to produce collagen and connective fibres (TGF, EGF). Simultaneously, the area becomes revascularised (FGF).

Epithelial cells at the edge of the wound begin to fill in the area under the scab and finally the new epidermis is formed and the wound is healed (EGF).

ANTIBODIES AND ANTIBODY THERAPY

What are antibodies?

Antibodies are immunoglobulin proteins, composed of four protein chains, two heavy chains (MW >53 000) and two light chains (MW *ca.* 23 000) linked together by S–S bridges. They constitute 20% of the proteins circulating in the blood. Antibodies are Y-shaped molecules having a constant region, which classifies the antibody as being of the IgA, IgD, IgE, IgG or IgM type (the effector domain) and a variable or idiotype region which is responsible for recognition and binding to a specific antigen (Fig. 27.18). The idiotype region is within the arms of the Y and an antigen binds in a lock-and-key fashion to the sites at the end of each arm. An antigen tagged in this way is recognised as foreign by the immune system and destroyed. The constant region determines the function

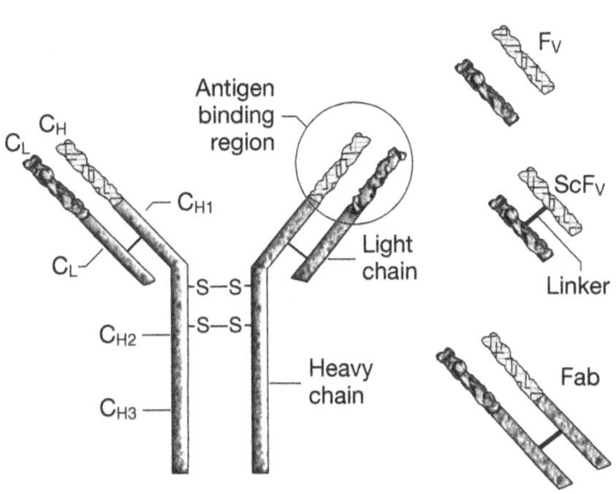

Figure 27.18 The structure of an antibody and some antibody fragments.

carried out by the antibody as detailed below. Antibodies are produced by B lymphocytes and there are five types:

- IgG has the highest circulating levels (12 mg/mL in serum) and is involved in triggering the binding of the complement system of enzymes to an antigen and triggering macrophage activity against the antigen, resulting in its destruction. The levels of IgG rise greatly in response to antigenic challenge.
- IgA is produced in tears and mucosal coatings. It mediates mucosal immunity by binding to antigens entering the mucosa. It has the second highest circulating levels (2 mg/mL) and is important for the effectiveness of oral vaccination. It can be transported from the serum into the mucosal layers.
- IgM is present in serum at 1 mg/mL. It binds very strongly to antigens and is the first antibody produced in an antigenic response. It triggers complement binding and macrophage activity.
- IgD, the role of which has not been completely elucidated, it is present only in trace levels in serum (0.03 mg/mL). It may be involved in the recognition of antigens by B cells.
- IgE is present at very low levels (0.0003 mg/mL) in serum but is found in higher amounts in tissues. IgE triggers histamine release from basinophil and mast cells and, if released too readily, triggers allergic reactions such as asthma and hay fever.

Production of antibodies

Antibodies are produced by B lymphocytes which circulate in the blood stream. The B cells are responsible for recognising antigens and tagging them so that they can be destroyed by white blood cells and by T lymphocytes.

Antibodies contain a number of discrete regions (Fig. 27.18), each of which is composed of about 110 amino acids, and the biotechnology of antibody production has developed through expression of parts of the antibody in various different cell systems. The various regions of importance are summarised in Table 27.2.

Therapeutic antibodies in the BNF

Antisera

Antibodies can be seen immediately to represent a method for therapeutic intervention since in cases of infection they can cause the body to recognise the infective agent and destroy it. Perhaps their use is most familiar in the dramatic circumstances of the use of antisera against snakebite. In

Table 27.2 Antibody regions

Region	Function	Comments
V_L	Variable region responsible for antigen recognition at the N-terminus of the light chain	Composed of four β-pleated sheets joined by 3 loops referred to as hypervariable loops or complementarity determining regions Two types of light chain are coded for by κ or λ genes About 60% of human antibodies contain κ chains
V_H	Variable region responsible for antigen recognition at the N-terminus of the heavy chain	As for the light chain composed of four β-pleated shoots joined by 3 loops V_H displays even greater diversity V_L
C_L	Single constant region of the light chain	Invariant part of the κ or λ gene sequence
C_H^1	First of three constant regions within the heavy chain above the hinge region	
C_H^2	Second of the constant regions of the heavy chain Contains glycosylation sites with sugar chains N-linked to asparagine residues	Glycosylation pattern may be important for the structural integrity of the antibody and for its effector functions such as recruitment of immune cells and complement activation
C_H^3	Third constant region of the heavy chain containing the C-terminus region	Contains the effector binding sites
V_L V_H C_L C_H^1	The Fab′ fragment is half of the antigen recognition site plus part of the constant chain	Has one antigen binding site
V_L V_H	The ScF_V fragment consisting of the variable regions of the light and heavy chains	Retains the full binding capacity of the antibody but lacks the effector functions Joined together with a linker sequence

this case, a fairly crude preparation containing antibodies prepared from the serum of animals exposed to the toxin is used to trigger the body into rapidly recognising and destroying the toxin. Such antisera are available for treatment of serious infectious diseases such as botulism and diphtheria. The use of antibodies is distinct from vaccination, which is discussed later in this chapter, in that the treatment is not dependent on stimulation of B cells to produce antibodies but immediately provides the body with a means of recognising the infection. They are only used in serious conditions since the antisera are produced in animals and have a high potential for triggering an allergic reaction to the animal protein.

Immunoglobulins

The use of partially fractionated human immunoglobulins (IgGs) represents a more refined approach to passive vaccination than the use of antisera. Normal immunoglobulin is harvested from pooled serum and confers immunity to a number of common infectious diseases, most prominently hepatitis A, measles and rubella. For many years it was the only source of protection against hepatitis A before the advent of a vaccine against the virus. More specific IgGs are prepared from pooled serum from selected donors with a high level of an antibody against a particular condition. More specific IgGs are available against hepatitis B, tetanus, rabies, tetanus, cytomegalovirus and varicella-zoster. Prophylaxis using IgGs is particularly effective because IgGs have a circulating half-life of several weeks. Of course, vaccination offers much longer-term protection.

MONOCLONAL ANTIBODIES

Introduction

Since antibodies are able to recognise and modulate the activity of other proteins within the body, they have great therapeutic potential. In 1975, Kohler and Milstein in a remarkable experiment showed that antibody-producing B lymphocytes could be fused with malignant rapidly proliferating myeloma cells (i.e. which contain oncogenes conferring immortality) and the hybrid myeloma cells or hybridomas could both express lymphocyte-specific antibodies and continue to proliferate. This provided the biotechnological basis for producing antibodies on a large scale.

Processes used for monoclonal antibody production (e.g. production of an antibody to tumour necrosis factor)

In the original experiment leading to monoclonal antibody (MAb) production the antibody-producing B lymphocytes were obtained by injecting a rabbit or mouse with the appropriate antigen (Fig. 27.19). For example, an antibody to tumour necrosis factor, a peptide involved in the autoimmune response, might be required. The spleen of the animal was removed and lymphocytes isolated from the spleen were fused with mouse myeloma cells by treatment with polyethylene glycol or Sendai virus.

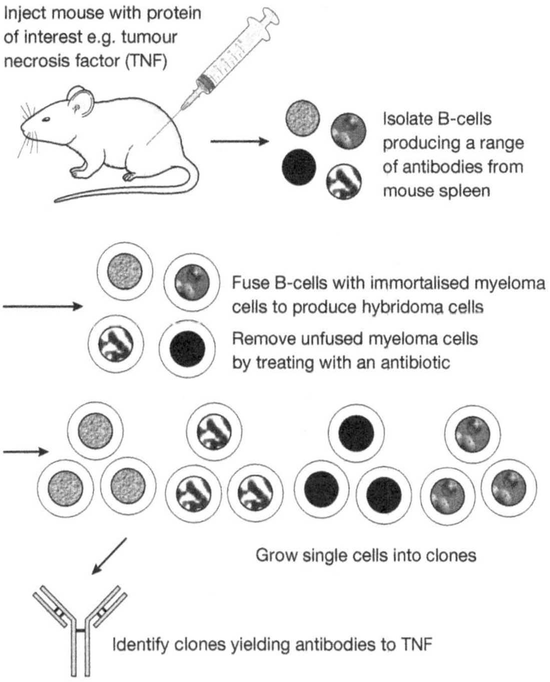

Figure 27.19 Process used for monoclonal antibody production.

The hybridoma cells were selected by poisoning any remaining unfused myeloma cells with aminopterin, which selectively blocked their DNA synthesis. The hybridoma cells survived the antibiotic treatment and single cells were then grown into clones and these clones were screened for production of the required antibody (a range of antibodies will be expressed by the mixture of lymphocytes originally isolated). In the example shown, clone 1 is selected as the one producing TNF antibodies. MAbs could then be produced on a large scale in air-lift fermentors of up to 10 000 litres. This volume of culture can produce up to 1 kg of MAb. Now the methodology for producing MAbs is more variable and in part depends on the application for which the antibody is required. In recent years there has been a move away from this type of production process towards the genetic engineering processes, described below, where the monoclonal antibodies are produced in mammalian cell lines such as CHO cells.[4]

Chimaeric antibodies

Pure murine antibodies produced as described above are allergenic in humans and thus are either toxic or have reduced half-lives in the body. In order to reduce these effects, chimaeric antibodies are produced where the constant regions of the heavy and light chains are replaced by human protein. The genes for all the human immunoglobulin subtypes have been cloned and this allows the replacement of all the genetic material coding for a murine antibody, apart from that coding for the variable region, with DNA coding for human protein. These hybrid genes can be expressed in a number of different cell cultures including mammalian and insect cell cultures. The most complete replacement of murine protein with human protein is in the humanised antibodies, where all the genetic material coding for the antibody is replaced with human gene sequence apart from the hypervariable regions. The disadvantage of replacing all but the hypervariable regions with human protein is that some binding specificity may be lost since the conformation of the β-pleated sheets present in the variable region of the original murine antibody may be optimal for binding of the hypervariable regions to the antigen. One way around this is to introduce the gene coding for human IgG into mouse embryos. When the mice developed from these embryos are challenged with an antigen, they produce B cells secreting fully human antibodies. These B cells may be isolated and fused with myeloma cells, thus producing human monoclonal antibodies.

Phage display technology

Phage display technology and related techniques such as ribosomal and yeast display systems form the basis of modern monoclonal antibody production.[5–9] Bacteriophages are viruses that infect a range of bacteria. They only have 11 genes. Figure 27.20 shows a schematic

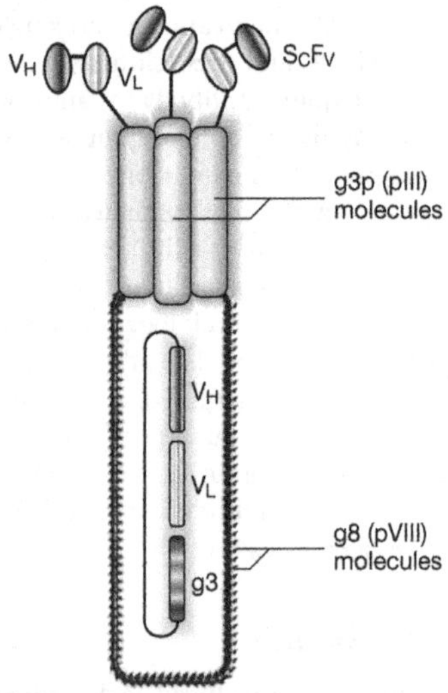

Figure 27.20 Phage display of ScFv.

diagram of a phage. The genetic material which is to be expressed as a protein is incorporated into the phage genetic material. A typical sequence involved in genetic engineering of a monoclonal antibody is as follows:

1. Inoculate a mouse with an antigen, e.g. the protein of a mutant receptor expressed on the surface of a cancer cell. Repeat the inoculation if necessary.
2. Isolate the spleen of the mouse and then the B cells from the spleen. Purify the mRNA from the B cells. Antibodies are assembled from several distinct proteins coded by separate mRNA molecules.
3. Produce a library of cDNA molecules using reverse transcriptase.
4. The cDNA molecules are then specifically amplified using primers which are specific for the VH and VL regions of the antibody.
5. A repertoire of VH/VL cDNAs (ScFvs) is produced by separating the cDNA strands and using a linking sequence which ligates to the ends of the DNA coding for VH and VL single chains. The linked VH/VL cDNA is then amplified by PCR.
6. The VH/VL cDNA is ligated into the phagemid vector which contains DNA coding for the pIII coat protein. The vector is then introduced into *E. coli*. The transformed bacterial cells are cultured and then infected with helper phage, resulting in incorporation of the phagemid vector into the phage DNA.
7. The transformed phages then express the linked VH and VL chains on the surface of the phage (Fig. 27.20) linked in the form of a fusion protein with the pIII coat protein. The surface expression of the ScFv does not compromise the ability of phage to replicate since the pIII coat protein is a minor coat protein when compared with the pVIII coat protein and not all of the pIII proteins are fused with the ScFv because there is also non-phagemid DNA in the phage which codes for pIII.
8. The surface expression of the ScFv is crucial so that the phage can be easily 'panned' using immobilised antigen. Phage expressing high-affinity antigens can be thus isolated. Sometimes, antigen is immobilised on magnetic beads to facilitate isolation of ScFv expressing phage. The clones expressing the high-affinity antibody variable regions can then be grown from single phage. The selection process can then be repeated if required. The DNA coding for a high-affinity ScFv can then be isolated from the phage and introduced into an expression vector which includes DNA coding for the IgG constant region, a gene to enable selection of successfully transfected cells, e.g. the dihydrofolate reductase gene and a promoter gene to drive expression of the humanised antibody. The expression vector is introduced into a suitable cell line such as CHO cells or murine lymphoid cell lines.

Fab′ fragments

Fab′ fragments lack the Fc chain and thus do not stimulate the immune response in the same way as antibodies which have the Fc chain to act as an effector. In some cases binding affinity with a lack of immune response is an advantage, e.g. where it is preferable to block a receptor protein on cell surface but not stimulate the immune system to destroy the cell. Expression of the smaller Fab′ fragments is much simpler than the expression of a full antibody. These fragments can be produced using phage display technology.

Types of MAb

There are currently 18 monoclonal antibodies which have been licensed for therapeutic use and this therapeutic category is expanding rapidly. The majority of these antibodies have been produced by recombinant DNA technology such as the phage display system but there are three which are produced by the more old-fashioned murine antibody technology produced in hybridomas. There is currently quite a number of Fab′ fragments in clinical trials.

Monoclonal antibodies targeted against receptor proteins

The most successful application of MAbs is in the targeting of receptor proteins on particular cell types. The result of the binding of the MAb may be blocking of the cell's function or destruction of the cell.

Anticancer antibodies

Rituximab (MabThera™) targets CD20 receptors on B lymphocytes causing their lysis through generation of an immune response. It is used in the treatment of chemotherapy resistant advanced follicular lymphoma. It is a chimaeric antibody containing murine light and heavy chain variable sequences and human constant region sequences. It is produced by genetically transformed CHO cells.
Cetuximab (Ebritux™) is used in the treatment of advanced colorectal cancer. It is a chimaeric antibody produced in a murine myeloma cell line.
Alemtuzumab (MabCampath™) is also used to target the CDw52 receptor (CAMPATH1 antigen) on B lymphocytes, thus reducing their numbers in cases of chronic lymphocytic leukaemia. It is a humanised antibody where the some of the murine protein in the variable region has been replaced by human protein. It is produced by genetically transformed CHO cells.
Trastuzumab (Herceptin™) blocks the human growth factor 2 (HER-2) receptor which is overexpressed in about 25% of breast cancer patients. The HER-2 receptor also occurs in other tumours such as ovarian and gastric cancers and is believed to be the cause of the tumour as well as an indicator of poor prognosis. Trastuzumab is the first example of a drug which has been found to be active against solid tumours. Trastuzumab is a humanised murine MAb expressed in CHO cells. It blocks the ability of the HER2 receptor to initiate growth signals and may also cause cell lysis through initiation of complement activity and consequent recruitment of cytotoxic cells. It is used in conjunction with conventional chemotherapy.
Bevacizumab (Avastin™) is a humanised antibody produced in CHO cells used as first-line treatment for patients with colorectal cancer.
Panitumumab (Vectibix™) is used in the treatment of epidermal growth factor expressing metastatic colorectal carcinoma. This is the first fully human antibody.

Immunosuppressive antibodies

Graft rejection occurs when organs are transplanted between humans, e.g. kidney transplant, or between animals and humans, and the immune system of the recipient of the transplant recognises the transplanted organ as being antigenic. The immune response can be suppressed by conventional drugs and a combination of ciclosporin and corticosteroids is used to prevent graft rejection. However, ciclosporin is quite toxic to the kidney. Another strategy is to target the immune response more directly. However, in summary, a major cause of rejection is that the body directs cytotoxic T lymphocytes against the transplanted tissue in order to destroy it. The cytotoxic T-lymphocyte response is triggered by another type of T cell called a T-helper lymphocyte. The T-helper cells are responsible for immune surveillance and they have several receptors on their surfaces which are sensitive to antigens. These receptors are known as cell differentiation clusters (CDs). One particular receptor on the surface of the T-helper cells, the CD3 receptor, is a useful target for reducing the T-helper cell response (which in turn triggers the cytotoxic T cells). The specificity of monoclonal antibodies means that they can be directed to very specifically bind to a particular antigen, and in order to modulate the immune response in transplant rejection the monoclonal antibody OKT3 was produced which binds the CD3 receptor. OKT3 is a first-generation MAb and was produced using hybridoma cells which were screened for OKT3 antibody production by measuring the strength of binding of the antibodies they were producing to mature T-helper cells. High-yielding hybridoma clones were cultured in the peritoneal cavities of mice, which resulted in a very high-yielding system where the OKT3 is produced at a level of 12–15 mg/mL. OKT3 is purely based on murine protein and as a consequence there is the risk of human anti-mouse antibody (HAMA) formation in patients. The consequence of the administration of OKT3 is that the levels of T-helper cells in the body are reduced through the immune system removing them from the circulation. There are, of course, side effects since the agent compromises the natural immune response, but in the specific case of kidney transplant the benefits can outweigh the side effects because the effects of ciclosporin on the kidney cause some confusion since it is difficult to tell whether a poorly functioning transplanted kidney results from rejection or is due to the toxicity of ciclosporin. The main indications of the drug are in the early stages after transplant or as rescue therapy after standard immunosuppressant therapy has failed to prevent rejection. The risk of HAMA has meant that the use of OKT3 has declined. Two antibodies with similar indications have recently been licensed. *Darlizumab* (Zenopax™) is used to reduce the likelihood of rejection following kidney transplantation. It binds to part of the IL-2 receptor produced on the surface of activated T cells, thus interrupting their role in tissue rejection. It has a very good side effect profile and a circulating half-life of 20 days. *Basiliximab* (Simulect™) has a similar effect to Darlizumab, acting on T cells to reduce their activity in tissue rejection.

Anticlotting

Abciximab (ReoPro™) is used to prevent platelet aggregation and consequent clot formation in unstable angina and during angioplasty. It binds to the GPIIb/IIIa receptors on platelets, blocking the binding of fibrinogen, which acts to bind the platelets together into a plug that results in clot formation. The drug was developed from antiplatelet antibodies which were generated in mice. It consists of the Fab fragment of a human/murine MAb which is produced using a hybridoma cell line into which the gene for a chimaeric antibody has been inserted. The Fab fragment is released by treatment with papain, followed by chromatographic purification. It consists of *ca.* 50% murine and 50% human amino acid sequences.

Monoclonal antibodies targeted against protein mediators

Infliximab (Remicade™) is one of the most commercially successful MAbs. It is used in a combination with methotrexate to treat rheumatoid arthritis.[10–12] It is a chimaeric MAb and thus has a complete Fc chain which is necessary for stimulating an immune response. The MAb binds to TNF-α, which is a protein involved in the inflammatory processes of the autoimmune response, thus causing a reduction in the levels of this protein and a reduction of the symptoms of the disease. Infliximab is also used to treat severe Crohn's disease since TNF-α is also involved in the aetiology of this disease.

Adalimumab (Humira™) is a humanised anti-TNF antibody produced by phage display technology. It is given in combination with methotrexate in treatment of rheumatoid arthritis.

Natalizumab (Tysabri™) is used to treat relapsing multiple sclerosis by targeting an integrin protein which enables leucocytes, which are a factor in the disease, to attach themselves to cell surfaces.

Efalizumab (Raptiva™) is humanised antibody used to treat psoriasis which binds to the LFA-1 integrin protein which is expressed on all leucocytes, thus inhibiting adhesion of leucocytes to the walls of blood vessels.

Problems can occur in the use of antiprotein antibodies due to the following factors:

1. Antibody may be antigenic and be destroyed by the body's enzymes before reaching the target.
2. The peptide targets are required for the normal functioning of the body and thus the body may self-compensate by increasing the rate of production of the peptide, leaving the disease unmodulated.
3. The receptor for the peptide target may become up-regulated as a compensation mechanism.

Monoclonal antibodies used as passive vaccines

The most widely used monoclonal antibody in this category is *palivizumab* (Synagis™) which is used in the prevention of lower respiratory tract infection caused by respiratory syncytial virus in premature infants, which can prove fatal.[13,14] As yet, there is no successful vaccine against infection. Palivizumab is a humanised mouse MAb which binds to the RSVF protein which is present on the surface of the virus. Binding to the virus stimulates the immune response to remove the virus.

Monoclonal antibodies used in targeted therapy

Work has been carried out on the conjugation of toxic agents to antibodies for directed targeting of particular cell types. The only licensed product so far is a conjugate of the complex oligosaccharide calicheamicin and a humanised monoclonal antibody (*gemtuzumab-ozogamicin* or Mylotarg™) to the CD33 receptor which is present on myeloid leukaemia cells but is not present on normal stem cells, which are needed to provide a supply of blood cells. Thus the drug acts as a selective toxin against the cancerous cells.

A conjugate between *Rituximab* and iodine-131 (Bexxar™) is in the final stages of clinical trials for treatment, as is the indication for Rituximab itself, advanced follicular lymphoma. A similar conjugate between Rituximab and yttrium-90 is also undergoing clinical trials.

> **Q** Self Test 27.3
>
> Explain in more detail the nature of the following MAbs which have entered clinical trials. For example, in the light of the modes of action discussed in the previous pages, what is the likely mode of action for these antibodies?
>
> *LymphoCide:* A humanised MAb which binds to the CD22 receptor found on some B-cell leukaemias.
>
> *Vitaxin:* A humanised MAb which binds to a vascular integrin (a protein which is expressed on endothelial cells and required for angiogenesis) found on the blood vessels of tumours but not on normal blood vessels.
>
> *Anti-hepatitis B monoclonal antibody.*
>
> *Anti-CD5:* An antibody linked to the toxic peptide ricin with specific affinity for the CD5 receptor which is present on T cells which are overproduced in T-cell lymphoma.

VACCINES

Introduction

Vaccines provide the most cost-effective method of disease prevention. Even during the mid 1960s fifteen million cases of smallpox occurred. The disease was finally eradicated, apart from the threat of bioterrorism, in the 1970s. The goal of vaccination is to generate memory cells from B lymphocytes that enable a heightened immune response to occur upon exposure to the pathogen. There are still many infectious diseases in the world that are not adequately controlled. These diseases include: malaria, 270 million cases worldwide, 2 million deaths per annum with 2 billion at risk from the disease; tuberculosis, 20 million of those infected have symptoms of the disease and it is projected that 30 million will die this decade from TB; trypanosomiasis, 20 million infected, mainly in South America; and schistosomiasis, 200 million infected worldwide. Biotechnology has brought with it the prospect of the improvement of existing vaccines and the development of new ones against the remaining serious infectious diseases.

Box 27.3 gives a brief summary of the immune system.

> Box 27.3 **The immune system in brief**
>
> Aspects of the immune system have been covered in relation to the action of monoclonal antibodies. There is a range of non-specific immune defences based on the action of immune defence cells such as macrophages. The specific immune response that recognises a particular antigen is based on the activities of T and B lymphocytes. A brief summary of the immune response required for the understanding of vaccine action is given below.
>
> **B cells**
>
> B cells circulate in the blood. Their surfaces have a number of receptors (CD35, CD21, etc.) and also immunoglobulins are present on the surface of the cell. Each 'naive' B cell expresses an immunoglobulin (Ig) that is fairly specific for a particular antigen. If the B cell encounters the antigen that binds to its Ig it will form a clone of plasma cells, which are rapidly dividing and which secrete large amounts of the specific Ig; the ability of the Ig to recognise its antigen will be refined as the plasma cells continue to divide. As part of the immune response, a subpopulation of B cells forms memory cells, and these circulate for a very long time after the antigen has disappeared and retain the ability to recognise antigens more rapidly than the 'naive' B cells.
>
> **T cells**
>
> The function of the immune system is complex and thus it is difficult to determine where recognition of an antigen begins. T cells have a surveillance role and it is easiest to cast the T-helper cells as the front line of the defence. T-helper cells have a receptor called the CD4 receptor that binds to the complexes formed between the major histocompatibility complex II (MHCII) and foreign peptides that have been partially digested by antigen-presenting cells. Complexes formed with the T cells and recognised as non-self persist and cause the T-helper cells to multiply, secrete cytokines and thus trigger the division of B cells and cytotoxic T cells.

Types of vaccine

Attenuated live vaccines

These were the first type of vaccine. The attenuated organism has much in common with the infective form but due to genetic alterations it is no longer pathogenic. Genetic alterations are produced by selection of non-virulent strains upon repeated culturing of the organism or by chemical treatment. Examples include the bacille Calmette-Guérin (BCG) tuberculosis vaccine, mumps, rubella, polio and measles vaccines. The live organism gives a full immune response, penetrating into cells to produce tissue immunity as well as humoral immunity in the blood stream. Live organisms persist in the body long enough to produce both T- and B-memory cells. The organism could revert to its virulent form and those with compromised immune systems may be challenged even by the weakened pathogen. Nowadays, genetic engineering techniques can be used to specifically delete specific virulence genes.

Inactivated (dead) pathogen vaccines

The pathogen is inactivated by heat or chemicals such as formaldehyde or glutaraldehyde while ensuring that the surface antigens remain intact. Examples include cholera, whooping cough, influenza, rabies and polio vaccines. With these vaccines there is no risk of pathogenicity developing. Complex immune response can be induced by multiple antigens. Such vaccines are not necessarily completely safe; e.g. the whooping cough vaccine has occasionally produced hypersensitive responses. These vaccines do not enter cells and thus do not produce cellular immunity; they only confer humoral immunity.

Purified subunit vaccines

The major determinants of the immune response are extracted from the organism and purified. For example, some organisms such as those causing tetanus and diphtheria produce toxins and the main defence of the body against these organisms is the production of antibodies against these toxins. Treatment of these toxins with formaldehyde (Box 27.4) to produce toxoids renders them safe for use as vaccines while preserving their ability to induce an immune response. A similar approach has been used in attempting to reduce the risks of the whole cell pertussis vaccine but without a wholly successful vaccine being produced. Another approach is to utilise the surface polysaccharides from bacteria. On their own, such polysaccharides are poorly immunogenic, and thus their immunogenicity is increased by conjugating them to tetanus or diphtheria toxoids. Some of the vaccines against meningitis are based on such polysaccharide–toxoid conjugates. The advantage of these types of vaccine is that there is no risk of pathogenicity and hypersensitivity, but the vaccine may only stimulate humoral immunity and is expensive to produce.

> **Box 27.4 Formaldehyde inactivation**
>
> The process of toxin inactivation by formaldehyde treatment is poorly understood. However, it does involve the formation of a Schiff's base, either with lysine or arginine residues in the protein, followed by cross-linking to residues such as tyrosine, lysine and tryptophan. The quality control for this reaction is bioassay of the resultant toxoid using an animal model but there is the possibility of using mass spectrometry to follow the modification (Fig. 27.21).[15]

Advances in oral vaccination

The development of oral vaccines for stimulation of mucosal immunity is an important goal because of the simplicity of administration. The mucosal system is the first barrier a pathogen has to penetrate, and mucosal immunity is based on the production of IgA antibodies. The oral polio vaccine was an early example. The types of vaccines used for oral dosage are the same as those available for administration by injection. Formulation of oral vaccines presents a particular challenge for the pharmacist and is likely to see major progress in the future.

Licensed vaccines

Live attenuated

Poliomyelitis (oral vaccine), measles, mumps, rubella (the attenuated virus strains are now combined in a single vaccine), tuberculosis (BCG vaccine), varicella-zoster, yellow fever.

Inactivated

Influenza (inactivated by formaldehyde or propiolactone treatment), hepatitis A (inactivated by formaldehyde treatment), pertussis (inactivated by formaldehyde treatment, usually combined with diphtheria and tetanus toxins into a single vaccine), rabies, tick-borne encephalitis (formaldehyde inactivated).

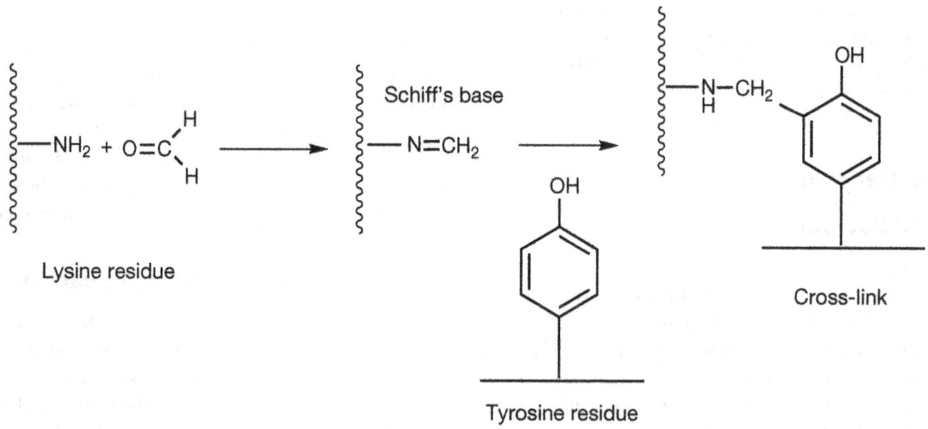

Figure 27.21 Formaldehyde inactivation.

Purified subunit

Influenza (formaldehyde treated haemagglutinin and neuraminidase antigens) and tetanus (formaldehyde treated tetanus toxin), diphtheria (formaldehyde treated diphtheria toxin).

Conjugated polysaccharide

Meningitis C (capsular polysaccharide conjugated to inactivated diphtheria toxin), meningitis A and C, pneumococcal vaccines (capsular polysaccharide conjugated to inactivated diphtheria toxin), typhoid (capsular polysaccharide alone).

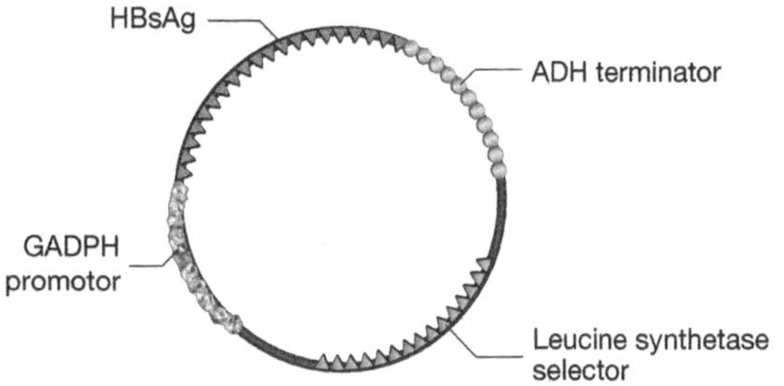

Figure 27.22 pBR322 based expression vector used to transform yeast cells so that they produce a hepatitis B vaccine.

Applications of biotechnology to vaccine production

A logical extension of the use of purified subunit vaccines is to try to produce antigenic components which are capable of producing an immune response using biotechnology. The first successful example of this was the hepatitis B subunit vaccine which has been very successful. The production of this is described in detail below.

The hepatitis B vaccine and example in detail

Hepatitis B virus infects the liver and causes progressive liver disease and ultimately liver cancer. There are about 250 million sufferers worldwide. Unlike hepatitis A, which can be contracted from contaminated food, hepatitis B is predominantly maternally or sexually transmitted or is transmitted by intravenous drug use. Infection can also arise from contact with physiological fluids and people working with these materials, e.g. in biochemistry labs, would be advised to receive vaccination against it. The first hepatitis B vaccines based on Dane particles were derived from plasma from human carriers of the disease, but supply was limited by the availability of such plasma. In addition, extensive processing of the material extracted from plasma was necessary to ensure its non-infectivity. From the point of view of patients, there was a reluctance to accept a vaccine derived from human plasma. The biotechnologically produced hepatitis B coat protein is now the most commonly used vaccine.

The vaccine is based on a surface glycoprotein of the virus coat and is thus an antigenic component vaccine as opposed to a live vaccine. Since the vaccine is not live it does not invade tissues and thus tissue immunity is not stimulated. Despite some limitations, the antigenic component hepatitis B vaccine does appear to be a highly effective vaccine.

The biotechnological process leading to the production of a hepatitis B vaccine

1. The primary structure of a surface glycoprotein (HBsAg) from the hepatitis B virus was determined. A preliminary selection of DNA coding for HBsAg was carried out using transformed *E. coli* cultures to amplify the viral DNA, and oligonucleotide probes were used to identify the required gene. The selected DNA was then inserted into a plasmid (pBR322) which in turn was ligated into a yeast expression vector (Fig. 27.22). Yeast was selected as a suitable organism for expression of a hepatitis B vaccine because of rapid growth characteristics in combination with production of the correctly folded protein. *E. coli* bacteria did not produce a correctly folded protein. The composite expression vector incorporated promoter and selection genes. The selection gene in this case was leucine synthetase which permits growth of transformed cultures in the absence of the amino acid leucine, and the promoter gene used to 'turn on' the expression of the HBsAg gene was glyceraldehyde 3-phosphate dehydrogenase (GAPDH). The alcohol dehydrogenase gene (ADH) was used to terminate transcription.
2. The incorporation of a leucine synthesising gene enabled selection of transformed yeast cells on the basis that they were able to grow in leucine-free medium. High-yielding colonies were selected and used as the basis of the production process. The coat protein is harvested by disrupting the yeast cells and, in the first instance, adsorbing the protein onto silica gel. The surface protein is produced in unglycosylated form but the lack of glycosylation does not appear to make it less effective as a vaccine.

Hepatitis B vaccines have also been produced by genetically transformed Chinese hamster ovary (CHO) cells. These vaccines contain both glycosylated and unglycosylated forms of the coat protein and are thus indistinguishable from the natural antigen. However, it has not been established that glycosylation is important with regard to antigenicity. A CHO-derived HBV (GenHevac B) is licensed for use in France.

Other recombinant vaccines

There have been no major developments in recombinant vaccine production since the hepatitis B vaccine. Recombinant vaccines were produced against Lyme disease and rotavirus but have been subsequently withdrawn from the market. Recently, an oral cholera vaccine (Dukoral) based on mixture on inactive cholera bacteria and a cholera toxin B subunit produced by recombinant technology has been launched.

Licensed recombinant vaccines

Engerix B. HBS Ag expressed in yeast cells 20 μg/mL absorbed onto aluminium hydroxide.
HBvaxPRO. HBS Ag expressed in yeast cells. Vials containing 5, 10 and 40 μg adsorbed onto aluminium hydroxphosphate sulphate.
Dukoral. Oral suspension. Inactivated cholera + recombinant cholera toxin B subunit.

Recent developments in vaccine production by biotechnology

There still remain many challenges in vaccine development and the examples discussed below indicate strategies provided by biotechnology which are being used to develop new vaccines.

Approaches to the development of an AIDS vaccine

No safe attenuated form of the virus has been recognised and thus a live attenuated vaccine is unlikely to be developed. The most promising approach is based on subunit vaccines based on the viral glycoproteins gp 160 and gp 120. These recombinant proteins have been expressed in a number of systems including yeast and mammalian cells. In order to stimulate T as well as B cell response, the genes coding these subunit vaccines have been coupled to the vaccinia virus, which has a track record of use in humans since it was used as a smallpox vaccine. A number of AIDS vaccines have undergone small-scale clinical trials.

Approaches to the development of a malaria vaccine

Vaccination against malaria is difficult because of the three stages in the development of the parasite. An effective vaccine might need to contain antigens from each stage. Examples of vaccines which have been tested have been based on: three merozite stage surface proteins, a seven-antigen vaccine containing proteins from each stage of the life cycle and a recombinant vaccine consisting of an antigen found in the sporozite stage fused with a hepatitis B antigen producing overall a stronger immune response than the antigen on its own.

Anticancer vaccines

The difficulty in developing this type of vaccine is in finding immunogens since cancers are often not recognised by the immune system as being foreign. There are three categories of tumour associated antigen: tumour-specific antigens, tumour-associated differentiation antigens which are found in normal tissues but are overexpressed in cancer cells, and antigenic peptides which are involved in the development of the cancer. A number of vaccines based on these approaches have been tested.

A Self Test 27.1

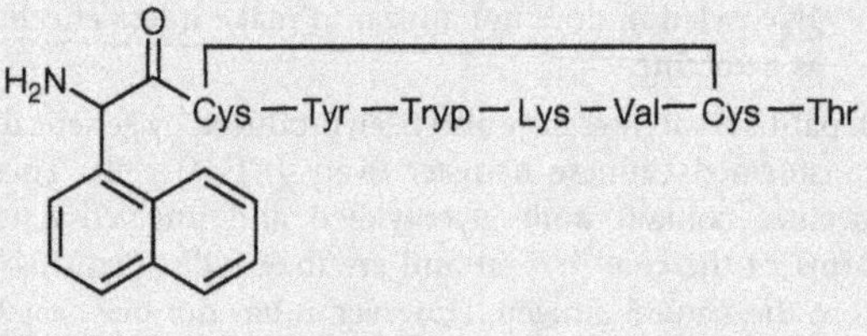

Lanreotide

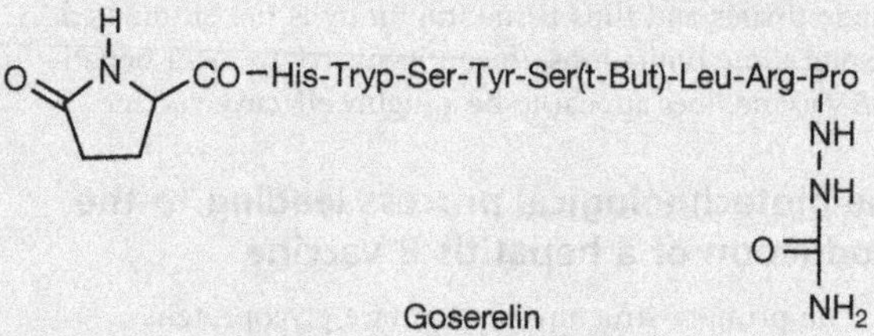

Goserelin

Self Test 27.2

1.
$$-HC-CO-NH-CH-COOH \xrightarrow{H_2O} -HC-COOH + NH_2-CH-COOH$$

with side chains:

$$
\begin{array}{cccc}
CH_2 & CH_2 & CH_2 & CH_2 \\
S & CONH_2 & S & CONH_2
\end{array}
$$

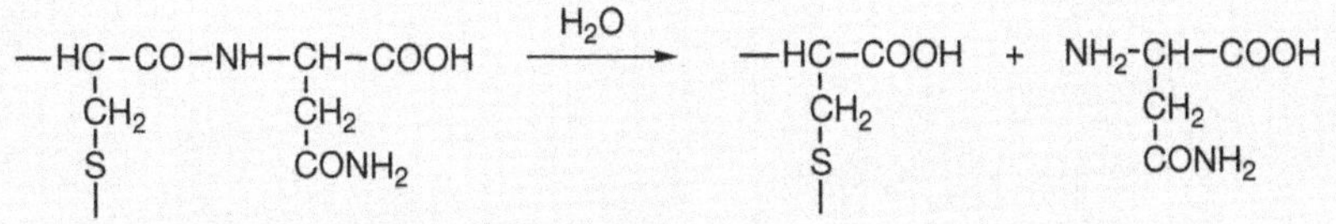

2. T. The single amino acid threonine is released from the C-terminal of the B-chain.
3. Six charges in total. Two on histidine, one on arginine, one on lysine and two at the N-terminus of the A and B chains.
4. Insulin has four aspartate residues and two terminal carboxyl groups making a total of six acidic residues. This is balanced by six basic residues. Thus the p*I* value = (3+8)/2 = 5.5, i.e. that insulin will be charge neutral at that pH with the acids and bases carrying equal charges.

Self Test 27.3

LymphoCide: Promotes lysis of malignant B lymphocytes by binding to a specific receptor on their surface.
Vitaxin: Binds to vascular integrin protein thus promoting its removal by the immune system and reducing angiogenesis in tumours.

Anti-hepatitis B monoclonal antibody: Binds to hepatitis B thus promoting removal of the virus, acting as a passive vaccine.
Anti-CD5: Toxic antibody targeted therapy specifically aimed at the T-cells overproduced in T-cell lymphoma.

REFERENCES

1. Bhatnagar S, Srivastava D, Jayadev MSK, Dubey AK. Molecular variants and derivatives of insulin for improved glycemic control in diabetes. *Progress Biophys Mol Biol.* 2006;91:199–228.
2. Roberts MJ, Bently MD, Harris JM. Chemistry for peptide and protein PEGylation. *Adv Drug Deliv Rev.* 2002;54:459–476.
3. Pradhananga S, Wilkinson I, Ross RJM. Pegvisomant: structure and function. *J Mol Endocrinol.* 2002;29:11–14.
4. Birch JR, Rachner AJ. Antibody production. *Adv Drug Del Rev.* 2006;58:671–685.
5. Popov S, Hubbard JG, Ward ES. Novel and efficient method for the isolation of antibodies that recognise T cell receptor Vαs. *Mol Immunol.* 1996;33:493–502.
6. Azzazy HME, Highsmith WE. Phage display technology: clinical applications and recent innovations. *Clin Biochem.* 2002;35:425–455.
7. Ladner RC, Sato AK, Gorzelany J, de Souza M. Phage display-derived peptides as therapeutic alternatives to antibodies. *Drug Discov Today.* 2004;9: 525–529.
8. Kehoe JW, Kay BK. Filamentous phage display in the new millennium. *Chem Rev.* 2005;105:4056–4072.
9. Nishbori N, Hiroyuki H, Furusawa S, Matsuda H. Humanisation of chicken monoclonal antibody using phage-display system. *Mol Immunol.* 2006; 43:634–642.
10. Vilcek J, Feldmann M. Historical review: cytokines as therapeutics and targets of therapeutics. *Trends Pharmacol Sci.* 2004;25:201–209.
11. Taylor PC. Antibody therapy for rheumatoid arthritis. *Current Opinion Pharmacol.* 2003;3:323–328.
12. Bayry J, Siberil S, Triebel F, et al. Rescuing CD4+CD25+ regulatory T-cell functions in rheumatoid arthritis by cytokine-targeted monoclonal antibody therapy. *Drug Discov Today.* 2007;12:548–552.
13. Wu H, Pfarr DS, Johnson S, et al. Development of Motavizumab, an ultra-potent antibody for the prevention of respiratory syncytial virus infection in the upper and lower respiratory tract. *J Mol Biol.* 2007; 368:652–665.
14. Bussel JB, Giulino L, Lee S, et al. Update on therapeutic monoclonal antibodies. *Curr Probl Pediatr Adolesc Health Care.* 2007;37:118–135.
15. Thaysen-Andersen M, Jørgensen SB, Wilhelmsen ES, et al. Investigation of the detoxification mechanism of formaldehyde-treated tetanus toxin. *Vaccine.* 2007;25:2213–2227.

Chapter **28**

Drug and gene delivery systems

Christine Dufès

CHAPTER CONTENTS

INTRODUCTION

Over the recent years, advances in biotechnology and molecular biology have led to the production of highly promising new drugs; however, such new drugs are often associated with drug delivery challenges. It is estimated that more than 40% of recently discovered drugs have delivery problems as the result of poor biopharmaceutical properties and need new delivery approaches. In order to overcome this problem, advanced drug delivery systems have been developed as strategies to overcome many of the delivery limitations associated with these novel drugs. They have been designed with the objective of developing 'magic bullets' as described by Paul Ehrlich, able to provide site-specific delivery of the drug to the disease site. This chapter is primarily designed to highlight some of the most exciting developments in the field of drug and gene delivery. This topic is extensive and, as such, only a general overview will be detailed here. It is hoped that this chapter will provide the reader with a basic understanding of the principal approaches to drug and gene delivery and of the potentially crucial role of the described systems as drug carriers.

LIPOSOMES

Liposomes are self-assembling vesicular structures based on one or more lipid bilayers encapsulating an aqueous core (Fig. 28.1).

Although a variety of amphipathic molecules can be used to form the bilayer, the major lipidic components of liposomes are usually phospholipids, amphiphilic moieties with a hydrophilic head group and two hydrophobic chains. The phospholipid molecules form a closed bilayer

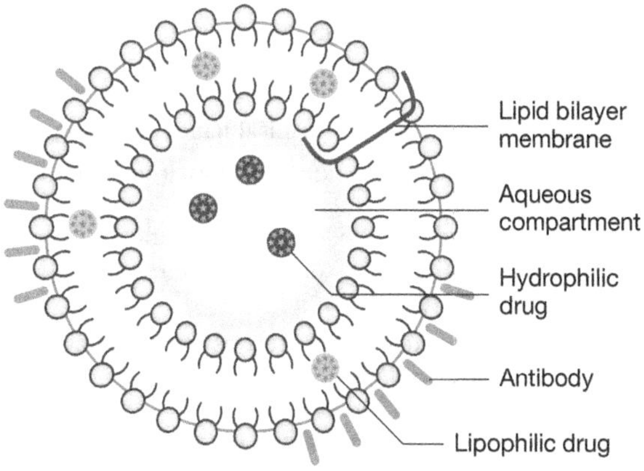

Figure 28.1 Structure of a liposome.

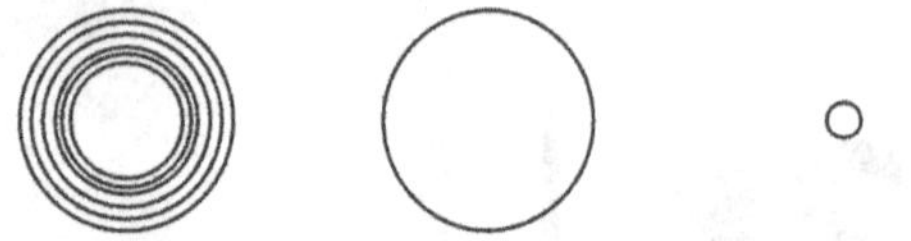

Figure 28.2 Typical morphology and size range of common types of liposomes.

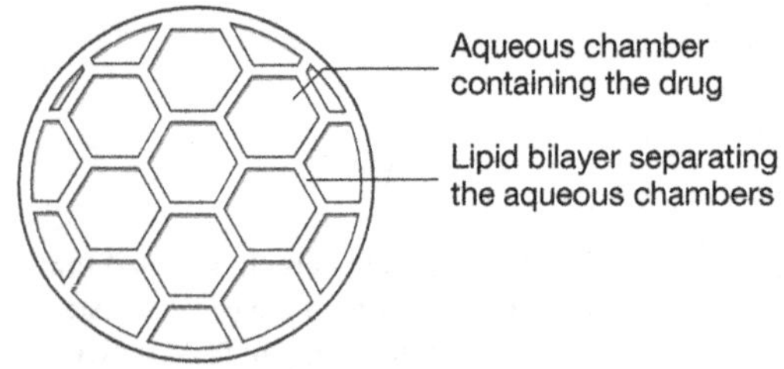

Figure 28.3 Cross-sectional structure of a DepoCyte® liposome.

sphere in an attempt to shield their hydrophobic groups from the aqueous environment while still maintaining contact with the aqueous phase via the hydrophilic head group.

On the basis of their size and their number of lipid bilayers, liposomes are classified into multilamellar vesicles (MLVs, diameter >200 nm), large unilamellar vesicles (diameter 100–1000 nm) and small unilamellar vesicles (diameter <100 nm) (Fig. 28.2). However, other structures have also been described. For example, DepoCyte®, a liposomal formulation of the anti-cancer drug cytarabine, can be described as a multivesicular liposome (Fig. 28.3).

If multilamellar vesicles are formed, water is present in the core of the liposome as well as between the lipidic bilayers.

Depending on its physicochemical nature, the drug can:

- be encapsulated in the aqueous phase (hydrophilic drugs)
- be intercalated into the bilayer (lipophilic drugs).
- interact with the surface of the liposome (through electrostatic interactions).

Liposomes can therefore be used as carriers for both hydrophilic and lipophilic drugs.

The composition of liposomes largely dictates their stability *in vivo*. Liposomes are generally made of two main types of chemicals: phospholipids and sterols. As phospholipids are the most abundant component

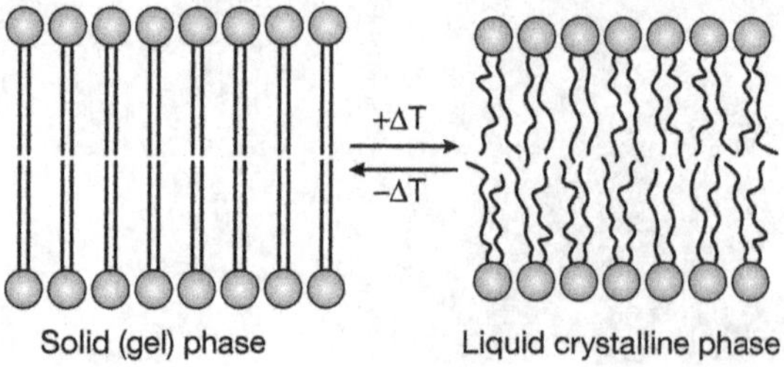

Figure 28.4 Modifications of membrane permeability following from variations in phase transition temperature.

in mammalian cell membranes, they are used as the major building block of liposomes. The choice of the phospholipid to be used in the formulation is important since this will determine the physical state of the liposome and therefore the permeability of the liposomal bilayer.

Formation of stable liposomes from phospholipids is only possible at temperatures above the gel to liquid-crystalline phase transition temperature (T_c) which represents the melting point of the acyl chains. All phospholipids have a characteristic T_c, which depends on the nature of the polar head group and on length and degree of unsaturation of the acyl chains (T_c increases with increasing chain length and with increasing saturation). Above T_c, phospholipids are in the liquid-crystalline phase, characterised by an increase in the mobility of the acyl chains (Fig. 28.4). Under these conditions the bilayer is more permeable and this may allow the escape of any drug dissolved in the aqueous solution or entrapped within the bilayer structure. A decrease in temperature to below T_c induces a transition to a more rigid state (gel state) resulting in restrained mobility due to tightly packed acyl chains. As drug permeability is reduced in the 'gel' state compared to the 'fluid' state, the stability of liposomal entrapment can be maximised by selecting high-phase transition phospholipids. For example, distearoyl phosphatidylcholine has long and saturated fatty acid acyl chains which remain in a gel state at physiological temperature (Fig. 28.5). Phosphatidylcholine has been used individually or in combination with cholesterol to prepare liposomes.

Sterols are steroid-based alcohols, the most commonly employed of which is cholesterol (Fig. 28.6). Cholesterol when used in equimolar proportions with a phospholipid is known to condense the packing of the phospholipids in bilayers above T_c, thereby reducing their permeability to encapsulated drugs. However, it has been shown that the inclusion of cholesterol in the liposome significantly decreases the solubilisation of hydrophobic drugs in the inlayers.

Liposomes can be subdivided into four groups:

- conventional liposomes
- sterically stabilised ('stealth') liposomes

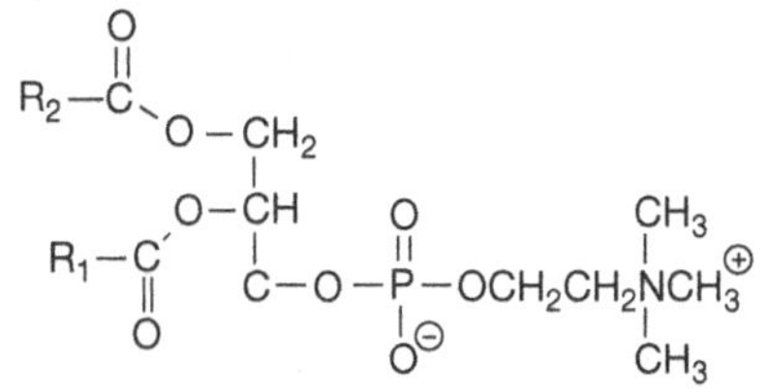

Common name: (prefix) – phosphatidylcholine

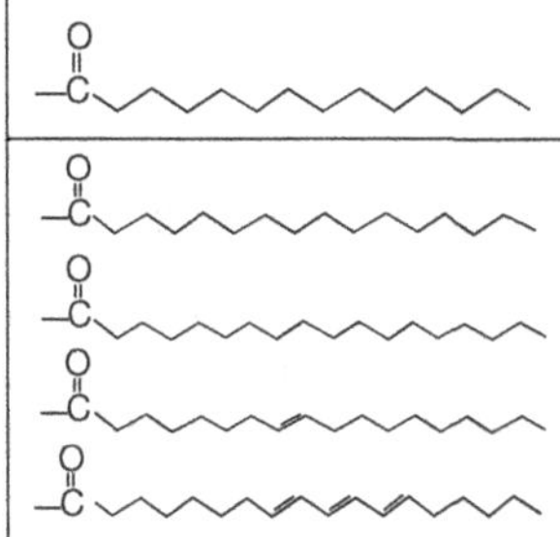

Where R_1 and R_2 are:	*Name of fatty acid*	*Phospholipid name*
	Myristic	Dimyristoyl phosphatidylcholine
	Palmitic	Dipalmitoyl phosphatidylcholine
	Stearic	Distearoyl phosphatidylcholine
	Oleic	Dioleoyl phosphatidylcholine
	Linolenic	Dilinoleoyl phosphatidylcholine

Figure 28.5 Common phospholipids used for liposomal manufacture.

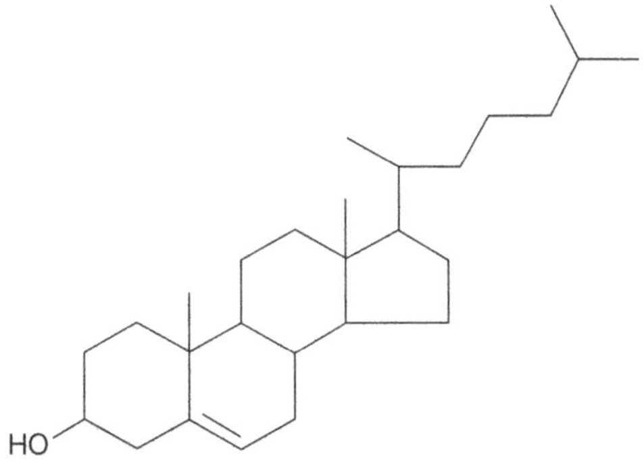

Figure 28.6 Structure of cholesterol.

- immunoliposomes (antibody-targeted liposomes)
- cationic liposomes.

Conventional liposomes

Conventional liposomes are typically composed of only phospholipids and/or cholesterol. This 'first generation' of liposomes is generally used for passive targeting: they tend to be phagocytosed by the cells of the mononuclear phagocyte system (MPS) and therefore accumulate in organs such as the liver and the spleen. Based on this property, a conventional liposome formulation of the antifungal drug amphotericin B (initially marketed under the name AmBisome®) has been shown to dramatically reduce the toxicity of the drug, thus improving its clinical efficacy.

Sterically stabilised liposomes

Conventional liposomes are generally rapidly cleared from the circulation following phagocytosis by cells of the reticuloendothelial system. The circulation time of the liposomes can be increased by covalently linking polyethylene glycol (PEG) to the liposome surface, therefore providing steric hindrance on the bilayer surface which inhibits phagocytosis. The prolongation of the residence time of the liposomes should encourage drug accumulation within regions of increased permeability, such as tumours. This passive targeting property is sometimes called the 'enhanced permeability and retention' (EPR) effect. As an example, Doxil® has been commercialised as a PEGylated long-circulating liposome encapsulating the anticancer drug doxorubicin. Its long circulation time, conjugated to the EPR effect, facilitates its accumulation in the tumours.

Immunoliposomes

Immunoliposomes can be targeted to specific cell populations, such as cancer cells, via incorporation of a targeting moiety. The targeting ligands can be a lipid-anchored antibody, an antibody fragment, or ligands such as transferrin and folate, for example.

Cationic liposomes

Positively charged cationic liposomes can form electrostatic complexes with negatively charged plasmid DNA, neutralising the charges and therefore facilitating gene transfer. For example, the transfection agent Lipofectin® is a cationic liposome composed of the cationic lipid N [1-(2,3-dioleyloxy)propyl]-N,N,N-trimethylammonium chloride) (DOTMA) and the co-lipid dioleoylphosphatidylethanolamine (DOPE). The hydrophobic moieties ensure that the cationic lipids assemble into bilayer vesicles, while exposing the positively charged amine group to the aqueous medium. The amine group is the DNA binding moiety, interacting electrostatically with the negatively charged phosphate groups of the DNA. This electrostatic interaction protects DNA from degradation. Plasmids may also be incorporated within the cationic liposomes to ensure protection against *in vivo* degradation; however, their encapsulation efficiency is very low.

Q Self Test 28.1

Describe the formulation approach used to increase the blood circulation time of liposomes.

What is the main use of a cationic liposome?

Explain the role played by the liquid-crystalline phase transition temperature Tc on the stability of liposomal entrapment.

NIOSOMES

Niosomes, also named non-ionic surfactant vesicles, are unilamellar or multilamellar vesicles prepared by the aqueous dispersion of synthetic, non-ionic amphipathic molecules. They have been developed as alternatives to phospholipid-based liposomes, with which they share the same structures shown in Figure 28.1. Niosomes are formed by the self-assembly of non-ionic amphiphiles in aqueous media resulting in closed bilayer structures. The assembly into closed bilayers is usually not spontaneous and requires the input of some form of energy, such as physical agitation or heat. The resulting vesicles shield their hydrophobic groups from the aqueous environment while maintaining maximum contact with the aqueous phase via the hydrophilic head groups.

Depending of its physicochemical nature, the drug can:

- be encapsulated in the aqueous phase (hydrophilic drugs)
- be intercalated into the bilayer (lipophilic drugs)
- interact with the surface of the niosome (through electrostatic interactions).

Like the liposomes, niosomes can be used as carriers for both hydrophilic and lipophilic drugs. The release of the encapsulated drug is influenced by the composition, the size and the number of bilayers in the vesicles. The properties of liposomes and niosomes are therefore largely similar; however, niosomes present several advantages over the phospholipids-based liposomes:

- Higher chemical stability. Niosomes are in most case prepared from saturated alkyl chains containing ether linkages. This results in a higher stability of the surfactant in comparison to phospholipids, which are easily hydrolysed due to the presence of ester bonds in their structure.
- Low cost. The synthetic surfactants are tailor-made compounds, generally made in large quantities and therefore generally cheaper than phospholipids.

Niosomes are formed mainly by self-assembly of synthetic non-ionic surfactants with the optional combination of cholesterol and charged surfactants. In order to form niosomes, the amphiphilic molecules must possess a hydrophilic head group and a hydrophobic tail. Many surfactants have been used in the preparation of niosomes, i.e. cholesteryl poly (24) oxyethylene ether, alkylglucoside, cetyl lactoside, polyoxyethylenealkyl ether, and cetyl diglycerolester. Additives are often required in the formulation to increase the stability of the vesicles. Cholesterol is the most commonly used additive found in niosomes. The addition of charged molecules, such as dicetylphosphate, cholesteryl sulphate and cholesteryl phosphate, to the bilayer may also be needed to stabilise the formulation. Niosomes have shown great potential for many applications in pharmacology, being equivalent to liposomes regarding their non-toxicity and administration efficiency of entrapped hydrophilic or lipophilic drugs, but with the advantage of a higher chemical stability (Fig. 28.7).

Q Self Test 28.2

Which of the following statements are *true*? (Answer below)

A. The assembly of the amphiphilic molecules into vesicles is spontaneous.
B. Niosomes can encapsulate lipophilic as well as hydrophilic drugs.
C. Niosomes are more stable than liposomes.
D. Cholesterol may be found only in liposomes.
E. Sterols increase the mechanical strength of the bilayer.
F. Phospholipids are major structural components of the niosomes.
G. Charged molecules may be added to the formulation of non-ionic surfactant vesicles.

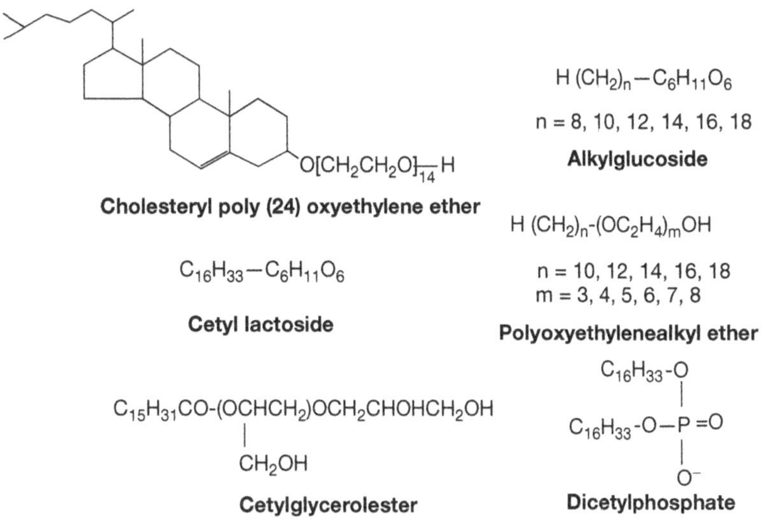

Figure 28.7 Chemical structure of non-ionic surfactants and associated compounds used in the preparation of niosomes.

POLYMERIC MICELLES

Amphipathic molecules such as phospholipids placed in an aqueous solution can also form micelles, which are small spherical structures with the hydrophilic heads of the molecules on the surface and a dense core region consisting of the hydrophobic tails (Fig. 28.8). Polymeric micelles are typically 5–100 nm in diameter. They are spontaneously formed above a certain critical concentration, the critical micelle concentration (CMC), by surfactants or block copolymers composed of hydrophilic and hydrophobic regions. The stability of the micelles depends on the CMC. Micelles with high CMC are unstable: they may dissociate into unimers and their content may precipitate out. By contrast, micelles with low CMC are more stable. As micelles must be stable upon dilution with a large volume of blood *in vivo*, their CMC must be very low for them to be effective drug carriers. The hydrophobic core region serves as a reservoir for hydrophobic drugs, whereas the hydrophilic outer shell prevents undesirable phenomena such as aggregation, precipitation, protein adsorption or cell adhesion. As a consequence, micelles are thought to have excellent water solubility irrespective of hydrophobic drug loading.

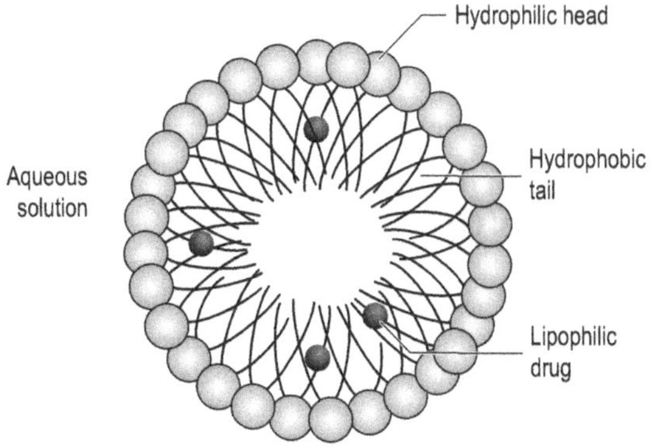

Figure 28.8 Structure of a micelle.

Micellar formulations present the following advantages:

- Ability to solubilise hydrophobic molecules
- Preservation of drug activity during delivery to the target since the drug in the hydrophobic core is protected from exposure to aqueous degradation processes
- Good water solubility
- Good structural stability if the CMC of the polymers is low
- High drug-loading capacity
- Small particle size, appropriate for long circulation in the blood compartment. The diameter of the micelles should be small enough to allow passive targeting due to the EPR effect (<0.2 μm) while remaining large enough to prevent penetration through normal endothelium. As a result, polymeric micelles will be able to slowly accumulate in malignant or inflamed tissues. However, their eventual instability upon dilution limits their pharmaceutical applications. Another limitation is that micellar formulations cannot be used for entrapping water-soluble drugs.

Generally, the amphiphilic core/shell structure of polymeric micelles is formed from block polymers. Polyethylene glycol (PEG) and polyethylene oxide (PEO) are often used as the hydrophilic blocks. They have been shown to prevent recognition by the reticuloendothelial system and increase circulation time *in vivo*. As in the case of liposomes and niosomes, the grafting of specific ligand molecules on the surface of the polymeric micelles allows

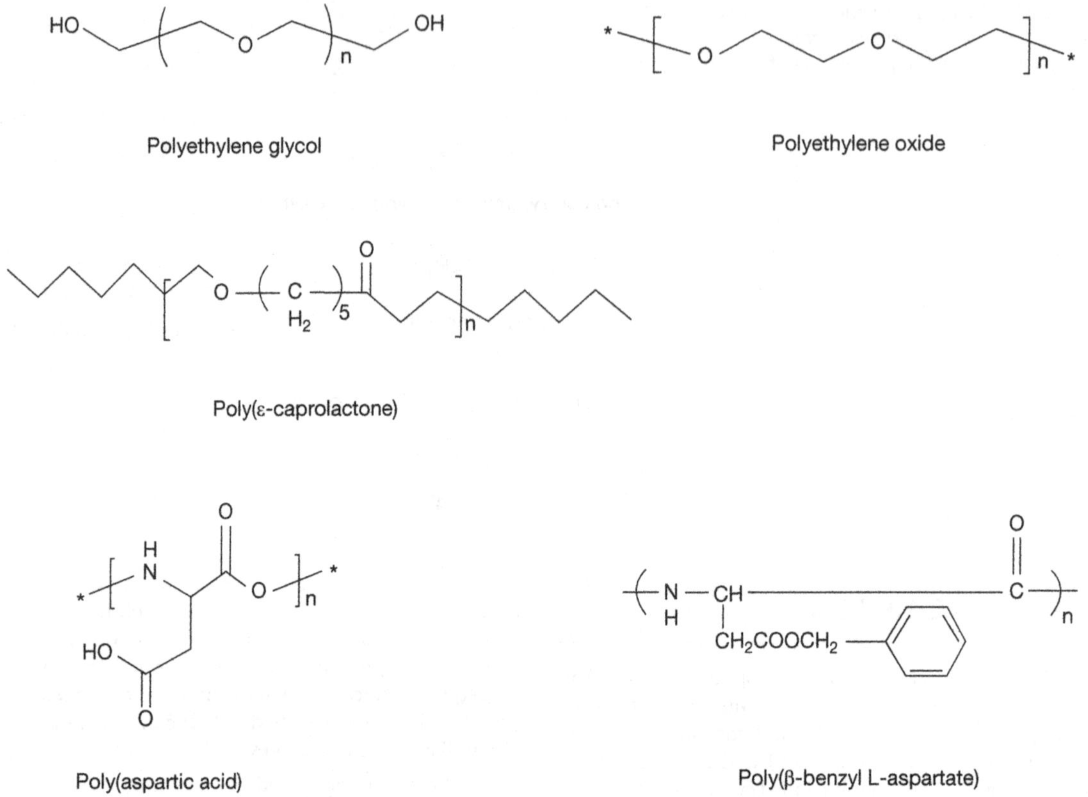

Figure 28.9 Chemical structure of hydrophilic and hydrophobic entities used in block polymers.

a specific and enhanced cellular uptake at the target tissue, thus reducing the administered dose and side effects. Many types of end-functionalised PEG-based block copolymers have been prepared to date using hetero-bifunctional PEG as the macroinitiator.

Poly(ϵ-caprolactone), poly(aspartic acid), poly(β-benzyl L-aspartate) and poly(ortho esters) are polymers popular for use as the dense micellar core, due to their hydrophobic nature and favourable interactions with poorly soluble hydrophobic drugs (Fig. 28.9). In particular, poly(aspartic) polymer is hydrolysable and possesses carboxyl groups for binding amino group-bearing drugs to form biodegradable amide linkages. The drug can be loaded into the micelle either by encapsulation or chemical covalent binding. Many groups have investigated polymeric micelles for drug and gene delivery. Micellar formulations have, for example, been used for the delivery of the anticancer drugs paclitaxel and doxorubicin, as well as the immunosuppressant drug ciclosporin.

PEG-polyelectrolyte block polymers were also found to form polyion complex (PIC) micelles with negatively charged DNA through electrostatic interactions. This is particularity important in the field of gene and DNA/RNA delivery, as the PIC micelles exhibit an excellent solubility in aqueous media and protect the carried DNA against enzymatic degradation.

> **Q Self Test 28.3**
>
> Name the similarities and the differences between liposomes and micelles.
>
> Give an example of a hydrophilic and a hydrophobic entity commonly used in the preparation of polymeric micelles.
>
> Explain the two drawbacks regarding the use of micelles as delivery systems.

NANOPARTICLES

Nanoparticles are colloidal, polymeric colloidal spheres ranging in size from 10 to 1000 μm. They are made of natural or artificial polymers. The term 'nanoparticles' encompasses both nanospheres and nanocapsules. Nanospheres are made of a continuous matrix, whereas nanocapsules have a core-shell structure (Fig. 28.10).

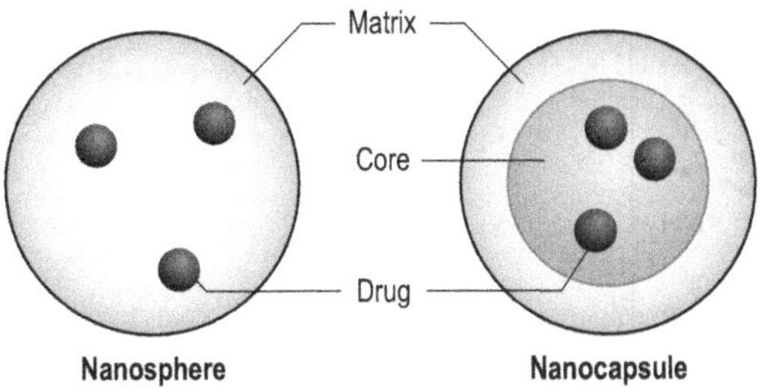

Figure 28.10 Structure of a nanosphere and a nanocapsule.

Depending of the method of preparation, the active principle (drug or oligonucleotide) can be:

- entrapped within the polymer matrix (in the case of a nanosphere)
- encapsulated within the core of the nanocapsule by its polymeric shell
- adsorbed or covalently bound to the surface of the nanoparticle.

Many techniques have been successfully used to prepare nanoparticles. They either use preformed polymers or involve the polymerisation of monomers.

Nanoparticles present many advantages, among these are:

- ability to carry a wide variety of drugs and oligonucleotides
- sustained delivery of the active principle for an extended period of time
- stability
- good tolerability of the components
- simplicity of the manufacturing process.

The release of the carried drug depends of the nature of its containment by the nanoparticle:

- Nanospheres entrap the drug within the matrix in a uniform manner. The release of the drug from the matrix may occur by diffusion through the nanoparticle matrix.
- In the case of the nanocapsules, the drug is encapsulated within the core of the nanoparticle and is released by diffusion through the polymer shell.
- Drugs can be released by erosion of the nanoparticle itself.
- A combination of diffusion–erosion mechanisms of release may also occur.
- Covalent coupling of the drug to the surface of the nanoparticle leads to a slower release rate than non-covalent binding.

Parameters such as size, density and molecular weight will influence the release of the carried drug. Due to their small size, nanoparticles degrade faster than larger microspheres. Degradation of the nanoparticles can occur either by erosion of the polymer backbone or cleavage of the ester bonds, for example in the case of the polyalkylcyanoacrylate nanoparticles. The mechanism of degradation of the nanoparticle may also be polymer-dependent. For example, polylactic acid-based microspheres degrade from their centre by hydrolysis. Human serum albumin nanoparticles also degrade from their centre, but only after their phagocytosis by macrophages.

Depending on their surface charge, nanoparticles may also interact by direct contact with biological membranes, thus resulting to an enhanced delivery of drugs through these membranes in comparison to a simple solution.

Nanoparticles may be used for similar purposes as liposomes. However, they present the advantage of a higher stability, leading to longer shelf-life.

Like other colloidal carriers, nanoparticles are rapidly taken up by the reticuloendothelial system after intravenous administration and therefore mainly accumulate within organs such as liver, spleen and lungs. Nanoparticles also exhibit a tendency to accumulate in tumours, and can thus be used to enhance the efficacy of the carried anticancer drugs. The mechanism producing this accumulation is still unknown and occurs even without tumour-targeting ligands being attached to the nanoparticle. Importantly, the improved efficacy of a given anticancer drug on a given type of tumour may depend on the delivery system carrying it. As a result, optimised cancer treatment may require an 'à la carte' choice of the drug delivery system depending on the tumour being treated.

It is also important to note that peptide drugs can be bound efficiently to nanoparticles. For example, insulin can be bound by surface adsorption to polyalkylcyanoacrylate nanoparticles or can be encapsulated into these nanoparticles. A subcutaneous injection of insulin in these two formulations led to an extended control of the blood glucose level compared to the free drug. Nanoparticles are prepared using various types of natural or synthetic polymers (Fig. 28.11).

Polymers used to prepare nanoparticles

Natural polymers

Natural polymers such as chitosan and gelatin have often been a material of choice for the delivery of oligonucleotides and proteins as well as drugs.

Chitosan

Chitosan, a naturally derived polysaccharide obtained by deacetylation of chitin, which occurs in crab and lobster shells, has been extensively studied for delivering anticancer drugs, genes and vaccines. This polymer presents numerous properties favourable to drug delivery applications, such as its biocompatibility, positive charge allowing DNA condensation via interactions with the phosphate groups of DNA, abundance of amine groups available for cross-linking and mucoadhesiveness. Interestingly, chitosan was also found to have antitumour activity by itself. The release of a drug

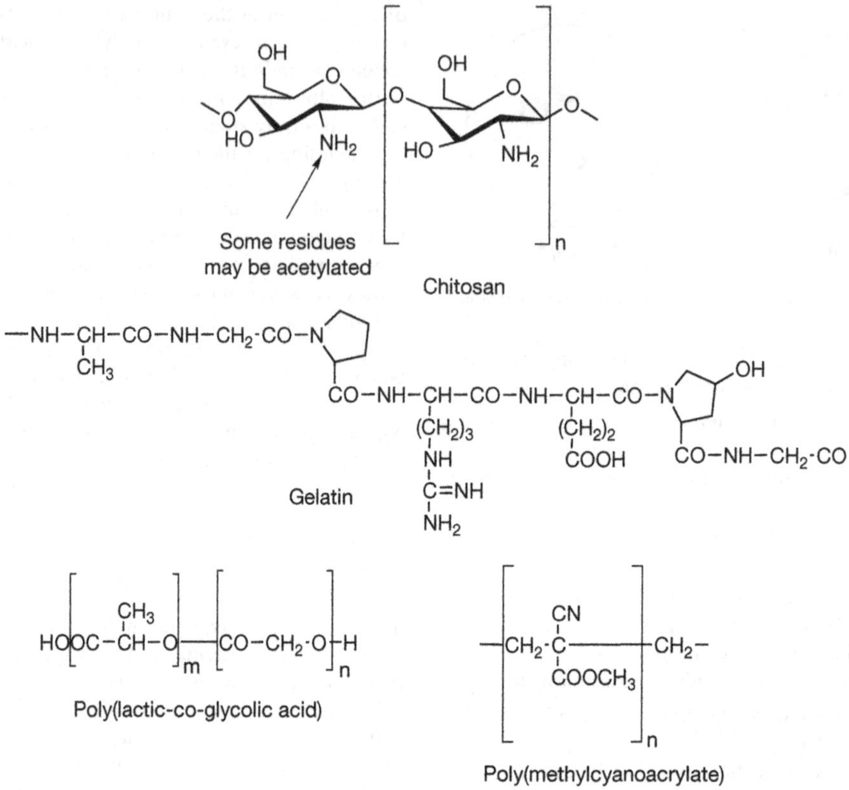

Figure 28.11 Chemical structure of polymers used as drug carriers.

from chitosan nanoparticles depends from the molecular weight of chitosan, its degree of deacetylation and the extent of cross-linking. Chitosan nanoparticles have been used, for example, to encapsulate a doxorubicin-dextran conjugate and for the transfection of numerous cancer cell lines.

Gelatin

Gelatin, a hydrophilic polymer derived from collagen, has been used for many years in the pharmaceutical industry for the preparation of capsules. Like albumin, gelatin presents properties favourable to drug delivery applications, such as being non-toxic, biocompatible and a stabiliser with sustained drug release characteristics. Gelatin nanoparticles have been used, for example, to entrap the anticancer drug paclitaxel and cycloheximide, a protein synthesis inhibitor used in cancer treatment. Gelatin nanoparticles were also cationised in order to be able to carry negatively charged DNA bound onto their surface. They led to an efficient gene transfection in a melanoma cell line.

Synthetic polymers

Numerous synthetic polymers have been used for preparing nanoparticles, including polyesters, polyorthoesters, polyanhydrides and polyamides. Poly(lactic-co-glycolic acid) (PLGA) and poly(alkylcyanoacrylate) are two examples of synthetic polymers that are widely used for the preparation of nanoparticles:

PLGA

Polylactic acid (PLA) and PLGA are polymers from the polyester group that is the most studied and best characterised class of polymers used for controlled release. They are prepared from lactide and glycolide, which are cyclic esters of lactic and glycolic acids. PLGA is one of the polymers most commonly used in nanoparticle preparation due to its biodegradability, biocompatibility and the fact that it is FDA-approved for human use. Upon absorption into the body, PLGA degrades by hydrolysis into lactic and glycolic acids, which are easily removed from the body. PLGA-based nanoparticles degrade through erosion at a uniform rate throughout the matrix. This degradation is highly dependent on the ratio of lactide to glycolide moieties, as lactide is more hydrophobic and thus reduces the rate of degradation. PLGA nanoparticles have been used to carry numerous drugs and genes for many therapeutic applications. They have been studied, for example, for delivering the anticancer drugs paclitaxel and doxorubicin to tumours.

Poly(alkylcyanoacrylate)

The alkyl cyanoacrylate monomers, well known for their use as haemostatic and tissue adhesives, can be polymerised to form nanoparticles for drug delivery. Drug loading within the nanoparticles is generally optimum for un-ionised, lipophilic drugs. These nanoparticles are rapidly biodegraded by surface erosion, with degradation kinetics depending on the nature of the alkyl chain of the polymer: poly(butylcyanoacrylate) nanoparticles are degraded within one day, whereas poly (hexylcyanoacrylate) nanoparticles take a number of days to degrade. Poly(alkylcyanoacrylate) nanoparticles tend to accumulate in the liver and the spleen following intravenous injection. They have been used for delivering doxorubicin to tumours, for example.

Polymers for gene delivery

Polymers and dendrimers bearing groups which are protonated at physiological pH can be used as gene carriers. The electrostatic interaction between the cationic charges on the polymer and the negatively charged DNA results in an electrostatic complex called polyplex in the case of polymers and dendriplexes in the case of dendrimers.

Polyethylenimine

Polyethylenimine (PEI) is a polycationic molecule that has been shown to produce efficient gene transfection in numerous cell lines *in vitro* without the need for an endosomolytic agent (Fig. 28.12). Every third atom of PEI is a nitrogen atom, leading to a densely positively charged backbone necessary for an efficacious DNA binding. PEI enhances the cellular endocytosis of plasmids but also facilitates their endosomal escape by buffering the endosomal compartments, leading to lysosomal osmotic swelling and disruption. Although PEI is an efficient gene transfer polymer *in vitro*, its cytotoxicity needs to be improved for widening its use *in vivo*.

Dendrimers

A dendrimer is a synthetic polymeric macromolecule of nanometre size, composed of multiple branched monomers that radiate from the central core. The resulting spherical polymers have their surface charge, density and diameter determined by the number of synthetic steps used, called generation. Dendrimers can condense plasmids through electrostatic interactions of their terminal primary amines with the DNA phosphate groups. Due to their unusual structure, dendrimers are characterised by the following properties, which differentiate them from other polymers and make them attractive for gene delivery: monodisperse size, modifiable surface functionality, multivalency, water solubility and available internal cavity suitable for drug delivery. The abundance of amino groups on their surface enables them to be simultaneously conjugated with various targeting ligands while still being able to carry DNA, yielding a dendrimer-based multifunctional gene delivery system. Upon cellular uptake, the release of the dendrimer-DNA complex from the endosome has been attributed to the protonation of the internal tertiary amino groups which then results in a swelling of the endosome

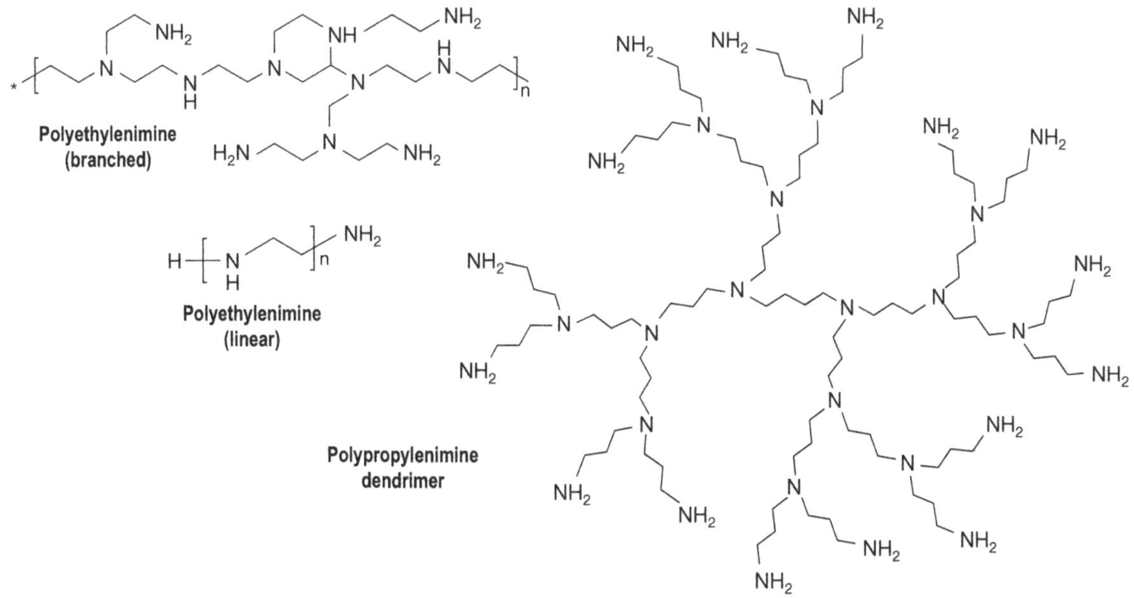

Figure 28.12 Chemical structure of polymers used for gene delivery.

due to electrostatic repulsion followed by the release of the DNA to the cytoplasm.

Poly(amidoamine) and poly(propylenimine) dendrimers (Fig. 28.12) have been shown to efficiently deliver nucleic acids in numerous cell lines. Their ability to transfect cells increases with the generation, unfortunately as does their toxicity, which is directly related to molecular weight. It is therefore necessary to find a compromise situation allowing transfection enhancement without toxic effects. Such a balance was found in the lower-generation 3 poly(propylenimine) dendrimers.

The choice of the appropriate polymer to be used for a given therapeutic application will depend on the chemical properties of the drug being delivered and on the therapeutic goal to be reached.

Q Self Test 28.4

Which of the following statements are *true*? (Answer below)

A. Drugs can exclusively be carried by nanoparticles via entrapment within the polymer matrix.
B. Nanocapsules have a core-shell structure.
C. Nanoparticles are generally more stable than liposomes.
D. A combined diffusion-erosion mechanisms of drug release from the nanoparticles may occur.

Give two examples of natural polymers and synthetic polymers used in the preparation of nanoparticles for controlled drug delivery

CONCLUSION

This chapter has highlighted the significant advances in drug delivery over the past three decades. Several of the drug delivery systems described have entered the marketplace and many more are in clinical trials. One common point of these systems is their indication for the treatment of life-threatening diseases, such as cancer and severe infectious diseases. As a consequence, these delivery systems have the potential to considerably contribute to the therapeutic *armamentarium* currently available.

As drug delivery technologies advance, the requirements for the next generation of advanced drug delivery systems grows increasingly more demanding. It is likely that during the next few years, extensive work in this rapidly expanding field will result in the development of even more sophisticated delivery systems.

A Self Test 28.2

B, C, E, G

A Self Test 28.4

B, C, D

FURTHER READING

Barenholz Y, Crommelin DJA. Liposomes as pharmaceutical dosage forms. In: Swarbrick J, Boylan JC, eds. *Encyclopedia of pharmaceutical technology*. Vol 9: New York: Marcel Dekker; 1991:1–39.

de Villiers MM, Aramwit P, Kwon GS. *Nanotechnology in drug delivery*. New York: AAPS Press, Springer; 2009.

Dufès C, Uchegbu IF, Schätzlein AG. Dendrimers in drug and gene delivery. In: Schätzlein AG, Uchegbu IF, eds. *Polymers in drug delivery*. CRC Press; 2006:199–235.

Dufès C, Uchegbu IF, Schätzlein AG. Dendrimers in gene delivery. *Adv Drug Deliv Rev*. 2005;57:2177–2202.

Gregoriadis G. *Liposomes technology*. Vols 1, 2 and 3. Boca Raton: CRC Press; 1984.

Kreuter J. *Colloidal drug delivery systems*. New York: Marcel Dekker, Inc; 1994.

Kumar MNVR. *Handbook of particulate drug delivery*. Vols 1 and 2. Stevenson Ranch: American Scientific Publishers; 2008.

Lasik DD, Templeton NS. Liposomes in gene therapy. *Adv Drug Del Rev*. 1996;20:221–266.

Ranade VV, Hollinger MA. *Drug delivery systems*. 2nd ed. Boca Raton: CRC Press; 2004.

Saltzman WM. *Drug delivery*. Oxford: Oxford University Press, Inc; 2001.

Thassu D, Deleers M, Pathak Y. *Nanoparticulate drug delivery systems*. New York: Informa Healthcare; 2007.

Uchegbu IF. *Synthetic surfactant vesicles: niosomes and other non-phospholipid vesicular systems*. Amsterdam: Harwood Academic Publishers; 2000.

Uchegbu IF, Dufès C, Kan PL, Schätzlein AG. Polymers and dendrimers for gene delivery in gene therapy. In: Templeton NS, Dekker M, eds. *Gene and cell therapy: therapeutic mechanisms and strategies*. 3rd ed. Taylor and Francis; 2009:321–339.

Zanthopoulos K. *Gene therapy*. New York: Springer-Verlag; 1998.

Chapter | 29 |

The tonic and toxic effects of alcohol and its metabolites

John Connolly

CHAPTER CONTENTS

INTRODUCTION

Traces of alcoholic beverages made from rice, honey and fruit have been found in 9000-year-old Neolithic pottery in China.[1] However, there have also been well-documented instances of wild animals, such as pentailed shrew monkeys, for whom substantial quantities of naturally fermented, fallen fruit containing 3.8% alcohol is a staple of their diet.[2] Thus it seems likely that people have been ingesting alcohol in one form or another for as long as human-like animals have roamed the Earth. As a result, alcohol consumption has become an integral part of the social and economic fabric of many societies, even in those societies which attempt to prohibit it.

Despite our familiarity with alcohol, it should still be classed as a drug. In fact, it is a very powerful drug. Even small amounts of alcohol can have profound pharmacological effects.[3] Such low doses can promote a socially convivial atmosphere, but unfortunately, misuse of alcohol can have the reverse effect and addiction to alcohol is currently having a very deleterious impact on individual lives and on society. For example, the immediate effects of binge drinking contribute heavily to statistics for accidents (11% of Accident and Emergency admissions in 2007–2008 in Scotland) and violence (70% of assault cases attending A&E are thought to be alcohol related[4]) and an even greater drain on the response capacity of the emergency services. Alcohol is also a factor in both the commission of, and vulnerability to, crime. Forty-nine per cent of Scottish prisoners have claimed that they were drunk at the time of their offence, although it is a common mitigating plea in defence arguments. The total cost of alcohol misuse to Scotland's legal, social, health and emergency services is estimated to be £2.5 billion annually,[5] and if one adds in lost productivity in the workplace and family strife the toll is probably even higher. Worldwide, the problem probably costs hundreds of millions of dollars.[6]

These are devastating statistics. To help explain them, we need to understand how alcohol is distributed within the bodies of men and women, how patterns of drinking may affect this distribution, and how alcohol produces its acute physiological effects. Over the longer term, we additionally need to understand the mechanisms through which chronic alcohol misuse results in damage to practically every major organ system and increases the risks of life-threatening illness.

Despite incontrovertible evidence of the damaging effects of alcohol abuse, health-promoting qualities are claimed for moderate alcohol consumption. To reconcile these seemingly contradictory views requires an understanding of the indirect actions of ethanol, the chemistry of the metabolic by-products of alcohol, as well as knowledge of the additional biologically active molecules that are found within the wide range of alcoholic beverages which are available. It also requires an examination of what the term 'moderate' really means.

ALCOHOL: PROPERTIES, INTAKE, DISTRIBUTION AND ELIMINATION

The physical properties of alcohol

Ethanol (Fig. 29.1 (ethyl alcohol, C_2H_5OH, molecular mass 46.07 $gmol^{-1}$) is the second member of the aliphatic (alkane) series of alcohols. In pure form, ethanol is a clear, colourless liquid at room temperature and has a distinctive smell that is perhaps associated with disinfection, one of many non-food uses of this substance.

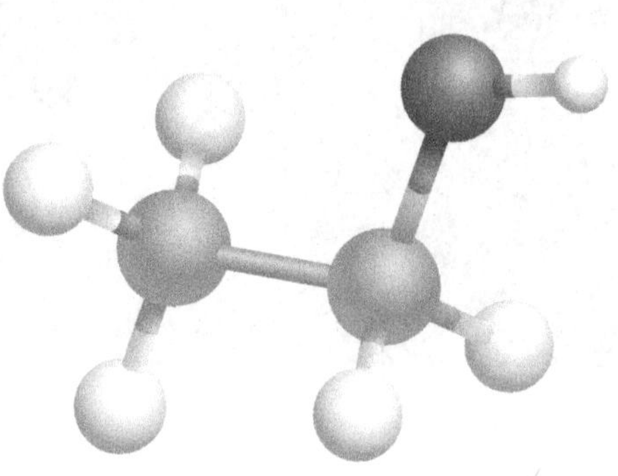

Figure 29.1 Ethanol.

Ethanol is less dense than water (0.789 g mL^{-1} at room temperature) and is completely miscible with it - unlike alcohols with a longer carbon backbone. Surprisingly, after combining ethanol and water in a 1:1 mixture, the resultant volume is only 1.92 of the sum of the individual starting volumes of water and alcohol. Heat is also released during this mixing process (777 J/mol^{-1} at 298K[7]). Once ethanol is combined with water, it is difficult for the two to be completely separated again. Ethanol is hygroscopic, and when alcohol/water mixtures are distilled, the percentage of alcohol never exceeds 95% in the distillate. During the distillation process, ethanol and water form an azeotropic or 'constant boiling' mixture, i.e. one which has a constant composition at a given constant temperature and pressure.

As suggested by its ease of distillation when mixed with water, ethanol is a very volatile liquid (boiling point 78.3°C, freezing point approximately −114°C). It also reduces the surface tension of water. These two properties combine to create the 'tears of wine' effect seen when wine is swirled around the upper walls of a large glass. At first the wine forms a thin film all over the wetted surface, but as the alcohol evaporates, the residual solution is left with lower alcohol content. As the alcohol content diminishes, the surface tension of the remaining liquid increases and beads of wine are formed. More concentrated alcoholic beverages such as whisky do not bead up, but instead form sturdy 'legs' upon the side of the glass.

Despite its miscibility with water, ethanol is also useful as an organic solvent. This is because the ethanol molecule has both a polar end due to its hydroxyl group and a non-polar end formed by the methyl group. This allows it to mix with non-polar solvents such as benzene and hexane. It can also dissolve the non-polar compounds found in some paints, varnishes, perfumes, hairsprays, mouth washes, cough treatments and medicines. Less happily, it can also contribute to the solubility of ingested or inhaled carcinogens. This ability to dissolve non-polar substances also contributes to the usefulness of alcohol as a disinfectant reagent. A 70% solution of ethanol will dissolve the lipids in the cell walls of bacteria, protozoans, and fungi. It will also denature proteins such as those found in viruses and this general ability to discourage cellular and viral growth has led to its use by biologists as a preservative for specimens. Despite these deleterious effects on living organisms, alcohol is, of course, also is used in beverages.

Another consequence of ethanol being an organic compound is that it has high energy content (1409 KJ mol^{-1}), and will burn with a translucent blue flame to produce carbon dioxide and water:

$$C_2H_5OH + 3\,O_2 \rightarrow 2\,H_2O + 2\,CO_2$$

Ethanol mixtures are thus a useful fuel source for lamps, cooking, fuel cells, cars, planes and even space rockets (with liquid oxygen). However, as discussed below, this high energy content may also have nutritional consequences.

Production of alcohol

For the kind of fuel and solvent uses mentioned above, industrial alcohol has traditionally been made by the addition reaction of steam (H_2O) with ethylene (C_2H_4). However, alcohol which is drunk by humans is produced by fermentation of plant sugars by yeast (*Saccharomyces cerevisiae*). This is usually a two stage process:

1.

$$\underset{\text{sucrose}}{C_{12}H_{22}O_{11} + H_2O} \xrightarrow{\text{invertase}} \underset{\text{glucose + fructose}}{C_6H_{12}O_6 + C_6H_{12}O_6}$$

2.

$$\underset{\text{glucose}}{C_6H_{12}O_6 + 2Pi + 2ADP + 2H^+} \xrightarrow{\text{zymase}} \underset{\text{ethanol}}{2\,C_2H_5OH + 2\,CO_2 + 2\,ATP + 2\,H_2O}$$

More recently, in the search for alternative ways of preparing biofuels, many other substrates for alcohol production, such as manure and sawdust, and other facilitating organisms, such as genetically engineered bacteria and algae, have been used to produce alcohol.

Estimation of alcohol content of beverages and monitoring of intake

Regardless of the fermentation substrate which is used to produce an alcoholic beverage, it is important to be able to estimate its alcohol content. An early way of doing this was to use the 'Proof Spirit' system. This is the weakest dilution of an alcoholic drink which will still allow gunpowder to be ignited when the two are mixed together. If the drink, such as rum, still allowed ignition to take place, it would 'prove' the drink had reasonable alcohol content. In terms of physical chemistry, a 'Proof Spirit' can be defined as one which at 51°F weighs 12/13 of an equal volume of distilled water. Such a spirit would contain around 57.10% of ethanol, volume/volume (v/v), and have a specific gravity of about 0.92 at 60°F. The percentage volume of water which needs to be added or subtracted from a liquor in order to turn it into a 'Proof Spirit' containing 57.10% ethanol then defines the number of degrees the beverage is 'under' or 'over' proof. For example, whisky contains around 40% alcohol by volume. To be 100 degrees proof it would need to contain 57.1% alcohol. The whisky would therefore need 30% of its water to be removed in order to make it concentrated enough to be a Proof Spirit of 100°. It is therefore 30° 'under Proof'. Usually, however, whisky's alcoholic strength is defined more directly as being 70° Proof (70% of full Proof strength).

However, the way alcohol content is usually described in health-promotion literature is in terms of units. A unit of pure ethanol is defined as a volume of 10 mL, which, because of its low density compared to water, weighs only 7.9 g. This is approximately the amount of alcohol that can be found in 0.5 of a pint (284.13 mL) of 3.5% (volume/volume) beer, or a 25 mL measure of 40% spirit.

To estimate the number of units in a bottle of beer or wine, the total volume of alcohol within the beverage is first calculated by multiplying the percentage alcohol (v/v) in it by the total number of millilitres in the bottle and then dividing by 100. This number (the number of millilitres of pure ethanol) can then be further divided by 10 (the number of millilitres of ethanol in one unit) to yield the number of units. This can be rearranged to:

$$\left[\frac{\textit{volume of drink (mL)}}{1000}\right] \times \%\ \textit{alcohol (vol./vol.)} = \textit{no. of units}$$

Thus a standard 330 mL bottle of 5% lager contains (330/1000) × 5 = 1.65 units.

In the Americas, health literature often talks about alcohol in terms of 'drinks'. Usually, this refers to the amount of alcohol in a standard 12 fluid ounces (USA) or 355 mL bottle of beer. At a typical alcoholic strength of 5%, one such beer would contain 1.78 units, almost the entire maximum daily allowance recommended for a woman. Two such beers would take a man over the recommended level for his maximum daily intake. However, the size of a 'drink' can vary in different studies, and so alcohol consumption will be described in units here. The alcohol unit contents of common beverages are shown in Table 29.1.

Absorption of alcohol

Once an alcoholic beverage has made its way from the bottle to the stomach, it is rapidly absorbed. If the stomach is empty, peak alcohol concentrations in the bloodstream will occur about 30–45 minutes after ingestion of a single alcoholic drink. However, fatty foods, such as milk, can slow the absorption rate from the stomach by about threefold. For spirits and other strong drink, food also diminishes the alcohol concentration gradient across the intestinal mucosa of the gut wall. However, this concentration effect is not really significant for weaker drinks like beer.

Alcohol not absorbed in the stomach tends to be absorbed across the gut wall in the small intestines and the

Table 29.1 Relative amounts of various beverages required to provide 1 unit of alcohol

Class of beverage	Dispensed form	Percentage alcohol (vol/vol)	Amount of beverage per unit of alcohol (10 mL)	Number of units in a typical measure
Beers, cider and alcopops	Bottle of alcopops (275 mL)	5%	200 mL (≈ 4/5 bottle)	1.4 per bottle
	Bottle of lager (330 mL)	5%	200 mL (≈ 1/3 pint)	1.7 per bottle
	Bottle of USA beer (355 mL/12 fluid oz)	5%	200 mL (≈ ½ bottle)	1.8 per bottle
	Can of lager (440 mL)	5%	200 mL (< ½ can)	2.2 per can
	Draught bitter (pint/568 mL)	4%	250 mL (< ½ pint)	2.3 per pint
	Draught cider (pint/568 mL)	6%	167 mL (< 1/3 pint)	3.4 per pint
	Can of strong cider (440 mL)	7.5%	133 mL (< 1/3 can)	3.3 per can
	Can of super-lager (440 ml)	9%	110 mL (¼ can)	4.0 per can
Wines (9–15 units in a 750 ml bottle)	Bottle of wine (750 mL, 9–11.3 units)	12–15%	67–83 mL (< ½ glass)	2.1–2.6 per 175 mL large glass
	Bottle of Buckfast wine (750 mL, 11.3 units)	15%	67 mL (< ½ glass)	2.6 units per 175 mL large glass
	Sherry/port/vermouth (750 mL, 15 units)	20%	50 mL (1 sherry glass)	1.0 unit per 50 mL measure
Spirits (28 Units in a 70 cl bottle)	Whisky, vodka, brandy, rum, gin (25 mL measure)	40%	25 mL (single measure)	1.0 per single measure

colon where the rate of transfer into the bloodstream is even faster. Since the presence of food in the stomach will inhibit gastric emptying, food can also slow the rise in alcohol concentrations in the bloodstream by hindering the transit of alcohol into the more quickly absorbing small intestines. Conversely, carbonation of drinks, as in champagne, can increase the rate of alcohol concentration by promoting gastric empyting. Thus drinking alcohol on an empty stomach is liable to lead to a rapid rise in blood level alcohol measurements. However, opioid analgesics, as well as diabetes treatments such as exenatide and liraglutide, can also inhibit gastric emptying. Thus medications can also affect the rate of rise of blood alcohol concentrations.

Distribution of alcohol within the body and blood concentrations

After alcohol has been absorbed into the bloodstream, it tends to stay within the aqueous compartments of the body. This is because the partition coefficient between tissue water and lipids heavily favours water by 25:1. This does not stop alcohol crossing cell membranes, which it can readily do, but the alcohol will not be concentrated within the bulk of the lipid bilayer. This partitioning characteristic dictates that alcohol will eventually be distributed evenly throughout the body tissues in proportion to their water content. Contrary to popular tourist belief, this fact makes it unlikely that elephants, with their vast body water content, are able to get drunk on ingested fermented fruit.[8]

This aqueous distribution of ethanol has particular consequences for women. In general, women tend to have higher lipid content within their bodies than men of an equal weight. Thus, on average, a man's total body water is about 68% of his total weight, while for a woman it is only 55%. Since alcohol is mainly found in tissue water, an identical amount of alcohol imbibed by a man or woman of equal weight will result in the woman having a higher whole blood alcohol concentration.

However, the first place that alcohol arrives after absorption from the gut and entry into the hepatic portal vein is the liver. There, a small amount of it is metabolised during the first pass before it travels on to other well-vascularised organs such as the brain, lungs and kidneys. Equilibration within these major organs is very rapid, but slightly slower than within muscle tissues unless the person is undergoing heavy exercise. Thus under resting conditions there can be a slight overshoot of alcohol concentrations in the brain just after drinking (more pronounced if the stomach is empty and absorption is rapid). This overshoot dissipates as the alcohol is slowly redistributed into the muscle tissue.

The 'overshoot' phenomenon also helps to explain why injection of even a small amount of alcohol into the bloodstream can be fatal. When injected directly into the bloodstream, alcohol rapidly makes its way to the brain without having the chance to be slowly equilibrated throughout the body. As a result, the initial alcohol concentration experienced by the brain following injection of less than a single measure of whisky can be seven times higher than if the alcohol was simply drunk in the normal way. This can cause medullary paralysis, with its associated depression of the respiratory and vasomotor centres. Severe depression results in the cessation of breathing and death can ensue. There are sporadic outbreaks of the misuse of alcoholic beverages by injection but they tend to be self-limiting. Apart from the vascular pain that occurs during injection, some of the abusers will collapse and die even before the syringe of alcohol is empty. Death is even more likely if the alcoholic drink is carbonated!

There is thus a relatively small concentration ratio (4) between levels of alcohol which cause inebriation and those which cause death. This risk is particularly strong for children or pre-adolescent teenagers, as it takes fewer drinks compared to adults for their blood alcohol levels to reach very high levels.[9] They may thus be more likely to unintentionally slip into medullary paralysis. Along with a risk of thrombosis or phlebitis and a severe drop in body temperature, the narrow therapeutic index of ethanol compared to modern anaesthetic agents makes it an unfavourable candidate as a general anaesthetic. For this and other reasons it has also been displaced as a smooth muscle relaxant during premature labour by calcium blockers such as nifedipine and adrenergic β_2 agonists such as ritodrine.

Elimination

Even while alcohol concentrations in the bloodstream are rising, alcohol is beginning to be eliminated. The average (70 kg) person will eliminate just less than 1 unit of alcohol an hour, but the range in the general population will be between 0.8 and 1.5 units per hour. Blood alcohol concentrations fall on average by about 15 mg/dL per hour (0.15 mg/mL) in a linear manner with approximately zero-order kinetics.[10]

This reduction in blood alcohol concentration occurs via several routes. Ethanol is eliminated through the lungs but since the partition coefficient between blood and air is 2100:1, this only represents a very small fraction of the total. Another consequence of the relatively low amount of ethanol in alveolar air is that it reduces the reliability of breath tests as a way of estimating blood alcohol concentrations. They are even more unreliable if other alcohol-containing substances such as mouthwashes have been present in the mouth but not ingested. Ethanol partitions on a more equal basis into urine, saliva and sweat, but again there is substantial individual variation in the range of the partition coefficients amongst the general population. This variability weakens the trustworthiness of deduced estimates of blood alcohol concentrations using these fluids also.

However, the above routes of elimination only play a minor role in the removal of ethanol from the body. Over 90% of ingested ethanol is eliminated by metabolism in the liver (see below), although metabolism is not completely restricted to this organ. Since most elimination occurs through liver metabolism, activities such as exercise which increase sweating and respiration rates do not have much effect on the equilibrated high blood alcohol concentration.

METABOLISM OF ALCOHOL

As noted above, ethanol makes use of endogenous biochemical pathways in the liver, and to a lesser extent in the brain and stomach, for its elimination. However, overloading any of the metabolic pathways with alcohol can lead to disequilibrium and redirection of normal metabolic processes. This usually results in the accumulation of harmful by-products.

Metabolism by alcohol dehydrogenase (ADH) and aldehyde dehydrogenase (ALD)

There are two main routes for ethanol metabolism in the liver. The first and most important of these begins with the zinc-containing, cytoplasmic, alcohol dehydrogenase (ADH) group of enzymes (especially alcohol dehydrogenase 1B). These enzymes are not particularly specific as they can also metabolise longer-chain alcohols produced in the ω-oxidation pathway for fatty acids. ADH converts alcohol to acetaldehyde with a K_M of 1.6 mmol/L:

$$\underset{\text{ethanol}}{CH_3CH_2OH + NAD^+} \xrightarrow{\text{alcohol dehydrogenase}} \underset{\text{acetaldehyde}}{CH_3CHO + NADH + H^+}$$

This conversion of ethanol to acetaldehyde is the rate-limiting step in alcohol metabolism, as the equilibrium for the reaction is far to the left. While it is possible for the reverse reaction to occur with acetaldehyde that has been produced by other metabolic pathways within the body, this only occurs at a pharmacologically insignificant level (2 mg/100 mL blood at most).

The activity of alcohol dehydrogenase varies both between individuals and during life. Activity is low in infants up to the age of 5 and levels of ADH are lower in the stomachs of women compared to men, in whose stomachs some metabolism takes place. In contrast, individuals suffering from glycogen storage disease may metabolise alcohol more quickly.

Table 29.2 Genetic polymorphisms of alcohol metabolising enzymes[9–11]

Enzyme	Polymorphism	Other names	Relative effect on function	Metabolic effect
Alcohol dehydrogenases (ADH)				
Alcohol dehydrogenase 1B	Normal Arg48, Arg370	ADH1B*1	1×	Normal clearance of alcohol
Alcohol dehydrogenase 1B	Arg48His,	ADH1B*2	40×	Rapid clearance and aldehyde production
Alcohol dehydrogenase 1B	Arg370Cys	ADH1B*3	90×	Rapid clearance and aldehyde production
Alcohol dehydrogenase 1C	Normal Arg272, Iso350	ADH1C*2	1×	
Alcohol dehydrogenase 1C	Arg272Gln; Iso350Val	ADH1C*1	2.5×	
Aldehyde dehydrogenases				
Aldehyde dehydrogenase H2	Normal E487	ALDH2*1	Normal function	Aldehyde converted to acetate at normal rate
Aldehyde dehydrogenase H2	E487K	ALDH2*2	Homozygous: enzyme inactive heterozygous: enzyme activity much reduced.	Aldehyde not cleared from elimination pathways

Several genetic polymorphisms of alcohol dehydrogenase have been identified (Table 29.2) which are associated with an increased rate of alcohol metabolism of up to 90× normal. Individuals with the ADH 1B and 1C polymorphisms, which result in slower alcohol metabolism, tend to have higher levels of alcohol consumption and an increased risk of alcoholism.[11] Since 90% of the white population of Europe (compared to less than 10% of East Asians) have the slower ADH1B*1 genotype, this may mediate a greatly increased risk of alcoholism for this group. However, even at normal levels of activity of ADH, heavy drinking can lead to problems with acetaldehyde accumulation. This accumulation is problematic because acetaldehyde is a very reactive molecule and can cause deleterious changes in proteins, nucleic acids and neurotransmitters (see below for examples of adducts).

The second step of this first route of degradation takes place in the mitochondria, where the acetaldehyde is converted to acetate by aldehyde dehydrogenase enzymes:

$$\underset{\text{acetaldehyde}}{CH_3CHO} + NAD^+ + H_2O \xrightarrow{\text{aldehyde dehydrogenase}} \underset{\text{acetate}}{CH_3COO^-} + NADH + H^+$$

In both steps NAD^+ is reduced to NADH. As discussed below, this overproduction of NADH, as well as the production of acetate, can lead to disturbances in other metabolic pathways. There are 19 aldehyde dehydrogenases in the human genome but from the point of view of ethanol detoxification, the most important of these is aldehyde dehydrogenase H2 (ALDH2).[12] This enzyme is a homomeric tetramer located in the mitochondrial matrix of cells in the liver, kidney, heart, lung and brain. Normally glutamate is present at position 487 of the mature ALDH2 protein. This glutamate (E) residue helps maintain the architecture of the enzyme so that the catalytic and co-factor domains can work together to oxidise acetaldehyde to acetate with a K_m of <1 μM. However, if lysine (K) is present in position 487, the subunit is inactive. Even if only one subunit of the four contains the lysine polymorphism, the effect is dominant and the activity of the enzyme is greatly reduced.[13,14] This ALDH2*2 E487K lysine polymorphism is present in 40–50% of people of Asian descent. If affected individuals drink alcohol, they are slow to clear acetaldehyde and consequently suffer from the effects of acetaldehyde toxicity. This may contribute to the low rates of alcoholism amongst this population, but also to higher rates of liver disease and certain cancers. It may also explain why nitroglycerin used for treating angina and heart failure is less effective amongst Chinese patients, as ALDH2 is needed for the activation of nitroglycerin.

In fact, the more active polymorphisms of alcohol dehydrogenase 1B and the less active forms of aldehyde dehydrogenase H2 are commonly found together among East Asian populations. This combination results in poor tolerance of alcohol and sustained levels of acetaldehyde. These sustained acetaldehyde levels lead to facial flushing in affected individuals as well as nausea and headache.

Metabolism by the microsomal ethanol oxidising system

An alternative route of ethanol metabolism is provided by the microsomal ethanol oxidising system (MEOS).[15] The oxidation is mediated by the P450 family of cytochromal enzymes. These enzymes and their polymorphisms are encoded by a large gene family which has arisen by gene duplication.[16] The P450 enzymes get their name from the wavelength (450 nm) at which they maximally absorb light when bound to carbon monoxide. These membrane-bound enzymes are located mainly on the smooth endoplasmic reticulum (which appears in the microsomal cell fraction upon ultracentrifugation) and are particularly abundant in the liver and small intestine where they can provide a first line of defence against toxic xenobiotic agents which gain entry to the body. They depend upon an intercalated haem group for their oxidising action in which molecular oxygen and NADPH are consumed and acetaldehyde is produced:

$$\underset{\text{ethanol}}{CH_3CH_2OH + NADPH + H^+ + O_2} \xrightarrow{\text{MEOS}} \underset{\text{acetaldehyde}}{CH_3CHO + NADP^+ + 2H_2O}$$

The P450 enzymes have a lower affinity for alcohol (about 1/5, K_M 8 mmol/L) compared to ADH and are less readily accessible. Therefore they are only responsible for 10–25% of total ethanol metabolism, being relatively unimportant at low blood alcohol concentrations but becoming more important at higher levels 100 mg/100 mL, just above the drink-drive limit. The main cytochrome P450 enzyme involved in ethanol metabolism is CYP2E1, although CYP1A2 and CYP3A4 can also oxidise ethanol.

In chronic alcoholics, the amounts of smooth endoplasmic reticulum and their associated P450 enzymes are markedly increased. In fact, a significant increase can occur with as little as 40 g of alcohol (approx 5 units) daily of alcohol for 1 week.[17] The MEOS enzymes are therefore inducible. In addition to alcohol, enzymes like CYP2E1 are also responsible for the metabolism of several prescribed drugs. For example, phenobarbital is hydroxylated by these enzymes to create a product which has increased solubility and speed of elimination. Caffeine, ibuprofen and warfarin are other examples of drugs metabolised by P450 enzymes. Over the short term, alcohol will compete directly with the drugs for degradation by the P450 enzymes and so the blood levels of such drugs may remain high in the presence of alcohol. Over the longer term, this increased elimination capacity of the MEOS enzymes creates a cross-tolerance in chronic alcohol abusers not just for alcohol, but for other drugs it metabolises too. Thus occasional or binge drinking may inhibit warfarin degradation, thereby increasing its blood concentration and anticoagulant effects. In turn, this would increase the risk of haemorrhagic stroke. In contrast, a habitual heavy drinker with an enhanced P450 enzymatic capacity may require a higher level of warfarin medication to achieve satisfactory protection against the formation of blood clots. However, sudden cessation of drinking by such an individual can put them at risk of bleeding.

In addition to its detoxifying role for ethanol, drugs and other xenobiotic agents, the MEOS can also produce harmful reagents. Polycyclic aromatic hydrocarbons and nitrosamines such as those found in tobacco smoke can be hydroxylated. This enables them to react with polar groups, making these carcinogens more soluble. Organic solvents such as carbon tetrachloride and benzene are also more toxic to alcoholics with increased levels of MEOS enzymes. Drugs too can be converted into harmful species. Normally therapeutic and harmless amounts of paracetamol can be converted by the enhanced CYP2E1 levels in an alcoholic into a toxic metabolite which can cause serious liver damage. Anaesthetics such as enflurane and halothane can also be metabolised into harmful species in alcoholics.

The increased activity of P450 enzymes also leads to an enhanced production of free radicals. Ethanol can scavenge hydroxyl radicals (OH°) to form hydroxyethyl free radicals during MEOS activity but other free radicals such as $O_2{}^\circ$ are also produced. These reactive oxygen species will bind to DNA, RNA and proteins, thus compromising DNA and protein function and potentially stimulating production of autoantibodies which are found in higher levels in alcoholics.

Polymorphisms of alcohol induced P-450 enzymes such as 2E1 have been identified, but the functional consequences of these polymorphisms are not clear. As with ADH, most of the acetaldehyde produced by MEOS is metabolised to acetate by the ALD pathway within the liver, but the more widely spread aldehyde oxidase can also be utilised:

$$\underset{\text{aldehyde}}{CH_3CHO + O_2 + NADPH} \xrightarrow{\text{aldehyde oxidase}} \underset{\text{acetate}}{CH_3COO^- + NADP^+ + H_2O}$$

Metabolism by catalase

One other system which can metabolise ethanol is catalase. It has little importance in liver but does play a more significant role in ethanol metabolism in the brain. In addition to ethanol, it requires hydrogen peroxide as a substrate. The hydrogen peroxide is usually produced during the oxidation of hypoxanthine and NADPH by xanthine oxidase and NADPH oxidase respectively:

$$\underset{\text{ethanol}}{CH_3CH_2OH} + H_2O_2 \xrightarrow{\text{catalase}} \underset{\text{acetaldehyde}}{CH_3CHO} + 2H_2O$$

Male/female sex differences

As mentioned above, women have less gastric ADH in their stomachs. Furthermore, the MEOS system in women is less able to metabolise fatty acids than that in men, and their cytoplasmic binding proteins are less able to bind esterified fatty acids. Thus fatty acids tend to accumulate in the livers of women, making them more prone to alcohol-related liver disease than men. Women are also more vulnerable to heart and brain damage from alcohol than men. These factors, along with the higher percentage lipid content in women, mean that the maximal limits for safe consumption of alcohol by women is lower than it is for men.

ACUTE SYSTEMIC EFFECTS OF ALCOHOL

Acute metabolic impact of ethanol metabolites

Terrestrial organisms live in an oxygen-rich environment and so the ubiquitous driving forces for their biosynthetic pathways are reducing power, in the form of NADH and NADPH (nicotinamide adenine dinucleotide phosphate). and energy, in the form of ATP (adenosine triphosphate). Homeostatic control of the redox levels of these molecules is therefore critical to normal physiological function. However, an excess of alcohol disturbs the balance between oxidised and reduced species and therefore disturbs many biochemical equilibria within cells.

For example, the NADH excess produced by the actions of alcohol and aldehyde dehydrogenases depletes NAD^+ levels and thus inhibits gluconeogenesis by the tricarboxylic acid (TCA) cycle by blocking conversion of lactate to pyruvate. In fact, the reverse reaction can be favoured, leading to accumulation of lactate. The overall effect of this is a lowering of blood pH and hypoglycaemia. This becomes more pronounced in individuals with low levels of stored glycogen.

The conversion of NAD^+ to NADH during alcohol oxidation also impacts on the oxidation of fatty acids. Not only do fatty acids no longer need to be oxidised to produce NADH, but fatty acid and triglyceride synthesis can be promoted. This can contribute to the early stages of liver disease.

In contrast, MEOS consumes NADPH during its oxidation of ethanol, thereby diminishing NADPH availability. This can be partially offset by the action of a transhydrogenase which couples this usage to the production of NADH by alcohol dehydrogenase. However, one of the many duties of NADPH is to maintain the sulphydryl group of glutathione (GSH) in a singular, reduced state. In this state, GSH is able to protect against the damaging effects of reactive oxygen species such as peroxides. GSH does this by creating a larger 'dimeric' molecule in which two singular glutathione residues are connected by a disulphide bridge (Fig. 29.2). Glutathione is particularly important for protection against reactive oxygen species produced in the liver, where alcohol is mainly metabolised, and in red blood cells and in the brain. Unfortunately, since alcohol reduces the availability of NADPH, regeneration of glutathione is diminished following consumption of ethanol. Thus protection against oxidative stress is compromised at the very time it is most needed.

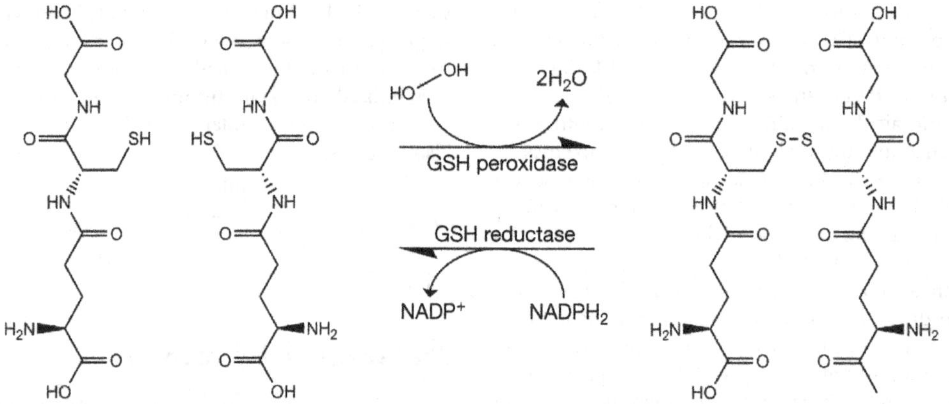

Figure 29.2 Illustration of the neutralising role of glutathione (GSH) on reactive oxygen species such as hydrogen peroxide, and its regeneration by the consumption of NADPH. NADPH is consumed by MEOS during alcohol metabolism, thus increasing susceptibility to oxidative stress.

Regardless of whether ethanol is metabolised by alcohol dehydrogenases, MEOS or catalase, the initial reaction product is acetaldehyde. Increased levels of aldehyde are dangerous as aldehydes react with many proteins, including those involved in mitochondrial function. This can compromise mitochondrial function within the liver and worsen the shortage of $NADPH_2$ and thereby the availability of reduced glutathione.

The secondary product of alcohol elimination is acetate. Acetate can be converted inside mitochondria into acetyl coenzyme A (acetyl CoA) by a thiokinase in a reaction which consumes ATP and yields AMP and diphosphate:

$$CH_3COOH + \text{coenzyme A} + ATP \rightarrow \text{acetylCoA} + AMP + P - P$$

In a normal situation, much of the acetyl CoA required by the body would be produced by β-oxidation of lipids within mitochondria, or decarboxylation of pyruvate from glycolysis. This product would go into the citric acid cycle and be metabolised to CO_2. However, in the mitochondria of hepatocytes in an alcohol-metabolising liver, the function of the citric acid cycle is inhibited by the abundance of NADH. This abundance blocks the citric acid cycle at the key points where NAD^+ is required for the decarboxylation of isocitrate to α-ketoglutarate by isocitrate dehydrogenase, and in the following step where α-ketoglutarate is decarboxylated by α-ketoglutarate dehydrogenase to succinyl CoA. The metabolism of pyruvate is also redirected towards lactate, thus lowering blood pH.

That portion of acetyl CoA which has been already been converted into citrate may be exported into the cytoplasm where it will act as a substrate for fatty acid synthesis. As mentioned above, this may be followed by increased hepatic triglyceride synthesis and lead to hypertriglyceridaemia. Alternatively, some of the excess acetyl CoA may be incorporated into 3-hydroxy-3-methylglutaryl CoA which is a starting point for cholesterol synthesis or the formation of ketone bodies that may increase acidosis. This acidosis can inhibit urea excretion by the kidney which in turn may exacerbate symptoms of gout. A summary diagram of the main effects of ethanol on metabolism is shown in Figure 29.3.

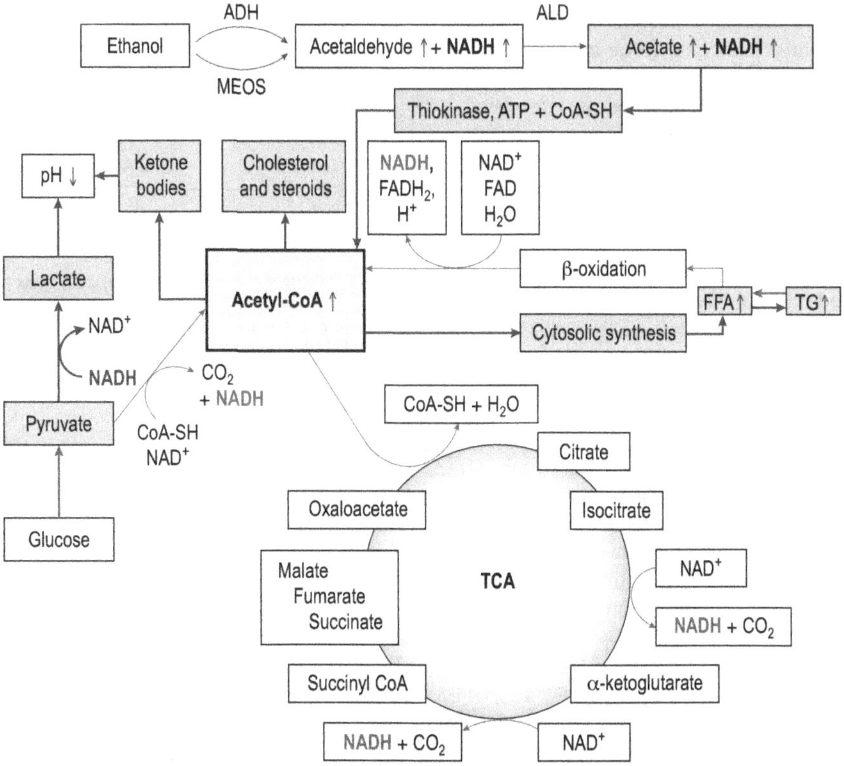

Figure 29.3 Summary diagram of major impacts of ethanol on metabolic pathways. An influx of ethanol disturbs the balance of carbohydrate and fatty acid metabolism. As a result of the oxidation of ethanol, concentrations of NADH and acetyl CoA are increased. Steps in the tricarboxylic acid cycle (TCA) and the mitochondrial pathway for β-oxidation of free fatty acids (FFA) which produce these species are inhibited (blue). At the same time, the excess amounts of NADH and acetyl CoA create conditions in which the fatty acid synthesis and acidosis are favoured (red). The abundance of acetyl CoA means alcohol precursor metabolites accumulate. See text for a detailed explanation. Abbreviations: ADH, alcohol dehydrogenase; MEOS, microsomal endoplasmic oxidising system; ALD, aldehyde dehydrogenase; TG, triglycerides; TCA, tricarboxylic acid cycle; FFA, free fatty acids.

As the ability of the TCA cycle to provide an elimination route for acetate is compromised, this will in turn inhibit the elimination of the acetaldehyde from which it is derived, leading to an increase in acetaldehyde levels. This increase in acetaldehyde levels can lead to competition for enzymes with acetaldehyde intermediates in other biodegradation pathways. For example, ethanol can redirect degradation of serotonin and catecholamines such as dopamine into alcohol rather than acid metabolites (see Ch. 3). Some of these metabolites may be pharmacologically active.

In addition, ethanol can alter metabolic pathways by altering the levels of expression of the proteins which carry them out. Ethanol alters the transcription and translation of hundreds of genes, most of which are associated with neuroplasticity, metabolism and stress responses. The metabolites of ethanol, in particular acetaldehyde, can also have epigenetic effects on DNA. Acetaldehyde inhibits methionine synthase, which utilises tetrahydrofolate and vitamin B_{12} to remethylate homocysteine to methionine. Activated methionine in the form of S-adenosylmethionine is a substrate for the methyltransferases which add methyl groups to CG base pairs in DNA. Genes containing many such methylated pairs tend to be inactive. In alcoholics, levels of homocysteine are increased, and gene expression can be affected. One gene whose expression is affected is that which leads to synthesis of α-synuclein, a protein which is strongly expressed in dopaminergic pathways[18] and which also accumulates in Parkinson's disease. Acetaldehyde itself can also directly form adducts which bind to DNA. Hence the alteration of gene expression is an important route through which ethanol achieves its advantageous and harmful effects on cellular metabolism.

Acute molecular effects of alcohol on ion channels and receptors

In addition to the impact of alcohol on cellular metabolism, ethanol can also impact on whole cell function through its action on particular proteins. Examples of this occur within the nervous system, where alcohol can directly affect the activity of excitable proteins such as voltage activated Ca^{2+} channels and the widely distributed ligand-gated ion channels that are activated by γ-aminobutyric acid (GABA) or glutamate.[19] Alcohol acts directly at particular allosteric sites within these proteins, rather than indirectly through disruption of overall membrane fluidity. Ethanol can enhance the function of chloride-permeable $GABA_A$ receptors, thus increasing entry of these negative ions into neurons and inhibiting their activity. Conversely, inhibition of cation-permeable glutamate receptors reduces their excitatory influence on nerve cells. Inhibition of calcium entry through voltage-gated calcium channels in nerve terminals leads to reduced transmitter release. The overall effect is a dampening of neuronal activity.

However, another important route through which effects on the function of the nervous system may be mediated is through nicotinic acetylcholine receptors. These receptors act as presynaptic 'gatekeepers' or filters at many synapses (including dopaminergic and gluatamatergic synapses) which mediate psychological and motor functions.[20] Manipulation of nicotinic receptor activity can lead to radical changes in the firing patterns of nerve cells and the kinds of information those patterns convey. Particular subtypes of nicotinic receptors can also be extremely sensitive to ethanol concentrations well below the drink-drive limit[3] (Fig. 29.4).

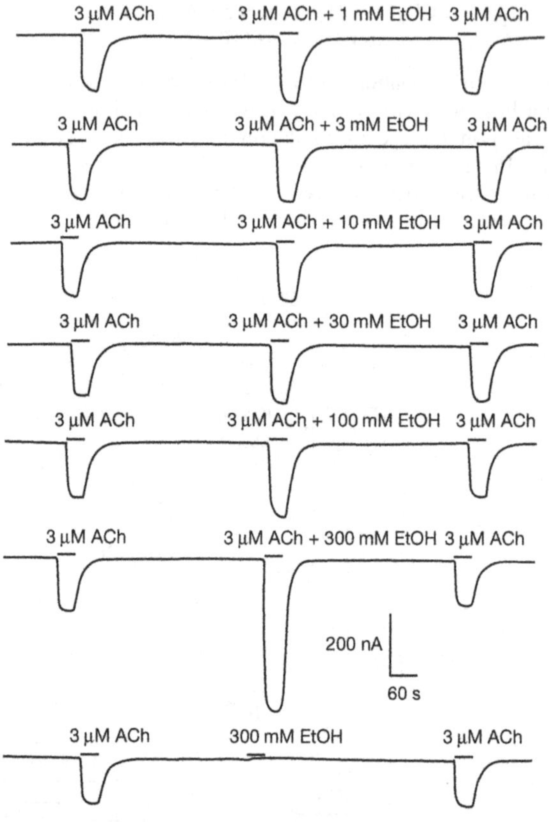

Figure 29.4 Nicotinic receptors are amongst those ligand-gated ion channels which mediate physiological responses to ethanol. Current responses from a single, voltage-clamped *Xenopus* oocyte previously injected with RNA encoding the α3β4 neuronal nicotinic receptor subunits are shown. This particular oocyte reveals a potentiating effect of ethanol on the responses of these receptors to 3 μM acetylcholine at both very low and high concentrations of ethanol. Some of the effects are seen below the drink-drive limit (17.4 mM ethanol). All responses run sequentially from top to bottom. Solutions: Current pipette, CsF 0.25 M, CsCl 0.25 M, 100 mM EGTA pH 7.2. Voltage pipette, 3 M KCl. External recording solution: NaCl 115 mM, BaCl2 1.8 mM, KCl 2.5 mM, HEPES 10 mM (pH7.2), and 1 mM atropine. (Connolly and Covernton, unpublished results; see also Reference 3).

Thus nicotinic receptors within the nervous system and ganglia may be significant mediators of the effects of ethanol.

One of the main results of the effects of ethanol on multiple receptor systems is the increased release of dopamine within the reward pathways of the brain, although endogenous opioids may also be involved in mediating the pleasurable effects of drinking.[19] Activation of D1 and D5 dopamine receptors in turn triggers activation of adenlyl cyclase whereas activation of D2 receptors inhibits it. Thus alcohol alters the activity of cAMP-dependent protein kinase A in many neuronal circuits. Stimulation of glutamate receptors can lead to Ca^{2+} entry into cells and also to NO release. This in turn can lead to elevation of cGMP. Protein kinase C activity may also be increased in the presence of alcohol. Thus the presence of alcohol in the nervous system and in somatic tissues can alter the status of a great many neurotransmitter and signalling systems. Even more directly, alcohol metabolites can react with the neurotransmitter compounds themselves. Box 29.1 shows some of the reaction products produced by acetaldehyde to produce compounds with neurological effects.[21]

Acute central nervous system effects of alcohol

As explained above, ethanol is essentially a central nervous system (CNS) depressant drug although mesolimbic dopamine neurones display increased activity. The effect in this latter case may be through inhibition of an inhibitory pathway. Generally however, alcohol depresses higher cortical function which in turn leads to a sense of relaxation, a loss of self restraint and uninhibited behaviour. This initial effect is followed by progressively increasing depression of all neuronal activity. Higher mental functions mediated by areas like the frontal cortex are affected first. Thus processes modified by learning such as training and education are affected before 'mechanical' performance. Therefore performance requiring skill does not improve, despite subjective impressions.

The effects of acute ethanol intoxication are well known: slurred speech, impairment of motor coordination, increased self-confidence and euphoria. Mood varies among individuals, most becoming more outgoing but some become morose and withdrawn. Heavy drinking can also be associated with antisocial behaviour and aggression, and a variety of psychological states ranging from anxiety and panic to psychosis and delusions can occur.

Sexual desire is also increased by alcohol, with both the drinker and their romantic target appearing to be more attractive in the drinker's mind. However, this increase in libido can be frustrated as alcohol tends to diminish penile erection, probably due to vasodilatation. In the words of Shakespeare's porter in MacBeth: Drink 'provokes the desire, but it takes away the performance, therefore much drink may be said to be an equivocator with lechery,' (Act 2, Scene 3, Lines 30–32).

Heavier drinking results in even more physical incapacity, until at levels around 300 mg/100 mL, the person can enter a comatose state. This may last for several hours, but there is also a danger that if the respiratory centres in the medulla oblongata become severely depressed, breathing stops and death may ensue. The average blood alcohol level noted in alcohol overdose fatalities is about 400 mg/100 mL, but lethal concentrations of alcohol can be significantly lower or higher depending upon individual variation in alcohol history. There have been reports of men and women surviving blood alcohol concentrations in excess of 1000 mg/100 mL of blood. However, individuals who survive significantly higher blood alcohol concentrations are usually chronic alcoholics with enhanced alcohol tolerance who have built up the blood alcohol concentration slowly. They are only able to survive with

Box 29.1

It has been speculated that tetrahydoisoquinolone adducts formed between acetaldehyde and neurotransmitters such as dopamine and serotonin are neurologically active and reinforce the addictive potential of alcohol.[18]

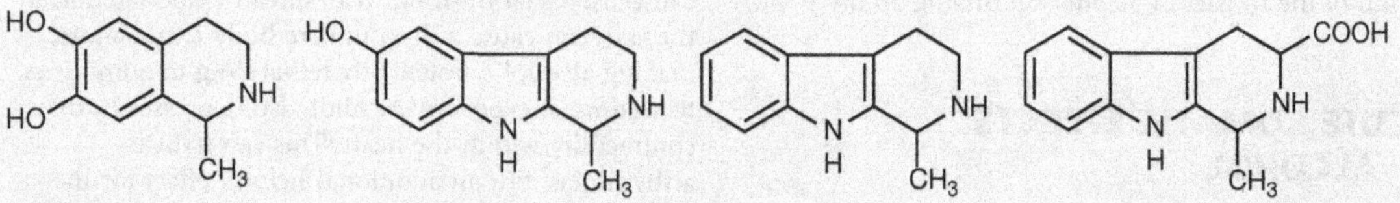

Salsoninol formed from dopamine

Hydroxymethyl tetrahydro beta carboline formed from serotonin

Methyltetrahydro beta carboline formed from tryptamine.

Carboxy methyltetrahydro beta carboline formed from tryptamine.

Table 29.3 The effects of alcohol on behaviour with dose

Plasma (EtOH) mg/100 mL	Units drunk males	Units drunk females	Effects
0–50	0–3	0–2.5	Loss of inhibitions and judgement, excitement, slurring & swaying
50–100	3–6	2.5–5	Impaired driving ability and reaction time
100–200	6–12	5–9.5	Staggering gait, inability to operate a car
200–300	12–18	9.5–14.5	Respiratory depression, danger of death with other CNS depressants, blackout
>300	>18	>14.5	Unconsciousness, coma, severe respiratory and cardiovascular depression, death

Box 29.2 **Drink driving**

In the UK, the drink-drive limit expressed in terms of the blood alcohol level (BAL) is 80 mg/100 mL plasma (17.4 mmol/L). This is equivalent to 0.08 g% using USA terminology for the Blood Alcohol Concentration (BAC).

This level can be reached if 4–5 units of alcohol are rapidly drunk by 70 kg males and 3–4 units by 70 kg females, although depending on one's individual build and metabolism, it is possible to be over the limit having ingested less alcohol. As explained above, the intoxication limits are different for men and women, mainly because of differences in the percentage of body fat and the capacity of women to metabolise alcohol.

The simultaneous use of medication exacerbates drowsiness and loss of driving skill. Medications which may adversely interact with alcohol include antidepressants, antihistamines, some cardiovascular medications, some antipsychotic medications and pain killers containing codeine.

However, although the drink-drive limit is set at 80 mg/100 mL (or 80 mg/dL), general driving skills deteriorate below 50 mg/100 mL. Furthermore, some skills such as ability to divide attention deteriorate at 20 mg/100 mL (less than 1/2 pint of beer). As a result, the relative risk of an accident rises with alcohol consumption, and can double well below the UK legal limit.[22] Therefore being within the drink-drive limit does not automatically mean one is safe to drive.

Perhaps because driving skills deteriorate below the 80 mg/100 mL level, some countries have set lower levels for the 'drink-drive' limit. In Brazil, Hungary, Ukraine, Slovakia, Barbados, Japan and many Middle Eastern and African countries, there is a policy of zero tolerance. Guyana has set the limit at 10 mg/100 mL, China and Poland at 20 mg/100 mL, India at 30 mg/100 mL and Australia between 20 and 50 mg/100mL depending upon which state one is driving in. Much of Europe, including Spain, Germany, Italy and France, operate a 50 mg/100 mL limit, while Ireland, Mexico, the United States and Canada have, like the UK, adopted an 80 mg/100 mL legal limit for blood alcohol concentration when in control of a motor vehicle.

the assistance of medical intervention. The immediate priorities in cases of severe intoxication are to support breathing and prevent aspiration of vomit. Such patients may also benefit from administration of glucose and electrolytes. The various stages of alcohol intoxication are shown in Table 29.3. (See also the Box 29.2 for a discussion of the impact of alcohol on driving ability.)

ACUTE SOMATIC EFFECTS OF ALCOHOL

In addition to the effects on the nervous system described above, alcohol also has profound effects on other body systems.

Cardiovascular effects: Following on from the depression of the vasomotor centre in the brain, vascular tone is further diminished by acetaldehyde. This can cause vasodilatation in the skin and gut. In individuals carrying the ALDH2*2 allele described above, vasodilatation caused by the failure to clear accumulated acetaldehyde can cause facial flushing. Widespread vasodilatation in the skin can cause a drop in core body temperature, making alcohol a potentially lethal drug to administer to victims of exposure. Alcohol also depresses cardiac contractility within the heart. This can reduce arrhythmias, but an additional helpful effect for the cardiovascular system is a transiently raised level of HDLs with moderate consumption of alcohol which may assist in reducing cholesterol deposition in blood vessel walls.

Endocrine effects: One of the most well-known effects of drinking alcohol is increased urine production. This diuresis is due to the inhibitory action of alcohol on the release of antidiuretic hormone from the pituitary gland. This diminishes the stimulatory effect of the hormone on water resorption within the kidney, and thus diuresis results. The levels of many other hormones, including oestrogen, insulin and growth hormone, are also altered by alcohol use.

Gastric and pancreatic secretions: Low levels of alcohol can stimulate the secretion of gastrin and histamine within the gut, but higher levels above 20% tend to inhibit secretion and spirits can irritate gastric mucosa. Alcohol has been used as an appetite stimulant, but this is contraindicated in patients suffering from gastric ulceration or hyperacidity. Pancreatic secretions are also increased by ethanol, and chronic oversecretion can lead to pancreatitis.

After-effects of drinking: Some individuals take a small drink of alcohol just before sleep as a nightcap. Although alcohol can initially help induce sleep, the quality of sleep is compromised by later restlessness and a suppression of REM stage sleep. Upon waking the following morning, drinkers may experience a range of unpleasant side effects which come under the general heading of a 'hangover'. Symptoms can include thirst, sweating, pale pallor, nausea, vertigo, increased heart rate, nystagmus and a pounding headache. Most of these effects are due to the effects of residual aldehyde intoxication, but dehydration and low blood sugar can add to feelings of discomfort. Rehydration with sugary drinks is a popular initial remedy after overindulgence. However, it should be noted that although a small quantity of alcohol ('hair of the dog') can also alleviate some hangover symptoms, this is the first step to alcoholism. It is worth noting that because physiological tolerance to the presence of alcohol increases with time after consumption, it is possible the morning after a heavy drinking session to feel sober but nonetheless still be over the drink-drive limit.

These acute somatic effects of ethanol explain another observation of the porter in Shakespeare's MacBeth (Act 2, Scene 3, Lines 28–29) that 'Drink is a great promoter of three things: nose painting (i.e. facial flushing), sleep and urine'.

LONG-TERM EFFECTS OF ETHANOL CONSUMPTION

Heavy drinking over an extended period of time can damage almost every organ system in the body. Chronic illness is almost inevitable following prolonged alcohol abuse and the risk of cancer is increased, often in a linear, dose-dependent manner. Unfortunately, women are more prone to alcohol-related liver, heart and brain damage than men, as well as certain types of cancer.

Liver

Alcoholic liver disease is a major and increasing cause of debilitating illness and death throughout the world.[23] It can proceed unnoticed for several years, until symptoms of fatigue and weight loss herald its arrival. Between 10% and 15% of heavy drinkers will go on to develop cirrhosis in their lifetimes. The earliest, and reversible, condition on the pathway to cirrhosis is 'fatty liver' or steatosis. As described above, a major impact of alcohol on lipid metabolism is the inhibition of fatty acid degradation by β-oxidation and a concurrent enhancement of fatty acid synthesis and esterification. Triglyceride synthesis is subsequently increased but the export of lipids from the liver through very low density lipoprotein chylomicrons is diminished. With nowhere else to go, the excess lipid is stored within the hepatocytes in small globules, creating the condition known as steatosis.

However, this may not be the only mechanism, as alcohol induces cytokines such as tumour necrosis factor (TNF) which can mobilise fatty acids and lipids whilst inhibiting β-oxidation. Alcohol also inhibits adenosine monophosphate kinase, an enzyme which promotes β-oxidation and inhibits the breakdown of lipids.

Following on from steatosis is the condition steatohepatitis, in which injury to the liver becomes apparent and its functional capacity is diminished as hepatocytes are lost. Critical to this step in the disease pathway is inflammation. Apart from mediators of inflammation by cytokine mediators such as TNF, reactive oxygen species are important contributors to this state of chronic inflammation. These are derived from many sources during alcohol abuse, including activation of Kupffer cells, overactivity of mitochondrial respiratory chain enzymes and the metabolism of alcohol to aldehyde by CYP2E1. This leads to an effectively continuous condition of oxidative stress for the liver, which is worsened by the accumulation of the highly reactive alcohol metabolite acetaldehyde. Iron overload in the liver, associated with raised levels of hydrogen peroxide (and again, a shortage of reduced GSH), are thought to be additional factors which add to the stressed status of the liver.

Following widespread cell death amongst hepatocytes, there is scarring and fibrosis within the liver accompanied by collagen deposition. This collagen first appears in the form of fine fibres surrounding liver cells close to the draining venules of the liver. Hepatic stellate cells are particularly affected and their collagen production is increased by acetaldehyde. However, as the liver cells die, the fibres become thickened into fibrous bands. The remaining liver cells still divide, but the tissue cannot adopt its normal architecture because of the fibrous bands and so nodules appear. Blood flow can become obstructed or rerouted, leading to portal hypertension. The danger of portal hypertension is that it leads to back pressure on the thin-walled blood vessels of the oesophagus, stomach and intestines. These can burst, leading to a catastrophic loss of blood.

If drinking continues, for example 8 units of alcohol daily for 10 years for men, 5.5 units for women, more and more fibrotic scar tissue is formed and the liver loses its normal structure. The condition of cirrhosis then occurs although, as noted below, it now seems that there is no clear threshold below which alcohol does not increase the risk of cirrhosis to some extent. This risk is greatly increased if the person has also suffered from viral hepatitis. Once cirrhosis has become established, the risk of also developing hepatocellular carcinoma (HCC) rises to 1–2% per year.

Nutrition

It is hypothesised that another condition which predisposes to the development of HCC is malnutrition. Alcohol can affect the blood levels and metabolism of a variety of other species important for biochemical synthesis and physiological function. DNA methylation can be affected by diminished absorption and metabolism of micronutrients such as folate and vitamins B_{12} and B_6. Vitamin A and β-carotene can also be present at below normal levels in alcoholics.

These deficiencies can arise because chronic alcoholics are often malnourished. Since ethanol has a high calorific value, alcoholics can rely on it as an energy source and do not eat a balanced diet. In those who do have a balanced diet but also drink to excess, the high calorific value of ethanol can lead to obesity. However, the effects of alcohol consumption on weight gain are controversial.[24]

In moderate drinkers, alcohol metabolism can inhibit β-oxidation of fatty acids, enhance appetite and contribute to the total calorie intake, although alcohol also increases thermogenesis. Weight gain, especially around the waist, may occur. In heavy drinkers, the MEOS system of the hepatocytes is much induced, and alcohol metabolised by this route may not be as available as a source of energy. Weight gain solely due to alcohol consumption may be less likely to occur.

The poor diet and food absorption of a chronic alcoholic can also cause vitamin deficiencies. These can result in neurological disorder Wernicke's encephalopathy, as described below. Alcohol abuse also worsens psoriasis, though this may be difficult to separate from vitamin deficiency.

Heart and cardiovascular system

Drinking more than 5–6 units of alcohol daily is associated with increased blood pressure. This brings associated risks of coronary artery disease, stroke and heart attacks. Heavy alcohol use is also associated with cardiomyopathy. The left ventricle can become enlarged and fibrotic while the myocardium itself can become prone to arrhythmias. These arrhythmias are particularly prevalent during binge drinking (sometimes defined as 2 × maximum recommended daily intake), but may also be seen in chronic alcoholics during withdrawal. An unusual finding in many alcoholics is mild anaemia. This may be partly due to folate deficiency and/or iron loss due to gastrointestinal bleeding, but may also be due to the myelosuppressive effect of alcohol on bone marrow.

Gastrointestinal tract and associated organs

Although alcohol does increase gastric secretions, it is thought to be the direct irritant effect of alcohol itself and its bacterial metabolites (which include acetaldehyde) which cause inflammation and damage to gastric mucosa and well as diminishing their protective barriers. The result is erosive gastritis, which can lead to ulcers and bleeding. In addition to the problem of anaemia mentioned above, gastritis can also affect the absorption of vitamins, thus worsening the already weak nutritional status of some alcoholics.

Secretions of the pancreas are also enhanced by alcohol and again alcohol and its metabolites can cause the organ to be inflamed. In common with organ diseases initiated by alcohol, the condition of pancreatitis is associated with fibrosis. This can lead to subsequent obstruction of the pancreatic duct and eventual destruction of the organ.

Sexual function

In addition to the transient deleterious effects of alcohol on sexual performance, there can be long-term damage to the sexual organs. In males, there can be damage to the Leydig cells of testis and a reduction in sperm production. Circulating testosterone levels are reduced, which in turn leads to reduced libido and can even cause breast enlargement. In women, oestrogen levels are also altered. This can lead to missed periods or even amenorrhea.

Neurotoxic effects

The long-term effects of alcohol on the nervous system can be debilitating and irreversible. In the periphery, there can be a loss of sensation, or paraesthesia, which begins in the extremities of the limbs. Depression can also be found in chronic alcoholics but a more severe central effect is Wernicke's encephalopathy. This acute condition, associated with thiamine deficiency, is characterised by relaxation of eye muscles, confusion and ataxia. It can be fatal if untreated but can be partially reversed by thiamine injections. However, a degree of memory impairment and confusion can be permanent and form part of the syndrome called Korsakoff's psychosis. Alcoholics may also suffer from dementia in the later stages of their illness.

Alcohol also compromises a patient's ability to recover from brain injuries. Alcoholics are more likely to enter a coma after a subdural haematoma, while neuronal regeneration from stem cells in the brain is suppressed by alcohol. It could be that this suppression of neuronal regeneration contributes to the brain atrophy seen with alcoholics.[25] Alcoholics also suffer from an impairment of olfaction, a factor which may lead to a lack of awareness of the amount of drinking taking place.[26]

Pregnancy

Chronic alcohol abuse, especially binge drinking, is associated with birth abnormalities. These can include small size and microcephaly, joint and facial anomalies, mental retardation, learning difficulties and poor coordination. These symptoms are collectively known as fetal alcohol syndrome and it is associated with improper neuronal migration during development. Other risks of alcohol abuse during pregnancy are spontaneous abortion and premature birth, as well as unplanned pregnancy itself.

Immune system

Alcoholics are more prone to infections, such as TB and pneumonia, than non-alcoholics. Many of the cellular components of the immune system, such as T cells and natural killer cells which are involved in immune surveillance, are reduced in number and responsiveness. This causes the immune system to be compromised in alcoholism, and cancer surveillance is thereby also reduced.

Alcohol and the risk of cancer

Although ethanol itself is not a carcinogen, there is very strong evidence that ethanol consumption is associated with an increased risk of certain types of cancer.[27,28]

These include cancers of the mouth, oesophagus, colon and rectum, liver cancer, and, in women, breast cancer.

The presence of nitrosamines in some beers and aromatic hydrocarbons in some drinks may be a contributory factor to this increased risk. Dual abuse of tobacco and alcohol synergistically increases the risk of cancer. This is because the increased activity of microsomal liver enzymes turns more of the tobacco tars into carcinogenic chemicals. The ability of alcohol to solubilise some of these carcinogens worsens this synergistic effect. In the retina, enhanced retinoic acid metabolism leads to the production of polar metabolites which can damage both the retina and the optic nerve. However, the main culprits in the increased risk for cancer are thought to be acetaldehyde and the range of highly reactive free radicals generated directly by the metabolism of alcohol and indirectly by the increased activity of the MEOS.

Along with reactive oxygen species produced by MEOS, reactive nitrogen species are released by activated Kupffer cells and free radical forms of ethanol are also produced during ethanol metabolism. These reactive species can lead directly to cell injury and also to lipid peroxidation. Lipid peroxidation yields additional aldehyde species such as 4-hydroxyl-2-nonenal (4HNE) and malondialdehyde. Such molecules can then form adducts with DNA, RNA and protein (Fig. 29.5). Acetaldehyde itself which has been produced by the oxidation of ethanol is also electrophilic and it too reacts directly with DNA. These aldehyde adducts inhibit DNA methylation as well as impairing the function of DNA repair enzymes.

Bacteria can also oxidise alcohol to acetaldehyde. It is thought that in smokers and others with poor oral hygiene, bacterial production of acetaldehyde from ingested alcohol may increase the risk of oral cancer. This has led to some recent concerns about the safety of alcohol-containing mouth washes. Examples of adducts associated with alcohol abuse are shown in Figure 29.5.

The likelihood of alcohol associated cancer can be further increased by factors that may not be directly related to the formation of DNA adducts. Aldehydes cause acceleration of cell proliferation in the colon, and this may play a role in the development of colorectal cancer. Ethanol leads to an elevation of the level of oestrogens which may contribute to the risk of breast cancer. This risk of breast cancer in women has a very low threshold, and the increased risk of breast cancer is estimated to be 7.1% for every 10 g per day of alcohol intake.[29] The physical proximity of a tissue to ingested alcohol (for example the tongue and hypopharynx) also appears correlated with increased cancer risk. A schematic diagram of some of the routes through which alcohol may trigger cancer is depicted in Figure 29.6.

While these routes may increase the risk of cancer in the general population, genetic polymorphisms in the genes encoding proteins mediating alcohol metabolism can also affect the risks of cancer. The ALDH2*2 polymorphism described above, which results in a reduced capacity to oxidise aldehyde to acetate, has been repeatedly associated with an increased risk of cancer in the oral cavity, larynx and oesophagus in Japanese populations.[30] Since this polymorphism is also associated with facial flushing following ingestion of alcohol, it has been suggested that this sign is a simple indicator to affected individuals that they have an increased cancer risk from alcohol use.[31]

TOLERANCE AND DEPENDENCE

Even very light use of ethanol can lead to the development of several different kinds of tolerance which can partially offset the effects of increased blood alcohol concentrations and therefore reduce its potency. Behavioural tolerance allows affected individuals to learn how to cope with the effects of alcohol on their motor coordination. Underlying this behavioural tolerance is the development

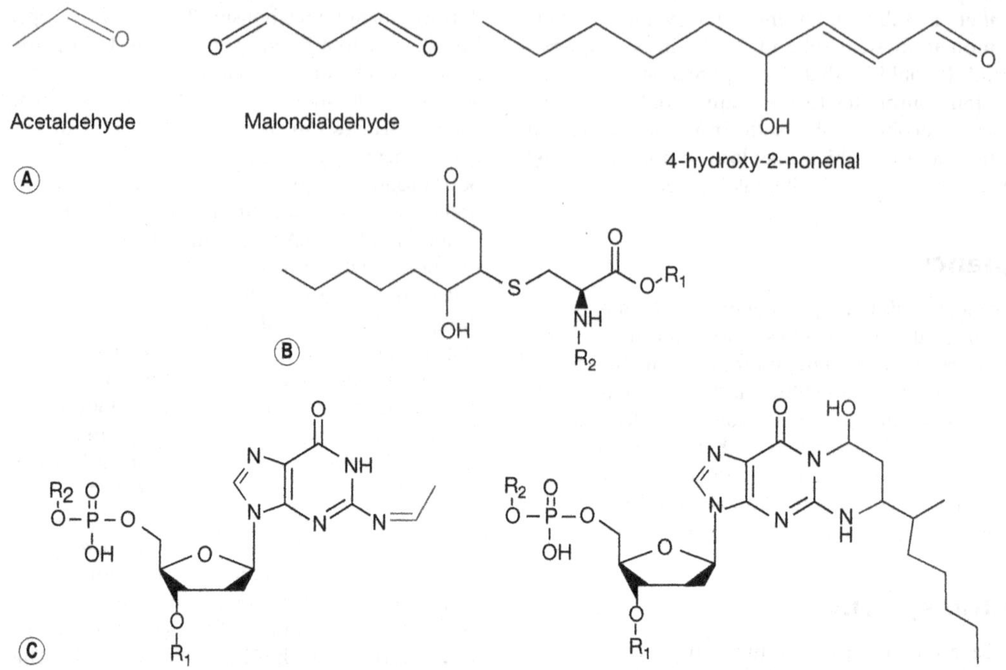

Figure 29.5 (**A**) Examples of aldehydes produced either directly (acetaldehyde) or indirectly, e.g. 4-hydroxy-2-nonenal from lipid peroxidation, which can form adducts with (**B**) sulphydryl groups on amino acids on proteins as well as amino groups on proteins, DNA (**C**) and RNA.

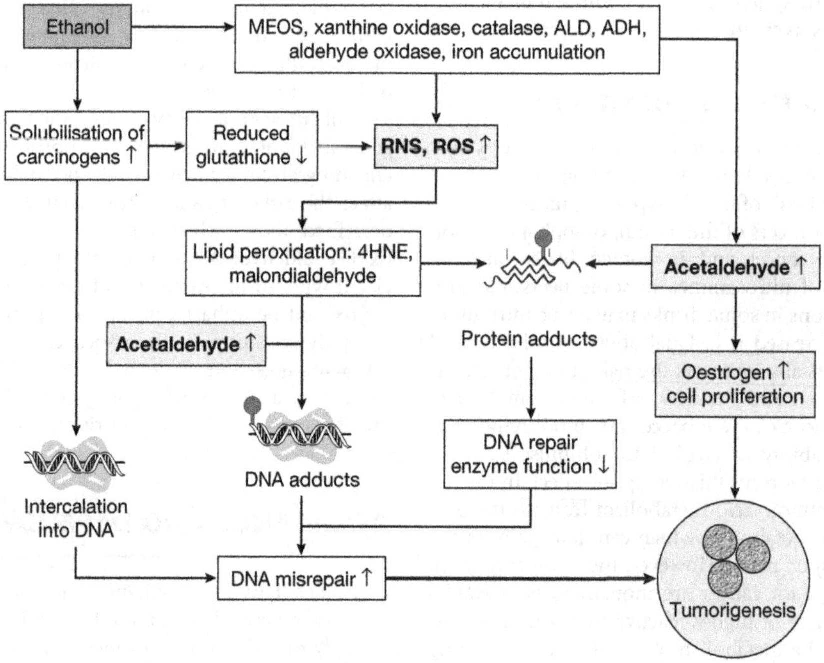

Figure 29.6 Possible routes of ethanol to cancer. This schematic diagram shows some of the ways in which it is suspected that ethanol may promote carcinogenesis. Although not carcinogenic itself, ethanol can solubilise organic carcinogens that can intercalate between the bases of DNA and cause it to be misread. The metabolism of alcohol generates large amounts of free radicals and reactive oxygen species. These cause peroxidation of lipids and the products of lipid peroxidation can form adducts with DNA and its repair enzymes. The acetaldehyde produced by alcohol oxidation can also do this, but can also induce cell proliferation in some tissues as well as altering the levels of steroid hormones upon which some tumours depend.

of tolerance at the neuronal level. The mechanisms of this tolerance are not completely understood, but can involve changes in the number of receptors and other excitable proteins so as to combat the effects of ethanol on their function. At the same time, metabolic tolerance, such as the induction of liver microsomal enzymes, enables alcohol users to metabolise ethanol more quickly than a naive drinker. However, as mentioned earlier, heavy drinkers may also metabolise other drugs, including anaesthetics, more rapidly and develop cross-tolerance to them.

Physical tolerance can slide into dependence. The CAGE Questionnaire asks: (1) Have you ever felt you should CUT down on your drinking? (2) Have people ANNOYED you by criticising your drinking? (3) Have you ever felt bad or GUILTY about your drinking? (4) Have you ever had an EARLY drink first thing in the morning to steady your nerves or get rid of a hangover? While a lot of people may answer yes to one of those questions on at least one occasion in their lives, the questionnaire suggests that people who have several such experiences may be heading for, or already showing, alcohol dependence. Established alcohol dependence is characterised by the ability to drink large quantities without getting drunk, irritability and tremulousness in the morning relieved by drink – possibly accompanied by nausea and retching, and increasing memory lapses.

Once dependence is entrenched, abstinence from it leads to the symptoms of ethanol withdrawal. In mild form this is characterised by agitation, anxiety, wakefulness and a lowering of seizure threshold about 6–8 hours after withdrawal. In more severe cases, tremor (known as delirium tremens) and hallucinations can also be manifested and will continue for the first 24–48 hours. This stage is followed by a period of confusion and aggression along with a continued higher risk of convulsions and arrhythmias.

Pharmacological management of withdrawal aims to reduce these risks of seizures and heart complications. To lower seizure threshold, long-acting benzodiazepines, e.g. chlordiazepoxide, are used, although short-acting drugs may be preferred if liver function is compromised, followed by gradual drug withdrawal. To help stabilise heart rate and oppose increased sympathetic activity, beta-blockers such as propanolol can be useful, while the adrenergic α_2-antagonist clonidine can inhibit the exaggerated release of neurotransmitters which occurs once the 'brake' provided by alcohol has been removed.

Of course, these symptoms can also be cured by ethanol itself and relapse is common in the first few months after withdrawal. To help avoid relapse, acamprosate, a weak NMDA antagonist, is sometimes used. This drug appears to help diminish feelings of craving. Naltrexone, an opioid receptor antagonist, can block reward pathways that are activated by alcohol and so break the link between alcohol and its reinforcing effects. An alternative approach of aversion therapy is provided by the drug disulfiram. This drug inhibits aldehyde dehydrogenase and so the aldehyde produced by alcohol dehydrogenase is not cleared. If a patient taking disulfiram also drinks alcohol, they experience all the unpleasant effects of aldehyde toxicity, including severe nausea.

BENEFICIAL EFFECTS OF ALCOHOL

Although the harmful effects of alcohol have been well documented, there is also evidence that light drinking may be beneficial for health.[32] Drinking less than three units per day reduces mortality compared to non-drinkers by about 25%. In addition, such light drinking can lead to increased insulin sensitivity, bone density, and cholesterol sequestering HDLs. Studies have also suggested that with light drinking, the risks of diabetes, gallstones, rheumatoid arthritis, artery spasm, thrombosis, silent infarcts and dementia are all decreased. Thus there do appear to be beneficial effects of light drinking, although the positive effects are rapidly outweighed by negative ones as the amount of drinking rises above three units per day for men or two for women. In terms of mortality, the greatest protective benefit is achieved below this consumption level from just under one unit a day to just under two units per day. However, for reducing the risk of type 2 diabetes,[33] maximum benefit is seen around three units per day for both men and women. This benefit is not completely lost until almost twice that amount of alcohol is consumed although most of it can be gained within the recommended maximum guidelines of two units per day for women.

IS ETHANOL ALWAYS THE ACTIVE AGENT?

The beneficial effects mentioned above may not be mediated by alcohol itself but perhaps by the congeners present in alcoholic beverages. In particular, it is thought that amongst the wide range of alcoholic beverages, red wine in particular may be protective for the cardiovascular system. Red wine is thought to be responsible for the 'French paradox' which refers to the relatively low incidence of cardiovascular disease amongst the residents of south-western France despite relatively high consumption of saturated fats. While a complex drink like red wine may contain thousands of different chemical compounds which may be biologically active, many of the beneficial effects of red wine have been attributed to presence of resveratrol which is found in the skin, seeds and stems of red grapes.[34] This has led to the study of the antioxidant resveratrol as a potential therapeutic agent for both cardiac and neuroprotection, diabetes, inflammation and cancer. Other compounds such as monomeric and polymeric flavan-3-ols, anthocyanins and phenolic acids are also found in abundance in red wine, and more recently the procyanidins have been proposed as important in mediating the longevity-enhancing properties of red wine.[35]

In addition to these beneficial components in alcoholic beverages, there are also some which may be harmful. Nearly every fermentable plant product has been used as a starting material for making alcoholic drinks. Also, during their distillation into spirits, a huge variety of herbs have been added. Thus many alcoholic beverages contain a wide range of potentially active components other than ethanol. Perhaps an extreme example of this is absinthe, which used to contain the convulsant thujone extracted from the herb wormwood (*Artmesia absinthum*). While aniseed has replaced wormwood in modern equivalents of this drink, modern alcoholic beverages, apart from vodka, can still contain a great variety of additional chemicals, some of which may be toxic.

For example, a Polish study of home-made alcoholic beverages revealed that many contained significant levels of methanol, propanol, isobutanol and 2/3 methyl-1-butanol.[36] These additional constituents, or congeners such as the higher alcohols in fusel oil, can slow metabolism by competing with ethanol for alcohol dehydrogenase. Thus drinkers of vodka, which is almost pure ethanol and water, tend to sober up slightly faster than imbibers of other drinks. An additional problem with unlabelled bottles was that some contained 70–85% alcohol by volume, while several 'fruit wines' derived from stone fruits contained unsafe levels of the carcinogen ethyl carbamate.

Occasionally, alcoholic beverages are illegally adulterated with methanol or ethylene glycol. Both of these additives are extremely dangerous. Methanol, for example, is first metabolised to formaldehyde by ADH and then to formic acid. This is toxic to the liver. However, in the brain and retina, metabolism by CYP2E1 and catalase contributes to the metabolism of methanol. In these tissues, the formaldehyde produced can form adducts with protein, and the formate can be converted into a free radical form. Severe acidosis as well as impairment of glycolysis and mitochondrial function results and even a relatively small amount of methanol (10 g) can cause total blindness. Ethylene glycol is also very toxic when ingested, and can cause renal failure due to the deposition of oxalate crystals in the kidney. Ethanol can be used therapeutically in cases of methanol or ethylene glycol poisoning. It binds more strongly to ADH than methanol or ethylene glycol, allowing more of the noxious substances to be eliminated by excretion in breath, sweat and urine before they are metabolised to even more dangerous metabolites. In some such cases, plasmapheresis and/or dialysis may be required.

CONCLUSION

Ethanol is such an accepted drug in society it sometimes is easy to overlook how powerful and wide reaching its effects are. It is still heavily promoted in advertising in the way tobacco products were until recently, and has been recommended as a social lubricant, for relaxation, and more recently for prevention of heart disease, diabetes and stroke when used in moderation. The beneficial effects are not, however, strong and are lost by heavy drinking. Such heavy use of ethanol quickly overloads the liver's capacity to metabolise and increases the risks of many adverse health and social effects. Women are especially at risk, and for breast cancer there seems to be no threshold level below which alcohol is completely safe. A recent Danish study[37] suggests the same may be true for liver disease, and that there is increased risk of cirrhosis (two- to sixfold) even at levels of drinking below the current health guidelines of 21 units for men and 14 for women, with two alcohol-free days per week.

Such guidelines inevitably represent a compromise between the evidence of beneficial effects of alcohol and known risks of adverse effects. They are designed for the general population, but for an individual the levels may be slightly different, according to their general genomic and health status. Perhaps for many it is only very light drinking (1–2 units, 3–4 days a week) or barely more than 1 'drink' a day on average (actually about 1.5 units) that may do as much or more good than harm overall. The problem for public health is many view existing guidelines as too abstemious, and well below what they consider to be moderate.

ACKNOWLEDGEMENT

The authors would like to thank Dr P.J.O. Covernton for permission to use the data in Figure 29.3 and also for valuable comments on the draft manuscript.

REFERENCES

1. McGovern PE, Zhang J, Tang J, et al. Fermented beverages of pre- and proto-historic China. *Proc Natl Acad Sci USA*. 2004;101:17593–175938.
2. Wiens F, Zitzmann A, Lachance MA, et al. Chronic intake of fermented floral nectar by wild treeshrews. *Proc Natl Acad Sci USA*. 2008;105:10426–10431.
3. Covernton PJO, Connolly JG. Subunit specific actions of ethanol on neuronal nicotinic acetylcholine receptor subtypes. *Br J Pharmacol*. 1997;122:1661–1668.

4. Alcohol: Statistical Publication Notice. NHS in Scotland. http://www.isdscotland.org/isd/5905.html; 2009.
5. Cost to society of alcohol abuse in Scotland. ISBN 978 0 7559 7105 3 (web only publication) http://www.scotland.gov.uk/Publications/2008/05/06091510/0; 2008.
6. Rehm J, Mathers C, Popova S, Thavorncharoensap M, Teerawattananon Y, Patra J. Global burden of disease and injury and economic cost attributable to alcohol use and alcohol-use disorders. *Lancet*. 2009;373:2223–2233.
7. Lide DR. *CRC Handbook of Chemistry and Physics*. 81st ed. CRC Press; 2000 ISBN 304184.
8. Morris S, Humphreys D, Reynolds D. Myth, marula, and elephant: an assessment of voluntary ethanol intoxication of the African elephant (*Loxodonta africana*) following feeding on the fruit of the marula tree (*Sclerocarya birrea*). *Physiol Biochem Zool*. 2006;79:363–369.
9. Donovan JE. Estimated blood alcohol concentrations for child and adolescent drinking and their implications for screening instruments. *Pediatrics*. 2009;123:e975–e981.
10. Bowman WC, Rand MJ. *Textbook of Pharmacology*. 2nd ed. Blackwell Scientific Publications; 1980.
11. Tolstrup JS, Nordestgaard BG, Rasmussen S, Tybærg-Hansen A, Grønbæk M. Alcoholism and alcohol drinking habits predicted from dehydrogenase genes. *Pharmacogenomics J*. 2008;8:220–227.
12. Marchitti SA, Brocker C, Stagos D, Vasiliou V. Non-P450 aldehyde oxidizing enzymes: the aldehyde dehydrogenase superfamily. *Expert Opin Drug Metab Toxicol*. 2008;4:697–720.
13. Xiao Q, Weiner H, Johnston T, Crabb DW. The aldehyde dehydrogenase ALDH2*2 allele exhibits dominance over ALDH2*1 in transduced HeLa cells. *J Clin Invest*. 1995;96:2180–2186.
14. Chen Y-C, Peng GS, Wang MF, Tsao TP, Yin SJ. Polymorphism of ethanol-metabolism genes and alcoholism: Correlation of allelic variations with the pharmacokinetic and pharmacodynamic consequences. *Chem Biol Interact*. 2009;178:2–7.
15. Lieber CS. Microsomal ethanol-oxidizing system – The first 30 years (1968–1998). A review. *Alcohol Clin Exp Res*. 1999;23:991–1007.
16. Zhou SF, Liu JP, Chowbay B. Polymorphism of human cytochrome P450 enzymes and its clinical impact. *Drug Metab Rev*. 2009;41:89–295.
17. Oneta CM, Lieber CS, Li JJ, et al. Dynamics of cytochrome P4502E1 activity in man: induction by ethanol and disappearance during withdrawal phase. *J Hepatol*. 2002;36:47–52.
18. Liang T, Spence J, Liu L, et al. α-Synuclein maps to a quantitative trait locus for alcohol preference and is differentially expressed in alcohol-preferring and -nonpreferring rats. *Proc Natl Acad Sci USA*. 2003;100:4690–4695.
19. Spanagel R. Alcoholism: A systems approach from molecular physiology to addictive behavior. *Physiol Rev*. 2009;89:649–705.
20. Wonnacott S. Gates and filters: Unveiling the physiological roles of nicotine receptors in dopaminergic transmission. *Br J Pharmacol*. 2008; 153:S2–S4.
21. Quertemont E, Didone V. Role of acetaldehyde in mediating the pharmacological and behavioural effects of alcohol. *Alcohol Res Health*. 2006;29:258–265.
22. Blomberg RD, Peck RC, Moskowitz H, Burns M, Fiorentino D. The Long Beach/Fort Lauderdale relative risk study. *J Safety Res*. 2009;40:285–292.
23. Breitkopf K, Nagy LE, Beier JI, et al. Current experimental perspectives on the clinical progression of alcoholic liver disease. *Alcohol Clin Exp Res*. 2009;33:1–9.
24. Suter PM, Tremblay A. Is alcohol consumption a risk factor for weight gain and obesity? *Crit Rev Clin Lab Sci*. 2009;42:197–227.
25. Nixon K, Kim DH, Potts EN, He J, Crews FT. Distinct cell proliferation events during abstinence after alcohol dependence: Microglia proliferation precedes neurogenesis. *Neurobiol Dis*. 2008;31:218–229.
26. Rupp CI, Kurz M, Kemmler G, et al. Reduced olfactory sensitivity, discrimination, and identification in patients with alcohol dependence. *Alcohol Clin Exp Res*. 2003;27: 432–439.
27. Boffetta P, Hashibe M. Alcohol and cancer. *Lancet Oncol*. 2006;7:149–156.
28. Homann N, Seitz HK, Wang XD, Yokoyama A, Singletary KW, Ishii H. Mechanisms in Alcohol-Associated Carcinogenesis. *Alcohol Clin Exp Res*. 2005;29:1317–1320.
29. Hamajima N, Hirose K, Tajima K, et al. Alcohol, tobacco and breast cancer—collaborative reanalysis of individual data from 53 epidemiological studies, including 58 515 women with breast cancer and 95 067 women without the disease. *Br J Cancer*. 2002;87:1234–1245.
30. Yokoyama A, Omori T. Genetic polymorphisms of alcohol and aldehyde dehydrogenases and risk for esophageal and head and neck cancers. *Jpn J Clin Oncol*. 2003;33:111–121.
31. Brooks PJ, Enoch MA, Goldman D, Li TK, Yokoyama A. The alcohol flushing response: an unrecognized risk factor for esophageal cancer from alcohol consumption. *PLoS Med*. 2009;6(3):e50.
32. Collins MA, Neafsey EJ, Mukamal KJ, et al. Alcohol in moderation, cardioprotection, and neuroprotection: epidemiological considerations and mechanistic studies. *Alcohol Clin Exp Res*. 2009;33:206–219.
33. Baliunas DO, Taylor BJ, Irving H, et al. Alcohol as a risk factor for type 2 diabetes. *Diabetes Care*. 2009;32: 2123–2132.
34. Brown L, Kroon PA, Das DK, et al. The biological responses to resveratrol and other polyphenols from alcoholic beverages. *Alcohol Clin Exp Res*. 2009;33:1513–1523.
35. Corder R, Mullen W, Khan NQ, et al. Oenology: red wine procyanidins and vascular health. *Nature*. 2006; 444:566.
36. Lachenmeier DW, Ganss S, Rychlak B, et al. Association between quality of cheap and unrecorded alcohol products and public health consequences in Poland. *Alcohol Clin Exp Res*. 2009;33:1–13.
37. Tolstrup JS, Grønbæk M, Tybærg-Hansen A, Nordestgaard BG. Alcohol intake, alcohol dehydrogenase genotypes, and liver damage and disease in the Danish general population. *Am J Gastroenterol*. 2009; advanced publication on line doi:10.1038/ajg.2009.370.

Index

Note: Page numbers followed by a *b* indicate boxes, *f* indicate figures and *t* indicate tables.

B

C

D

E

F

G

H

J

K

L

M

O

P

Q

R

S

T

U